TEXTBOOK OF CLINICA
AND FUNCTIONAL MEDICINE, VOLUME 2

PROTOCOLS FOR COMMON INFLAMMATORY DISORDERS

FUNCTIONAL INFLAMMOLOGY & INFLAMMATION MASTERY, VOL 2

The Colorful and Definitive Guide *toward* Health and Vitality and *away from* the Boredom, Risks, Costs, and Inefficacy of Endless Analgesia, Immunosuppression, and Polypharmacy: A Three-Part Learning System of Text, Images, and Video

ALEX VASQUEZ D.C. N.D. D.O. F.A.C.N.

* Doctor of Osteopathic Medicine, graduate of University of North Texas Health Science Center, Texas College of Osteopathic Medicine (2010)
* Doctor of Naturopathic Medicine, graduate of Bastyr University (1999)
* Doctor of Chiropractic, graduate of University of Western States (1996)
* Fellow of the American College of Nutrition (2013-present)
* Former Overseas Fellow of the Royal Society of Medicine
* Editor, *International Journal of Human Nutrition and Functional Medicine* IntJHumNutrFunctMed.org. Former Editor, *Naturopathy Digest*; Former/Recent Reviewer for *Journal of Naturopathic Medicine, Alternative Therapies in Health and Medicine, Autoimmune Diseases, International Journal of Clinical Medicine, PLOS One* and *Neuropeptides*
* Private practice of integrative and functional medicine in Seattle, Washington (2000-2001), Houston, Texas (2001-2006), Portland, Oregon (2011-2013), consulting practice (present)
* Consultant Researcher and Lecturer (2004-present), Biotics Research Corporation
* Teaching and Academics:
  o Director of Programs, International College/Conference on Human Nutrition and Functional Medicine ICHNFM.ORG
  o Founder and Former Program Director of the world's first accredited university-affiliated graduate-level program in Functional Medicine
  o Adjunct Professor, Integrative and Functional Nutrition in Immune Health, Doctor of Clinical Nutrition program
  o Former Adjunct Professor (2009-2013) of Laboratory Medicine, Master of Science in Advanced Clinical Practice
  o Former Faculty (2004-2005, 2010-2013) and Forum Consultant (2003-2007), The Institute for Functional Medicine
  o Former Professor (2011-2013) of Pharmacology, Evidence-Based Nutrition, Immune and Inflammatory Imbalances, Principles of Functional Medicine, Psychology of Wellness
  o Former Adjunct Professor of Orthopedics (2000), Radiographic Interpretation (2000), and Rheumatology (2001), Naturopathic Medicine Program, Bastyr University
* Author of more than 100 articles and letters published in *JAMA—Journal of the American Medical Association, BMJ—British Medical Journal, TheLancet.com, JAOA—Journal of the American Osteopathic Association, Annals of Pharmacotherapy, Journal of Clinical Endocrinology and Metabolism, Alternative Therapies in Health and Medicine, Nutritional Perspectives, Journal of Manipulative and Physiological Therapeutics, Integrative Medicine, Current Allergy and Asthma Reports, Nutritional Wellness, Evidence-based Complementary and Alternative Medicine, Nature Reviews Rheumatology* and *Arthritis & Rheumatism*: Official Journal of the American College of Rheumatology

INTERNATIONAL COLLEGE OF HUMAN NUTRITION & FUNCTIONAL MEDICINE

ICHNFM.ORG

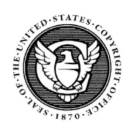
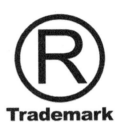

Chapter and Introduction	*Page*
Preamble	i

Volume 1

1. Patient Assessments, Laboratory Interpretation, Clinical Concepts, Patient Management, Practice Management and Risk Reduction: *This chapter introduces/reviews/updates patient assessments, laboratory interpretation, musculoskeletal emergencies, healthcare paradigms; the common and important conditions hemochromatosis and hypothyroidism are also included in this chapter since these need to be considered on a frequent basis in clinical practice* — 1

2. Wellness Promotion & Re-Establishing the Foundation for Health: *Reviewed here are diet, lifestyle, psychosocial health, and—given the pervasiveness of persistent organic pollutants and their increasingly recognized clinical importance—an introduction to environmental medicine* — 187

3. Basic Concepts and Therapeutics in (Nondrug) Musculoskeletal Care and Integrative Pain Management: *Nonpharmacologic management of musculoskeletal problems is preferred over pharmacologic (e.g., NSAID, Coxib, steroid, opioid) management because of the collateral benefits, safety, and cost-effectiveness associated with manual, dietary, botanical, and nutritional treatments. A brief discussion of the current crisis in musculoskeletal medicine is provided for contextualization and emphasis of the importance of expanding clinicians' knowledge of effective nondrug treatments* — 243

4. The Major Modifiable Factors in Sustained Inflammation: *Major components of the "Functional Inflammology Protocol" are reviewed here, from concepts and molecular biology to an emphasis on practical clinical applications* — 303

1) Food & Basic Nutrition	307
2) Infections: Dysbiosis / Viral	396 / 540
3) Nutritional Immunomodulation	609
4) Dysmetabolism, Mitochondrial Dysfunction, ERS/UPR, mTOR	622
5) Special Considerations: Sleep, Sociopsychology, Stress, Surgery	674
6) Endocrine Imbalances	688
7) Xenobiotic Immunotoxicity	699

Volume 2: Chapter 5—Clinical Applications of the Functional Inflammology Protocol — 713

1) Hypertension	727
2) Diabetes Mellitus	819
3) Migraine & Headaches	863
4) Fibromyalgia	901
5) Allergic Inflammation	984
6) Rheumatoid Arthritis	1019
7) Psoriasis and Psoriatic Arthritis	1038
8) Systemic Lupus Erythematosus	1053
9) Scleroderma & Systemic Sclerosis	1074
10) Vasculitic Diseases	1094
11) Spondyloarthropathies & Reactive Arthritis	1108
12) Sjögren Syndrome/Disease	1119
13) Raynaud's Syndrome/Phenomenon/Disorder	1127
14) Clinical Notes on Additional Conditions: Behçet's Disease, Sarcoidosis, Dermatomyositis and Polymyositis	1131

Index & Appendix — 1154

Dedications: I dedicate this book to the following people in appreciation for their works, their direct and indirect support of this work, and for their contributions to the advancement of true healthcare.

- **To the students and practitioners of naturopathic/functional medicine**, those who continue to learn so that they can provide the best possible care to their patients; **and to their oft-underpaid and underappreciated professors**
- **To the researchers** whose works are cited in this text
- **To Dr Alan Gaby and Dr Jeffrey Bland,** my most memorable and influential *personal* professors and mentors
  - Dr Gaby's diligent scholarship of the medical nutrition literature laid the evidence-based foundation for nearly all of us; his *Nutritional Medicine* is an excellent companion text to compliment this volume
  - Dr Bland deserves credit for being the primary developer of the American rendition of "functional medicine", a conceptual framework and clinical model used and discussed in this text. While development and continuous maturation of the functional medicine model has depended upon numerous researchers and clinicians, Dr Bland was clearly the pioneer for this concept circa 1993 and the nucleus around which many of us have worked (at least initially) in this regard.
- **To Henry Rollins**, in particular for his prose book *One from None*, which completely changed my life in 1991
- **To Dr Linus Pauling**, for modeling the combination of scientific scholarship (Nobel Prize in Chemistry 1954) and social engagement (Nobel Peace Prize 1962)
- **To Dr Friedrich Nietzsche and Dr Noam Chomsky,** my most memorable and influential *virtual* professors and mentors, both of whom exemplify profound scholarship and intellectual independence in favor of developing the highest possible human culture on earth
- **To Dr Robert Richard**, my clinical mentor in general outpatient medicine—a truly exemplary clinician
- **To Dr Bruce Ames**[1] **and Dr Roger J Williams**[2], for proving the importance of biochemical individuality
- **To Dr Chester Wilk**[3,4] **and important others**[5,6,7] for documenting and resisting the organized oppression of natural, non-pharmaceutical, non-surgical healthcare
- **To Jorge Strunz and Ardeshir Farah,** for daily artistic inspiration since my first listen of *Primal Magic* in 1992

Acknowledgments for Peer and Editorial Review of Earlier Versions of This Work: Most of the sections that comprise the current work have been previously reviewed/published/presented; peer/editorial reviews are acknowledged below. Acknowledgement here does not imply that the reviewer fully agrees with or endorses the material in this text but rather that they were willing to review specific sections of the book for clinical applicability and clarity and to make suggestions to their own level of satisfaction.

- 2016 Edition of *Inflammation Mastery* and the excerpt *Pain Revolution for Migraine and Fibromyalgia*: Sabrina Piper BSc (2016 ND candidate), John Bartemus DC BCIM CFMP DACBN, Elizabeth Busetto DC ND, Kenneth Cintron MD
- 2015 Edition of *Human Microbiome and Dysbiosis in Clinical Disease*: Julie Jean BS BSN RN, Joseph Iaccino DC MSc
- 2014 Edition of *Antiviral Strategies and Immune Nutrition*: Annette D'Armata ND, Elizabeth Busetto DC ND
- 2014 Edition of *Naturopathic Rheumatology*: Annette D'Armata ND
- 2012 Edition of *Fibromyalgia in a Nutshell*: Lisa Scholl BA, Annette D'Armata ND
- 2012 Edition of *Migraine Headaches, Hypothyroidism, and Fibromyalgia*: Holly Furlong DC
- 2011 Edition of *Integrative Chiropractic Management of High Blood Pressure and Chronic Hypertension*: Barry Morgan MD, Holly Furlong DC, Kris Young DC, Erika Mennerick DC, and J William Beakey DOM
- 2011 Edition of *Integrative Medicine and Functional Medicine for Chronic Hypertension*: Erika Mennerick DC, JoAnn Fawcett DC, Ileana Bourland MSOM LAc, James Bogash DC, J William Beakey DOM
- 2010 Edition of *Chiropractic Management of Chronic Hypertension*: Joseph Paun MS DC, David Candelario OMS4 (TCOM c/o 2010), James Bogash DC, Bill Beakey DOM, Robert Richard DO
- 2009 Edition of *Chiropractic and Naturopathic Mastery of Common Clinical Disorders*: Heather Kahn MD, Robert Richard DO, James Leiber DO, David Candelario (UNT-HSC TCOM OMS4)
- 2007 Edition of *Integrative Orthopedics*: Barry Morgan MD, Dennis Harris DC, Richard Brown DC (DACBI candidate), Ron Mariotti ND, Patrick Makarewich MBA, Reena Singh (SCNM ND4), Zachary Watkins DC, Charles Novak MS DC, Marnie Loomis ND, James Bogash DC, Sara Croteau DC, Kris Young DC, Joshua Levitt ND, Jack Powell III MD, Chad Kessler MD, Amy Neuzil ND
- 2006 Edition of *Integrative Rheumatology*: Amy Neuzil ND, Cathryn Harbor MD, Julian Vickers DC, Tamara Sachs MD, Bob Sager BSc MD DABFM (Clinical Instructor in the Department of Family Medicine, University of Kansas), Ron

---

[1] Ames BN, et al. High-dose vitamin therapy stimulates variant enzymes with decreased coenzyme binding affinity (increased K(m). *Am J Clin Nutr*. 2002 Apr;75:616-58
[2] Williams RJ. *Biochemical Individuality: The Basis for the Genetotrophic Concept*. Austin and London: University of Texas Press; 1956
[3] Wilk CA. *Medicine, Monopolies, and Malice: How the Medical Establishment Tried to Destroy Chiropractic*. Garden City Park: Avery, 1996
[4] Getzendanner S. Permanent injunction order against AMA. *JAMA*. 1988 Jan 1;259(1):81-2
[5] Carter JP. *Racketeering in Medicine: The Suppression of Alternatives*. Norfolk: Hampton Roads Pub; 1993
[6] Morley J, Rosner AL, Redwood D. A case study of misrepresentation of the scientific literature: recent reviews of chiropractic. *J Altern Complement Med*. 2001;7:65-78
[7] Terrett AG. Misuse of the literature by medical authors in discussing spinal manipulative therapy injury. *J Manipulative Physiol Ther*. 1995 May;18(4):203-10

Mariotti ND, Titus Chiu (DC4), Zachary Watkins (DC4), Gilbert Manso MD, Bruce Milliman ND, William Groskopp DC, Robert Silverman DC, Matthew Breske (DC4), Dean Neary ND, Thomas Walton DC, Fraser Smith ND, Ladd Carlston DC, David Jones MD, Joshua Levitt ND

- 2004 Edition of *Integrative Orthopedics*: Peter Knight ND, Kent Littleton ND MS, Barry Morgan MD, Ron Hobbs ND, Joshua Levitt ND, John Neustadt (Bastyr ND4), Allison Gandre BS (Bastyr ND4), Peter Kimble ND, Jack Powell III MD, Chad Kessler MD, Mike Gruber MD, Deirdre O'Neill ND, Mary Webb ND, Leslie Charles ND, Amy Neuzil ND

Format and Layout: The format/layout of this book is designed to efficiently take the reader through the clinically relevant spectrum of considerations for each condition that is detailed. Important topics are given their own section within each chapter, while other less important or less common conditions are only described briefly in terms of the four "clinical essentials" of 1) definition/pathophysiology, 2) clinical presentation, 3) assessment/diagnosis, and 4) treatment/management. Each of the expanded sections that details the more important/common conditions maintains a consistent format, taking the reader through the spectrum of primary clinical considerations: definition/pathophysiology, clinical presentations, differential diagnoses, assessments (physical examination, laboratory, imaging), complications, management, and treatment. As my books have progressed, I am increasingly using an article-by-article review format (especially in the sections on management and treatment) so that readers have more direct access to the information so as to understand and *incorporate* more deeply what the research actually states; the goal and general approach here is to use a *representative sampling* of the research literature.

References and Citations: Citations to articles, abstracts, texts, and personal communications are footnoted throughout the text to provide supporting information and to provide interested readers the resources to find additional information. Many of the cited articles are available on-line for free, and often I have included the website addresses so that readers can easily access the complete article.

Peer-review and Quality Control: Peer-review is essential to help ensure accuracy and clinical applicability of health-related information. Consistent with the importance of these goals, I have employed several "checks and balances" to increase the accuracy and applicability of the information within my textbooks:

- Reliance upon authoritative references: Nearly all important statements are referenced to peer-reviewed biomedical journals or authoritative texts, examples of the latter include *The Merck Manual, Current Medical Diagnosis and Treatment,* and *5-Minute Clinical Consult.* Each citation is provided by a footnote at the bottom of each page so that readers will know quickly and easily exactly where the information was obtained.
- Extensive cross-referencing: Readers will notice the supranormal number of references and citations. Many important statements have several references. Many references (especially textbooks) are referenced several times even on the same page; the purpose of this extensive referencing is three-fold: 1) to guide you—the reader—to additional information, 2) to help me (as writer) stay organized, and 3) to help you and me (the practicing physicians) employ this information with confidence. In more recent updates/revisions, I have started shortening the number of listed authors by frequent use of *et al* with an interest in keeping each citation to one line of text on the page, likewise reducing mental and eye strain; quite obviously I respect each of the authors—even those whose names are not listed in the citation—and am implementing this solely for the sake of efficient book formatting (aiming for one citation per line) and information density (fewer lines dedicated to citations allows more space for text and images). Given hundreds of pages and thousands of citations, formatting considerations such as these are summatively significant.
- Periodic revision: Any significant errors that are discovered will be posted at InflammationMastery.com/volume1 (...volume2, etc); please check these folders periodically to ensure that you are working with the most accurate information of which I am aware.
- Peer-review: The peer-review process for my books takes several forms. First, colleagues and students are invited to review new and revised sections of the text before publication; every section of the book that you are holding has been independently reviewed by health science students and/or practicing clinicians from various backgrounds: allopathic, chiropractic, osteopathic, naturopathic. Second, you - the reader - are invited to provide feedback about the information in the book, typographical errors, syntax, case reports, new research, etc. If your ideas truly change the nature of the material, I will be glad to acknowledge you in the text (with your permission, of course). If your contribution is hugely significant, such as reviewing three or more chapters or helping in some important way, I will be glad to not only acknowledge you, but to also send you the next edition at a discount or courtesy when your ideas take effect. Third, I keep abreast of new literature by constantly perusing new research and advancements in the health sciences. Having been successful in three separate doctoral programs in the health sciences, I have learned not only to master large amounts of material but to also separate and integrate different viewpoints as appropriate. I also "field test" my protocols with patients in the various clinical arenas in which I work and also with professionals and

academicians via presentations and critical dialogue. By implementing these quality control steps, I hope to create a useful text and advance our professions and practices by improving the quality of care that we deliver to our patients.

How to Use This Book Most Effectively: Ideally, these books should be read cover-to-cover within a context of coursework that is supervised by a clinically experienced professor. For post-graduate professionals, they might consider forming a local or virtual "book club" and meeting for weekly or monthly discussions to check their understandings and share their clinical experiences to refine the application of clinical knowledge, perceptions, and skills. Virtual groups and internet forums—such as those hosted by International College of Human Nutrition and Functional Medicine at ICHNFM.ORG—can provide access to an assembly of international professional peers wherein sharing of clinical questions and experiences are synergistic. This book is not intended to extensively cover all aspects of clinical medicine, such as clinical pharmacology and prescribing (for which I recommend *Epocrates.com* and its associated app) and medical management (for which I recommend *5-Minute Clinical Consult* via book, website, and app).

Video access: Video access is provided via notices and footnotes appropriately placed and indicated throughout the book. Readers actually have to read the book to access the information and gain knowledge.

- Sample: vimeo.com/ichnfm/drv-functional-inflammology-intro2013
- Password: DrVprotocol

Notices: The intention and scope of this text are to provide health science students and doctorate-level clinicians with useful information and a familiarity with available research and resources pertinent to the management of patients in integrative primary care and specialty care settings. Specifically, the information in this book is intended to be used by licensed healthcare professionals who have received hands-on/residential clinical training and supervision at accredited health science colleges. Additionally, information in this book should be used in conjunction with other resources, texts, and in combination with the clinician's best judgment and intention to *"first, do no harm"* and second to provide effective healthcare. Information and treatments applicable to a specific *condition* may not be appropriate for or applicable to a specific *patient* in your office; this is especially true for patients with multiple

> **Purpose, scope, recommended companion resources**
>
> The purpose of this book is not to serve as a stand-alone "recipe book" for the complete management of all reviewed conditions; rather the focus of this book is the delivery of clinically important concepts and facts to enhance the management of various clinical disorders, in particular by documenting and explicating this author's naturopathic, allopathic, integrative and functional medicine approach. Readers and instructors using this book are encouraged to use whichever additional resources they choose, including but not limited to the supporting videos at Vimeo.com/DrVasquez and Vimeo.com/ICHNFM; in particular, *5-Minute Clinical Consult* and *Epocrates* are excellent and strongly advised companion guides for overall medical diagnosis/management and clinical pharmacology/prescribing, respectively. Clinicians need to have a good understanding of clinical medicine before applying many of the approaches described in this book; cross-referencing and double-checking management strategies and drug doses are essential components of quality care. Both *5-Minute Clinical Consult* and *Epocrates* are available as point-of-care references, and their use is advised.
>
> This work is best used with the relevant videos from DrV available online, some of which are linked and made password-accessible via this book; additional videos by Dr Vasquez are available online (occasionally with accompanying printed presentation slides); please see the following examples and locations:
> - vimeo.com/ichnfm
> - vimeo.com/drvasquez

comorbidities and those taking pharmaceutical medications with potential for multiple adverse effects and drug/nutrient/herb interactions. In my books and articles, I describe treatments—manual, dietary, nutritional, botanical, pharmacologic, and occasionally surgical—and their research support for the clinical condition being discussed; each practitioner must determine appropriateness of these treatments for his/her individual patient and with consideration of the doctor's scope of practice, education, training, skill, and—occasionally—the appropriateness of "off label" use of medications and treatments. This book has been carefully written and checked for accuracy by the author and professional colleagues. However, in view of the possibility of human error and new discoveries in the biomedical sciences, neither the author nor any party associated in any way with this text warrants that this text is perfect, accurate, or complete in every way, and we disclaim responsibility for harm or loss associated with the application of the material herein. With all conditions/treatments described herein, each physician must be sure to consider the balance between what is best for the patient and the physician's own level of ability, expertise, and experience. When in doubt, or if the physician is not a specialist in the treatment of a given severe condition, referral is appropriate. These notes are written with the routine "outpatient" in mind and are not tailored to severely injured patients or "playing field" or "emergency response" situations; consult your First Aid and Emergency Response texts and course materials for appropriate information. These notes represent the author's perspective based on academic education, experience, and post-graduate continuing education and are not inclusive of every fact that a clinician may need to know. This is not an "entry level" book except when used in an academic setting with a knowledgeable professor who can explain the concepts, tests, physical exam procedures, and treatments; this book requires a certain level of knowledge from the reader and familiarity with clinical concepts, laboratory assessments, and physical examination procedures. Suggested doses—if any—are for adults (not infants and children) unless otherwise specified in context; the responsibility for appropriate dosing is of course that of the prescribing clinician in view of the patient's age, weight, overall state, hepatic and renal function, comorbidities, polypharmacy, etc.

Updates, Corrections, and Newsletter: When and if omissions, errata, and the need for important updates become clear, I will post these at the website InflammationMastery.com. A reader might access this page periodically to ensure staying informed of any corrections that might have clinical relevance. This book consists not only of the text in the printed pages you are holding, but also the footnotes and any updates at the website. If any clinically important corrections are made, they will be distributed by newsletter InflammationMastery.com/join_email.html and/or placed in the folder FunctionalInflammology.com/volume1/ (with analogous folders for subsequent volumes, e.g., volume2, etc) for constant availability. Be alerted to new integrative clinical research, updates to this textbook and other news/publications/conferences/videos by registering for the free newsletter at ICHNFM.ORG.

Language, Semantics, and Perspective: As a diligent student who previously aspired to be an English professor, I have written this text with great (though inevitably imperfect) attention to detail. Individual words were chosen with care. I confess to knowing, pushing, and creatively breaking several rules of grammar and punctuation. With regard to the he/she and him/her debacle of the English language, I've occasionally mixed singular and plural pronouns for the sake of being efficient and so that the images remain gender-neutral to the extent reasonable. In several previous publications, the subtitle *The art of creating wellness while effectively managing acute and chronic musculoskeletal/health disorders* was chosen to emphasize the intentional creation of wellness rather than a limited focus on disease treatment and symptom suppression; for the 2009 printing of *Chiropractic and Naturopathic Mastery of Common Clinical Disorders*, this subtitle was slightly modified from "creating" to "co-creating" to emphasize the team effort required between physician and patient. *Managing* was chosen to emphasize the importance of treating-monitoring-referring-reassessing, rather than merely *treating*. *Disorders* was chosen to reflect the fact that a distinguishing characteristic of *life* is the ability to regularly create *organized structure* and *higher order* from chaos and *disorder*. For example, plants organize the randomly moving molecules of air and water into the organized structure of biomolecules which eventually take shape as plant structure—fiber, leaves, flowers, petals. Similarly, the human body creates organized structure of increased complexity from consumed plants and other foods; molecules ingested and inhaled from the environment are organized into specific biochemicals and tissue structures with distinct characteristics and definite functions. Injury and disease *result in* or *result from* a lack of order, hence my use of the word "disorders" to characterize human illness and disease. For example, a motor vehicle accident that results in bodily injury, for example, is an example of an external chaotic force, which, when imparted upon human body tissues, results in a disruption (disorder) of the normal structure and organization that previously defined and characterized the now-damaged tissues of the body; likewise, an autoimmune disease process that results in tissue destruction is an *anti-evolutionary* process that takes molecules of higher complexity and reverts them to simpler, fragmented, and non-functional forms. From the perspective of "health" as *organized structure and meaningful function* and "disease" as *the reversion to chaos, destruction of structure, and the loss of function*, the task of healthcare providers is essentially to restore order, and to acutely reduce and proactively prevent/eliminate clinical-biochemical-biomechanical-emotional chaos insofar as it adversely affects the patient's life experience as an individual and our collective experience as an interdependent society. What is required of clinicians then is the ability *first* to create conceptual order from what appears to be chaotic phenomena, and then *second* to materialize—make real and practically applied for patients/people seeking improved health—that conceptual order into our physical world; this is our task, and no small task it is. Also under this heading of Semantics and Language, I will make readers aware of the following additional facts. First, I tend to write very long sentences, both in general and at times when I want to connect two or more complex ideas; rather than be dismayed or discouraged by this occurrence, readers are encouraged to read these longer sentences more than just once and to engage actively, perhaps by asking, "*Why is DrV making an effort to connect these ideas*?" "**What is the conceptual advantage to the binding of these ideas together?**" I am aware of most of the rules of grammar, and I am generally—but not always—compliant. Second, I create new words and phrases as needed; an index of some of these is provided toward the back of the book, whereas some of these new terms are self-explanatory, e.g., *hypoinsulinreception*—underreception or lack of receptor responsiveness to insulin. When possible, I strongly prefer to use single words when discussing concepts, rather than multiple disparate words for singular concepts. I have started to prefer using *italics* rather than "quotation marks" when introducing new terms or when using terms/phrases/words with emphasis; the main purpose of this is to reduce the number of punctuation marks and character spaces, both of which over the course of a multi-volume work of 2,000 pages and hundreds of thousands of words are numerically significant. Last for this section, the *colorization* process that I began in April 2014 for my (larger) books is intended to 1) bring out more detail in my increasingly complex diagrams, 2) bring emphasis and highlighting to areas of particular interest, 3) make the work more visually stimulating/pleasing over the previous black/white/grayscale versions, and—relatedly—4) to keep the work interesting as readers tread through a remarkable amount of complex and detailed information; I realize that some readers may at times find the colorization to be a small distraction, but I think this is better than the alternative of monotony induced by several hundred dense pages of grayscale.

Integrity and Creativity: I have endeavored to accurately represent the facts as they have been presented in texts and research, and to specifically resist any temptation to embellish or misrepresent data as others have done.[8,9] Conversely, I have not endeavored to make this book appeal to the "average" student or reader; my goal is to write and teach to the students at the top of the class, thereby affirming them and pulling the other students forward and upward. While I offer *explanations*, I intentionally resist *simplifications*, except when one simplification might facilitate the comprehension of a more complex phenomenon, or when such a simplification might facilitate the conveyance of information from clinician to patient. I have allowed this text to be unique in format, content, and style, so that the personality of this text can be contrasted with that of the instructor and reader, thus enabling the learner to at least benefit from an intentionally different – and intentionally honest – perspective and approach. Students using this text with the guidance of a qualified professor will benefit from the experience of "two teachers" rather than just one.

Linearity, Nonlinearity, Redundancy, Asynchronicity: Although the overall flow of the text is highly linear and sequential, occasionally I place a conclusion before its introduction for the sake of foreshadowing and therefore for preparing the reader for what is to come. The purpose of this is not simply one of preparation for the sake of allowing the reader to know what is already lying ahead on the path, but more to begin creating new "shelf space" in the reader's intellectual-neuronal "library" so that when the new—particularly if *neoparadigmatic*—information is encountered, a space will already exist for it; in other words: the intent is to make learning easier. Likewise, for the sake of *information retention*— or what is physiologically understood as synaptogenesis—important points are presented more than once, either identically or variantly. Given that *"No one ever reads the same book twice"*[10] (because the "person who starts" the reading of a meaningful book is changed into the "person who finishes" the reading of that book (assuming proper intentionality and application of one's "self"), the person reading these words might consider a second glace after the first. For the sake of efficient use of space I have tried to minimize redundancy; however, in a few locations, redundancy of text and images proved necessary as—for example—viewing the same diagram within two different conversations allows the reader to gain a more profound understanding of the concepts by viewing them from two different contexts.

Bon Voyage: All artists and scientists—regardless of genre—grapple with the divergent goals of *perfecting* their work and *presenting* their work; the former is impossible in the ultimate sense, while the latter is the only means by which the effort can create the desired effect in the world, whether that is pleasure, progress, or both. At some point, we must all agree that it is "good enough" and that it contains the essence of what needs to be communicated. While neither this nor any future edition of this book is likely to be "perfect", I am content with the literature reviewed, presented, and the new conclusions and implications which are described—many for the first time ever—in this text. Firstly in and progressively from my *Integrative Rheumatology* (2006), each chapter achieved/achieves a paradigm shift which distanced/distances us farther from the simplistic pathocentric and pharmacocentric model and toward one which authentically empowers both practitioners and patients. With time, I will make future editions more complete, consistently passionate, and either more or less polemical. I hope you are able to implement these conclusions and research findings *into your own life* and into the *treatment plans for your patients*. Hopefully this work's value and veracity will promote patients' vitality via the vigilant and virtuous clinicians viewing this volume; to the more attentive and thoroughgoing reader, more is revealed (for example, the last sentence is a reference to the descriptive and prophetic movie *V for Vendetta* (2006).

Thank you for engaging with this work, and I wish you and your patients the best of success and health.

Alex Vasquez, D.C., N.D., D.O., F.A.C.N.
March 23, 2016

---

[8] Vasquez A. Zinc treatment for reduction of hyperplasia of prostate. *Townsend Letter for Doctors and Patients* 1996; January: 100
[9] Broad W, Wade N. _Betrayers of the Truth: Fraud and Deceit in the Halls of Science_. New York: Simon and Schuster; 1982
[10] Davies R. _Reading and Writing_. Salt Lake City: University of Utah Press; 1992, page 23

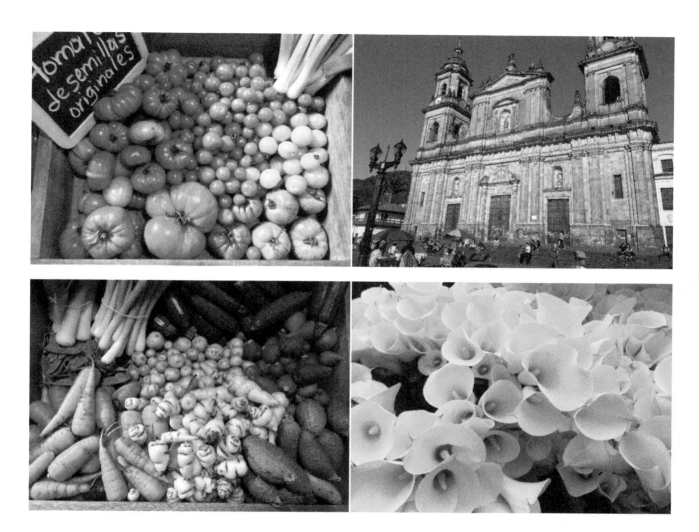

Living color, more vitality: The "colorization" process for the interior of this book began in April 2014 in Bogota (above) and Cartagena Colombia (below).

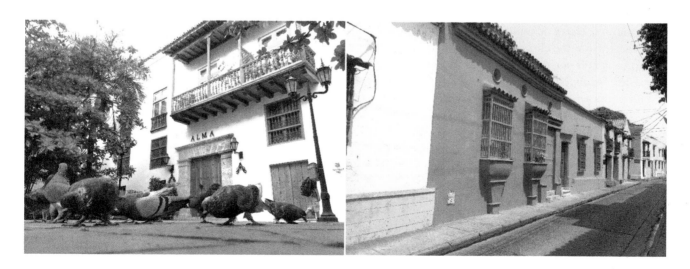

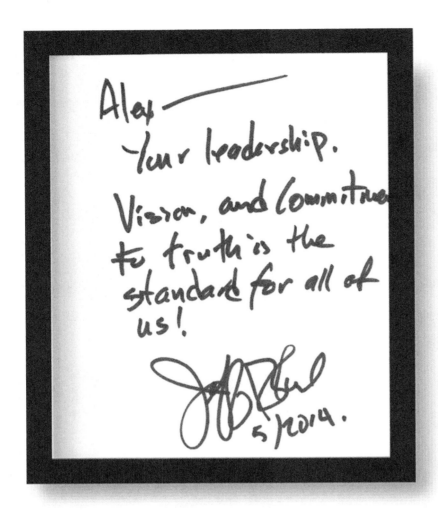

Pictured above—Personal inscription from Dr. Jeffrey Bland at a book signing event for his book *Disease Delusion*: My inclusion of Dr Bland's personal note above is not meant to imply that he is endorsing this book; he might very well reject any or all of it. Further, this inclusion does not imply that he carries those same sentiments beyond the day that he wrote them to me in May of 2014. Rather, my inclusion signifies our mutual respect as colleagues, and my personal respect for his thought and demeanor, and his influence on my life and work. I have respectfully honored him in this book as the founder of what most clinicians in America know as Functional Medicine, and I have developed and extended my own version of his concept—that disease states are *malleable* rather than *destined*—to the clinical management of inflammatory disorders under the name of Functional Inflammology. Importantly and personally—but not paradoxically if one understands the true goals of mentorship, affiliation, and friendship—due to the support of friends and colleagues, this book also represents a departure from concern that I had for endorsement from or agreement with other people, professions, universities, or organizations. In this book, I have presented the truth as I see it—without apology—and without any filtering other than as the limitations imposed by time, space, my own abilities, and limitations imposed by human physiology. This work—now published as *Inflammation Mastery, 4th Edition* —has been "in progress" since its origin as course notes for Orthopedics and Rheumatology which I taught at Bastyr University in Seattle in 2000-2001 and through its previous publications in many books starting with *Integrative Orthopedics* (2004) and *Integrative Rheumatology* (2006) and peer-reviewed publications in journals such as *Annals of Pharmacotherapy* (2005), *Alternative Therapies in Health and Medicine* (2004, 2014), *British Medical Journal* (2005), and *Nature Reviews Rheumatology* (2016). In addition to spanning more than 16 years, this work has also spanned various countries and cultures—including Houston, Fort Worth, Austin (Texas), Seattle (Washington), Portland (Oregon) in the United States, then to Bogota Colombia and Barcelona Spain. I consider this volume to be my highest presentation of truth, accuracy, clinical application and—most importantly for me: contextualization—that I could humanly muster while maintaining my own health, relationship, and other obligations. I will remain open to the correction and the updating of this work as the weight of evidence indicates. The goals of healthcare should be the optimization of physical health and psychosocial-intellectual freedom.

Reviews of previous and recent works:

- "Alex is the master of painful conditions and metabolic treatments." *Public comment by an award-winning neurosurgeon and functional medicine practitioner, 2016*

- "I love this course and your approach to the material. I am learning so much. Each article you assigned was strategically chosen and offered support and insight. I was pleasantly surprised by the exam and thought it was very fair. ... Thank you for sharing your knowledge and experience with us!" *Doctorate Student under Dr Vasquez, 2016*

- "I appreciate the lecture yesterday and I am truly fascinated by your topic and your vast knowledge. ... I for one feel having people like you on our faculty can only strengthen the credibility of our school. ... I appreciate your education, knowledge and clearly you are the authority in your field. I have listened to all your lectures on YouTube - fantastic!" *University Faculty and Doctorate Student under Dr Vasquez, 2016*

- "Thank you most kindly for your incredible dedication and kindness in sharing your knowledge with us. I am due to start med school next semester and thanks to you and all those who have taught you, I'll be way ahead of the curve." *Premedical/Medical student 2015*

- "Dr Vasquez, I have followed your work extensively and admire your intellect and passion. Thank you for your passion for teaching with integrity!" *Chiropractic doctor 2015*

- "I just wanted to tell you how much I appreciate the information I have received from you. I am still digesting most of it. I feel I have learned quite a bit already yet also feel I have barely scratched the surface." *Doctor and Graduate student under Dr Vasquez, 2013*

- "Dr. Vasquez, Thank you for all you do. **Your conference was simply amazing**. No one wanted to leave the room. I met medical professionals and very interesting lay people who were stimulated and invigorated to change their lives and the lives of others. **I am in awe at your intellectual integrity and veracity.** Best of luck to you in all of your future endeavors." *Medical physician and ICHNFM 2013 Conference Attendee*

- **2014 review of Functional Inflammology, Volume 1: "A truly comprehensive text on the vast subject of inflammation. I consider this book to be an essential addition to any health care practitioner who wishes to operate within the realm of Function Medicine. Please be aware that this book is dense in its content, and its 700 plus pages are full of deeply insightful information. I think Dr. Vasquez is one of the most prolific functional medicine contributors and books such as this should cement his reputation as such."**

- "I attended the last ICHNFM conference in Portland (and am still basking in the amazing information received)." *Email from Clinical Oncology Dietitian, in late February 2014*

- "Thanks for a fantastic conference!" *ICHNFM 2013 Conference Attendee*

- "Your discourse today reflected not only your passion and commitment to the wellness of our planet but most importantly the clarity and sincerity of your spirit/ heart/ mind. Always good to be with you and look forward to seeing you soon. Hope we can spend more time then." *Medical physician attendee 2014*

- "I was so refreshed by the 'unfiltered excellence.' What humanness. Breaths of fresh air." *ICHNFM 2013 Attendee*

- "Keep in mind Alex, that humanity is a better place because of you. I know you can't undo it all, but think about how many people would be worse off if it wasn't for your wonderful knowledge being shared with all us docs. Things that I have learned from you have changed peoples' lives for the better." *Naturopathic physician, 2014*

- "Just got back to Guam. Great experience at the International Conference on Human Nutrition and Functional Medicine. Exciting concepts on functional medicine. Thanks Dr Alex Vasquez and team!" *ICHNFM 2013 Conference Attendee*

- "Already waiting in line to buy next year's ticket! **Dr. Vasquez you crushed it!** The future is looking fun already ☺" *ICHNFM 2013 Conference Attendee*

- "Had an incredible time at the 2013 International Conference on Human Nutrition and Functional Medicine. Got to meet some amazing people and hear from some of the top researchers/health professionals about human nutrition and functional medicine approaches. It was definitely worth every penny and can't wait to go back next year!" *ICHNFM 2013 Conference Attendee*

- "I miss you! Your confidence in a program you believed in. I miss your live classes where we would get off topic on a clinical pearl. I miss your way of teaching in a laid back atmosphere that made me feel comfortable, not intimidated. I just needed to let you know, this program is not the same, I am almost done, otherwise, I would have bailed out! I am grateful for the last 18 months I did have with you at the helm. ... You ignited in me my passion for learning again. You sparked the minds of all of us with your enthusiasm. Don't ever let anyone take that away. It has given birth to your new endeavor, and we will follow where you lead. Enjoy your new surroundings and celebrate your new beginnings. I know I look forward to what is ahead." *Doctor and Graduate student under Dr Vasquez, 2013*

- "Wonderful conference! Thanks so much." *ICHNFM 2013 Conference Attendee*

- "Really wonderful conference! Lots of material ready to implement Monday morning! **Congrats to Alex Vasquez on a herculean job very well done!**" *ICHNFM 2013 Conference Attendee*

- "Thanks for a great conference. I really enjoyed all of the speakers, but your lectures were by far the most useful for implementing ideas into my clinical practice. And the most entertaining." *ICHNFM 2013 Conference Attendee*

- "Thank you for your life-changing work." *Physician, 2011*
- "I want Dr. Vasquez to know that I have just received his book, *Chiropractic and Naturopathic Mastery of Common Clinical Disorders*. **It is a treasure. The best book in my library.** Thank you for the contribution that you are giving to the world of health care." *Clinician, 2010*
- "I appreciate the resources you offer the profession. I use your books and articles regularly." *Doctor, 2011*
- "Dr. Vasquez, I greatly appreciate your efforts. I am a student at ___, 8th trimester, and would like to express my gratitude for your research and works. After coming across your texts in the library, **I quickly found your insight and explanations of the current health care crisis, and in depth coverage and algorithms for inflammatory diseases as a profound inspiration and call to action. I appreciate your attention to detail, and have been taken back several times by the potency and meaning of your sentences. Thank you for your hard work, I will enjoy these books and will surely share with those that have the same drive for true and competent patient care.**" *Health Sciences Student, 2008*
- "I never told you this, but whenever I need to research a particular disease, **besides going on Pubmed and checking some classic Pathophysiology and Clinical Nutrition books, I use your books and I find them extremely well organized, concise, and up-to-date and with the functional/integrative medicine thinking I enjoy and believe it is the future of Health Care.**" *Nutrition Research Consultant and University Faculty in Europe, 2009*
- "Thanks so much. You are a great asset to our profession." *Doctor, 2010*
- "As a 7th trimester student quickly approaching 8th trimester and student clinic, I know I will be utilizing your books often. **Your "Chiropractic and Naturopathic Mastery of Common Clinical Disorders" book is referenced very frequently by many clinicians and faculty members at [our university]. Your work is highly regarded**, and I look forward to clinically utilizing the information I will obtain from your writings." *Health Sciences Student, 2011*
- "I am a chiropractic student at ___ Chiropractic College. I just wanted to drop a quick line thanking you for your thorough and accessible textbook Integrative Orthopedics. We are using it in our Differential Diagnosis class, and **it is the best book I've come across in Chiropractic College bar none. The writing is concise, informative and refreshingly eloquent. The material is super practical. I hope you continue putting out great resources.**" *Health Sciences Student, 2011*
- "I appreciate the resources you offer the profession. **I use your books and articles regularly.**" *Doctor, 2011*
- "**Your Integrated Orthopedics book is magnificent**. I wish all textbooks were structured and as thoughtful as that one." *Health Sciences Student, 2008*
- "By reading the introduction I realize that calling it an orthopedics book; does not do it justice. **It is far more than that. It looks to me that you have created, or are creating, the bible of Integrative Orthopedics and physical medicine.** *Physician, 2007*
- "First of all let me say how honored I am that you have allowed me to review this work. You have done an amazing job! In my opinion **every healthcare provider SHOULD have this on their bookshelf.**" *Physician, 2007*
- "Your work on Chapter 12: Hip and Thigh is very good. The chapter is inclusive of the typical pathologies seen in private practice and I particularly liked the separation of juvenile from adult pathologies. Your choice of tests to assess hip and thigh pathology on page 320 is very nice and inclusive. I appreciate your use of algorithms and find them very useful in teaching and in practice. In general, **I thought this chapter represents a quality, state of the art presentation**!" *Clinician and Professor in Clinical Sciences, 2007*
- "I saw your books in a colleague's office and was really impressed. Really appreciate the thoroughness you've put into them." *Doctor, 2010*
- "**It is with great interest and fascination that I have been reading your material both in your two books (Integrative Orthopedics and Integrative Rheumatology) and online. I consider myself very fortunate to have come across your work**, as many of the basic elements of health which you discuss I never learnt or even heard about while in chiropractic college." *Doctor, 2010*
- "I appreciate the resources you offer the profession. I use your books and articles regularly." *Doctor, 2011*
- "**I'm so pleased with your books and was inspired to let you know they have already been incredibly useful! Good index; well organized algorithms. Sometimes I buy educational material and it just sort of sits there... Your books now live on my main desk. Thanks.**" *Physician and Journal Editor, 2009*
- "I just wanted to let you know how much I am enjoying reading **your book Integrative Rheumatology. It is having an extremely positive impact in the way I view health and am having a tough time putting it down. It is very inspirational.** I have long felt that it is very important to set a good example for your patients and now try my best to be one for my future patients. I like how you stress this in your book. In order to be the best example for my patients I am going to need to address some problems with my own health. I look healthy from the outside but I have been suffering from fatigue for about 4 years. It has a very negative impact on my health. People say that doing the same thing and expecting different results is the definition of insanity so I think it is time that I attempt to make some

changes. ... **Thanks again for writing such a great book. I feel it is a must have for anyone in a musculoskeletal practice.**" *Health Sciences Student, 2010*

- "My name is [recent graduate], and I've been a fan of your books since I was in chiropractic college at [university] campus. Dr. [Author, Presenter] made your book, Integrative Rheumatology, required reading for his 9th quarter nutrition class. I never looked back, and have since purchased Chiropractic & Naturopathic Mastery of Common Clinical Disorders as well as Chiropractic Management of Chronic Hypertension." *Doctor, 2010*

- "I saw your books in a colleague's office and was really impressed. Really appreciate the thoroughness you've put into them." *Doctor, 2010*

- "Reading the new integrative management of high blood pressure book and I am thoroughly enjoying it; excellent job. **I am feeling so empowered I'm opening another office focusing on 'restoring the foundations of health' for the community** that I open it in. I am looking for a location and networking to find an internist and cardiologist that are forward thinking; I'm very excited!" *Doctor, 2011*

- "Thank you for the presentation at [the university] this past weekend. **My horizons about what can be done to help people were greatly expanded. I am now still studying the notes from the seminar and am looking forward to more study and learning on how to** *correctly* **manage diabetes and hypertension.**" *Doctor, 2011*

- "Thank you for exposing so many people to the results of our research on the treatment of hypertension. I hope you can pay us a visit during your next trip to our area so we can give you the tour of our new 50+ bed inpatient facility." *Dr Alan Goldhamer, Chief of Health Promoting Clinic, 2010*

- "**I always enjoy reading your work.** I personally gain a lot of knowledge through being a peer-reviewer for you and am better because of it!" *Doctor, Faculty Member, and Postgraduate Instructor, 2011*

- "**I attended your seminar at [University] in June and have been utilizing your hypertension protocols. In that short time, I have seen some marked progress with various patients.**" *Doctor, 2010*

- "I want to personally thank you for your expertise and books on...everything. I'm in my last year at SCNM (taking rheumatology right now) and I truly admire your research and ability to compile valuable information. Thank you." *Naturopathic Medical Student, 2014*

- "Doc, I really want to thank you for sharing some of the most important-relevant Facebook posts. **If we had more doctors, leaders and informed human beings (like yourself) our world would be a better place. Thank you for your commitment to truth and doing the right thing.**" *Doctorate Clinician, 2016*

- "I love your No BS approach to everything you do. I loved it in 2013 when you hosted the most informative conference I have ever had the opportunity to attend (because I could afford it at the time thank you). I wish there were more scientists/authors/academics/doctors like you! You are a breath of fresh air among the smell of BS and one can almost "smell" your intolerance to corruption. Please don't ever stop speaking your mind, disseminating information, and rebutting the "experts" because sadly, you're a rare breed." *Doctorate Clinician, 2016*

Work as love made tangible

"You work that you may keep pace with the earth and the soul of the earth.
For to be idle is to become a stranger unto the seasons, and to step out of life's procession. ...
Work is love made visible."

Kahlil Gibran (1883-1930). *The Prophet*, 1973

Begin at the beginning

"He who wishes one day to *fly*, must first learn *standing*
and *walking*
and *running*
and *climbing*
and *dancing*.
One does not *fly* into *flying*."

Friedrich Nietzsche (1845-1900). *Thus Spoke Zarathustra—A Book for All and None*, 1883-1885

Neuroinflammation in fibromyalgia and CRPS is multifactorial

Alex Vasquez

In his Review article (Neurogenic neuroinflammation in fibromyalgia and complex regional pain syndrome. *Nat. Rev. Rheumatol.* 11, 639–648; 2015)[1], Geoffrey Littlejohn ascribes neuroinflammation to a "neurogenic" origin, presumably triggered by pain and stress. However, attribution of neuroinflammation and central sensitization to a primary neurogenic origin is premature without integrating the well-documented coexistence of small intestine bacterial overgrowth (SIBO, one type of gastrointestinal dysbiosis), vitamin D deficiency, and mitochondrial dysfunction.

Littlejohn[1] notes that chronic pain has been associated with lipopolysaccharide (LPS)–stimulated proinflammatory cytokines (particularly IFN-γ and TNF); however, he does not pursue this line of thought to connect it to relevant literature showing clear evidence of gastrointestinal dysbiosis and increased intestinal permeability in patients with fibromyalgia and complex regional pain syndrome (CRPS). The gastrointestinal tract is the most abundant source of LPS, systemic absorption of which is increased by SIBO and increased intestinal permeability. In 1999, Pimentel *et al.*[2] showed that oral administration of antibiotics led to alleviation of pain and other clinical measures of fibromyalgia. In 2004, Pimentel *et al.*[3] showed that among 42 fibromyalgia patients, all (100%) showed laboratory evidence of SIBO, severity of which correlated positively with severity of fibromalgia. In that same year, Wallace and Hallegua[4] showed that eradication of SIBO with antimicrobial therapy led to clinical improvements in fibromyalgia patients in direct proportion to antimicrobial efficacy. In 2008, Goebel *et al.*[5] documented that patients with fibromyalgia and CRPS have intestinal hyperpermeability; mucosal "leakiness" was highest in patients with CRPS, indicating a strong gastrointestinal component to the illness. In 2013, Reichenberger *et al.*[6] showed that CRPS patients have a distinct alteration in their gastrointestinal microbiome characterized by reduced diversity and significantly increased levels of Proteobacteria. LPS from Gram-negative bacteria is powerfully proinflammatory and is known to trigger microglial activation via Toll-like receptor 4; experimental studies have shown that LPS promotes muscle mitochondrial impairment, peripheral hyperalgesia, and central sensitization[7].

Vitamin D deficiency is prevalent in chronic pain and fibromyalgia patients and promotes pain sensitization, myalgia and bone pain (osteomalacia)[8]. Human clinical trials have shown that vitamin D supplementation can alleviate inflammation[9], intestinal hyperpermeability[10], fibromyalgia pain[11] and other neuromusculoskeletal pain. Vitamin D reduces experimental microglial activation[12], a component of neuroinflammation and central sensitization.

Mitochondrial dysfunction, noted in fibromyalgia[13] and CRPS[14], may be triggered by gastrointestinal dysbiosis via LPS, D-lactate, hydrogen sulfide, and inflammation; mitochondrial dysfunction exacerbates and perpetuates microglial activation and glutaminergic neurotransmission[15], thereby promoting pain sensitization centrally while also contributing to muscle pain peripherally[7]. Treatment of mitochondrial dysfunction with ubiquinone alleviates many biochemical and clinical manifestations of fibromyalgia[13].

Thus, neuroinflammation in fibromyalgia and CRPS has biological contributions including gastrointestinal dysbiosis, vitamin D deficiency, and mitochondrial dysfunction. These independent contributions commonly coexist, and each of these is additive/synergistic with the others in the promotion of peripheral and central hyperalgesia. The consistent pain-alleviating benefits of treatments for intestinal dysbiosis (antibiotics), vitamin D deficiency (supplementation) and mitochondrial dysfunction (ubiquinone) establish that these painful conditions are multifactorial and maintained by ongoing physiologic insults, each of which is treatable.

Alex Vasquez is at the International College of Human Nutrition and Functional Medicine, Calle Balmes 184, 3° 3ª, Barcelona, Spain 08006.
avasquez@ichnfm.org

doi:10.1038/nrrheum.2016.25
Published online 3 Mar 2016

1. Littlejohn, G. Neurogenic neuroinflammation in fibromyalgia and complex regional pain syndrome. *Nat. Rev. Rheumatol.* 11, 639–648 (2015).
2. Pimentel, M. *et al.* Improvement of symptoms by eradication of small intestinal overgrowth in FMS: a double-blind study [abstract]. *Arthritis Rheum.* 42, S343 (1999).
3. Pimentel, M. *et al.* A link between irritable bowel syndrome and fibromyalgia may be related to findings on lactulose breath testing. *Ann. Rheum. Dis.* 63, 450–452 (2004).
4. Wallace, D. J. & Hallegua, D. S. Fibromyalgia: the gastrointestinal link. *Curr. Pain Headache Rep.* 8, 364–368 (2004).
5. Goebel, A., Buhner, S., Schedel, R., Lochs, H. & Sprotte, G. Altered intestinal permeability in patients with primary fibromyalgia and in patients with complex regional pain syndrome. *Rheumatology* 47, 1223–1227 (2008).
6. Reichenberger, E. R. *et al.* Establishing a relationship between bacteria in the human gut and complex regional pain syndrome. *Brain Behav. Immun.* 29, 62–69 (2013).
7. Vasquez, A. *Human Microbiome and Dysbiosis in Clinical Disease 2015* (International College of Human Nutrition and Functional Medicine, 2015).
8. von Känel, R., Müller-Hartmannsgruber, V., Kokinogenis, G. & Egloff, N. Vitamin D and central hypersensitivity in patients with chronic pain. *Pain Med.* 15, 1609–1618 (2014).
9. Timms, P. M. *et al.* Circulating MMP9, vitamin D and variation in the TIMP-1 response with VDR genotype: mechanisms for inflammatory damage in chronic disorders? *QJM* 95, 787–796 (2002).
10. Raftery, T. *et al.* Effects of vitamin D supplementation on intestinal permeability, cathelicidin and disease markers in Crohn's disease: results from a randomised double-blind placebo-controlled study. *United European Gastroenterol. J.* 3, 294–302 (2015).
11. Wepner, F. *et al.* Effects of vitamin D on patients with fibromyalgia syndrome: a randomized placebo-controlled trial. *Pain* 155, 261–268 (2014).
12. Hur, J., Lee, P., Kim, M. J. & Cho, Y. W. Regulatory effect of 25-hydroxyvitamin D$_3$ on nitric oxide production in activated microglia. *Korean J. Physiol. Pharmacol.* 18, 397–402 (2014).
13. Cordero, M. D. *et al.* Oxidative stress correlates with headache symptoms in fibromyalgia: coenzyme Q$_{10}$ effect on clinical improvement. *PLoS One* 7, e35677 (2012).
14. Tan, E. C. *et al.* Mitochondrial dysfunction in muscle tissue of complex regional pain syndrome type I patients. *Eur. J. Pain* 15, 708–715 (2011).
15. Nguyen, D. *et al.* A new vicious cycle involving glutamate excitotoxicity, oxidative stress and mitochondrial dynamics. *Cell Death Dis.* 8, e240 (2011).

Competing interests statement
The author declares that he has worked as a consultant for Biotics Research Corporation (a nutraceutical company based in the USA), and that he has lectured and written for this company on various topics, including fibromyalgia.

2016 publication in *Nature Reviews Rheumatology* substantiating the model (at least partly, per the space limitations) of fibromyalgia described in this text: Provided here in printed format in accord with publisher's copyright agreement ("Authors retain the following nonexclusive rights to reproduce the contribution in whole or in part in any printed book of which they are the author"). The article needed to be added to this preface rather than deeper into the text in order to avoid the massive task of renumbering/indexing the entire book, and it serves as a validating foreshadowing of several of the concepts and clinical approaches contained herein. *Citation details*: Vasquez A. Neuroinflammation in fibromyalgia and CRPS is multifactorial. *Nat Rev Rheumatol.* 2016 Mar 3. doi: 10.1038/nrrheum.2016.25. PMID: 26935282. *Publisher site*: nature.com/nrrheum/journal/vaop/ncurrent/full/nrrheum.2016.25.html

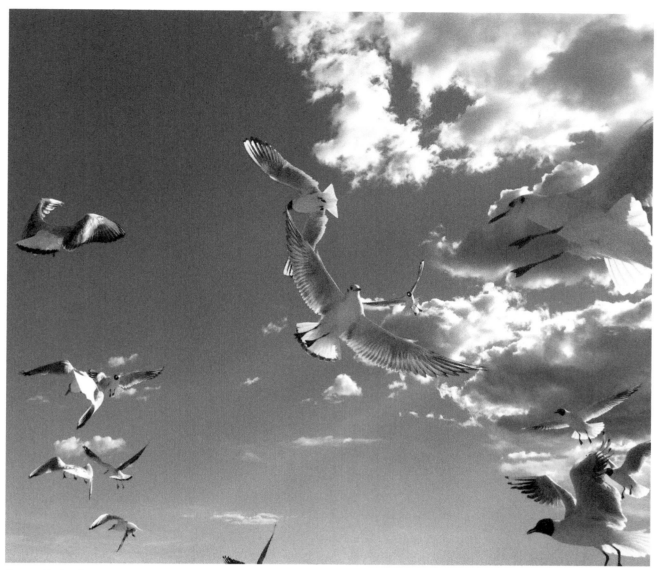

Seagulls in Sitges, Spain (2016 photo by DrV): "Most gulls don't bother to learn more than the simplest facts of flight — how to get from shore to food and back again." … "One school is finished, and the time has come for another to begin." … "We can lift ourselves out of ignorance, we can find ourselves as creatures of excellence and intelligence and skill." Richard Bach. *Jonathan Livingston Seagull*.1972

In 2016, ICHNFM initiated several new means by which students, clinicians, and benefactors can contribute to our ongoing efforts, ranging from supporting the Editorial and Review Staff of the *International Journal of Human Nutrition and Functional Medicine* (IntJHumNutrFunctMed.Org) to continue the free distribution of our publication and associated videos and interviews, to underwriting our ongoing certification efforts and joining as members to access the growing video archive and attend our webinars of case reports and research reviews. Support can also be sent directly via PayPal.com account admin@ichnfm.org; additionally, all of the ICHNFM print and ebook publications are available on Amazon.com listed under International College of Human Nutrition and Functional Medicine.

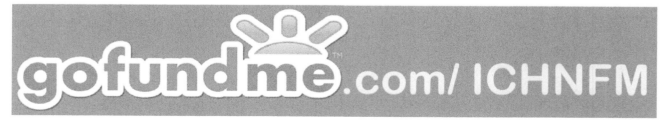

Orientation to Excerpts from *Inflammation Mastery*:
Introduction to DrV's Functional Inflammology Protocol:
The Seven Major Modifiable Factors in
Systemic Inflammation, Allergy, and Autoimmunity

Major Modifiable Influences on Immune and Inflammatory Balance

Chapter 4 of the larger textbooks—*Inflammation Mastery* (630 pages printed in 2014; 1,200 pages printed in 2016) and *Functional Inflammology* (700 pages printed in 2014)—details and organizes a massive amount of information, organized in my "functional inflammology protocol." I have developed this clinical protocol over many years of working with patients clinical practice, teaching at the graduate, doctorate, and post-graduate levels since 2000, publishing more than 110 articles and letters, and writing and re-writing more than a dozen books, the largest of which—*Inflammation Mastery, 4th Edition*—reached for the publisher's limit of 1,200 pages. I anticipate that my books are a bit of a challenge to read although I make no effort to make them unduly complicated; I simply write the information as it occurs to me, trying to add what I consider to be necessary explanations while not dumbing-down the information nor defining every term. The purpose of reading is, or at least traditionally has been, the quest for new views and information; occasionally we all have to reach for the dictionary or do some background work to enhance our understanding while exploring a new subject. Not everyone needs to or wants to read a textbook of 900 pages; hence, I occasionally excerpt sections that can stand alone as separate books.

However and obviously, these excerpted sections do not and by definition cannot contain all of the previous materials (ie, clinical overview in Chapter 1, wellness promotion and lifestyle medicine in Chapter 2, nonpharmacologic pain management in Chapter 3, the entire functional inflammology protocol in Chapter 4) that leads to the conclusions and clinical applications in Chapter 5, which details the assessment and treatment of a variety of inflammatory disorders, which I categorize as ❶ metabolic inflammation—hypertension, diabetes, migraine, fibromyalgia, ❷ allergic inflammation—allergies in general and asthma in particular, and ❸ autoimmune inflammation—all of the rheumatic conditions ranging from rheumatoid arthritis to lupus/SLE to spondylitis, psoriasis, and vasculitis. The only way to understand the foundational information in Chapters 1,2,3 and 4 is to read those chapters; the most efficient way to grasp an introductory understanding to the overall clinical approach is to see my presentation videos, two of which from the 2013 International Conference on Human Nutrition and Functional Medicine are available per these links and passwords:

* Protocol introduction, part 1: https://vimeo.com/100089988 Password: "DrVprotocol_volume1"
* Protocol introduction, part 2: https://vimeo.com/99857164 Password: "DrVprotocol_volume1"

Following my review and perusal of thousands of research articles in addition to the attentive application of my interest in these conditions throughout three doctoral programs, I have come to appreciate seven major modifiable factors that are chiefly relevant for the initial and long-term management of patients with inflammatory conditions and rheumatic diseases. These seven factors are:

1. Food intake and nutritional status: The pro/anti-inflammatory effects of diet, including food allergies and intolerances, nutrient deficiencies and dependencies,
2. Infections and dysbiosis: Chronic exposure to microbial effectors/effects,
3. Nutritional modulation of the immune system: Nutrigenomic modification of immunocyte phenotype,
4. Dysmetabolism and Dysfunctional organelles, most notably mitochondria: Especially the pro-inflammatory, pro-oxidant, and anti-apoptotic consequences of dysfunctional mitochondria (DysMito or MitoDys); more recently the conversation has extended beyond mitochondrial dysfunction to include endoplasmic reticulum stress/dysfunction (ERS) and resultant unfolded protein response (UPR),
5. Stress, sleep deprivation vs sleep sufficiency, spinal health, social and psychological considerations: Included in this section is a collection of important considerations which—in the first draft of this acronym—started with stress management, sleep hygiene, and pSychological and social factors. Later versions have included spinal health (chiropractic model), somatic dysfunction (osteopathic model), surgery, specialized supplementation, and "stamp your passport"—sometimes we all just need to vacate for a while and implement some *geographic cure* for the sake of inspiration, life enhancement, exposure to new ideas and lifestyles, and the breaking of (dysfunctional) thought patterns and routines,
6. Endocrine imbalances: Hormones can promote or retard the genesis and perpetuation of inflammation/allergy/autoimmunity; therapeutic correction with prescription or nonprescription interventions can have a profound anti-inflammatory benefit.
7. Xenobiotic immunotoxicity: Exposure to and accumulation of toxic chemicals and/or toxic metals can alter immune responses toward allergy and autoimmunity and away from immunosurveillance against infections and cancer.

The above-listed seven modifiable factors—Food, Infections, Nutri-immunology, Dysmetabolism, Society, Endocrine, Xenobiotics—can be recalled by my FINDSEX® acronym which outlines and organizes my Functional Inflammology Protocol. The overall model is represented graphically in the image below.

    With regard to the model and my books as a whole, readers should appreciate that the information in various sections likely applies either conceptually or specifically to conditions described in other sections and that therefore the best way to understand inflammatory/allergic/autoimmune disorders in their totality is to appreciate the nuances of each and the common themes among all.

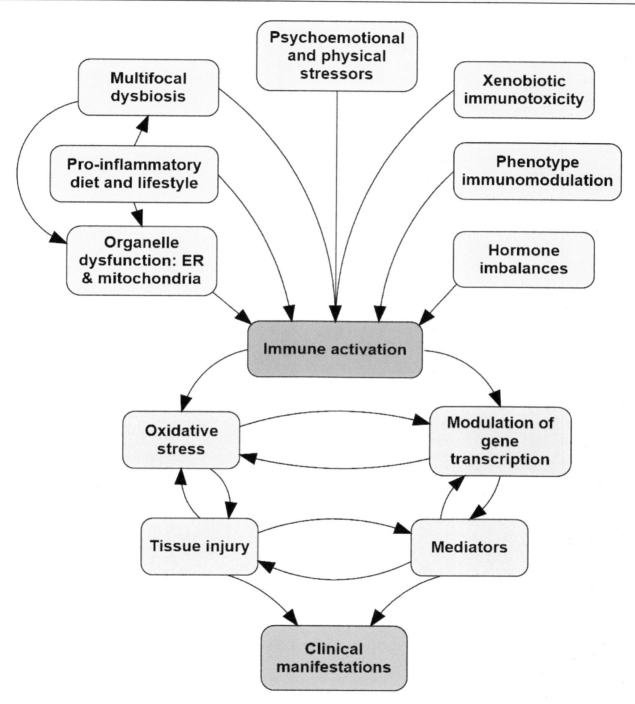

Inflammation in a simple cause-and-effect diagram: The major causative factors amenable to clinical implementation are represented, along with the pathophysiologic consequences and clinical effects. Molecular details, clinical assessments, and therapeutic interventions are introduced/reviewed in this chapter; in later volumes of this work, clinical protocols detail the drugs and doses, etc.

Affirmation and consistency of common themes in an interconnected reality; the importance of transitioning from reception to comprehension to conception to behavior

"The fact that today I still stand by these ideas, **that in the intervening time they themselves have constantly become more strongly associated with one another, even to the point of growing into each other, intertwining, and becoming *one*,** that has reinforced in me the joyful confidence that they may not have originally developed in me as single, random, or sporadic ideas, but up out of common roots, from some fundamental *will for knowledge* ruling from deep within, always speaking with greater clarity, always demanding greater clarity.

In fact, this is the only thing appropriate and proper for a philosopher. **We have no right to be isolated in any way: we are not permitted to make isolated mistakes or to run into isolated truths**. Our ideas, our values, our affirmations and denials, our *if*s and *but*s—these rather grow out of us from the same necessity which makes a tree bear its fruit—totally related and interlinked amongst each other: witnesses of one will, one health, one soil, one sun."

Nietzsche FW. *On the Genealogy of Morals*, 1887, Preface essay #2

"In order for a particular species to maintain itself and increase its power, **its conception of reality must comprehend enough of the calculable and constant** for it to **base a scheme of behavior on it.**"

Nietzsche FW. *Will to Power*,1901, #480

Infection, dysbiosis

Nutritional immunomodulation

Functional Inflammology
F.I.N.D.S.E.X.® acronym

Food, Nutrition

Dysmetabolism, dysfunctional mitochondria

"enough of the calculable and constant to base a scheme of behavior"

Style of living (lifestyle): psychology, sociology, politics, sweat/exercise, stress, sleep, special considerations such as surgery

© ICHNFM.org

Xenobiotic load

Endocrine

This work is a stand-alone monograph and yet at the same time is an updated excerpt from Dr Vasquez's larger works *Functional Inflammology* (700 pages) and *Inflammation Mastery, 4th Edition* (1,180 pages). While this monograph is complete in itself, reference is made to other sections and chapters for those who have or might be interested in the complete model and "functional inflammology protocol."

Nutrition & FxMed for chronic immune-inflammatory disorders

Causes of Inflammation-Immune-Metabolic Imbalance:

1. Food, Lifestyle

2. Infection, Dysbiosis

3. Nutritional Immunomodulation

4. Dysfunctional mitochondria

5. Stress, Emotions, Psychology, Sociology, Lifestyle

6. Endocrine, Hormones

7. Xenobiotics, Toxins

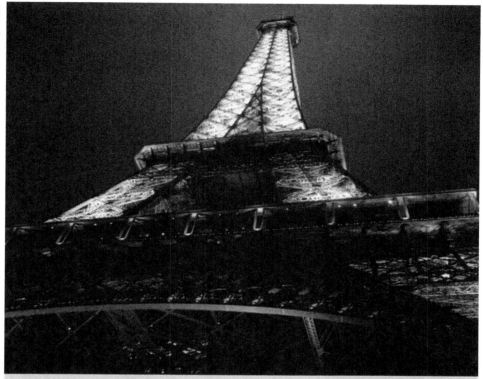

Notice that these 7 factors can be remembered by the acronym: **F.I.N.D. S.E.X.**
♥ First presented in Paris in 2012 ♥

The "Functional Inflammology Protocol" and FINDSEX® acronym: As the clinical protocol expanded from five components (diet, dysbiosis, xenobiotics, hormones, and stress) published in 2006 and 2007 to seven components (adding nutritional immunomodulation and mitochondrial dysfunction) in 2012, I realized that the time had come to attempt an acronym in order to facilitate student memorization and clinician application. I applied some priority to the sequence of the categories, and then experimented with a few acronyms. The rest, as is said, is history. This occurred just before a series of presentations in France (starting in Paris), Holland, and Belgium in March of 2012. The FINDSEX acronym is a registered trademark (e.g., ® and ™) in association with *Functional Immunology and Nutritional Immunomodulation*[11], *F.I.N.D.S.E.X. The Easily Remembered Acronym for the Functional Inflammology Protocol*[12], *Integrative Rheumatology and Inflammation Mastery, Third Edition*[13], and other books, videos[14], audios[15], and presentations by Dr Vasquez since 2012. One of the more recent introductions to this protocol was delivered at the International Conference on Human Nutrition and Functional Medicine in Portland Oregon in September 2013 and is posted here vimeo.com/ichnfm/drv-functional-inflammology-intro2013 and accessed with the password "DrVprotocol"; access to new videos, book updates, and articles are periodically distributed by email newsletter from ICHNFM.ORG.

[11] Published Jun 2012, ISBN-10: 1477603859, ISBN-13: 978-1477603857
[12] Published Apr 2013, ISBN-10: 1484046765, ISBN-13: 978-1484046760
[13] Published Jan 2014, ISBN-10: 1495272621, ISBN-13: 978-1495272622
[14] vimeo.com/drvasquez and vimeo.com/ichnfm
[15] itunes.apple.com/us/artist/dr-alex-vasquez/id475526413 and cdbaby.com/Artist/DrAlexVasquez

Examples of commonly used abbreviations:

- **25-OH-D** = serum 25-hydroxy-vitamin D(3)
- **ACEi** = angiotensin-2 converting enzyme inhibitor
- **Alpha-blocker** = alpha-adrenergic antagonist
- **ANA** = antinuclear antibodies
- **ARB** = angiotensin-2 receptor blocker/antagonist
- **ARF** = acute renal failure
- **BB** = beta blocker or beta-adrenergic antagonist
- **bHB, BHB** = beta-hydroxy-butyrate
- **BMP** = basic metabolic panel, includes serum Na, K, Cl, CO2, BUN, creatinine, and glucose
- **BP** = blood pressure, relatedly **HBP** = high blood pressure
- **BUN** = blood urea nitrogen
- **C and S** = culture and sensitivity
- **CAD** = coronary artery disease
- **CBC** = complete blood count
- **CCB** = calcium channel blocker/antagonist
- **CE** = cardiac enzymes, including creatine kinase (CK), creatine kinase myocardial band (CKMB), and troponin-1, with the latter being the most specific serologic marker for acute myocardial injury; for the evaluation of acute MI, these are generally tested 2-3 times at 6-hour intervals with ECG performed at least as often.
- **CHF** = congestive heart failure
- **CHO, carb** = carbohydrate
- **CK** = creatine kinase, historically named creatine phosphokinase (CPK)
- **CKD** = chronic kidney disease, generally stratified into five stages based on GFR of roughly <90, 90-60, 60-30, 30-15, and >15, respectively
- **CMP** = comprehensive metabolic panel, also called a chemistry panel, includes the BMP along with markers of hepatic status albumin, protein, ALT, AST, may also include alkaline phosphatase and rarely GGT; panels vary per laboratory and hospital.
- **CNS** = central nervous system
- **COPD** = chronic obstructive pulmonary disease
- **CRF, CRI** = chronic renal failure/insufficiency
- **CVD** = cardiovascular disease

- **CRP** = c-reactive protein, hsCRP = high-sensitivity c-reactive protein **CT** = computed tomography
- **CXR** = chest X-ray
- **DM** = diabetes mellitus
- **DMARD** = disease-modifying antirheumatic drugs
- **ECG** or **EKG** = electrocardiograph
- **Echo** = echocardiography
- **ERS** = endoplasmic reticulum stress
- **GFR** = glomerular filtration rate
- **HDL** = high density lipoprotein cholesterol
- **HTN** = hypertension
- **Ig** = immune globulin = antibodies of the G, A, M, E, or D classes.
- **IHD** = ischemic heart disease
- **I+D** = incision and drainage
- **IM, IV** = intramuscular, intravenous
- **LPS** = bacterial lipopolysaccharide, endotoxin
- **MCV** = mean cell volume
- **MI** = myocardial infarction
- **Mito** = mitochondria(l)
- **MRI** = magnetic resonance imaging, **MRA** = magnetic resonance angiography
- **mTOR** = mechanistic or mammalian receptor of rapamycin; **TOR** is also reasonable
- **NFkB** = nuclear transcription factor kappa beta
- **PNS** = peripheral nervous system
- **PRN** = from the Latin "pro re nata" meaning "on occasion" or "when necessary"
- **PTH** = parathyroid hormone, iPTH = intact parathyroid hormone
- **PVD** = peripheral vascular disease
- **RA** = rheumatoid arthritis
- **RAD** = reactive airway disease, asthma
- **SIBO** = small intestine bacterial overgrowth
- **SLE** = systemic lupus erythematosus
- **TLR** = Toll-like receptor
- **TRIG(s)** = serum triglycerides
- **UA** = urinalysis
- **UPR** = unfolded protein response
- **US** = ultrasound

Dosing shorthand:
- **bid** = twice daily
- **cc** = with meals
- **hs** = at bedtime
- **ic** = between meals
- **po** = per os = by mouth

- **prn** = as needed (additional details above)
- **qd** = each day, also /d or /day
- **qid** = four times per day
- **tid** = thrice daily
- **yo** = years old

Read, pause, consider, struggle, think, grow

"If this book is incomprehensible to anyone and jars on his ears, the fault, it seems to me, is not necessarily mine. It is clear enough, assuming, as I do assume, that one has first read my earlier writings and has not spared some trouble in doing so: for they are, indeed, not easy to penetrate. Regarding my _Zarathustra_, for example, I do not allow that anyone knows the book who has not at some time been profoundly wounded and at some time profoundly delighted by every word in it; for only then may he enjoy the privilege of reverentially sharing in the halcyon element out of which that book was born and in its sunlight clarity, remoteness, breadth, and certainty. In other cases, people find difficulty with the aphoristic form: this arises from the fact that today this form is not taken seriously enough. An aphorism, properly stamped and molded, has not been "deciphered" when it has simply been read; rather, one has then to begin its exegesis—its explanation, its extraction, for which is required an art of deciphering.

To be sure, one thing is necessary above all if one is to practice reading as an art in this way, something that has been unlearned most thoroughly nowadays—something for which one has almost to be a cow and in any case not a "modern man": _rumination_—taking time to pause, to reflect, to consider...

Friedrich Nietzsche, _On the Genealogy of Morals_, Preface, Section #8, Sils-Maria, Upper Engadine, July 1887

Chapter 5: Clinical Applications of the Functional Inflammology Protocol

---

Introduction

- <u>The functional inflammology protocol is a decipherative technology for understanding complex chronic illnesses and for organizing an effective treatment approach</u>: The functional inflammology protocol is a decipherative technology for understanding complex chronic illnesses and for organizing an effective treatment approach; the FINDSEX ® acronym reminds clinicians of the most important lifestyle, nutritional, environmental, and (patho)physiologic contributors and interventions

- <u>History of this Chapter</u>: The bulk of this chapter was updated for *Rheumatology v3.5* (2014); an appendix of less common autoimmune/rheumatic disease has been added at the end of this chapter, imported with minimal revision from *Integrative Rheumatology v2* (2007) and *Integrative Rheumatology and Inflammation Mastery v3* (2014). Sections on migraine, hypertension, diabetes and allergy were imported from previous publications, specifically *Chiropractic and Naturopathic Mastery of Common Clinical Disorders* (2009). The section on fibromyalgia has been completely restructured for this publication and embellished with new diagrams and new information, especially on glial activation and central sensitization which also applies to migraine and other disorders of sustained inflammation and secondary pain sensitization. The detailed information in Chapter 4 and the clinical applications in Chapter 5 are more than sufficient for application to the newly imported conditions from previous publications, even while the FINDSEX ® acronym and structured protocol were developed in 2012.

- <u>Foundational Belief in a Comprehensible and Rational/Orderly Universe</u>: Rheumatologic disorders are multifactorial, not idiopathic. The Functional Inflammology Protocol reviewed in Chapter 4 covers the most important concepts; in this chapter those concepts will encounter opportunities for clinical application in the management/comanagement of rheumatologic diseases, better described as rheumatologic/autoimmune disease *states*, with the latter added to imply their temporal and potentially escapable nature. Stated differently, let us begin with the assumption that we are intelligent and capable, and that while we do not now and never will have "all of the answers", we have enough talent and information within our current grasp to allow us to rationally approach these multifactorial conditions and address the largest components, as outlined by the FINDSEX® acronym. Knowledge is—commonly if not generally— asymptotic; we get closer and closer to the truth without actually touching all components at all times; but this is no rationale for us either as humans generally or clinicians specifically to languish in nihilistic repose. We are obligated to act on what we know and to orchestrate rational treatment.

- <u>Comanagement and Risk Management</u>: A wise clinical strategy when managing any serious or potentially-life threatening condition is for the clinician to arrange for co-management with a specialist, and this is particularly true for conditions that might necessitate hospitalization or acute immunosuppression. Autoimmune diseases such as lupus are notorious for acute flares that can cause permanent damage (e.g., transverse myelitis resulting in paralysis); likewise, giant cell arteritis is notorious for causing rapid-onset visual loss, which is generally permanent and thus debilitating. Reviews of patient management, risk management, and common musculoskeletal emergencies are provided in Chapter 1—this information should be reviewed prior to the reading of this chapter and implementation of the clinical applications herein. Pharmaceuticalization of these patients offers no chance of cure but is useful for "controlling" inflammation with limited efficacy and numerous adverse long-term effects. The best general approach is one that is etiotherapeutic/polyetiotherapeutic—directed at treating the cause(s) of the disorder while accessing pharmacoimmunosuppression on an "as needed" basis.

- <u>Video Presentations and Tutorials</u>: These are provided to help reinforce—*not replace*—the written material in this chapter, and these additional videos should be viewed *following* the videos corresponding to the overall protocol (Chapter 4), mitochondrial dysfunction (Chapter 4), the detailing of dysbiosis (Chapter 4 plus additional presentation slides—see presentation slides for video access). One of the major goals with these videos, in addition to simply providing more information and reinforcing the material in the text, is that these will promote learning of the material in a conversational style, because ultimately the material must be understood in words and communicable in words in order to be understood and applied: vimeo.com/album/3000884, password: DrV_Allergy_Rheum. Updates and sample syllabi: InflammationMastery.com/books/rheum/

- <u>Understanding autoimmunity as "patterns of inflammation"</u>: My perspective for years—supported by the phrase "patterns of inflammation" by WG Meggs MD PhD—is that autoimmune disorders as we appreciate them (phenomenonistically and diagnostically) are simply "variations on the theme" of the seven factors I've identified via the FINDSEX® acronym and functional inflammology protocol. As such, readers should note the consistency of the pattern, and also how research "specific" for one disease might well apply to a particular autoimmune/inflamed/autoinflammed patient even if he/she has a different diagnostic label; such is the rule, rather than the exception. As such, the information in this textbook needs to be appreciated and integrated in its entirety, not simply accessed for information on a specific topic without consideration of the provided—and synergistic—context.

Clinical Topics—following this introduction: Note that immediately before the start of the clinical topics is a summary outline of the functional inflammology protocol otherwise detailed in Chapter 4.

❶ Metabolic inflammation, mitochondrial dysfunction
  1. Hypertension
  2. Diabetes
  3. Migraine
  4. Fibromyalgia
❷ Allergic inflammation
  5. Allergy (general), asthma and reactive airway disease—note that allergy in general and eczema is covered in several locations of the book, particularly Chapter 4, Sections 1 and 3

❸ Autoimmune/rheumatic inflammation
  6. Rheumatoid arthritis
  7. Psoriasis and psoriatic arthritis
  8. Systemic lupus erythematosus
  9. Scleroderma, systemic sclerosis Vasculitic diseases
  10. Spondyloarthropathies
  11. Sjögren syndrome/disease
  12. Raynaud's syndrome/phenomenon/disorder
  13. Clinical Notes on Additional Conditions: Behçet's Disease, Sarcoidosis, Dermatomyositis and Polymyositis

Layout of each section—listed once here to avoid unnecessary repetition at each section:

- Introduction and Overview
- Clinical Presentation
- Prevalence, Symptoms, and Clinical Findings
- Pathophysiology
- Differential Diagnosis
- Diagnosis
- Standard Medical Treatment
- Therapeutic Interventions—Clinical Application of the Functional Inflammology Protocol via FINDSEX™ acronym

---

The Functional Inflammology Protocol is a decipherative clinical approach—"a scheme of behavior"—for the understanding and treatment of complex inflammatory-metabolic disorders implemented via the F.I.N.D.S.E.X.® mnemonic acronym

"In order for a particular species to maintain itself and increase its power, its conception of reality **must comprehend enough of the calculable and constant** for it to base a **scheme of behavior** on it."

Nietzsche FW. *Will to Power*, 1901, #480

Factors that are "calculable and constant" in sustained inflammatory diseases: F.I.N.D.S.E.X.®

- **F**ood and nutritional variables
- **I**nfections, dysbiosis
- **N**utritional (deficiency) alternations in immune phenotype and function
- **D**ysmetabolism of mitochondria, ER
- **S**leep disturbance, social stressors, sweating deficiency (lack of exercise)
- **E**ndocrine imbalances
- **X**enobiotic immunotoxicity

Twilight of the Idiopathic Era and the Dawn of New Possibilities in Health and Healthcare

This article was originally published in *Naturopathy Digest* in 2006; minor edits were made in 2010 and 2014
naturopathydigest.com/archives/2006/mar/idiopathic.php

Among the perplexing paradoxes that exist in healthcare is coexistence of our adoration of allopathy for its "scientific method" along with the description of most chronic diseases as "idiopathic." If the allopathic use of the scientific method were so adroit, then why are so many conditions described as having "no known cause"? Is the scientific method inadequate, or is the allopathic lens incapable of bringing disease causation into focus? Perhaps a third option exists: that some groups—namely the medical profession generally and the pharmaceutical companies specifically—benefit by convincing us that most diseases have "no known cause" and that therefore the best that doctors and patients can hope for is additive and endless pharmaceuticalization of all health problems. When the cause of our health problems is "unknown", we are disempowered, and we must depend on "experts" and those who have "the cure" to help us and save us. When the causes of our problems are known, we are empowered to take effective action. Certainly, some groups have financial and political interests in keeping us *as professionals* and *as patients* confused and disempowered.

  The End of the Idiopathic Era: A stark contrast exists between primary research literature and the "facts" that are selectively reported in medical textbooks and which are used to buttress "conventional wisdom" and the resultant status quo. While I have been aware of this contrast for many years, the divergence was impressed upon me with renewed vigor during the preparation of a recent article[1] and the completion of my 2006 textbook *Integrative Rheumatology*.[2] Arthritis in general and autoimmune and rheumatic diseases in particular are frequently described as "idiopathic" and as having "no known cause" by most mainstream medical books like *The Merck Manual* and *Current Medical Diagnosis and Treatment*; these contentions are inconsistent with the abundant and diverse research showing that—rather than being *idiopathic*—most chronic musculoskeletal disorders are *multifactorial*. When a disease is codified as *idiopathic*, doctors lose their incentive to look for and treat the *causes* [plural] of the disease because the codified conventional wisdom has already stated that "The cause [singular] of the disease has not been identified." Similarly, patients are convinced to give up their hope of ever being *cured*; they chose what appears to be the second best option: lifelong medicalization. In these instances, acceptance of the codified conventional wisdom benefits doctors and patients by freeing them of the obligation to think, to mobilize their consciousness; the price paid for this exoneration from consciousness is perpetuated unconsciousness and drug dependence for doctors and patients. Being told by powerful institutions and ensconced authorities that "There's nothing else you can do, and nothing more to think about" lulls us all into apathy and conformity at the price of our individual and collective lives and consciousness.

 Multifactorial—not idiopathic: Let's look at psoriasis and rheumatoid arthritis as two shining examples of *idiopathicity*. If one looks into a standard medical textbook, one sees that these conditions have *no known cause* and *therefore* the lifelong prescription of anti-inflammatory medications is presumptively justified. On the contrary, if one spends a few days in any medical library, one can find articles that point to the causes of these diseases and which then illuminate the path (and paths) by which doctors and patients can arrive at authentic improvement or permanent cure. Most patients can be cured of psoriasis, and a large percentage of rheumatoid arthritis patients can avoid the complications and medicalization associated with their disease, particularly if *the causes* of their condition are treated early. We now know that most autoimmune diseases are caused by and/or perpetuated by ~~chronic~~ sustained infections, phenotypic/epigenetic immune imbalances, a proinflammatory lifestyle, hormonal imbalances, and exposure to chemicals and metals that cause immune dysfunction/activation. When the cause(s) of the disease is treated, the disease has the potential to be cured, provided that it is treated comprehensively and hopefully before the onset of irreversible damage. When the disease is cured, lifelong medicalization becomes unnecessary, the patient is free to fully resume his/her life, and doctors are liberated from their roles as drug representatives and can resume their proper positions as healers and creative free-thinking individuals.

 Asserting an empowered stance toward disease prevention and treatment carries implications beyond those for the doctor and the patient. These implications also point to new ways of living and stewarding the world. When we look at a disease like Parkinson's disease and then determine that it is *idiopathic*, then nothing happens to change or shape our view of the world, our place in it, and the interconnected components of health and disease. Everyone agrees that that clinical manifestations of Parkinson's disease result from the death (or perhaps impairment?) of dopaminergic neurons. From the allopathic perspective, the disease is *idiopathic*, while from an integrative naturopathic perspective, we see Parkinson's disease as a *multifaceted disorder* associated with defective mitochondrial function, impaired xenobiotic detoxification, and occupational and/or recreational exposure to toxicants, particularly pesticides. These associations align to create a new model for the illness based on exposure to neurotoxicants such as pesticides[3] which are ineffectively detoxified[4] and then accumulate in the brain[5] and induce mitochondrial dysfunction[6] and resultant oxidative stress[7] which leads to impairment/death of dopaminergic neurons. Therefore, from the perspective of both prevention and treatment, the clinical approach to Parkinson's disease should include pesticide avoidance and optimization of detoxification to prevent the cellular accumulation of neurotoxic mitochondrial poisons. The plan must also include optimization of nutritional status, antioxidant capacity, and mitochondrial function.[8] Further, if our goal is to reduce the societal prevalence of

[1] Vasquez A. Nutritional and Botanical Treatments against "Silent Infections" and Gastrointestinal Dysbiosis. *Nutritional Perspectives* 2006; January
[2] Vasquez A. *Integrative Rheumatology*. First Edition. 2006
[3] Ritz B, Yu F. Parkinson's disease mortality and pesticide exposure in California 1984-1994. *Int J Epidemiol*. 2000 Apr;29(2):323-9
[4] Menegon A, Board PG, Blackburn AC, et al. Parkinson's disease, pesticides, and glutathione transferase polymorphisms. *Lancet*. 1998;352(9137):1344-6
[5] Kamel F, Hoppin JA. Related Articles, Association of pesticide exposure with neurologic dysfunction and disease. *Environ Health Perspect*. 2004;112(9):950-8
[6] Parker WD Jr, Swerdlow RH. Mitochondrial dysfunction in idiopathic Parkinson disease. *Am J Hum Genet*. 1998;62(4):758-62
[7] Davey GP, Peuchen S, Clark JB. Energy thresholds in brain mitochondria. Potential involvement in neurodegeneration. *J Biol Chem*. 1998;273(21):12753-7
[8] Kidd PM. Parkinson's disease as multifactorial oxidative neurodegeneration: implications for integrative management. *Altern Med Rev*. 2000 Dec;5(6):502-29

Parkinson's disease, then we must begin living in better harmony with nature and thinking of ways to reduce our use of pesticides and herbicides, the chemicals that are consistently shown to cause premature neuronal death and which are increasingly pervasive in our home, work, and outdoor environments.

The Dawn of New Possibilities in Health and Healthcare: The time is now past when credible physicians can assert that most diseases are "of unknown origin." The truth is that we already have access to the information we need to help our patients. The truth is that we can often offer our patients the *probability of cure* rather than *lifelong and endless prescriptions for symptom-modifying drugs*. These truths imply that healthcare and our systems of healthcare delivery must change, because the pharmaceutical and medical icons that stand before us were built upon feet and legs of clay and interspersed lead. We stand at the dawn of a new era in healthcare—one in which patients with chronic diseases in general and autoimmune diseases in particular—have a tangible and authentic opportunity to regain their health.

Higher education
"Our real problem is to determine: *what is the goal of education?*
Are we forming children who are only capable of learning what is already known?
Or should we try to develop creative and innovative minds, capable of discovery from the preschool age onward, throughout life?"
Jean Piaget (1896-1980), Swiss developmental psychologist and philosopher known for his epistemological studies with children

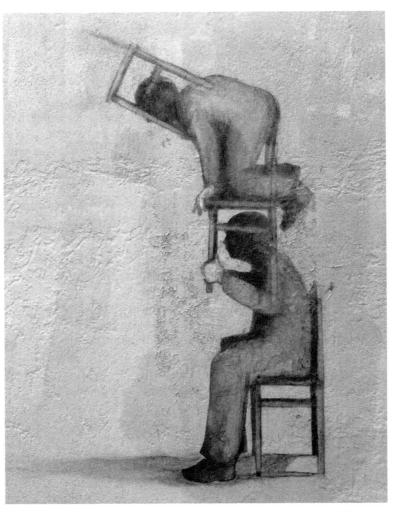

Anonymous art-quality graffiti in Paris, France—photo by Dr Vasquez in 2013: This image reminds me of the (common, American) educational process, which is often stupefying and *stupidifying*. Throughout most of my educational experience—including 12 years of doctorate-level study—I found that most schools have impressively little commitment to *instruction* (Latin: *instruere*: to pack in, to load) and even less to *education* (Latin: *educare*: to lead out); in fact, most "professional" academicians and so-called "administrators" do not appreciate these words or concepts for their meanings nor their implications. In my experience as a Professor and Director at various schools, I frequently found so-called "senior administrators" to be completely incompetent in their roles, and completely corrupt in their willingness to literally sell-out quality faculty for personal gain and financial advantage, even at major cost to students, programs, courses, and the institution—I have seen this in various schools in various professions, including professions and some schools which I previously cherished. The pervasiveness and high level of incompetence and corruption in healthcare professions and institutions is bewildering. What I strive for with my books and courses is to resist the "dumbing down" of students and the dehumanization and eunuchification of academia in general and intellectuality in particular.

Review of the Functional Inflammology Protocol and each of the FINDSEX® Components:
Summarized here to reduce redundancy and repeated citations throughout the clinical application subsections

---

The Functional Inflammology Protocol is reviewed and substantiated in Chapter 4; the protocol is reviewed/outlined here with the most important components cited. In the clinical application sections that follow, the protocol is applied, and its disease-specific implications are emphasized; the abbreviated overview/summary is included in each subsection with nuances noted and citations omitted to enhance safety/efficacy/applicability and space/time efficiency, respectively.

- **FOOD & NUTRITION** The 5-part "supplemented Paleo-Mediterranean diet" (SPMD—reviewed in Chapter 4, Section 1) consists of ❶ <u>foundational plant-based low-carbohydrate diet of fruits, vegetables, nuts, seeds, berries and lean sources of protein</u>: the plant-based diet optimizes antioxidant and phytonutrient intake[9] while promoting favorable modification of gastrointestinal flora for a systemic anti-inflammatory benefit[10]; carbohydrate intake is minimized and tailored per individual need for weight maintenance and exercise recovery/compensation; maintaining mild ketosis via low carbohydrate intake helps maintain optimal body weight, mitochondrial efficiency, bHB's antioxidant function and a rejuvenative phenotype via histone acetylation[11]; plant-based diets promote alkalinization and counteract the Western diet's promotion of diet-induced acidosis[12]; renal insufficiency mandates vigilance for hyperkalemia, especially when considering implementation of a potassium-rich diet ❷ <u>multivitamin and multimineral supplementation</u>: this component serves to correct pandemic nutritional deficiencies[13], prevent long-latency deficiency diseases[14], improve mood[15], reduce systemic inflammation[16], and provide some/partial/complete compensation for genotropic metabolic defects[17], ❸ <u>physiologic doses of vitamin D3 (range 2,000-10,000 IU/d)</u>: vitamin D3 supplementation[18] alleviates pain, improves mood, reduces inflammation, enhances immunity, normalizes hypertension, ❹ <u>combination fatty acid therapy (CFAT) with n3-ALA, n6-GLA, n3-EPA, n3-DHA, and phytochemical-rich olive oil which contains n9-oleate</u>: anti-inflammatory, mood-enhancing, and cardioprotective benefits are conclusively documented, ❺ <u>probiotics</u>: probiotics promote immunotolerance via several mechanisms including induction of Treg; probiotic supplementation helps prevent and treat insufficiency dysbiosis, which causes 1) decreased colonization resistance, 2) increased bacterial translocation, and 3) failure of optimal Treg induction. Per "Expert consensus document: The International Scientific Association for Probiotics and Prebiotics consensus statement" published in *Nature Reviews Gastroenterology and Hepatology* 2014 Aug[19], probiotics—by definition—require administration of at least one billion (1,000,000,000 or 1×10^9) colony forming units (CFU); many probiotic nutritional supplements in the form of powders and capsules contain 1-20 billion organisms yet not all organisms are viable at time of consumption and not all viable organisms become CFU. Importantly, some benefits of probiotic supplementation are not dependent on viable microorganisms but rather on the molecular signature of the microbe; other—and obviously more complete—benefits require microbial viability and are mediated via metabolites, which are themselves interdependent on microbes and the host's diet. Bertazzoni et al[20] extensively reviewed the issue of microbial/CFU count number and concluded that the appropriate dose is patient-dependent, disease-dependent, and strain-dependent and thus cannot be generalized; their review included several studies that safely and effectively used varying doses, e.g., 1, 30, 70,

---

[9] Liu RH. Health benefits of fruit and vegetables are from additive and synergistic combinations of phytochemicals. *Am J Clin Nutr.* 2003 Sep;78(3 Suppl):517S-520S

[10] Peltonen R et al. Faecal microbial flora and disease activity in rheumatoid arthritis during a vegan diet. *Br J Rheumatol.* 1997 Jan;36(1):64-8

[11] Shimazu T, Hirschey MD, et al. Suppression of oxidative stress by β-hydroxybutyrate, an endogenous histone deacetylase inhibitor. *Science* 2013 Jan;339:211-4. To access more of Dr Matt Hirschey's work and video presentations, please see ichnfm.org/events/MitochondrialMedicine. For additional information on the rejuvenative effect of histone acetylation, see: Matuoka et al. Rapid reversion of aging phenotypes by nicotinamide through possible modulation of histone acetylation. *Cell Mol Life Sci.* 2001 Dec;58:2108-16

[12] Adeva et al. Diet-induced metabolic acidosis. *Clin Nutr.* 2011 Aug;30:416-21. Cordain et al. Origins and evolution of the Western diet. *Am J Clin Nutr.* 2005 Feb;81(2):341-54

[13] Fletcher RH, Fairfield KM. Vitamins for chronic disease prevention in adults: clinical applications. *JAMA.* 2002 Jun 19;287(23):3127-9

[14] Heaney RP. Long-latency deficiency disease: insights from calcium and vitamin D. *Am J Clin Nutr.* 2003 Nov;78(5):912-9

[15] Benton D, Haller J, Fordy J. Vitamin supplementation for 1 year improves mood. *Neuropsychobiology.* 1995;32(2):98-105

[16] Church TS, Earnest CP, Wood KA, Kampert JB. Reduction of C-reactive protein levels through use of a multivitamin. *Am J Med.* 2003 Dec 15;115(9):702-7

[17] Ames BN, et al. High-dose vitamin therapy stimulates variant enzymes with decreased coenzyme binding affinity (increased K(m)). *Am J Clin Nutr.* 2002 Apr;75(4):616-58

[18] See discussion and citaitons throughout Chapter 4. Vasquez A, Manso G, Cannell J. The clinical importance of vitamin D (cholecalciferol): a paradigm shift with implications for all healthcare providers. *Altern Ther Health Med.* 2004 Sep-Oct;10(5):28-36 ichnfm.academia.edu/AlexVasquez /

[19] Hill et al. Expert consensus document: The International Scientific Association for Probiotics and Prebiotics consensus statement on the scope and appropriate use of the term probiotic. *Nat Rev Gastroenterol Hepatol.* 2014 Aug;11(8):506-14

[20] Bertazzoni et al. Probiotics and clinical effects: is the number what counts? *J Chemother.* 2013 Aug;25(4):193-212

300 billion CFU/d. Per expert clinical opinion, a clinician might use one billion [units = microbes or CFU] for a small or young child, and a starting dose of 10 billion scaling up to 90 billion per day for adults.[21]

- o Additional details—implementation of the "low-carbohydrate (low fermentation) supplemented Paleo-Mediterranean diet" ("low-carb SPMD"): The diet should be plant-based, but not necessarily vegan or vegetarian; I refer to this diet at "plant-based Paleo" since "the Paleo diet" as commonly discussed is simply a diet of whole natural foods which can generally be consumed without cooking or processing. For purposes of meeting physiologic expectations and attaining the highest satiety, weight optimization, and nutrient density with a phytonutrient-dense low-fermentation diet, the diet should primarily consist of fruits, vegetables, nuts, seeds, berries, and lean sources of protein; carbohydrate intake is modulated per caloric and carbohydrate needs while protein intake is tailored to lean body mass, exercise and healing/recuperation needs. Preferred sources of protein are grass-fed land animals as well as wild-caught cold-water fish, both of which are low in total fat and high in the anti-inflammatory and immunomodulatory omega-3 fatty acids, especially EPA and DHA. Whey protein isolate can also be used as it is an inexpensive convenient source of high-quality protein well-tolerated for most patients and as it also contains many functional components such as glutathione precursors, tryptophan, immunoglobulins, and growth factors anti-gastrin effects which help to heal/protect damaged intestinal mucosa. Plant-based diets, which can be further phyto-supplemented with food concentrates and fruit/vegetable smoothies/juices, provide the greatest dietary density and diversity of phytonutrients which generally have antioxidant and anti-inflammatory effects; also very important is the highly important modulation of gastrointestinal flora by plant-based diets which serves as a major mechanism by which such diets exert their clinically significant systemic anti-inflammatory benefits. I have detailed this diet—"the Supplemented Paleo-Mediterranean diet" as a combination of the "Paleolithic" or "Paleo diet" and the well-known "Mediterranean diet", both of which are well described in peer-reviewed journals and the lay press. (See Chapter 2 and my other publications[22,23] for details). This diet is the most nutrient-dense diet available, and its benefits are further enhanced by supplementation with vitamins, minerals, and the health-promoting fatty acids: ALA, GLA, EPA, DHA, and oleic acid. Vitamin and mineral supplementation is warranted in the general population and even more so among patients[24], who are more likely to be nutrient deficient due to their disease processes, mediations, and concomitant problems such as mild metabolic acidosis, malabsorption, and drug-induced nutrient depletions. Beyond routine vitamin-mineral supplementation, additional vitamin D3 supplementation is generally needed to meet the physiologic requirement of approximately 4,000 IU per day and to achieve the physiologic and clinical benefits including prevention/alleviation of depression, chronic pain, diabetes mellitus, hypertension, immunosuppression, immune activation, and cancer.[25] Likewise, absolute or relative deficiencies/insufficiencies of health-promoting anti-inflammatory fatty acids—namely: ALA, GLA, EPA, DHA, and oleic acid—are common and clinically consequential insofar as these deficiencies/insufficiencies promote chronic/sustained inflammation, pain, and neuroemotional impairment; thus, combination fatty acid therapy/replacement/supplementation (CFAT) is indicated based on its physiological effects and clinical benefits. Probiotics, especially when consumed in conjunction with a plant-based diet which promotes an enhanced milieu for their growth and effect, provide clear clinical benefits which are both local to the gut (e.g., reduced incidence of opportunistic infections/colonizations, prevention/amelioration of increased intestinal permeability) and systemic via the anti-inflammatory benefits of enhanced induction of Treg cells at the reciprocal expense of Th-17 cells. This "supplemented Paleo-Mediterranean diet" obviates overconsumption of chemical preservatives, artificial sweeteners, and carbohydrate-dominant foods such as candies, pastries, breads, potatoes,

---

[21] Conversation and personal communication 2014 Aug with my friend and colleague Mike Ash DO ND, an international expert on probiotics and mucosal immunology, "But some studies suggest 1 billion is the number needed to generate an effect (of clinical relevance), and this may suit a small or young child. I tend to start at 10 billion and rarely ever exceed 90 billion in a day [for adults]."

[22] Vasquez A. A Five-Part Nutritional Protocol that Produces Consistently Positive Results. *Nutritional Wellness* 2005 September

[23] Vasquez A. Implementing the Five-Part Nutritional Wellness Protocol for the Treatment of Various Health Problems. *Nutritional Wellness* 2005 November

[24] "However, suboptimal intake of some vitamins, above levels causing classic vitamin deficiency, is a risk factor for chronic diseases and common in the general population, especially the elderly. ... Most people do not consume an optimal amount of all vitamins by diet alone. Pending strong evidence of effectiveness from randomized trials, it appears prudent for all adults to take vitamin supplements. ... Physicians should make specific efforts to learn about their patients' use of vitamins to ensure that they are taking vitamins they should, ..." Fletcher RH, Fairfield KM. Vitamins for chronic disease prevention in adults: clinical applications. *JAMA.* 2002 Jun 19;287(23):3127-9

[25] Vasquez et al. The clinical importance of vitamin D (cholecalciferol): a paradigm shift. *Altern Ther Health Med.* 2004 Sep-Oct;10(5):28-36

grains, and other foods with a high glycemic load and high glycemic index (from a practical and conceptual standpoint: glycemic load x glycemic index = glycemic impact = more oxidative stress, antioxidant depletion, immunosuppression, and mitochondrial impairment).

- Supplemented Paleo-Mediterranean diet / Specific Carbohydrate Diet: The specifications of the *specific carbohydrate diet* (SCD) detailed by Gottschall[26] are met with adherence to the Paleo diet by Cordain.[27] The combination of both approaches and books will give patients an excellent combination of informational understanding and culinary versatility.

- The use of a low starch diet in the treatment of patients suffering from ankylosing spondylitis: alleviation of dysbiosis and immune complex formation via nutritional intervention (*Clin Rheumatol* 1996 Jan[28]): "The majority of ankylosing spondylitis (AS) patients not only possess HLA-B27, but during active phases of the disease have elevated levels of total serum IgA, suggesting that a microbe from the bowel flora is acting across the gut mucosa. .... Furthermore AS patients from 10 different countries have been found to have elevated levels of specific antibodies against Klebsiella bacteria. It has been suggested that these Klebsiella microbes, found in the bowel flora, might be the trigger factors in this disease and therefore reduction in the size of the bowel flora could be of benefit in the treatment of AS patients. Microbes from the bowel flora depend on dietary starch for their growth and therefore a reduction in starch intake might be beneficial in AS patients. A "low starch diet" involving a reduced intake of "bread, potatoes, cakes and pasta" has been devised and tested in healthy control subjects and AS patients. The "low starch diet" leads to a reduction of total serum IgA in both healthy controls as well as patients, and furthermore to a decrease in inflammation and symptoms in the AS patients."

  o Celiac disease and autoimmunity (*J Gastroenterol Hepatol* 2013 Jan[29]): 356 patients with CD participated in this study. "Autoimmune thyroiditis (10.6% vs 0.4%), insulin dependent diabetes mellitus (IDDM) (2.2% vs 1.7%), systemic lupus erythematosus (SLE) (1.1% vs 0), and psoriasis (12.9% vs 5.5%) occurred more frequently in CD patients."

  o Refractory immune thrombocytopenia successfully treated with high-dose vitamin D supplementation and hydroxychloroquine: two case reports (*J Med Case Rep.* 2013 Apr[30]): "In our two case reports, we found an association between vitamin D deficiency and immune thrombocytopenia where platelet levels responded to vitamin D treatment and hydroxychloroquine but not to prednisone. We believe there may be synergism between vitamin D supplementation and hydroxychloroquine."

- INFECTIONS & DYSBIOSIS Essentially all autoimmune/rheumatic disorders are associated with microbial colonization and intolerance to same; the presence of persistent microbial colonization is *prima facie* evidence of immunosuppression, commonly due to nutritional deficiencies, psychoemotional stress, sleep deprivation, overconsumption of simple carbohydrates, or—most commonly since all of these are common—a combination of all of these. The eight areas of dysbiosis (multifocal)—listed here from head to toe and inside out—are: ❶ sinorespiratory, ❷ orodental, ❸ gastrointestinal, ❹ urogenital/genitourinary, ❺ parenchymal/tissue, ❻ microbial (dysbiosis within microbes, e.g., bacteriophages), ❼ dermal/cutaneous, and ❽ environmental. Patients with low mucosal sIgA levels, recurrent mucosal infections, or autoimmunity are candidates for serum IgA testing to evaluate for genotropic selective secretory IgA deficiency.

  o Interventions and antimicrobial agents for gastrointestinal dysbiosis:

    - *Saccharomyces boulardii*: A non-colonizing, non-pathogenic yeast that increases sIgA production and can aid in the elimination of pathogenic/dysbiotic yeast, bacteria, and parasites. It is particularly useful during antibiotic treatment to help prevent secondary *Candida* and *Clostridium difficile* infections. Common dose is 250 mg thrice daily for adults and twice daily for children.

[26] Gotschall E. *Breaking the Vicious Cycle: Intestinal health though diet*. Kirkton Press; Rev edition (August, 1994) scdiet.com/
[27] Cordain L. *The Paleo Diet*. John Wiley & Sons Inc., New York 2002 thepaleodiet.com/
[28] Ebringer A, Wilson C. The use of a low starch diet in the treatment of patients suffering from ankylosing spondylitis. *Clin Rheumatol*. 1996 Jan;15 Suppl 1:62-66
[29] Iqbal et al. Celiac disease arthropathy and autoimmunity study. *J Gastroenterol Hepatol*. 2013 Jan;28(1):99-105
[30] Bockow et al. Refractory immune thrombocytopenia successfully treated with high-dose vitamin D supplementation and hydroxychloroquine. *J Med Case Rep*. 2013 Apr 4;7:91

- Berberine (generally available as generic berberine hydrochloride or as a plant-based standardized extract with synergistic phytochemicals[31]) 1,000-1,500 mg/d in divided doses PO for up to 3 months: Berberine is a botanical alkaloid extracted from plants such as *Berberis vulgaris,* and *Hydrastis canadensis* with millennia of clinical use for various conditions and also specifically for the treatment of infectious diseases, such as those caused by *E coli, Giardia lamblia* (comparable to metronidazole), *Entamoeba histolytica, Streptococcus* and *Chlamydia trachomatis.*[32] Many clinicians use berberine as a standard treatment for gastrointestinal dysbiosis due to bacteria, yeast, and/or other microbes; it is very safe and has a wide range of antimicrobial action. Oral dose of 400 mg per day has been traditionally common for adults[33]; however newer clinical research has shown that berberine 1,000-1,5000 mg/d for three months provides major clinical benefits and is effective treatment for dyslipidemia, insulin resistance, diabetes mellitus type-2 (comparable to metformin), and overweight/obesity.[34,35,36,37] Berberine is available in a "generic" form from many companies.

- Oregano oil (time-released emulsified preparation named "ADP" from Biotics Research Corporation) 600 mg/d generally given as 200 mg/d PO TID for 6 weeks: Oil of Mediterranean oregano *Oreganum vulgare* was orally administered to 14 adult patients whose stools tested positive for enteric parasites, *Blastocystis hominis, Entamoeba hartmanni* and *Endolimax nana.* Six weeks of supplementation with 600 mg emulsified oil of oregano daily resulted in complete disappearance of *Entamoeba hartmanni* (four cases), *Endolimax nana* (one case), and *Blastocystis hominis* in eight cases. *Blastocystis hominis* scores declined in three additional cases.[38] An *in vitro* study[39] and clinical experience support the use of emulsified oregano against *Candida albicans* and various gastrointestinal microbes. Many clinicians use ADP as a standard treatment for gastrointestinal dysbiosis due to bacteria, yeast, and/or other microbes; it is very safe and has a wide range of antimicrobial action.

- Undecylenic acid (also known as 10-undecenoic acid, available as "Formula SF722" from Thorne Research, each gelcap contains 10-undecenoic acid 50 mg) dosed at "450-750 mg undecylenic acid daily in three divided doses"[40] equates to 10-15 capsules per day, or 5 capsules 2-3 times per day: An eleven-carbon monounsaturated fatty acid found naturally in the body (occurring in sweat) and produced commercially by the vacuum distillation of castor bean oil, undecylenate shows laboratory and clinical human-trial effectiveness against *Herpes Simplex, Candida albicans,* and tinea pedis caused by *Trychophyton rubrumor* and *Trychophyton mentagrophytes.*

- Combination botanical antimicrobials ("Tricycline" from Allergy Research Group; "Dysbiocide" and "FC-Cidal" from Biotics Research Corporation): Tricycline contains black walnut, artemesinin, berberine, and citrus seed extract; in the early days of my clinical practice, I used this product routinely with a standard dosing of 2 capsules BID for 2-4 weeks. Two capsules BID each of Dysbiocide and FC-Cidal for 4 weeks is effective—more effective than rifaxamin—against SIBO.[41]

- DrV's (in)famous "vitamin C purge"—the author's perspective and rationale: Generally when I lecture on the topic of dysbiosis to post-graduate audiences, I mention one of my preferred

[31] Stermitz et al. Synergy in a medicinal plant: antimicrobial action of berberine potentiated by 5'-methoxyhydnocarpin. *Proc Natl Acad Sci U S A.* 2000 Feb 15;97(4):1433-7

[32] [No authors listed]. Berberine. *Altern Med Rev.* 2000 Apr;5(2):175-7

[33] Berberine. *Altern Med Rev.* 2000 Apr;5(2):175-7 thorne.com/altmedrev/.fulltext/5/2/175.pdf

[34] Kong et al. Berberine is a novel cholesterol-lowering drug working through a unique mechanism distinct from statins. *Nat Med.* 2004 Dec;10(12):1344-51

[35] "...obese human subjects (Caucasian) were given 500 mg berberine orally 3 times a day for 12 weeks. ... Results demonstrate that berberine treatment produced mild weight loss (average 5 lb/subject) in obese human subjects. But more interestingly, treatment significantly reduced blood lipid levels (23% decrease of triglyceride and 12.2% decrease of cholesterol levels) in human subjects." Hu et al. Lipid-lowering effect of berberine in human subjects and rats. *Phytomedicine* 2012 Jul;19:861-7

[36] "In study A, 36 adults with newly diagnosed type 2 diabetes mellitus were randomly assigned to treatment with berberine or metformin (0.5 g 3 times a day) in a 3-month trial. The hypoglycemic effect of berberine was similar to that of metformin. Significant decreases in hemoglobin A1c (from 9.5% to 7.5%), fasting blood glucose (from 10.6 mmol/L to 6.9 mmol/L), postprandial blood glucose (from 19.8 to 11.1 mmol/L), and plasma triglycerides (from 1.13 to 0.89 mmol/L) were observed in the berberine group. In study B, 48 adults with poorly controlled type 2 diabetes mellitus were treated supplemented with berberine in a 3-month trial. Berberine acted by lowering fasting blood glucose and postprandial blood glucose from 1 week to the end of the trial. Hemoglobin A1c decreased from 8.1% to 7.3%." Yin J, Xing H, Ye J. Efficacy of berberine in patients with type 2 diabetes mellitus. *Metabolism.* 2008 May;57(5):712-7

[37] "One hundred sixteen patients with type 2 diabetes and dyslipidemia were randomly allocated to receive berberine (1.0 g daily) and the placebo for 3 months. ... In the berberine group, fasting and postload plasma glucose decreased from 7.0 +/- 0.8 to 5.6 +/- 0.9 and from 12.0 +/- 2.7 to 8.9 +/- 2.8 mm/liter, HbA1c from 7.5 +/- 1.0% to 6.6 +/- 0.7%, triglyceride from 2.51 +/- 2.04 to 1.61 +/- 1.10 mm/liter, total cholesterol from 5.31 +/- 0.98 to 4.35 +/- 0.96 mm/liter, and low-density lipoprotein-cholesterol from 3.23 +/- 0.81 to 2.55 +/- 0.77 mm/liter,..." Zhang et al. Treatment of type 2 diabetes and dyslipidemia with the natural plant alkaloid berberine. *J Clin Endocrinol Metab.* 2008 Jul;93(7):2559-65

[38] Force M, Sparks WS, Ronzio RA. Inhibition of enteric parasites by emulsified oil of oregano in vivo. *Phytother Res.* 2000 May;14(3):213-4

[39] Stiles JC, Sparks W, Ronzio RA. The inhibition of Candida albicans by oregano. *J Applied Nutr* 1995;47:96–102

[40] [No authors listed] Undecylenic acid. Monograph. *Altern Med Rev.* 2002 Feb;7(1):68-70

[41] Chedid et al. Herbal therapy is equivalent to rifaximin for the treatment of small intestinal bacterial overgrowth. *Glob Adv Health Med.* 2014 May;3(3):16-24

treatments for GI dysbiosis, for which I seem to be either famous or infamous, namely the "vitamin C purge." The application is essentially as straightforward as the underlying logic: the *per os* use of vitamin C (20-60 grams in 1 liter of water, preferably with two cups of coffee) for its osmotic laxative effect to rapidly reduce the quantity of bacteria/microorganisms throughout the gut by introduction of a cleansing water bolus; while the vitamin C and water serve as an osmotic nonstimulant laxative (perhaps with some antimicrobial effect), the coffee/caffeine serves as a bowel stimulant. I have used this treatment empirically with great success in achieving rapid quantitative reductions in gastrointestinal microbes. For many years plain ascorbic acid was used at doses of 20-60 grams 20,000-60,000 mg) to induce therapeutic laxation (occasionally described as "do-it-yourself top-to-bottom gastrointestinal lavage") with onset of action generally within 30-60 minutes following consumption of powered ascorbate in approximately one liter of water, preferably *and often necessarily* with a bowel peristalsis stimulant such as coffee. The goal and purpose are to achieve a cleansing water bolus that purges the bowels of dysbiotic microbes and their pro-inflammatory debris and mitochondria-impairing metabolites. The use of therapeutic laxatives for the treatment of intestinal parasitic disease is well represented in the Infectous Disease and Tropical Medicine literature; in this instance, we are using ascorbic acid as an osmotic laxative and the coffee as a bowel stimulant. In high concentrations, ascorbic acid is directly microbicidal, at least against *E coli* (per Gaby, c 1993). The vitamin C can be administered as ascorbic acid—perfectly fine but very acidic, Ca/Mg/K buffered ascorbate—same laxative effect with the additional nutritive or laxative effect of minerals, or as home-made buffered ascorbate by mixing—per my own use—one heaping teaspoon or tablespoon of ascorbic acid with 1/2-one teaspoon baking soda (sodium bicarbonate). Additional agents can be ingested simultaneously for additional antimicrobial effect (e.g., iodine-iodide 12-48 mg [given that the standard antimicrobial dose for systemic/dermal infections usually starts at 1,000mg/d]) or intraluminal adsorption (e.g., activated charcoal). Patient selection excludes those who are generally frail and those with renal impairment, cardiac arrhythmia, bowel obstruction, electrolyte imbalance, dementia/psychosis, postural instability and/or reduced mobility to attend the toilet promptly, etc; patients with iron overload are reasonably be excluded—thus serum ferritin should be tested as described in Chapter 1—given that oral vitamin C administration may lead to clinical deterioration in patients with hemochromatosis, per a single case report.[42] As a general rule, the vitamin C purge is initiated only in the morning 1-2 hours before the first meal and is followed later in the day—especially when used for several days consecutively—some effective form of electrolyte replacement, whether in supplemental pill/powder form or as salted vegetable juice; patients can use this treatment PRN, at the beginning of antimicrobial therapy especially to break the vicious cycle of SIBO and resultant GI stasis resulting from microbial methane and H2S, or consecutively; when the latter, periodic assessment of serum electrolytes is reasonable, with one standard interval for monitoring dietary intervention being weekly.

Coffee as a gastrointestinal stimulant

"Coffee stimulates gastrin release and gastric acid secretion... Coffee induces cholecystokinin release and gallbladder contraction... Coffee increases rectosigmoid motor activity within 4 min after ingestion in some people. Its effects on the colon are found to be comparable to those of a 1000 kCal meal. ... Coffee promotes gastro-esophageal reflux, but is not associated with dyspepsia. Coffee stimulates gallbladder contraction and colonic motor activity.

Boekema et al. Coffee and gastrointestinal function: facts and fiction. *Scand J Gastroenterol.* 1999;230:35-9

"Caffeinated coffee, decaffeinated coffee and meal induced more activity in the colon with a greater area under the curve of pressure waves and a greater number of propagated contractions when compared with water. Caffeinated coffee, decaffeinated coffee and meal induced greater motor activity in the transverse/descending colon when compared with the rectosigmoid colon. ... Caffeinated coffee stimulates colonic motor activity. Its magnitude is similar to a meal, 60% stronger than water and 23% stronger than decaffeinated coffee."

Rao et al. Is coffee a colonic stimulant? *Eur J Gastroenterol Hepatol.* 1998 Feb;10(2):113-8

---

[42] "We describe rapidly fatal cardiomyopathy in a young man. He had for twelve months ingested large amounts of ascorbic acid and was admitted with severe heart failure having been symptomatic for two months. He died after eight days. Idiopathic haemochromatosis was diagnosed at autopsy." McLaran et al. Congestive cardiomyopathy and haemochromatosis--rapid progression possibly accelerated by excessive ingestion of ascorbic acid. *Aust N Z J Med.* 1982 Apr;12(2):187-8

> **Laxatives promote eradication of intestinal microbes and are especially useful in patients with stasis/constipation**
>
> "Our case shows that although the dose of praziquantel is an important issue, supportive care, including the optimal use of an oral laxative and enemas to ensure smooth evacuation of the worm, is also important. This is especially true for young patients who are usually constipated or who cannot evacuate feces intentionally.
>
> <div align="right">Fujita et al. A 2-year-old girl with <i>Diphyllobothrium nihonkaiense</i> infection
treated with oral praziquantel and a laxative. <i>J Nippon Med Sch</i>. 2008 Aug</div>
>
> For irritable bowel syndrome with constipation: "Treatment with osmotic laxatives (milk of magnesia or polyethylene glycol) may increase stool frequency, improve stool consistency, and reduce straining."
>
> <div align="right">Papadakis M, McPhee SJ, Rabow MW (eds). <i>Current Medical Diagnosis and Treatment</i>, 2014</div>

- *Artemisia annua*: Artemisinin has been safely used for centuries in Asia for the treatment of malaria, and it also has effectiveness against anaerobic bacteria due to the pro-oxidative sesquiterpene endoperoxide.[43,44] This author has commonly used artemisinin at 200 mg per day in divided doses for adults with dysbiosis. Given its pro-oxidative mechanism, treatment should probably be of limited duration, i.e., 1-2 months; concomitant neuroprotection with CoQ-10 (et al) would be reasonable.

- St. John's Wort (*Hypericum perforatum*): Hyperforin from *Hypericum perforatum* shows impressive antibacterial action *in vitro*, particularly against gram-positive bacteria such as *Staphylococcus aureus*, *Streptococcus pyogenes*, *Streptococcus agalactiae*[45] and perhaps gram-negative *Helicobacter pylori*.[46] Up to 600 mg three times per day of a 3% hyperforin standardized extract is customary in the treatment of depression.

- Bismuth: Bismuth is commonly used in the empiric treatment of diarrhea (e.g., "Pepto-Bismol") and is commonly combined with other antimicrobial agents to reduce drug resistance and increase antibiotic effectiveness.[47]

- Peppermint (*Mentha piperita*): Peppermint shows antimicrobial and antispasmodic actions and has demonstrated clinical effectiveness in patients with bacterial overgrowth of the small bowel.

o Commonly used antibiotic/antifungal drugs: The most commonly employed drugs for intestinal bacterial overgrowth are described here.[48] Treatment duration is generally at least 2 weeks and up to 8 weeks, depending on clinical response and the severity and diversity of the intestinal overgrowth. With all anti*bacterial* treatments, use empiric anti*fungal* treatment to prevent yeast overgrowth; some patients benefit from antifungal treatment that is continued for *months* and occasionally *years*. Probiotic yeast and bacteria are generally appropriate except in patients with hypersensitivity, severe immunosuppression, or extreme or recalcitrant bacterial overgrowth of the intestines. Drugs can generally be co-administered with natural antibiotics/antifungals for improved efficacy. Treatment can be guided by identification of the dysbiotic microbes, results of culture and sensitivity tests, and response to treatment. Examples of doses are provided below, but clinicians must choose dose and duration per their judgment, experience, and the patient's situation, comorbidity, age, hepatic and renal function, and accompanying polypharmacy; the use of dosing and drug-interaction data (e.g., *Epocrates*) is strongly recommended.

- Metronidazole: 250-500 mg BID-QID (generally limit to 1.5-2 g/d); metronidazole has systemic bioavailability and effectiveness against a wide range of dysbiotic microbes, including protozoans, amebas/Giardia, *H. pylori*, *Clostridium difficile* and most anaerobic gram-negative bacilli.[49] Adverse effects are generally limited to stomatitis, nausea, diarrhea, and—rarely and/or with long-term use—peripheral neuropathy, dizziness, and metallic taste; the drug must not be consumed with alcohol. Metronidazole resistance by *Blastocystis hominis* and other parasites has been noted.

- Erythromycin: 250-500 mg TID-QID; this drug is a widely used antibiotic that also has intestinal promotility benefits (thus making it an ideal treatment for intestinal bacterial overgrowth associated

[43] Dien et al. Effect of food intake on pharmacokinetics of oral artemisinin in healthy Vietnamese subjects. *Antimicrob Agents Chemother*. 1997 May;41(5):1069-72

[44] Giao et al. Artemisinin for treatment of uncomplicated falciparum malaria: is there a place for monotherapy? *Am J Trop Med Hyg*. 2001 Dec;65(6):690-5

[45] Schempp et al. Antibacterial activity of hyperforin from St John's wort, against multiresistant Staphylococcus aureus and gram-positive bacteria. *Lancet*. 1999 Jun 19; 2129

[46] "A butanol fraction of St. John's Wort revealed anti-Helicobacter pylori activity with MIC values ranging between 15.6 and 31.2 microg/ml." Reichling J, Weseler A, Saller R. A current review of the antimicrobial activity of Hypericum perforatum L. *Pharmacopsychiatry*. 2001 Jul;34 Suppl 1:S116-8

[47] Veldhuyzen van Zanten SJ, Sherman PM, Hunt RH. Helicobacter pylori: new developments and treatments. *CMAJ*. 1997;156(11):1565-74 cmaj.ca/cgi/reprint/156/11/1565.pdf

[48] Saltzman JR, Russell RM. Nutritional consequences of intestinal bacterial overgrowth. *Compr Ther*. 1994;20(9):523-30

[49] Tierney ML. McPhee SJ, Papadakis MA. *Current Medical Diagnosis and Treatment 2006. 45th edition*. New York; Lange Medical Books: 2006, pages 1578-1577

with or caused by intestinal dysmotility/hypomotility such as seen in scleroderma[50,51]). Do not combine erythromycin with the promotility drug **cisapride** due to risk for serious cardiac arrhythmia.

- Tetracycline: 250-500 mg QID
- Ciprofloxacin: 500 mg BID, Caution: tendonopathy and tendon rupture can occur within 72 hours; new data connects fluoroquinolone with aortic aneurysm.[52]
- Cephalexin/Keflex: 250 mg QID
- Minocycline: Minocycline (200 mg/day)[53] has received the most attention in the treatment of rheumatoid arthritis due to its superior response (65%) over placebo (13%)[54]; in addition to its antibacterial action, the drug is also immunomodulatory and anti-inflammatory. Ironically, minocycline can cause drug-induced autoimmunity, especially lupus.[55,56]
- Nystatin: Nystatin 500,000 units BID-TID with food; duration of treatment begins with a minimum duration of 2-4 weeks and may continue as long as the patient is deriving benefit.

o Antiviral (phyto)nutrition: Antiviral therapeutics should include those with the greatest safety, efficacy, synergistic/additive/collateral benefits, most obviously—per my antiviral protocol[57]—1) 5pSPMD discussed previously, 2) vitamin D3 2,000-10,000 IU/d for its tolerogenic (via Treg) and antimicrobial (via AMP) benefits, 3) vitamin A 25,000 IU/d with discussion and monitoring for toxicity; particularly important given the high percentage of (female) patients who cannot effectively convert carotene to retinol, 4) selenium 600 mcg/d to retard viral mutagenesis and replication, 5) melatonin 2-20 mg nightly for antioxidant, immunostimulatory, antiinflammatory, and mitochondrial-protective benefits, 6) NAC 1,500 mg TID for antioxidant, GSH-promoting, anti-mTOR, anti-NFkB and antiviral benefits, to be used with 7) lipoic acid 400 mg TID for antioxidant, GSH-preserving, anti-IL-17, anti-NFkB and antiviral benefits, 8) zinc 20-50 mg/d for immunosupportive, pro-thymulin, anti-NFkB, and direct antiviral effects in its ionized form, 9) glycyrrhizin from licorice—doses of glycyrrhizin in the treatment of human viral diseases can be set at 40 mg per day, 5 mg/kg, or dosed reasonably from tea and supplements with periodic monitoring for hypokalemia and hypertension; the generally accepted safe daily dose of glycyrrhizin is 0.2 mg/kg[58], 10) lysine 2-3 g/d is effective and perhaps specific for HSV infections but may be generalizable for all herpes virus infections; generally, the treatment is administered along with a low-arginine diet but arginine itself is necessary for immunocompetence, 11) additional antiviral treatments include injectable adenosine monophosphate, oral/topical lemon balm (*Melissa officinalis*), and oral/topical lithium.

- **NUTRITIONAL IMMUNOMODULATION** Nutrients and therapeutic approaches that promote Treg or IL-10 induction and/or Th-17, IL-17 suppression include 1) mitochondrial optimization and mTOR suppression, 2) biotin, 3) vitamin E, 4) sodium avoidance, 5) transgenic/GMO food avoidance, 6) probiotics, 7) lipoic acid, 8) vitamin A, 9) inflammation reduction, 10) vitamin D, 11) fatty acid supplementation with GLA and n3, 12) infection and dysbiosis remediation, 13) green tea EGCG. Readers should recall the MiBESTPLAIDFIG acronym outlined in Chapter 4.

---

[50] "Prokinetic agents effective in pseudoobstruction include metoclopramide, domperidone, cisapride, octreotide, and erythromycin. ... The combination of octreotide and erythromycin may be particularly effective in systemic sclerosis." Sjogren RW. Gastrointestinal features of scleroderma. *Curr Opin Rheumatol.* 1996 Nov;8(6):569-75
[51] "Erythromycin accelerates gastric and gallbladder emptying in scleroderma patients and might be helpful in the treatment of gastrointestinal motor abnormalities in these patients." Fiorucci et al. Effect of erythromycin administration on upper gastrointestinal motility in scleroderma patients. *Scand J Gastroenterol* 1994 Sep:807-13
[52] Fluoroquinolone use associated with aortic aneurysm. *Pharmaceutical Journal* 2015 Nov pharmaceutical-journal.com/news-and-analysis/research-briefing/fluoroquinolone-use-associated-with-aortic-aneurysm/20200171.article
[53] "...48-week trial of oral minocycline (200 mg/d) or placebo." Tilley et al. Minocycline in rheumatoid arthritis. A 48-week, double-blind, placebo-controlled trial. MIRA Trial Group. *Ann Intern Med.* 1995 Jan 15;122(2):81-9
[54] "In patients with early seropositive RA, therapy with minocycline is superior to placebo." O'Dell et al. Treatment of early rheumatoid arthritis with minocycline or placebo: results of a randomized, double-blind, placebo-controlled trial. *Arthritis Rheum.* 1997 May;40(5):842-8
[55] "...many cases of drug-induced lupus related to minocycline have been reported. Some of those reports included pulmonary lupus..." Christodoulou et al. Respiratory distress due to minocycline-induced pulmonary lupus. *Chest.* 1999 May;115(5):1471-3 chestjournal.org/cgi/content/full/115/5/1471
[56] Lawson TM, Amos N, Bulgen D, Williams BD. Minocycline-induced lupus: clinical features and response to rechallenge. *Rheumatology* (Oxford). 2001 Mar;40(3):329-35
[57] Chapter 4, Section 2b, "Antiviral Protocol" in *Inflammation Mastery, 4th Edition* (2015) and *Antiviral Strategies and Immune Nutrition: Against Colds, Flu, Herpes, AIDS, Hepatitis, Ebola, Dengue, and Autoimmunity* (2014). Digital book ASIN: B00OPJXMTS; Printed book ISBN: 1502894890
[58] Fiore et al. Antiviral effects of Glycyrrhiza species. *Phytother Res.* 2008 Feb;22(2):141-8

o   Altered Th17 cells and Th17/regulatory T-cell ratios indicate the subsequent conversion from undifferentiated connective tissue disease [UCTD] to definitive systemic autoimmune disorders (*Hum Immunol.* 2013 Dec[59]): "Th17-cells were increased in UCTD vs. controls, which further increased in those, whom developed SAIDs eventually. The Th17/nTreg ratio gradually increased from controls through UCTD patients, reaching the highest values in SAID-progressed patients. The derailed Th17/Treg balance may contribute to disease progression therefore could function as a prognostic marker."

- DYSMETABOLISM & DYSFUNCTIONAL MITOCHONDRIA The major clinical considerations in this section are mitochondrial dysfunction, endoplasmic reticulum stress, unfolded protein response, TLR activation, and the dysmetabolic effects of sustained hyperglycemia and hyperinsulinemia and resultant oxidative stress, inflammation, RAGE activation, and accumulation of AGE, palmitate and ceramide. The review of this information in Chapter 4 covered approximately 30 interventions relevant to dysmetabolism, mitochondrial dysfunction, ERS-UPR, etc; these will not be reviewed here except to mention those most commonly, easily, empirically, synergistically, and effectively used: 1) low-carbohydrate diet with 2) moderate exercise, 3) CoQ-10, 4) acetyl-carnitine with 5) lipoic acid, 6) NAC, 7) resveratrol, and 8) melatonin.

- STYLE OF LIVING (LIFESTYLE) & SPECIAL CONSIDERATIONS This is a buffet of mostly lifestyle-based interventions yet also including: sleep optimization, sociopsychology, stress management/avoidance, somatic/spinal treatments, special supplementation, sweat/exercise, sauna/detoxification, surgery, stamp your passport and vacate current reality, and sensory deprivation therapy.

- ENDOCRINE IMBALANCE & OPTIMIZATION Common hormonal imbalances seen among autoimmune/inflammatory patients and which contribute to the genesis and perpetuation of these same autoimmune/inflammatory diseases are easily assessed with standard serum laboratory measurements; conveniently, three hormones tend to be elevated, and three tend to be reduced: ❶ *elevated* prolactin, ❷ *elevated* estrogen, ❸ *elevated* insulin—as a surrogate marker (insulin itself actually appears to have an anti-inflammatory effect, counteracting the effect of excess glucose; however the net effect of hyperglycemia-hyperinsulinemia is conclusively pathogenic) for excess carbohydrate intake, insufficient exercise, sarcopenia, mitochondrial dysfunction, nutrient deficiencies, xeobiotic exposure, palmitate and ceramide accumulation, etc, ❹ *reduced* DHEA, ❺ *reduced* cortisol, and ❻ *reduced* testosterone; see Chapter 4 for discussion of these hormones and respective interventions. Thyroid evaluation (history + exam + labs + response to treatment) should be comprehensive, as discussed in Chapter 1, with a low threshold for empiric treatment.

- XENOBIOTIC ACCUMULATION & DETOXIFICATION The clinical relevance and pathogenic mechanisms of xenobiotic accumulation are irrefutably well documented and described. Population-wide toxin accumulation results from corporate irresponsibility and government collusion with industry via lax regulations; at times the situation is so grave that one might wonder if corporations and government are intentionally trying to poison the population (e.g., glyphosate application to water supply, rivers, and population-wide food despite consistently documented adverse effects[60]). These persistent organic pollutants (POPs) promote disease primarily via mitochondrial dysfunction and endoplasmic reticulum stress (thus directly promoting ATP production failure, oxidative injury, insulin resistance, antioxidant nutrient depletion, inflammation and promotion of Treg/Th-17 imbalance) and via additional immunogenic effects including bystander activation and haptenization—see discussion and review in Chapter 4. Clinical assessments include history, physical examination, and laboratory assessment (using serum, whole blood, urine or—rarely yet accurately—fat biopsy), and response to treatment. Treatments include nutritional support for Phases 1 and 2 of detoxification (e.g., oxidation and conjugation) and excretion via bile and urine; for the latter, urinary alkalinization is generally recommended. Chemical toxins can be bound in the gut using activated charcoal[61],

---

[59] Szodoray et al. Altered Th17 cells and Th17/regulatory T-cell ratios indicate the subsequent conversion from undifferentiated connective tissue disease to definitive systemic autoimmune disorders. *Hum Immunol.* 2013 Dec;74(12):1510-8
[60] Krüger et al. Detection of glyphosate residues in animals and humans. *J Environ Anal Toxicol* 2014, 4:2 omicsonline.org/open-access/detection-of-glyphosate-residues-in-animals-and-humans-2161-0525.1000210.pdf
[61] Goel et al. Pesticide poisoning. *Nat Med J India* 2007:20;182-191

cholestyramine[62], or Chlorella (6 g/d [2g TID cc] taken after breakfast, lunch, and dinner)[63]—all of these three treatments have documented safety and effectiveness; clinically and empirically, phytochelatin (plant-derived peptides that bind toxic metals[64]) concentrates appear safe and effective despite lack of conclusive published data supporting clinical use.

- o Chlorella pyrenoidosa on fecal excretion and liver accumulation of polychlorinated dibenzo-p-dioxin in mice. (*Chemosphere* 2005 Apr[65]): "Among mice fed the 10% *C. pyrenoidosa* diet, cumulative fecal excretion of H6CDD over the first week following administration was significantly greater (9.2-fold) than that observed among mice fed the basal diet. Moreover, excretion during the fifth week following administration of H6CDD was still significantly greater (3.1-fold) among mice fed the 10% C. pyrenoidosa diet than among mice fed the basal diet. Five weeks after administration of H6CDD, liver accumulation of H6CDD in mice fed the 10% C. pyrenoidosa diet was significantly less than that observed among mice fed either the basal diet and the Spinach diet (by 27.9% and 34.8%, respectively). These findings suggest that C. pyrenoidosa may be useful in inhibiting the absorption of dioxins via food and the reabsorption of dioxins stored already in the body in the intestinal tract, thus preventing accumulation of dioxins within the body."

- o Chlorella (Chlorella pyrenoidosa) supplementation decreases dioxin and increases immunoglobulin a concentrations in breast milk (*J Med Food* 2007 Mar[66]): "The present results suggest that Chlorella supplementation not only reduces dioxin levels in breast milk, but may also have beneficial effects on nursing infants by increasing IgA levels in breast milk."

- o Maternal-fetal distribution and transfer of dioxins in pregnant women in Japan, and attempts to reduce maternal transfer with Chlorella (Chlorella pyrenoidosa) supplements (*Chemosphere* 2005 Dec[67]): "Concentrations of 28 dioxin (polychlorinated dibenzo-p-dioxins, polychlorinated dibenzofurans, and co-planar polychlorinated biphenyls) congeners in blood, adipose tissue, breast milk, cord blood and placenta collected from 44 pregnant Japanese women were measured. … Correlations were observed between dioxin total toxic equivalents (total TEQ) in blood and total TEQ in adipose tissue (r=0.913, P<0.0001), breast milk (r=0.695, P=0.0007), and cord blood (r=0.759, P<0.0001). Dioxin levels transferred to fetuses and nursing infants reflect cumulative maternal concentrations of dioxins. … Total TEQ in breast milk were approximately 30% lower in the Chlorella group than in controls. This finding suggests that maternal transfer of dioxins can be reduced using dietary measures such as Chlorella supplements."

Corporate-derived government-enabled pollution: Now broadly acknowledged as a major contributor to disease and rising healthcare expenses

Humans in the general population worldwide have become living repositories for industrial pollutants and environmental contaminants, generally referred to in contemporary literature as POPs—persistent organic pollutants. POP retention/accumulation is causatively associated with induction of insulin resistance and the resulting hyperinsulinemia and hyperglycemia via suppression of GLUT-4 receptor expression via xenobiotic-induced activation of the aryl hydrocarbon receptor. Additively or synergistically, POP-induced mitochondrial dysfunction retards insulin secretion from the pancreas and insulin reception in the periphery, thereby synergizing to create the essential pathophysiology that characterizes type-2 diabetes.

"Health care spending in the U.S. has surged more than eightfold since the 1960s. Skyrocketing in that same time: Rates of chronic disease, use of synthetic chemicals, and evidence that many of these widely used substances may be wreaking havoc on human health. … The use of bisphenol A, or BPA, in food and beverage containers, according to the study, is responsible for an estimated $3 billion a year in costs associated with childhood obesity and adult heart disease."

Peeples L. BPA among Toxic Chemicals Driving Up Health Care Costs. 2014 Jan huffingtonpost.com/2014/01/22/bpa-health-care-costs_n_4644372.html

[62] Cohn WJ et al. Treatment of chlordecone (Kepone) toxicity with cholestyramine. Results of a controlled clinical trial. *N Engl J Med.* 1978 Feb 2;298(5):243-8
[63] Nakano S, Takekoshi H, Nakano M. Chlorella (Chlorella pyrenoidosa) supplementation decreases dioxin and increases immunoglobulin a concentrations in breast milk. *J Med Food.* 2007 Mar;10(1):134-42. Nakano S, Noguchi T, Takekoshi H, Suzuki G, Nakano M. Maternal-fetal distribution and transfer of dioxins in pregnant women in Japan, and attempts to reduce maternal transfer with Chlorella (Chlorella pyrenoidosa) supplements. *Chemosphere.* 2005 Dec;61(9):1244-55
[64] Cobbett CS. Phytochelatin biosynthesis and function in heavy-metal detoxification. *Current Opinion in Plant Biology* 2000, 3:211–216. Cobbett CS. Phytochelatins and their roles in heavy metal detoxification. *Plant Physiology* 2000 Jul; 825–832. Readers should have noticed that these are plant physiology journals—not clinical journals. These articles substantiate that phytochelatins are plant-produced metal-binding peptides; in clinical practice, extracts from certain vegetables rich in phytochelatins are used to bind heavy metals in the gut to reduce absorption and enterohepatic recirculation and promote fecal excretion, in a manner analogous to that of cholestyramine and chlorella.
[65] Takekoshi et al. Effect of Chlorella pyrenoidosa on fecal excretion and liver accumulation of polychlorinated dibenzo-p-dioxin in mice. *Chemosphere.* 2005 Apr;59(2):297-304
[66] Nakano et al. Chlorella pyrenoidosa supplementation decreases dioxin and increases immunoglobulin a concentrations in breast milk. *J Med Food* 2007 Mar;10(1):134-42
[67] Nakano et al. Maternal-fetal distribution and transfer of dioxins in pregnant women in Japan, and attempts to reduce maternal transfer with Chlorella (Chlorella pyrenoidosa) supplements. *Chemosphere.* 2005 Dec;61(9):1244-55

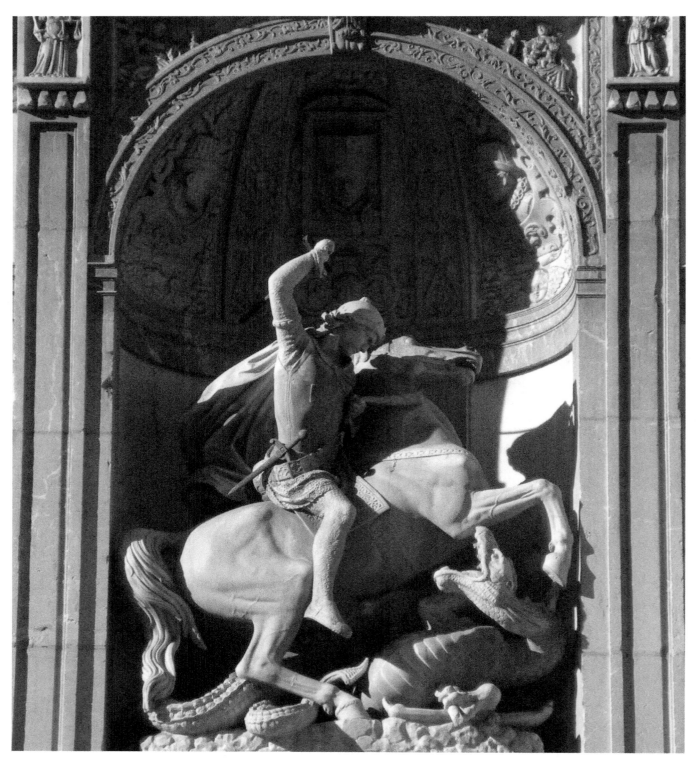

Palau de la Generalitat de Catalunya: In Western societies, one of the dominating paradigms has been that of "man versus nature", which is commonly represented in history, myth, and art as humanity's combat with and attempts at dominance over nature, commonly viewed as hostile or at the very least mysterious, therefore unknown, therefore uncontrollable. As such, nature—despite its beauty and life-giving properties—is often represented as monstrous and demonic, as in the sculpture above. We continue to see this "combat" in science and medicine. Especially in Western/pharmacocentric medicine, the body is depicted as chaotic and in need of outside control and "medical management", and diseases are described as "idiopathic"—from an unknown source. Indeed, Western medicine is full of its own myths, not appreciated as such, which continue to drive thought and action. Wiser approaches to both life and medicine encourage synergy, acceptance, nurturance, and orchestration rather than attempts to outwardly dominate and artificially—and therefore temporarily—control. Photo and caption by DrV, 2016.

High Blood Pressure (HBP) & Hypertension (HTN)

Introduction:

This section reviews clinically relevant information related to chronic hypertension—its cause(s), its social and economic impacts, selected aspects of its pathophysiology and complications, differential diagnosis, assessments, overall management and specific treatments. This chapter is a stand-alone clinical monograph detailing the clinical considerations and etiologic contributors necessary for an accurate multidimensional grasp of this phenomenon and its effective management, both at the level of the individual patient and also at the level of public health and population-wide disease prevention. This chapter also includes the most (or at least one of the most) comprehensive list of differential diagnoses for hypertension that has ever been published. An easy-to-implement clinical approach rooted in the functional inflammology FINDSEX® protocol is detailed, followed by an overview of drug treatments, followed by additional considerations and previously published articles. Throughout, emphasis is placed—not on simply clinical accuracy, therapeutic efficacy, and patient safety—but on the patient-centered rather than disease-centered goal of the best possible outcome for the patient, which is health preservation and optimization, not simply the lowering of arterial pressure.

   Treatment options reviewed include drugs, diet, lifestyle, metabolic modifications such as weight loss and improvement in insulin sensitivity, nutritional supplementation, manipulative therapeutics and surgical treatment for the alleviation of medullary neurovascular compression. Recent updates to the clinical approach include the focus on alleviating mitochondrial dysfunction and the restoration of immune and inflammatory balance via nutritional immunomodulation; these newer considerations are clearly relevant for the treatment of hypertension as an isolated finding and are even more relevant for the treatment of cardiometabolic syndrome, of which hypertension is merely one component.

   Clearly, most of the non-drug non-surgery treatments reviewed here are natural, non-patentable, and widely available; they work with the body's physiology to improve metabolic function and to thereby improve overall health and cardiovascular, endothelial, endocrine and neuroregulatory homeodynamics. As with most nutritional and natural interventions, side-effects are minimal, and collateral benefits are many; therefore, as overall health improves, various complaints and disorders are alleviated, vitality is enhanced, and patient compliance increases while the need for medical management of other issues decreases.

   A quantitative compilation can effect a qualitative transformation in the reader's perception of the nature of the disease and its place in clinical care and healthcare policy; such is the goal of this section on ~~chronic~~ *sustained* hypertension. The strength of the evidence supporting this disease model and the treatment approach is consistent, robust, and much more attractive—both clinically and intellectually—than is the ascribing of hypertension to some "idiopathic" cause which somehow evades biomedical science and the collective human intellect except for the extent to which it allows itself to be appropriately targeted by population-wide polypharmacy. Hypertension is only "chronic" when its causes are ignored and/or not effectively treated; as such, a more accurate descriptor is "sustained." This review of contributors to ~~chronic~~ *sustained* hypertension will provide patients and clinicians a conceptual and factual framework from which to perceive and address the causes of sustained elevations in arterial pressure.

   Sustained hypertension is a major risk factor for cardiovascular disease, exacerbated by hyperglycemia and other metabolic factors such as hypercholesterolemia and hyperhomocysteinaemia, all of which are reviewed in the following section on diabetes, obesity, and insulin resistance.

<u>Description, Pathophysiology, and Key Concepts</u>:

- <u>Sustained/chronic high blood pressure—the most common clinical diagnosis</u>: High blood pressure (chronic hypertension) is the most common disease diagnosis encountered in clinical practice worldwide. As such, the diagnosis and successful integrative management of chronic hypertension represents an opportunity for clinicians to achieve higher levels of practice success and for patients to receive the healthcare that they need. In America, 30% of adults have hypertension. For those of us specializing in adult healthcare, these hypertensive adults in the population can be thought of as belonging to two categories: ❶ patients receiving comprehensive integrative functional medicine care (very small minority), and ❷ patients who are either undiagnosed, untreated, or treated only with drugs and therefore in need of comprehensive integrative functional medicine care for optimal hypertension management, disease prevention, and wellness promotion (the vast majority of hypertensive patients).

   Most hypertensive patients have no symptoms of their disorder and are therefore reliant upon a competent clinician to reveal the problem and to provide the appropriate education and the motivation to initiate and maintain compliance with treatment. Clinicians have the responsibility to detect and effectively manage high blood pressure. High blood pressure accelerates the development of cardiovascular disease and additional complications including stroke, heart attack (myocardial infarction), heart failure, renal failure, blindness, peripheral vascular disease and endothelial dysfunction which can contribute to (for example) lower leg amputation and sexual dysfunction[1] in both men and women.

> **1 in 3 US adults has hypertension; the vast majority of these cases have no clear "medical" cause**
>
> "In the United States, one in three adults has hypertension. Most of these patients have no clear etiology and are classified as having essential hypertension."
>
> Viera AJ, Neutze DM. Diagnosis of secondary hypertension: an age-based approach. *Am Fam Physician* 2010 Dec

Clinicians have three core responsibilities related to hypertension management. First, the condition must be diagnosed by the clinician; this is a simple physical exam procedure. Second, the patient must be assessed for underlying causes and disease complications. Third, the patient must be enrolled in a treatment program to ensure proper lowering of elevated pressures; this is best accomplished with diet optimization, nutritional supplementation, therapeutic lifestyle changes, spinal manipulation, and—rarely—use of medications.

- Overview and perspective: The emphasis of this section will be the integrative management of so-called "primary" or "essential" hypertension (HTN), which is generally considered "idiopathic" from an outdated medical perspective that has failed to appreciate and integrate the research that has clarified the numerous causes of and contributors to HTN. From the allopathic medical perspective, >90-95% of HTN is considered idiopathic and thus by definition "of no known cause" and therefore appropriate for treatment with drugs. Most (more than 70%) medically managed patients with HTN take two or more antihypertensive drugs from the time of diagnosis until the end of their lives; these drugs commonly cause adverse effects, are relatively devoid of collateral benefits, and do not address the underlying causative physiologic imbalances. Patients managed with nutritional and lifestyle modifications must likewise remain compliant with the prescribed health-promoting treatment-diet-lifestyle, but they generally experience clinically and statistically meaningful *collateral benefits*; for example, ❶ **correction of vitamin D deficiency can alleviate hypertension**[2] and musculoskeletal pain[3] while improving mood[4,5]; ❷ **fish oil supplementation slightly lowers blood pressure** but tremendously and safely lowers cardiovascular mortality and all-cause mortality[6] while also improving mental health[7] and alleviating pain and inflammation[8,9]; ❸ **CoQ10 is very effective for the treatment of HTN**[10] while also restoring lost renal function[11,12], alleviating migraine headaches[13], and helping to control asthma.[14] The exemplary nutritional interventions listed in the previous sentence are virtually devoid of adverse effects when employed with a modicum of competence, and each of these natural and nonpatentable interventions is widely available. Furthermore, **their clinical benefit (in this case, the reduction of elevated blood pressure) is derived from their ability to restore proper physiologic function** rather than—as with most pharmaceutical drugs—the blockade of normal physiology. If the routine outpatient medical treatment of HTN were to shift away from synthetic chemical drugs that function by interfering with normal physiology (e.g., beta-adrenergic

---

[1] "Available data indicate that essential hypertension is a risk factor for sexual dysfunction, as male and female sexual dysfunction is more prevalent in hypertensive patients than normotensive individuals. Several mechanisms have been implicated in the pathogenesis of sexual dysfunction in hypertensive patients, and major determinants include severity and duration of hypertension, age, and antihypertensive therapy. Female sexual dysfunction, although more frequent than its male counterpart, remains largely under-recognized." Manolis A, Doumas M. Sexual dysfunction: the 'prima ballerina' of hypertension-related quality-of-life complications. *J Hypertens*. 2008 Nov;26(11):2074-84

[2] "A short-term supplementation with vitamin D(3) and calcium is more effective in reducing SBP than calcium alone. Inadequate vitamin D(3) and calcium intake could play a contributory role in the pathogenesis and progression of hypertension and cardiovascular disease in elderly women." Pfeifer et al. Effects of a short-term vitamin D(3) and calcium supplementation on blood pressure and parathyroid hormone levels in elderly women. *J Clin Endocrinol Metab*. 2001 Apr;86(4):1633-7

[3] "Findings showed that 83% of the study patients (n = 299) had an abnormally low level of vitamin D before treatment with vitamin D supplements. After treatment, clinical improvement in symptoms was seen in all the groups that had a low level of vitamin D, and in 95% of all the patients (n = 341). CONCLUSIONS: Vitamin D deficiency is a major contributor to chronic low back pain in areas where vitamin D deficiency is endemic." Al Faraj S, Al Mutairi K. Vitamin D deficiency and chronic low back pain in Saudi Arabia. *Spine*. 2003;28:177-9

[4] Vieth R, Kimball S, Hu A, Walfish PG. Randomized comparison of the effects of the vitamin D3 adequate intake versus 100 mcg (4000 IU) per day on biochemical responses and the wellbeing of patients. *Nutrition Journal* 2004, 3:8 nutritionj.com/content/3/1/8

[5] Lansdowne AT, Provost SC: Vitamin D3 enhances mood in healthy subjects during winter. *Psychopharmacology* (Berl) 1998, 135:319-323

[6] GISSI-Prevenzione Investigators. Dietary supplementation with n-3 polyunsaturated fatty acids and vitamin E after myocardial infarction: results of the GISSI-Prevenzione trial. Gruppo Italiano per lo Studio della Sopravvivenza nell'Infarto miocardico. *Lancet*. 1999 Aug 7;354(9177):447-55

[7] Peet M, Stokes C. Omega-3 fatty acids in the treatment of psychiatric disorders. *Drugs*. 2005;65(8):1051-9

[8] Maroon JC, Bost JW. Omega-3 fatty acids (fish oil) as anti-inflammatory: alternative to nonsteroidal anti-inflammatory drugs for discogenic pain. *Surg Neurol*. 2006 Apr:326-31

[9] "Many of the placebo-controlled trials of fish oil in chronic inflammatory diseases reveal significant benefit, including decreased disease activity and a lowered use of anti-inflammatory drugs." Simopoulos AP. Omega-3 fatty acids in inflammation and autoimmune diseases. *J Am Coll Nutr*. 2002 Dec;21(6):495-505

[10] Singh et al. Hydrosoluble coenzyme Q10 on blood pressures and insulin resistance in hypertensive patients with coronary artery disease. *J Hum Hypertens* 1999 Mar;13:203-8

[11] Singh et al. Randomized, double-blind placebo-controlled trial of coenzyme Q10 in chronic renal failure: discovery of a new role. *J Nutr Environ Med* 2000;10:281-8

[12] Singh et al. Randomized, Double-blind, Placebo-controlled Trial of Coenzyme Q10 in Patients with Endstage Renal Failure. *J Nutr Environ Med* 2003; 13 (1): 13–22

[13] Rozen et al. Open label trial of coenzyme q10 as a migraine preventive. *Cephalalgia* 2002;22(2):137-41

[14] Gvozdjáková et al. Coenzyme Q10 supplementation reduces corticosteroids dosage in patients with bronchial asthma. *Biofactors*. 2005;25(1-4):235-40

blockers, calcium channel *blockers*, ACE *inhibitors*, angiotensin-2 receptor *blockers*, etc) and toward the favor of natural treatments—diet optimization, body weight reduction/optimization, and evidence-based nutritional supplementation—that promote normalization of blood pressure by helping restore balance to the body's physiology (i.e., by facilitating the restoration of homeostasis), then meaningful and authentic progress in the otherwise never-ending "fight against hypertension" would be made. (For more discussion, see "Thinking Outside the (Pill) Box" at the end of this chapter.)

> ### "Prehypertension" is deadly: mortality increases starting at 115/75 mm Hg
>
> "Hypertension-related diseases are the leading causes of morbidity and mortality in industrially developed societies. Surprisingly, **68% of all mortality attributed to high blood pressure (BP) occurs with systolic BP between 120 and 140 mm Hg and diastolic BP below 90 mm Hg.** Dietary and lifestyle modifications are effective in the treatment of borderline hypertension."
>
> Goldhamer et al. Medically supervised water-only fasting in the treatment of borderline hypertension. *J Altern Complement Med.* 2002 Oct

- Blood pressure and mortality: Increased risk for cardiovascular mortality begins with blood pressures that are still well within the accepted normal range; therefore blood pressure that is consistent with an official diagnosis of hypertension—blood pressure consistently greater than 140 mm Hg systolic and/or greater than 90 mm Hg diastolic—is clearly worthy of treatment if part of the clinical goal is—*as it should be*—to reduce unnecessary morbidity and early mortality. Benowitz[15] wrote, "Starting at 115/75 mm Hg, cardiovascular risk doubles with each increment of 20/10 mm Hg throughout the blood pressure range." Thus, from both *wellness-centered* as well as *disease-prevention* perspectives, pro-active integrative clinicians can define mild HTN as > 115/75 mm Hg. Data from the Framingham study showed that sustained BP > 140/90 induces left ventricular hypertrophy.[16] A reduction of systolic BP (sBP) of -5 mm Hg correlates with a -7% reduction in cardiovascular mortality[17]; thus, patients must be encouraged to take HTN and its effective treatment seriously, since even small numerical decrements in BP can have impressive ameliorating effects on the risk for cardiovascular complications. Except in younger age groups, sBP is more predictive of adverse cardiovascular outcomes than is diastolic BP. Systolic hypertension indicates the presence of vascular abnormalities including reductions in elasticity/compliance of large and medium arteries; thus, the finding of systolic HTN simultaneously indicates *current* vascular abnormalities and *future* cardiovascular disease (CV) risk elevation.

> ### Affective interpretations: emotional needs influence intellectual perspectives
>
> "...to see differently in this way for once, to *want* to see differently, is no small discipline and preparation of the intellect for its future "objectivity"—the latter understood not as "contemplation without interest" (which is a nonsensical absurdity), but as the ability *to control* one's Pro and Con and to dispose of them, so that one knows how to employ a *variety* of perspectives and *affective interpretations* in the service of knowledge."
>
> Nietzsche FW. *Genealogy of Morals*, 1887. Essay #3, section #12.

- Hypertension and vascular disease: Sustained HTN accelerates the development of CVD and end-organ damage by several mechanisms including promotion of endothelial damage resulting in accelerated atherosclerosis (e.g., stroke, myocardial infarction, peripheral vascular disease), direct pressure (e.g., retinal hemorrhages, aortic aneurysm), hyperplastic arteriolosclerosis and occlusive vasculopathy due to smooth muscle proliferation, fibrosis, and hyaline deposition (e.g., hypertensive nephrosclerosis), interstitial edema (e.g., cerebral edema, peripheral edema), and pathologic myocardial adaptation (e.g., hypertrophic cardiomyopathy, hypertensive heart disease, congestive heart failure). Hyperplastic arteriolosclerosis causes hypertensive nephrosclerosis, characterized by renal ischemia which triggers release of renin and increased formation of angiotensin-2 which exacerbates renal ischemia and systemic hypertension.[18]

- Medical physiology-pharmacology of hypertension: Drug treatment of hypertension must have some physiologic basis, even if this basis is simplistic, limited, and outdated by current research and emerging paradigms that might surpass and supplant previous and well entrenched models. In the medical/allopathic paradigm, "physiology" must be tailored to support pharmacology, since the latter is the profession's primary intervention. Thus, the study of physiology must be made to fit pharmacology by limiting the variables

---

[15] Benowitz NL. "Antihypertensive Agents." In Katzung BG (editor). *Basic and Clinical Pharmacology. 10th Edition*. New York: McGraw Hill Medical; 2007, 159
[16] Kumar V, Abbas AK, Fausto N (Editors). *Robbins and Cotran Pathologic Basis of Disease. 7th Edition*. Philadelphia: Elsevier; 2005, 587
[17] Nahas R. Complementary and alternative medicine approaches to blood pressure reduction: An evidence-based review. *Can Fam Physician.* 2008 Nov;54(11):1529-33
[18] Kumar V, Abbas AK, Fausto N (Editors). *Robbins and Cotran Pathologic Basis of Disease. 10th Edition*. Philadelphia: Elsevier; 2005, 1007-8

considered to those which are amenable to drug intervention. Thus, per medical pharmacology textbooks[19], the primary variables considered for the support of antihypertensive pharmacotherapy are ❶ cardiac output ("to be controlled with beta-blockers"), ❷ peripheral resistance ("to be treated with vasodilators such as ACEi and CCB"), and ❸ blood volume ("to be reduced by the first-line use of diuretics"). While this perspective is necessarily limited in the service of the medical paradigm, it is also useful for provisionally grasping a view of some of the key factors involved in blood pressure regulation, including those that are relevant for drug intervention in the acute care setting as well as the long-term nondrug treatment of HTN. Given that this text details the "functional" and "integrative" management of HTN and must therefore provide a variety of perspectives, a concise review of medical physiology is appropriate. The medical paradigm views

Antihypertensive drugs function by blocking *normal* physiology (rather than by *correcting* dysfunctional physiology)
"All antihypertensive [drugs]... produce their effects by interfering with normal mechanisms of blood pressure regulation."   Benowitz NL. "Antihypertensive Agents." In Katzung BG (editor). *Basic and Clinical Pharmacology. Tenth Edition*. New York: McGraw Hill Medical; 2007, p159
"In Western medicine, because of the prevailing mechanistic view, we treat our bodies as dumb machines. We move in with surgery and drugs to make them do what we want [a reflection of the *power-over model*, or the *control paradigm*], bypassing strategies that support the body's capacity to solve its own problems, learn, and regenerate itself."   Breton D, Largent C. *The paradigm conspiracy: why our social systems violate human potential and how we can change them*. Hazelden Publishing; 1998, pages 147-148

most HTN as idiopathic and "somehow" resulting from a complex dysregulation of normal physiology; thereby, the "appropriate" intervention is to interfere with the normal physiologic mechanisms that have gone astray. One interconnecting theme in this paradigm is that of activation of the sympathetic nervous system by some unknown insult or combination thereof. Whether due to "stress", faulty disinhibition of baroreceptors in the aortic arch, carotid sinuses, or renal juxtaglomerular cells, sympathetic activation increases cardiac output via increased rate and contractility, increases peripheral resistance via vasoconstriction, and increases blood volume via aldosterone-enhanced sodium retention. The enzyme renin converts angiotensinogen into angiotensin-1, which is converted via angiotensin converting enzyme (ACE) into angiotensin-2, which is a powerful vasoconstrictor and trigger for the release of aldosterone, which promotes sodium reabsorption and thus sodium-water retention. With this simple and simplistic model, one can grasp the rationale employed for antihypertensive pharmacotherapeutics as well as some of the natural and *eu*physiologic[20] interventions detailed in this text; drug treatments for HTN are detailed toward the end of this chapter.

- Acceleration of atherogenesis and atherosclerosis: HTN is the single most important risk factor for the development of CVD. On a population-wide basis, achieving the target of ≤ 140 mmHg systolic would result in a 28-44% reduction in stroke and a 20-35% reduction in ischemic heart disease (IHD). In describing these benefits for the United Kingdom (population ~60 million in 2005), Tomson and Lip[21] noted in 2005 that control of HTN would prevent approximately 42,800 strokes and 82,800 IHD events per year.

- Basic pathology: Reviewed here are several of the more direct and salient effects of high blood pressure on important organs, the most relevant of which are brain, eye, heart, and kidney.

  - Brain—intracerebral hemorrhage, lacunar infarcts, slit hemorrhages, hypertensive encephalopathy: HTN can cause intracerebral hemorrhage and cerebellar hemorrhage. Arteriolar sclerosis of small vessels can lead to ischemia of the basal ganglia, cerebral white matter, and brainstem. Cavitary lacunar ("lake-like") infarcts classically affect the lenticular nucleus, thalamus, internal capsule, caudate nucleus, and pons. Rupture of small vessels can leave a slit-like cavity of discoloration, cell destruction, and gliosis termed a *slit hemorrhage*. Hypertensive encephalopathy presents with headache, confusion, vomiting, seizure, and/or coma; cerebral edema, petechiae, and transtentorial or tonsillar herniation may be noted at autopsy.[22]

  - Eye—ocular vascular disease and hypertensive retinopathy: Hypertensive sclerosis of arteries and arterioles serving the eye results in the "copper wire" then "silver wire" fundoscopic changes that occur as

---

[19] Harvey RA, Champe PC (eds). *Lippincott's Illustrated Reviews: Pharmacology, 3rd Edition*. Philadelphia, Lippincott Williams and Wilkins; 1997
[20] The prefix "eu" means good or beneficial. The term "euphysiologic" was used more commonly in medical literature of the early 1900's than it is today. Here, euphysiologic means "properly-working physiology" or "beneficial to physiology" in contrast to interventions that are contrary to normal physiology ("antiphysiologic" or—per Greenblatt [*Obstet Gynecol Clin North Am.* 1987;14:251-68]—"contraphysiologic") such as enzyme-blocking drugs which have their therapeutic and adverse effects by working against normal physiology and enzyme function.
[21] Tomson J, Lip GY. Blood pressure demographics: nature or nurture...genes or environment? *BMC Med.* 2005;3:3 biomedcentral.com/1741-7015/3/3
[22] Frosch et al. "Chapter 28: Central nervous system." in Kumar, Abbas, Fausto (eds). *Robins and Cotran Pathologic Basis of Disease. 7th Edition*. Elsevier; 2005, 1368-1369

the arteriole wall thickens and obscures visualization of luminal blood. Within the nerve fiber layer of the retina, "cotton-wool spots" are infarcts, and "flame hemorrhages" are due to vascular rupture. Retinal exudates secondary to vascular leak due to severe hypertension may induce retinal detachment and acute vision loss. Occlusion of retinal arterioles causes retinal infarction.[23]

- Heart—hypertensive cardiomyopathy and cardiac hypertrophy: HTN increases the work demands placed on the heart and leads to myocyte hypertrophy followed by altered proportions of cardiac anatomy as well as functional abnormalities: left atrial enlargement leads to conduction defects such as atrial fibrillation; ventricular walls thicken and encroach upon intraventricular volume leading to reduced ejection volume. Adaptations to chronically increased blood pressure lead to alterations in cardiac anatomy, histology, physiology, and gene expression that—if persistent and progressive—eventually culminate in cardiac failure.[24] Acute-onset hypertension can induce oxygen/nutrient delivery-demand mismatch resulting in myocardial infarction.

- Kidney—malignant hypertension and accelerated nephrosclerosis: Malignant hypertension—the full syndrome of which includes diastolic pressure > 130 mm Hg, papilledema/retinopathy, encephalopathy, renal failure, and cardiovascular complications—occurs in 1-5% of hypertensive patients; it is more common in patients who are male, young, and of African descent. Risk factors include pre-existing chronic hypertension (whether primary or secondary), scleroderma, and preexisting renal disease such as reflux nephropathy or glomerulonephritis. The main pathophysiologic sequence appears to include intrarenal vascular damage followed by vascular occlusion secondary to intimal smooth muscle hypertrophy and hyperplastic arteriolosclerosis; eventually this leads to renal hypoperfusion and ischemia. Renal hypoperfusion, besides leading to azotemia and oliguria in acute severe hypertension, leads to activation of the renin-angiotensin-aldosterone system (RAAS) which leads to additional vasoconstriction and the cascade of events (including sodium and water retention) which leads to further elevations in blood pressure. Histologic changes in the kidney include fibrinoid necrosis of the arterioles, hyperplastic arteriolitis, intrarenal arterial thrombosis, and glomerular necrosis.[25]

• Treatment-resistant hypertension: "Resistant hypertension" was defined in a December 2010 review as "elevated blood pressure despite patient adherence to optimal dosages of three antihypertensive agents, including a diuretic."[26]

• Obesity, type-2 diabetes mellitus, and hypertension—*unnecessary epidemics*: **In the United States (population ~300 million in 2005), 65% of adults are overweight or obese,** generally as a direct result of *overconsumption malnutrition* and physical inactivity). In the US, the number of deaths attributable to obesity is greater than 280,200 yearly. At least 11 million Americans have type-2 diabetes mellitus, while **50 million Americans have hypertension.**[27]

Prevalence of HTN
• 50 million people in the U.S.
• 1 billion worldwide
• European Americans:
o 15% of women,
o 25% of men > age 45 years
• African Americans:
o 35% of women,
o 40% of men > age 45 years
Villela T. Hypertension: Diagnosis and Management. University of California, San Francisco-San Francisco General Hospital. Family and Community Medicine Residency Program. July 2010

• Hypertension diagnosis and control—an international health priority: Control of HTN is a worldwide healthcare priority. According to a 2001 editorial by Chobanian[28] in *New England Journal of Medicine*, "…more than one-fourth of the estimated 42 million people with hypertension in the United States remain unaware that they have the disorder, and approximately three-fourths of those with known hypertension have blood pressure that exceeds recommended levels." Dr Chobanian goes on to note that the prevalence and severity of the problem is comparable in the rest of the world, where approximately 20% of the adult population (more than 800 million people) are hypertensive, and rates of control are even worse than in the United States. According to an extensive review of international data published in *The Lancet* in 2005, the global prevalence of HTN was 26.4% (972 million people) in 2000 and is projected to increase to

[23] Folberg R. "Chapter 29: The eye." in Kumar V, Abbas AK, Fausto N (eds). *Robins and Cotran Pathologic Basis of Disease. 7th Ed*. Elsevier; 2005, 1436-1437
[24] Schoen FJ. "Chapter 12: The heart" in Kumar V, Abbas AK, Fausto N (eds). *Robins and Cotran Pathologic Basis of Disease. 7th Ed*. Elsevier; 2005, 560-562
[25] Alpers CE. "Chapter 20: The kidney" in Kumar V, Abbas AK, Fausto N (eds). *Robins and Cotran Pathologic Basis of Disease. 7th Ed*. Elsevier: Philadelphia; 2005, 1007-1008
[26] Viera AJ, Neutze DM. Diagnosis of secondary hypertension: an age-based approach. *Am Fam Physician*. 2010 Dec 15;82(12):1471-8
[27] Cordain L, Eaton SB, Sebastian A, Mann N, Lindeberg S, Watkins BA, O'Keefe JH, Brand-Miller J. Origins and evolution of the Western diet: health implications for the 21st century. *Am J Clin Nutr*. 2005 Feb;81(2):341-54 ajcn.org/cgi/content/full/81/2/341 This will forever be an important publication and landmark in nutritional science.
[28] Chobanian AV. Control of hypertension--an important national priority. *N Engl J Med*. 2001 Aug 16;345(7):534-5

29.2% (1.56 billion people) by the year 2025; the authors concluded, "Hypertension is an important public-health challenge worldwide."[29]

- Hypertension—a multifaceted entity with clinical, political, social, and economic components and implications: First, as previously noted, HTN is a treatable and therefore avoidable contributor to CVD and other forms of end-organ damage—stroke, myocardial infarction, congestive heart failure, peripheral vascular disease, renal failure, and hypertensive retinopathy. Second, HTN as a clinical manifestation is *always* a sign of underlying dysfunction or disease; HTN does not cause itself (at least initially) and therefore the "treatment of hypertension" should focus on the identification and "treatment of underlying dysfunction" rather than simply suppressing the visible manifestation of this dysfunction—the elevated blood pressure. **The finding of HTN is a sign to the clinician that one or more underlying physiologic imbalances are present and in need of detection and/or corrective intervention.** The environmental-social factors that predispose toward the development of HTN—including overconsumption malnutrition, lack of exercise, and psychoemotional stress—tend to disproportionately affect people of lower socioeconomic status. Third, HTN is not merely a disease; it is a *business* (leading diagnosis in Family Medicine practices[30]), and an industry (direct costs approach $200 billion per year in the United States). Among allopathic and osteopathic physicians, HTN is the most common clinical diagnosis in Family Medicine practice. For the medical profession and pharmaceutical industry, antihypertensive medications and services are a major source of revenue. Direct annual medical expenses related to HTN exceed $185 billion per year in the United States. Most patients treated exclusively with drugs require *multiple drugs* for adequate BP control[31], and—from the day of diagnosis—they are prescribed to take these drugs for the rest of their lives. **Thus, the term "hypertension" describes much more than one individual patient's elevated blood pressure; the term refers to an entity that spans and interconnects clinical, political, social, and economic phenomena and institutions.** To change the management of hypertension is to change—or at least begin changing in an important way—the practice of medicine as previously known. By perceiving high blood pressure as a barometer of poor health rather than as an isolated clinical entity, clinicians have license to intervene in numerous ways to improve each patient's overall health, thereby reducing suffering and death *beyond that attributable to hypertension-related illness* because most of the natural interventions described in this chapter provide clinically meaningful collateral benefits and reduce blood pressure *en passant*.[32]

- Hypertension—primarily a "disease of Western civilization": The prevalence of HTN among hunter-gatherer societies is virtually zero.[33] Contrasting the absence of CVD noted in *physically active* societies that consume *natural diets* against the pandemics of HTN and CVD seen in Westernized/industrialized nations, O'Keefe and Cordain[34] wrote, "**The lifetime incidence of hypertension [among Americans] is an astounding 90%,** and the metabolic syndrome is present in up to 40% of middle-aged American adults. **Cardiovascular disease remains the number 1 cause of death,** accounting for 41% of all fatalities, and the prevalence of heart disease in the United States is projected to double during the next 50 years." In industrialized nations, the prevalence of HTN in adults is approximately 1 per 4-5 (20-25%) with the vast majority of these considered idiopathic, chronic, and unresponsive to diet and lifestyle improvements from the dominant allopathic medical perspective. Integrative clinicians who appreciate the broad range of causes of and *synergistic contributors to hypertension* do not generally view this disorder as *idiopathic,* nor as necessarily *chronic,* nor as *unresponsive,* but rather find it *understandable* and *highly amenable* to numerous interventions—necessarily specific for each patient (e.g., food allergies and/or hypothyroidism and/or nutrient deficiencies)—supported by publications in peer-reviewed biomedical journals. **The high prevalence of primary hypertension seen in industrial "Westernized" societies does not necessarily imply that the people in these societies are as a group genetically defective and**

[29] Kearney PM, Whelton M, Reynolds K, Muntner P, Whelton PK, He J. Global burden of hypertension: analysis of worldwide data. *Lancet.* 2005 Jan 15-21;365(9455):217-23
[30] Sloane PD, Slatt LM, Ebell MH, Jacques LB, Smith MA (Eds). *Essentials of Family Medicine, 5th Edition.* Lippincott Williams & Wilkins, 2007
[31] Domino FJ (editor in chief). *The 5-Minute Clinical Consult. 2010. 18th Edition.* Philadelphia; Wolters Kluwer: 2009, 656-7
[32] French: *in passing* or *in passage*. Capturing "en passant" is a strategy used in the game of chess wherein a player is allowed to capture an opponent's pawn in an adjacent row after the opponent has moved the pawn forward by two spaces. In this context, I use the phrase *en passant* to denote that most of the natural treatments detailed in the following pages do not directly and intentionally target hypertension *per se* but rather reduce hypertension *in passing* as overall health is improved.
[33] Eaton SB, Shostak M, Konner M. *The Paleolithic Prescription.* New York: Harper and Row Publishers; 1988, 49
[34] O'Keefe JH Jr, Cordain L. Cardiovascular disease resulting from a diet and lifestyle at odds with our Paleolithic genome. *Mayo ClinProc* 2004;79:101-8

therefore **"in need of medical intervention"** but perhaps **rather that the industrialized/Westernized lifestyle is inherently adverse to the preservation of human health, well-being, and longevity.**[35] In early biomedical and socioanthropologic literature such as Dr Weston Price's *Nutrition and Physical Degeneration: A Comparison of Primitive and Modern Diets and Their Effects*[36] published in 1945, hypertension—just like diabetes mellitus, dental carries, malocclusion, chronic dermatopathies such as acne, eczema, and psoriasis, and a myriad of clinical and subclinical neuropsychiatric problems—was often described as one of the "diseases of Western civilization", i.e., a disease that did not generally exist within primitive hunter-gatherer societies until such societies were infiltrated with white flour, white sugar, alcohol, salt [sodium chloride], and other aspects of the Western/industrialized way of existing and surviving.

- The clinician's responsibilities: The obligations imposed upon clinicians in the management of hypertension include:

  o Comprehensive clinical assessment: Assess for urgent situations (BP > 210/120 mm Hg) and end-organ damage, particularly of the **eyes** (fundoscopic examination), **kidneys** (measure serum BUN and creatinine; determine GFR; obtain UA, perhaps also look for albumin:creatinine ratio to detect early proteinuria), and **cardiovascular system** (cardiopulmonary auscultation and blood pressure measurement with every visit; consider bruit screening, ECG, echocardiography, ankle-brachial index, and assessment for other cardiovascular risk factors such as hyperglycemia, dyslipidemia, and inflammation with hsCRP. Assessing for other risk factors such as n-3 fatty acid insufficiency (generally dietary history is sufficient for assessment; laboratory analysis is expensive and generally not required), vitamin D3 insufficiency, serum cystatin C, serum ferritin, lipoprotein a (Lp-a), aldosterone, renin, and fibrinogen can also be performed.

"Diseases of Western civilization"

- Primary hypertension
- Diabetes mellitus, type-2
- Metabolic syndrome
- Dental carries and malocclusion
- Common neuropsychiatric problems
- Obesity
- Dermatopathies: eczema, psoriasis, and acne

"Diseases of Western civilization" can be understood by appreciation of the physiologic effects caused by the lifestyle and dietary changes historically imposed upon indigenous hunter-gather societies from incoming Westerners/Europeans. These changes include what was *added* (white flour, grains, table salt, white sugar, alcohol, and other so-called "refined" foods, which were poor in substance and vitality compared to their more "natural" and "primitive" counterparts) and what was *removed* (exercise, whole fruits, vegetables, nuts, seeds, berries, roots [i.e., fiber and phytonutrients], multigenerational community, natural living, full-body exposure to sunshine and therefore ensured adequacy of vitamin D). Important to appreciate is that these diseases were once exceedingly rare but are now commonplace. The fact that most of these conditions are common these days in children dispels the shibboleth espoused by pharmacosurgical proponents that these diseases have become more common simply because people are living longer due to "advances in medicine." Quite to the contrary, medicine as generally practiced has reinforced and abetted the conditions which generate many of these illnesses; thankfully, we are seeing positive changes in medicine, but only recently, and mainly due to outside pressures and the popularity of and market demand for open-mindedness toward healthy living.

The classic text on this subject is Price WA. *Nutrition and Physical Degeneration: A Comparison of Primitive and Modern Diets and Their Effects*. 1945

---

  o Differential diagnosis: Competently assess for and exclude genuine causes of HTN before ascribing HTN to a "genetic" or familial cause requiring perpetual medicalization; detailed information on assessment (e.g., physical exam, lab tests, and diagnostic/therapeutic interventions) is reviewed later in this chapter.

  o Effective treatment: Effective intervention must be prescribed by the physician and implemented by the patient; results must be documented in the patient's chart. The clinician has the responsibility to effect improved outcome, document patient noncompliance, and/or initiate a *complete referral* to a specialist for recalcitrant cases, for additional testing, advanced treatment, and/or liability defense.

  o Patient education: Because hypertension—like diabetes and hemochromatosis—is generally asymptomatic in its early stages and in milder cases, doctors (derived from the Latin *docere*, which means "to teach"[37]) have the responsibility to instruct patients on the nature of their disorder, its effects and treatment options, and the consequences of nontreatment. Patients have the responsibility to comply with the treatment plan, implement an effective alternate plan, or absorb the consequences of noncompliance and disease progression.

---

[35] O'Keefe JH Jr, Cordain L. Cardiovascular disease resulting from a diet and lifestyle at odds with our Paleolithic genome. *Mayo ClinProc* 2004;79:101-8
[36] Price WA. *Nutrition and Physical Degeneration: A Comparison of Primitive and Modern Diets and Their Effects*. Price-Pottinger Nutrition Foundation, 1945
[37] Prakash R, Misra R, Misra R. Doctors as Teachers. *Psychiatric News* 2002; 37: 37 pn.psychiatryonline.org/content/37/9/37.1.full

- o <u>Implement a follow-up plan</u>: Doctors must (pre)schedule patients for follow-up in-office visits to monitor treatment adherence and therapeutic effectiveness.
- o <u>Complete referral for nonresponsive or noncompliant patients</u>: "Complete referral" includes a professional letter of referral including the patient's history, examination findings, lab results, and any imaging and other assessments that are within the referring clinician's scope of competence/practice. Generally, the referring clinician's office should call the specialist's office to make the appointment for the patient, then provide the appointment time and address to the patient; the components of this complete referral are then documented in the patient's chart. Simply telling a patient, "You need to see a specialist" is often insufficient because doing so places the burden of responsibility onto the patient, and many of our patients lack the sophistication and knowledge to successfully navigate various overlapping healthcare systems. By ensuring that the patient's appointment is made with the specialist, the physician facilitates patient care and protects herself/himself from undue liability.

Consequences of failing to adequately manage hypertension
• Accelerated atherosclerosis, CVD
• Hemorrhagic and ischemic stroke,
• Peripheral arterial disease,
• Mesenteric ischemia,
• Erectile dysfunction in men,
• Myocardial infarction,
• Heart failure,
• Cerebral and aortic aneurysm,
• Nephropathy, dialysis, transplant,
• Retinopathy, intra ocular hemorrhage, vision loss,
• Patient dissatisfaction
• Physician dissatisfaction, malpractice litigation

Clinical Presentations:

- Clearly the vast majority of clinical presentations of HTN are silent, discovered only when the clinician finds elevated blood pressure on routine examination. This underscores the importance of hypertension screening among asymptomatic patients. The second and remaining group of clinical presentations of HTN includes those of end-organ damage: nephropathy, retinopathy, cardiomyopathy, and the consequences of HTN-accelerated CVD including stroke, myocardial infarction, aortic dissection, and rupture of an enlarged (generally >5.5 cm) abdominal aortic aneurysm.
- Typical clinical presentations of the hypertensive patient can range from incidental to catastrophic and include the following:
  - o Asymptomatic: incidental finding during presentation and evaluation for another concern such as routine examination, injury, or infection
  - o Headache, altered mental status
  - o Congestive heart failure presenting with fatigue, lower extremity edema, or dyspnea
  - o Retinopathy, vision impairment
  - o Myocardial infarction or sudden death due to accelerated CVD complicated by cardiac hypertrophy (i.e., supply-demand mismatch)
  - o Hypertensive nephropathy presenting with renal insufficiency: azotemia, edema, malignant hypertension, anuria/oliguria

Major Differential Diagnoses: Characteristics of secondary hypertension include therapeutic recalcitrance (defined as inefficacy or subefficacy of simultaneous use of three or more drugs[38]), onset at an early age (< 30y) or at a more advanced age (>50y), and the typical associated features of the causative disorder, such as hypokalemia with hyperaldosteronism, depression or musculoskeletal pain with hypovitaminosis D, and cold intolerance, bradycardia, and delayed Achilles reflex return with hypothyroidism. Listed below are most of the primary causes of hypertension with a brief sketch of their classic clinical characteristics, including physical examination and laboratory findings. Additionally, the December 2010 review by Vierra and Neutze[39] recommends an age-based approach which will also be included in the following descriptions of differential diagnoses; of note, 70-85% of hypertension in children is secondary to an identifiable primary disorder. While the purpose of this text is to focus on *adult* hypertension, many of the diagnostic and treatment considerations are appropriately applicable to children. Normal and abnormal values for blood pressure in infants and children differ from those of adults and are stratified based on age, gender, and height in a chart from the International Pediatric Hypertension Association available at PediatricHypertension.org.

---

[38] Viera AJ, Neutze DM. Diagnosis of secondary hypertension: an age-based approach. *Am Fam Physician*. 2010 Dec 15;82(12):1471-8
[39] Viera AJ, Neutze DM. Diagnosis of secondary hypertension: an age-based approach. *Am Fam Physician*. 2010 Dec 15;82(12):1471-8

- <u>Aortic coarctation</u>: Coarctation of the aorta is the second most common cause of HTN in children. (Kidney disease is the most common cause of HTN in children, as reviewed later.) Aortic coarctation is 2-5x more common in males, and typical age of diagnosis is 5 years. Classic presentation includes upper extremity hypertension with lower extremity hypotension/hypoperfusion/claudication, with or without discrepancies in bilateral brachial pressure, in a child or young adult; secondary activation of the renin-angiotensin system due to renal hypoperfusion exacerbates the HTN and complicates this *focal* anatomic disorder by adding a *systemic* neurohormonal component. Physical examination findings may include leg blood pressure at least 20 mm Hg less than arm blood pressure, delayed or absent femoral pulses, and an audible murmur or bruit. Imaging modalities of choice are transthoracic ultrasonography for children and MRI for adults; computed tomography (CT), magnetic resonance angiography/aortography (MRA) may also be used. Treatment includes antihypertensive interventions (reviewed in the section on *Therapeutic Considerations*) to manage the hypertension until surgery corrects the coarctation.

- <u>Cocaine use</u>: Cocaine use can cause acute and chronic elevations in blood pressure. Drug cessation is the key to treatment; urine drug testing is appropriate for patients suspected of undisclosed drug use or noncompliance with cessation. In hospital practice, patients presenting with hypertensive disorders, chest pain, and other cardiovascular syndromes are routinely tested for acute (serum drug screen) and chronic (urine drug screen) drug exposure; an impressive number of these tests come back positive even among patients who swear to have never used or not recently used recreational drugs.

- <u>Cushing's disease/syndrome, hypercortisolism</u>: Excess glucocorticoids whether endogenous or exogenous promote sodium retention directly via their mineralocorticoid effect and by causing hyperinsulinemia via induction of peripheral insulin resistance; both of these pathophysiologic processes contribute to HTN. Determination of iatrogenic hypercortisolism can be determined by reviewing the patient's medication intake. Endogenous hypercortisolism (2-5 diagnoses per million patients per year) can be assessed with measurements of serum adrenocorticotropic hormone (ACTH), 24-hour urinary free cortisol, nighttime salivary cortisol, and the low-dose dexamethasone suppression test in addition to looking for the clinical characteristics of moon facies, striae, sarcopenia, and abdominal obesity. Treatment is withdrawal of exogenous steroids (if possible) for iatrogenic Cushing's syndrome, or surgical removal of the ACTH-producing pituitary corticotroph adenoma (classically) in cases of endogenous Cushing's disease. An additional type of Cushing's syndrome can result from ectopic ACTH production from tumors such as small cell carcinoma of the lung or a carcinoid tumor.

- <u>Drug side-effect</u>: Many pharmaceutical drugs can cause an elevation in blood pressure. Reviewing the adverse effects of each drug that a patient is taking may be sufficient to identify the offending agent; a clinical trial of discontinuation may be appropriate to determine if a drug causes or contributes to elevated blood pressure in a particular patient. Many options to the use of pharmaceutical drugs exist, allowing the prevention and alleviation of many diseases and disorders commonly encountered in clinical practice. Several common hypertension-inducing drugs are listed in separate paragraphs within this section on differential diagnosis; drugs worthy of specific mention include amphetamines, buspirone, carbamazapine, clozapine, fluoxetine, lithium, tricyclic antidepressants, prednisone and methylprednisolone, and sympathomimetic decongestants.[40]

- <u>Estrogen, oral contraceptives</u>: As a group of various hormones with divergent effects, estrogens generally tend to promote sodium and water retention, which promotes volume overload and the development of HTN. For women with "estrogen dominance" due to excess endogenous production or exogenous administration of estrogens, supplementation with pyridoxine 50-250 mg/d (nearly always co-administered with magnesium 600-1,200 mg/d or to bowel tolerance; pyridoxal-5-phosphate [p5p] might also be used) and/or natural progesterone (rather than a synthetic progestin, since many of these preparations have inherent glucocorticoid/mineralocorticoid activity) can frequently offset the HTN-inducing effects of estrogens. Clinicians desiring a more comprehensive anti-estrogen protocol within a context of practical hormone optimization ("orthoendocrinology") may find helpful the review in chapter 4.

- <u>Ethanol overconsumption</u>: Excess ethanol consumption raises blood pressure and makes HTN more difficult to treat. Many patients fail to accurately disclose the extent and duration of their alcohol consumption. In acute

---

[40] Viera AJ, Neutze DM. Diagnosis of secondary hypertension: an age-based approach. *Am Fam Physician*. 2010 Dec 15;82(12):1471-8

care and hospital settings, plasma ethanol (blood alcohol concentration, BAC) can be measured, along with either serum toxicology screening for acute/recent intoxication or urinary toxicology screening for chronic/past drug use. Many patients who claim to have not used drugs ever or recently will be found to have positive drug tests with replicable results. Clues to occult alcoholism may include socioeconomic problems and elevations of serum AST (aspartate transaminase) greater than ALT (alanine transaminase), along with elevations of GGT (gamma glutamyl transpeptidase) and triglycerides; hepatic cirrhosis, splenomegaly, and pancytopenia may also be noted among patients with chronic alcoholism, even among patients who deny alcohol use. Differential diagnosis of occult alcoholism includes chronic viral hepatitis B or C, hemochromatosis and other forms of iron overload, overuse of other drugs or medications, and psychiatric disorders.

Rapid-onset HTN must be managed early and assertively
Rapid-onset HTN of 160 mm Hg systolic or 110 mm Hg diastolic requires urgent treatment. *Rapid-onset* HTN can cause stroke at pressures generally tolerated in *chronic* HTN because, in the latter, the vasculature has time to adapt to the higher pressures, while in the former, the cardiovascular system has not had time to adapt, thus leaving the patient particularly vulnerable to hemorrhagic stroke. Acute-onset HTN *from any cause* should be treated urgently when pressures approximate or exceed 160-180 mm Hg systolic or 110 mm Hg diastolic, especially *but not exclusively* if accompanied by complications such as angina (test serum cardiac enzymes), shortness of breath (consider pulmonary edema and auscultate for crackles), vision changes, papilledema, headache/ confusion/ seizures (which suggest cerebral edema or cerebral vasospasm), proteinuria, or edema of the face, peripheral extremities, or of the general body (anasarca, check for sacral edema and weight gain).

- Gestational hypertension and preeclampsia: Pregnancy-induced (after week 20 of gestation) hypertension without proteinuria is termed *gestational hypertension*; gestational hypertension with concomitant proteinuria is termed *preeclampsia*, while the addition of seizures advances the diagnosis to *eclampsia*—all of these pregnancy-related hypertensive syndromes can present with acute HTN. Preeclampsia can accelerate rapidly and cause life-threatening complications for the mother and/or fetus; treatment requires parenteral therapy (intravenous magnesium sulfate for seizure prophylaxis; hydralazine and/or labetolol for HTN control) and/or emergency interventions—namely, delivery.[41] Some evidence suggests that the incidence of preeclampsia can be reduced via increased intake of aspirin, ascorbate, calcium, tocopherol(s), and magnesium[42], and by pre-pregnancy treatment/cure of obesity, diabetes mellitus, and HTN.

- Hypercalcemia: Easily diagnosed by routine laboratory testing, hypercalcemia may be caused by hyperparathyroidism, malignancy, Paget's disease of bone, sarcoidosis, or rarely by nutritional excesses of calcium and/or vitamin D. Most hypercalcemia (80-90%) is due to hyperparathyroidism or malignancy; the most common cause of hypercalcemia in the outpatient setting is hyperparathyroidism, while in the hospital setting the most common cause is malignancy, particularly multiple myeloma, lymphoma, lymphosarcomas, and metastatic disease.[43] While other differential diagnoses also need to be considered, some endocrinologist particularly advocate testing 24-h urinary calcium levels as a test for familial hypocalciuric hypercalcemia. When primary hyperparathyroidism is suspected, the serum level of intact parathyroid hormone (iPTH) is tested. When malignancy is suspected (particularly from the finding of an unexplained serum calcium > 13 mg/dL [> 3.25 mmol/L]), patient-centered evaluation is performed, which often includes initial chest radiograph followed by *pan-scanning* with CT for occult malignancies in the thorax (e.g., lung cancers), abdomen and pelvis (e.g., gastrointestinal tumors).

- Insulin resistance and hyperinsulinemia: Insulin promotes renal retention of sodium which leads to water retention and the subsequent volume overload and systemic hypertension which logically follow in sequence. This explains the well proven and replicable benefit of low-carbohydrate diets in treating "idiopathic" HTN in the general population. Elevated or high-normal serum insulin along with chronic hyperglycemia is most suggestive of insulin resistance; the most effective treatments for insulin resistance are integrative nutritional interventions.[44]

- Licorice (*Glycyrrhiza glabra*) over-consumption: Used medicinally for thousands of years with excellent safety and effectiveness, *Glycyrrhiza glabra* is particularly useful against several common human viral infections. The active constituent glycyrrhizin (also known as glycyrrhizic acid, the hydrolysis product of which is

[41] Wagner LK. Diagnosis and management of preeclampsia. *Am Fam Physician*. 2004 Dec 15;70(12):2317-24
[42] Domino FJ (editor in chief). *The 5-Minute Clinical Consult, 2010, 18th Edition*. Philadelphia; Wolters Kluwer: 2009, 1062
[43] Bent S, Gensler LS, Frances C. *Saint-Frances Guide: Clinical Clerkship in Outpatient Medicine, 2nd Edition*. Philadelphia; Wolters Kluwer: 2008, 490
[44] Vasquez A. *Chiropractic and Naturopathic Mastery of Common Clinical Disorders*. IBMRC 2009. And later versions published in the Inflammation Mastery series.

glycyrrhetinic acid) can cause clinically severe hypertension with hypokalemia via potentiation of endogenous mineralocorticoids leading to clinical syndrome called "pseudo-hyperaldosteronism." More specifically, glycyrrhizin inhibits 11-beta hydroxysteroid dehydrogenase thus preventing cortisol's inactivation to cortisone in the kidney; this potentiates the mineralocorticoid effect of endogenous cortisol leading to sodium retention and potassium excretion. The hypertension resolves following discontinuation of the excess licorice.

- Mercury toxicity: Mercury is an established neurotoxin, immunotoxin, and nephrotoxin. Because pathophysiologic effects are noted even with very small doses of exposure, one could reasonably argue that no safe amount exists and therefore that any detected mercury is an indication for therapeutic intervention to remove this toxicant. According to an article by Schober et al[45] published in *JAMA—Journal of the American Medical Association* in 2003, "Approximately 8% of [1,709 American] women had [blood mercury] concentrations higher than the US Environmental Protection Agency's recommended reference dose (5.8 µg/L), below which exposures are considered to be without adverse effects." Sources of exposure include dental amalgams, vaccinations, airborne pollution, and fish; recently, high-fructose corn syrup was shown to contain mercury.[46] Mercury impairs catecholamine degradation and can thereby cause a clinical syndrome that can include hypertension, tremor, tachycardia, diaphoresis, and neurocognitive changes.[47] Per Shih and Gartner[48], "Mercury combines with the sulfhydryl group of S-adenosylmethionine, which is a cofactor for catecholamine-O-methyltransferase (COMT), and this inhibition of COMT allows accumulation of norepinephrine, epinephrine, and dopamine." The clinical presentation of mercury toxicity can include any of the following: diffuse erythematosus rash, dermatitis (acrodynia), anorexia, malaise, fatigue, muscle pain, proximal and/or distal muscle weakness, tremor, weight loss, insomnia, night sweats, burning peripheral neuropathy (axonal neuropathy), renal insufficiency/failure, inattention, neurocognitive compromise, personality changes, depression, diaphoresis, tachycardia, and hypertension. Differential diagnoses for mercury toxicity are numerous, including pheochromocytoma, hyperthyroidism, conversion disorder, viral infection, toxic shock syndrome, and Kawasaki disease. Laboratory assessment can include 24-hour urinary catecholamines, random urine mercury, and whole blood mercury; these tests are particularly appropriate for acute and subacute intoxications. For distant and chronic mercury intoxications, many clinicians including this author prefer to use dimercaptosuccinic acid (DMSA) dosed orally at 10 mg per kilogram of body weight to enhance the sensitivity of urine toxic metal testing. The use of DMSA for children and adults is supported by peer-reviewed literature[49,50,51,52,53] and has been reviewed in more detail by this author in *Integrative Rheumatology*[54] and to a lesser extent in *Musculoskeletal Pain: Expanded Clinical Strategies*.[55] DMSA chelation is approved by the US Food and Drug Administration (FDA) for the treatment of lead toxicity in children.[56]

- Neurogenic hypertension: In the context of discussing HTN, "neurogenic" was historically interchangeable with "essential", "primary", and "idiopathic." Since *neurogenic* is no longer

> **Physiologic irritation of the nucleus tract solitarius (NTS) and other nearby structures in the brainstem appears to contribute to some cases of hypertension**
>
> "Impaired NTS (CNS) function can produce an amplification of the action of the environmental stresses on blood pressure. Thus environmental stimuli or the expression of behaviors which normally result in trivial elevations of blood pressure will, after the NTS is perturbed, result in marked elevations (of blood pressure)."
>
> Reis DJ. The nucleus tractus solitarius and experimental neurogenic hypertension. *Adv Biochem Psychopharmacol* 1981

---

45 Schober et al. Blood mercury levels in US children and women of childbearing age, 1999-2000. *JAMA*. 2003 Apr;289:1667-74 jama.ama-assn.org/content/289/13/1667.long

46 "Average daily consumption of high fructose corn syrup is about 50 grams per person in the United States. With respect to total mercury exposure, it may be necessary to account for this source of mercury in the diet of children and sensitive populations." Dufault R, LeBlanc B, Schnoll R, Cornett C, Schweitzer L, Wallinga D, Hightower J, Patrick L, Lukiw WJ. Mercury from chlor-alkali plants: measured concentrations in food product sugar. *Environ Health*. 2009 Jan 26;8:2. See also: "High fructose corn syrup has been shown to contain trace amounts of mercury as a result of some manufacturing processes, and its consumption can also lead to zinc loss." Dufault et al. Mercury exposure, nutritional deficiencies and metabolic disruptions may affect learning in children. *Behav Brain Funct*. 2009 Oct 27;5:44.

47 Wössmann W, Kohl M, Grüning G, Bucsky P. Mercury intoxication presenting with hypertension and tachycardia. *Arch Dis Child*. 1999 Jun;80(6):556-7

48 Shih H, Gartner JC Jr. Weight loss, hypertension, weakness, and limb pain in an 11-year-old boy. *J Pediatr*. 2001 Apr;138(4):566-9

49 Bradstreet et al. A case-control study of mercury burden in children with autistic spectrum disorders. *J Am Physicians Surg* 2003; 8: 76-79 jpands.org/vol8no3/geier.pdf

50 Crinnion WJ. Environmental medicine, part three: long-term effects of chronic low-dose mercury exposure. *Altern Med Rev*. 2000 Jun;5(3):209-23

51 Forman J, Moline J, Cernichiari E, Sayegh S, Torres JC, Landrigan MM, Hudson J, Adel HN, Landrigan PJ. A cluster of pediatric metallic mercury exposure cases treated with meso-2,3-dimercaptosuccinic acid (DMSA). *Environ Health Perspect*. 2000 Jun;108(6):575-7 ehp.niehs.nih.gov/docs/2000/108p575-577forman/abstract.html

52 Miller AL. Dimercaptosuccinic acid (DMSA), a non-toxic, water-soluble treatment for heavy metal toxicity. *Altern Med Rev*. 1998 Jun;3(3):199-207

53 DMSA. *Altern Med Rev*. 2000 Jun;5(3):264-7

54 Vasquez A. *Integrative Rheumatology*. IBMRC 2006, 2007 and all future editions, most recently updated as *Inflammation Mastery, 4th Edition* (2016).

55 Vasquez A. *Musculoskeletal Pain: Expanded Clinical Strategies*. Institute for Functional Medicine (2008), most recently updated as *Inflammation Mastery, 4th Edition* (2016).

56 "The Food and Drug Administration has recently licensed the drug DMSA (succimer) for reduction of blood lead levels >/= 45 micrograms/dl. This decision was based on the demonstrated ability of DMSA to reduce blood lead levels. An advantage of this drug is that it can be given orally." Goyer et al. Role of chelating agents for prevention, intervention, and treatment of exposures to toxic metals. *Environ Health Perspect*. 1995 Nov;103(11):1048-52 ehp.niehs.nih.gov/docs/1995/103-11/meetingreport.html

generally used for this purpose, and because new research advocates the term's reinstitution, *neurogenic hypertension* should be exonerated from its previous identification with *idiopathicity* and given revised meaning. For the purposes of this discussion and as detailed later in this chapter, **the term "neurogenic hypertension" will mean what its name implies,** namely **chronic HTN induced principally by the nervous system due to** *irritation* or *functional disturbance* **rather than overt pathology**. Given its basis in physiology rather than pathology per se, the term "functional neurogenic hypertension" would serve to further emphasize the functional and therefore largely reversible mechanism of the disorder. Foci of neurogenic hypertension can reside in the central nervous system (CNS) or peripheral nervous system (PNS). In this text, **"central neurogenic hypertension"** describes hypertensive states induced by irritation of the central nervous system, in particular at the level of the brainstem (i.e., medulla oblongata in general and the root entry zones [REZ] of cranial nerves 9 and 10 as well as the nucleus tract solitarius [NTS] in particular) as will be reviewed in a following section on surgical interventions for the treatment of medullary neurovascular compression. The first use of the term "central neurogenic hypertension" of which this author is aware was published by Reis[57] in a 1981 review, mostly of animal research. In this review, Reis included the hypothesis that irritation of the CNS by either mechanical or neurochemical means could serve as a predisposition or antecedent to the manifest development of clinical HTN. The diagnosis of central neurogenic hypertension is generally based upon ❶ MRI/MRA or CT findings of neurovascular compression of the left medulla oblongata in conjunction with ❷ reduction in blood pressure following decompressive intervention.

> **Facilitation: chronic low-threshold nerve discharge**
>
> "Previous studies have indicated the existence, in man, of pools of spinal extensor motoneurons which are in a state of enduring excitation, as reflected in low reflex thresholds. ... The data indicate that differences in pressure thresholds reflect differences in central facilitation, and that the facilitation is due to a bombardment of the motoneurons by impulses originating, in part at least, from points other than the spinous process which was the site of stimulation."
>
> Denslow, Korr, et al. Quantitative studies of chronic facilitation in human motoneuron pools. *Am J Physiology* 1947

"**Peripheral neurogenic hypertension**" as an entity is more theoretical, less studied, and might be exemplified by irritation of spinal nerve roots and sympathetic ganglia as discussed primarily in the chiropractic[58,59,60,61,62] and osteopathic literature.[63,64] Functional compromise in general and **facilitation**[65] in particular of the nerve roots and sympathetic ganglia as a potential *cause of* or *contributor to* chronic HTN supports the rationale for the use of spinal manipulation and manual medicine for the treatment of HTN and other nonmusculoskeletal disorders. Peripheral neurogenic hypertension may be diagnosed based on clinical/electrographic/vasodynamic evidence of functional PNS compromise/ facilitation/ irritation and alleviation of HTN following appropriate regional intervention such as manual manipulative treatment of the spine and adjacent neuromusculoskeletal structures applied to effect restoration of proper nervous system function and balance. Central and peripheral types of neurogenic HTN will be discussed in more detail later in this chapter within the context of their surgical and manipulative treatments, respectively.

- Nonsteroidal anti-inflammatory drugs (NSAIDs): NSAIDs in general such as ibuprofen and naproxen and COX-2 inhibitors (coxibs) in particular reduce endogenous production of vasodilating prostacyclin and thus cause pharmacologic/iatrogenic renal artery constriction, which leads to varying degrees of HTN via activation of the renin-angiotensin system. This explains, in part, the increased cardiovascular mortality due to overutilization of coxibs such as rofecoxib/Vioxx, withdrawn from the US market in 2005 by the US FDA due to its causal role in increasing cardiovascular deaths.[66] Evidence of increased cardiovascular morbidity and mortality secondary to coxib use was widely publicized for several years before rofecoxib/Vioxx and a similar

---

[57] "The abnormalities of pressure control resulting from abnormal transmission in NTS met most of the criteria of an animal model of central neurogenic hypertension. ... Impaired NTS function can produce an amplification of the action of the environmental stresses on blood pressure." Reis DJ. The nucleus tractus solitarius and experimental neurogenic hypertension: evidence for a central neural imbalance hypothesis of hypertensive disease. *Adv Biochem Psychopharmacol*. 1981;28:409-20

[58] Bakris et al. Atlas vertebra realignment and achievement of arterial pressure goal in hypertensive patients: a pilot study. *J Hum Hypertens*. 2007 May;21(5):347-52

[59] Plaugher G, Bachman TR. Chiropractic management of a hypertensive patient. *J Manipulative Physiol Ther*. 1993 Oct;16(8):544-9

[60] Yates et al. Effects of chiropractic treatment on blood pressure and anxiety: a randomized, controlled trial. *J Manipulative Physiol Ther*. 1988 Dec;11(6):484-8

[61] Plaugher et al. Practice-based randomized controlled-comparison clinical trial of chiropractic adjustments and brief massage treatment at sites of subluxation in subjects with essential hypertension: pilot study. *J Manipulative Physiol Ther*. 2002 May;25:221-39

[62] Crawford et al. Management of hypertensive disease: review of spinal manipulation and the efficacy of conservative therapeusis. *J Manipulative Physiol Ther* 1986 Mar ;:27-32

[63] Celander E, Koenig AJ, Celander DR. Effect of osteopathic manipulative therapy on autonomic tone as evidenced by blood pressure changes and activity of the fibrinolytic system. *J Am Osteopath Assoc*. 1968 May;67(9):1037-8

[64] Fichera AP, Celander DR. Effect of osteopathic manipulative therapy on autonomic tone as evidenced by blood pressure changes and activity of the fibrinolytic system. *J Am Osteopath Assoc*. 1969 Jun;68(10):1036-8

[65] Denslow JS, Korr IM, Krems AD. Quantitative studies of chronic facilitation in human motoneuron pools. *Am J Physiol*. 1947 Aug;150(2):229-38

[66] Topol EJ. Failing the public health—rofecoxib, Merck, and the FDA. *N Engl J Med*. 2004 Oct 21;351(17):1707-9

drug valdecoxib/Bextra were belatedly withdrawn from the consumer market.[67,68] The multiple failures involved in this politicopharmaceutical phenomenon include ❶ failure of Merck to act on data showing that its popular and profitable new drug was harming and killing an unacceptable proportion of patients who took it, ❷ failure of the US FDA to regulate the pharmaceutical industry, ❸ failure of the medical profession as a whole to police itself and call for a ban on the use of this drug before either Merck or the FDA took action. See Topol's "Failing the public health— rofecoxib, Merck, and the FDA" published in the October 21, 2004 issue of *New England Journal of Medicine* for authoritative discussion.

> **Fraudulent marketing of valdecoxib/Bextra contributed to the largest healthcare fraud settlement in the history of the US Department of Justice—US $2.3 billion**
>
> Pharmacia and Upjohn Company, a subsidiary of Pfizer Inc, pled guilty to a felony violation of the Food, Drug & Cosmetic Act for misbranding the drug Bextra with the intent to defraud or mislead. Pharmacia and Upjohn Company admitted to its criminal conduct in the promotion of Bextra and agreed to pay a criminal fine of $1.195 billion, the largest criminal fine ever imposed in the United States for any matter. Pharmacia and Upjohn Company also agreed to forfeit $105 million, for a total criminal resolution of $1.3 billion. In addition Pfizer agreed to pay an additional $1 billion plus interest to settle civil allegations that it fraudulently promoted and marketed Bextra, as well as three other drugs in its portfolio, Geodon, an anti-psychotic drug, Zyvox, an antibiotic, and Lyrica, an anti-epileptic drug, as well as claims that it paid kickbacks for these, as well as other drugs, to induce physician prescribing.
>
> justice.gov/usao/ma/Press Office Press Release Files/Sept2009/PharmaciaPlea.html. Posted September 15, 2009. Accessed November 23, 2010. See also news.bbc.co.uk/2/hi/business/8234533.stm

- Pheochromocytoma: An exceedingly rare cause of secondary HTN (0.5%) in contrast to the high frequency with which it is covered in textbooks and licensing board exams, pheochromocytoma's classic presentation includes episodic HTN, headache, tremor, and diaphoresis. Pheochromocytoma is diagnosed with increased 24-hour urinary catecholamines, metanephrines, and vanillylmandelic acid with or without plasma free metanephrines followed by CT/MRI to localize the secreting neuroendocrine tumor. Mercury intoxication whether acute or chronic must be considered in the differential diagnosis of pheochromocytoma and similar clinical presentations.[69,70] Treatment is surgical excision of the adrenal/extra-adrenal catecholamine-producing tumor.

- Primary hyperaldosteronism (Conn's syndrome): Primary hyperaldosteronism is caused by a unilateral adrenal adenoma or bilateral adrenal hyperplasia; this condition accounts for approximately 6% of adult HTN and 10-20% of cases of treatment-resistant HTN.[71] The classic finding is HTN with hypokalemia (30%), occasionally with slight hypernatremia, and the diagnosis is established by documentation of an elevated serum aldosterone:renin ratio. Importantly, aldosterone must be tested with renin (i.e., plasma renin activity) since measurement of serum aldosterone alone is insensitive; 25% of patients with hyperaldosteronism will have a normal serum aldosterone level.[72] Per *The Merck Manual*:

> "Initial laboratory testing consists of plasma aldosterone levels and plasma renin activity (PRA). Ideally, tests are done with the patient off of drugs that affect the renin-angiotensin system (e.g., thiazide diuretics, ACE inhibitors, angiotensin antagonists, β-blockers) for 4 to 6 wk. PRA is usually measured in the morning with the patient recumbent [or upright[73]]. Patients with primary aldosteronism typically have plasma aldosterone > 15 ng/dL (> 0.42 nmol/L, [or > 416.10 pmol/L[74]]) and low levels of PRA, with a ratio of plasma aldosterone (in nanograms/dL) to PRA (in nanograms/mL/h) > 20."[75]

Diagnosis is confirmed by an endocrinologist performing a salt-suppression test. CT imaging is insensitive for detecting microadenomas and milder degrees of glandular hyperplasia. Curative treatment is laparoscopic removal/resection of the hypersecreting adrenal tumor; for patients who are not surgical candidates, drug treatment with an aldosterone-blocking drug (e.g., spironolactone or eplerenone) is used.

[67] "The results from VIGOR showed that the relative risk of developing a confirmed adjudicated thrombotic cardiovascular event (myocardial infarction, unstable angina, cardiac thrombus, resuscitated cardiac arrest, sudden or unexplained death, ischemic stroke, and transient ischemic attacks) with rofecoxib treatment compared with naproxen was 2.38 (95% confidence interval, 1.39-4.00; P =.002)." Mukherjee et al. Risk of cardiovascular events associated with selective COX-2 inhibitors. *JAMA* 2001 Aug 22-29;286(8):954-9
[68] "Systolic blood pressure increased significantly in 17% of rofecoxib- compared with 11% of celecoxib-treated patients (P = 0.032) at any study time point. Diastolic blood pressure increased in 2.3% of rofecoxib- compared with 1.5% of celecoxib-treated patients (P = 0.44)." Whelton et al; SUCCESS VI Study Group. Cyclooxygenase-2--specific inhibitors and cardiorenal function: a randomized, controlled trial of celecoxib and rofecoxib in older hypertensive osteoarthritis patients. *Am J Ther* 2001 Mar-Apr;8(2):85-95
[69] Wössmann W, Kohl M, Grüning G, Bucsky P. Mercury intoxication presenting with hypertension and tachycardia. *Arch Dis Child.* 1999 Jun;80(6):556-7
[70] Shih H, Gartner JC Jr. Weight loss, hypertension, weakness, and limb pain in an 11-year-old boy. *J Pediatr.* 2001 Apr;138(4):566-9
[71] Viera AJ, Neutze DM. Diagnosis of secondary hypertension: an age-based approach. *Am Fam Physician.* 2010 Dec 15;82(12):1471-8
[72] Viera AJ, Neutze DM. Diagnosis of secondary hypertension: an age-based approach. *Am Fam Physician.* 2010 Dec 15;82(12):1471-8
[73] Viera AJ, Neutze DM. Diagnosis of secondary hypertension: an age-based approach. *Am Fam Physician.* 2010 Dec 15;82(12):1471-8
[74] Viera AJ, Neutze DM. Diagnosis of secondary hypertension: an age-based approach. *Am Fam Physician.* 2010 Dec 15;82(12):1471-8
[75] unboundmedicine.com/merckmanual/ub/view/Merck-Manual-Pro/503850/all/Primary_Aldosteronism Accessed October 2, 2010

Pseudohyperaldosteronism can be caused by overconsumption of *Glycyrrhiza glabra* (licorice) and by Liddle's syndrome, a genotropic disorder causing increased sodium reabsorption, characterized by early onset (<35y) HTN with hypokalemia, low urinary sodium levels, and normal serum aldosterone levels.

- Renal artery (renovascular) stenosis: Partial obstruction of the renal arteries whether by thrombus (rare), atherosclerosis, or fibromuscular dysplasia causes renal hypoperfusion and activation of the renin-angiotensin system. Accounting for approximately 10% of renal artery stenosis (RAS), fibromuscular dysplasia is the most common cause of renovascular stenosis in young adults (19-39 years of age); women are affected much more commonly than are men. The other 90% of renovascular

> **Clinical pearl: Increase in serum K, BUN, or creatinine following ACEi or ARB treatment suggests RAS**
>
> An increase in serum creatinine (0.5-1.0 mg/dL [44.2-88.4 micromol/L]) following initiation of ACEi or ARB treatment suggests renal artery stenosis (RAS). Additional considerations include heart failure, renal insufficiency, dehydration, and drug intolerance with secondary acute renal injury. The drug does not necessarily have to be stopped until the creatinine has increased >30% over baseline or unless another compelling reason exists; monitor serum K and recheck GFR within 10 days.

stenosis is caused by atherosclerosis and is therefore mostly seen in older adults (>50y), particularly those with clinically significant CVD risk factors such as smoking and dyslipidemia and/or already established vascular disease. Renovascular stenosis is suggested by elevation of serum potassium, BUN, and/or creatinine following administration of an ACEi or an ARB; a high-pitched holosystolic renal artery bruit may be heard upon careful physical examination. The diagnosis of renal artery stenosis, per review by Zhang et al[76] in December 2009, can be made via imaging or invasive procedures, each with distinct advantages, disadvantages, safety profiles and costs. Catheter angiography with pressure gradient measurements is the definitive gold standard but is invasive, expensive, and thus reserved for surgical revascularization candidates. Ultrasonography is safe and inexpensive but the least accurate. Contrast-enhanced computed tomographic angiography and magnetic resonance angiography are intermediate in safety and accuracy. Magnetic resonance angiography *without any contrast* has become progressively more accurate and can rival contrast-enhanced techniques in its clinical utility, thereby making it the preferred imaging assessment for patients with renal insufficiency. Captopril-augmented renography lacks sensitivity and specificity and is no longer recommended. Treatment options are generally surgical (e.g., stent placement, angioplasty, or other revascularization technique) and/or pharmaceutical, with surgical approaches generally preferred for fibromuscular dysplasia and pharmaceutical treatment preferred for atherosclerotic renovascular stenosis.

- Renal parenchymal disease (nephrogenic hypertension): Renal disease can both lead to and result from HTN. Kidney diseases are the most common cause of hypertension in childhood; the leading primary etiologies are glomerulonephritis, congenital abnormalities, and reflux nephropathy. Over time and especially in adults, chronic HTN causes renal parenchymal damage, and parenchymal damage (whether due to HTN or another cause such as glomerulonephritis, pyelonephritis, polycystic kidneys, etc) leads to water retention and activation of the renin-angiotensin-aldosterone system, thus promoting a vicious cycle of progressive HTN and renal failure. The clinical picture commonly includes edema, elevated BUN and creatinine, proteinuria, anemia due to insufficient production of erythropoietin, and osteomalacia and osteodystrophy due to hyperphosphatemia, hypocalcemia, and insufficient renal formation of 1,25-dihydroxyvitamin D3. The diagnosis of renal disease is suggested by the finding of elevated BUN and creatinine on routine chemistry/metabolic panel blood tests; the diagnosis is further verified and refined by the use of CT, MRI, or US imaging, followed if necessary by renal biopsy. The Cockcroft-Gault formula has commonly been used for bedside estimation of renal function based on the patient's age, weight, gender, and serum creatinine (sCr); the formula is provided below in two versions, one using American-favored mg/dL as the unit for sCr, and the other using the international units of micromol/L—note that the latter formula employs a different constant value per gender in the numerator of the equation. The Cockcroft-Gault formula estimates creatinine clearance, which in turn is an estimate of the glomerular filtration rate (GFR), a measure of kidney function; thus creatinine clearance and GFR are somewhat interchangeable from a practical clinical perspective. Clinicians should appreciate the importance of the patient's age in determining GFR; sCr in the upper end of the normal range may indicate renal insufficiency in a patient of advanced age. Variants can be used per units in mg/dL or micromol/L, as shown in the following formulas:

---

[76] Zhang HL, Sos TA, Winchester PA, Gao J, Prince MR. Renal artery stenosis: imaging options, pitfalls, and concerns. *Prog Cardiovasc Dis*. 2009 Nov-Dec;52(3):209-19

Estimated Creatinine Clearance =	$\dfrac{(140 - \text{age in years}) \times \text{Weight in kilograms} \times (0.85 \text{ if female})}{72 \times \text{serum } \textbf{creatinine in mg/dL}}$

Estimated Creatinine Clearance =	$\dfrac{(140 - \text{age in years}) \times \text{Weight in kilograms} \times (1.23 \text{ for men or } 1.04 \text{ for women})}{72 \times \text{serum } \textbf{creatinine in micromol/L}}$

Although the Cockcroft-Gault formula is the *best-known* and *longest-used* formula for the estimation of GFR, currently the *best* equation for *more accurately* estimating GFR from serum creatinine is the Modification of Diet in Renal Disease (MDRD) Study equation, available on-line: nkdep.nih.gov/professionals/gfr_calculators/.[77]

Finally on this topic of renal disease, clinicians should be aware of measuring serum cystatin C to assess renal function. Cystatin C is a cysteine protease inhibitor produced by all nucleated cells, and its serum level is not affected by diet or muscle mass (unlike serum creatinine). The normal range for cystatin C when measured by particle-enhanced nephelometric immunoassay (PENIA) is <0.28 mg/L or <0.95 mg/L when measured by other immunologic methods. Cystatin C is a more sensitive indicator of declining renal function than is serum creatinine, and—like elevating serum creatinine or declining GFR (or elevated CRP for that matter)—cystatin C predicts risk and severity of CVD, CHF, and CKD; furthermore, cystatin C is directly involved in the pathogenesis of atherosclerosis.[78]

> **Clinical pearls for managing the patient with declining renal function**
>
> - **When the GFR < 60 (CKD stage 3)**, modify dosages or withdraw certain drugs. Treat the causative problem and/or begin specialist co-management. Avoid intravenous contrast agents and other nephrotoxic drugs when feasible. Blood pressure and glucose control are important; initiation of ACEi or ARB should be considered.
> - **When the GFR < 30 (CKD stage 4)**, the patient needs to consult a nephrologist.
> - **When the GFR < 15 (CKD stage 5)**, the patient needs transplant or dialysis.

- Sleep apnea: Obstructive sleep apnea (OSA) is a risk factor for HTN, and treatment for OSA with continuous positive airway pressure (C-PAP) can produce modest reductions in BP that are proportionate to the severity of the HTN and compliance with treatment. Diagnosis is suggested by history of unrestful sleep, fatigue, depression, and/or a spouse's report of interrupted nighttime breathing. Physical exam may show obesity and impairment of upper airway airflow. An overnight sleep study (polysomnography) provides data on sleep, respiratory effort, and blood oxygenation and has been considered the standard for the diagnosis of sleep apnea; however, nocturnal pulse oximetry may be sufficient for the diagnosis in selected high-index patients and is less cumbersome and less expensive.

- Systemic sclerosis: HTN in general and treatment-resistant HTN in particular are seen in systemic sclerosis, a disease in which cardiopulmonary disease (e.g., pulmonary hypertension, congestive heart failure) and renal compromise (e.g., acute renal crisis heralded by nephrogenic hypertension) are the most common causes of death. Abnormalities disclosed on history and physical exam may include Raynaud's phenomenon, sclerodactyly, mask-like face, telangiectasia, and esophageal dysfunction. Laboratory findings typically include some combination of positive antinuclear antibodies (ANA), anticentromere antibodies, anti-SCL-70 antibodies, and (more rarely) anti-fibrillarin antibodies. Treatment for scleroderma and other common autoimmune disorders is reviewed in *Integrative Rheumatology*.[79]

- Thyroid disease, including both hyperthyroidism and hypothyroidism: Hypothyroidism generally causes diastolic HTN, whereas hyperthyroidism generally causes systolic HTN and widened pulse pressure. Assess clinically (e.g., pulse rate, physical exam, weight loss/gain, Achilles reflex return speed, body temperature), and with laboratory testing. A low TSH and elevated free T4 is sufficient to diagnose hyperthyroidism. The diagnosis of hypothyroidism is indicated by any one or more of the following: elevated TSH, low free T4, low free T3 and/or total T3. Elevated titers of antithyroid antibodies (e.g., either anti-thyroid peroxidase or anti-thyroglobulin) can provide sufficient indication for treatment with thyroid hormone to prevent overt hypothyroidism from developing. Elevated reverse T3 and/or a ratio of total T3 to reverse T3 less than 10:1 indicates impaired peripheral metabolism of thyroid hormones; many integrative clinicians—including this

---

[77] National Kidney Disease Education Program, National Institutes of Health (NIH). nkdep.nih.gov/professionals/gfr_calculators/

[78] "Prospective studies have shown in various clinical scenarios that patients with increased cystatin C are at a higher risk of developing both CVD and CKD. Importantly, cystatin C appears to be a useful marker for identifying individuals at a higher risk for cardiovascular events among patients belonging to a relatively low-risk category as assessed by both creatinine and estimated glomerular filtration rate values." Taglieri N, Koenig W, Kaski JC. Cystatin C and cardiovascular risk. *Clin Chem.* 2009 Nov;55(11):1932-43

[79] Vasquez A. *Integrative Rheumatology.* IBMRC 2006, 2007 and all future editions, most recently updated as *Inflammation Mastery, 4th Edition* (2016).

author—hold that the ratio of total T3 to reverse T3 should be > 10:1 to ensure proper peripheral thyroid metabolism.[80]

- Tobacco use: Tobacco smoke constituents cause arterioconstriction which promotes HTN. Constituents and free radicals in tobacco smoke are more pathogenic than nicotine, while the latter in isolation indeed causes adverse cardiovascular effects via vasoconstriction. Conversely, nicotine (*sin* tobacco smoke) provides synaptogenic and anti-inflammatory benefits.

- Upper cervical spine dysfunction/subluxation: A remarkable clinical trial published in *Journal of Human Hypertension* in 2007 by Bakris et al[81] showed that **correction of upper cervical spine subluxation/dysfunction by chiropractic spinal manipulation causes "marked and sustained reductions in BP [blood pressure] similar to the use of two-drug combination therapy."** These results suggest and perhaps indicate that subtle biomechanical dysfunction of the upper cervical spine can cause hypertension, perhaps via neuronal reflex mechanisms or possibly—as suggested by Bakris et al—by alleviating neurovascular compression and/or by alleviating circulatory compromise of the vertebral artery.

- Vitamin D deficiency: Vitamin D deficiency is common in the general population—often up to 90-100% of subjects in large population-based studies—and causes intracellular hypercalcinosis[82] via elevated PTH levels and contributes to chronic HTN[83] via endothelial dysfunction, systemic inflammation, insulin resistance, and activation of the renin-angiotensin-aldosterone system.[84] **Correction of vitamin D deficiency can cause a reduction in elevated blood pressure comparable to that which can be achieved by single-drug oral antihypertensive medication[85] while also providing numerous collateral benefits (including reductions in depression, pain, and risks for autoimmune and malignant diseases) at lower cost and greater safety than can be achieved with pharmaceutical drugs.[86,87]**

Clinical Assessments:

- **History/subjective**: As stated previously, **most patients with HTN are asymptomatic** and only become symptomatic as a result of severe HTN which results in end-organ compromise, such as renal insufficiency, cerebral edema, or transient myocardial ischemia. The clinical history should include inquiry about chest pain, shortness of breath, family history of CVD or diabetes mellitus (DM), morning occipital headaches, new stressors, tobacco/caffeine use, and current medications/drugs including antihypertensives, nonsteroidal anti-inflammatory drugs (NSAIDs), estrogens, ethanol, cocaine, sympathomimetics and decongestants. During this standard *history of the present illness* (HPI) which all clinicians are taught to master before graduation from their respective colleges, astute clinicians have already begun the psychographic assessment (described hereafter as "BVG-LOC profiling") which will enable them to couch the treatment objectives and details in a manner tailored for that particular patient. In this context, the patient's BVG-LOC profile (i.e., personal profile of beliefs, values, goals, and locus of control) must be appreciated by the clinician since each aspect is essential to the understanding needed by the clinician in order to address or "speak to" the patient in such a way as to improve treatment compliance—these concepts are discussed more under the section *Clinical Management* below.

- **Physical Examination/Objective**: A screening physical examination is necessary (with details emphasized below) along with documentation of findings and vital signs, including blood pressure, pulse rate, breathing rate, temperature, pain level; weight and body mass index should be noted. Auscultation of the heart, lungs, carotid and renal arteries is performed, and cranial nerves are screened.
  - Blood pressure measurement: Screening for HTN should be performed at least once every two years starting at 18 years of age. The blood pressure cuff must be at heart level and properly fitted to the patient; the patient should be seated and relaxed for 5-10 minutes prior to blood pressure measurement. At initial

[80] McDaniel AB. Thyroid Assessment: Controversies and Conundrums. Institute for Functional Medicine 14th International Symposium. Tuscon, Arizona, 2007. Detailed in: Vasquez A. *Musculoskeletal Pain: Expanded Clinical Strategies*. Institute for Functional Medicine (2008), most recently updated as *Inflammation Mastery, 4th Edition* (2016).
[81] Bakris et al. Atlas vertebra realignment and achievement of arterial pressure goal in hypertensive patients: a pilot study. *J Hum Hypertens.* 2007 May;21(5):347-52
[82] Vasquez A. Intracellular Hypercalcinosis: A Functional Nutritional Disorder with Implications Ranging from Myofascial Trigger Points to Affective Disorders, Hypertension, and Cancer. *Naturopathy Digest* 2006 Previously published in-print and on-line at naturopathydigest.com/archives/2006/sep/vasquez.php and included in this book.
[83] Vasquez A. Nutritional Treatments for Hypertension. *Naturopathy Digest* 2006. Previously published in-print and on-line at naturopathydigest.com and included herein.
[84] Pilz S, Tomaschitz A, Ritz E, Pieber TR; Medscape. Vitamin D status and arterial hypertension: a systematic review. *Nat Rev Cardiol.* 2009 Oct;6(10):621-30
[85] "Inadequate vitamin D(3) and calcium intake could play a contributory role in the pathogenesis and progression of hypertension and cardiovascular disease in elderly women." Pfeifer M, Begerow B, Minne HW, Nachtigall D, Hansen C. Effects of a short-term vitamin D(3) and calcium supplementation on blood pressure and parathyroid hormone levels in elderly women. *J Clin Endocrinol Metab.* 2001 Apr;86(4):1633-7
[86] Vasquez et al. The clinical importance of vitamin D: a paradigm shift with implications for all healthcare providers. *Altern Ther Health Med.* 2004 Sep-Oct;10(5):28-36
[87] Faloon B. Millions of Needless Deaths. *Life Extension Magazine.* 2009 January lef.org/magazine/mag2009/jan2009_Millions-of-Needless-Deaths_01.htm

evaluation and periodically thereafter, blood pressure should be assessed in both the right and left arms; a significant side-to-side discrepancy > 20/10 mm Hg suggests a partial unilateral occlusion and is worthy of further evaluation. The two measurements upon which the diagnosis of HTN is being considered should occur on different visits at least 3 days apart; alternatively, if the blood pressure is >160/100 mm Hg on any one visit, then a presumptive diagnosis of HTN can be made and treatment initiated—in the pharmaceutical paradigm, treatment for BP >160/100 mm Hg is often initiated with two drugs. Blood pressure 120/80-139/89 mm Hg is considered "prehypertension" and is observed for progression without drug treatment in standard allopathic medicine[88] but is obviously a prime opportunity to intervene with nutritional and lifestyle improvements for those clinicians more progressively inclined. Blood pressure ≥140/90-160/100 is considered "stage 1 hypertension" and in the medical model is initially treated with one drug—generally a thiazide—while blood pressure ≥160/100-210/120 ("stage 2 hypertension") is often treated initially with a two-drug combination, with one of those drugs generally being a thiazide and the other drug selected based on patient characteristics. (Antihypertensive drug treatments are summarized at the end of this chapter). Blood pressures ≥210/120 are worthy of urgent or emergency treatment, based on the absence or presence of symptoms or organ damage, respectively, in an emergency hospital setting—additional details are provided in a following section on *Clinical Management*.

- Cardiopulmonary examination: Auscultation for rate, rhythm, rales/crackles; localize the cardiac point of maximal impulse (PMI) for evidence of lateral displacement or increased intensity which could indicate cardiomegaly or left ventricular hypertrophy.

- Eye and fundoscopic examination: Look for cotton-wool spots, retinal/flame hemorrhages, arteriovenous nicking, and papilledema; manifestations of diabetic retinopathy may also be seen if DM is concomitant. Patients with DM are referred for ophthalmologic evaluation at the time of diagnosis and annually/biannually thereafter depending on severity and compliance with and effectiveness of treatment.

- Inspection for diagonal ear lobe crease: Numerous studies have shown that the diagonal ear lobe crease is one of the easiest and most sensitive (~75%) and specific (~80%) physical examination findings to correlate with advanced atherosclerosis and cardiovascular disease.[89,90]

- Examination of the extremities: Assess pulse strength, arm:leg blood pressure differences[91] (ankle:brachial index should be > 1), lower extremity edema, capillary refill/perfusion and trophic changes consistent with peripheral vascular disease.

- Renal disease survey: Renal diseases are the most common causes of secondary hypertension. No physical examination finding correlates specifically with renal disease; peripheral edema is correlative but not indicative. Laboratory assessments include serum BUN, serum creatinine, serum cystatin C, and urine albumin:creatinine ratio (microalbuminuria) and/or urine albumin (proteinuria).

- Auscultation for bruits: Use the stethoscope bell over the carotid arteries (atherosclerosis) and renal arteries (renovascular hypertension due to atherosclerosis or fibromuscular dysplasia). Occasionally, an aortic bruit may be heard, particularly in cases of malformation or dissection. Higher degrees of arterial occlusion may reduce blood flow to such an extent that no bruit is heard.

- Neurologic examination: Observation for facial symmetry, inquiry about headache and mental status, and quick screening for symmetric and normal extremity muscle strength and reflexes may be sufficient for "low index" cases of mild hypertension in middle-aged patients without concomitant disease, such dyslipidemia or diabetes mellitus. However, as the number and severity of risk factors accumulate, the case becomes progressively worthy of a "high index" examination to establish a comprehensive assessment of baseline status and to screen for underlying causes or contributors to the HTN, as well as for other risk factors for CVD and complications from HTN. Situations indicating the appropriateness of a more thorough examination include younger or older patients in whom the HTN is more likely to be secondary to an underlying cause, patients with comorbidities or increased risk for complications, patients with more severe hypertension, and in patients with possible or impending complications from chronic HTN. Deep

---

[88] Le T, Dehlendorf C, Mendoza M, Ohata C. *First Aid for the Family Medicine Boards*. New York: McGraw-Hill Medical; 2008, 50
[89] Edston E. The earlobe crease, coronary artery disease, and sudden cardiac death: an autopsy study of 520 individuals. *Am J Forensic Med Pathol*. 2006 Jun;27(2):129-33
[90] Motamed M, Pelekoudas N. The predictive value of diagonal ear-lobe crease sign. *Int J Clin Pract*. 1998 Jul-Aug;52(5):305-6
[91] Ankle-brachial index test. webmd.com/heart-disease/ankle-brachial-index-test Referenced January 2010

tendon reflexes are checked for hyperreflexia (particularly with preeclampsia), and the Achilles reflex return is assessed for noteworthy delay that can indicate hypothyroidism[92], a well-documented cause of HTN and dyslipidemia. All patients deserve a thorough exam, whether for the assessment of baseline status, complications, contributions, or for the reassurance (for both doctor and patient) that is attained after a competent professional evaluation reveals no abnormalities.

- Body mass index (BMI) for assessing current BMI and predicting amount and duration of weight loss: Given that the average citizen of industrialized nations is overweight, nearly all patients can benefit from developing a specific goal-oriented and time-oriented plan for the achievement of weight optimization. **Contrasting current BMI with optimal BMI** clarifies the **amount of weight** that needs to be lost and provides an estimate of the **duration of the weight loss program**, given that adherent patients can lose an average of 4-8 lbs (~9-15 kg) per month. Although some patients can achieve highly significant improvements in various parameters such as glycemic control and blood pressure *without* significant weight loss, the fact remains that obesity (more specifically, abdominal obesity) is a **risk**

> **Clinical wisdom**
>
> Patients with lifestyle-generated diseases should be coached in the reversal of the patterns that have caused their disease rather than being enabled to pursue their disease-promoting lifestyles while surrogate markers of metabolic-physiologic dysfunction (e.g., hypertension) are pharmacologically suppressed.

factor and often the **primary determinant** for CVD-HTN-dyslipidemia-hyperglycemia-inflammation as well as osteoarthritis, many types of cancer, and significant but immeasurable (and generally unspoken) suffering associated with diminished self-esteem, inefficacy, social isolation, and depression. Patients have a myriad of reasons and rationalizations for maintaining their overweight status quo—every excuse from being "big boned" to "big framed" to "I've always been big" to "Everyone in my family is big" to "I don't have time to take care of myself" to "I don't know how to cook" to "I simply cannot [eat right, exercise, say 'no' to candy, give up wheat, give up ice cream, drink coffee without sugar and cream, etc]." Clinicians need to anticipate this resistance and have a diverse array of techniques—ranging from patient to insistent, from gentle to confrontational, from emotional to intellectual— to use *as appropriate to the individual patient's needs* to coax, inspire, lead, or push the patient who will benefit from weight loss. Elevated BMI correlates with numerous biochemical risk factors for CVD—progressively elevated levels of blood glucose, insulin, triglycerides, increasing

> **How to measure waist circumference**
>
> "To measure your waist circumference, place a tape measure around your bare abdomen just above your hip bone. [Waist circumference is the distance around your natural waist (just above the navel).*] Be sure that the tape is snug (but does not compress your skin) and that it is parallel to the floor. Relax, exhale, and measure your waist."
>
> Weight and Waist Measurement: Tools for Adults. win.niddk.nih.gov/Publications/tools.htm
> * Body Composition Tests.
> americanheart.org/presenter.jhtml?identifier=4489
> Accessed February 2009

severity of insulin resistance, and progressively lower levels of beneficial high-density lipoprotein (HDL) cholesterol—and an increased risk for cardiovascular death, various cancers, psychosocial problems including low self-esteem, reduced academic performance, and impaired interpersonal relationships, e.g., being a target for prejudice.[93] Elevated BMI is a preventable and treatable condition; physicians should not ignore this problem simply because it is common or difficult for some patients to acknowledge and effectively address. Relatedly, BMI should be viewed in context, especially with that of cardiovascular fitness, patient's symptoms (or lack thereof) of pain (joint pain and inflammatory diseases such as asthma and psoriasis are more common among the obese) and shortness of breath (dyspnea on exertion); also and importantly, several studies have shown that xenobiotic load is a more powerful predictor of insulin resistance than is obesity/BMI. Not surprisingly, the combination of obesity with either/both 1) lack of cardiovascular fitness and/or 2) elevated xenobiotic load is more problematic than obesity by itself. Obesity and elevated BMI are the easiest to detect and most obvious to discuss; patients and doctors alike need to be aware of the importance of enhancing both cardiovascular fitness (e.g., increasing the level of activity and exercise) and reducing the total xenobiotic load (e.g., avoiding exposure, promoting detoxification/depuration, and supporting governmental regulations to protect the public) rather than focusing solely on the obvious and easy: obesity and BMI.

---

[92] Degowin RL. *DeGowin and DeGowin's Diagnostic Evaluation. 6th Edition*. New York: McGraw Hill: 1994, 900. See also Khurana AK, Sinha RS, Ghorai BK, Bihari N. Ankle reflex photomotogram in thyroid dysfunctions. *J Assoc Physicians India*. 1990 Mar;38(3):201-3

[93] Costa et al. Body mass index has a good correlation with proatherosclerotic profile in children and adolescents. *Arq Bras Cardiol*. 2009 Sep;93(3):261-7

Laboratory Assessments:

- **Chemistry/metabolic panel:** Heightened attention is given to glucose, BUN, creatinine, calcium, and potassium. To screen for a renal cause of HTN, test serum BUN and creatinine and check urine albumin:creatinine ratio on a random urine sample; these tests are generally sufficient to confirm or refute a renal etiology of HTN. Renal US or CT imaging can be used for further renal evaluation. Glomerular filtration rate (GFR) can be estimated by the Cockcroft-Gault equation (DrV's tutorial: vimeo.com/152296851) and should be used by clinicians to monitor renal function in patients at risk for renal insufficiency, namely patients with HTN, diabetes mellitus, advanced age, and known renal disease. **Estimated GFR = (140 - age) x weight (kg) / (72 x serum creatinine); in women, multiply this result by .85.** GFR values consistently less than 60 for 3 months are consistent with chronic kidney disease and approximately 50% loss of renal function; at this level of impaired renal function, drug doses need to be modified. Hypercalcemia is a rare cause of HTN and requires evaluation for underlying cause, such as hyperparathyroidism, hyperthyroidism, malignancy (especially multiple myeloma, lymphoma, or cancer of the breast, lung, or kidney), granulomatous diseases such as sarcoidosis, vitamin D or vitamin A excess, adverse drug effect (especially lithium or thiazide diuretics), Paget disease of bone, adrenal insufficiency, or genotropic metabolic disorder such as familial hypocalciuric hypercalcemia.

- **Renal assessment, urinalysis (UA):** Test for hematuria, proteinuria, and glucosuria; random albumin:creatinine ratio to assess for microalbuminuria. See Chapter 1 (lab interpretation), video archive vimeo.com/152293616.

- **Thyroid assessment—glandular function, peripheral metabolism, and autoimmunity:** The purpose of thyroid assessment is to determine the overall functionality of the pituitary-thyroid-metabolic axis, and therefore thyroid testing should be comprehensive and include TSH, free T4, free or total T3, and reverse T3, and the antibodies directed against thyroid peroxidase (anti-TPO) and thyroglobulin (anti-thyroglobulin). Overt or imminent hypothyroidism is suggested by TSH greater than 2 mU/L[94] or 3 mU/L[95], low T4 or T3, and/or the presence of anti-thyroid peroxidase antibodies.[96] Objective laboratory abnormality suggesting hypothyroidism in a patient with compatible clinical symptomatology or objective findings is sufficient justification to warrant a clinical trial of thyroid hormone supplementation provided that no contraindications are present and that the apparent hypothyroidism is not due to another cause such as hyperestrogenemia, which reduces thyroid hormone cellular bioavailability due to increased production of thyroxine binding globulin (TBG). Common clinical manifestations of hypothyroidism include fatigue, depression, cold hands and feet, dry skin, constipation, bradycardia, adult acne, hypertension, head hair loss, hypercholesterolemia, dysthymia/anhedonia, menstrual irregularities in women, and hypogonadism and subfertility in both men and women. Several approaches to the treatment of hypothyroidism are described in the section of *Therapeutic Considerations*.

- **Serum 25-hydroxy-vitamin D:** In 2004, Vasquez, Manso, and Cannell[97] proposed a "paradigm shift" for clinicians' appreciation of vitamin D that summarized new applications for the clinical use of this nutrient beyond its application in patients with osteoporosis or malabsorption. A novel concept at its time, our article admonished clinicians to use empiric supplementation and/or laboratory assessment of all patients seen in clinical practice. The goal with vitamin D supplementation is to get serum 25-hydroxy-vitamin D (25-OH-D) levels into the optimal range, as currently defined in the illustration. As the cardioprotective role of vitamin D becomes more clear, the peer-reviewed

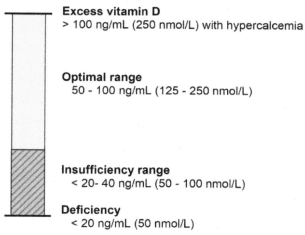

Excess vitamin D
> 100 ng/mL (250 nmol/L) with hypercalcemia

Optimal range
50 - 100 ng/mL (125 - 250 nmol/L)

Insufficiency range
< 20- 40 ng/mL (50 - 100 nmol/L)

Deficiency
< 20 ng/mL (50 nmol/L)

---

[94] Weetman AP. Hypothyroidism: screening and subclinical disease. *BMJ*. 1997 Apr 19;314(7088):1175-8 bmj.bmjjournals.com/cgi/content/full/314/7088/1175

[95] "Now AACE encourages doctors to consider treatment for patients who test outside the boundaries of a narrower margin based on a target TSH level of 0.3 to 3.0. AACE believes the new range will result in proper diagnosis for millions of Americans who suffer from a mild thyroid disorder, but have gone untreated until now." American Association of Clinical Endocrinologists (AACE). 2003 Campaign Encourages Awareness of Mild Thyroid Failure, Importance of Routine Testing aace.com/pub/tam2003/press.php November 26, 2005

[96] Beers MH, Berkow R (eds). *Merck Manual. 17th Edition*. Whitehouse Station: Merck Research Laboratories; 1999, Page 96

[97] Vasquez et al. The clinical importance of vitamin D: a paradigm shift with implications for all healthcare providers. *Altern Ther Health Med*. 2004 Sep-Oct;10(5):28-36

medical research increasingly advocates that **"vitamin D supplementation should be prescribed to patients with hypertension and 25-hydroxyvitamin D levels below target values."**[98]

- Uric acid: Many years ago uric acid was generally included in the standard chemistry/metabolic panel; these days it has to be ordered as a separate test. For at least a decade, "a strong, specific, stepwise, independent association of increasing serum uric acid and cardiac morbidity and mortality" has been noted[99], and recent research has shown that inhibition of uric acid production with allopurinol prevents fructose-induced urate-mediated metabolic disturbances that contribute to CVD, HTN, and the metabolic syndrome.[100] The roles of fructose and uric acid are discussed in greater detail in a following section.

- Urine pH: Urine pH can easily be monitored in-office or at home with the use of simple pH strips. Urine pH fluctuates throughout the day and therefore the most reliable evaluations are made with multiple daily assessments (easy and practical) and/or 24-h urine collections (cumbersome, inconvenient, and relatively impractical); an additional and important advantage to using multiple daily assessments of urine pH is that it allows the patient and doctor to observe how dietary and lifestyle fluctuations alter the whole-body biochemical-physiologic milieu. A urine pH of 7.0-8 is desirable as an indicator of dietary compliance and avoidance of the acidogenic Western diet, which is generally HTN-inducing due to its content of sodium, chloride, simple sugars and insufficiency of magnesium, potassium, calcium, and phytonutrients. Mild urinary alkalosis is the natural and optimal state of human physiology[101,102,103], and its induction is therefore simply a restoration of normalcy rather than an intervention or treatment per se. Caution might be employed when using this (or any other) treatment in patients with severe hepatorenal disease (who have lost the ability to buffer efficiently) and in patients with pre-existing electrolyte disturbances. Patients susceptible to urinary tract infections (UTIs) might experience an increased frequency of UTIs due to urinary alkalinization and may need to improve hygiene, supplement with additional ascorbic acid to prevent urine from becoming excessively alkaline, and/or correct gastrointestinal dysbiosis—this latter point is particularly important for women who experience recurrent UTIs, since urovaginal flora is strongly influenced by intestinal flora.[104]

- Urine sodium and potassium: Urine sodium (Na) and potassium (K) can be measured as markers for dietary intake and therefore as direct markers for compliance with dietary optimization. Urinary Na excretion ranges widely (thousand-fold) between human populations and individuals based mostly on dietary intake; among Yanomamo Indians in Brazil uNa is 0.2 mmol/24 h while among the northern Chinese the uNa is 242 mmol/24 h.[105] Very obviously, the general therapeutic goal in the treatment of HTN is to increase intake of potassium and reduce intake of sodium; the inverse ratio of these two cations positively correlates with blood pressure and other metabolic markers such as insulin sensitivity and endothelial function; thus measurement of urine sodium/potassium is more than a marker for nutritional compliance since is reflective and predictive of key aspects of cardiovascular health. Excepting sodium and potassium losses through perspiration, emesis, and diarrhea the urinary measurement of these minerals is clinically meaningful and correlates with dietary intake; the large Intersalt Study[106] involving 52 population samples in 32 countries for a total of 10,074 men and women aged 20-59 showed that higher urinary sodium excretion correlated positively and directly with systolic and diastolic blood pressures. While patient/physician-estimated potassium intake correlates with 24-h urinary K excretion, "patients tend to underestimate their sodium intake by 30% to 50%; therefore, urinary sodium excretion is more accurate to assess sodium intake."[107] Per the clinical trial by McCullough et al[108], patients on a low-Na diet (10 mEq/d) with excellent compliance have 24-hr Na excretion of approximately 4.6 - 13.4 mEq (outpatients and inpatients, respectively), compared with 24-hr Na excretion of 184.5 - 195.3 mEq for patients

[98] Pilz S, Tomaschitz A, Ritz E, Pieber TR; Medscape. Vitamin D status and arterial hypertension: a systematic review. *Nat Rev Cardiol.* 2009 Oct;6(10):621-30

[99] Alderman M. Uric acid in hypertension and cardiovascular disease. *Can J Cardiol* 1999 Nov;15 Suppl F:20F-2F

[100] News release from American Heart Association's 63rd High Blood Pressure Research Conference. High-sugar diet increases men's blood pressure; gout drug protective. Abstract P127. Sept. 23, 2009. americanheart.mediaroom.com/index.php?s=43&item=829 Accessed December 19, 2009

[101] Sebastian et al. Estimation of the net acid load of the diet of ancestral preagricultural Homo sapiens and their hominid ancestors. *Am J Clin Nutr.* 2002 Dec;76(6):1308-16

[102] Maurer et al. Neutralization of Western diet inhibits bone resorption independently of K intake and reduces cortisol secretion in humans. *Am J Physiol Renal Physiol.* 2003 Jan;284(1):F32-40

[103] Frassetto L, Morris RC Jr, Sellmeyer DE, Todd K, Sebastian A. Diet, evolution and aging--the pathophysiologic effects of the post-agricultural inversion of the potassium-to-sodium and base-to-chloride ratios in the human diet. *Eur J Nutr.* 2001 Oct;40(5):200-13

[104] Miles MR, Olsen L, Rogers A. Recurrent vaginal candidiasis. Importance of an intestinal reservoir. *JAMA.* 1977 Oct 24;238(17):1836-7

[105] Intersalt Cooperative Research Group. Intersalt: an international study of electrolyte excretion and blood pressure. Results for 24 hour urinary sodium and potassium excretion. Intersalt Cooperative Research Group. *BMJ.* 1988 Jul 30;297(6644):319-28

[106] Elliott et al. Intersalt revisited: further analyses of 24 hour sodium excretion and blood pressure within and across populations. *BMJ.* 1996 May 18;312(7041):1249-53

[107] Leiba et al. Does dietary recall adequately assess sodium, potassium, and calcium intake in hypertensive patients? *Nutrition.* 2005 Apr;21(4):462-6

[108] McCullough ML, Swain JF, Malarick C, Moore TJ. Feasibility of outpatient electrolyte balance studies. *J Am Coll Nutr.* 1991 Apr;10(2):140-8

on a higher Na diet (200 - 250 mEq/d); the differences seen here in 24-hr Na excretion of approximately 9 mEq in low-Na groups compared to approximately 190 mEq in high-Na groups is plain to see, even for the mathematically impaired and those stalwart skeptics who continue to resist appreciating the ability of dietary modification to have measurable and meaningful effects. The urinary sodium:creatinine (uNa/uCr) ratio can be assessed; for example, in the study by Kwok et al[109] among 111 ambulatory vegetarians, hypertensives had uNa/uCr ratio of 32.6 compared with a ratio of 12.4 among normotensives. In this same study, the urinary sodium:potassium (uNa/uK) ratio was 4.7 for hypertensives and 3.4 for normotensives; blood pressure also correlated with calcium intake, and the review by Ruilope et al[110] showed that calcium increases renal excretion of sodium (in a prostaglandin-dependent mechanism). With this latter data in mind, a clinician might speculate that part of vitamin D3's HTN-ameliorating effect may be derived *in part* from its ability to increase intestinal absorption of calcium and thereby promote renal loss of sodium.

- <u>Fasting serum insulin</u>: A direct relationship exists between elevated serum insulin, peripheral insulin resistance, and cardiovascular mortality.[111,112] Insulin promotes renal retention of sodium which leads to water retention and the subsequent volume overload and systemic hypertension. Clinicians can consider testing fasting serum insulin in patients likely to have hyperinsulinemia and insulin resistance; this can be used to tailor treatment, monitor benefit and compliance, and as a teaching aid for patients requiring or requesting additional details and insight. One of the largest medical laboratories in the US uses a reference range of "0.0-24.9 µIU/mL" (micro-IU [international units] per milliliter) for insulin.[113] Elevated fasting insulin concentration is generally defined as > 100 pmol/L (16.6 mU/L); however, leaning toward 60 pmol/L (10 mU/L)—or more conservatively 90 pmol/L (15 mU/L)—as the upper acceptable limits would provide for more sensitive detection of insulin resistance *as a marker for metabolic dysfunction* in appropriate clinical settings.[114] Per Vølund[115], the correct conversion factor for human insulin is 1 mU/L = 6 pmol/L.

- <u>Hemoglobin A1c (Hgb-A1c)</u>: Hgb-A1c is also known as glycosylated hemoglobin, levels of which increase in direct proportion to average blood glucose levels. Thus, Hgb-A1c can be used on random blood samples to estimate blood glucose levels to establish or exclude a diagnosis of prediabetes or diabetes mellitus. Interpretation of Hgb-A1c levels is as follows:

A1c Percentage	Description
<5.7	<u>Normal</u>:
5.7 - 6.4	<u>Prediabetic</u>: Interestingly, the phrase "prediabetic" reflects the allopathic medical paradigm of the unidirectionality and unavoidability of diabetes. A more proper term could be "borderline diabetes" indicating that the patient is *not* diabetic but showing a tendency toward *insulin resistance* or *glucose intolerance*—note that either of the two latter phrases are better and more "actionable" than the pseudoprophetic phrase *prediabetic*. Unlike *"insulin resistance"*, the phrase *"glucose intolerance"* is actionable because the common-sense implication is that if a patient has a metabolic impairment to the efficient utilization and metabolism of glucose then this substance should be avoided. By popularizing the phrases insulin resistance and—even worse—*metabolic syndrome*, physicians and patients alike are distracted from the importance of reducing carbohydrate intake in the treatment of these conditions.
>6.5	<u>Diabetes mellitus</u>: Diabetes mellitus and insulin resistance are reviewed elsewhere.

---

[109] Kwok TC, Chan TY, Woo J. Relationship of urinary sodium/potassium excretion and calcium intake to blood pressure and prevalence of hypertension among older Chinese vegetarians. *Eur J Clin Nutr*. 2003 Feb;57(2):299-304

[110] "...calcium influences renal function and enhances renal sodium excretion. The intrarenal effects of low doses of calcium are dependent on the renal production of prostaglandins." Ruilope LM, Lahera V, Araque A, Suarez C, Rodicio JL, Romero JC. Electrolyte excretion and sodium intake. *Am J Med Sci*. 1994;307 Suppl 1:S107-11

[111] "The magnitude and direction of the relationship between insulin concentration and incident CVD were similar. CONCLUSIONS: We found a significant association between HOMA-IR and risk of CVD after adjustment for multiple covariates." Hanley AJ, Williams K, Stern MP, Haffner SM. Homeostasis model assessment of insulin resistance in relation to the incidence of cardiovascular disease: the San Antonio Heart Study. *Diabetes Care*. 2002 Jul;25(7):1177-84

[112] "Hyperinsulinemia was associated with increased all-cause and cardiovascular mortality in Helsinki policemen independent of other risk factors,..." Pyörälä et al. Plasma insulin and all-cause, cardiovascular, and noncardiovascular mortality: the 22-year follow-up results of the Helsinki Policemen Study. *Diabetes Care*. 2000;23(8):1097-102

[113] Insulin. Test Number: 004333 CPT Code: 83525. https://labcorp.com Accessed November 24, 2010

[114] Personal communications, November 2010. I am grateful to Bill Beakey of Professional Laboratory Co-Op, James Bogash DC, Kara Fitzgerald ND, Dan Lukaczer, and Todd Lepine MD for their conversations with me about serum insulin.

[115] Vølund A. Conversion of insulin units to SI units. *Am J Clin Nutr*. 1993 Nov;58(5):714-5

- Tests for lead accumulation: In the United States, a consistent correlation has been found between body burden of lead and HTN, even when blood lead levels are well below the current US occupational exposure limit guidelines (40 microg/dl).[116] Harlan et al[117] analyzed data from the second National Health and Nutrition Examination Survey (1976-1980) and thereby found a direct relationship between blood lead levels and systolic and diastolic pressures for men and women and for white and black persons aged 12 to 74 years; they concluded, "Blood lead levels were significantly higher in younger men and women (aged 21 to 55 years) with high blood pressure, but not in older men or women (aged 56 to 74 years). In multiple regression analyses, the relationship of blood lead to blood pressure was independent of other variables for men, but not for women. Dietary calcium and serum zinc levels were inversely related to blood pressure." Schwartz and Stewart[118] contrasted blood lead, dimercaptosuccinic acid (DMSA)-chelatable lead, and tibial lead to find that blood lead was the assessment that most strongly correlated with HTN; they concluded, "**Systolic blood pressure was elevated by blood lead levels as low as 5 microg/dl.**" Thus, clinicians might first measure blood lead levels, which do not measure total body burden but rather the lead that is mobile or *in transit* within the body and which appears to have the best correlation with HTN; the finding of normal blood lead results could then be followed with the more sensitive DMSA-provoked heavy metal testing before concluding that heavy metals are noncontributory to that particular patient's HTN. For heavy metal testing in various clinical scenarios, this author's preference is to use DMSA-provoked measurement of urine toxic metals. After a minimal test dose of DMSA (e.g., in the range of 50-100 mg) to screen for hypersensitivity, patients take oral DMSA 10 mg/kg as a single oral dose in the morning on an empty stomach after emptying the bladder and send a sample from the next urination for laboratory analysis; follow laboratory protocol if different from these instructions. Use of DMSA for lead and mercury chelation/detoxification and for diagnostic purposes is generally safe and effective[119,120,121,122,123]; see Chapter 4 of *Functional Inflammology* / *Inflammation Mastery* (2014 and later).
- Plasma aldosterone-to-renin ratio: As the screening blood test for primary hyperaldosteronism, this test is indicated in any hypertensive patient with unexplained hypokalemia. When the plasma aldosterone measured in ng per dL is > 20 times the level of plasma renin activity in ng *per* mL *per* hour, hyperaldosteronism is suspected, confirmatory testing can be performed by an endocrinologist using an available salt-suppression test.[124]
- Plasma and urine levels of epinephrine and norepinephrine: Plasma and urine levels of epinephrine and norepinephrine can be measured while the patient is on a stable low-sodium diet. In a review and exemplary case report summarized in a following section, Morimoto *et al*[125] describe the use of plasma and urine epinephrine and norepinephrine as markers of sympathetic nervous system activity in a patient treated with neurovascular decompression (detailed later in this chapter); their strategy employed a sodium intake of 120 mmol/d with fasting blood samples taken via indwelling catheter at 7:30am after the patient had rested for 30 minutes in the supine position. Over the course of four months following surgical neurovascular decompression of the left ventrolateral medulla oblongata, Morimoto *et al* report the following postsurgical changes:
  - Plasma epinephrine: Reduced from 0.22 to <0.05 (reference range <0.93 nmol/L).
  - Plasma norepinephrine: Reduced from 0.95 to 0.30 (range 0.89 - 3.37 nmol/L).
  - Urine epinephrine: Reduced from 83.5 to 26.2 (range 5.5 – 76.4 nmol/d).
  - Urine norepinephrine: Reduced from 0.52 to 0.39 (range 0.06 – 0.024 mmol/d).

The importance of their case report is, among other considerations, that it shows that a post-intervention reduction in sympathetic nerve activity can be documented objectively, and that antihypertensive benefits can

[116] Nash et al. Blood lead, blood pressure, and hypertension in perimenopausal and postmenopausal women. *JAMA.* 2003 Mar 26;289(12):1523-32 jama.ama-assn.org
[117] Harlan et al. Blood lead and blood pressure. Relationship in the adolescent and adult US population. *JAMA.* 1985 Jan 25;253(4):530-4
[118] "Systolic blood pressure was elevated by blood lead levels as low as 5 microg/dl." Schwartz BS, Stewart WF. Different associations of blood lead, meso 2,3-dimercaptosuccinic acid (DMSA)-chelatable lead, and tibial lead in 543 former organolead manufacturing workers. *Arch Environ Health.* 2000 Mar-Apr;55(2):85-92
[119] Bradstreet J, Geier DA, Kartzinel JJ, Adams JB, Geier MR. A case-control study of mercury burden in children with autistic spectrum disorders. *Journal of American Physicians and Surgeons* 2003; 8: 76-79 jpands.org/vol8no3/geier.pdf
[120] Crinnion WJ. Environmental medicine, part three: long-term effects of chronic low-dose mercury exposure. *Altern Med Rev.* 2000 Jun;5(3):209-23
[121] Forman J, Moline J, Cernichiari E, Sayegh S, Torres JC, Landrigan MM, Hudson J, Adel HN, Landrigan PJ. A cluster of pediatric metallic mercury exposure cases treated with meso-2,3-dimercaptosuccinic acid (DMSA). *Environ Health Perspect.* 2000 Jun;108(6):575-7 ehp.niehs.nih.gov/docs/2000/108p575-577forman/abstract.html
[122] Miller AL. Dimercaptosuccinic acid (DMSA), a non-toxic, water-soluble treatment for heavy metal toxicity. *Altern Med Rev.* 1998 Jun;3(3):199-207
[123] DMSA. *Altern Med Rev.* 2000 Jun;5(3):264-7
[124] Viera AJ, Neutze DM. Diagnosis of secondary hypertension: an age-based approach. *Am Fam Physician.* 2010 Dec 15;82(12):1471-8
[125] Morimoto S, Sasaki S, Takeda K, Furuya S, Naruse S, Matsumoto K, Higuchi T, Saito M, Nakagawa M. Decreases in blood pressure and sympathetic nerve activity by microvascular decompression of the rostral ventrolateral medulla in essential hypertension. *Stroke.* 1999 Aug;30(8):1707-10

be significant and associated with *relative* reductions in catecholamine levels that may be *within* or *outside of* the normal reference range. With the awareness that reference ranges for plasma and urine levels of epinephrine and norepinephrine were established exclusively for the detection of *overt pathology* (i.e., autonomic failure at the bottom of the range and pheochromocytoma at the top of the range) rather than for *functional disorders* such as neurogenic hypertension, clinicians may judiciously utilize measurements of plasma and urine epinephrine and norepinephrine to assess for hypersympathotonia and to monitor patient's response to treatment by documenting reductions in catecholamine production after intervention.

Applied physiology
Epinephrine levels reflect activity of the adrenal medulla, while norepinephrine levels are a more general indicator of overall sympathetic nervous system activity. Post-intervention reductions in epinephrine and norepinephrine indicate reduced sympathetic activity, generally an important benefit in patients with hypertensive and cardiovascular diseases.

- Other cardiovascular risk factors: Lipids (and an increasing number of lipid fractions), homocysteine, high-sensitivity C-reactive protein (hsCRP) can also be assessed to evaluate overall long-term cardiovascular risk.

Imaging:
- Electrocardiography (ECG, EKG): To assess for injury or pathophysiologic adaptation, ECG is appropriate for patients with HTN[126] and those at high risk for or with evidence of CVD, MI, PVD, CHF, chest pain (CP, including angina), or shortness of breath (SOB).
- Upper cervical radiographs: Clinicians highly skilled in manual manipulative therapeutics might choose to radiograph the upper cervical spine as a means to determine the appropriateness and application of spinal manipulative therapy to effect "marked and sustained reductions in BP similar to the use of two-drug combination therapy."[127] Generally however, radiographs prior to spinal manipulative therapy are not advised unless indicated by specific clinical characteristics such as recent trauma, neurologic deficit, or increased possibility for congenital anomaly (e.g., Sprengel's deformity), atlantoaxial instability (e.g., Down syndrome, rheumatoid arthritis, ankylosing spondylitis), or underlying disease (e.g., suspicion of malignant disease).
- Other imaging: CT, US, and angiographic techniques are commonly used to assess for HTN-related tumors, vascular anomalies/occlusion, and renal abnormalities. More specifically, US or IV contrast CT assessment for abdominal aortic aneurysm is indicated for hypertensive patients with any history of smoking aged >65yo and patients with documented CAD/CVD.[128]
- Biopsy/Procedure: Tissue biopsy is generally not required except when investigating a specific pathoetiologic consideration. Angioplasty and stent placement for the treatment of renal artery stenosis, and aldosterone measurement in the adrenal vein to lateralize the side of an aldosterone-secreting tumor are examples of procedures used in some cases of HTN. Renal biopsy specifies type and severity of intrinsic renal disease when history, labs, and imaging are inconclusive.

Establishing the Diagnosis of Hypertension in Adults: The diagnosis of adult hypertension is established after at least two measurements of blood pressure with either component greater than 140/90 mm Hg. Patients with systolic blood pressure 120-139 mm Hg or diastolic blood pressure 80-89 mm Hg are considered "prehypertensive"[129] and should be differentially diagnosed then treated with lifestyle and non-pharmacologic measures unless a *true primary cause* of the hypertension is discovered. Patients with diabetes mellitus, renal disease, or CVD should have their blood pressure controlled to ≤ 130/80 mm Hg. Patients with elevated systolic and normal diastolic pressures have **isolated systolic hypertension**, which in adults indicates an increased risk for stroke, heart failure, myocardial infarction, and overall mortality that can be ameliorated by effective intervention.[130] Given that mortality increases with chronic blood pressures greater than 115/75 mm Hg[131], progressive clinicians should appreciate 115/75 mm

[126] Bent S, Gensler LS, Frances C. *Saint-Frances Guide: Clinical Clerkship in Outpatient Medicine. 2ⁿᵈ Edition*. Philadelphia; Wolters Kluwer: 2008, 90
[127] Bakris et al. Atlas vertebra realignment and achievement of arterial pressure goal in hypertensive patients: a pilot study. *J Hum Hypertens*. 2007 May;21(5):347-52
[128] "In-hospital screening of AAA is very efficient among patients with coronary artery disease. Therefore, patients with CAD may be considered for routine AAA screening." Monney et al. High prevalence of unsuspected abdominal aortic aneurysms in patients hospitalised for surgical coronary revascularisation. *Eur J Cardiothorac Surg* 2004 Jan:65-8
[129] Bent S, Gensler LS, Frances C. *Saint-Frances Guide: Clinical Clerkship in Outpatient Medicine. 2ⁿᵈ Edition*. Philadelphia; Wolters Kluwer: 2008, 87
[130] Chobanian AV. Control of hypertension—an important national priority. *N Engl J Med*. 2001 Aug 16;345(7):534-5
[131] Benowitz NL. "Antihypertensive Agents." In Katzung BG (editor). *Basic and Clinical Pharmacology. 10ᵗʰ Edition*. New York: McGraw Hill Medical; 2007, 159

Hg as the upper end of the ideal range; from this perspective, the diagnostic threshold of 140/90 mm Hg for hypertension is appropriately seen as a great deviation from normal.

- <u>Hypertension in infants, children, and adolescents</u>: As previously mentioned, normal and abnormal values for blood pressure in infants and children are different from those of adults and are stratified based on age, gender, and height in a chart from the International Pediatric Hypertension Association. Please see their website at PediatricHypertension.org for downloadable charts and additional information helpful when dealing with childhood hypertension.

Blood pressure description and clinical considerations

BP in mm Hg	Description and clinical considerations
<u>115/75</u> or slightly lower	<u>Optimal blood pressure</u>: "Starting at 115/75 mm Hg, cardiovascular risk doubles with each increment of 20/10 mm Hg throughout the blood pressure range."[132]
<u>120/80</u> to <u>139/89</u>	<u>Prehypertension</u>: Elevated risk for adverse cardiovascular outcomes; begin assessment and assertive lifestyle and nutritional interventions.
≤ <u>130/80</u>	<u>Blood pressure goal for patients with diabetes mellitus, renal disease, or CVD</u>: Patients with multiple risk factors for adverse cardiovascular outcomes must have each variable treated to more assertively than if only one risk factor was present.
<u>140/90</u> to <u>159/99</u>	<u>Stage 1 hypertension</u>: Implement effective treatment and management strategies and reviewed here and elsewhere. Drug-treated patients are generally started with **one** medication, most commonly hydrochlorothiazide. See the concise pharmacotherapy review at the end of this chapter for more information on drug therapy.
<u>160/100</u> or greater	<u>Stage 2 hypertension</u>: Implement effective treatment and management strategies and reviewed here and elsewhere. Drug-treated patients are generally started with **two** medications, most commonly hydrochlorothiazide plus another medication prescribed based on the patient's comorbidities and tolerance. See the concise pharmacotherapy review at the end of this chapter for more information on drug therapy. The *acute onset* of blood pressures greater than 160/100 – 160/110 must be treated as a potentially life-threatening emergency, because *acute* onset hypertension by definition of its acute onset poses a higher risk of complications because physiologic adaptations have not had time to accommodate the higher pressures. In inpatient hospital settings, sBP > 160 is commonly used as a threshold for use of hydralazine, generally administered as 10 mg IV PRN each 1-2 hours.
<u>200/120</u> or greater *without* complications	<u>Hypertensive urgency</u>: Severe HTN *without* symptoms or evidence of end-organ damage. These patients are appropriately treated in the emergency department with *orally administered* medications—see details that follow.
<u>200/120</u> or greater *with* complications	<u>Hypertensive emergency</u>: Severe HTN with symptoms or evidence of end-organ damage such as headache, blurred vision, chest pain, shortness of breath, or renal insufficiency. Must be treated in an intensive/critical care setting with *intravenous* antihypertensive medications—see details that follow.

<u>Disease Complications</u>:
- The increased morbidity and mortality of HTN can manifest as any of the following:
  - Congestive heart failure presenting with fatigue, lower extremity edema, rales, dyspnea or orthopnea
  - Retinopathy and visual impairment
  - Hypertensive nephropathy presenting as azotemia, edema, recalcitrant HTN
  - Stroke—hemorrhagic or ischemic
  - Atrial fibrillation due to atrial enlargement
  - Myocardial infarction or sudden death due to accelerated CVD complicated by cardiac hypertrophy (i.e., supply-demand mismatch)
  - Abdominal aortic aneurysm, especially with HTN plus tobacco smoking

---

[132] Benowitz NL. "Antihypertensive Agents." In Katzung BG (editor). *Basic and Clinical Pharmacology. 10th Edition*. New York: McGraw Hill Medical; 2007, 159

Clinical Management: For routine outpatients, the obvious goal is to get the blood pressure down below 140/90 mm Hg as quickly, safely, and cost-effectively as possible while treating any primary underlying disorders; treatments that provide *collateral benefits* are preferred over those which cause *side effects*. Attention to naturopathic medicine's "hierarchy of therapeutics"[133] is important here in order to prioritize the implementation of therapeutic interventions. Correction of nutritional deficiencies (e.g., vitamin D, magnesium, potassium, calcium,

> **The physician's judgment remains paramount**
>
> "Positive experiences, trust in the clinician, and empathy improve patient motivation and satisfaction. This report serves as a guide, and the committee continues to recognize that the responsible physician's judgment remains paramount."
>
> Seventh Report of the Joint National Committee on Prevention, Detection, Evaluation and Treatment of High Blood Pressure [JNC 7]

phytonutrients), nutritional imbalances (e.g., insulin resistance and hyperglycemia, diet-induced metabolic acidosis), and hormonal imbalances (e.g., thyroid deficiency/excess, estrogen excess, aldosterone excess) should take precedence over the simple utilization of **antihypertensive drugs which suppress the manifestation of underlying dysfunction and thus allow it to perpetuate**; because of the latter, pharmacotherapy often abets rather than abates chronic disease. Following the exclusion of pathologic causes of HTN, the diagnosis of HTN should be explained to the patient as a sign of internal (e.g., nutritional, hormonal, metabolic, or structural) imbalance or otherwise as an opportunity to use this marker (blood pressure) as a barometer of overall health and compliance with a health-promoting lifestyle, including optimization of diet, exercise, relationships, and nutritional intake.

- Stratification of HTN management: Factors that direct the management of HTN include severity, manifestations of associated organ damage, and the patient's general condition and comorbidities.
    - Hypertensive emergency = >200/120 mm Hg *with evidence of end-organ damage* or *symptoms possibly attributable to the hypertension such as headache, blurred vision, chest pain, or shortness of breath*: Accompanying clinical manifestations may include renal failure, hematuria, proteinuria, altered mental status, papilledema, retinal vascular changes, MI, angina, stroke, aortic dissection, and pulmonary edema. Treat in intensive/critical care setting with *intravenous* antihypertensive medications such as nitroprusside, nitroglycerine, esmolol, hydralazine, labetolol, nicardipine then transition to oral beta-blockers and ACEi (angiotensin converting enzyme inhibitor) drugs. Add diuretics such as furosemide/Lasix as needed to alleviate volume overload, pulmonary edema, HTN, and heart failure. The initial drop in blood pressure should not exceed 25% in order to prevent precipitation of organ ischemia due to reflexive arteriospasm.
    - Hypertensive urgency = blood pressure >220/120 mm Hg[134] or >220/125 mm Hg[135] *without end-organ damage* and *without symptoms*: These patients are appropriately treated in the emergency department with *orally administered* medications such as nifedipine (oral, not sublingual), clonidine, and/or captopril. Patients can be discharged following normalization of blood pressure, but these patients require timely follow-up with a primary care provider. Complicating factors and concomitant disease may necessitate hospital admission.
    - Acute-onset HTN: Acute HTN in a previously normotensive patient can lead to stroke and other complications at pressures of 160 mm Hg systolic or 110 mm Hg diastolic. Acute-onset HTN can cause stroke at pressures generally tolerated in chronic cases because in the latter vascular adaptations accommodate higher pressures. **Acute-onset HTN** *from any cause* **should be treated emergently/urgently when pressures approximate or exceed 160-180 mm Hg systolic or 110 mm Hg diastolic**, especially but not exclusively if accompanied by complications such as angina, shortness of breath, vision changes, papilledema, headache/confusion/seizures (which suggest cerebral edema or cerebral vasospasm), proteinuria, or edema of the face, peripheral extremities, or of the general body (anasarca, check for sacral edema and weight gain).
    - Malignant HTN: Severe, intractable, and generally progressive HTN characterized by diastolic HTN > 130 mm Hg with clinical complications including renal failure, encephalopathy, or papilledema. Treat in hospital setting with intravenous antihypertensive medications (reviewed above for hypertensive emergency).

---

[133] The "hierarchy of therapeutics" is a guiding principle of naturopathic medicine providing a conceptual framework for prioritization and sequencing of therapeutic interventions, reviewed in the section on "Naturopathic Medicine" in Chapter 1 and—in concepts and applications—throughout Chapter 2.
[134] Bent S, Gensler LS, Frances C. *Saint-Frances Guide: Clinical Clerkship in Outpatient Medicine. 2nd Edition*. Philadelphia; Wolters Kluwer: 2008, 89
[135] McPhee SJ, Papadakis MA (editors). *Current Medical Diagnosis and Treatment. 2009. 48th Edition*. New York; McGraw Hill Medical: 401

- Routine recommendations that should be communicated then documented in the patient's chart: These include ❶ encouragement of smoking cessation, ❷ a minimum of 30 minutes of exercise per day (for patients healthy enough to exercise), ❸ weight loss/optimization, ❹ limit alcohol intake to no more than 1-2 drinks per day, ❺ restrict sodium to ≤ 2,400 mg/d (i.e., ≤ 6 grams/d of sodium chloride), ❻ increase intake of fruits and vegetables, and ❼ reduce intake of total and saturated fat in order to promote weight loss and optimize serum lipids.[136] In the allopathic model, these lifestyle recommendations are used for three months before initiating drug treatment of HTN.

- Drug management and comanagement of HTN may be required. Drug management is appropriate in urgent situations, recalcitrant cases, patients with initial BP > 160/100 mm Hg, and for patients who are noncompliant with treatment. Patients and clinicians can facilitate progression through the "stages of change"[137] by appreciating the barriers and requirements that characterize the overcoming of each stage until the final stage of termination/integration is achieved. In common medical practice, lifestyle interventions, the processes of change, nutritional supplementation, and spinal manipulation are almost never given their full due consideration; thus, by default, drug treatment of hypertension is the allopathic standard of care because it is the only treatment given priority. Failure to discuss nondrug treatments with hypertensive patients is unethical because many nondrug treatments are superior in safety, affordability, and effectiveness when compared with drug treatments; failure to discuss nondrug treatments is also a violation of medical ethics' principles of beneficence, autonomy and informed consent.

> **Clinical insight**
> Patients with lifestyle-generated diseases should be coached in the reversal of the patterns that have caused their disease rather than being enabled to pursue their disease-promoting lifestyles while surrogate markers of metabolic-physiologic dysfunction (e.g., hypertension) are pharmacologically suppressed.

- Tailor treatment recommendations and goals to the patient's specific psychographics and BVG-LOC profile. More than 90-95% of HTN patients will be found to have no pathologic/medical cause of their HTN, thus implicating diet and lifestyle as the most responsible factors. In some situations, the resolution of the patient's HTN comes expeditiously through the simple and imperfect implementation of weight loss, diet modification, correction of nutritional deficiencies, and avoidance or reduced intake of infamous triggers such as tobacco, alcohol, and excess caffeine. **For many patients with HTN— especially when the HTN is part of a larger cluster of clinical findings such as type-2 diabetes mellitus or the metabolic syndrome—the successful management of their HTN will rely on the implementation of numerous changes in various aspects of "lifestyle" including diet, preparation/procurement of food, social interactions, core relationships, exercise involvement, time and money allocation, and—most importantly— changes in self-image, and the establishment and "affirmation-through-action" of core values.** These issues can appear complex to the point of being "too complicated" for doctors and patients who are not personally accustomed to living consciously and for whom dispensing and consuming pills, respectively, are easier than the consciousness-raising and the self-disciplined and self-directed living required to advocate and manifest a health-centered life. Complexity and convenience should not be the determinants of care. Patients with lifestyle-generated diseases should be coached in the reversal of the patterns that have caused their disease rather than being enabled to pursue these disease-promoting lifestyles while surrogate markers of metabolic-physiologic dysfunction are pharmacologically suppressed. Therapeutic lifestyle changes must be merged with the patient's **beliefs** (important but changeable paradigms), **values** (subjective-objective rules), and **goals** (conscious and subconscious aspirations and trajectory). In order to facilitate this merger, the clinician must— first—understand the patient's position on these variables, then—second—deliver the treatment plan in such a way as to "speak to" the patient's beliefs, values, and goals. Most people do not have consciously-chosen and declarable beliefs, values, and goals for their lives; thus, this process of the physician's gaining an understanding of the patient's unconscious psychographic details is generally not completed on the first visit and may not be completed until the patient has done the requisite "homework" (perhaps facilitated by a professional therapist or lay counselor/coach) and has thereafter returned with a perceptible level of self-awareness. Clinicians who **seek first to understand, then to be understood**[138] will have advantages over clinicians who steamroll patients with lifestyle impositions and a "to do" list that is foreign to the patient's

---

136 Bent S, Gensler LS, Frances C. *Saint-Frances Guide: Clinical Clerkship in Outpatient Medicine. 2nd Edition*. Philadelphia; Wolters Kluwer: 2008, 90
137 Prochaska, JO, Norcross, JC, and DiClemente, CC. *Changing for Good*. NY, William Morrow and Company; 1994
138 Covey SR. *The Seven Habits of Highly Effective People* (1989); see also *The 8th Habit: From Effectiveness to Greatness* (2004).

inner and previous experiences. With regard to psychographic information, clinicians are wise to remember the three tenets of evidence-based medicine, one of which rests upon this psychographic information: ❶ published research, ❷ the clinician's experience and expertise, and ❸ the patient's preferences and goals.

Psychographic profiling: Understanding patients to help them connect personal goals with health goals

- <u>Beliefs</u>: What are the fundamental beliefs and expectations that the patient has for his/her future? Is life merely "suffering and toil" or is it meant to be "a well of delight"? Patients who expect misery are generally successful in its attainment unless they are guided and provoked toward a more positive life expectancy. The clinician can correct errors in thought and information.

- <u>Values</u>: What does the patient value? "*Autonomy and independence*"—will this manifest as resistance to the clinician's advice or as a willingness to comply with treatment so as to avoid future disability? "*Strength*"—will this be resistance to the plan or disciplined adherence to the plan? "*Love*"—is this self-sacrificing 'love' for other people or is it a wholesome and healthy love that includes the self? "*My family*"—does this include avoiding disability, being alive to support and encourage family members and upcoming generations? "*Nothing really*"—what are the mental barriers and painful experiences that have resulted in this emotional numbness; what would his/her life be like if he/she were to engage in life consciously and with purpose? The clinician assigns homework for the patient to clarify—and later manifest in action—a list of personal values. Patients need to understand how their *personal* goals are connected to their *health* status and goals.

- <u>Goals</u>: What are the patient's social, physical, professional, personal, and spiritual goals? Is the current lifestyle and health/disease trajectory consistent with the attainment and extended enjoyment of these goals? Are the goals too limited, and has the patient accommodated small goals with small effort and the resulting lackluster results that reinforce self-depreciation and low self-esteem, thus perpetuating a vicious cycle? Goals are a reflection of core values and one's intimate belief about what is possible and what levels of success, love, and happiness are appropriate for one's life.

- <u>Locus of Control</u>: Does the patient view the world as chaotic and menacing (external locus of control), or as understandable and thus worthy of meaningful engagement (internal locus of control)? If the patient views him/herself as a victim, then compliance will be low because every and any excuse will serve as a rationalization for why he/she "couldn't" exercise, eat right, and take medications or nutrients as prescribed. Patients who experience their health problems as incomprehensible and "idiopathic" are less likely to engage in purposeful health activities and are more likely to be noncompliant with treatment(s) and more passive in their willingness to rely on "doctor's orders" and drug treatments. Physicians should encourage the best self-image in and self-efficacy from patients by reminding them by either Socratic-dialectic education or direct verbalization that the patient has the power and thus the "response-ability" to strongly influence his/her health outcomes via positive health expectations and behaviors.

- <u>Patients must receive instruction on at-home blood pressure monitoring and/or follow-up in-office assessments</u>: At the time of diagnosis, patients are instructed of the importance of proper treatment and follow-up visits (ranging from weekly to biweekly to monthly) to facilitate compliance and monitor treatment effectiveness. HTN must never be taken lightly by the clinician or the patient as it represents and indicates a significant departure from optimal health and the failure of internal homeostatic mechanisms; more concretely, HTN is generally a silent and progressive disorder which prematurely undercuts health and vitality and which tends to culminate in unnecessary morbidity (e.g., pain, suffering, loss of function, renal dialysis, and stroke) and early death. Patients can use office-calibrated home blood pressure monitoring equipment to self-monitor compliance, lifestyle effects, and effectiveness of treatment; patients are advised that at-home monitoring does not substitute for in-office visits and that in-office blood pressure measurements are the standard by which treatment decisions are made. "White coat hypertension" (WCH) is explained as an exaggerated stress response to innocuous stimuli that has parallels in other areas of the patient's life and is therefore not an excuse for normal at-home readings; accordingly, studies have shown that patients with WCH show increased risk for cardiovascular complications.[139,140] Depending on HTN severity and the protocol being followed, patients might be seen in the office for a quick follow-up assessment once every 2-7 days, or less frequently if BP checks are occurring reliably at home. Patients with metabolic syndrome, obesity, or who are likely to be noncompliant are followed-up more frequently than medically indicated in order to promote compliance and patient-physician alliance. Generally, after the normalization of blood pressure with treatment, patients are reevaluated every 3-6 months in the office. Laboratory tests are performed at least annually and can be performed on an as needed basis with any evidence or suspicion of problems such as nephropathy, dyslipidemia, DM, or drug side effects.

---

[139] "Coronary disease may be more severe among patients with WCH than among those without." Kostandonis et al. Topography and severity of coronary artery disease in white-coat hypertension. *Eur J Intern Med.* 2008 Jun;19(4):280-4

[140] "Our findings also further stress the interest of assessing the presence of a white-coat effect as a means to further identify patients at increased cardiovascular risk and guide treatment accordingly." Bochud et al. Association between White-Coat Effect and Blunted Dipping of Nocturnal Blood Pressure. *Am J Hypertens.* 2009 Oct;22(10):1054-61

- Patients already taking antihypertensive medications are likely to require a dosage adjustment or medication discontinuation after using diet, lifestyle, and nutritional interventions. Clinicians should anticipate this benefit and inform the patient and prescribing doctor appropriately. Failure to anticipate the normalization of blood pressure and to adjust medications appropriately may result in hypotension, most commonly manifested by fatigue and/or (pre)syncope.
- Document everything: Document all relevant clinical findings, laboratory/imaging results, treatments with rationale, patient education, plan of scheduled follow-up, and referal/comanagment. Ensure that chart notes document education, consent to treatment, and that "patient verbalizes understanding; all questions are answered and concerns addressed."

Clinical management of HTN

1. Assessment for urgency and end-organ damage
2. Differential diagnosis and comprehensive assessment
3. Effective treatment or appropriate referral
4. Patient education—legitimate, effective education, not simply drug indoctrination buttressed by ineffective diet and lifestyle advice
5. Scheduled follow-up
6. Monitor for compliance, treatment effectiveness, adverse effects, and new complications; clinicians have the responsibility to implement effective treatment or refer for effective treatment. Non-treatment is not an appropriate option. Nonresponsive and noncompliant patients need in-office and/or written information regarding risk; referrals need to include written letter to the other physician plus scheduling of the patient's appointment, with the patient clearly informed of the date, time, and location of the appointment.
7. Document all of the above in the patient chart, signed and dated.

Treatment Considerations for "Primary" Hypertension—An Evidence-based Article-by-Article Review with Commentary: Reviewed here are the most successful and/or most common treatments for HTN; these treatments can generally be categorized as **dietary** (i.e., foods consumed), **nutritional** (i.e., foods consumed plus the use of nutritional supplements), **hormonal** (e.g., correction of hypothyroidism, hyperaldosteronism, hyperparathyroidism), **surgical** (reviewed here: microvascular decompression of the left ventrolateral medulla oblongata), **manipulative** (reviewed here: spinal and paraspinal soft tissue manipulation), and **lifestyle intervention**, with the latter being a large general category that includes but is not limited to exercise, weight optimization (generally weight *loss* for the treatment of HTN), Qigong, controlled breathing, meditation, and acupuncture. Readers will be better able to appreciate the clinical significance of the blood pressure reductions achieved if they are aware that ❶ most blood-pressure-lowering drugs used chronically on an outpatient basis achieve reductions in the magnitude of approximately 12/6 mm Hg while reductions of 20/10 mm Hg generally require combination (i.e., at least two drugs) therapy[141], ❷ the vast majority (more than 70%) of medically-treated HTN patients take at least two blood-pressure-lowering drugs to achieve or approach their BP goal, and ❸ the criteria to establish efficacy of an antihypertensive effect as defined by the US Food and Drug Administration for approval of a new antihypertensive drug requires proof of both efficacy and safety in a blinded-design study; proof of efficacy is defined as a placebo-subtracted reduction in diastolic BP of 4-5 mm Hg or more, and "…most single agent antihypertensive [drugs] yield an 8 mm Hg drop in pressure in people with Stage 1 hypertension…"[142] Upon close reading of the following sections, readers will note that most of the nonpharmacologic therapeutics reviewed can achieve reductions greater than 5 mm Hg in BP.

FOOD & NUTRITION The first component of "DrV's functional inflammology protocol" recalled by the FINDSEX® acronym is the (re)establishment of nutritional sufficiency and nutrition-related biochemical balance via implementation of a healthy foundational diet and basic nutritional supplementation. Paleolithic diets—defined as those which emphasize fruits, vegetables, nuts, seeds, berries and sufficient intake of lean protein—are the most nutrient-dense, satiating, and neuro-enhancing diets available; the diet can be customized to meet the needs of all patients. Atop this foundational diet, supplementation of vitamins, minerals, fatty acids—specifically ALA, GLA,

---

[141] Magill MK, Gunning K, Saffel-Shrier S, Gay C. New developments in the management of hypertension. *Am Fam Physician*. 2003 Sep 1;68(5):853-8

[142] "The criteria used in this study to establish efficacy of an antihypertensive effect are those defined by the Food and Drug Administration for approval of a new antihypertensive drug. Specifically, it would require a blinded design with a placebo-subtracted reduction in diastolic BP of 5 mm Hg or more and be free of serious side effects to be approvable." Bakris et al. Atlas vertebra realignment and achievement of arterial pressure goal in hypertensive patients: a pilot study. *J Hum Hypertens*. 2007 May;21(5):347-52. See also information from the US FDA website (fda.gov/RegulatoryInformation/Guidances/ucm129461.htm, accessed June 12, 2010) which states, "…because the effect of active drugs is often small (diastolic blood pressure change of 4-5 mm Hg more than placebo), studies conducted in a blinded fashion and with placebo controls are essential."

EPA, DHA, and oleic acid, and probiotics provides the optimal base from which metabolic/physiologic balance and function can be restored/maintained, and from which balance and function can be further optimized by the skilled addition of other components of the protocol.

- **The supplemented Paleo-Mediterranean Diet**: The health-promoting diet of choice for the majority of people is a diet based on abundant consumption of fruits, vegetables, seeds, nuts, omega-3 and monounsaturated fatty acids, and lean sources of protein such as lean meats, fatty cold-water fish, soy and whey proteins. This diet prohibits and obviates overconsumption of chemical preservatives, artificial sweeteners, and carbohydrate-dominant foods such as candies, pastries, breads, potatoes, grains, and other foods with a high glycemic load and high glycemic index. This "Paleo-Mediterranean Diet"—first detailed by Vasquez[143] in 2005—is a combination of the "Paleolithic" or "Paleo diet" and the well-known "Mediterranean diet", both of which are well described in peer-reviewed journals and the lay press. The Paleo-Mediterranean Diet is wholly consistent with the "polymeal"—a multicomponent cardioprotective diet plan characterized by emphasis on phytonutrient-rich foods including fish, red wine, garlic, almonds, dark chocolate, and most (low-carbohydrate) fruits and vegetables—which is estimated to have the potential to lower the incidence of CVD by 76%.[144]

  In the subsections that follow, various studies related to dietary intervention for hypertension will be summarized; these dietary patterns can be viewed in a continuum ranging from the ❶ SAD diet to ❷ the DASH diet to ❸ the Paleo-Mediterranean diet. Also included is the fourth most common dietary pattern, that of ❹ the vegetarian diet and its related variants of veganism, pescovegetarianism, and lacto-ovo-vegetarianism.

> **Cardiovascular and metabolic benefits of the Paleolithic hunter-gatherer diet pattern**
> ☑ **Significant reductions in blood pressure**,
> ☑ Improved arterial distensibility,
> ☑ **Significant reduction in plasma insulin**,
> ☑ Large significant reductions in total cholesterol, low-density lipoproteins (LDL) and triglycerides,
> ☑ Consistently improved status of circulatory, carbohydrate and lipid metabolism/physiology.
>
> "Conclusions: Even **short-term consumption of a Paleolithic type diet improves BP and glucose tolerance, decreases insulin secretion, increases insulin sensitivity and improves lipid profiles without weight loss in healthy sedentary humans.**"
>
> Frassetto et al. Metabolic and physiologic improvements from consuming a Paleolithic, hunter-gatherer type diet. *Eur J Clin Nutr.* 2009 Feb

Combining the Paleo-Mediterranean diet with multivitamin/multimineral supplementation (including physiologic doses of vitamin D3 to optimize serum levels), with balanced combination fatty acid (ALA, GLA, EPA, DHA) supplementation and probiotics forms the "supplemented Paleo-Mediterranean diet" (sPMD)[145], the five basic components of which are outlined below:

1. Paleo-Mediterranean Diet: The most nutrient-dense diet available; more amenable to social integration and greater nutrient content compared to vegetarianism; provides sufficient protein to promote satiety and therefore reduced caloric intake. The importance of carbohydrate restriction is commonly underappreciated, and it provides an anti-hypertensive benefit regardless of weight change/loss; carbohydrate restriction provides numerous eumetabolic benefits such as promoting depletion of ceramide and promoting mitochondrial autophagy/biogenesis—ie, mitochondrial recycling. Importantly and very easy to understand mechanistically, low-carbohydrate diets lower blood glucose and thereby lower insulin levels; because (elevated) insulin serves to promote sodium and water retention, reducing insulin (in this case by reducing the carbohydrate load) reduces hypertension by reducing sodium and water retention, thereby functioning in a *poly*beneficial manner, one that is partly analogous to diuretic therapy.

2. Multivitamin and multimineral supplementation: Routine vitamin and mineral supplementation is warranted because dietary intake (based on SAD) is generally insufficient to provide sufficient vitamins and minerals[146]; supranutritional doses of vitamins and minerals stimulates variant/defective enzymes with decreased coenzyme binding affinity (increased K[m]).[147]

---

[143] Vasquez A. A Five-Part Nutritional Protocol that Produces Consistently Positive Results. *Nutritional Wellness* 2005 Sept. Vasquez A. Importance of Integrative Chiropractic Health Care in Treating Musculoskeletal Pain and Reducing the Nationwide Burden of Medical Expenses and Iatrogenic Injury and Death. *Original Internist* 2005; 12(4): 159-182

[144] Franco OH, Bonneux L, de Laet C, Peeters A, Steyerberg EW, Mackenbach JP. The Polymeal: a more natural, safer, and probably tastier (than the Polypill) strategy to reduce cardiovascular disease by more than 75%. *BMJ.* 2004 Dec 18;329(7480):1447-50

[145] Vasquez A. The Importance of Integrative Chiropractic Health Care in Treating Musculoskeletal Pain and Reducing the Nationwide Burden of Medical Expenses and Iatrogenic Injury and Death. *Original Internist* 2005; 12(4): 159-182

[146] Fletcher RH, Fairfield KM. Vitamins for chronic disease prevention in adults: clinical applications. *JAMA.* 2002 Jun 19;287(23):3127-9

[147] Ames BN, Elson-Schwab I, Silver EA. High-dose vitamin therapy stimulates variant enzymes with decreased coenzyme binding affinity (increased K(m)): relevance to genetic disease and polymorphisms. *Am J Clin Nutr.* 2002 Apr;75(4):616-58

3. <u>Vitamin D3 in physiologic doses to optimize serum 25-OH-D levels</u>: Vitamin D3 deficiency and insufficiency are common in the general population and are causatively and/or epidemiologically associated with HTN, CVD, CHF, type-1 and type-2 diabetes mellitus, mental depression and schizophrenia, systemic inflammation, and various cancers and autoimmune disorders. The physiologic requirement for vitamin D3 is approximately 4,000 IU per day for adult men. Dosages should be sufficient to effect serum 25-OH-D levels within the optimal range of 50-100 ng/ml.

4. <u>Balanced combination fatty acid supplementation with ALA, GLA, EPA, DHA, with dietary oleic acid</u>: Patients consuming the SAD may be presumed to have numerous fatty acid imbalances (e.g., excess arachidonate and *trans*-fatty acids) along with insufficiencies of ALA, GLA, EPA, DHA, and oleic acid. Hunter-gather intake of omega-3 fatty acids is approximately 7 grams per day contrasted to 1 gram per day provided by Westernized/industrialized diets. Fatty acid imbalances/deficiencies commonly seen in patients consuming Westernized/industrialized/SAD diets—similar to and probably additive to if not synergistic with vitamin D deficiency/insufficiency—contributes to HTN, CVD, CHF, type-1 and type-2 diabetes mellitus, mental depression and schizophrenia, systemic inflammation, and various cancers and autoimmune disorders.

5. <u>Probiotics</u>: Probiotics are safe and effective anti-inflammatory, immunoenhancing, and immunomodulating agents[148,149] and are—based on published research and clinical experience—suitable for routine use, ideally as a rotating combination of yogurts, kefir, other fermented foods, and—particularly for dairy-intolerant patients—supplements.

The Four Main Food-Consumption Patterns

Diet pattern	Characteristics
❶ SAD: Standard American Diet	<ul><li>Food choices in this diet are based on convenience, recent advertisements, coupons and cost, popular trends, social pressure, and instant gratification at the expense of the feeling of health or its authentic attainment.</li><li>This diet tends to be high in sucrose, fructose, sodium, chloride, and chemical colorants, preservatives, and artificial flavors. It is generally low in essential fatty acids, minerals, vitamins in their natural form, fiber and phytonutrients.</li><li>This diet is largely responsible for the modern epidemics of *overconsumption malnutrition* which causes obesity, hypertension, cardiovascular disease, and increased risk for various cancers and other chronic diseases.</li><li>Because the foods tend to be mass-produced, of low quality, and of durable shelf life due to lack of nutritional value, chemical preservatives, and packaging, the economics of these products is that of low cost for consumers and high profit for producers and sellers. Tertiary profitability is enjoyed by drug companies, so-called "health insurance" corporations, and hospital and clinic systems that have to implement the damage control and rescue remedies necessary to sustain life following long-term consumption of this diet.</li><li>If not for the SAD dietary pattern and the physical inactivity that generally accompanies it, hypertension would not exist as the epidemic that it currently is, and antihypertensive medications would be *orphan drugs*.</li><li>Because of the characteristic incorporation of "flavor enhancers" such as monosodium glutamate and carrageenan, and because of the high content of sodium and sugars, the *supranormal* stimulation provided to taste receptors downregulates the subtle perception of taste so that consumers become accustomed to (i.e., *addicted to*) the supranormal stimulation and are thereby disinclined to consume a normal natural diet due to its comparatively "bland" taste. **_Clinical pearl_**: Generally, 1-2 weeks are required following discontinuation of the SAD diet before gustatory sensitivity is restored so that foods in their natural state can be appreciated. Patients need to lean toward going "cold turkey" (pun intended) and thereby avoiding excess sugar, sodium, flavor-enhancers and other supranormal stimulation for 1-2 weeks so that they can thereafter consume and enjoy a *natural* whole foods diet.</li></ul>

148 Neish AS. Microbes in gastrointestinal health and disease. *Gastroenterology*. 2009 Jan;136(1):65-80
149 Galdeano et al. Proposed model: mechanisms of immunomodulation induced by probiotic bacteria. *Clin Vaccine Immunol*. 2007 May;14(5):485-92

The Four Main Food-Consumption Patterns—*continued*

Diet pattern	Characteristics
❷ DASH: Dietary Approaches to Stop Hypertension	<ul><li>*Better* food choices than the SAD diet, with emphasis placed on:</li><li>*Reduced* consumption of saturated fat, cholesterol, and total fat, red meat, sweets, added sugars, and sugar-containing beverages compared to the SAD.</li><li>*Increased* consumption of fruits, vegetables, and fat-free or low-fat milk and milk products, whole grain products, fish, poultry, and nuts.</li><li>Compared to the SAD, DASH provides more potassium, magnesium, calcium, protein, and fiber and less sodium and sugars such as sucrose and fructose.</li><li>In sum, the DASH diet a *better* diet pattern compared to the random and nonlogical convenience- and pleasure-based eating habits followed by most Americans and others seduced by the convenience, low cost, and supranormal stimulation of the SAD or "Westernized" diet. However, the inclusion of grains and excess carbohydrates makes it suboptimal, particularly when compared to diets based on vegetables, nuts, berries, seeds.</li></ul>
❸ Paleo-Mediterranean Diet	<ul><li>The Paleo-Mediterranean diet consists almost exclusively of unprocessed and as-fresh-as-possible and as-raw-as-possible fruits, vegetables, nuts, seeds, berries and lean sources of protein, especially fish, poultry, and lean grass-fed meats and game meats. A modern modification allows the inclusion of whey and soy protein isolates for their functional benefits beyond the mere provision of protein to include functionally active proteins, peptides, amino acid profiles, whey immunoglobulins and lactoferrin, and the soy phytonutrients genistein, daidzein, and beta-sitosterol. Dark chocolate, olive oil, and red wine are also accepted staples of this dietary pattern.</li><li>The Mediterranean diet as commonly described also includes "whole grains" such as wheat and starchy vegetables such as potatoes; these are best avoided. Knowledgeable clinicians will appreciate that the modern notion of "whole grains" is a farce because of mechanical processing which pulverizes the husk and bran of the grain into oblivion, rendering its natural-state physiochemical properties powerless.</li><li>In its highest form (i.e., excluding grains and other mechanically processed and overcooked food items), the Paleo-Mediterranean diet is the most nutrient-dense and physiologically appropriate diet for human beings with the greatest promise of health optimization and disease prevention.[150]</li></ul>
❹ Vegetarian diet, and related variants	<ul><li>Plant-based diets *should* consist of fruits, vegetables, nuts, seeds, berries consumed as raw and as fresh as possible; this might seem obvious except that many (pseudo)vegetarians rely on grains and processed foods and are thus only vegetarians to the extent that they avoid meat (perhaps "acarneists") and not to the extent that they rely on vegetables, as the term *vegeta*rianism implies. Consumption of legumes for their relatively higher protein content is common. Avoidance of grains due to their allergenicity and low phytonutrient and micronutrient content is advised.</li><li>The lack of sufficient vitamin B-12 along with the relatively higher content of anti-nutrients such as phytic acid makes a purely vegetarian diet of tenuous durability for the unskilled, unknowledgeable, and undisciplined consumer. Many people adopt a so-called vegetarian diet for sociopolitical reasons without becoming aware of its proper implementation; such persons can consume a protein-deficient diet consistent with "breaditarianism"[151]—which is basically equal to or worse than the SAD diet due to its lack of adequate protein and overreliance on simple carbohydrates</li><li><u>Vegan</u> = exclusive consumption of plant foods only.</li><li><u>Vegetarian</u> = reliance upon plant foods, with the occasional inclusion of diary, eggs, and fish.</li><li><u>Pescovegetarian</u> = consumption of plants and fish.</li><li><u>Lacto-ovo-vegetarian</u> = consumption of plants, milk, eggs (i.e., animal protein without the killing of animals).</li></ul>

[150] Cordain et al. Origins and evolution of the Western diet: health implications for the 21st century. *Am J Clin Nutr.* 2005 Feb;81(2):341-5 ajcn.org/cgi/content/full/81/2/341
[151] O'Keefe JH Jr, Cordain L.Cardiovascular disease resulting from a diet and lifestyle at odds with our Paleolithic genome. *Mayo Clin Proc* 2004;79:101-8

Most of the studies reviewed in the following section pertain to the Paleo-Mediterranean diet (PMD) and its optimized expression in the supplemented Paleo-Mediterranean diet (sPMD). Studies on the DASH diet generally showed benefit when contrasted to the SAD eating pattern which is the norm for most Americans and increasingly among other nationalities. In this text, the DASH diet is advocated only insofar as it is an improvement over the SAD eating pattern; it is secondary to the PMD and tertiary to the sPMD in its effectiveness for disease treatment and prevention.

- Small clinical trial: Metabolic and physiologic improvements from consuming a Paleolithic, hunter-gatherer type diet (*European Journal of Clinical Nutrition* 2009 Feb): Despite the small subject size (n = 9), this study demonstrates safety and beneficial effectiveness of the Paleolithic diet in addressing several of the perturbations that characterize the metabolic syndrome and lifestyle-induced predisposition to CVD. "Results: Compared with the baseline (usual) diet, we observed (a) **significant reductions in BP** associated with improved arterial distensibility; (b) **significant reduction in plasma insulin** vs time AUC [area under the curve], during the OGTT [oral glucose tolerance testing]; and (c) large significant reductions in total cholesterol, low-density lipoproteins (LDL) and triglycerides (-0.8, -0.7 and -0.3 mmol/l respectively). In all these measured variables, either **eight or all nine participants had identical directional responses when switched to Paleolithic type diet, that is, near consistently improved status of circulatory, carbohydrate and lipid metabolism/physiology.**"[152]

- Randomized 3-month cross-over pilot study: Beneficial effects of a Paleolithic diet on cardiovascular risk factors in type 2 diabetes (*Cardiovascular Diabetology* 2009 Jul): Although small (n=13), this study is impressive because it shows not only the benefits of the Paleolithic diet but also its superiority over the commonly recommended "diabetic diet" which is advocated by so-called conventional-standard-mainstream-government and medical groups that claim to advocate health and victory in the so-called war against obesity and diabetes mellitus. "Compared to the diabetes diet, the Paleolithic diet resulted in lower mean values of HbA1c (-0.4% units), triacylglycerol (-0.4 mmol/L), **diastolic blood pressure (-4 mmHg)**, weight (-3 kg), BMI (-1 kg/m2) and waist circumference (-4 cm), and higher mean values of high density lipoprotein cholesterol (+0.08 mmol/L)."[153]

- Randomized controlled trial: Effects of the DASH diet alone and in combination with exercise and weight loss on blood pressure and cardiovascular biomarkers in men and women with high blood pressure (*Archives of Internal Medicine* 2010 Jan): This publication reports results of a randomized controlled clinical trial among 144 overweight/obese hypertensive patients for 4 months; intervention was either DASH diet alone, DASH diet with a weight management program, or usual control diet.

Intervention	Results
DASH diet alone	☺ BP was reduced by -11.2/-7.5 mm Hg
DASH diet *with* aerobic exercise *and* caloric restriction	☺ BP was reduced by **-16.1/-9.9** mm Hg ☺ Greater improvement was noted in this group than with DASH alone for pulse wave velocity, baroreflex sensitivity, and left ventricular mass
Usual control (UC) diet	☺ Nonsignificant BP reduction of -3.4/-3.8 mm Hg

The authors reported the results and conclusion as follows: "Clinic-measured BP was reduced by 16.1/9.9 mm Hg (DASH plus weight management); 11.2/7.5 mm (DASH alone); and 3.4/3.8 mm (usual diet controls). … Greater improvement was noted for DASH plus weight management compared with DASH alone for pulse wave velocity, baroreflex sensitivity, and left ventricular mass. CONCLUSION: For overweight or obese persons with above-normal BP, the addition of exercise and weight loss to the DASH diet resulted in even larger BP reductions, greater improvements in vascular and autonomic function, and reduced left ventricular mass."[154]

[152] Frassetto et al. Metabolic and physiologic improvements from consuming a paleolithic, hunter-gatherer type diet. *Eur J Clin Nutr*. 2009 Feb 11.
[153] Jonsson et al. Beneficial effects of a Paleolithic diet on cardiovascular risk factors in type 2 diabetes: a randomized cross-over pilot study. *Cardiovasc Diabetol*. 2009;8:35.
[154] Blumenthal JA, Babyak MA, Hinderliter A, et al. Effects of the DASH diet alone and in combination with exercise and weight loss on blood pressure and cardiovascular biomarkers in men and women with high blood pressure: the ENCORE study. *Arch Intern Med*. 2010 Jan 25;170(2):126-35

- Randomized controlled trial with n=144: Effects of the Dietary Approaches to Stop Hypertension (DASH) diet alone and in combination with exercise and caloric restriction on insulin sensitivity and lipids (*Hypertension* 2010 May[155]): In this study lead by Blumenthal published in 2010, the authors examined the effects of the DASH diet on insulin sensitivity and lipids in a randomized controlled trial with 144 overweight (BMI: 25 to 40) men (n=47) and women (n=97) with BP up to 159/99 mm Hg. Study subjects were randomly assigned for 4 months to one of three groups with the following results (table below), respectively. Of important note is the worsening of glucose control and insulin sensitivity on the DASH diet; this suggests that the DASH diet may ultimately promote development of metabolic syndrome despite appearing to be cardioprotective based on short-term reductions in blood pressure. Note that the weight loss induced by *caloric restriction + exercise* of 19 lbs over 4 months equates to 4.75 lbs per month; this is consistent with what clinicians should expect in clinical practice, namely patients' weight loss of 4-8 lbs per month with dietary optimization plus increased physical activity.

Intervention	Results
DASH diet alone	☺ Weight loss: Imperceptible, only -0.3 kg ☺ Exercise capacity: No improvement ☹ Glucose control: Slight worsening of glucose levels after the oral glucose load; fasting serum insulin actually increased from 16.6 to 17.6 mcu/ml ☹ Lipids: No change; slight worsening of triglycerides ☺ Blood pressure: Clinically significant reductions in blood pressure
DASH diet *with* aerobic exercise *and* caloric restriction	☺ Weight loss: Clinically and statistically significant at -8.7 kg (-19.2 lbs) ☺ Exercise capacity: Significant increase in aerobic capacity ☺ Glucose control: Lower fasting glucose; lower glucose levels after the oral glucose load; improved insulin sensitivity; fasting serum insulin reduced from 18.1 to 12.5 mcu/ml ☺ Lipids: Meaningful reductions in total cholesterol, triglycerides, and low-density lipoprotein cholesterol (LDL) ☺ Blood pressure: Clinically significant reductions in blood pressure
Usual control (UC) diet	☹ Weight *gain*: +0.9 kg ☺ Exercise capacity: No improvement ☺ Glucose control: No improvement ☺ Lipids: No improvement ☺ Blood pressure: No improvement

- Randomized clinical trial: Effects of the dietary approaches to stop hypertension diet, exercise, and caloric restriction on neurocognition in overweight adults with high blood pressure (*Hypertension* 2010 Jun[156]): In this clinical trial, 124 subjects with either prehypertension or stage 1 hypertension (sBP 130 to 159 mm Hg or dBP 85 to 99 mm Hg) who were sedentary and overweight or obese (BMI: 25 to 40) were randomized to the DASH diet alone, DASH with exercise and caloric restriction, or a usual control (UC) diet group. Subjects completed tests of executive function, memory, and learning and psychomotor speed at baseline and at the end of the 4-month trial. Results showed the following: "Participants on the DASH diet combined with a behavioral weight management program exhibited greater improvements in executive function-memory-learning and psychomotor speed, and DASH diet alone participants exhibited better psychomotor speed compared with the usual diet control. Neurocognitive improvements appeared to be mediated by increased aerobic fitness and weight loss. ... In conclusion, combining aerobic exercise with the DASH diet and caloric restriction improves neurocognitive function among sedentary and overweight/obese individuals with prehypertension and hypertension." Specific to changes in blood pressure, the following results were noted (per Table 2 of the original article):

---

[155] Blumenthal et al. Effects of dietary approaches to stop hypertension diet alone and in combination with exercise and caloric restriction on insulin sensitivity and lipids. *Hypertension*. 2010 May;55(5):1199-205
[156] Smith et al. Effects of dietary approaches to stop hypertension diet, exercise, and caloric restriction on neurocognition in overweight adults with high blood pressure. *Hypertension*. 2010 Jun;55(6):1331-8

Intervention	Initial BP	Final BP	BP change
DASH diet alone	137.5/87.2	127.8/79.5	-9.7/-7.7
DASH diet *with* aerobic exercise *and* caloric restriction	138.6/85.4	125.1/77.2	**-13.5/-8.2**
Usual control (UC) diet	138.6/85.7	136.2/82.7	-2.2/-3

Thus, as we should expect, dietary improvement plus caloric restriction and exercise resulted in greater reductions in BP than diet improvement alone, which was better than no change at all. The neurocognitive improvements associated with improved diet and increased exercise are consistent with the previously documented neurogenic/neuroprotective/synaptogenic effects of exercise[157], as well as improved neuronal function seen with increased phytonutrient intake.[158] *Consider the implications: the "standard American diet" along with the standard American lifestyle of inactivity basically dumbs people down.* As discussed in Chapter 4.4, Kihn's 2013 essay "Political Roots of American Obesity" is an impressive alignment of compelling ideas.[159]

What might be the cumulative additive/synergistic neuro-intellectual results—on a personal, interpersonal, social, and national level—of dietary optimization, frequent exercise, decided application of one's efforts and abilities, and habitual exposure to complex neurointellectual phenomena—for example, the combination of humanistic psychology, authentic (not "pop") philosophy, and highly structured music?[160,161] Synergism of these events would likely elevate humanity toward its positive potential.

- Review: Effects of exercise, diet and weight loss on high blood pressure (*Sports Medicine* 2004[162]): The authors of this review note that HTN "is a major health problem in the US, affecting more than 50 million people" and that "anti-hypertensive medications are not effective for everyone, and may be costly and result in adverse effects that impair quality of life and reduce adherence. Moreover, abnormalities associated with high BP, such as insulin resistance and hyperlipidemia, may persist or may even be exacerbated by some anti-hypertensive medications." Thereafter, their expert review of the literature may be summarized in the table below. The benefits of exercise and weight loss extend beyond BP reduction to include reductions in left ventricular mass and wall thickness (i.e., reductions in left ventricular hypertrophy), reduced arterial stiffness and improved endothelial function.

Intervention	Blood pressure reduction
Exercise alone: without intentional weight loss or diet intervention	-3.5/-2.0 mm Hg
DASH diet	-5.5/-3.0 mm Hg
Weight loss of 17.6 lbs (8 kg)	-8.5/-6.5 mm Hg
Combined exercise & weight loss	-12.5/-7.9 mm Hg

- The 2009 Canadian Hypertension Education Program recommendations for the management of hypertension: Part 2—therapy (*Canadian Journal of Cardiology* 2009 May[163]): These are very conventional and standard recommendations from the medical community which are included here for the sake of completeness so that doctors have a recent reference guideline from which they can move beyond in the delivery of superior clinical care. "RECOMMENDATIONS: For lifestyle modifications to prevent and treat hypertension, restrict dietary sodium to less than 2300 mg (100 mmol)/day (and 1500 mg to 2300 mg [65 mmol to 100 mmol]/day in hypertensive patients); perform 30 min to 60 min of aerobic exercise four to seven days per week; maintain a healthy body weight (body mass index 18.5 kg/m(2) to 24.9 kg/m(2)) and waist circumference (smaller than 102 cm for men and smaller than 88 cm for women); limit alcohol consumption to no more than 14 units [drinks] per week in men or nine units per week in women; follow

[157] Cotman CW, Berchtold NC, Christie LA. Exercise builds brain health: key roles of growth factor cascades and inflammation. *Trends Neurosci.* 2007 Sep;30(9):464-72

[158] Spencer JP. The impact of fruit flavonoids on memory and cognition. *Br J Nutr.* 2010 Oct;104 Suppl 3:S40-7 and Spencer JP. Flavonoids and brain health: multiple effects underpinned by common mechanisms. *Genes Nutr.* 2009 Dec;4(4):243-50

[159] Kihn ED. The Political Roots of American Obesity. 2013 May truth-out.org/opinion/item/16149-the-political-roots-of-american-obesity

[160] Suda M, Morimoto K, Obata A,Koizumi H, Maki A.Cortical responses to Mozart's sonata enhance spatial-reasoning ability.*Neurol Res* 2008;30:885-8

[161] Jausovec N, Jausovec K, Gerlic I. The influence of Mozart's music on brain activity in the process of learning. *Clin Neurophysiol.* 2006;117:2703-14

[162] Bacon SL, Sherwood A, Hinderliter A, Blumenthal JA. Effects of exercise, diet and weight loss on high blood pressure. *Sports Med.* 2004;34:307-16

[163] Khan et al. 2009 Canadian Hypertension Education Program recommendations for the management of hypertension: Part 2—therapy. *Can J Cardiol.* 2009 May;25(5):287-98

a diet that is reduced in saturated fat and cholesterol, and that emphasizes fruits, vegetables and low-fat dairy products, dietary and soluble fiber, whole grains and protein from plant sources; and consider stress management in selected individuals with hypertension." These guidelines would have been better if they had advised complete avoidance of grains (sources of generally acidogenic phytonutrient-poor carbohydrates) and other sources of simple carbohydrate including candies and soft drinks in general and those pseudofoods laden with high-fructose corn syrup in particular.

- Meta-analysis: Adherence to Mediterranean diet and health status (*British Medical Journal* 2008 Sep[164]): "Greater adherence to a Mediterranean diet is associated with a significant improvement in health status, as seen by a **significant reduction in overall mortality** (-9%), mortality from **cardiovascular diseases** (-9%), incidence of or mortality from **cancer** (-6%), and incidence of **Parkinson's disease and Alzheimer's disease** (-13%). These results seem to be clinically relevant for public health, in particular for **encouraging a Mediterranean-like dietary pattern for primary prevention of major chronic diseases.**" The results of this meta-analysis have major implications for clinical practice and public health policy.

Lifestyle recommendations from the Canadian Hypertension Education Program

- Restrict dietary sodium to less than 2300 mg (100 mmol)/day (and 1500 mg to 2300 mg [65 mmol to 100 mmol]/day in hypertensive patients).
- Perform 30 min to 60 min of aerobic exercise four to seven days per week.
- Maintain a healthy body weight (body mass index 18.5 kg/m(2) to 24.9 kg/m(2)) and waist circumference (< 102 cm for men and < 88 cm for women).
- Limit alcohol consumption to no more than 14 units per week in men or nine units per week in women.
- Follow a diet that is reduced in saturated fat and cholesterol.
- Follow a diet that emphasizes fruits, vegetables and low-fat dairy products, dietary and soluble fiber, whole grains and protein from plant sources.
- Consider stress management in selected individuals with hypertension.

Khan NA, Hemmelgarn B, Herman RJ, et al. The 2009 Canadian Hypertension Education Program recommendations for the management of hypertension: Part 2—therapy. *Can J Cardiol.* 2009 May;25(5):287-98

- **Short-term water-only fasting**: The anti-hypertensive and anti-diabetic benefits of low-carbohydrate diets and short-term fasting have been substantiated in the research literature for several decades. However, the chiropractic physician Alan Goldhamer deserves credit for the most recent revival of short-term fasting as a therapeutic tool for chronic hypertension and diabetes mellitus.

Clinical Pearl: lowering plasma glucose → lower insulin levels → less sodium-water retention → alleviation of hypertension

Treatments that lower plasma glucose levels, either via reduced intake of carbohydrates or by increasing glucose disposal (i.e., increasing insulin sensitivity) have an anti-hypertensive effect via lowering insulin levels. **Because insulin promotes sodium-water retention, any treatment that lowers glucose-insulin levels will help correct the contribution of hyperinsulinemia to hypertension.** Likewise, avoidance of dietary fructose is now known to avoid the fructose-induced elevations in serum uric acid which contribute to endothelial dysfunction, hypertension, and the metabolic syndrome.

- Open clinical trial: Chiropractic-supervised water-only fasting in the treatment of hypertension (*Journal of Manipulative Physiological Therapeutics* 2001 Jun[165]): In this open trial, 174 consecutive hypertensive patients were treated in an inpatient setting under clinician supervision. The treatment program began with a short prefasting period (approximately 2 to 3 days on average) during which food consumption was limited to fruits and vegetables, followed by supervised water-only fasting (approximately 10 to 11 days on average) and a refeeding period (approximately 6 to 7 days on average) introducing a low-fat, low-sodium, vegan diet. "RESULTS: Almost 90% of the subjects achieved blood pressure less than 140/90 mm Hg by the end of the treatment program. **The average reduction in blood pressure was 37/13 mm Hg**, with the greatest decrease being observed for subjects with the most severe hypertension. **Patients with stage 3 hypertension (those with systolic blood pressure greater than 180 mg Hg, diastolic blood pressure greater than 110 mg Hg, or both) had an average reduction of 60/17 mm Hg at the conclusion of treatment**. All of the subjects who were taking antihypertensive medication at entry (6.3% of the total sample) successfully discontinued the use of medication. CONCLUSION: Medically supervised water-only fasting appears to be a safe and effective means of normalizing blood pressure and may assist in motivating health-promoting diet and lifestyle changes."

[164] Sofi F, Cesari F, Abbate R, Gensini GF, Casini A. Adherence to Mediterranean diet and health status: meta-analysis. *BMJ.* 2008 Sep 11;337:a1344
[165] Goldhamer et al. Medically supervised water-only fasting in the treatment of hypertension. *J Manipulative Physiol Ther* 2001 Jun;24(5):335-9

- Open clinical trial: Chiropractic-supervised water-only fasting in the treatment of borderline hypertension (*Journal of Alternative and Complementary Medicine* 2002 Oct[166]): 68 consecutive patients with borderline hypertension were treated in an inpatient setting under professional supervision. The treatment program consisted of a short prefasting period (approximately 1-2 days on average) during which food consumption was limited to fruits and vegetables followed by supervised water-only fasting (approximately 13.6 days on average). Fasting was followed by a refeeding period (approximately 6.0 days on average). The refeeding program consisted of a low-fat, low-sodium, plant-based, vegan diet. "RESULTS: Approximately 82% of the subjects achieved BP at or below 120/80 mm Hg by the end of the treatment program. **The mean BP reduction was 20/7 mm Hg,** with the greatest decrease being observed for subjects with the highest baseline BP. A linear regression of BP decrease against baseline BP showed that the estimated BP below which no further decrease would be expected was 96.0/67.0 mm Hg at the end of the fast and 99.2/67.3 mm Hg at the end of refeeding. These levels are in agreement with other estimates of the BP below which stroke events are eliminated, thus suggesting that these levels could be regarded as the "ideal" BP values. CONCLUSION: Medically supervised water-only fasting appears to be a safe and effective means of normalizing BP and may assist in motivating health-promoting diet and lifestyle changes."
- Retrospective analysis of the cost-effectiveness and clinical effectiveness of short-term fasting: Initial cost of supervised water-only fasting for treating high blood pressure and diabetes (*Journal of Alternative and Complementary Medicine* 2002 Dec[167]): In this brief report, Dr Goldhamer again reports success with the short-term fasting program in hypertensive patients as well as diabetic patients. Here, Goldhamer reports that the **average reduction in systolic blood pressure was 30/11 mm Hg at the completion of the program and 28/11 mm Hg on follow-up.** "Weight loss averaged 26 pounds after the program and was 28 pounds below baseline on follow-up. The average cost of medical care and drugs was $5,784.00 per year in the year(s) prior to participation and $3,000.00 in the year after participation for an average reduction of $2,784.00 per subject in the first year alone. This exceeded the cost of the entire program and compound savings are expected in the years to follow."

- **Specific food items to be avoided or reasonably minimized**: Clinicians and patients should be aware that dietary intake of food allergens, fructose, sodium chloride, and arachidonic acid can contribute to the development, perpetuation, and therapeutic recalcitrance of chronic HTN.
  - Food allergen avoidance, customized per patient (*The Lancet* 1979 May[168]): According to a clinical study of migraineurs (n = 60) published in *The Lancet*, identification and avoidance of food allergens can generally normalize blood pressure in migraine patients who have concomitant hypertension; findings of this study included, "The commonest foods causing reactions were wheat (78%), orange (65%), eggs (45%), tea and coffee (40% each), chocolate and milk (37%) each), beef (35%), and corn, cane sugar, and yeast (33% each). When an average of ten common foods was avoided there was a dramatic fall in the number of headaches per month, 85% of patients becoming headache-free. The 25% of patients with hypertension became normotensive."
  - Minimization of dietary sodium chloride: Excess sodium (Na) promotes water retention and subsequent volume expansion, while also contributing to vasoconstriction and arterial stiffness via enhanced adrenergic reactivity and via promotion of "intracellular hypercalcinosis" (per Vasquez[169]) possibly due to enhanced sodium-calcium exchange.[170] When consumed in common table salt, the chloride (Cl) anion promotes acidosis which results in the progression of CAD/CVD morbidity and mortality and the exacerbation of HTN with increased renal losses of magnesium, potassium, and calcium. These effects justify the advice for HTN patients to avoid dietary NaCl and also justify the use of drug diuretics that enhance Na excretion by the kidney. Clinical responsiveness to low-sodium diets ranges from clinically insignificant to a maximum reduction in the range of -22/-14 to -16/-9.[171] Contraindications to low-sodium

---

[166] Goldhamer et al. Medically supervised water-only fasting in the treatment of borderline hypertension. *J Altern Complement Med.* 2002 Oct;8(5):643-50

[167] Goldhamer AC. Initial cost of care results in medically supervised water-only fasting for treating high blood pressure and diabetes. *J Altern Complement Med.* 2002 Dec;8(6):696-7

[168] Grant EC. Food allergies and migraine. *Lancet.* 1979 May 5;1(8123):966-9

[169] Vasquez A. Intracellular Hypercalcinosis: A Functional Nutritional Disorder with Implications Ranging from Myofascial Trigger Points to Affective Disorders, Hypertension, and Cancer. *Naturopathy Digest* 2006 Previously published in-print and on-line at naturopathydigest.com/archives/2006/sep/vasquez.php and included in this book.

[170] Benowitz NL. "Antihypertensive Agents." In Katzung BG (editor). *Basic and Clinical Pharmacology. 10th Edition.* New York: McGraw Hill Medical; 2007, 163

[171] "The average fall in blood pressure from the highest to the lowest sodium intake was 16/9 mm Hg." MacGregor et al. Double-blind study of three sodium intakes and long-term effects of sodium restriction in essential hypertension. *Lancet.* 1989 Nov 25;2(8674):1244-7

diet are uncommon (e.g., hyponatremia, adrenal failure); low-sodium/NaCl diets should generally be a component of all anti-hypertensive treatment plans. Approximately 20% of patients will show antihypertensive benefit from sodium restriction.[172] As previously noted, Canadian guidelines published in 2009 support the restriction of dietary sodium to less than 2300 mg (100 mmol)/day and to less than 1500-2300 mg [65 mmol to 100 mmol]/day in hypertensive patients.[173] One might hope that readers would appreciate that human physiology developed over millennia wherein the addition of manufactured table salt was a logistical impossibility; in an excellent paradigm-shifting compilation and integration of research, Cordain and his pioneering expert co-authors[174] noted, "the addition of manufactured salt to the food supply and the displacement of traditional potassium-rich foods by foods introduced during the Neolithic and Industrial periods caused a 400% decline in the potassium intake while simultaneously initiating a 400%

The importance of potassium
"Adults should consume at least 4.7 grams of potassium per day to lower blood pressure, blunt the effects of salt, and reduce the risk of kidney stones and bone loss. However, most American women 31 to 50 years old consume no more than half of the recommended amount of potassium, and men's intake is only moderately higher. There was no evidence of chronic excess intakes of potassium in apparently healthy individuals and thus no UL [upper limit of intake] was established."
Food and Nutrition Board of the Institute of Medicine of the National Academies. "Dietary Reference Intakes: Water, Potassium, Sodium, Chloride, and Sulfate." Released: February 11, 2004 iom.edu/Reports/2004/Dietary-Reference-Intakes-Water-Potassium-Sodium-Chloride-and-Sulfate.aspx

increase in sodium ingestion. The inversion of potassium and sodium concentrations [dietary sodium-potassium ratio] in hominin diets had no evolutionary precedent and now plays an integral role in eliciting and contributing to numerous diseases of civilization." Adverse effects of NaCl can be at least partly offset by administration of calcium, vitamin D, magnesium, potassium, bicarbonate and citrate.

- Potassium supplementation, preferably via fruits, vegetables, and their juices: Antihypertensive mechanisms of potassium include vasodilator activity, diuretic and naturietic effects, and suppression of renin, angiotensin, and adrenergic tone.[175] In February 2004, the Institute of Medicine (IOM) set the Adequate Intake of potassium for adults at 4.7 grams a day—more than double previous recommendations; more than 90% of American adults do not meet these recommendations. If 90% of the population is not meeting recommended intakes of potassium, and these recommendations from the IOM come after an extensive review of the scientific literature, then potassium assessment and supplementation should be routine components of patient care; furthermore, this shows to the inadequacy of current laboratory assessments for evaluating potassium status and potassium balance. The commonly used "serum potassium" test detects only the most extreme potassium deficiency and is wholly and obviously insensitive for detection of subtle long-term potassium *insufficiency*.

An irony exists in the observations that 1) metabolic syndrome is a very common lethal condition with a hypertensive component, and 2) thiazide diuretics are first-line treatment for most cases of hypertension, and 3) thiazide diuretics exacerbate many CVD-inducing aspects of the metabolic syndrome, such as insulin resistance and dyslipidemia. A 2007 experimental [animal] study published in *Journal of the American Society of Nephrology* showed that potassium supplementation—alone or in combination with treatment to reduce fructose-induced hyperuricemia—can ameliorate exacerbation of metabolic syndrome caused by thiazide diuretics.[176] This is yet another example of nutritional intervention being used to treat the primary disease as well as alleviate the secondary metabolic disturbances caused by the current drug-of-choice.

True to what is to be expected from studies conducted by researchers with little or no previous training in clinical nutrition, most studies of potassium supplementation for the treatment of HTN have been methodologically flawed due to ❶ utilization of potassium in the form of potassium chloride (KCl), ❷ failure to simultaneously reduce intake of dietary NaCl so as to normalize the K:Na ratio and ❸ also reduce total Cl intake; furthermore, ❹ the notion that "potassium intake from foods is associated with reduced blood pressure and that potassium supplementation (e.g., KCl) could be equivalent to potassium intake from food" is a *colossal failure* to appreciate the manifold cardioprotective benefits of the phytonutrients *consumed along with potassium*

---

[172] Domino FJ (editor in chief). *The 5-Minute Clinical Consult. 2010. 18th Edition*. Philadelphia; Wolters Kluwer: 2009, 656-7
[173] Khan et al. 2009 Canadian Hypertension Education Program recommendations for the management of hypertension: Part 2—therapy. *Can J Cardiol*. 2009 May;25(5):287-98
[174] Cordain et al. Origins and evolution of the Western diet: health implications for the 21st century. *Am J Clin Nutr*. 2005 Feb;81(2):341-5 ajcn.org/cgi/content/full/81/2/341
[175] Patki et al. Efficacy of potassium and magnesium in essential hypertension: a double-blind, placebo controlled, crossover study. *BMJ*. 1990 Sep 15;301(6751):521-3
[176] Reungjui et al. Thiazide diuretics exacerbate fructose-induced metabolic syndrome. *J Am Soc Nephrol*. 2007 Oct;18(10):2724-31

when obtained from its richest natural food sources—fruits, vegetables, nuts, seeds, berries. Furthermore, reverence for KCl reveals ignorance of the cardiovasculotoxic and acidogenic effects of chloride. Respective amounts of potassium per serving of food or juice (1 cup = 8 fluid ounces =240 milliliters) are provided in the table below.

Potassium content of common foods

Food serving	Potassium in mg (sodium as available)
One papaya	780
One cup of mixed vegetable juice	740 (35 mg sodium, up to 630 mg sodium)
One cup of prune juice	700
One cup of carrot juice	520 (160 mg sodium)
One cup plain low-fat yogurt	510 (150 mg sodium)
One cup of cantaloupe	490
One cup of orange juice	470
One small banana	465
One cup of honeydew melon	460
One-third cup of raisins	365
One cup of carrot-orange juice	360 (35 mg sodium)
One medium mango	320
One medium kiwi	250
One small orange	240
One medium pear	210

Note again that the physiologic effect of potassium is influenced by the potassium:sodium ratio (sodium reduces effectiveness and retention of potassium), potassium:chloride ratio (chloride reduces effectiveness and retention of potassium), and the overall pH acid-base balance of the human host (i.e., metabolic acidosis reduces effectiveness and retention of potassium, while an alkaline state improves retention and effectiveness of potassium). Importantly, magnesium status is an important positive-direct determinant of potassium status, particularly in patients with recalcitrant hypokalemia and/or hyperaldosteronism.[177]

- Double-blind, placebo controlled, crossover study: Efficacy of potassium and magnesium in essential hypertension (*British Medical Journal* 1990 Sep[178]): The authors conducted a double-blind randomized placebo-controlled crossover trial of 32 weeks' duration among 37 adults with mild hypertension (diastolic blood pressure less than 110 mm Hg); patients received either placebo or potassium 60 mmol/day (approximately 2,250 mg/d) alone or in combination with magnesium 20 mmol/day (approximately 480 mg/d) in a crossover design without other intervention. More specifically, patients were treated with either placebo, K alone, or K+Mg for 8 weeks each with a 2-week washout period between treatments. While blood pressure in the placebo group did not change after 8 weeks of treatment, BP in the K group dropped from 157/101 to 143/85 (drop of **-14/-16 mm Hg**) and from 154/99 to 146/88 (drop of -8/-11) in the K+Mg group. The reduction in serum cholesterol was from the initial value of 7.5 mmol/l (290 mg/dL) to 6.0 mmol/l (232 mg/dL) and 6.1 mmol/l (235 mg/dL) in the K and K+Mg groups, respectively. The authors wrote, "RESULTS: **Potassium alone or in combination with magnesium produced a significant reduction in systolic and diastolic blood pressures** (p less than 0.001) and a **significant reduction in serum cholesterol concentration** (p less than 0.05); other biochemical variables did not change. Magnesium did not have an additional effect. … The drug was well tolerated and compliance was satisfactory. CONCLUSION: Potassium 60 mmol/day lowers arterial blood pressure in patients with mild hypertension. Giving magnesium as well has no added advantage." While the reduction in blood pressure by potassium is to be expected, two surprising findings in this study are 1) the reduction in serum cholesterol and 2) the

---

[177] "Magnesium deficiency is frequently associated with hypokalemia. Concomitant magnesium deficiency aggravates hypokalemia and renders it refractory to treatment by potassium. Herein is reviewed literature suggesting that magnesium deficiency exacerbates potassium wasting by increasing distal potassium secretion. A decrease in intracellular magnesium, caused by magnesium deficiency, releases the magnesium-mediated inhibition of ROMK channels and increases potassium secretion. Magnesium deficiency alone, however, does not necessarily cause hypokalemia. An increase in distal sodium delivery or elevated aldosterone levels may be required for exacerbating potassium wasting in magnesium deficiency." Huang CL, Kuo E. Mechanism of hypokalemia in magnesium deficiency. *J Am Soc Nephrol*. 2007 Oct;18(10):2649-52

[178] Patki et al. Efficacy of potassium and magnesium in essential hypertension: a double-blind, placebo controlled, crossover study. *BMJ*. 1990 Sep 15;301(6751):521-3

lack of additive benefit by the magnesium supplementation, particularly when other studies have shown antihypertensive benefit of magnesium when used alone. In this study, both the potassium and the magnesium were provided in a liquid form as KCl and MgCl, respectively; better sources would have been the citrate or malate chelates for alkalinization and enhanced bioavailability. Attentive readers might have also noted one additional curious finding from this study: none of the 37 patients were reported to have developed diarrhea or loose stools from the magnesium 480 mg/d; this may or may not be significant to the credibility of the study; in clinical practice, some patients will report loose stools with magnesium doses as low as 200 mg per day.

- **Meta-analysis: Potassium supplementation for the management of primary hypertension in adults** (*Cochrane Database of Systematic Reviews* 2006 Jul[179]): Using reasonable inclusion/exclusion criteria, the authors of this meta-analysis found that "Six RCT's (n=483), with eight to 16 weeks follow-up, met our inclusion criteria. Meta-analysis of five trials (n=425) with adequate data indicated that potassium supplementation compared to control resulted in a large but statistically non-significant reductions in **SBP** (mean difference: **-11.2**, 95% CI: -25.2 to 2.7) and **DBP** (mean difference: **-5.0**, 95% CI: -12.5 to 2.4)." The conclusion that potassium supplementation resulted in "large but statistically non-significant reductions" would appear to be an example of *statistical methodology* trumping *clinical practicality* insofar as a reduction of -11/-5 mm Hg is indeed clinically significant and also meets criteria for drug efficacy/approval per the US FDA (assuming that the difference is placebo subtracted). The authors reviewed "two high quality trials (n=138)" showing blood pressure reductions of **-7.1/-5.5** mm Hg but again concluded that these findings represented "non-significant reductions in blood pressure." Given the safety and *essentiality* of potassium, its inadequate consumption from Westernized diets, its facilitated urinary excretion due to consumption of salt/sugar/caffeine/alcohol and many diuretic drugs, and its demonstrated efficacy, clinicians are justified in utilizing potassium in the treatment of HTN especially when sourced from *natural whole foods* and fruit/vegetable juices; indeed, a recent clinical trial[180] utilizing the DASH diet (described previously) in all subjects showed that blood pressure reductions were enhanced among the subset of subjects consuming 8-16 ounces of vegetable juice daily, even when the sodium:potassium ratio was nonphysiologic at >1 since 8 ounces of the juice contained 480 mg of sodium and 470 mg of potassium.

- Randomized trial with 1-year follow-up and a title that says it all: Increasing the dietary potassium intake reduces the need for antihypertensive medication (*Annals of Internal Medicine* 1991 Nov[181]): The stated purpose of this study was "To determine whether an increase in dietary potassium intake from natural foods reduces the need for antihypertensive medication in patients with essential hypertension." Forty-seven patients with medication-controlled hypertension completed one year of dietary treatment (or control nonintervention) and follow-up; the dietary intervention focused on increasing intake of potassium-rich foods, with compliance monitored by 3-day food records and by measuring 24-hour urinary potassium excretion. Results showed the following: "After 1 year, the average drug consumption (number of pills per day) relative to that at baseline was 24% in group 1 (potassium-rich diet) and 60% in group 2 (control diet) (P less than 0.001). By the end of the study, blood pressure could be controlled using less than 50% of the initial therapy in 81% of the patients in group 1 compared with 29% of the patients in group 2 (P = 0.001). Patients in group 1 ended the study with a lower number of reported symptoms compared with patients in the control group (P less than 0.001). CONCLUSION: Increasing the dietary potassium intake from natural foods is a feasible and effective measure to reduce antihypertensive drug treatment." With powerful results such as these, world-wise clinicians will not be surprised that US National Heart, Lung, and Blood Institute (NHLBI)'s endorsed dietary program "Stay Young at Heart: Cooking the Heart-Healthy Way"[182] is notably low in potassium; this will be reviewed in a section toward the end of this chapter.

---

[179] Dickinson et al. Potassium supplementation for the management of primary hypertension in adults. *Cochrane Database Syst Rev*. 2006 Jul 19;3:CD004641
[180] Shenoy et al. The use of a commercial vegetable juice as a practical means to increase vegetable intake: a randomized controlled trial. *Nutr J*. 2010 Sep 17;9:38
[181] Siani et al. Increasing the dietary potassium intake reduces the need for antihypertensive medication. *Ann Intern Med*. 1991 Nov 15;115(10):753-9
[182] US National Heart, Lung, and Blood Institute (NHLBI). Stay Young at Heart: Cooking the Heart-Healthy Way. nhlbi.nih.gov/health/public/heart/other/syah/index.htm Accessed December 2009 and re-reviewed in November 2010.

- <u>Magnesium (Mg) dosed at 600 mg per day or to bowel tolerance</u>: Given the safety and low cost of magnesium, along with the high prevalence of magnesium deficiency in the general population, routine oral magnesium supplementation is warranted. The standard replacement dose for oral magnesium supplementation is 600 mg per day; some patients may tolerate less or need more, with a typical range of 200-1,800 mg/d being used in clinical practice. Insufficient doses are inefficacious, while excess doses are generally benign (causing only transient loose stools). Renal insufficiency and/or treatment with the magnesium-retaining diuretic spironolactone indicate the need for cautious dosing and more frequent clinical and laboratory monitoring. Measurement of *intracellular* Mg levels in erythrocytes or leukocytes is more accurate than is measurement of *serum* Mg levels.

  - <u>Oral magnesium supplementation reduces ambulatory blood pressure in patients with mild hypertension (*American Journal of Hypertension* 2009 Oct[183])</u>: For a 12-week period, 48 patients with mild uncomplicated hypertension were assigned either to treatment with 600 mg (25 mmol) of magnesium pidolate orally twice a day for 12 weeks + lifestyle recommendations (n=24) or to treatment with lifestyle recommendations only. "RESULTS: In the Mg(2+) supplementation group, **small but significant reductions in mean 24-h systolic and diastolic BP**

> **Key concept: Subphysiologic doses of nutrients are generally subtherapeutic**
>
> In order to obtain a physiologic effect and an optimal clinical benefit from nutritional supplementation, the supplementation must be of adequate *duration*, *dose*, and *bioavailability* to optimally supply cellular processes. *Cofactors*, *co-nutrients*, and the *proper biochemical milieu* (pH in particular) are also required for optimal effectiveness of the nutritional intervention.
>
> Vasquez A. **Subphysiologic doses of vitamin D are subtherapeutic**: comment on study by The Record Trial Group. *TheLancet.com.* Published online May 6, 2005

levels were observed, in contrast to control group (**-5.6** vs. -1.3 mm Hg, and **-2.8** vs. -1 mm Hg, respectively). These effects of Mg(2+) supplementation were consistent in both daytime and night-time periods. Serum Mg(2+) levels and urinary Mg(2+) excretion were significantly increased in the intervention group. Intracellular Mg(2+) and K(+) levels were also increased, while intracellular Ca(2+) and Na(+) levels were decreased in the intervention group. None of the intracellular ions were significantly changed in the control group. CONCLUSION: This study suggests that oral Mg(2+) supplementation is associated with small but consistent ambulatory BP reduction in patients with mild hypertension." Readers should note that magnesium supplementation in this study was shown to reduce intracellular calcium and to increase intracellular potassium simultaneously with the reduction in BP. These findings are consistent with my proposal for treatment of intracellular hypercalcinosis[184] published in 2006 and with the fact that magnesium sufficiency is mandatory for the intracellular uptake of potassium; **any patient with chronic hypokalemia should be tested and/or treated for magnesium insufficiency.** *How do we translate "600 mg (25 mmol) of magnesium pidolate orally twice a day" into an understanding of the clinical dosage which is generally expressed in milligrams of elemental Mg?* The physiologic action of magnesium supplements depends upon their content of magnesium ion. Magnesium pidolate is the magnesium salt of pidolic acid (pyroglutamic acid), which is only 8.7% Mg by weight. Thus, "600 mg (25 mmol) of magnesium pidolate orally twice a day" provides 1,200 mg of magnesium pidolate which provides 8.7% of 600 mg of elemental magnesium, which is only 104 mg of elemental Mg per day. Given that the standard replacement dose for Mg is 600 mg per day of elemental Mg, we see that the dose used in this study was suboptimally therapeutic (only 17% of the standard dose of Mg) and that therefore the clinical results are less impressive than those which would have likely been obtained if the study subjects had used a more substantial amount of Mg.

- <u>Fructose avoidance for caloric moderation and uric acid reduction (American Heart Association, news release 2009 Sep[185])</u>: Production of uric acid is stimulated by ingestion of fructose (most notoriously in the form of high-fructose corn syrup, common in many processed foods and cola drinks), and uric acid directly contributes to the development of insulin resistance and HTN and other classic features of the metabolic syndrome. In a clinical trial published in 2009, 74 adult men added fructose 200 g/d to their regular diet (typical American diet averages 50-70 g/d of fructose) for 2 weeks and experienced a 6/3 elevation in BP, elevations in serum triglycerides and LDL cholesterol, and a more than doubling of the incidence of metabolic syndrome from

---

[183] Hatzistavri et al. Oral magnesium supplementation reduces ambulatory blood pressure in patients with mild hypertension. *Am J Hypertens.* 2009 Oct;22(10):1070-5

[184] Vasquez A. Intracellular Hypercalcinosis: A Functional Nutritional Disorder with Implications Ranging from Myofascial Trigger Points to Affective Disorders, Hypertension, and Cancer. *Naturopathy Digest* 2006 Previously published in-print and on-line at naturopathydigest.com/archives/2006/sep/vasquez.php and included at the end of this chapter.

[185] News release from American Heart Association's 63rd High Blood Pressure Research Conference. High-sugar diet increases men's blood pressure; gout drug protective. Abstract P127. Sept. 23, 2009. americanheart.mediaroom.com/index.php?s=43&item=829 Accessed December 19, 2009

approximately 20% to 50% as determined by two sets of international criteria. The authors logically concluded, "These results suggest that fructose may be a cause of metabolic syndrome. They also suggest that excessive fructose intake may have a role in the worldwide epidemic of obesity and diabetes." Men in this trial who were randomized to receive the xanthine oxidase inhibitor allopurinol (dose not reported; common adult amount is 200-600 mg/d in divided doses, preferably with food) did not develop adverse effects from the increased fructose ingestion, thus clearly implicating fructose-induced hyperuricemia as the biochemical pathway involved. Clinicians should appreciate that the rapid (within 2 weeks) development of HTN and a doubling of the incidence of metabolic syndrome by the addition of fructose to the diet is of undeniably major importance as it clearly implicates high-fructose corn syrup as a major culprit in the burgeoning epidemics of HTN, type-2 diabetes mellitus, and the metabolic syndrome. In a study[186] involving adolescents with elevated uric acid levels (serum uric acid levels > or = 6 mg/dL), allopurinol 200 mg twice daily resulted in a reduction in blood pressure of approximately -7/-5 mm Hg (compared to approximately -2/-2 for placebo); this was a proof-of-concept study (i.e., that uric acid contributes to HTN) and not necessarily an endorsement to use allopurinol for the treatment of HTN. Adverse effects due to allopurinol can include skin rash that may be followed by more severe hypersensitivity reactions such as "exfoliative, urticarial and purpuric lesions as well as Stevens-Johnson syndrome (erythema multiforme exudativum) and/or generalized vasculitis, irreversible hepatotoxicity and on rare occasions, death."[187] Adherence to the Paleo-Mediterranean Diet in general and a low-fructose diet in particular can help reduce elevated serum uric acid levels without the use of drugs because this dietary profile is low in fructose and promotes urinary alkalinization; alkalinizing the urine via avoidance of acidogenic foodstuffs such as dairy and sodium chloride and by increased intake of fruits and vegetables (or supplemental forms of citrate and bicarbonate[188]) promotes renal excretion of uric acid, thus lessening the adverse metabolic effects of uric acid on insulin resistance and endothelial dysfunction. Clinicians should note that, as a result of the manufacturing process, high-fructose corn syrup contains mercury[189], a toxic metal for which no known "safe" and free-from-harm dose exists; adverse effects of mercury exposure include renal damage and clinical hypertension, the latter is promoted by the former while also being generated independently by increased catecholamine release (according to case reports[190]). Per the 2009 review by Houston[191], "The clinical consequences of mercury toxicity include hypertension, CHD, MI, increased carotid IMT [intima media thickness] and obstruction, CVA, generalized atherosclerosis, and renal dysfunction with proteinuria." Mercury contamination of corn syrup ranks among the better examples of how industrialization of the food supply causes untoward [i.e., unexpected and negative] effects; it also exemplifies how one problem (overconsumption of processed "junk" food which contains pro-hypertensive fructose in nonphysiologic/unnatural concentrations) can lead/contribute to other types of problems (adverse effects of mercury, neurotoxicity, nephrotoxicity, and chronic overstimulation of the sympathetic nervous system). Rapid induction of hypertension and the metabolic syndrome in humans by fructose consumption is almost certainly *not* mediated by the mercury content; the extent to which mercury from corn syrup contributes to hypertension is not known, but facts that are already established include the following: ❶ mercury is a known immunotoxin, nephrotoxin, and neurotoxin, ❷ mercury can cause hypertension in humans, ❸ mercury causes hypertension in humans via at least two mechanisms—inhibition of catecholamine breakdown, and induction of renal damage, ❹ corn syrup contains two agents known to cause hypertension in humans: mercury and fructose.

---

[186] "Allopurinol, 200 mg twice daily for 4 weeks,... For casual BP, the mean change in systolic BP for allopurinol was -6.9 mm Hg vs -2.0 mm Hg for placebo, and the mean change in diastolic BP for allopurinol was -5.1 mm Hg vs -2.4 for placebo. CONCLUSIONS: In this short-term, crossover study of adolescents with newly diagnosed hypertension, treatment with allopurinol resulted in reduction of BP." Feig et al. Effect of allopurinol on blood pressure of adolescents with newly diagnosed essential hypertension: a randomized trial. *JAMA.* 2008 Aug 27;300(8):924-32

[187] Brinker AD. Allopurinol and the role of uric acid in hypertension. [letter] *JAMA.* 2009 Jan 21;301(3):270

[188] "The treatment of uric acid stones should focus on alkalinization of the urine with citrate or bicarbonate salts." Liebman SE, Taylor JG, Bushinsky DA. Uric acid nephrolithiasis. *Curr Rheumatol Rep.* 2007 Jun;9(3):251-7

[189] "Average daily consumption of high fructose corn syrup is about 50 grams per person in the United States. With respect to total mercury exposure, it may be necessary to account for this source of mercury in the diet of children and sensitive populations." Dufault et al. Mercury from chlor-alkali plants: measured concentrations in food product sugar. *Environ Health.* 2009 Jan 26;8:2. See also: "High fructose corn syrup has been shown to contain trace amounts of mercury as a result of some manufacturing processes, and its consumption can also lead to zinc loss." Dufault et al. Mercury exposure, nutritional deficiencies and metabolic disruptions may affect learning in children. *Behav Brain Funct.* 2009 Oct 27;5:44.

[190] "Because of the clinical presentation [severe hypertension in children] and the finding of elevated catecholamines, most of the patients were first studied for possible pheochromocytoma. Subsequently, elevated levels of mercury were found." Torres AD, Rai AN, Hardiek ML. Mercury intoxication and arterial hypertension: report of two patients and review of the literature. *Pediatrics.* 2000 Mar;105(3):E34

[191] Houston MC. The role of mercury and cadmium heavy metals in vascular disease, hypertension, coronary heart disease, and myocardial infarction. *Altern Ther Health Med.* 2007 Mar-Apr;13(2):S128-33

- <u>Arachidonate avoidance</u>: Arachidonate promotes intracellular calcium accumulation which promotes the development of HTN. Avoidance of arachidonic acid helps restore intracellular ion homeostasis and results in reduction of elevated BP. Restoration of fatty acid balance via simultaneous reduced intake of arachidonate and increased intake of oleic acid (found in olive oil), gamma-linolenic acid (found in borage seed oil, hemp seed oil, black currant seed oil, and evening primrose oil), and eicosapentaenoic acid (EPA) and docosahexaenoic acid (DHA) (both from cold-water fish oil) helps reduce intracellular hypercalcinosis that promotes chronic HTN in addition to effecting beneficial changes in inflammatory, hemorrheologic, and coagulation indices.

- <u>Fish oil or combination fatty acid supplementation</u>: The cardioprotective benefits of fish oil are insufficiently represented by the minimal numerical reduction in blood pressure that is achieved with this intervention. Despite only lowering blood pressure by a few points (if at all), n-3 fatty acids are safer, less expensive, and more effective than statin and fibrate antihypercholesterolemic drug treatment for reducing total and cardiovascular mortality.[192] Thus, combination fatty acid supplementation should be used for its pronounced cardioprotective benefits regardless of its modest ability to reduce elevated blood pressure. The combination of EPA+DHA from fish oil and GLA from borage oil (or other source) in a ratio of approximately 2:1 (e.g., daily intake of 4 grams EPA+DHA along with 2 grams GLA) appears to provide the best cardioprotective benefit based on favorable changes in serum lipids, according to a speculative prospective clinical trial by Laidlaw and Holub.[193]

- <u>Correction of vitamin D deficiency</u>: Vitamin D3 (cholecalciferol)—with or without calcium supplementation—can reduce blood pressure in cholecalciferol-deficient hypertensive patients as effectively as the use of antihypertensive medication. As I have discussed in extensive detail elsewhere, a reasonable dose of vitamin D3 for adults is in the range of 4,000-10,000 IU per day, and doctors new to vitamin D therapy should read our clinical monograph published in 2004 and available on-line.[194] The most important drug interaction with vitamin D3 is seen with hydrochlorothiazide (HCTZ), a commonly-used antihypertensive diuretic that promotes hypercalcemia. Vitamin D supplementation in patients taking HCTZ must be implemented slowly, with professional supervision, and with laboratory monitoring of serum calcium at days 10, 30, and 60 following the use of combined cholecalciferol-HCTZ treatment. The goal of vitamin D3 supplementation is for serum 25-OH-vitamin D3 levels to reach the optimal range of 50-100 ng/ml, as shown in the diagram.

  - <u>Controlled clinical trial: Effects of short-term calcium supplementation with or without vitamin D3 supplementation on blood pressure and parathyroid hormone levels in elderly women.</u> (*Journal of Clinical Endocrinology and Metabolism* 2001 Apr[195]): In an 8-week study of 148 elderly women (average age 74 years) with a 25-hydroxycholecalciferol (25OHD(3)) level <20 ng/ml (<50 nmol/l), daily administration of 1200 mg calcium plus 800 IU vitamin D3 (note: very low dose of vitamin D) was superior to 1200 mg calcium without vitamin D. Vitamin D plus calcium resulted in an increase in serum 25OHD(3) of 72%, a decrease in serum PTH of 17%, a decrease in heart rate of 5.4%, and a decrease in blood pressure of approximately -13/-7 mm Hg. These results are clinically important because of the significant alleviation of hypertension that is noted, even despite the low dose of vitamin D3 that was used. Collateral benefits in muscle strength, mood, cognition, balance (and reduced falling), and enhanced resistance to infection are commonly noted with vitamin D3 supplementation; such benefits are not seen with antihypertensive drug use.

  - <u>Placebo-controlled clinical trial: Vitamin D improves endothelial function and reduces blood pressure in patients with Type 2 diabetes mellitus and low vitamin D levels</u> (*Diabetic Medicine* 2008 Mar[196]): In a double-blind, parallel group, placebo-controlled randomized trial, a single dose of 100,000 IU vitamin D2 (note the use of ergocalciferol, the less effective form of vitamin D compared with cholecalciferol, vitamin D3) or placebo was administered to patients with Type-2 diabetes mellitus (DM-2) who were vitamin D deficient

[192] "Compared with control groups, risk ratios for overall mortality were 0.87 for statins, 1.00 for fibrates, 0.84 for resins, 0.96 for niacin, 0.77 for n-3 fatty acids, and 0.97 for diet. Compared with control groups, risk ratios for cardiac mortality indicated benefit from statins (0.78), resins (0.70) and n-3 fatty acids (0.68)." Studer M, Briel M, Leimenstoll B, Glass TR, Bucher HC. Effect of different antilipidemic agents and diets on mortality: a systematic review. *Arch Intern Med.* 2005 Apr 11;165(7):725-30

[193] "A mixture of 4 g EPA+DHA and 2 g GLA favorably altered blood lipid and fatty acid profiles in healthy women. On the basis of calculated PROCAM values, the 4:2 group was estimated to have a 43% reduction in the 10-y risk of myocardial infarction." Laidlaw M, Holub BJ. Effects of supplementation with fish oil-derived n-3 fatty acids and gamma-linolenic acid on circulating plasma lipids and fatty acid profiles in women. *Am J Clin Nutr.* 2003 Jan;77(1):37-42

[194] Vasquez A, Manso G, Cannell J. The clinical importance of vitamin D (cholecalciferol). *Altern Ther Health Med.* 2004 Sep-Oct;10(5):28-36

[195] "A short-term supplementation with vitamin D(3) and calcium is more effective in reducing SBP than calcium alone. Inadequate vitamin D(3) and calcium intake could play a contributory role in the pathogenesis and progression of hypertension and cardiovascular disease in elderly women." Pfeifer et al. Effects of a short-term vitamin D(3) and calcium supplementation on blood pressure and parathyroid hormone levels in elderly women. *J Clin Endocrinol Metab.* 2001 Apr;86(4):1633-7

[196] Sugden et al. Vitamin D improves endothelial function in patients with Type 2 diabetes mellitus and low vitamin D levels. *Diabet Med.* 2008 Mar;25(3):320-5

with an average baseline 25-hydroxyvitamin D level <20 ng/ml (<50 nmol/l). Benefits of vitamin D supplementation included significantly improved flow mediated vasodilatation (FMD) of the brachial artery by 2.3% and significantly decreased systolic blood pressure by -14 mmHg compared with placebo. Total reduction in blood pressure for vitamin D compared to placebo (per Table 2 of the original article) was -13.9/-4.5 mm Hg.

- <u>Vitamin C (ascorbic acid) 3 g/d or bowel tolerance</u>: Since ascorbic acid is biochemically synthesized from glucose, these molecules remain structurally similar; not surprisingly therefore, an excess of glucose (i.e., as in hyperglycemia) reduces cellular uptake of ascorbic acid, leading to a relative "cellular scurvy" even in the absence of the classic presentation of scurvy. "In neutrophils from different volunteers, glucose inhibited uptake and accumulation of ascorbic acid by both transport activities 3-9-fold. ... Glucose-induced inhibition of both ascorbic acid transport activities occurred in neutrophils of all donors tested and was fully reversible."[197]

  - <u>Clinical trial: Vitamin C for refractory hypertension in elderly patients (*Arzneimittelforschung* 2006[198])</u>: Treatment with ascorbic acid 600 mg/d for 6 months was evaluated for effects on blood pressure and levels of C-reactive protein, 8-isoprostane, and malondialdehyde-modified low-density lipoproteins among 12 elderly patients (average age 78.3y) and 12 adult patients (average age 54.6y) with refractory hypertension. Treatment with ascorbic acid markedly reduced systolic blood pressure in the elderly group from 154.9 to 134.8 mmHg (p < 0.001); pulse pressure reduced from 79.1 to 63.4. These benefits of vitamin C supplementation were accompanied by an increase in the serum levels of ascorbic acid and decreases in the levels of C-reactive protein, 8-isoprostane, and malondialdehyde-modified low-density lipoproteins. In contrast, ascorbic acid did not affect blood pressure in the adult nonelderly group. These results suggest that ascorbic acid is useful for controlling blood pressure in elderly patients with refractory hypertension." Clinicians should appreciate that elevated systolic blood pressure is an important predictor of cardiovascular mortality in elderly patients, and that its ascorbate-induced reduction by -20 mmHg is highly clinically significant.

- <u>Urinary alkalinization</u>: In non-pathologic states, the pattern of dietary intake is the single most important determinant of systemic/urine acid-base balance.[199] The two main classes of acids of physiologic importance are 1) carbonic acid—formed when carbon dioxide (CO_2) from metabolism of carbohydrates and fatty acids combines with water (H_2O) to form carbonic acid (H_2CO_3), and 2) noncarbonic acids—these are primarily generated from the oxidation of sulfur-containing amino acids which results in the formation of sulfuric acid (H_2SO_4); avoidance of the former is mostly achieved via respiration (i.e., removal of CO_2) while elimination of the latter requires bicarbonate and renal excretion.[200] Average urine pH among societies consuming a Paleo-Mediterranean diet and obtaining daily physical exercise is 7.5-9; clearly this very alkaline state reflects a diet high in fruits and vegetables, and provides physiologic benefits including increased excretion of xenobiotics[201] and renal retention of potassium, magnesium, and calcium. For example, among New Guinean hunter-gatherer tribal groups living in the *primitive feral condition*, "urine pH of adults was usually between 7.5 and 9.0 because of potassium bicarbonate and carbonate excretion."[202] Excess urine alkalinity can predispose to urinary tract infections; thus some clinicians may be more comfortable with a urine pH goal of approximately 7.5-8.0.

  - <u>Clinical trial: Neutralization of Western diet inhibits bone resorption independently of K intake and reduces cortisol secretion in humans (*American Journal of Physiology - Renal Physiology* 2003 Jan[203])</u>: Acid-base neutralization by substituting equimolar amounts of sodium bicarbonate and potassium bicarbonate for NaCl and KCl "induced a significant cumulative calcium retention (10.7 +/- 0.4 mmol) and significantly reduced the urinary excretion of deoxypyridinoline, pyridinoline, and n-telopeptide. Mean daily plasma cortisol decreased from 264 to 232 nmol/l (P = 0.032), ... An acidogenic Western diet results in mild

---

[197] Washko P, Levine M. Inhibition of ascorbic acid transport in human neutrophils by glucose. *J Biol Chem*. 1992 Nov 25;267(33):23568-74

[198] Sato et al. Effects of ascorbic acid on ambulatory blood pressure in elderly patients with refractory hypertension. *Arzneimittelforschung*. 2006;56(7):535-40

[199] "Nutrition has long been known to strongly influence acid-base balance. Recently, we have shown that it is possible to appropriately estimate the renal net acid excretion (NAE) of healthy subjects from the composition of their diets." Remer T. Influence of nutrition on acid-base balance--metabolic aspects. *Eur J Nutr*. 2001 Oct;40(5):214-20

[200] Rennke HG, Denker BM. *Renal Physiology: The Essentials. 2nd Edition*. Philadelphia: Lippincott Williams and Wilkins; 2007, p129

[201] "Urine alkalinization is a treatment regimen that increases poison elimination by the administration of intravenous sodium bicarbonate to produce urine with a pH > or = 7.5." Proudfoot AT, Krenzelok EP, Vale JA. Position Paper on urine alkalinization. *J Toxicol Clin Toxicol*. 2004;42(1):1-26

[202] Sebastian et al. Estimation of the net acid load of the diet of ancestral preagricultural Homo sapiens and their hominid ancestors. *Am J Clin Nutr*. 2002 Dec;76(6):1308-16

[203] Maurer M, Riesen W, Muser J, Hulter HN, Krapf R. Neutralization of Western diet inhibits bone resorption independently of K intake and reduces cortisol secretion in humans. *Am J Physiol Renal Physiol*. 2003 Jan;284(1):F32-40

metabolic acidosis in association with a state of cortisol excess, altered divalent ion metabolism, and increased bone resorptive indices. Acidosis-induced increases in cortisol secretion and plasma concentration may play a role in mild acidosis-induced alterations in bone metabolism and possibly in osteoporosis associated with an acidogenic Western diet." Clinicians should appreciate that long-term reductions in cortisol along with renal retention of calcium would be expected to have a favorable effect on blood pressure.

- Review: Diet, evolution and aging—the pathophysiologic effects of the post-agricultural inversion of the potassium-to-sodium and base-to-chloride ratios in the human diet (*European Journal of Nutrition* 2001 Oct[204]): This excellent review article discusses the changes in mineral intake (i.e., less potassium complicated by more sodium) and the shift from a plant-based alkalinizing diet to a pseudo-food acidifying diet and the physiological ramifications of these dietary changes. Note their conclusion in the following quote which states that any level of acidosis may be unacceptable and that (conversely) a state of alkalinization is the normal and ideal human condition: "We argue that any level of acidosis may be unacceptable from an evolutionarily perspective, and indeed, that **a low-grade metabolic alkalosis may be the optimal acid-base state for humans.**"

- Clinical trial: Urine alkalization facilitates uric acid excretion (*Nutrition Journal* 2010 Oct[205]): Highly consistent with and positively affirming of the protocol and paradigm advocated in this text, this clinical trial published in *Nutrition Journal* in 2010, authors of this study note that "Increase in the incidence of hyperuricemia associated with gout as well as hypertension, renal diseases and cardiovascular diseases has been a public health concern." Their clinical trial therefore sought to increase renal excretion of uric acid by altering urine pH via dietary improvement, moving in the direction of a more plant-based and more Paleo-Mediterranean diet. The authors made recipes consisting of "protein-rich and less vegetable-fruit food materials" (acid diet) and of "less protein but vegetable-fruit rich food materials" (alkali diet). Urine pH reached a steady state 3 days after switching from ordinary daily diets to specified regimens. Results showed that H+ (acidity) in urine is directly affected by the metabolic degradation of food materials, and that uric acid and excreted urine pH retained a linear relationship; the higher

> **Diet optimization is the "safest and most economical" intervention to lower the total body load of uric acid**
>
> "This study has clarified that alkalization of urine by the manipulation of food materials promotes the removal of uric acid. When one pays enough attention to the construction of a nutritionally balanced menu, dietary intervention becomes the safest and the most economical way for the prevention of hyperuricemia."
>
> Kanbara et al. Urine alkalization facilitates uric acid excretion. *Nutrition Journal* 2010, 9:45 nutritionj.com/content/9/1/45

the pH (more alkaline), the greater the uric acid excretion. The authors concluded, "We conclude that alkalization of urine by eating nutritionally well-designed food is effective for removing uric acid from the body." Given the increasing evidence that intracellular urate directly contributes to microvascular disease and the anticipated pathological complications in the brain, kidneys, and cardiovascular system[206], reducing the total body load of uric acid (i.e., the composite load in intracellular and extracellular/plasma compartments) is justified and warranted.

- Cocoa & Dark Chocolate (*Theobroma cacao*): Cacao has been cultivated for thousands of years in South and Central America; currently most production comes from Africa as well as various other countries such as Belize. The word chocolate came into English from Spanish and entered Spanish either from the Aztecs ("chocolatl" or "chicolatl") or the Maya ("chokol"). Among its numerous constituents, alkaloids such as theobromine and phenethylamine and various antioxidants such as epicatechin and procyanidins have received the most attention. Dark chocolate *without added sugar* and *without the addition of excess fat or cow's milk* provides antioxidant, cardioprotective, neuroprotective, and anticancer benefits. People who regularly consume higher levels of cocoa (suggested range 10-30 grams up to 100 grams daily) have lower BP and a -50% relative reduction in cardiovascular and all-cause mortality; regarding the mechanism of action for the BP-lowering

---

[204] Frassetto L, Morris RC Jr, Sellmeyer DE, Todd K, Sebastian A. Diet, evolution and aging—the pathophysiologic effects of the post-agricultural inversion of the potassium-to-sodium and base-to-chloride ratios in the human diet. *Eur J Nutr*. 2001 Oct;40(5):200-13

[205] "We conclude that alkalization of urine by eating nutritionally well-designed food is effective for removing uric acid from the body." Kanbara A, Hakoda M, Seyama I. Urine alkalization facilitates uric acid excretion. *Nutrition Journal* 2010, 9:45 nutritionj.com/content/9/1/45

[206] "...dietary intake of sugars rich in fructose may be driving the development of microvascular disease as a consequence of raising intracellular uric acid." Kanbay M, Sánchez-Lozada LG, Franco M, Madero M, Solak Y, Rodriguez-Iturbe B, Covic A, Johnson RJ. Microvascular disease and its role in the brain and cardiovascular system: a potential role for uric acid as a cardiorenal toxin. *Nephrol Dial Transplant*. 2010 Oct 8. [Epub ahead of print]

effect of chocolate: flavonoids in cacao upregulate nitric oxide synthase in endothelial cells, and thus chocolate improves endothelial function.[207] The cocoa content should be at least 65% and preferably 85%-90%. In December 2009, MD Anderson Cancer Center endorsed dark chocolate for its probable cancer-preventive benefits.[208] Because of its stimulating effects, cocoa should be consumed in the earlier part of the day in order to avoid sleep disturbance.

- Systematic review and meta-analysis: Benefits of cocoa products on blood pressure (*American Journal of Hypertension* 2010 Jan[209]): For this systematic review, the authors performed a meta-analysis of randomized controlled trials assessing the antihypertensive effects of flavanol-rich cocoa products. They found that among 10 randomized controlled trials with a total of 297 individuals (either healthy normotensive adults or patients with prehypertension/stage 1 hypertension), systolic BP dropped -4.5 mm Hg while diastolic BP dropped -2.5 mm Hg following cocoa consumption for durations of 2-18 weeks. The authors concluded that "The meta-analysis confirms the BP-lowering capacity of flavanol-rich cocoa products...." Rather than rendering the typical cautionary note ("…questions such as the most appropriate dose and the long-term side effect profile warrant further investigation before cocoa products can be recommended as a treatment option in hypertension."), the authors might have been more wise to suggest increased consumption of chocolate for its antihypertensive and cardioprotective benefits and its greater safety profile compared to pharmaceutical drugs.

- Randomized controlled trial: Effects of habitual cocoa intake on blood pressure and bioactive nitric oxide (*JAMA—Journal of the American Medical Association* 2007 Jul[210]): The authors of this clinical trial review previously published research and note that regular intake of cocoa-containing foods is linked to lower cardiovascular mortality and that short-term interventions show that **high doses of cocoa can improve endothelial function and reduce BP due to the action of the cocoa polyphenols**. Their clinical trial design was a randomized, controlled, investigator-blinded, parallel-group trial involving 44 adults aged 56 through 73 years (24 women, 20 men) with untreated upper-range prehypertension or stage 1 hypertension without comorbidity; the treatment was 6.3 g (30 kcal) per day of dark chocolate containing 30 mg of polyphenols or a placebo of polyphenol-free white chocolate. Main outcome measures were ❶ BP, ❷ plasma markers of vasodilative nitric oxide (S-nitrosoglutathione), ❸ oxidative stress (8-isoprostane), and ❹ bioavailability of cocoa polyphenols. "RESULTS: From baseline to 18 weeks, **dark chocolate reduced mean systolic BP by -2.9 mm Hg and diastolic BP by -1.9 mm Hg** without changes in body weight, plasma levels of lipids, glucose, and 8-isoprostane. **Hypertension prevalence declined from 86% to 68%.** The BP decrease was accompanied by a sustained increase of S-nitrosoglutathione by 0.23 nmol/L, and a dark chocolate dose resulted in the appearance of cocoa phenols in plasma. White chocolate intake caused no changes in BP or plasma biomarkers. CONCLUSIONS: Data in this relatively small sample of otherwise healthy individuals with above-optimal BP indicate that **inclusion of small amounts of polyphenol-rich dark chocolate as part of a usual diet efficiently reduced BP and improved formation of vasodilative nitric oxide.**"

- Randomized controlled single-blind crossover trial: Benefits of acute dark chocolate and cocoa ingestion on endothelial function (*American Journal of Clinical Nutrition* 2008 Jul[211]): The purpose of this clinical trial (n = 45, BMI = 30, age = 53y) was to assess the acute effects of solid dark chocolate and liquid cocoa intake on endothelial function and blood pressure in overweight adults. First, subjects were randomly assigned to consume a solid dark chocolate bar (containing 22 g cocoa powder) or a cocoa-free placebo bar (containing 0 g cocoa powder). In the second part of the trial, subjects were randomly assigned to consume sugar-free cocoa (containing 22 g cocoa powder), sugared cocoa (containing 22 g cocoa powder), or a placebo (containing 0 g cocoa powder). "RESULTS: Solid dark chocolate and liquid cocoa ingestion improved endothelial function (measured as [ultrasound-visualized] flow-mediated dilatation) compared

[207] Nahas R. Complementary and alternative medicine approaches to blood pressure reduction: An evidence-based review. *Can Fam Physician.* 2008 Nov;54(11):1529-33

[208] "In addition to being delicious, moderate amounts of dark chocolate may play a role in cancer prevention. ... To get those cancer prevention benefits, the chocolate should contain at least 65% cocoa. Winters R. Focused on Health - December 2009. mdanderson.org/publications/focused-on-health/issues/2009-december/share-the-health.html Accessed January 15, 2010

[209] Desch et al. Effect of cocoa products on blood pressure: systematic review and meta-analysis. *Am J Hypertens.* 2010 Jan;23(1):97-103

[210] Taubert et al. Effects of low habitual cocoa intake on blood pressure and bioactive nitric oxide: a randomized controlled trial. *JAMA.* 2007 Jul 4;298(1):49-60

[211] Faridi et al. Acute dark chocolate and cocoa ingestion and endothelial function: a randomized controlled crossover trial. *Am J Clin Nutr.* 2008 Jul;88(1):58-63

with placebo (dark chocolate: 4.3% compared with -1.8% [for placebo]; sugar-free and sugared cocoa: 5.7% and 2.0% compared with -1.5%). Blood pressure decreased after the ingestion of dark chocolate and sugar-free cocoa compared with *placebo* (dark chocolate: systolic, -3.2 mm Hg compared with 2.7 mm Hg; and diastolic -1.4 mm Hg compared with 2.7 mm Hg; sugar-free cocoa: systolic, -2.1 mm Hg compared with 3.2 mm Hg; and diastolic: -1.2 mm Hg compared with 2.8 mm Hg. Endothelial function improved significantly more with sugar-free than with regular cocoa (5.7 % compared with 2.0%). CONCLUSIONS: The acute ingestion of both solid dark chocolate and liquid cocoa improved endothelial function and lowered blood pressure in overweight adults. Sugar content may attenuate these effects, and sugar-free preparations may augment them." The practical application of this research is important to communicate to patients: to obtain the cardioprotective benefits of chocolate, the chocolate must be consumed without added sugar, i.e., it must be **dark chocolate**, *not* sugar-sweetened milk chocolate.

- Population-based inception cohort study with 8-year follow-up: Chocolate consumption and mortality following a first acute myocardial infarction: the Stockholm Heart Epidemiology Program (*Journal of Internal Medicine* 2009 Sep[212]): Authors of this study followed 1,169 non-diabetic patients hospitalized with a confirmed first acute myocardial infarction (AMI) between 1992 and 1994. Participants self-reported usual chocolate consumption over the preceding 12 months with a standardized questionnaire distributed during hospitalization. Participants were followed for 8 years. "RESULTS: Chocolate consumption had a strong inverse association with cardiac mortality. When compared with those never eating chocolate, the multivariable-adjusted hazard ratios were 0.73 (95% confidence interval, 0.41-1.31) for those consuming chocolate less than once per month, 0.56 (0.32-0.99) for up to once per week, and 0.34 (0.17-0.70) and twice or more per week respectively. [Note: dose-response relationships suggest causality.] Chocolate consumption generally had an inverse but weak association with total mortality and nonfatal outcomes. In contrast, intake of other sweets was not associated with cardiac or total mortality. CONCLUSIONS: Chocolate consumption was associated with lower cardiac mortality in a dose dependent manner in patients free of diabetes surviving their first AMI. Although our findings support increasing evidence that chocolate is a rich source of beneficial bioactive compounds, confirmation of this strong inverse relationship from other observational studies or large-scale, long-term, controlled randomized trials is needed." The importance of this study is that it suggests that the cardioprotective benefits of cocoa are not limited to short-term alleviation of hypertension but extend to a more generalized cardioprotective benefit; beyond this, the reduction in all-cause mortality is what we would expect from a functional food rich in bioactive health-promoting constituents. Limitations to this study include the self-selected nature of the intervention and lack of randomization; however, the large number of subjects (n = 1,169) serves to mitigate these methodological limitations.

- **Whey peptides, casokinins, and lactokinins**: Yet another benefit of whey protein consumption is the salutary effect on blood pressure, probably mediated by whey protein's anti-stress, anti-oxidant/pro-glutathione, and ACE-inhibiting properties. Very interestingly, the anti-hypertensive effects of milk peptides may depend on their specific hydrolysation by lactic acid producing bacteria in the intestines; thus, clinical anti-hypertensive benefit of milk/whey peptides may require establishment of eubiosis, eradication of intestinal dysbiosis, and/or co-supplementation with probiotics. (For extensive reviews on the clinical consequences of dysbiosis and the [re]establishment of eubiosis, see monographs[213] and book chapters[214] by Vasquez). Whey protein is commonly consumed in doses that provide 20-80 grams of protein per day; individual antihypertensive responses will, of course, vary.

  - Clinical trial: The long-term effects of whey protein isolate on blood pressure, vascular function, and inflammatory markers in overweight individuals. (*Obesity* 2010 Jul[215]): This study evaluated the effects of whey protein isolate (27 grams twice daily) on blood pressure, vascular function and inflammatory markers compared to the effects of casein and glucose (control) supplementation in overweight/obese individuals. Seventy men and women with average BMI of 31.3 completed this 12-week study. Blood pressure

[212] Janszky et al. Chocolate consumption and mortality following a first acute myocardial infarction. *J Intern Med.* 2009 Sep;266(3):248-57
[213] Vasquez A. Reducing Pain and Inflammation Naturally - Part 6: Nutritional and Botanical Treatments against "Silent Infections" and Gastrointestinal Dysbiosis, Commonly Overlooked Causes of Neuromusculoskeletal Inflammation and Chronic Health Problems. *Nutritional Perspectives* 2006; 29 (January): 5-21
[214] Chapter Four in: Vasquez A. *Integrative Rheumatology*. IBMRC 2006, 2007 and all later versions.
[215] Pal S, Ellis V. The chronic effects of whey proteins on blood pressure, vascular function, and inflammatory markers in overweight individuals. *Obesity.* 2010 Jul;18(7):1354-9

reductions due to whey protein isolate were noted at 6 weeks and were significant for systolic and diastolic pressures at 12 weeks of supplementation. No significant changes in inflammatory markers were noted. This study demonstrated that supplementation with whey protein improves blood pressure and vascular function (assessed by the augmentation index) in overweight and obese individuals. Systolic blood pressure (SBP) decreased significantly by 3% at week 6 (115.5 mm Hg) and by 4% at week 12 (114.5 mm Hg) compared to baseline (119.3 mm Hg) in the whey protein group. A significant decrease of 3.3% in diastolic blood pressure (DBP) at week 12 (62.0 mm Hg) compared with baseline (64.1 mm Hg) in the whey protein group was noted. Thus, the total BP reduction by whey protein isolate in this study is approximately -4.8/-2.1 mm Hg.

- <u>Clinical trial: Effects of whey protein isolate on body composition, lipids, insulin and glucose in overweight and obese individuals. (*British Journal of Nutrition* 2010 Sep[216])</u>: Whey protein isolate supplementation in 70 men and women with a mean age of 48.4 years and a mean BMI of 31.3 for 12 weeks in a parallel study design resulted in no significant change in body composition or serum glucose at 12 weeks compared with the control (glucose) or casein group. A significant decrease in total cholesterol and LDL cholesterol at week 12 in the whey protein isolate group compared with the casein and control groups was noted. Fasting insulin levels and homeostasis model assessment of insulin resistance scores were also significantly decreased in the whey protein isolate group compared with the control group. The present study demonstrated that supplementation with whey protein isolate improves fasting lipids and insulin levels in overweight and obese individuals.

- <u>Randomized cross-over clinical trial: The acute effects of four protein meals on insulin, glucose, appetite, and energy intake in lean men. (*British Journal of Nutrition* 2010 Oct[217])</u>: The authors note that different dietary proteins vary in their ability to influence satiety and reduce food intake. The present study compared the effects of four protein meals—whey, tuna, turkey, and egg albumin—on postprandial glucose and insulin concentrations as well as on appetite measures and energy intake in 22 lean healthy men. Results showed that blood glucose response after the consumption of the test meal measured as area under the curve (AUC) was significantly lower with the whey meal and tuna meal than with the turkey and egg meals. The AUC blood insulin was significantly higher with the whey meal than with the tuna, turkey and egg meals; however, the AUC rating of hunger was significantly lower with the whey meal than with the tuna, turkey, and egg meals. Mean energy intake at the ad libitum meal following the protein meal was significantly lower with the whey meal than with the tuna, egg, and turkey meals. Results showed that whey protein meal produced a greater acute insulin response, reduced appetite and decreased ad libitum energy intake at a subsequent meal compared with the other protein meals, indicating a potential for appetite suppression and weight loss in overweight or obese individuals. This is a very interesting study showing that even though whey protein acutely elevates insulin levels postprandially, the reduced appetite and calorie intake induced by whey protein consumption may actually help patients lose weight.

- <u>Review: Lactokinins are whey protein-derived ACE inhibitory peptides (*Nahrung* 1999 Jun[218])</u>: Whey protein contains lactokinins, peptides that function as ACE-inhibitors. "Peptides derived from the major whey proteins, i.e. alpha-lactalbumin (alpha-la) and beta-lactoglobulin (beta-lg) in addition to bovine serum albumin (BSA), inhibit ACE. ... While they do not have the inhibitory potency of synthetic drugs commonly used in the treatment of hypertension, these naturally occurring peptides may represent nutraceutical/functional food ingredients for the prevention/treatment of high blood pressure."

- <u>Review: Milk protein-derived peptide inhibitors of angiotensin-I-converting enzyme (*British Journal of Nutrition* 2000 Nov[219])</u>: "Numerous casein and whey protein-derived angiotensin-I-converting enzyme (ACE) inhibitory peptides/hydrolysates have been identified. Clinical trials in hypertensive animals and humans show that these peptides/hydrolysates can bring about a significant reduction in hypertension. These peptides/hydrolysates may be classified as functional food ingredients and nutraceuticals due to

---

[216] Pal et al. Effects of whey protein isolate on body composition, lipids, insulin and glucose in overweight and obese individuals. *Br J Nutr.* 2010 Sep;104(5):716-23
[217] Pal S, Ellis V. The acute effects of four protein meals on insulin, glucose, appetite and energy intake in lean men. *Br J Nutr.* 2010 Oct;104(8):1241-8
[218] FitzGerald RJ, Meisel H. Lactokinins: whey protein-derived ACE inhibitory peptides. *Nahrung.* 1999 Jun;43(3):165-7
[219] FitzGerald RJ, Meisel H. Milk protein-derived peptide inhibitors of angiotensin-I-converting enzyme. *Br J Nutr.* 2000 Nov;84 Suppl 1:S33-

their ability to provide health benefits i.e. as functional food ingredients in reducing the risk of developing a disease and as nutraceuticals in the prevention/treatment of disease."

- Review: Hypotensive peptides from milk proteins (*Journal of Nutrition* 2004 Apr[220]): "Milk proteins, both caseins and whey proteins, are a rich source of ACE inhibitory peptides. Several studies in spontaneously hypertensive rats show that these casokinins and lactokinins can significantly reduce blood pressure. Furthermore, a limited number of human studies have associated milk protein-derived peptides with statistically significant hypotensive effects (i.e., lower systolic and diastolic pressures)."

- **L-Arginine**: L-arginine (Arg) is the amino acid precursor for the formation of vasodilating nitric oxide (NO) produced via the action of endothelial nitric oxide synthase. A significant number of hypertensive patients have impaired conversion of Arg into NO, and a subset of these patients benefit from oral Arg supplementation. As usual, amino acid supplementation is delivered between meals (empty stomach) to facilitate absorption, and coadministration of simple carbohydrate can facilitate insulin-mediated cellular amino acid uptake. Recently, asymmetric dimethylarginine (ADMA) has been identified as an independent cardiovascular risk factor; per the excellent review by Böger[221], clinicians should appreciate that ADMA—formed from degradation of methylated proteins and an endogenous competitive inhibitor of NO synthase (NOS)—is a vasoconstrictor found in elevated levels among patients with hypercholesterolemia, atherosclerosis, hypertension, chronic renal failure, chronic heart failure, hyperthyroidism, hyperhomocysteinemia and folate deficiency. As expected, administration of Arg has demonstrated antihypertensive benefit, particularly among patients with high ADMA levels; indeed, elevated ADMA may identify which patients are likely to respond to Arg supplementation via a more favorable Arg:ADMA ratio. Laboratory testing for ADMA is available now from some research centers (such as Baylor[222]) and will surely become more widely available in the future. The predictable clinical take-home messages are that ❶ intravenous Arg administration generally produces a greater response than does oral administration, ❷ the hypotensive benefits of Arg supplementation are short-lived, ❸ the hypotensive benefits of Arg are more consistently seen in the groups expected to have high ADMA levels as previous listed, and ❹ younger patients (with less atherosclerosis and arterial calcification) are more likely to respond. Clinicians should appreciate that the cardioprotective benefits of Arg extend beyond and are not entirely dependent upon its antihypertensive benefit; other benefits include decreased platelet aggregation and adhesion, decreased monocyte adhesion, antiproliferative effects on vascular smooth muscle, and improved endothelium-dependent vasodilation which can occur locally and systemically without an accompanying hypotensive effect. Very importantly, concomitant administration of the amino acid N-acetyl-cysteine (NAC) appears to enhance the cardioprotective efficacy of Arg according to recent research.[223] Aside from the possibility of promoting reactivation of herpes simplex outbreaks, Arg is remarkably safe and is commonly used in immunonutrition formulas as a life-saving treatment in critically ill patients; Zhou and Martindale[224] recently noted, "The numerous potential beneficial effects of arginine in the critically ill patient include: 1) stimulation of immune function via its influence on lymphocyte, macrophage, and dendritic cells; 2) improved wound healing; 3) increased net nitrogen balance; 4) increased blood flow to key vascular beds; and 5) decreased clinical infections and length of hospital stay." The doses employed have ranged widely from 1,200 mg/d to 30,000 mg/d, (i.e., 1.2-30 g/d) and have included both oral and intravenous administration. Of course, Arg can be used with other dietary and nutritional interventions and with drug treatments with the caveat that common sense is employed to minimize the risk of hypotension by not initiating too many new treatments simultaneously in a given patient. While oral administration of L-arginine is generally considered beneficial at best and benign at worst, a report published in 2009 by Jahangir et al[225] showed that L-arginine supplementation at 9 grams per day for 4 days did not alter vascular reactivity but did increase methylation demand (shown by increased homocysteine to methionine ratio); this study and its implications (namely that

---

[220] FitzGerald RJ, Murray BA, Walsh DJ. Hypotensive peptides from milk proteins. *J Nutr.* 2004 Apr;134(4):980S-8S

[221] Böger RH. Asymmetric dimethylarginine, an endogenous inhibitor of nitric oxide synthase, explains the "L-arginine paradox" and acts as a novel cardiovascular risk factor. *J Nutr.* 2004 Oct;134(10 Suppl):2842S-2847S jn.nutrition.org/cgi/content/full/134/10/2842S

[222] Institute of Metabolic Disease at Baylor Research Institute. Asymmetric dimethylarginine (ADMA). baylorhealth.edu/imd/researchtests/asymmetric.htm Accessed Dec 2009

[223] Martina V, Masha A, Gigliardi VR, et al. Long-term N-acetylcysteine and L-arginine administration reduces endothelial activation and systolic blood pressure in hypertensive patients with type 2 diabetes. *Diabetes Care.* 2008 May;31(5):940-4 care.diabetesjournals.org/content/31/5/940.long

[224] "The numerous potential beneficial effects of arginine in the critically ill patient include: 1) stimulation of immune function via its influence on lymphocyte, macrophage, and dendritic cells; 2) improved wound healing; 3) increased net nitrogen balance; 4) increased blood flow to key vascular beds; and 5) decreased clinical infections and length of hospital stay." Zhou M, Martindale RG. Arginine in the critical care setting. *J Nutr.* 2007 Jun;137(6 Suppl 2):1687S-1692S jn.nutrition.org/cgi/content/full/137/6/1687S

[225] Jahangir et al. The effect of L-arginine and creatine on vascular function and homocysteine metabolism. *Vasc Med.* 2009 Aug;14(3):239-48

methylation factors such as folate, betaine, pyridoxine, and cobalamin might be coadministered with L-arginine to optimize vascular health and endothelial function) are reviewed at the end of this section on L-arginine.

- Open clinical trial: The effects of sustained-release L-arginine on blood pressure and vascular compliance in 29 healthy individuals (normotensives and hypertensives) treated for one week (*Alternative Medicine Review* 2006 Mar[226]): Miller used 2.1 g/d Arg administered in two divided doses in a sustained release preparation to find that approximately 65% of hypertensive patients responded favorably with an average reduction of -4/-3.7 mm Hg for the group as a whole that included normotensives and hypertensives. Among patients who were "borderline or hypertensive" the average BP reduction was -11/-4.9 mm Hg. Vascular elasticity assessed by digital pulse wave analysis showed a significant increase in large artery compliance (mean 23% improvement). Given the low dose, the short duration, and the low cost and absence of adverse effects, these results are worthy of clinical consideration and additional study. Consistent with many studies in clinical nutrition, the intervention provided an *alterative*, homeostatic effect in that—in contrast to the effects of pharmaceutical drugs—the effects are benign and rather minimal in healthy-normotensive persons and are clinically significant and therapeutic in patients with the index disease.

- Randomized placebo-controlled trial with 123 patients: Effect of L-arginine on blood pressure in pregnancy-induced hypertension (*Journal of Maternal-Fetal and Neonatal Medicine* 2006 May[227]): Inclusion criteria for this trial included maternal age range 16-45 years, diagnosis of gestational hypertension without proteinuria (patients normotensive until the 20th week), and gestational age ranging between 24 and 36 weeks. Subjects were allocated to receive either Arg 20 g/500 mL intravenously or placebo treatment through an i.v. line. Treatment or placebo was administered in the morning from 8-10 a.m. and was repeated for four consecutive days. The final analysis was performed on 62 women in the Arg group and 61 in the placebo group. "RESULTS: Maternal clinical features such as age, height, weight, and gestational age at inclusion were similar between groups. Both systolic and diastolic blood pressures were reduced by treatment, the effect of L-arginine being significantly higher than that of the placebo (systolic values $F = 8.59$, $p < 0.005$; diastolic values $F = 3.36$; $p < 0.001$). ... CONCLUSIONS: In conclusion, these data support the use of L-Arg as an antihypertensive agent for gestational hypertension especially in view of the other beneficial effects nitric oxide donors display in pregnancy. Further, L-Arg seems well tolerated since in this sample none of the patients reported adverse effects requiring study interruption." According to Figure 4 of the article, BP reductions due to arginine supplementation were approximately -5/-8 mm Hg.

- Double-blind placebo-controlled clinical trial: Long-term N-acetylcysteine and L-arginine administration reduces endothelial activation and systolic blood pressure in hypertensive patients with type 2 diabetes (*Diabetes Care* 2008 May[228]): This double-blind trial included 24 male patients with type-2 DM and HTN divided into two groups of 12 patients that randomly received either placebo or NAC 1,200 mg/d and ARG 1,200 mg/d orally for 6 months. "RESULTS—The NAC + ARG treatment caused a reduction of both systolic and diastolic mean arterial blood pressure, total cholesterol, LDL cholesterol, oxidized LDL, high-sensitive C-reactive protein, intracellular adhesion molecule, vascular cell adhesion molecule, nitrotyrosine, fibrinogen, and plasminogen activator inhibitor-1, and an improvement of the intima-media thickness during endothelial postischemic vasodilation. HDL cholesterol increased. No changes in other parameters studied were observed. CONCLUSIONS—NAC + ARG administration seems to be a potential well-tolerated antiatherogenic therapy because it improves endothelial function in hypertensive patients with type 2 diabetes by improving NO bioavailability via reduction of oxidative stress and increase of NO production. Our study's results give prominence to its potential use in primary and secondary cardiovascular prevention in these patients." The **BP change in the treatment group was -5/-5 mm Hg**; the results of this study are remarkable considering the low dose of Arg employed and the manifold biochemical benefits attained.

---

[226] Miller AL. The effects of sustained-release-L-arginine formulation on blood pressure and vascular compliance in 29 healthy individuals. *Altern Med Rev*. 2006 Mar;11(1):23-9

[227] Neri et al. Effect of L-arginine on blood pressure in pregnancy-induced hypertension: a randomized placebo-controlled trial. *J Matern Fetal Neonatal Med*. 2006 May:277-81

[228] Martina V, Masha A, Gigliardi VR, et al. Long-term N-acetylcysteine and L-arginine administration reduces endothelial activation and systolic blood pressure in hypertensive patients with type 2 diabetes. *Diabetes Care*. 2008 May;31(5):940-4 care.diabetesjournals.org/content/31/5/940.long

- Review: L-arginine and cardiovascular system (*Pharmacological Reports* 2005 Jan-Feb[229]): "The majority of experimental and clinical studies clearly show a beneficial effect of L-arginine on endothelium in conditions associated with its hypofunction and thus with reduced NO synthesis. Some clinical studies involving healthy volunteers or patients suffering from hypertension and diabetes indicate that it may also regulate vascular hemostasis." The full text of this article goes on to itemize several clinical trials (at variable level of detail), the majority of these synopses related to HTN are summarized here:

Adverse effects of elevated homocysteine
• Activation of coagulation
• Stimulation of monocyte adhesion
• Enhanced oxidation of low density lipoprotein (LDL),
• Impairment of NO-mediated vascular responses (vasodilation)
• Adverse effects on bone health and increased risk for osteoporosis
• Neuroinflammation, activation of glutamate receptors
• Mitochondrial impairment
• Endothelial dysfunction, relative or absolute vasoconstriction

  - Placebo controlled trial of 30 g (thirty grams) Arg infused intravenously over 30 minutes to healthy volunteers: Diastolic BP was "markedly reduced" more than was systolic BP; another study conducted in women found similar results.
  - Consumption of an Arg-enriched diet by healthy volunteers: BP reduction.
  - Oral administration of 21g daily to healthy young men for 3 days: No correlation of Arg with blood pressure.
  - Oral administration of 20g daily to healthy men for 28 days: No reduction in BP.
  - Oral administration of 9g daily to healthy subjects for 6 months: No reduction in BP; however, "long-term administration of this amino acid had a favorable effect on endothelium, improving its function and reducing concentration of endothelin." (Endothelins are peptides that constrict blood vessels and contribute to HTN.)
  - Intravenous Arg given at a dose of 500 mg/kg in patients with primary and secondary hypertension: "Considerable reduction both in systolic and diastolic pressure in all the cases."
  - Intravenous Arg given at a dose of 30g over 60 minutes in patients with treated/untreated HTN: Previously untreated HTN patients had the best clinical response, followed by ACEi-treated patients, and a slight BP reduction in normal volunteers.
  - Oral Arg 5.6 or 12.6 g/day for 6 weeks in patients with heart failure: Reduction in arterial blood pressure.
  - Oral Arg 21 g for 3 days to young men with coronary artery disease: No changes in blood pressure despite improvement in brachial artery dilation.
  - Intravenous bolus of 3g Arg to healthy subjects and patients with insulin-independent diabetes, hypercholesterolemia and primary hypertension: Best response was seen in young healthy patients (response inverse to age), then hypertensives, and lastly in patients with hypercholesterolemia and DM.
  - Oral Arg 21 g/d for 4 weeks in young patients with hypercholesterolemia: Improved endothelium-dependent dilatation.
  - Intravenous infusion of Arg 30 g for 60 minutes in patients with limb ischemia: "Marked reduction in diastolic and systolic pressure and an increased blood flow in the femoral artery."
- Randomized placebo-controlled clinical trial: The effect of L-arginine and creatine on vascular function and homocysteine metabolism (*Vascular Medicine* 2009 Aug[230]): The authors introduce their study by noting that studies with L-arginine supplementation have shown inconsistent effects on endothelial function (readers will have noted this from the studies reviewed above). The authors point out that, while L-arginine is a nitric oxide precursor, it is also the precursor to guanidinoacetate (GAA), which leads to the formation of creatine and the consumption of methionine to produce homocysteine, thereby utilizing methyl groups and increasing methylation demand. The purpose of this study was to investigate the effect of supplementation with L-arginine and creatine (alone or in combination) on vascular function and methylation/homocysteine metabolism. Patients with documented CAD (n=109) were randomized to

[229] Cylwik D, Mogielnicki A, Buczko W. L-arginine and cardiovascular system. *Pharmacol Rep*. 2005 Jan-Feb;57(1):14-22 if-pan.krakow.pl/pjp/pdf/2005/1_14.pdf
[230] Jahangir et al. The effect of L-arginine and creatine on vascular function and homocysteine metabolism. *Vasc Med*. 2009 Aug;14(3):239-48

receive L-arginine (9gm/d), creatine (21gm/day), L-arginine plus creatine, or placebo for 4 days (n=26–29 per group); brachial artery flow-mediated dilation and plasma levels of L-arginine, creatine, homocysteine, methionine, and GAA were measured at baseline and follow up. Results of this study showed that L-arginine and creatine supplementation had no effects on vascular function; we could argue that 4 days is insufficient duration to produce changes in physiologic function. L-arginine increased GAA (P<0.01) and the ratio of homocysteine to methionine (from 0.7 to 0.9; P<0.01) suggesting increased methylation demand. Supplementation with L-arginine increased plasma homocysteine from 11.1 micromol/L to 11.2 micromol/L (P=0.006); one could easily argue that such a minute change is clinically insignificant, while one could also argue that a negative change within the span of 4 days of supplementation portends a potentially hazardous trend if carried out for months and years, especially in the large number of patients with defective or deficient methylation pathways.

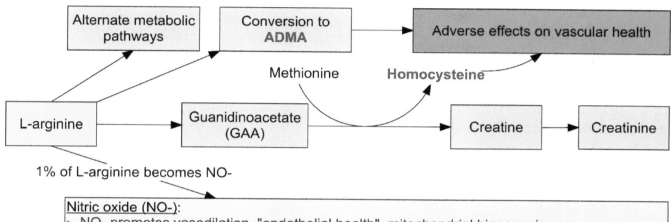

L-arginine conversion to nitric oxide and ADMA, effect on methionine-homocysteine metabolism: Beyond the lure and lore of biochemistry, this pathway shows that administration of arginine might promote depletion of methyl groups in patients deficient (nutritionally) or impaired (genetically, hormonally) in this pathway. Utilization of methyl groups via S-adenosyl methionine (SAMe) results in elevated homocysteine and depletion of methyl groups if methylation factors such as folate are in short supply. L-arginine (whether as an isolated supplement or as contained within dietary proteins) can be converted into asymmetric dimethylarginine (ADMA)—notably by Gram-negative and dysbiotic bacteria (or possibly via the inflammatory response thereto) such as *Helicobacter pylori*, but also endogenously (e.g., in adipocytes), especially in patients at heightened cardiometabolic risk—which, despite some antiinflammatory actions, appears mostly vasculotoxic. Thus, administration of arginine for the sake of vascular health for enhancement of endothelial function and nitric oxide production, can—depending on host factors of nutritional (in)sufficiency and/or dysbiosis—actually have vasculotoxic effects via homocysteine and ADMA, respectively. Administration of L-arginine can clearly lead to elevations of ADMA in humans.[231] Böger[232] summarized the "arginine paradox" as follows: "Asymmetric dimethylarginine (ADMA) is an endogenous competitive inhibitor of NO synthase. ADMA inhibits vascular NO production in concentrations found in pathophysiological conditions; ADMA also causes local vasoconstriction when it is infused intraarterially. Thus, elevated ADMA levels may explain the "L-arginine paradox," i.e., the observation that supplementation with exogenous L-arginine improves NO-mediated vascular functions in vivo, although its baseline plasma concentration is about 25-fold higher than the Michaelis-Menten constant K(m) of the isolated, purified endothelial NO synthase in vitro. ... Thus, ADMA may explain the discrepant results of clinical trials in which L-arginine sometimes improves endothelial function and sometimes does not—a discrepancy that has so far remained unexplained." Administration of L-citrulline as an L-arginine precursor might be preferred to use of L-arginine itself.

More important than the change in homocysteine levels is the more sensitive increase in the ratio of homocysteine to methionine, indicating increased methylation demand which is likely to have adverse effects in various metabolic pathways; the authors note, "Thus, it remains possible that L-arginine

---

[231] "Patients were later randomized to either L-arginine (2 g tid or 4 g tid) or placebo. ... Additionally plasma ADMA concentrations after 28 days of L-arginine supplementation significantly exceeded initial concentrations. CONCLUSIONS: L-arginine supplementation increases plasma arginine, citrulline and TAS in patients with mild arterial hypertension. It confirms the thesis that augmented concentrations of L-arginine stimulate NO biosynthesis which leads to reduction of oxidative stress. Increase of ADMA plasma level after L-arginine supplementation confirms correlation between ADMA and L-arginine." Jabecka et al. Oral L-arginine supplementation in patients with mild arterial hypertension and its effect on plasma level of asymmetric dimethylarginine, L-citruline, L-arginine and antioxidant status. *Eur Rev Med Pharmacol Sci.* 2012 Nov;16(12):1665-74
[232] Böger RH. Asymmetric dimethylarginine, an endogenous inhibitor of nitric oxide synthase, explains the "L-arginine paradox" and acts as a novel cardiovascular risk factor. *J Nutr.* 2004 Oct;134(10 Suppl):2842S-2847S

metabolism imposes a methylation demand that counterbalances the effects of NO generated despite the absence of a change in measured plasma homocysteine." The average GFR of patients in this study was 68 ml/min by the Cockcroft–Gault formula (consistent with stage 2—almost stage 3—kidney disease), and previous studies have shown that patients with kidney disease are less likely to respond to treatments that improve endovascular health, including L-arginine, due in part to higher levels of circulating ADMA and homocysteine. The combination of creatinine and L-arginine did not suppress GAA production or prevent the increase in homocysteine-to-methionine ratio. Unexpectedly, the authors found that creatine supplementation (alone or in combination with L-arginine) was associated with an 11 to 20% increase in plasma homocysteine; other studies *of longer duration* using *lower doses of creatine* (<5.5 gm/d for 4 weeks) have shown the opposite effect—namely that creatine supplementation lowers plasma homocysteine. Altogether, these findings raise the possibility that L-arginine's effects on vascular function may be dependent on the patient's methylation ability; patients with poor methylation ability may experience exacerbation of endothelial dysfunction via L-arginine's conversion to GAA and the increased production of homocysteine. When L-arginine is used, supplementation with methyl donors and homocysteine-lowering nutrients such as folic acid, pyridoxine, cobalamin, betaine, and N-acetyl-cysteine may improve the efficacy of L-arginine supplementation while additively or synergistically improving vascular reactivity and endothelial health; this underscores the importance of dietary optimization and foundational multivitamin/multimineral supplementation (as a component of the "5-part nutritional protocol" described previously in this text) and the general need to avoid single-intervention treatment approaches.

- **Garlic, *Allium sativum*:** As both food and medicine, garlic has a long history of use dating back thousands of years. Cardioprotective mechanisms are reported to include alleviation of hypertension, reduction in serum lipids, platelet aggregation, and improvements in insulin sensitivity and endothelial function; obviously these vasculoprotective effects would be expected to produce additive and perhaps synergistic clinical benefits. Accordingly, epidemiologic studies have shown inverse relationships between garlic consumption and cardiovascular disease prevalence; while various mechanisms are in effect, a recent *in vitro* study showed that human RBCs convert garlic-derived organic polysulfides (allyl-substituted sulfur compounds) into hydrogen sulfide (H_2S), an endogenous cell signaling molecule that exerts vasculoprotective effects in endothelial cells.[233] Per *in vitro* studies, extracts from garlic leaf and bulbs have shown ability to inhibit 5-lipoxygenase, cyclooxygenase, thrombocyte aggregation, and angiotensin-converting enzyme (ACE).[234] Garlic's antimicrobial properties and its numerous immune-enhancing effects might also be included in its spectrum of cardioprotective properties, since occult infections in general (i.e., multifocal polydysbiosis, particularly the orodental and gastrointestinal subtypes[235]) and bacterial lipopolysaccharide (LPS) in particular are correlated in humans with HTN, diabetes mellitus, and cardiovascular disease; additionally, garlic's ability to modulate cytokine expression and inhibit activation of NFkB could further mitigate the cardiovasculotoxic effects of inflammation and dysbiosis.

  - Critical review: Garlic and cardiovascular disease (*Journal of Nutrition* 2006 Mar[236]): The authors note that epidemiologic studies show an inverse correlation between garlic consumption and progression of cardiovascular disease and that garlic has many cardioprotective properties:
    - Garlic inhibits enzymes involved in lipid synthesis, most notably beta-hydroxy-beta-methylglutaryl-CoA (HMG-CoA) reductase, the rate limiting enzyme in cholesterol biosynthesis,
    - Garlic decreases platelet aggregation,
    - Garlic prevents lipid peroxidation of erythrocytes and LDL,
    - Garlic improves antioxidant status,
    - Garlic inhibits angiotensin-converting enzyme (ACE).

Garlic's inconsistent results on BP, the authors suggest, is due ❶ to a combination of usage of different garlic preparations, ❷ uncertainty about which active constituents should be provided, and their respective

---

[233] Benavides et al. Hydrogen sulfide mediates the vasoactivity of garlic. *Proc Natl Acad Sci* U S A. 2007 Nov 13;104(46):17977-82
[234] "The inhibition rates as IC50 values of both extracts for 5-LO, CO, and TA showed a good correlation with %-content of the major S-containing compounds (thiosulfinates and ajoenes) of the various extracts. … In ACE test, water extract of the leaves of wild garlic containing glutamyl-peptides showed the highest inhibitory activity followed by that of the garlic leaf and the bulbs of both drugs." Sendl et al. Comparative pharmacological investigations of Allium ursinum and Allium sativum. *Planta Med.* 1992 Feb;58(1):1-7
[235] Vasquez A. *Integrative Rheumatology*. IBMRC 2006, 2007 and all future editions. Vasquez A. Nutritional and Botanical Treatments Against "Silent Infections" and Gastrointestinal Dysbiosis, Commonly Overlooked Causes of Neuromusculoskeletal Inflammation and Chronic Health Problems. *Nutritional Perspectives* 2006; January
[236] Rahman K, Lowe GM. Garlic and cardiovascular disease: a critical review. *J Nutr.* 2006 Mar;136(3 Suppl):736S-740S

bioavailability, ❸ inadequate randomization, ❹ selection of inappropriate subjects, and ❺ insufficient duration of trials. However, the gestalt of garlic's cardioprotective benefits strongly suggest its value in dietary utilization for patients with elevated cardiovascular risk, which obviously includes patients with hypertension.

- Double-blind, placebo-controlled trial: Time-released garlic powder tablets lower systolic and diastolic blood pressure in men with mild and moderate arterial hypertension (*Hypertension Research* 2009 Jun[237]): This double-blind placebo-controlled trial with 84 hypertensive men employed either ❶ time-released garlic powder tablets (600-2400 mg Allicor) or ❷ "regular garlic pills" (900 mg Kwai). Allicor (600 mg daily) resulted in a reduction of both systolic and diastolic blood pressures by 7.0 mm Hg and 3.8 mm, respectively, with no advantage noted at the higher 2400 mg/d dose. Use of Kwai resulted in a similar decrease in systolic blood pressure (-5.4 mm Hg), but no decrease in diastolic blood pressure was observed with Kwai. Noting that both garlic preparations provided an antihypertensive benefit, the authors concluded, "The results of this study show that time-released garlic powder tablets are more effective for the treatment of mild and moderate arterial hypertension than are regular garlic supplements."[238] Of note, a different study by the same primary author (Igor Sobenin) also demonstrated lipid-modifying effects of time-released garlic powder tablets, (Allicor 600 mg daily) in a double-blinded placebo-controlled randomized study among 42 men: total cholesterol reduced by >7%, LDL cholesterol reduced by approximately 12%, and HDL cholesterol increased by 11.5%.

- Systematic review and meta-analysis: Effect of garlic on blood pressure (*BioMed Central - Cardiovascular Disorders* 2008 Jun[239]): The authors reviewed eleven criteria-selected studies published between 1955 and October 2007 identified from Medline and Embase databases. Results showed, "…the mean decrease in the hypertensive subgroup was 8.4 mm Hg for SBP (n = 4; $p < 0.001$), and 7.3 mm Hg for DBP (n = 3; $p < 0.001$). Regression analysis revealed a significant association between blood pressure at the start of the intervention and the level of blood pressure reduction (SBP: R = 0.057; $p = 0.03$; DBP: R = -0.315; $p = 0.02$). CONCLUSION: Our meta-analysis suggests that garlic preparations are superior to placebo in reducing blood pressure in individuals with hypertension."

- Meta-analysis: Effects of garlic on blood pressure in patients with and without systolic hypertension (*Annals of Pharmacotherapy* 2008 Dec[240]): For this meta-analysis, the authors performed a systematic search of MEDLINE, CINAHL, and the Cochrane Central Register of Controlled Trials to identify randomized controlled trials in humans evaluating garlic's effect on blood pressure; to this was added a manual search of published literature, and the complete search yielded 10 trials for review. The authors write, "Garlic reduced SBP by **16.3 mm Hg** (95% CI 6.2 to 26.5) and DBP by **9.3 mm Hg** (95% CI 5.3 to 13.3) compared with placebo in patients with elevated SBP. … This meta-analysis suggests that garlic is associated with blood pressure reductions in patients with an elevated SBP although not in those without elevated SBP. Future research should focus on the impact of garlic on clinical events and the assessment of the long-term risk of harm." While the authors' cautionary note is reasonable given the potential for adverse effects from nearly any agent, the risk-benefit scales appear to tip in favor of garlic's overall cardioprotective, antihypertensive, eulipidemic benefits in addition to its wide availability and low cost; indeed, given these results, an argument could be made that withholding garlic—like CoQ10 and fish oil and vitamin D3— could be unethical in patients at elevated CVD risk.

- Garlic (*Allium sativum* L.) modulates cytokine expression in lipopolysaccharide-activated human blood thereby inhibiting NF-kappaB activity (*Journal of Nutrition* 2003 Jul[241]): Given the well-established role of inflammation in CVD initiation and progression, and the potential role of occult infections (i.e., various types and locations of dysbiosis), an anti-inflammatory mechanism to garlic's cardioprotective benefits is intriguing. The authors write, "This paper shows that garlic powder extracts (GPE) and single garlic metabolites modulate lipopolysaccharide (LPS)-induced cytokine levels in human whole blood" and that

[237] Sobenin et al. Lipid-lowering effects of time-released garlic powder tablets in double-blinded placebo-controlled randomized study. *J Atheroscler Thromb*. 2008 Dec;15:334-8
[238] Sobenin et al. Time-released garlic powder tablets lower systolic and diastolic blood pressure in men with mild/moderate arterial hypertension. *Hypertens Res*. 2009 Jun:433-7
[239] Ried et al. Effect of garlic on blood pressure: a systematic review and meta-analysis. *BMC Cardiovasc Disord*. 2008 Jun 16;8:13
[240] Reinhart et al. Effects of garlic on blood pressure in patients with and without systolic hypertension: a meta-analysis. *Ann Pharmacother*. 2008 Dec;42(12):1766-71
[241] Keiss et al. Garlic modulates cytokine expression in lipopolysaccharide-activated human blood thereby inhibiting NF-kappaB activity. *J Nutr*. 2003 Jul;133(7):2171-5

these favorable modifications in GPE-altered cytokine levels "reduced nuclear factor (NF)-kappaB [NFkB] activity in human cells exposed to these samples." Pretreatment with garlic extracts reduced LPS-induced production of proinflammatory cytokines interleukin (IL)-1beta from 15.7 to 6.2 micro g/L (greater than 50% reduction) and tumor necrosis factor (TNF)-alpha from 8.8 to 3.9 micro g/L (greater than 50% reduction). In an additional experiment, exposure of human embryonic kidney cell line (HEK293) cells to GPE-treated blood sample supernatants reduced NFkB activity by 25% (unfertilized garlic) and 41% (sulfur-fertilized garlic). The authors conclude, "In summary, garlic may indeed promote an anti-inflammatory environment by cytokine modulation in human blood that leads to an overall inhibition of NFkB activity in the surrounding tissue." Beyond demonstrating an anti-inflammatory effect of garlic, this study also serves as a reminder that suppression of proinflammatory cytokines can favorably downregulate NFkB activity in a "retroactive" manner, since NFkB activation generally precedes elaboration of proinflammatory cytokines; thus, garlic extracts appear capable of breaking the proinflammatory vicious cycle.

- **Nattokinase**: Nattokinase is an enzyme extracted and purified from a Japanese food called Natto, a cheese-like food made from fermented soybeans.
  - Randomized, controlled trial: Effects of nattokinase on blood pressure (*Hypertension Research* 2008 Aug[242]): 86 participants with pre-hypertension or stage-1 hypertension received nattokinase (2,000 FU/capsule) or a placebo capsule for 8 weeks. **Net changes in systolic and diastolic blood pressure were -5.55 mmHg and -2.84 mmHg, respectively, after the 8-week intervention.** Renin activity levels dropped by -1.17 ng/mL/h for the nattokinase group compared with the control group. The authors concluded, "…nattokinase supplementation resulted in a reduction in SBP and DBP. These findings suggest that increased intake of nattokinase may play an important role in preventing and treating hypertension."

INFECTIONS/DYSBIOSIS Over the past many years—and perhaps due to changes in the environment such as the overuse of the antibiotic glyphosate and the superabundance of other metabolism-inhibiting corporate chemicals, all of which have culminated in increased metabolic fragility and pro-inflammatory tendencies—we have become increasingly aware of the role of the gut microbiome in mitochondrial dysfunction and the resulting insulin resistance, obesity, and hypertension.

- **Berberine**: Used for its health-promoting properties for thousands of years, berberine is a naturally-occurring plant alkaloid present in *Hydrastis canadensis* (goldenseal), *Coptis chinensis* (goldenthread), *Berberis aquifolium* (Oregon grape), *Berberis vulgaris* (barberry), and *Berberis aristata* (tree turmeric). Naturopathic physicians have commonly employed berberine-containing treatments for anti-infective benefits, particularly against gastrointestinal dysbiosis and respiratory tract infections. Within the past few years, numerous experimental studies in animals and clinical trials in humans have clearly demonstrated that berberine possesses many cardioprotective benefits, only one of which is its ability to promote normalization of elevated blood pressure. Given its well-documented antimicrobial effects, berberine quite likely improves overall health by reducing microbe-induced total inflammatory load (TIL) in addition to its direct benefits on metabolic and genomic processes. The current author appreciates berberine's numerous benefits demonstrated in clinical practice and in recent research, but prefers to limit its high-dose (1,000 mg/d) use to 3-6 months.
  - Clinical trial: Treatment of type 2 diabetes and dyslipidemia with the natural plant alkaloid berberine (*Journal of Clinical Endocrinology and Metabolism* 2008 Jul[243]): In this randomized placebo-controlled trial, 116 patients with diabetes mellitus type-2 and dyslipidemia were randomly allocated to receive berberine (1,000 mg/d) or placebo for 3 months. Significant benefits were shown by berberine in insulin sensitivity, glucose homeostasis, and plasma lipids; except for mild to moderate constipation in five subjects in the berberine group, no major adverse effects were observed. With regard to blood pressure, results showed that systolic blood pressure decreased from 124to 117 mm Hg and diastolic blood pressure decreased from 81 to 77 mm Hg in subjects treated with berberine (i.e., total reduction of -7/4 mm Hg); this effect was superior to that shown in patients treated with placebo, who showed reduction of -3/-3 mm Hg. Note that these patients—even though they were diabetic—were not hypertensive. The authors concluded the text of their article by stating, "Given the benefits of berberine in lowering blood glucose, lipids, body weight,

[242] Kim et al. Effects of nattokinase on blood pressure: a randomized, controlled trial. *Hypertens Res*. 2008 Aug;31(8):1583-8
[243] Zhang et al. Treatment of type 2 diabetes and dyslipidemia with the natural plant alkaloid berberine. *J Clin Endocrinol Metab*. 2008 Jul;93(7):2559-65

and blood pressures, we speculate that berberine may be used for patients with type-2 diabetes and metabolic syndrome."

- **Probiotics**: The term "probiotics" generally refers to beneficial microorganisms—most commonly bacteria but also including the probiotic yeast *Saccharomyces boulardii*—that are consumed either in the supplement/nutraceutical form of tablets, capsules, powders or as fermented foods such as yogurt, kefir, kombucha, miso, tempeh, cottage cheese (some types), and sauerkraut. Due to their numerous benefits, probiotics have been included as the fifth component of the 5-part nutritional protocol published by Vasquez[244] in 2005. As science has continued to progress (both qualitatively and quantitatively), so has our knowledge of the diversity and mechanisms of the health-promoting benefits of probiotic supplementation. This section reviews several of the mechanisms behind the antihypertensive (and also cardioprotective, antidiabetic, antidyslipidemic, and anti-inflammatory) benefits of probiotic supplementation. Starting with and strongly relying upon a review article by Lye et al[245] named "The improvement of hypertension by probiotics: effects on cholesterol, diabetes, renin, and phytoestrogens", this section will concisely review the more prominent antihypertensive benefits and mechanisms of probiotic supplementation. Lye et al emphasize the role of dyslipidemia in the genesis of HTN by stating, "…lipid metabolism disorders are often the causes of hypertension." Relevant to this paradigm, they review data from controlled studies in humans, rats, and/or pigs showing that antidyslipidemic benefits (reduction in total serum cholesterol, very low density lipoprotein, intermediate density lipoprotein, and LDL cholesterol and increase in HDL cholesterol) have been documented due to the use of *Lactobacillus acidophilus, Lactobacillus casei, Bifidobacterium longum*, and *Saccharomyces boulardii* (when used with bacterial probiotics). The antidyslipidemic benefit of supplementation with *L. acidophilus, B. breve, Lactococcus lactis* and other probiotics is mediated in part or in whole part via ❶ cholesterol assimilation during growth (i.e., the bacteria actively take up cholesterol for their own use), ❷ binding of cholesterol to the cellular surface, in part via exopolysaccharides (EPS) which adhere to the cell surface and absorb cholesterol, and ❸ probiotic elaboration of the enzyme bile salt hydrolase (BSH; cholyglycine hydrolase) which catalyzes the hydrolysis of glycine- and/or taurine-conjugated bile salts into amino acid residues and free bile acids, the latter of which contain cholesterol and are preferentially excreted in the feces rather than being reabsorbed in the intestines. Thus, probiotics function in part (mechanisms 1 and 2) similarly to the anticholesterolemic drug cholestyramine, which exerts its cholesterol-lowering effect via enhanced fecal excretion of cholesterol. Also, the authors note the correlation between diabetes mellitus, insulin resistance, and HTN, and that probiotics may also mediate an antihypertensive benefit by ❹ ameliorating diabetes and insulin resistance; in their words, "The consumption of probiotics is a new therapeutic strategy in preventing or delaying the onset of diabetes and subsequently reducing the incident of hypertension." With regard to this fourth mechanism, the postulated mechanism of the antihypertensive and antidiabetic benefit is worthy of appreciation both as a mechanism and as an independent benefit. The authors state that the antidiabetic benefit of probiotics is due to the reduction in systemic inflammation mediated via improvements in intestinal microecology which effect a reduction in systemic absorption of intestinally-derived bacterial lipopolysaccharides [LPS], which are inherently proinflammatory; the authors write, "…the composition of natural intestinal gut microflora often determine the degree of inflammation contributing to the onset of diabetes and obesity. The concentration of plasma lipopolysaccharides, the proinflammatory factor, is inversely correlated with the population of *Bifidobacterium* spp. … Several studies have also shown that bifidobacteria can reduce the intestinal endotoxin levels and improve mucosal barrier thus reducing systemic inflammation and subsequently reduced the incidence of diabetes." This **systemic anti-inflammatory benefit derived from the (re)establishment of eubiosis** is wholly consistent with the model of dysbiosis-induced systemic inflammation and autoimmunity detailed in both the 2006 and 2007 editions of *Integrative Rheumatology*.[246] In summarizing this mechanism, we must (again) conclude that probiotics are antidysbiotic and anti-inflammatory (dependent on and independent from LPS reduction) and that ❺ the antihypertensive benefit of probiotic supplementation is mediated at least in part via reducing systemic LPS-induced inflammation and thus subsequent insulin resistance and endothelial dysfunction, which independently and synergistically promote HTN. In either *in vitro*, animal, or human studies, the

[244] Vasquez A. A Five-Part Nutritional Protocol that Produces Consistently Positive Results. *Nutritional Wellness* 2005 September
[245] Lye et al. The improvement of hypertension by probiotics: effects on cholesterol, diabetes, renin, and phytoestrogens. *Int J Mol Sci.* 2009 Aug 27;10(9):3755-75
[246] Vasquez A. *Integrative Rheumatology*. IBMRC 2006, 2007 and all future editions

beneficial effects of probiotic supplementation have been demonstrated (in descending order of efficacy) from the use of living and growing probiotic populations, non-growing probiotics, and dead cells. Finally but not exhaustively, we should appreciate as mentioned previously that ❻ probiotic bacteria interact with dietary components—especially proteins from cow's milk—to produce antihypertensive peptides which, in particular, have ACE-inhibiting functions. As summed by Lye et al, "Probiotics are able to grow in milk products because they possess a proteolytic system that degrades casein along with lactose hydrolyzing enzymes. Upon fermentation, the proteinases of various probiotics are capable of releasing ACE inhibitory peptides and thus a blood-pressure lowering effect can be derived from the milk proteins. Several studies have demonstrated that *Lactobacillus helveticus* are capable of releasing antihypertensive peptides which are ACE inhibitory tripeptides Val-Pro-Pro (VPP) and Ile-Pro-Pro (IPP) from milk protein casein."

- Randomized, placebo-controlled, double-blind study: Effect of powdered fermented milk with *Lactobacillus helveticus* on subjects with high-normal blood pressure or mild hypertension (*Journal of the American College of Nutrition* 2005 Aug[247]): This study used a randomized, placebo-controlled, double-blind design in 40 subjects with high-normal blood pressure (HN group: SBP 130–139 mm Hg and DBP 85–89 mm Hg) and 40 subjects with mild hypertension (MH group: SBP 140–159 mm Hg and DBP 90–99 mm Hg). Each subject ingested 12 g of powdered fermented milk (in tablet form) with *L. helveticus* CM4 daily for 4 weeks (test group) or the same amount of placebo tablets for 4 weeks (placebo group). The authors noted that **among the patients with high-normal blood pressure, the change in SBP in the test group was 3.2 mm Hg lower than that in the placebo group, and DBP decreased more in the test group than in the placebo group during treatment, by 5.0 mm Hg** at the end of week 4. Further, they write, "**In the [Mild Hypertension] group, SBP decreased by 11.2 mm Hg and there was a statistically non-significant decrease in DBP of 6.5 mm Hg** compared with the placebo group." Their conclusions read, "Daily ingestion of the tablets containing powdered fermented milk with *L. helveticus* CM4 in subjects with high-normal blood pressure or mild hypertension reduces elevated blood pressure without any adverse effects." Readers should appreciate that this group with mild hypertension (SBP 140–159 mm Hg and DBP 90–99 mm Hg) represents the largest group of HTN patients and that this benefit of peptides from fermented milk—a reduction in blood pressure of -11.2/-6.5—is on par with the antihypertensive effect derived from many commonly used FDA-approved pharmaceutical drugs.

NUTRITIONAL IMMUNOMODULATION Evidence is accumulating that proinflammatory immune imbalances contribute to sustained hypertension.[248] What is becoming more and more clear—to the amazement of many of us—is the interrelationship between mitochondrial dysfunction and immunophenotype imbalance: **clearly at this time we must acknowledge that a bidirectional relationship exists between mitochondria and the immune system**—a fact that is not commonly within the curriculum of most medical schools nor the intellectual armamentarium of most clinicians. Per the illustration that follows, this section will discuss the role of immunophenotype imbalance in the genesis and perpetuation of sustained hypertension; therapeutic correction of immunophenotype imbalance—simplified as "excess Th17 and insufficient Treg"—is discussed in Chapter 4. I call this the "mito-immunologic model of hypertension."

- Evidence for immunophenotype imbalance—functional usurpation by Th1, Th2, and Th17 with functional abdication of Treg—in sustained hypertension: See section on Nutritional Immunomodulation in Chapter 4 for important pathophysiologic details and therapeutic interventions; this section serves solely to describe and substantiate the causal connection between immunophenotype imbalance and sustained hypertension. In sum, mitochondrial ROS (mtROS) directly contribute to the pro-hypertensive response of immune cells[249], mediated significantly by Th17 cells and their signature cytokine IL-17. [250]
  - The immune system in in hypertension (*Can J Cardiol* 2013 May[251]): The author of this article provides an efficient review and summary by reminding us that various lymphocyte subsets and their respective cytokines are involved in vascular remodeling, hypertensive renal disease, and cardiovascular disease.

[247] Aihara K, Kajimoto O, Hirata H, Takahashi R, Nakamura Y. Effect of powdered fermented milk with Lactobacillus helveticus on subjects with high-normal blood pressure or mild hypertension. *J Am Coll Nutr.* 2005 Aug;24(4):257-65
[248] Schiffrin EL. The immune system: role in hypertension. *Can J Cardiol.* 2013 May;29(5):543-8
[249] Nazarewicz RR, Dikalov SI. Mitochondrial ROS in the prohypertensive immune response. *Am J Physiol Regul Integr Comp Physiol.* 2013 Jul 15;305(2):R98-100
[250] Wang J et al. Elevated Th17 and IL-23 in hypertensive patients with acutely increased blood pressure. *American Journal of Immunology* 2012: 8: 27-32
[251] Schiffrin EL. The immune system: role in hypertension. *Can J Cardiol.* 2013 May;29(5):543-8

Among the effector lymphocytes, Th1 produce interferon-γ, Th2 produce IL-4, Th17 produce IL17), and Tregs are anti-inflammatory and express the FoxP3 transcription factor. **These immune cells mediate the cardiovascular effects of angiotensin-2 and mineralocorticoids.** Further, "....neoantigens could be generated by elevated blood pressure through damage-associated molecular pattern [DAMP] receptors [rDAMP] or other mechanisms. When activated, Th1 may contribute to blood pressure elevation by affecting the kidney, vascular remodeling of blood vessels directly via effects of the cytokines produced, or through their effects on perivascular fat. **T regulatory cells protect from blood pressure elevation** acting on similar targets. These novel findings may open the way for new therapeutic approaches to improve outcomes in hypertension and cardiovascular disease in humans."

> **Immune activation and pro-inflammatory cytokines are "essential" for the sustenance of "essential HTN"**
>
> "**T-cells are critical for hypertension**; however, the exact mechanism of T-cell activation in hypertension has not been fully understand. Once activated, T-cells intensively proliferate, produce cytokines that further stimulate immune system, **alter vascular function** and stimulate ROS production. **MtROS regulates cellular signaling, cell functions, and metabolism.**" Inhibition of NOX2 prevents production of **TNFα, a cytokine that is critical for the development of hyp**ertension. Inhibition of TNFα mutes hypertension; thus, scavenging ROS in immune cells may attenuate their pro-hypertensive effect.
>
> Nazarewicz RR, Dikalov SI. Mitochondrial ROS in the prohypertensive immune response. *Am J Physiol Regul Integr Comp Physiol* 2013 Jul

- Elevated Th17 and IL-23 in hypertensive patients with acutely increased blood pressure (*American Journal of Immunology* 2012[252]): "The involvement of **immune activation in hypertension has been well demonstrated** by many research groups... **Th17**, a recently discovered subset of CD4+T cells, is believed to play a role in the **pathogenesis of vascular dysfunction and hypertension**. In the current study, demonstrated an increased level of Th17 and IL-17 in hypertensive patients with acute increases of blood pressure..."

- Mitochondrial ROS in the prohypertensive immune response (*Am J Physiol Regul Integr Comp Physiol* 2013 Jul[253]): This nice article provides insight into the connection between mitochondrial dysfunction and the immune system's role in sustaining hypertension. In a nutshell, evidence supports circular and bidirectional connections between mitochondrial dysfunction and proinflammatory and immunodysfunctional contributions to sustaining the hypertensive phenotype. Mechanistically, intramitochondrial and intracellular ROS function as intracellular signals independent from systemic oxidative stress to induce additional mitochondrial dysfunction, dependence on glycolysis, inhibition of mitochondrial electron transport chain (ETC) function, additional mtROS formation, enhanced elaboration of pro-inflammatory cytokines, and increased hypertensive sensitivity to angiotensin. Cutting to the clinical chase, these authors state that "... angiotensin II-induced hypertension leads to endothelial dysfunction dependent on mtROS and NADPH oxidases. These pathological conditions can be reversed by preventing mitochondrial superoxide production. ... It is conceivable that mitochondria-targeted antioxidants interfere with signal transduction in vascular cells; resulting in protection against the development of hypertension." Inhibition of NOX2 prevents production of TNFα, a cytokine that is critical for the development of hypertension. Inhibition of TNFα mutes hypertension; thus, scavenging ROS in immune cells may attenuate their pro-hypertensive effect. I think this likely explains the extraordinary effectiveness of CoQ10 in the treatment *and reliable clinical cure* of HTN, the mechanism being the mitochondria-specific sequestration of ROS with the simultaneous enhancement/support of ETC complexes 1, 2, and 3.

- T-cells in the genesis of angiotensin-2-induced hypertension and vascular dysfunction (*J Exp Med* 2007 Oct[254]): Experimental studies show that hypertension is blunted in animals lacking T-cells and/or the oxidant-producing enzyme nicotinamide adenosine dinucleotide phosphate (NADPH) oxidase discussed previously (see diagram). In fact, the pro-hypertensive effect of the prototypic prohypertensive hormone angiotensin-2 appear to be mediated via activity of nicotinamide adenosine dinucleotide phosphate (NADPH) oxidase via the resultant oxidant stress which mediates changes in (pro)inflammatory immune function resulting in the hypertensive clinical phenotype. Angiotensin-2 causes immune activation which

---

[252] Wang J et al. Elevated Th17 and IL-23 in hypertensive patients with acutely increased blood pressure. *American Journal of Immunology* 2012: 8: 27-32

[253] Nazarewicz RR, Dikalov SI. Mitochondrial ROS in the prohypertensive immune response. *Am J Physiol Regul Integr Comp Physiol*. 2013 Jul 15;305(2):R98-100

[254] Guzik TJ et al. Role of the T cell in the genesis of angiotensin II induced hypertension and vascular dysfunction. *J Exp Med*. 2007 Oct 1;204(10):2449-60

is dependent upon ROS produced via nicotinamide adenosine dinucleotide phosphate (NADPH) oxidase. Thus, we see a tripartite overlapping and vicious cycle via which ❶ angiotensin-2 activates NADPH oxidase to produce ROS which then leads to immune activation (i.e., angiotensin-2 is proinflammatory, and its hypertensive effects are ROS-dependent and immunocytes-dependent), and ❷ heightened immune activation leads to increased secretion of IL-17 and TNFa, both of which promote hypertension, and ❸ hypertension itself leads to immune activation. These authors articulated part of the vicious cycle as follows, "Hypertension also increased T lymphocyte production of tumor necrosis factor (TNF) alpha, and treatment with the TNFalpha antagonist etanercept prevented the hypertension and increase in vascular superoxide caused by angiotensin II. These studies identify a previously undefined role for T cells in the genesis of hypertension and support a role of inflammation in the basis of this prevalent disease. T cells might represent a novel therapeutic target for the treatment of high blood pressure."

Hypertensive immune imbalance via deficient Treg and excess Th17, IL-17, TNFa

Material/physical (not simply biochemical) predisposition toward inflammation, allergy, and autoimmunity; overproduction of pro-inflammatory and tissue-damaging cytokines which lead to synergistic production of ROS as well as alteration of native molecules and the activation of DAMP receptors (rDAMP), thereby promoting a vicious cycle of tissue damage, metabolic dysfunction, and "inflammation dysfunction."

Immunophenotype imbalance promotes hypertension

Mechanisms include inflammation-driven 1) insulin resistance, 2) endothelial dysfunction, 3) phagocytic production of NADPH oxidase (Nox2) augments mtROS pro-hypertensive cell signaling. Prohypertensive actions of angiotensin-2 are largely dependent on Nox2-mediated ROS production, which augments prohypertensive cytokine (TNFa) production. Hypertensive HTN patients show elevations in Th17 cells and the proinflammatory cytokines IL-6, IL-17, and TNFa.

Vicious cycles: mtROS is produced by immune activation and also leads to immune activation; immunocyte involvement is significant for the induction of the hypertensive response promoted by angiotensin-2 and mineralocorticoids

1) mtROS-induced mtROS production
2) Immune-driven immunoactivation
3) mtROS-induced immune-mediated mitochondrial dysfunction and immunoimbalance which promotes dysmetabolism, dysinsulinism, hypertension, autoimmunity, etc.
4) Hypertension is itself pro-inflammatory, and the resulting inflammation and ROS sustain the HTN.

Mitochondrial dysfunction promotes HTN

Mitochondrial dysfunction promotes HTN via dysinsulinism, endothelial dysfunction, altered intracellular signaling mediated by mtROS, and via enhanced elaboration of prohypertensive cytokines, especially IL-17 and TNFa. Mitochondrial dysfunction promotes prohypertensive "priming" of the immune system toward an exaggerated hypertensive response to glucocorticoids and angiotensin-2. Excessive mtROS from the ETC in the form of superoxide leads directly to neutralization of vasodilating nitric oxide and formation of peroxinitrite

Mitochondrial dysfunction

Mitochondrial hyperpolarization, activation of mTOR, and increased mitochondrial ROS production function *independently* and *synergistically* to inhibit Treg maturation, to promote Th17 maturation, and to promote molecular damage which provokes additional unnecessary/nonproductive immune responsiveness and inflammation. Superoxide radical combines with and therefore neutralizes what would otherwise be vasodilating nitric oxide, resulting in the production of the aggressive free radical peroxinitrite.

The mitoimmunology and mitoinflammology model: Immune phenotype imbalance and mitochondrial dysfunction can exist independently (at least initially) but eventually become interconnected and pathosynergistic: Proinflammatory cytokines are—in many experimental models—either necessary or sufficient for the establishment of sustained hypertension, and recent evidence shows elevated Th17 cells and serum IL-17 in acutely hypertensive patients. Elaboration of prohypertensive cytokines is increased by mitochondrial dysfunction; simultaneously, immune-mediated damage and resultant release of DAMP and activation of rDAMP likely perpetuates the cycle. rDAMP = receptor for damaged associated molecular pattern (DAMP), mtROS = mitochondrial reactive oxygen species. Nox2 = nicotinamide adenosine dinucleotide phosphate (NADPH) oxidase or NADPH oxidase, a ROS-generating enzyme in phagocytes and also in nonphagocytic tissues such as renal parenchyma and vascular endothelium

- Therapeutic nutritional immunomodulation and immunophenotype (im/re)balance in hypertension: Briefly, we can surmise that the "immune system" and inflammatory responses are necessary for the maintenance of the hypertensive clinical phenotype. Prohypertensive hormones such as glucocorticoids and angiotensin-2 effect elevated blood pressure through various means, some of which are completely dependent on induction of mitochondrial oxidative stress and the resultant pro-inflammatory immune response; I have termed this interdependency "**mitoimmunology**" and "**mitoinflammology**."

   Correction of **mitochondrial dysfunction** and **immunophenotype imbalance** are both now-appreciated means by which clinicians can modulate dysfunctional pro-hypertensive pathophysiologic tendencies; furthermore, we must now appreciate the intimate connection between mitochondrial dysfunction (especially the role played by intramitochondrial ROS as cell signaling molecules that promote inflammation, hypertension, and autoimmunity) and the immune system, which can now be seen as the effector of the mitochondria's direction. Stated more plainly: Mitochondrial signals (e.g., mtROS) direct the proinflammatory and hypertensive response of the immune system (which will "over-react" if already in a state of pro-inflammatory imbalance) to promote harmful inflammation, which I categorize as ❶ metabolic (e.g., hypertension), ❷ allergic, and ❸ autoimmune. These insights provide access to "new" and nonpharmaodependent means by which clinicians can address hypertension via correction and optimization of physiologic function rather than dependence on pharmacomonkeywrenching—using drugs to interfere with a system that is already dysfunctional.

   Clinicians have generally considered oxidative stress to be "bad" and antioxidants to be "good" and while this is generally true in a quantitative sense, we as intellectually competent clinicians should discern more than such broad categories of "good and bad" given that the information is now available to us thanks to the efforts of innumerable named/unnamed researchers, their students, and assistants. Further to this deepening understanding, we need to discern the names and characteristics, roles and functions, location and compartmentalization of ROS to better appreciate their participation in health and disease; with this knowledge we will be better able to help our patients and strengthen the science of our healthcare and art.

MITOCHONDRIA/METABOLIC IMPAIRMENT CoQ10 is the most safe, effective, and reliable nutritional/physiological treatment for hypertension; its nearest competitors (and biochemical synergists) are potassium, magnesium, and vitamin D3). Not too many years ago, we were not perfectly clear on the mechanism of action, and indeed many different antihypertensive actions exist, including antioxidant, antiinflammatory, and mitochondrial. However, at this time, the mitochondrial mechanism clearly prevails: CoQ10 facilitates electron transfer in the electron transport chain, reducing free radical elaboration: notably reducing superoxide production and thereby reducing the binding of nitric oxide with superoxide which thereby leads to inhibited vasodilation, endothelial dysfunction, and the relative/absolute vasoconstriction that promotes vascular resistance and the resultant hypertension.

   In a personal communication by email in which the current author corresponded with world-renowned CoQ10 researcher Peter Langsjoen MD FACC (citations[255,256]) about CoQ10's mechanism of action in the treatment of hypertension, the following reply was received, as quoted in the textbox, with permission:

Personal communication from Peter H. Langsjoen, MD, FACC
January 25, 2011
Dear Alex,
In regards to the antihypertensive effect of coenzyme Q10, I do have a couple of thoughts.
The first theory is that coenzyme Q10 (CoQ10) has some influence on endothelial function, which may thereby have some benefit in hypertension. There is one thing that is quite clear, and that is that CoQ10 cannot have any direct vasodilator function because we never see a decrease in blood pressure in patients who already have low-normal blood pressures.
My own theory on this subject is that the decrease in blood pressure from CoQ10 supplementation is a secondary phenomenon. We have observed that patients with established hypertension quite frequently have underlying diastolic dysfunction and it is clear that CoQ10 supplementation improves diastolic function because this is in large part an active process requiring a large amount of ATP to re-establish calcium gradients such that the actin and myosin fibrils can uncouple. When diastolic function improves, there is a secondary gradual decrease in hypertension. The theory is that the

[255] Langsjoen PH, Langsjoen AM. Supplemental ubiquinol in patients with advanced congestive heart failure. *Biofactors*. 2008;32(1-4):119-28
[256] Langsjoen P, Langsjoen P, Willis R, Folkers K. Treatment of essential hypertension with coenzyme Q10. *Mol Aspects Med*. 1994;15 Suppl:S265-72

diastolic dysfunction actually occurs first as a result of CoQ10 decrease, which occurs beginning in early-middle age and can certainly be aggravated by a variety of factors including stress and poor diet. One of the first adaptive responses that we have from impairment in the filling phase, or diastole phase, of the cardiac cycle is an increase in catecholamines, and these patients almost always have a tendency for an increase in both blood pressure and heart rate. It is my theory that when we improve the diastolic dysfunction, the adaptive high catecholamine state gradually subsides, and with this, there is frequently a decrease in blood pressure and a decreased need for antihypertensive medication.

…Additional correspondence February 17, 2011: "QH (ubiquinol) is 2-3x better absorbed than QX (ubiquinone). Some promotional materials have exaggerated this. Also, since QX is promptly reduced to QH after absorption, there is no difference in antioxidant effect of supplemental QH vs QX. The only difference is the improved absorption." …

My very best regards,
Peter
Peter H. Langsjoen, MD, FACC

CoQ10's safety and efficacy in the treatment of hypertension are very well established, and the mechanism(s) of action are manifold rather than singular. CoQ10 has been shown to improve glycemic control, reduce serum insulin levels, promote beneficial redistribution of adipose, provide anti-inflammatory and anti-allergy benefits, and to improve mitochondrial bioenergetics. Peer-reviewed articles on the use of CoQ10 for cardiovascular health are reviewed and summarized in the sections that follow.

- **Coenzyme Q-10 (CoQ10) with doses ranging from 100-300 mg per day**: Average dietary intake of CoQ10 is 2-5 mg/d. CoQ10 is made endogenously; however, some patients—particularly those with migraines, asthma, hypertension, allergies, heart failure and idiopathic dilated cardiomyopathy—may have an inborn or acquired error of metabolism that prevents them from making sufficient amounts of this vitally important substance. Hypertensive patients generally have lower serum CoQ10 levels than normotensive persons. **Typical blood levels of CoQ10 range from 0.7-1 mcg/ml; however clinical benefit in CVD may require serum levels of 2-3 and up to 4 mcg/ml to attain maximal clinical benefit.**[257] Testing of serum CoQ10 levels is not necessary before starting treatment; however, patients who do not benefit as expected should have their CoQ10 levels measured and supplementation increased to attain optimal serum levels before deciding that treatment is inefficacious. While clinical benefit may occur within the first week of supplementation, maximal improvement generally takes 4-8 weeks in order to obtain tissue saturation and beneficial changes in cell physiology. CoQ10 is clearly one of the most powerful and broadly-beneficial nutritional supplements on the nutrition-healthcare market; research literature shows clinically meaningful benefit of CoQ10 supplementation in patients with myocardial infarction, HTN, heart failure, renal failure, allergies, asthma, migraine, Parkinson's disease, and chronic viral infections such as HIV. CoQ10 has generally been produced and studied in its oxidized form as "ubiquinone" however more current research and clinical trends suggest that the reduced form "ubiquinol" is better absorbed (perhaps 3x); a small clinical trial (n=7) showed impressive improvements in serum CoQ10 and clinical status followed by ubiquinol treatment compared to ubiquinone treatment in CHF patients with malabsorption-inducing bowel wall edema.[258] Whether ubiquinol has clinical advantage over ubiquinone to such an extent that the higher cost is justified in other clinical scenarios—especially those which are not associated with malabsorption and/or the bowel wall edema seen in severe heart failure—remains to be determined. **In hypertensive patients, CoQ10 doses of 60-120 mg/d can typically lower BP by about -15/-9 mm Hg.** CoQ10 can be safely used with antihypertensive medications and is generally safer than all antihypertensive medications. CoQ10 may rarely interfere with coumadin/warfarin action in some patients; a cross-over study of 24 patients on chronic warfarin showed that neither CoQ10 nor *Ginkgo biloba* affected coagulation indices nor warfarin dosage.[259] More frequent monitoring of INR is routinely advised following any change in diet or medication. CoQ10 supplementation provides numerous collateral benefits; research literature shows clinically meaningful benefit of CoQ10 supplementation in patients with myocardial infarction, HTN, heart failure, renal

[257] Kumar A, Kaur H, Devi P, Mohan V. Role of coenzyme Q10 (CoQ10) in cardiac disease, hypertension and Meniere-like syndrome. *Pharmacol Ther*. 2009 Dec;124(3):259-68
[258] "Patients with CHF, NYHA class IV, often fail to achieve adequate plasma CoQ10 levels on supplemental ubiquinone at dosages up to 900 mg/day. These patients often have plasma total CoQ10 levels of less than 2.5 microg/ml and have limited clinical improvement. It is postulated that the intestinal edema in these critically ill patients may impair CoQ10 absorption. … Ubiquinol has dramatically improved absorption in patients with severe heart failure and the improvement in plasma CoQ10 levels is correlated with both clinical improvement and improvement in measurement of left ventricular function." Langsjoen PH, Langsjoen AM. Supplemental ubiquinol in patients with advanced congestive heart failure. *Biofactors*. 2008;32(1-4):119-28
[259] "The study indicated that Coenzyme Q10 and Ginkgo biloba do not influence the clinical effect of warfarin." Engelsen J, Nielsen JD, Hansen KF. [Effect of Coenzyme Q10 and Ginkgo biloba on warfarin dosage in patients on long-term warfarin treatment. A randomized, double-blind, placebo-controlled cross-over trial]. [Article in Danish] *Ugeskr Laeger*. 2003 Apr 28;165(18):1868-71. See also Engelsen et al. The healthcare products coenzyme Q10 and ginko biloba do not interact with warfarin. Abstracdt P796. *Thrombosis and Haemostasis*. 2001: July Presented at Eighteenth Congress of the International Society on Thrombosis and Haemostasis, July 6-12, 2001 in Paris, France.

failure, allergies, asthma, migraine, fibromyalgia, gingivitis, male infertility/subfertility, Parkinson's disease, and chronic viral infections.

- Correlational study: CoQ10 is an independent predictor of mortality in chronic heart failure (*Journal of the American College of Cardiology* 2008 Oct[260]): Plasma samples from 236 patients admitted to the hospital with heart failure were assayed for LDL and total cholesterol, and total CoQ10. "CONCLUSIONS: Plasma CoQ10 concentration was an independent predictor of mortality in this cohort. The **CoQ10 deficiency might be detrimental to the long-term prognosis of CHF [chronic heart failure]**, and there is a rationale for controlled intervention studies with CoQ10."

- Review: Role of coenzyme Q10 (CoQ10) in cardiac disease, hypertension and Meniere-like syndrome (*Pharmacology and Therapeutics* 2009 Dec[261]): In this excellent review that covers the role of CoQ10 in the treatment of cardiovascular diseases—heart failure, HTN, myocardial infarction, arrhythmia—and Meniere syndrome and hearing loss, Kumar et al review the literature to conclude that CoQ10 provides major clinical benefit in all of these conditions and without adverse effects. Cardioprotective properties of CoQ10 include its role as an antioxidant, vasodilator, and membrane stabilizer in addition to its ability to decrease blood viscosity, proinflammatory cytokines, endothelial dysfunction, insulin resistance, and to promote proper diastolic and systolic function of the myocardium. Additional functions of CoQ10 specific to its benefit in HTN appear related to the ability of CoQ10 to antagonize aldosterone and/or angiotensin; if confirmed, these functions would support the concept that CoQ10 functions in part like an aldosterone antagonist (such as spironolactone) and/or an angiotensin 2 receptor blocker (such as losartan). **Typical blood pressure reduction with use of CoQ10 can be as high as -18/-11 mm Hg,** depending on dose, attained serum levels; other common nutritional deficiencies such as magnesium, potassium, and vitamin D can also be addressed to improve efficacy. Maximal improvement might take 4-8 weeks; however, some patients will respond more quickly—within the first week—and this observation underscores the importance of frequent BP monitoring and the need to adjust doses of antihypertensive drugs as needed to avoid hypotension and its complications such as syncope.

- Randomized, double-blind, placebo-controlled trial of coenzyme Q10 in isolated systolic hypertension (*Southern Medical Journal* 2001 Nov[262]): Twice daily administration of 60 mg of oral CoQ10 was given to 46 men and 37 women with isolated systolic hypertension in a 12-week randomized, double-blind, placebo-controlled trial. "**RESULTS: The mean reduction in systolic blood pressure of the CoQ-treated group was 17.8 mm Hg**. None of the patients exhibited orthostatic blood pressure changes. CONCLUSIONS: Our results suggest CoQ may be safely offered to hypertensive patients as an alternative treatment option."

- Open clinical trial: Coenzyme Q-10 in essential hypertension (*Molecular Aspects of Medicine* 1994[263]): In this open trial with no comparative placebo group, 26 patients with essential hypertension received oral CoQ10 50 mg twice daily for 10 weeks. Results of this study showed the following:
  - Systolic BP decreased from 164.5 to 146.7 mmHg (reduction of -17.8 mmHg).
  - Diastolic BP decreased from 98.1 to 86.1 mmHg (reduction of -12 mmHg).
  - Plasma CoQ10 values increased from 0.64 mcg/ml to 1.61 mcg/ml. Of particular note is that eight of 26 patients (30%) had baseline values of plasma CoQ10 that were subnormal before treatment and which normalized with supplementation.
  - Serum total cholesterol decreased from 222.9 mg/dl to 213.3 mg/dl.
  - Serum HDL cholesterol increased slightly from 41.1 mg/dl to 43.1 mg/dl.

NYHA Stages of Heart Failure
1. **Class 1**: Comfortable at all times. No limitation of physical activity. Ordinary activity does not cause undue fatigue, palpitation, dyspnea or anginal pain.
2. **Class 2**: Comfortable at rest. Slight limitation of physical activity. Ordinary activity causes fatigue, palpitation, dyspnea, or anginal pain.
3. **Class 3**: Comfortable at rest. Marked limitation of physical activity. Less than ordinary activity causes fatigue, palpitation, dyspnea or anginal pain.
4. **Class 4**: Symptomatic at rest. Cannot perform any physical activity without progressive discomfort.
American Heart Association. 1994 Revisions to Classification of Functional Capacity and Objective Assessment of Patients with Diseases of the Heart. http://americanheart.org Accessed Nov 2010.

[260] Molyneux et al. Coenzyme Q10: an independent predictor of mortality in chronic heart failure. *J Am Coll Cardiol*. 2008 Oct 28;52(18):1435-41

[261] Kumar A, Kaur H, Devi P, Mohan V. Role of coenzyme Q10 (CoQ10) in cardiac disease, hypertension and Meniere-like syndrome. *Pharmacol Ther*. 2009 Dec;124(3):259-68

[262] Burke et al. Randomized, double-blind, placebo-controlled trial of coenzyme Q10 in isolated systolic hypertension. *South Med J*. 2001 Nov;94(11):1112-7

[263] Digiesi et al. Coenzyme Q10 in essential hypertension. *Mol Aspects Med*. 1994;15 Suppl:s257-63

- Plasma renin activity, urinary aldosterone, serum and urinary sodium and potassium, plasma endothelin, electrocardiographic and echocardiographic findings and did not change.
- In a subgroup of 5 patients tested, peripheral vascular resistances were 2,283 dyne·s·cm−5 before treatment and 1,627 dyne·s·cm−5 after treatment, thus indicating a clear reduction in peripheral resistance by CoQ10. The authors concluded that the antihypertensive effect of CoQ10 is probably mediated by reduction in peripheral resistance.

These anti-hypertensive results, the collateral benefits, and the absence of adverse effects make CoQ10 superior to drug treatment for the treatment of chronic/persistent/sustained HTN.

- Clinical trial with water-soluble CoQ10: Effect of hydrosoluble coenzyme Q10 on blood pressures and insulin resistance in hypertensive patients with coronary artery disease (*J Hum Hyperten* 1999 Mar[264]): In this randomized double-blind placebo-controlled trial among patients receiving antihypertensive medication and with coronary artery disease (n=59: 30 in treatment group, 29 in placebo group), patients received oral coenzyme Q10 (60 mg twice daily) for 8 weeks. **In the coenzyme Q10 group, beneficial reductions were noted in systolic and diastolic blood pressures (average 168/106 reduced to 152/97 [-16/-9] mm Hg),** heart rate, **waist–hip ratio**, fasting and 2-h plasma insulin and glucose levels, triglyceride levels and angina; CoQ10 supplementation raised HDL-cholesterol. The authors concluded, "These findings indicate that treatment with coenzyme Q10 decreases blood pressure possibly by decreasing oxidative stress and insulin response in patients with known hypertension receiving conventional antihypertensive drugs."
- Open trial using average dose of CoQ10 225 mg/d for the treatment of essential hypertension (*Molecular Aspects of Medicine* 1994[265]): This study was one of the first to use dosage adjustments to attain serum CoQ10 levels of at least 2 mcg/ml. "A total of 109 patients with symptomatic essential hypertension presenting to a private cardiology practice were observed after the addition of CoQ10 (average dose, 225 mg/day by mouth) to their existing antihypertensive drug regimen. … A definite and gradual improvement in functional status was observed with the concomitant need to gradually decrease antihypertensive drug therapy within the first one to six months. Thereafter, clinical status and cardiovascular drug requirements stabilized with a significantly improved systolic and diastolic blood pressure. Overall New York Heart Association (NYHA) functional class improved from a mean of 2.40 to 1.36 (P < 0.001) and 51% of patients came completely off of between one and three antihypertensive drugs at an average of 4.4 months after starting CoQ10. … In the 9.4% of patients with echocardiograms both before and during treatment, we observed a highly significant improvement in left ventricular wall thickness and diastolic function."

- **Acetyl-L-carnitine and L-carnitine**: Acetyl-L-carnitine (ALC) first made its impression on clinicians when it was found to be effective treatment for Alzheimer's disease; later research found application for this nutrient in the treatment of hepatic coma, Peyronie's disease, male sexual dysfunction, various types of peripheral neuropathy, dysthymia, fibromyalgia, and various types of physical and mental fatigue. The primary mechanism of action is most likely the support/enhancement of mitochondrial function, while other mechanisms clearly exist and are additive/synergistic. Common therapeutic doses are 1,500-3,000 mg per day of either or both of ALC and/or L-carnitine, taken orally, between meals; clinicians should appreciate that amino acid therapy is generally administered between meals to avoid problems arising from competitive blockade among amino acids as they are absorbed/utilized. L-carnitine and ALC can be administered together; use of one does not necessarily preclude use of the other. For example in the study by Cavallini et al[266] among aging men, L-carnitine 2 g/day plus acetyl-L-carnitine 2 g/day proved significantly more effective than testosterone in improving nocturnal penile tumescence and International Index of Erectile Function score.
  - Review: Carnitine insufficiency caused by aging and overnutrition compromises mitochondrial performance and metabolic control (*Journal of Biological Chemistry* 2009 Jun[267]): The authors wrote, "…we hypothesized that **carnitine insufficiency might contribute to mitochondrial dysfunction and obesity-related impairments in glucose tolerance.** Consistent with this prediction, whole body carnitine diminution was identified as a common feature of insulin resistant states such as advanced age, genetic

[264] Singh et al. Hydrosoluble coenzyme Q10 on blood pressures and insulin resistance in hypertensive patients with coronary artery disease. *J Hum Hypertens.* 1999 Mar;13:203-8
[265] Langsjoen P, Langsjoen P, Willis R, Folkers K. Treatment of essential hypertension with coenzyme Q10. *Mol Aspects Med.* 1994;15 Suppl:S265-72
[266] Cavallini et al. Carnitine versus androgen administration in the treatment of sexual dysfunction, depressed mood, fatigue associated with male aging. *Urology.* 2004 Apr:641-6
[267] Noland et al. Carnitine Insufficiency Caused by Aging and Overnutrition Compromises Mitochondrial Performance and Metabolic Control. *J Biol Chem.* 2009 Jun 24

diabetes and diet-induced obesity." This impressive study documented that carnitine deficiency is noted in patients with obesity and insulin resistance; thus, carnitine supplementation—either as L-carnitine or acetyl-L-carnitine, or a combination of the two—appears warranted in such groups simply from the standpoint of correcting this nutrient deficiency/insufficiency.

- Clinical trial: Ameliorating hypertension and insulin resistance in subjects at increased cardiovascular risk. Effects of acetyl-L-carnitine therapy (*Hypertension* 2009 Sep[268]): In a previous trial, acetyl-L-carnitine infusion acutely ameliorated insulin resistance in type-2 diabetics. In this sequential off-on-off pilot study, the authors prospectively evaluated the effects of 24-week oral acetyl-L-carnitine (1 g twice daily) therapy on the glucose disposal rate (GDR), assessed by hyperinsulinemic euglycemic clamps, and components of the metabolic syndrome in nondiabetic subjects at increased cardiovascular risk. "Acetyl-L-carnitine increased GDR from 4.89+/-1.47 to 6.72+/-3.12 mg/kg per minute (P=0.003, Bonferroni-adjusted) and improved glucose tolerance in patients with GDR </=7.9 mg/kg per minute, whereas it had no effects in those with higher GDRs. ... Systolic blood pressure

> ### Acetyl-L-carnitine increases adiponectin: clinical significance and mechanism of action against hypertension
>
> Discovered in 1996, adiponectin is a beneficial protein hormone secreted from adipose tissue, and as such it is an adipokine (adipocyte-derived hormone). Adiponectin is secreted in two forms: a low molecular weight form and a more metabolically active high molecular weight (HMW) multimer. Adiponectin is unique among adipokines in that its effects are largely beneficial; it has anti-diabetic, anti-atherogenic, and anti-inflammatory properties. Another unique feature of adiponectin is that—even though it is made in adipose tissue—its production is inversely proportional to the total load of visceral fat. Per Matsuzawa: "Hypoadiponectinemia induced by visceral fat accumulation is closely associated with type 2 diabetes, lipid disorders, **hypertension** and also certain inflammatory diseases."
>
> Metabolic effects of adiponectin include:
> - Decreases gluconeogenesis and reduces serum glucose,
> - Increases peripheral glucose uptake, indicating improved insulin sensitivity,
> - Enhances β-oxidation of fatty acids, promotes triglyceride clearance,
> - Protects from endothelial dysfunction and atherosclerosis,
> - Promotes weight loss.
>
> Matsuzawa Y. Adiponectin. *Curr Pharm Des.* 2010 Jun

decreased from 144.0 to 135.1 mm Hg and from 130.8 to 123.8 mm Hg in the lower and higher GDR groups, respectively... Acetyl-L-carnitine safely ameliorated arterial hypertension, insulin resistance, impaired glucose tolerance, and hypoadiponectinemia in subjects at increased cardiovascular risk. Whether these effects may translate into long-term cardioprotection is worth investigating." Total adiponectin increased from 4.7 to 6.0 meq/L, while HMW adiponectin increased from 2.2 to 3.0 meq/L (p<0.05 for both changes). The finding of relative carnitine deficiency in patients with HTN and DM along with the finding that acetyl-L-carnitine supplementation raises adiponectin in these patient groups suggests that the hypoadiponectinemia in HTN and DM may be a direct result from hypocarnitinemia.

- Randomized placebo-controlled double-blind crossover study: Effect of combined treatment with alpha-lipoic acid (400 mg/d) and acetyl-L-carnitine (1,000 mg/d) on vascular function and blood pressure in patients with documented coronary artery disease (*Journal of Clinical Hypertension* 2007 Apr[269]): The authors note that mitochondria produce reactive oxygen species that may contribute to vascular dysfunction, and that both oxidative stress and mitochondrial dysfunction can be ameliorated by alpha-lipoic acid and acetyl-L-carnitine. Among 36 subjects with coronary artery disease, active treatment for 8 weeks increased brachial artery diameter by 2.3%, consistent with reduced arterial tone. "Active treatment **decreased systolic blood pressure** for the whole group and had a significant effect in the subgroup with blood pressure above the median (151 to 142 mm Hg) and in the subgroup with the metabolic syndrome (139 to 130 mm Hg)." Although this study used low-modest doses of acetyl-carnitine and lipoic acid, it showed that antihypertensive benefits were greatest in patients with systolic blood pressure >135 mm Hg—blood pressure was reduced by approximately -9/-5 mm Hg—and in patients with metabolic syndrome—blood pressure was reduced by approximately -7/-3 mm Hg. More significant results probably would have been obtained with higher doses, but these results are still statistically and clinically significant.

---

[268] Ruggenenti et al. Ameliorating Hypertension and Insulin Resistance in Increased Cardiovascular Risk. Effects of Acetyl-L-Carnitine Therapy. *Hypertension*. 2009 Sep:567-74
[269] McMackin et al. Combined treatment alpha-Lipoic acid and acetyl-L-carnitine on vascular function and blood pressure in coronary disease. *J Clin Hypertens* 2007 Apr:249-55

SOMATIC, SOCIAL, (LIFE)STYLISTIC, SURGICAL AND OTHER SPECIAL CONSIDERATIONS Lifestyle and other considerations are listed here, notably including surgery (for reduction of neurovascular compression) and spinal manipulation.

- **Exercise**: Current guidelines indicate that everyone should obtain 30-60 minutes of exercise 4-7 times per week unless specific contraindications exist. Patients with or at risk for CAD should receive baseline and stress/exercise ECG before commencing vigorous exercise; if ECG abnormalities are detected or if angina is reported, then stress echocardiography and/or perfusion scan should be considered.

- **Weight optimization**: All patients *and doctors* should maintain a healthy body weight. Canadian guidelines published in 2009 specify a body mass index 18.5-24.9 and waist circumference (<102 cm [40.2 inches] for men and <88 cm [34.6 inches] for women).[270] In most patients and clinical situations, body weight and body mass can be used as an indicator of compliance with a health-promoting diet and plan of regular *sufficiently intense* exercise. Exercise sufficiency can be assessed by the ability of the activity to produce mild breathlessness, diaphoresis, and changes in or favorable maintenance of body composition and optimal weight.

> **Weight loss for overweight patients provides numerous psychosocial and physical benefits**
>
> "With a substantial weight loss of 35 kg and 42% loss of excessive weight, and correction of disturbed metabolic parameters, they significantly improved in general well-being, health distress, and perceived attractiveness, approaching halfway the values of a normal-weight reference group. ... In physical activity, they bypassed the reference group. Days of sick leave decreased to the level of the reference group. **Improvements in HRQL [health-related quality-of-life] paralleled the rate of weight loss."**
>
> Mathus-Vliegen et al. Health-related quality-of-life in patients with morbid obesity after gastric banding for surgically induced weight loss. *Surgery.* 2004 May

- **Mind-Body Approaches including Qigong, controlled breathing, transcendental meditation, and acupuncture**: Traditional therapeutics and lifestyle activities such as Qigong, controlled breathing, meditation, and acupuncture can effect statistically and clinically significant reductions in BP among hypertensive patients. Mechanisms of action include induction of beneficial neurohormonal responses (e.g., increased dehydroepiandrosterone and melatonin levels following meditation) as well as induction of a relaxed state. Avoidance of physiological stressors can play a role in blood pressure control and should be implemented on an as-appropriate basis. Sympathetic neural activity via beta-adrenergic receptors in the kidney stimulates release of renin, which is a peptidase enzyme that converts angiotensinogen to angiotensin-1 and thereby expedites the formation of angiotensin-2 in the lungs; angiotensin-2 is a vasoconstrictor and stimulates aldosterone production which increases sodium resorption and thus water retention.[271]; Thus, the net effect of sympathetic nervous activation is increased volume within a constricted vasculature, thus causing HTN. Data on therapeutic interventions in the following four subsections are derived from the review by Nahas[272] (*Canadian Family Physician* 2008 Nov) unless otherwise noted.

  - Qigong: A Chinese medicine form of movement, breathing, and meditation: As a part of traditional Chinese medicine (TCM), Qigong incorporates movement, breathing, and meditation. Two systematic reviews involving hundreds of patients (n = > 900 to > 1,200 subjects) have examined the role of Qigong in the treatment of hypertension. Despite some methodological shortcomings, evidence shows that Qigong can reduce BP among hypertensives by -12 to -17 mm Hg systolic and -8.5 to -10 mm Hg diastolic. Thus, the BP-lowering results obtained by Qigong are comparable to drug treatment of HTN.

  - Controlled breathing: Most studies (4 of 5) using slow controlled breathing have shown an antihypertensive benefit presumably mediated through increased parasympathetic and reduced sympathetic activity; as expected, diabetics with autonomic dysfunction tend to receive less benefit.

  - Transcendental meditation: Twice-daily sessions of sitting quietly while repeating a specific mantra can effect a BP-lowering effect of approximately -4.7/-3.2 mm Hg.

  - Acupuncture: Acupuncture is difficult to study in a placebo-controlled manner due to the physical, individualized, and experiential nature of the treatment. Antihypertensive benefits of acupuncture have ranged from no different from the so-called placebo to reductions of -6 to -14 mm Hg for systolic BP and -3 to -7 mm Hg for diastolic BP.

---

[270] Khan et al. 2009 Canadian Hypertension Education Program recommendations for the management of hypertension: Part 2—therapy. *Can J Cardiol.* 2009 May;25(5):287-98

[271] Benowitz NL. "Antihypertensive Agents." In Katzung BG (editor). *Basic and Clinical Pharmacology. 10th Edition*. New York: McGraw Hill Medical; 2007, 161

[272] Nahas R. Complementary and alternative medicine approaches to blood pressure reduction: An evidence-based review. *Can Fam Physician.* 2008 Nov;54(11):1529-33

- **Treatment of "central neurogenic hypertension" with surgical techniques—focus on neurovascular (de)compression at the level of the left ventrolateral medulla oblongata**: Physical compression or mechanical irritation of neuronal structures can result in systemic hypertension through a variety of mechanisms; these mechanisms have been most thoroughly described in the biomedical research literature under the disciplines of Surgery as well as of Manipulative Medicine and Spinal Manipulation. Readers should appreciate the basic commonality between surgical intervention and physical manipulation: both interventions have the potential to change physiological relationships experienced between two or more anatomical components via either direct means (i.e., physical alteration) or indirect mechanisms (e.g., reflexive or adaptive changes). Several studies describing surgical alleviation of neurogenic hypertension will be reviewed and summarized here, while those focusing on manipulative treatments will be discussed in the subsection immediately following. Dr Peter Jannetta (MD) is generally attributed with the origination of the concept of medulla oblongata vascular compression by the vertebral artery as one of the causes of hypertension; he has demonstrated that neurovascular compression can be surgically treated by microvascular decompression (MVD) with resultant antihypertensive benefits.[273] Initially, patients selected for surgery (generally either left retromastoid craniectomy or lateral suboccipital craniectomy) were chosen for their cranial nerve deficits such as trigeminal neuralgia, hemifacial spasm, glossopharyngeal neuralgia, Bell's palsy, and spasmodic torticollis, and alleviation of HTN was a "side benefit" of the surgery. Later, severe recalcitrant HTN alone without overt CN deficits has become sufficient basis for surgery in carefully selected patients in appropriate treatment centers, perhaps within a prospective research protocol (per Geiger *et al* in 1998, reviewed below). Also, as stated in a previous section, the perspectives offered by Reis[274] is worthy of recall because of the two truths contained therein, namely that neurogenic contributors to HTN can be ❶ *omnipotent* (Reis: "A neural or neurochemical imbalance in brain **can produce** hypertension"), or ❷ *contributory/amplificatory* (Reis: "Impaired NTS [nucleus tract solitarius] function can produce an **amplification** of the action of the environmental stresses on blood pressure. Thus environmental stimuli or the expression of behaviors which normally result in trivial elevations of blood pressure will, after the NTS is perturbed, result in marked elevations [of blood pressure])." Per descriptions in the literature, central neurogenic hypertension is typically difficult to control, chronic, and progressive.

  - Review and case series: Neurogenic hypertension etiology and surgical treatment: observations in 53 patients (*Annals of Surgery* 1985 Mar[275]): Among 53 patients with simultaneous cranial nerve (CN) dysfunctions and systemic hypertension, 51 of these 53 patients were noted to have arterial compression of the **left lateral medulla oblongata** by looping arteries at the base of the brain (note: neurovascular compression was *not* noted in *normotensive* patients); all 53 patients underwent left retromastoid craniectomy and microvascular decompression (MVD) for treatment of the cranial nerve dysfunctions. More specifically, treatment by vascular decompression of the medulla was performed in 42 of the 53 patients. Relief in the hypertension was seen in 32 of 42 (76% of total) patients and improvement in four; "improvement" was defined in this article as "more than a 20-mm drop in both systolic and diastolic pressures", and thus the total number of patients with a highly meaningful antihypertensive response was 36 of 42 (85% of total). Generally, the problem appears localized to the left vagal nerve and the left lateral medulla oblongata (more specifically between the inferior olive anteriorly and the root entry zone (REZ) or CN 9 and CN 10 posteriorly) and is most commonly caused by arteriosclerosis and arterial ectasia which contribute to arterial elongation and looping, which can eventually lead to pulsatile compression of the left lateral medulla; hypertension can then develop from compromise of the balance in the neural control systems that regulate blood pressure. Because systemic HTN can further contribute to arterial elongation, a vicious cycle of HTN followed by progressive arterial ectasia followed by additional neuronal compromise which results in additional HTN may be established. Specific arteries that can contribute to medulla and/or cranial nerve neurocompression include the left vertebral artery (due to normal anatomy, ectasia, or severe atherosclerosis), posterior inferior cerebellar artery, superior cerebellar artery, basilar

[273] See "Discussion": ncbi.nlm.nih.gov/pmc/articles/PMC1346999/pdf/annsurg00224-0102.pdf
[274] Reis DJ. Nucleus tractus solitarius and experimental neurogenic hypertension: central neural imbalance hypothesis of hypertensive disease. *Adv Biochem Psychopharmacol.* 1981;28:409-20
[275] Jannetta PJ, Segal R, Wolfson SK Jr. Neurogenic hypertension: etiology and surgical treatment. I. Observations in 53 patients. *Ann Surg.* 1985 Mar;201(3):391-8

artery, and anterior inferior cerebellar artery. Neural pathways involved in BP control relevant to this discussion as reviewed by Jannetta *et al* include ❶ carotid baroreceptors with afferents traveling in CN 9 to the nucleus tractus solitarius, ❷ aortic baroreceptors with afferents traveling in CN 10 (i.e., aortic vagal afferents), ❸ cardiac vagal afferents, ❹ descending sympathetic output to vascular smooth muscle; of these, *vasodepressive* cardiac vagal afferent fibers are unmyelinated and are thus most susceptible to compression (per Jannetta *et al*, 1985) thus neurovascular compressive compromise at the REZ of the medulla likely causes HTN (at least in large part) by disinhibition, i.e., impairment of vasodepressive cardiac vagal afferent input. Furthermore, the pulsatile nature of arterial compression may cause greater damage than constant pressure and may desynchronize neural cardiac-pressor control centers. Following surgical displacement of the offending artery away from the brainstem by use of an implant of plastic sponge, muscle, or synthetic felt, many of these patients with chronic systemic HTN who had been taking "large doses of strong medications" were able to reduce or altogether discontinue their drug dependency over the course of days to months following the surgical microvascular decompression. Thus, neurovascular decompression of the left medulla oblongata is a treatment option worth considering in affected and appropriately selected patients with chronic hypertension.

- Exemplary case report: Decreases in blood pressure and sympathetic nerve activity by microvascular decompression of the rostral ventrolateral medulla in essential hypertension (*Stroke* 1999 Aug[276]): The authors of this report begin by noting that neurovascular compression of the rostral ventrolateral medulla, a major center regulating sympathetic nerve activity, may be causally related to essential hypertension, and that microvascular decompression of the rostral ventrolateral medulla decreases elevated blood pressure in some patients. A 47-year-old male with "essential hypertension" and hemifacial nerve spasms was found to have neurovascular compression of the rostral ventrolateral medulla and facial nerve; **microvascular decompression of the rostral ventrolateral medulla successfully reduced blood pressure from 152/110 mm/Hg** while on amlodipine, quinapril, and doxazosin **to 108/74** with only low-dose quinapril (the authors note that quinapril was being tapered to discontinuation at time of publication). Microvascular decompression of the rostral ventrolateral medulla also reduced plasma and urine norepinephrine levels, and reduced other markers of excessive sympathetic nerve activity. Reductions in plasma and urine epinephrine and norepinephrine following MVD in their case report were listed previously in this chapter and are included here again in context to show that post-intervention reduction in sympathetic nerve activity can be documented objectively, and that clinical antihypertensive benefits (BP reductions of 10–30% at 48h postsurgery) can be associated with *relative* reductions in catecholamine levels that may be *within* or *outside of* the normal reference range:
  - Plasma epinephrine: Reduced from 0.22 to <0.05 (reference range <0.93 nmol/L).
  - Plasma norepinephrine: Reduced from 0.95 to 0.30 (range 0.89 - 3.37 nmol/L).
  - Urine epinephrine: Reduced from 83.5 to 26.2 (range 5.5 – 76.4 nmol/d).
  - Urine norepinephrine: Reduced from 0.52 to 0.39 (range 0.06 – 0.024 mmol/d).
- Prospective study (n=14) with long-term follow-up: Temporary reduction of blood pressure and sympathetic nerve activity in hypertensive patients after microvascular decompression (*Stroke* 2009 Jan[277]): Fourteen patients with essential hypertension underwent microvascular decompression of the brain stem. Vasoconstrictor muscle sympathetic nerve activity (recorded by microneurography: burst frequency, bursts/min) and blood pressure (24-hour profiles) were measured before surgery and 7 days, 3 months, and every 6 months postoperatively. **Muscle sympathetic nerve activity** decreased from preoperative levels (35 bursts/min) a nadir of 19 bursts/min before spontaneously rising again to 34 bursts/min; in more detail, the sympatholytic benefits were noted as follows: a reduction from preoperative levels of 35 bursts/min to 19 bursts/min (at 3 months postoperatively), 19 bursts/min (at 6 months), and 23 bursts/min (at 12 months) but were minimized to statistical and clinical insignificance to 28 bursts/min (at 18 months) and 34 bursts/min (at 24 months). **Systolic and diastolic blood pressure** decreased from 162/98 mm Hg preoperatively to 133/85 mm Hg (at 7 days postoperatively), 136/86 mm Hg (at 3 months), 132/85 mm Hg

[276] Morimoto S, Sasaki S, Takeda K, Furuya S, Naruse S, Matsumoto K, Higuchi T, Saito M, Nakagawa M. Decreases in blood pressure and sympathetic nerve activity by microvascular decompression of the rostral ventrolateral medulla in essential hypertension. *Stroke*. 1999 Aug;30(8):1707-10
[277] Frank H, Heusser K, Geiger H, Fahlbusch R, Naraghi R, Schobel HP. Temporary reduction of blood pressure and sympathetic nerve activity in hypertensive patients after microvascular decompression. *Stroke*. 2009 Jan;40(1):47-51 stroke.ahajournals.org/cgi/content/full/40/1/47

(at 6 months), 132/85 mm Hg (at 12 months), and then increased to 158/96 mm Hg at 24 months; thus both blood pressure and hypersympathotonia were reduced by MVD surgery but both returned many months thereafter. The fact that hypersympathotonia returned before HTN would appear to indicate that the former caused the latter despite the fact that the latter can cause the former as discussed in a preceding section. (For review: hypersympathotonia causes HTN via vasoconstriction and activation of the renin-angiotensin system, while HTN causes activation of the sympathetic nervous system when chronic HTN induces elongation and tortuosity of the arteries [left vertebral artery, posterior inferior cerebellar artery, superior cerebellar artery, basilar artery, and anterior inferior cerebellar artery] that are in close proximity to the nucleus tract solitarius and related pressure-controlling neurologic structures.) The authors of the study conclude that, "The data are a hint for sympathetic overactivity as a pathomechanism in this subgroup of patients" while also noting that in the patients selected for this study, the life-threatening severity of their hypertension was probably of such an extent that end-organ damage and various neurohormonal vicious cycles had probably already been established so as to make long-term suppression of HTN particularly challenging. The authors of this paper, published in 2009 in the American Heart Association's journal *Stroke*, close with the following four main conclusions:

- Neurovascular compression of the RVLM causes neurogenic hypertension mediated by a central sympathetic hyperactivity.
- Surgical microvascular decompression reduces central sympathetic outflow and reduces blood pressure, at least temporarily.
- In this study, neither blood pressure improvement nor sympathetic deactivation was sustained effectively for the long-term.
- Until more conclusions are established regarding appropriate imaging and patient selection, MVD is not recommended as cure for HTN and should be performed only in prospective study protocols.

o Case series (n=8) using microvascular decompression as therapy for severe chronic HTN: Decrease of blood pressure by ventrolateral medullary decompression in essential hypertension (*The Lancet* 1998 Aug[278]): Previously, this group of authors showed that 83% of patients with primary HTN, 24% of patients with secondary HTN, and 7% of normotensive controls showed evidence of looping vessels at the left ventrolateral medulla consistent with neurovascular compression as seen on magnetic resonance imaging. In this study, the authors investigated whether neurosurgical microvascular decompression substantially decreases blood pressure long-term in patients with severe essential hypertension. Eight patients—all of whom had experienced one or more life-threatening hypertensive crises—who had received *three or more* antihypertensive drugs without adequate control of blood pressure, intolerable side-effects, or both, underwent microvascular decompression at the root-entry zone (REZ) of cranial nerves 9 and 10 after neurovascular compression of the ventrolateral medulla oblongata was seen with magnetic resonance angiography (MRA). Three months after surgery, blood pressure and antihypertensive drug regimens had decreased substantially in 7 of 8 patients. Four patients who were followed up for more than 1 year became normotensive. No complications associated with decompression occurred except that one patient experienced a transient vocal-cord paresis after the laryngeal part of the vagus nerve was maneuvered during surgery. The authors concluded, "We showed a direct causal relation between raised blood pressure and irritation of cranial nerves 9 and 10. A subgroup of patients with essential hypertension may exist who have secondary forms of hypertension related to neurovascular compression at the ventrolateral medulla and who may be successfully treated with decompression."

- **Treatment of "central and peripheral neurogenic hypertension" with chiropractic and osteopathic manipulative techniques**: Spinal manipulative therapy has proven safe and effective for musculoskeletal spinal pain as well as some extra-spinal disorders, notably asthma.[279] Chiropractic manipulation differs from the types of manipulation provided by other professions (e.g., osteopathic, naturopathic) and thus research substantiating the effectiveness of chiropractic manipulation may not be applicable to different manipulative approaches. Based on the material reviewed in the previous section, readers should already have some

---

[278] Geiger et al. Decrease of blood pressure by ventrolateral medullary decompression in essential hypertension. *Lancet.* 1998 Aug 8;352(9126):446-9
[279] Mein et al. Manual medicine diversity: research pitfalls and the emerging medical paradigm. *J Am Osteopath Assoc.* 2001 Aug;101(8):441-4

appreciation of the rationale, potential benefits, and potential limitations of upper cervical spinal manipulation for the treatment of HTN via reduction of **central neurogenic hypertension** (i.e., potentially via reduction in medullary compression and NTS irritation) as well as via reduction of **peripheral neurogenic hypertension** insofar as upper cervical and cranial/occipital manipulation has been suggested—mainly by theory, extrapolation of anatomy, and less so by strong clinical trials—to potentially decompress, de-facilitate, or otherwise generally relieve from mechanical (and thus physiologic) irritation CN 9, CN 10, and the cervical sympathetic ganglia, all of which are involved in regulation of blood pressure, heart rate, and/or peripheral resistance.

- Double-blind, placebo-controlled pilot study of chiropractic upper cervical manipulation for treatment of hypertension: Atlas vertebra realignment and achievement of arterial pressure goal in 50 *pain-free* hypertensive patients (*Journal of Human Hypertension* 2007 May[280]): The authors introduce this study by writing, "Anatomical abnormalities of the cervical spine at the level of the Atlas vertebra are associated with relative ischemia of the brainstem circulation and increased blood pressure (BP). Manual correction of this mal-alignment has been associated with reduced arterial pressure." The authors used a double-blind, placebo-controlled design at a single center among 50 *pain-free* drug-naïve (n=26) or washed-out (n=24) patients with Stage 1 hypertension; patients were randomized (n=25 in each treatment or placebo group) to receive a National Upper Cervical Chiropractic (NUCCA) procedure or a sham

> ### Cervical spine manipulation for chronic hypertension
>
> "At week 8, there were differences in **systolic BP (-17 mm Hg, NUCCA [chiropractic]** versus -3 mm Hg, placebo) and **diastolic BP (-10 mm Hg, NUCCA [chiropractic]** versus -2 mm Hg). ... No adverse effects were recorded. We conclude that restoration of Atlas alignment is associated with marked and sustained reductions in BP similar to the use of two-drug combination therapy.
>
> ... most single agent antihypertensive [drugs] yield an 8 mm Hg drop in pressure in people with Stage 1 hypertension..."
>
> Bakris et al. Atlas vertebra realignment and achievement of arterial pressure goal in hypertensive patients: a pilot study. *J Hum Hypertens.* 2007 May.

procedure. Significant findings included the following, "At week 8, there were differences in **systolic BP (-17 mm Hg, NUCCA** versus -3 mm Hg, placebo) and **diastolic BP (-10 mm Hg, NUCCA** versus -2 mm Hg [placebo]). ... No adverse effects were recorded. We conclude that restoration of Atlas alignment is associated with marked and sustained reductions in BP similar to the use of two-drug combination therapy." Because the patients were pain-free at the start of the study, relief of neck pain due to treatment with chiropractic manipulation does not explain antihypertensive benefit. Pretreatment patient assessment for NUCCA-specific chiropractic treatment (rather than all forms of chiropractic treatment, of which exist many different techniques) includes ❶ assessment for dynamic functional leg-length discrepancy in the supine position while the patient actively rotates the neck left and right in the transverse/horizontal plane, ❷ paracervical skin temperature measurement, ❸ postural analysis with a proprietary device named Anatometer[281] for precise static biomechanical measurements, and ❹ craniocervical radiographs which are then assessed with NUCCA-specific roentgenometric techniques. As with any procedure involving exposure to ionizing radiation, long-term risk-to-benefit ratios need to be determined and compared to the risk-to-benefit ratios of other treatments; if radiographic evaluation could be eliminated from the assessment protocol without compromising treatment safety efficacy then both costs and risks would be reduced. Impressively, **85% of patients in the chiropractic-treated group required only one treatment to maintain the antihypertensive benefit during the study's duration of two months.** NUCCA treatment of the atlas vertebra resulted in significant measurable changes in atlas lateral and rotational positioning (measured by the pre- and post-treatment radiographs), lateral displacement of C-7 vertebra, frontal-plane pelvic distortion, and lateral-plane pelvic distortion which correlated with the reductions in blood pressure. Lastly for this discussion, readers should appreciate that the NUCCA chiropractic technique uses a gentle direct technique of spinal manipulation which is not the typical, more forceful, high-velocity low-amplitude (HVLA) type which is more commonly used by the majority of chiropractic and (to a lesser extent) osteopathic clinicians; in the current article, NUCCA treatment was described as "A series of precise, subtle, external nudges causes Atlas to recoil into normalized alignment, reseating occipital

---

[280] Bakris et al. Atlas vertebra realignment and achievement of arterial pressure goal in hypertensive patients: a pilot study. *J Hum Hypertens.* 2007 May;21(5):347-52
[281] Anatometer is manufactured by Benesh Corporation: anatometer.com

condyles into Atlas' lateral masses", and the technique's delivery can be observed in the video hyperlinks provided and specifically at nucca.org. Readers of this section may have—hopefully—seen beyond the "data" of this study to appreciate the paradigm shifts implied, which are built upon and/or include but are not limited to the following: ❶ a single gentle musculoskeletal manipulation delivered to the atlas vertebra can lower blood pressure just as effectively as the use of two-drug antihypertensive treatment; ❷ a single gentle musculoskeletal manipulation delivered to the atlas vertebra can affect the positioning of the C-7 vertebra as well as pelvic positioning in the frontal and lateral planes; ❸ subtle changes (invisible to the naked eye) in the positioning of the atlas vertebra, the C-7 vertebra, and pelvis correspond to clinically and statistically significant changes in arterial pressure that can be sustained for at least two months; ❹ individually and collectively, these findings present us with paradigm shifts regarding the local effects of spinal manipulation, body-wide musculoskeletal effects of spinal manipulation, and the systemic nonmusculoskeletal effects of spinal manipulation.

- Case report: Chiropractic management of a hypertensive patient (*Journal of Manipulative and Physiological Therapeutics* 1993 Oct[282]): In this single illustrative case report, the clinician authors describe their experience with a 38-year-old male previously diagnosed with and medicated for chronic essential HTN; the patient's presenting complaints were HTN, drug-related side effects, and low back pain. Chiropractic treatment emphasized specific contact, short lever arm spinal adjustments as the primary mode of chiropractic care. The authors noted, "**During the course of chiropractic treatment, the patient's need for hypertensive medication was reduced.** The patient's medical physician gradually withdrew the medication over 2 months." Appreciating the BP-normalizing benefits of chiropractic manipulation and how these benefits may—paradoxically—lead to iatrogenic complications in patients whose physiologic homeostasis is restored, the authors caution that "specific contact short lever arm spinal adjustments may cause a hypotensive effect in a medicated hypertensive patient that may lead to complications (e.g., hypotension). Since a medicated hypertensive patient's blood pressure may fall below normal while he or she is undergoing chiropractic care, it is advised that the blood pressure be closely monitored and medications adjusted, if necessary, by the patient's medical physician." This point about the very real potential of drug-induced iatrogenic hypotension is analogous to the drug-induced iatrogenic hypoglycemia that can occur when patients' utilization of non-drug integrative treatments overlaps with their previously prescribed drug treatments. When working with medicated and particularly *polymedicated* HTN patients, clinicians have the responsibility to implement treatment in such a way as to minimize the risk for hypotension (and other complications, such as hypoglycemia, respectively)—for example, by starting with lower doses of nutritional supplements, implementing treatment in a step-wise manner, coordinating modifications/reductions in drug doses, and having the patient use more frequent self-monitoring (of blood pressure, blood glucose [etc], respectively); patient education and documentation of informed consent are standards of care for all interventions.

- Randomized, controlled trial (active treatment, placebo treatment, or no treatment): Effects of chiropractic treatment on blood pressure and anxiety (*Journal of Manipulative and Physiological Therapeutics* 1988 Dec[283]): This study (n=21) differs from the previously cited article "Atlas vertebra realignment and achievement of arterial pressure goal in hypertensive patients" in that ❶ the thoracic spine (T1-T5) rather than the upper cervical spine was the area of treatment, ❷ the treatment used a mechanical chiropractic adjusting device rather than manual manipulation, and ❸ the study included assessment for anxiety as well as for changes in BP, rather than BP alone. The mechanical chiropractic adjusting device used in this study is the Activator Adjusting Instrument[284], which delivers a highly-localized 28-pound thrust within 1/300 of a second. The authors concluded, "Results indicated that systolic and diastolic blood pressure decreased significantly in the active treatment condition, whereas no significant changes occurred in the placebo and control conditions. State anxiety significantly decreased in the active and control conditions. Results provide support for the hypothesis that blood pressure is reduced following chiropractic treatment."[285]

[282] Plaugher G, Bachman TR. Chiropractic management of a hypertensive patient. *J Manipulative Physiol Ther*. 1993 Oct;16(8):544-9
[283] Bakris et al. Atlas vertebra realignment and achievement of arterial pressure goal in hypertensive patients: a pilot study. *J Hum Hypertens*. 2007 May;21(5):347-52
[284] Activator Methods International, Ltd. (AMI) produces the Activator Adjusting Instrument. See also activatoronline.com
[285] Yates et al. Effects of chiropractic treatment on blood pressure and anxiety: a randomized, controlled trial. *J Manipulative Physiol Ther*. 1988 Dec;11(6):484-8

Cervical Spine: Rotation Emphasis

Patient:
- Supine, neck slightly flexed

Doctor position:
- At 45° angle from head of table; may also be in a more lateral position aside the patient's head and neck; while it is acceptable to assess and set-up with straight legs, at the time of impulse, doctor's legs should be bent to provide the doctor with greater power, stability, and biomechanical safety

Assessment:
- <u>Subjective</u>: neck pain, headaches
- <u>Motion palpation</u>: rotation restriction; primary or compensatory hypermobile segments may be detected above or below the restricted segment
- <u>Static palpation</u>: vertebra may feel relatively posterior on the side opposite the rotational restriction, e.g., a right rotational restriction may present with a relative left rotational malposition that brings the vertebral lamina and articular pillars posterior on the left
- <u>Soft tissue</u>: tenderness, may also have muscle spasm

Treatment contact:
- Doctor uses either an index or proximal phalange contact on the posterior aspect of the transverse process and/or articular pillar
- The doctor's vector and hence the positioning of the forearm of the contact hand must change depending on the level of the cervical spine that is being treated
- Notice in this photograph that the thumb of the doctor's contact hand is placed on the angle of the mandible, this is more to help anchor the contact and stabilize the doctor's wrist than to assist with the manipulation; very little pressure and zero thrust are applied to the mandible

Supporting contact:
- Head is held into rotation and slight flexion; as with all techniques, nuanced adjustments in flexion-extension, rotation, and side-bending are made until the premanipulative tension is localized to the specific direction/tissue of restriction

Pretreatment positioning:
- Slight flexion and extension may be used below and above the treatment contact to create motion restriction at the adjacent motion segments; this helps to focus the motion and therapeutic force at the specific; importantly the support hand is largely responsible for proper positioning with the correct amount of nuanced flexion-extension and side-bending so that the rotational force is accurately delivered

Thrust:
- Rotational thrust with contact hand; support hand keeps head off table allowing rotation

Image:

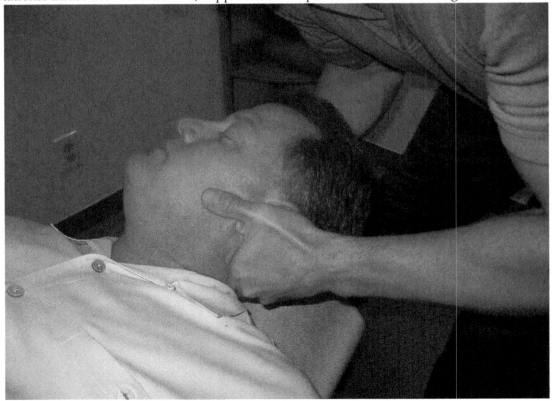

INFLAMMATION MASTERY & FUNCTIONAL INFLAMMOLOGY © ICHNFM.ORG

Cervical Spine: Lateral Flexion (Side-Bending) Emphasis; Treatment of Lateral Malposition

Patient position:	• Supine, head is neutrally placed—neither flexed nor extended; slight flexion is allowed; this technique can also be adapted for use in a seated position
Doctor position:	• At 45° angle from head of table; may also be in a more lateral position aside the patient's head and neck
Assessment:	• <u>Subjective</u>: neck pain, headaches
	• <u>Motion palpation</u>: lateral flexion restriction
	• <u>Static palpation</u>: vertebra may *feel* laterally displaced
	• <u>Soft tissue</u>: tenderness, may also have muscle spasm
Treatment contact:	• Using an index (metacarpal-phalangeal) contact at the tip of the transverse process or slightly posterior to the transverse process; an index phalangeal contact can also be used on the articular pillars as long as doctor is careful not to thrust in a rotational direction; notice in this picture how Dr Harris has the forearm of his contact hand perfectly aligned in the treatment vector, which is almost purely in the patient's transverse/horizontal plane; notice also that Dr Harris has his knees bent and is forward flexed to bring his torso closer to his contact and thereby minimize stress and strain on his own shoulders; with slight modifications in vector direction, this technique can be applied throughout the cervical spine from C0-C7
Supporting contact:	• Lateral aspect of head, opposite contact; generally the supporting hand is neutral, however it can supply some traction and can help induce lateral flexion at impulse; with more aggressive adjustments, the supporting hand can supply a counterforce to minimize motion following the application of a faster and more powerful thrust
Pretreatment positioning:	• Lateral flexion at the targeted segment; the slightest amount of contralateral rotation is applied
Therapeutic action:	• Establish minimal premanipulative tension once the end range of motion has been reached, then use quick and very shallow trust to induce lateral flexion
Image:	

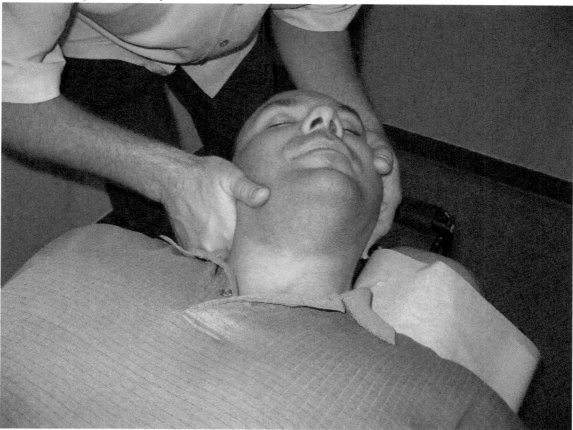

- Pilot study to determine the feasibility of a practice-based randomized controlled clinical trial with three parallel groups: Chiropractic adjustments and brief massage treatment at sites of subluxation in subjects with essential hypertension (*Journal of Manipulative and Physiological Therapeutics* 2002 May[286]): Treatment groups in this study consisted of ❶ chiropractic manipulation, ❷ brief soft tissue massage, or ❸ nontreatment control group. The patient group consisted of 23 subjects, 24-50 years of age, with systolic or diastolic primary HTN. In the active chiropractic treatment group, the intervention consisted of 2 months of full-spine chiropractic care using Gonstead technique, described as specific-contact, short-lever-arm adjustments delivered at motion segments exhibiting signs of subluxation. The massage group received brief effleurage at localized regions of the spine believed to be exhibiting signs of subluxation. The nontreatment control group rested alone for a period of approximately 5 minutes in a treatment room. In both the chiropractic and massage therapy groups, all subjects were classified as either overweight or obese; in the control group, only 2 subjects were overweight—these baseline differences in the study groups are important as they suggest that more patients in the chiropractic treatment group probably had HTN as a component of the metabolic syndrome rather than HTN due specifically and solely to a musculoskeletal lesion. The authors report that at the end of the study period, the BP change was -6.3 mm Hg in the chiropractic group, -1.0 mm Hg in the massage group, and -7.2 mm Hg in the relaxation "control" group. The authors of this pilot feasibility study noted several methodological shortcomings and logistical complications of their study, most notably the limited subject pool of patients who have hypertensive disease but who are not taking medications for its control. A larger study group would have allowed improved randomization and thus equilibration of baseline patient characteristics such as body mass index, which shows a strong correlation with severity of HTN.

- Review: Spinal manipulation and the efficacy of conservative therapeusis for the treatment of hypertension (*Journal of Manipulative and Physiological Therapeutics* 1986 Mar[287]): These authors review relevant chiropractic and osteopathic literature of the day (published in 1986) and conclude that manipulative therapy has a rational basis in the treatment of HTN based on the potential for spinal manipulation to promote restoration of homeostasis via reducing excess sympathetic tone and effecting a relative increase in parasympathetic tone. Spinal regions that are emphasized are ❶ the upper cervical spine (occiput-atlas) which correlates anatomically with the superior cervical sympathetic ganglia, ❷ the upper thoracic spine (T1-T6, especially T2-T3) which correlates with the thoracic sympathetic ganglia, and ❸ the lower thoracic spine (T11-T12) which correlates with sympathetic innervation via the renal ganglia/plexus that services the kidney. Clinicians should recall that sympathetic activation of the kidney increases production of renin (the enzyme), angiotensin-2 (the product of renin acting upon angiotensin-1), and aldosterone (produced by the adrenal cortex in response to stimulation by angiotensin-2) to effect systemic vasoconstriction and retention of sodium and water to increase blood volume and blood pressure. Comprehensive chiropractic treatment should include (but not be limited to) manipulation of spinal segments, massage and manipulation of regional soft tissues, mobilization of the ribs, and the implementation of dietary, nutritional, exercise/lifestyle, sleep pattern, and psychoemotional interventions. The authors conclude that alleviating HTN via resolution of musculoskeletal dysfunction and restoration of homeostasis is a more logical and ethical approach than is the suppression of HTN with the use of drugs that commonly have iatrogenic consequences.

- Review: Effect of osteopathic manipulative therapy on autonomic tone as evidenced by blood pressure changes and activity of the fibrinolytic system (*JAOA—Journal of the American Osteopathic Association* 1968 May[288]): The authors describe their prior research experience with humans and animals in the investigation of the effects of osteopathic manipulation on blood pressure and activation of the sympathetic nervous system as evaluated by changes in the fibrinogen/fibrinolytic system; they wrote, "In research which has been conducted in this laboratory to date, the relationship between changes in blood pressure and the manipulative therapeutic approach not only has been validated in human beings with hypertension, but

[286] Plaugher et al. Practice-based randomized controlled-comparison clinical trial of chiropractic adjustments and brief massage treatment at sites of subluxation in subjects with essential hypertension: pilot study. *J Manipulative Physiol Ther.* 2002 May;25(4):221-39
[287] Crawford et al. Management of hypertensive disease: spinal manipulation and the efficacy of conservative therapeusis. *J Manipulative Physiol Ther* 1986 Mar ;9(1):27-32
[288] Celander E, Koenig AJ, Celander DR. Effect of osteopathic manipulative therapy on autonomic tone as evidenced by blood pressure changes and activity of the fibrinolytic system. *J Am Osteopath Assoc.* 1968 May;67(9):1037-8

has also been demonstrated in normal persons as well as in experimental dogs. **Soft tissue manipulation of the upper thoracic and cervical vertebrae leads in almost every case to a decrease in blood pressure.**" These authors go on to note that "…a cumulative effect does occur, four or five treatments accomplishing a greater effect than a single treatment…" and that a reduction in pro-coagulative tendency occurs as evidenced by reductions in fibrinogen and other serum levels of coagulation factors.

- <u>Clinical trial: Effect of osteopathic manipulative therapy on autonomic tone as evidenced by blood pressure changes and activity of the fibrinolytic system</u> (*JAOA—Journal of the American Osteopathic Association* 1969 Jun[289]): The authors describe the use of an interventional protocol consisting of ❶ 15 minutes of rest in the supine position during measurement of blood pressure and laboratory indices, ❷ 5 minutes of soft tissue manipulation in the prone position ("The patient then assumes the prone position for 5 minutes. During this time soft tissue manipulation is applied equally to the left and right posterior cervical and thoracic areas. In the control experiment, no soft tissue manipulation is performed during this time interval.", and ❸ 15 minutes of rest in the supine position during measurement of blood pressure and laboratory indices. The authors wrote, "In our study after an initial rest period followed by manipulation there was a significant decrease (p<0.01) in both diastolic and systolic pressure in the hypertensive group." Furthermore, they noted laboratory evidence of reduced hemoconcentration, erythrocyte sedimentation rate, and a reduction in fibrinogen levels in 96% of patients with hypertension; among normotensive patients, fibrinogen levels decreased in 32% and increased in 51%.

- <u>Blinded randomized clinical trial using chiropractic and diet to treat hypertension: Treatment of Hypertension with Alternative Therapies (THAT) Study</u> (*Journal of Hypertension* 2002 Oct[290]): Given the potential implications of the use of "chiropractic spinal manipulation and diet" for the treatment of HTN, this study is potentially important and therefore worthy of detailed analysis; this is even more true when we appreciate that the authors titled this study "Treatment of Hypertension with Alternative Therapies" and thus broadened the implications of this article to all modes, genres, professions, and interventions that might fall under the rubric of "alternative medicine." The authors begin their abstract by stating that the objective of the study is to "To examine the effect of spinal manipulation on blood pressure" and then go on to describe the design of the study to be "This randomized clinical trial compared the effects of chiropractic spinal manipulation and diet with diet alone for lowering blood pressure in participants with high-normal blood pressure or stage I hypertension."; thus, from the outset, the study was not designed to truly investigate "alternative therapies" *per se* as the term should be applied (if it is to be used at all[291]) but rather only "chiropractic spinal manipulation" (within which many techniques exist) and "diet" (which can mean different things to different clinicians and can be variously applied to and implemented by diverse groups of patients). Per the study description, "One hundred and forty men and women, aged 25-60 years, with high-normal blood pressure or stage I hypertension, were enrolled. One hundred and twenty-eight participants completed the study. INTERVENTIONS: (i) A dietary intervention program administered by a dietitian [Diet] or (ii) a dietary intervention program administered by a doctor of chiropractic in conjunction with chiropractic spinal manipulation [DC+diet]. The frequency of treatment for both groups was three times per week for 4 weeks, for a total of 12 visits"; this might appear to be a reasonable study design insofar as it distinguishes the effectiveness of Diet from the effectiveness of DC+diet however the comparison is not balanced insofar as the Diet group was seen by a full-time dietician (who focuses only on nutrition) versus the diet advice administered by a full-time clinician with a broader range of responsibilities and daily actions who then by definition has less time to dedicate to dietary advice. Results of the study showed that "Average decreases in systolic/diastolic blood pressure were -4.9/5.6 mmHg for diet group and -3.5/4.0 mmHg for the chiropractic group. Between group changes were not statistically significant. CONCLUSIONS: For patients with high normal blood pressure or stage I hypertension, chiropractic spinal manipulation in conjunction with a dietary modification program offered

---

[289] Fichera AP, Celander DR. Effect of osteopathic manipulative therapy on autonomic tone as evidenced by blood pressure changes and activity of the fibrinolytic system. *J Am Osteopath Assoc.* 1969 Jun;68(10):1036-8

[290] Goertz et al. Treatment of Hypertension with Alternative Therapies (THAT) Study: a randomized clinical trial. *J Hypertens.* 2002 Oct;20(10):2063-8

[291] MacIntosh A. "Understanding the Differences between Conventional, Alternative, Complementary, Integrative and Natural Medicine" *Townsend Letter* 1999 July tldp.com/medicine.htm This is a brilliant -- if not obvious -- explanation that was powerful for the time it was written, and beyond. This article should be required reading for politicians, clinicians, and policy-makers and others with a stake in so-called "CAM."

no advantage in lowering either diastolic or systolic blood pressure compared to diet alone." This conclusion could easily be interpreted to imply that chiropractic manipulation is inefficacious and/or that the dietary advice given by the chiropractic doctors in this study was of poor quality or that it even negated the potential benefits of spinal manipulation (or vice versa). For many clinicians and policy-makers, this is probably as far as they might go with this study, with the take-away message being that both diet and spinal manipulation are essentially inefficacious for the treatment of hypertension. However, detailed reading of the article reveals several study

characteristics that may have contributed to the report of inefficacy, which is suspiciously noteworthy for its severity in both groups treated with diet therapy. Critique of the article follows:

❶ Participants in this study did not have hypertension to begin with. Participants for this study were relatively healthy with systolic pressures below 160 mmHg and diastolic pressures of 85–99 mmHg. Since patients with less severe degrees of hypertension would be expected to show less numerical improvement, this study's use of subjects with average blood pressure of 135/88 mm Hg—a level which is considered nonhypertensive—slanted the scales toward a conclusion of inefficacy because the subjects had no disease. In a very real sense therefore, the title of this article "Treatment of Hypertension with Alternative Therapies" is doubly misleading; first, the subjects did not have hypertension to begin with, and second, among the hundreds of "alternative therapies" available, only two were chosen for this study. A more accurate title of this article (as will become more clear in the following discussion) would have been "Treatment of nonhypertensive patients with weak dietary advice and nonspecific chiropractic manipulation lowers blood pressure by approximately 4/5 mm Hg."

❷ The diet advice given was standardized rather than customized. The study reads "DC/Diet patients received all of the written diet information received by the Diet group, but from the chiropractor. In addition, DC/Diet participants received chiropractic spinal manipulation." Regardless of whether the information was delivered by a chiropractic doctor or an experienced registered dietitian, the information was "prefabricated" rather than customized per patient. Better results are obtained when treatments are customized per patient; thus, this study failed to offer optimal diet therapy and not surprisingly found lackluster results.

❸ The study prohibited the use of several of the most effective "alternative therapies" for hypertension despite being titled "Treatment of Hypertension with Alternative Therapies". The requirement that "All treating clinicians agreed not to offer dietary advice other than that included in the standard diet instructions (e.g. supplements), aerobic exercise advice, acupuncture or activator treatment to participants" was good for the standardization of the study but it eliminates the possibility of implementing some of the most valuable "alternative therapies" that exist for the treatment of HTN, such as vitamin D3, CoQ10, exercise, and weight loss. Again, the study was given a misleading title.

❹ The "specific diet intervention instructions" used in this study were suspiciously inefficacious and were not disclosed in the materials and methods. The authors fail to disclose the details of their diet intervention, thus ensuring that their study can never be subjected to scientific scrutiny by replication. Further, the only details provided are that subjects were given "written instructions on how to modify their current diet and were also given diet sheets, which included low-fat, low-salt recipes. The nutritionist explained the diet and covered a pre-set list of topics." The low-fat aspect of the diet strongly suggests that the diet was low in the health-promoting cardioprotective fatty acids previously reviewed, namely ALA, GLA, EPA, DHA, and oleic acid; the diet pattern suggested was probably neither Paleo nor Mediterranean. Diets that are relatively lower in fat tend to be by default relatively higher in carbohydrates, which leads to insulin release, retention of sodium and water, systemic inflammation, endothelial dysfunction, and the perpetuation of hypertension. That the diet was highly inefficacious is made obvious by the results provided in Table @ of their study, which shows that participants in both groups lost essentially zero weight (-0.8 lbs) during the 4-week study duration; this proves the inappropriate design of the intervention diet provided to both groups because clinical experience and clinical trials have repeatedly demonstrated that patients on effective optimized diets generally lose 4-8 lbs per month. Failure of the diet intervention to effect weight loss in both therapeutic groups

having an average BMI of 30.5 *which clearly shows that most patients in this study met objective criteria for obesity* provides objective proof that the interventional diet was of faulty design; again, these patients should have lost 4-8 lbs during the study period had the diet been appropriately designed, delivered, and implemented.

❺ The subjects in the chiropractic group were healthier than those in the diet group. "The diet group overall weighed more than the chiropractic group at 200 versus 187 lbs, and this difference was borderline significant (P = 0.06)." Regardless of statistical significance, the clinical significance of a 13-pound weight difference is noteworthy. Because the DC+diet group was healthier from the start of the study, less improvement would have been expected. The DC+diet group also had fewer smokers and fewer patients taking medications; these differences between groups were not mathematically significant, but they may have been additively or synergistically clinically significant.

❻ Exclusion of patients with pain negates the recognition of chiropractic's probable antihypertension-via-analgesia benefit from spinal manipulation. The authors acknowledge, "Because spinal manipulation has been reported to lower pain levels for individuals with back pain, and there is a correlation between pain levels and blood pressure, participants reporting average pain levels of five or above on a 0–10 point visual analog type scale were also excluded." In the real world, if a patient with pain and hypertension has both conditions relieved via spinal manipulation's antinociceptive benefits, then this would be documented as a dual benefit from a single therapy. This study's design eliminated the possibility of detecting and documenting this benefit.

❼ Positive selection of subjects likely confused the findings of the study. Recruitment methods quite likely selected patients already using "alternative therapies" and who may have already been "maximally improved" from their former baseline of hypertension severity. "All methods [of subject recruitment] incorporated the same message and highlighted the alternative therapy aspect of the study."; this would have resulted in positive selection of patients interested in and perhaps already using CAM treatments including nutritional supplements and exercise. Since the authors did not include use of nutritional supplements, exercise, acupuncture, diet therapy (etc) in their exclusion criteria, some of the test

subjects may have already been maximally treated with self-selected or professionally-directed treatments. The exclusion criteria failed to control for this important variable.

❽ With all of these problems invalidating the design, implementation, and conclusions of the study, its publication calls into question the intent and/or the wakefulness of the journal's editorial board. Supposedly, the purpose of having an Editor and an Editorial Board is to create what is called the "peer-review" process by which an article undergoes at least some modicum of scientific *or perhaps even intellectual* scrutiny prior to publication so that drivel is not incorporated into our collective body of knowledge that we use to direct patient care. Bad research is bad enough, but when it becomes codified by publication in a journal such as *Journal of Hypertension* and then indexed into Medline by the US National Library of Medicine, then it has the power to influence the healthcare received by thousands of patients, nationally and internationally. The publication of articles such as this calls into question the value and reliability of the peer-review process, the quality and intent of journal editors and editorial boards, and the value of doctorate-level training *prima facie* if its results are such as these. In sum, this study had numerous flaws—the three most important are ❶ the patients were nonhypertensive from the start, ❷ the dietary intervention was standardized (rather than individualized) and was clearly inefficacious as demonstrated by its inability to effect weight loss in a group of obese patients, and ❸ the interventional diet was prefabricated rather than reflecting the type of dietary intervention that a chiropractic doctor might actually use in real clinical practice. Thus, this study completely failed to offer any legitimate insight into the "treatment of hypertension with alternative therapies" and it unscientifically and inaccurately slanders both chiropractic manipulation and dietary intervention for the treatment of hypertension.

Clinical pearls: Ways to objectively assess treatment involvement (compliance)

1. **Vitamin D levels**: Serum 25-OH-cholecalciferol can be tested as a surrogate marker for compliance with nutritional supplementation (detailed later); levels should rise within one month and plateau at the optimal range within 2-3 months if dose and compliance are appropriate. Since most patients will have low levels of 25-OH-D at initial assessment, retesting serum levels after 1-2 months of supplementation is an easy way to assess compliance with and effectiveness of this aspect of the treatment plan.
2. **Recall**: Patients should be able to recite their daily regimen of nutritional supplementation, pharmaceutical drugs, dietary prescriptions/proscriptions, and exercise-lifestyle habits. *If the patient cannot recall their daily health-promoting activities, then compliance is likely either low or nonexistent.*
3. **Consciousness**: Ideally, patients should be able to recite their personal values and goals, as these are the driving forces that either *support* or *subvert* their daily health-related behaviors. Conscious physicians should encourage consciousness-raising in their patients.
4. **Weight optimization**: Often, the "scale of truth" can be used for objective determination of compliance with the Paleo-Mediterranean Diet and particularly its low-carbohydrate and ketogenic variants. Overweight patients who comply with dietary optimization and lifestyle modification can generally achieve weight loss of 4-8 lbs (13-18 kg) per month. Certainly not all benefits of diet optimization are mediated through weight loss; however, the fact remains that weight loss is an important goal for the majority of hypertensive patients. Failure of weight loss can also be used to assess compliance and effectiveness of clinical trials involving dietary intervention; obviously, those trials that fail to effect weight loss were affected by inadequate compliance on behalf of the group of subjects (unlikely) or failure to design an appropriate dietary intervention on behalf of the researchers (more likely).
5. **Urinary sodium and potassium**: With a decided and consistent shift away from the Standard American-type diet (SAD) and toward the health-promoting Paleo-Mediterranean Diet (PMD) and particularly with its supplemented version (sPMD), the urinary sodium:creatinine ratio will decrease, as will the urinary sodium:potassium ratio.

ENDOCRINE Generally speaking: estrogen promotes water retention and thus hypertension; an excess or deficiency of thyroid hormone/function can lead to systolic or diastolic hypertension, respectively. Melatonin is an antioxidant (among its many functions) and can help reduce elevated blood pressure; obviously, melatonin is take only at night.

- **Treatment of hypothyroidism**: Obviously, HTN caused by primary, secondary, or peripheral/metabolic hypothyroidism is not primary/essential HTN because it is due to the thyroid hormone disorder/dysfunction. Clinicians can choose any of several—or a combination thereof—methods to correct thyroid dysfunction, not the least of which are gluten avoidance in gluten-intolerant patients[292], zinc[293] and selenium supplementation[294,295,296,297], administration of *inactive* T4 (levothyroxine) and/or T3 (liothyronine, the most active thyroid hormone[298,299]), or the use of bovine/porcine-sourced glandular thyroid products—the latter should be avoided in patients with antibody-positive thyroid autoimmunity.
- **Melatonin**: Melatonin is an endogenously produced hormone from the pineal gland that plays numerous physiologic roles beyond its sedative effect for sleep promotion. Trace amounts of melatonin are found in food;

---

[292] "In most patients who strictly followed a 1-yr gluten withdrawal (as confirmed by intestinal mucosa recovery), there was a normalization of subclinical hypothyroidism. ... CONCLUSIONS: The greater frequency of thyroid disease among celiac disease patients justifies a thyroid functional assessment. In distinct cases, gluten withdrawal may single-handedly reverse the abnormality." Sategna-Guidetti et al. Prevalence of thyroid disorders in untreated adult celiac disease patients and effect of gluten withdrawal: an Italian multicenter study. *Am J Gastroenterol.* 2001 Mar;96(3):751-7

[293] "RESULTS: Thirteen had low levels of serum free T3 and normal T4. ... After oral supplementation of Zn sulphate (4-10 mg/kg body weight) for 12 months, levels of serum free T3 and T3 normalized, serum rT3 decreased, and the TRH-induced TSH reaction normalized. ... CONCLUSION: Zn may play a role in thyroid hormone metabolism in low T3 patients and may in part contribute to conversion of T4 to T3 in humans." Nishiyama et al. Zinc supplementation alters thyroid hormone metabolism in disabled patients with zinc deficiency. *J Am Coll Nutr.* 1994 Feb;13(1):62-7

[294] Duntas et al. Effects of a six month treatment with selenomethionine in patients with autoimmune thyroiditis. *Eur J Endocrinol.* 2003 Apr;148(4):389-93

[295] Gartner R, Gasnier BC, Dietrich JW, Krebs B, Angstwurm MW. Selenium supplementation in patients with autoimmune thyroiditis decreases thyroid peroxidase antibodies concentrations. *J Clin Endocrinol Metab.* 2002 Apr;87(4):1687-91 jcem.endojournals.org/cgi/content/full/87/4/1687

[296] "We recently conducted a prospective, placebo-controlled clinical study, where we could demonstrate, that a substitution of 200 wg sodium selenite for three months in patients with autoimmune thyroiditis reduced thyroid peroxidase antibody (TPO-Ab) concentrations significantly." Gartner R, Gasnier BC. Selenium in the treatment of autoimmune thyroiditis. *Biofactors.* 2003;19(3-4):165-70

[297] "A highly significant linear correlation between the T3/T4 ratio and indices of Se status was observed in the older group of subjects. Indices of Zn status did not correlate with thyroid hormones, ... We concluded that reduced peripheral T4 conversion is related to impaired Se status in the elderly." Olivieri et al. Selenium, zinc, and thyroid hormones in healthy subjects: low T3/T4 ratio in the elderly is related to impaired selenium status. *Biol Trace Elem Res.* 1996 Jan;51(1):31-41

[298] McDaniel AB. Thyroid Assessment: Controversies and Conundrums. Institute for Functional Medicine Fourteenth International Symposium. Tuscon, Arizona. May 23-26, 2007. Reviewed in more detail in: Vasquez A. *Integrative Rheumatology.* IBMRC 2006, 2007 and all future editions and Vasquez A. *Musculoskeletal Pain: Expanded Clinical Strategies.* Institute for Functional Medicine. May 2008

[299] Friedman et al. Supraphysiological cyclic dosing of sustained release T3 in order to reset low basal body temperature. *P R Health Sci J.* 2006 Mar;25(1):23-9

when taken as a dietary supplement, melatonin demonstrates chronobiologic, sedative, antioxidant, antitumor, and immunomodulatory benefits.

- Double-blind placebo-controlled clinical trial: Melatonin reduces night blood pressure in patients with nocturnal hypertension (*American Journal of Medicine* 2006 Oct[300]): The authors begin by noting that "Nocturnal hypertension is associated with a high risk of morbidity and mortality." In this study, 38 adult patients medicated for HTN were randomized to receive melatonin 2 mg or placebo for 4 weeks. The results read as follows, "Melatonin treatment reduced nocturnal systolic BP significantly from 136 to 130 mm Hg (P=.011), and diastolic BP from 72 to 69 mm Hg (P=.002), whereas placebo had no effect on nocturnal BP." Thus, the authors concluded, "**Thus, an addition of melatonin 2 mg at night to stable antihypertensive treatment may improve nocturnal BP control in treated patients with nocturnal hypertension.**" This study showed that the addition of melatonin to standard drug treatment for HTN resulted in a **decrease in nighttime blood pressure of -6/-3 mm Hg** among patients with nocturnal HTN.

- Randomized placebo-controlled double-blind crossover study: Blood pressure response to melatonin in type 1 diabetes (*Pediatric Diabetes* 2004 Mar[301]): Eleven normotensive adolescent patients with type 1 diabetes of average 7-year duration and 10 healthy controls aged 14-18y participated in a randomized placebo-controlled double-blind crossover study of 5 mg melatonin for 1 week followed by a 1-week washout. Results showed that, "In the patients with type 1 diabetes, the decline in **diastolic blood pressure during sleep was significantly greater on melatonin (17.8 mmHg) than on placebo (16.0 mmHg, p < 0.01)."** This study showed use of melatonin 5 mg resulted in a **decrease in nighttime diastolic pressure of -1.6 mm Hg** among type-1 diabetic patients.

- Randomized, double-blind, placebo-controlled, crossover trial: Daily nighttime melatonin reduces blood pressure in male patients with essential hypertension (*Hypertension* 2004 Feb[302]): The authors of this study show uncommon insight in their introduction which partly reads: "Our objective was to determine whether enhancement of the functioning of the biological clock by repeated nighttime melatonin intake might reduce ambulatory blood pressure in patients with essential hypertension." Sixteen men with untreated essential HTN were given oral melatonin 2.5 mg at 1 hour before sleep, while 24-hour ambulatory blood pressure and actigraphic estimates of sleep quality were measured. Results showed that **repeated melatonin intake reduced systolic and diastolic blood pressure during sleep by -6 and -4 mm Hg, respectively**, with no effect on heart rate.

| XENOBIOTICS | Xenobiotics and "toxins" such as lead, mercury, and the wide range of POPs—persistent organic pollutants—such as dioxin have a long record of causing or contributing to hypertension and many other health problems; these facts are so well established that citation to research is not necessary for this section—see details in Chapter 2 and Chapter 4, Section 7. As such, all patients need to live a "detoxification lifestyle" including the following:

> **Xenobiotic-induced HTN**
>
> Pesticides and other pollutants commonly induce mitochondrial dysfunction, thereby contributing to insulin resistance and vasoconstriction, both of which promote HTN.

1. Organic diet
2. Political activism—the only way to stop the daily chemical assault is to get governments to *write* and *enforce* pollution-control and to deter corporate irresponsibility. Failure to effect political and social change will lead to continued poisoning of the population, while partially salvaging only the more affluent and educated portions of the population able to afford and knowledgeable about detoxification; we are witnessing negative selection of the entire population, with only the more educated and affluent able to avoid or detoxify chemicals that are poisoning everyone. In the United States for example, large portions of the population are exposed to glyphosate in air and water; clearly eating "an organic diet" is only of partial help if the air is contaminated.

   - **America's air and (rain) water are contaminated with pesticides** (*Environ Toxicol Chem* 2014 Jun[303]): "Seven compounds in 1995 and 5 in 2007 were detected in ≥50% of both air and rain samples. Atrazine, metolachlor,

---

[300] Grossman et al. Melatonin reduces night blood pressure in patients with nocturnal hypertension. *Am J Med.* 2006 Oct;119(10):898-902

[301] Cavallo A, Daniels SR, Dolan LM, Khoury JC, Bean JA. Blood pressure response to melatonin in type 1 diabetes. *Pediatr Diabetes.* 2004 Mar;5(1):26-31

[302] Scheer et al. Daily nighttime melatonin reduces blood pressure in male patients with essential hypertension. *Hypertension.* 2004 Feb;43(2):192-7

[303] Majewski et al. Pesticides in Mississippi air and rain: a comparison between 1995 and 2007. *Environ Toxicol Chem.* 2014 Jun;33(6):1283-93

and propanil were detected in ≥50% of the air and rain samples in both years. Glyphosate and its degradation product, aminomethyl-phosphonic acid (AMPA), were detected in ≥75% of air and rain samples in 2007… The 1995 seasonal wet depositional flux was dominated by methyl parathion (88%) and was >4.5 times the 2007 flux. Total herbicide flux in 2007 was slightly greater than in 1995 and was dominated by glyphosate."

3. Avoid exposure, e.g., plastics and consumption of foods from cans lined with BPA—bisphenol A.
4. Establish and maintain urine pH of ~7.5-8 to promote reductions in cortisol, retention of magnesium and potassium, and urinary excretion of toxins/xenobiotics.
5. Optimization of gut flora to avoid LPS inhibition of detoxification.
6. Exercise to promote lipolysis, circulation of toxins (for hepatic and renal clearance), and sweating/diaphoresis for dermal clearance of toxins.
7. Basic mitochondrial and detoxification support with NAC and CoQ10 at the very least.

The connection between xenobiotic exposure and mitochondrial dysfunction is so strong and consistent that the former term is becoming synonymous with the latter. Xenobiotic-induced mitochondrial dysfunction promotes ROS production, persistent systemic inflammation, pro-inflammatory phenotype, insulin resistance, and vasoconstriction—any one of which independently and all of which additively/synergistically promote HTN.

| Using models of interconnection to understand chronic hypertension | Among variations on this theme, this diagram provides a reasonable representation of several of the key factors that generate and perpetuate the common clinical syndromes of overweight-obesity, hypertension, insulin resistance and diabetes type-2.

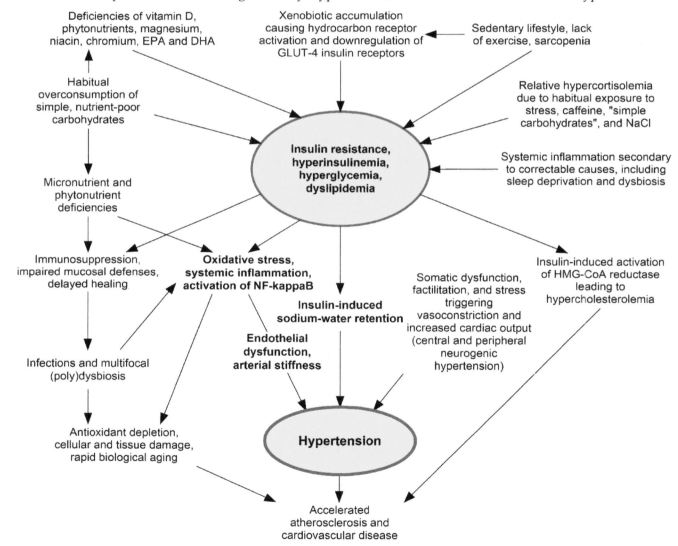

Simple Integrated Model of "Primary Hypertension": Interconnected lifestyle-physiologic mechanisms contribute to the hyperinsulinemia-inflammation-hypertension syndrome commonly known as "idiopathic hypertension" and metabolic syndrome.

- **Decipherative contextualization**: The social (and therefore political and economic) context in which "hypertension" exists is of supreme and generally neglected importance. Hypertension as a common disease does not exist in cultures that follow healthy lifestyles, particularly characterized by sufficient physical activity, Paleo-Mediterranean diets, and low to moderate societal stress; in sharp contrast, hypertension is an epidemic in countries like the United States where the social scene is littered with physical inactivity, unhealthy processed-food diets including overconsumption of high-fructose corn syrup and underconsumption of micronutrients (including vitamins [e.g., vitamin D], minerals [e.g., magnesium and potassium], and phytonutrients), and high levels of psychosocial and political stress coupled with epidemic individual isolation and pervasive social fragmentation.[304] I consider this fact self-evident: "hypertension" as we generally "know"/perceive it in the industrialized world would not exist in its epidemic form were it not for the social context and corporate-political climate which synergistically nurture it. This does not imply the need necessarily for political change to precede the treatment of hypertension, nor is such necessary in order to quantitatively reduce the number of affected individuals; what it does imply is that we as healthcare providers will be more successful in the achievement of our goals—if those goals are the beneficent alleviation of individual and societal disease burden and the optimization of individual and societal health—if we attend to the social-political-paradigmatic environment that contributes to patterns of disease pathogenesis. The goal here is to contextualize hypertension so thoroughly that the "disease" itself—as it exists in industrialized societies (pandemic) and we have been taught to see it (idiopathic, and therefore drug-dependent)—vanishes into comprehensibility and manageability and therefore loses its enigmatic power. I call this approach "decipherative contextualization" from the perspective that describing the disease as an extension of the social context from which it arises allows us to conceptually and intellectually apprehend the condition and thus decipher/decode/deflate its illusory enigmacity; of course, this model and each component therein has to be based on verified facts, as are readily abundant. My "decipherative contextualization" seeks to explain—to a sufficiently thorough degree—these enigmatic diseases so that they lose their phenomenalistic luster and can thereafter be managed dexterously, hopefully with ease, eventually with pleasure.

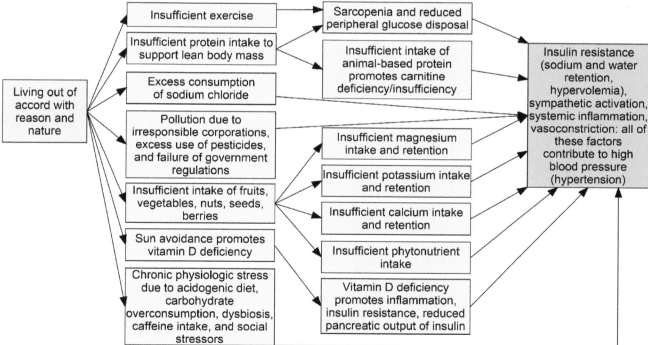

HTN—a singular etiology, multiple etiologies, or both?: Failure to meet nature-based physiologic expectations is a major cause of different secondary causes of hypertension: The above diagram shows how the simple act of what is referred to here as "living out of accord with nature" sets the stage for numerous biochemical and physiologic factors which contribute to HTN. Thus, this singular etiology or cause leads to numerous secondary etiologies or causes which all culminate in volume

[304] Kihn, E Douglas.The Political Roots of American Obesity. truth-out.org/opinion/item/16149-the-political-roots-of-american-obesity. 2013 May. Excellent article.

overload, sympathetic activation, systemic inflammation, and vasoconstriction. "Living out of accord with nature" has been a theme of so-called modernized/ Westernized/ industrialized societies since their subtle and progressive development. Dr Price's *Nutrition and Physical Degeneration: A Comparison of Primitive and Modern Diets and Their Effects*[305] documented in 1945 the effects that this "progress" was having on the health of societies that became "modernized"—their health status and social structures fell into decline, often complete ruin. More recently, O'Keefe and Cordain[306] wrote in their review article entitled *Cardiovascular disease resulting from a diet and lifestyle at odds with our Paleolithic genome: how to become a 21st-century hunter-gatherer* that, "Accumulating evidence suggests that this mismatch between our modern diet and lifestyle and our Paleolithic genome is playing a substantial role in the ongoing epidemics of obesity, hypertension, diabetes, and atherosclerotic cardiovascular disease. ... Although the human genome has remained largely unchanged (DNA evidence documents relatively little change in the genome during the past 10,000 years), our diet and lifestyle have become progressively more divergent from those of our ancient ancestors." Whether we call the problem "living out of accord with nature" or "the mismatch between our modern diet and lifestyle and our Paleolithic genome" the concept is the same, and the biophysiologic and social results are obviously negative. America's social fabric has deteriorated to the point that most Americans have only 2-3 friends and no confidants[307], and the progressively larger epidemics of obesity, depression, cancer, diabetes mellitus, and cardiovascular disease are well publicized and known to all.

- **Drug treatments for chronic HTN**: From a practical standpoint, the many drugs used for the suppression of HTN can be placed in one of five categories; the mnemonic offered in the *Saint-Frances Guide*[308] is "A.B.C.D.E." which stands for ❶ ACEis (angiotensin converting enzyme inhibitors) and ARBs (angiotensin II Receptor Blockers), ❷ BBs (beta-blockers), ❸ CCBs (calcium channel blockers), ❹ diuretics, and ❺ everything else (e.g., central alpha-agonists, alpha-blockers, vasodilators). For uncomplicated HTN, the initial treatment is a diuretic, generally hydrochlorothiazide (HCTZ), since the thiazide diuretics have the best cost-effectiveness of various drug classes; as noted by Howland and Mycek[309], "Current treatment recommendations are to **initiate therapy with a thiazide diuretic unless there are compelling reasons to employ other drug classes**. ... Recent data suggest that diuretics are superior to beta-blockers in older adults." For complicated HTN (resistant to treatment or with concomitant illness), a different first-line or additive second drug is chosen from a different class based on patient characteristics, as outlined below. While clinicians might choose a higher initial dose based on HTN severity or the doctor's experience and preference, as a general rule the most reasonable course is to start with a single drug at a low dose in order to minimize risk for adverse effects and to readily determine the offending agent in the event of an expected or idiosyncratic side effect. In the outline below, patient profiles are matched to drug classes; when specific drugs are listed, they are chosen based on general frequency of use with preference for those administered once daily due to improved compliance. If drug treatment is well tolerated but insufficient to achieve BP goal,

> **Analogy: "Treating hypertension" simply by using drugs to lower blood pressure is like turning off a smoke alarm and then letting the fire continue to blaze.**
>
> High blood pressure is a manifestation of dysfunction. Rather than directing treatment toward the manifestation (i.e., the blood pressure elevation), clinicians would be more wise to address the nature and cause of the imbalance that is causing the elevation in blood pressure.
>
> If the metabolic-physiologic fire is extinguished, then the smoke alarm will silence itself though autoregulation, and spending billions of dollars and work-hours on alarm silencers (i.e., drugs) and alarm specialists will thereby become largely unnecessary. The results will include enhanced health via collateral benefits of natural treatments, reductions in costly and dangerous adverse drug effects, patient liberation from drug dependency, authentic patient empowerment, and improved fulfillment of medicine's purported tenets of beneficence, autonomy, and nonmalfeasance.

then *treatment compliance is verified* before increasing the dose and eventually adding a second drug from a different class. For the patient-centered and drug-centered tables that follow, primary sources of information are *Lippincott's Illustrated Reviews: Pharmacology, Third Edition*[310] for pharmacology and The 5-Minute Clinical Consult, 18th Edition[311] for more clinical information and doses; Ebell's review and clinical worksheet ("Hypertension Encounter Guide") published in "Initial evaluation of hypertension" in *American Family Physician* (March 2004)[312] was also used as a very practical point-of-care guide. The tables that follow were

[305] Price WA. *Nutrition and Physical Degeneration: A Comparison of Primitive and Modern Diets and Their Effects*. Price-Pottinger Nutr Foundtn: 1945
[306] O'Keefe JH Jr, Cordain L. Cardiovascular disease resulting from a diet and lifestyle at odds with our Paleolithic genome. *Mayo Clin Proc*. 2004 Jan;79(1):101-8
[307] McPherson et al. Social Isolation in America: Changes in Core Discussion Networks over Two Decades. *American Sociological Review* 2006; 71: 353-75 asanet.org
[308] Bent S, Gensler LS, Frances C. *Saint-Frances Guide: Clinical Clerkship in Outpatient Medicine. 2nd Edition*. Philadelphia; Wolters Kluwer: 2008, 90
[309] Howland RD, Mycek MJ. *Lippincott's Illustrated Reviews: Pharmacology, 3rd Edition*. Baltimore: Lippincott Williams and Wilkins; 2006, 213-226
[310] Howland RD, Mycek MJ. *Lippincott's Illustrated Reviews: Pharmacology, 3rd Edition*. Baltimore: Lippincott Williams and Wilkins; 2006, 213-226
[311] Domino FJ (editor in chief). *The 5-Minute Clinical Consult. 2010. 18th Edition*. Philadelphia; Wolters Kluwer: 2009, 656-7
[312] Ebell MH. Initial evaluation of hypertension. *Am Fam Physician*. 2004 Mar 15;69(6):1485-7 aafp.org/afp/2004/0315/p1485.html

originally written by Alex Vasquez and reviewed by Robert Richard DO[313] in January 2010 for the publication of *Chiropractic Management of Chronic Hypertension* (from which this more current text is derived); later editions of this publication have undergone additional professional and peer review.

- The medical profession's near-exclusive reliance upon drug treatments for HTN is fraught with problems, particularly including adverse drug effects, failure to address the underling primary cause(s) of the metabolic disturbance(s), of which, HTN is only the tip of the proverbial iceberg, and patient noncompliance. According to a 2001 editorial published in the *New England Journal of Medicine*, "Approximately one-half of patients who are prescribed antihypertensive medications discontinue therapy by the end of the first year."[314]

- In representative medical pharmacology textbooks[315] the primary variables considered for the support of antihypertensive pharmacotherapy are ❶ cardiac output (controlled with beta-blockers), ❷ peripheral resistance (treated with vasodilators such as ACEi and CCB), and ❸ blood volume (reduced by the first-line use of diuretics). One interconnecting theme in this paradigm is that of activation

Sequential HTN Drug Protocol
1. **Thiazide diuretic: Hydrochlorothiazide 12.5-25 mg/d po** initially for most patients, not with renal insufficiency. For patients with DM or proteinuria, start with ACEi. Add **spironolactone 25-50 mg/d** if hypokalemia develops.
2. **ACEi: Lisinopril 10-40 mg/d po**, give the first dose in the office to monitor for hypotensive syncope or angioedema. If cough or angioedema develop, switch to ARB, particularly **losartan 25-100 mg/d** due to modest uricosuric effect. ACEi and ARB are contraindicated in pregnancy.
3. **CCB: Amlodipine 2.5-10 mg/d po**, particularly for patients with migraine, COPD, asthma.
4. **BB: Metoprolol 50-100 mg/d po** (up to bid), especially with angina or MI; not with bradycardia, insulin-requiring DM, depression, or sexual dysfunction.
5. **Loop diuretic: Furosemide 20-320 mg/d po** if patient has severe volume overload; effective with renal insufficiency.
Ebell MH. Initial evaluation of hypertension. *Am Fam Physician.* 2004 Mar 15;69:1485-7 aafp.org/afp/2004/0315/p1485.html Domino FJ (editor-in-chief). *The 5-Minute Clinical Consult. 2010. 18th Edition*: 2009, 656-7

of the sympathetic nervous system by some unknown insult or combination thereof. Whether due to "stress", faulty disinhibition of baroreceptors in the aortic arch, carotid sinuses, or renal juxtaglomerular cells, sympathetic activation increases cardiac output via increased rate and contractility, increases peripheral resistance via vasoconstriction, and increases blood volume via aldosterone-enhanced sodium (and thus water) retention. The enzyme renin converts angiotensinogen into angiotensin-1, which is converted via angiotensin converting enzyme (ACE) into the vasoconstrictor and trigger for aldosterone release angiotensin-2.

- Suggested doses of course need to be tailored to individual patient needs; doses suggested are for adults of average adult size and are administered by mouth (per os, p.o.) unless otherwise indicated. Note that IV and IM doses are generally much smaller than oral doses.

Comorbidity profile suggesting specific first- or second-line treatment of hypertension

- **Tailoring drug selection per comorbidities:** Although the first choice for an antihypertensive drug is generally hydrochlorothiazide, the second drug and occasionally the first-line drug are selected based on patient tolerance and co-morbidities. The following quote by Chobanian[316] summarizes the general approach: "…for those who have had a heart attack, beta blockers and ACE inhibitors are preferred; for those at high risk for coronary heart disease, ACE inhibitors, beta blockers, calcium channel blockers, as well as diuretics are recommended; and for chronic kidney disease, ACE inhibitors and angiotensin receptor blockers are drugs of first choice." Additional details are provided below:

  o **Uncomplicated:** Thiazide diuretics (especially **HCTZ**) are first choice (can worsen gout and dyslipidemia); BB have historically been a common second choice, but recently atenolol has fallen out of favor[317] and with the increasing prevalence of DM which indicates ACEi and ARB treatment, these

---

[313] Robert Richard DO is Medical Director of the John Peter Smith Polytechnic Clinic and Chair of Community Medicine at Texas College of Osteopathic Medicine. Dr Richard's review of these tables does not imply his endorsement of their content nor of the content of this document as a whole. Furthermore, Dr Richard's review does not imply endorsement by JPS Health Network or Texas College of Osteopathic Medicine.
[314] Chobanian AV. Control of hypertension—an important national priority. *N Engl J Med.* 2001 Aug 16;345(7):534-5
[315] Harvey RA, Champe PC (eds). *Lippincott's Illustrated Reviews: Pharmacology, 3rd Edition*. Philadelphia, Lippincott Williams and Wilkins; 1997
[316] Chobanian AV. Press Conference Remarks: The Seventh Report of the Joint National Committee on Prevention, Detection, Evaluation, and Treatment of High Blood Pressure (JNC 7). May 14, 2003. nhlbi.nih.gov/guidelines/hypertension/speaker2.htm Accessed November 2010
[317] Domino FJ (editor in chief). *The 5-Minute Clinical Consult. 2010. 18th Edition*. Philadelphia; Wolters Kluwer: 2009, 656-7

medications may become the preferred second line; the ARB **losartan** would seem particularly favorable in patients with metabolic syndrome and type-2 DM due to its uricosuric effect.

- o **Diabetes mellitus**: ACEis are renoprotective (but not used with renovascular disease), ARB's are second choice due to cost and less historical use; beta-blockers are generally avoided in insulin-requiring DM due to blunting of protective responses to hypoglycemia.
- o **Renal disease**: ACEis are renoprotective (but not used with renovascular disease), ARBs are second choice. Nondihydropyridine CCBs reduce intrarenal filtration pressure thus reducing proteinuria. Thiazides require renal function and are generally not useful if creatinine is >2 mg/dl.
- o **African American**: African-Americans tend to respond better to diuretics and CCB than to BB or ACEi.[318]
- o **Asthma and COPD**: Use a CCB. Generally avoid beta-blockers with any airway disease, B1-selective metoprolol might be considered
- o **Angina**: BB and CCB improve outcomes independent of BP-lowering; when BB and CCB are combined, the CCB should be a dihydropyridine (i.e., from the class of "-pyridines" or "-pines"). Do not combine a BB with a negative inotropic non-dihydropyridine CCB so as to avoid inducing heart block.
- o **Erectile dysfunction**: Avoid beta-blockers; thiazides may exacerbate. Consider concomitant administration of arginine and/or a phosphodiesterase-5 inhibitor; also consider treatment for excess estrogen in men with a serum estradiol greater than 30 picogram/mL (for details see the anti-estrogen protocol outlined in chapter 4 of *Integrative Rheumatology/ Inflammation Mastery*[319]). Implement diet and lifestyle modification for weight optimization; optimize endothelial health.
- o **Systolic HTN**: Dihydropyridine CCB ("-pyridines" or "-pines") are preferred because of their relative selectivity for the peripheral vasculature—the vascular *tree*.
- o **CAD or prior MI**: BB are top choice if not contraindicated by problematic asthma, COPD, or DM.
- o **Pregnancy**: Use methyldopa, hydralazine, magnesium; pregnancy contraindicates ACEi and ARB due to teratogenic effects.
- o **CHF**: BB are particularly useful for diastolic CHF to slow heart rate and allow greater filling time: Carvedilol is BB of choice in this situation. Monitor for signs of excessive cardiosuppresion such as edema, SOB, rales, bradycardia. Carvedilol is a non-selective beta blocker/alpha-1 blocker indicated in the treatment of mild to moderate CHF. Do not use BB or CCB with bradycardia; generally do not use verapamil (negative inotrope CCB) with CHF. Diuretics such as Lasix are mainstays of CHF treatment, particularly for exacerbations. ACEi and ARB drugs are also routinely used in CHF.
- o **Bradycardia**: Do not use BB or CCB with bradycardia.
- o **Edema**: Sodium and water restriction along with use of loop diuretics (e.g., furosemide/Lasix) is common treatment. Lasix is generally dosed "to effect."

The next several pages provide a review of each drug class. Preferred/representative drugs are listed based on the author's experience, training (especially observed prescribing patterns by attending physicians) and research; following the so-called preferred drug is optional at the discretion of the clinician.

ACEi: angiotensin-2 converting enzyme inhibitors

- Pharmacology and introduction: Blocking formation of angiotensin-2 reduces peripheral vascular resistance and aldosterone secretion; vasodilation is effected by reduced breakdown of bradykinin; sympathetic tone may be reduced. For best safety, the initial dose of an ACEi can be given in the office under supervision due to risks for first-dose syncope and life-threatening angioedema; this advised practice is rarely followed.
- Unique benefits of class: ACE inhibitors provide renoprotection, hence their routine use in patients with DM, with or without HTN. Thiazide, BB, and ACEi can be safely used together. As summarized by Domino (editor, *5-Minute Clinical Consult*), "ACE inhibitors should be used in patients with diabetes, proteinuria, atrial fibrillation, or CHF but not in pregnancy."
- Unique adverse effects and contraindications: Not used with **renal artery stenosis** (can cause acute renal failure) or **pregnancy** (teratogenic); may cause **cough (10%) and angioedema** due to reduced breakdown of bradykinin. Reduced aldosterone secretion promotes hypotension and **hyperkalemia—potassium levels should be monitored**

---

[318] Howland RD, Mycek MJ. *Lippincott's Illustrated Reviews: Pharmacology, 3rd Edition*. Baltimore: Lippincott Williams and Wilkins; 2006, 213-226
[319] Vasquez A. *Integrative Rheumatology*. IBMRC 2006, 2007 and all future editions.

especially in diabetic **patients and those with renal insufficiency and/or renal vascular stenosis; coadministration of ACEi and spironolactone is generally contraindicated** due to risk of hyperkalemia.
- Representative drug of class (dose range): Lisinopril 10 mg/d—see table

ARB: angiotensin-2 receptor blocker/antagonist

- Pharmacology and introduction: ARBs block reception of angiotensin-2 and thus reduce vasoconstriction and aldosterone secretion; risk-benefit profile is similar to ACEi except that bradykinin-mediated benefits (vasodilation) and risks (cough, angioedema) are not seen. ARBs improve endothelial dysfunction in patients with HTN and/or CAD, reduce cardiovascular mortality and morbidity, and have anti-inflammatory benefits.
- Unique benefits of class: Hypotensive and renoprotective benefits without the risks of cough and angioedema compared with ACEi.
- Unique adverse effects and contraindications: Fetotoxicity contraindicates ARB use in pregnancy—this is a black box warning.
- Representative drug of class (dose range): Losartan 50 mg/d—see table

BB: beta-adrenergic receptor blockers, "beta blockers"

- Pharmacology and introduction: Primary mechanism of drug action is via blockade of B1 receptors; this reduces cardiac output, sympathetic tone, and renin secretion. Major adverse effects include bradycardia, fatigue, depression, sexual dysfunction, exacerbation of asthma and COPD, and **rebound hypertension with rapid discontinuation of drug.**
- Unique benefits of class: Thiazide, BB, and ACEi can be safely used together. BB considered more effective in Caucasians than Africans, more effective in young than elderly. BB are particularly used in HTN patients who also have **supraventricular tachyarrhythmia, previous MI, angina, migraine, and anxiety.**
- Unique adverse effects and contraindications: Do not use BB or CCB with **bradycardia** due to potential for inducing **heart block or hypotension.** Nonselective BB such as propranolol which target B1 (heart) and B2 (lungs) have potential to **exacerbate asthma and COPD**; however, **propranolol's B1 blockade helps reduce renin levels.** Patients with PVD may have a worsening of limb ischemia secondary to reduced perfusion. **Hypotension, fatigue, depression, sexual dysfunction,** and **rebound hypertension** are common adverse BB effects; lowering of HDL and elevation of TRIGs has also been noted. Sudden discontinuation of BB can result in **rebound hypertension** (presumably due to upregulation of beta-adrenergic receptors under prolonged suppression). Of note, **atenolol** is no longer considered first-line treatment due to recent evidence of **inefficacy** in preventing HTN complications.[320]
- Representative drug of class (dose range): Metoprolol in extended release (Toprol-XL) 25 mg/d—see table

CCB: calcium channel blockers (dihydropyridine class)

- Pharmacology and introduction: The "-pyridines" block calcium entry into vascular smooth muscle and thus cause relative arterial dilation and thus a reduction in peripheral resistance. *Memory tool*: Remember that *pyridines* sounds like *pines* and that these drugs work on the *vascular tree* to lower blood pressure via systemic arterial dilation.
  - Not detailed here are the non-dihydropyridine class of CCB (i.e., including diltiazem/Cardizem and Verapamil) which are not used for HTN but rather are used for their cardioselective effects. *Memory tool*: Remember that the *non*-dihydropyridine CCBs are cardiosuppressive via a *negative* inotropic effect.
- Unique benefits of class: Generally safe in HTN patients with asthma, DM, angina, and PVD.
- Unique adverse effects and contraindications: Do not use BB or non-dihydropyridine CCB with bradycardia. Adverse effects include constipation (10%, especially with nifedipine), headache, and fatigue.
- Representative drug of class (dose range): Amlodipine 5 mg/d, or start with 2.5 mg/d—see table

Diuretic—loop class: furosemide /Lasix

- Pharmacology and introduction: A key mechanism of action of most diuretics is enhanced excretion of sodium. Sodium (Na) retention promotes water retention and subsequent volume expansion, while also contributing to vasoconstriction

Loop diuretics infamously cause electrolyte and thiamine loss

Loop diuretics such as furosemide/Lasix are commonly used in the treatment of heart failure and other edematous states in elderly patients, but the depletion of thiamine, magnesium, potassium, and calcium can exacerbate heart failure and contribute to co-morbidity such as depression, delirium, and dementia.

Felípez et al. Drug-induced nutrient deficiencies. *Pediatr Clin North Am.* 2009

[320] Domino FJ (editor in chief). *The 5-Minute Clinical Consult. 2010. 18th Edition*. Philadelphia; Wolters Kluwer: 2009, 656-7

and arterial stiffness via enhanced adrenergic reactivity and via promotion of intracellular hypercalcinosis (possibly due to enhanced sodium-calcium exchange).[321]

- Unique benefits of class: Fast action even in patients with renal insufficiency; efficacy of Lasix is via diuresis and venodilation.
- Unique adverse effects and contraindications: Chronic use promotes depletion of potassium, magnesium, and thiamine. Diuretic effect is potent and acute.
- Representative drug of class (dose range): Furosemide 20 mg/d po is reasonable starting dose—see table

Diuretic—thiazide class: hydrochlorothiazide (HCTZ)

- Pharmacology and introduction: Drug of choice for initial treatment of HTN. Sulfa sensitivity does not necessarily contraindicate thiazide use, even though thiazides are sulfa derivatives; use with caution. Thiazide diuretics are ineffective in patients with renal insufficiency; the loop diuretic furosemide is effective in patients with renal insufficiency.
- Unique benefits of class: Thiazide, BB, and ACEi can be safely used together. Particularly beneficial in elderly (as long as renal function is intact) and Africans. Promotion of calcium retention may benefit osteoporosis and reduce calcium nephrolithiasis. Thiazide diuretics reduce peripheral vascular resistance, perhaps via sodium elimination.
- **Unique adverse effects and contraindications**: Not useful in patients with renal insufficiency (creatinine clearance < 50 mL/min).
  - o Thiazide diuretics can worsen **hyperuricemia** (70% of patients) and **gout** due to competition for renal excretion (organic acids).
  - o **Hypokalemia** (70%)—potassium levels should be monitored in patients predisposed to cardiac arrhythmia and those treated with digitalis. Coadministration with ACEi/lisinopril helps negate the tendency toward hypokalemia.
  - o **Hyperglycemia (10%), dyslipidemia, hypomagnesemia**
  - o Promotion of calcium retention can promote **hypercalcemia** when HCTZ is combined with vitamin D3, even with the use of modest doses of vitamin D (e.g., 2,000 IU/d).[322]
  - o Exacerbation of (fructose-induced) metabolic syndrome was recently proven experimentally [animal study] and published in a peer-reviewed journal[323]; this effect is mediated at least in part due to potassium depletion.
- Representative drug of class (dose range): Hydrochlorothiazide, started at 12.5-25 mg/d—see table

Diuretic—potassium-sparing: spironolactone

- Pharmacology and introduction: Potassium-sparing diuretics are weak diuretics; **spironolactone** is the prototype and also has anti-androgen action and is therefore used in hirsutism.
- Unique benefits of class: Spironolactone is commonly used with HCTZ; it beneficially diminishes cardiac remodeling seen in CHF. Spironolactone reduces incidence of spontaneous bacterial peritonitis (SBP) in patients with cirrhosis.
- Unique adverse effects and contraindications: Spironolactone has antiandrogen effects, can promote sexual dysfunction in men and gynecomastia; can precipitate hyperkalemia and hypermagnesemia.
- Representative drug of class (dose range): Spironolactone, start HTN dose at 12.5 mg/d—see table

Alpha-1-blocker: alpha-adrenergic receptor type-1 antagonist

- Pharmacology and introduction: Reduce BP via relaxation of venous and arterial smooth muscle. These drugs are certainly not used as first-line treatments for HTN, generally speaking.
- Unique benefits of class: Can be used when other drugs have not been effective; can benefit men with prostatic hyperplasia.
- Unique adverse effects and contraindications: Sodium-water retention, hypotension, syncope, and reflex tachycardia are common; reflex tachycardia can be prevented with BB.
- Representative drug of class: Prazosin, start with 1 mg/d—see table

Alpha-2 agonists: alpha-adrenergic receptor class-2 agonist

- Pharmacology and introduction: Centrally acting drugs reduce sympathetic output via central feedback inhibition. Rebound hypertension with clonidine withdrawal mandates tapering discontinuation.
- Unique benefits of class: Safe for use in renal disease; generally used with diuretic.

---

[321] Benowitz NL. "Antihypertensive Agents." In Katzung BG (editor). *Basic and Clinical Pharmacology. 10th Edition.* New York: McGraw Hill Medical; 2007, 16
[322] Vasquez et al. The clinical importance of vitamin D: a paradigm shift with implications for all healthcare providers. *Altern Ther Health Med.* 2004 Sep-Oct;10(5):28-36
[323] Reungjui et al. Thiazide diuretics exacerbate fructose-induced metabolic syndrome. *J Am Soc Nephrol.* 2007 Oct;18(10):2724-31

- <u>Unique adverse effects and contraindications</u>: Generally used with a diuretic to counteract the sodium-water retention. Sedation and dry nose may occur. Rebound hypertension mandates *tapering* discontinuation. **Alpha-2 agonists are best avoided due to high risk of rebound HTN following noncompliance or missed/skipped dose.**
- <u>Representative drug of class</u>: Clonidine, start at 0.1 mg bid—see table

---

Vasodilators: Direct-acting smooth muscle relaxants: hydralazine

- <u>Pharmacology and introduction</u>: Vasodilators are used for treatment-resistant HTN, acute severe HTN, and pregnancy-related HTN. During my hospital training, we used these drugs commonly in emergency settings and in obstetrics; generally these drugs were administered intravenously at 10 mg per dose repeated as needed for HTN control. Hydralazine's mechanism of action includes limiting calcium release from the sarcoplasmic reticulum of smooth muscle thereby resulting in relaxation of arterioles and veins; hydralazine recently has been identified as a nitric oxide donor.
- <u>Unique benefits of class</u>: Rapid onset of action; safe for use during pregnancy.
- <u>Unique adverse effects and contraindications</u>: Sodium-water retention can be avoided with BB and diuretic. BB can be used to avoid vasodilator-induced tachycardia.
- <u>Representative drug of class</u>: Hydralazine—see table

<u>**Common anti-hypertensive drugs listed in alphabetical order per class**</u>: ACE-inhibitor, ARB, Beta-blocker, Calcium channel blocker, Diuretics, Extra (less commonly used) drugs: alpha1-blocker, alpha2-agonist, Vasodilators (ie, direct-acting vasodilators)

Drug, starting dose, comments	Benefits	Risks
Lisinopril: 10 mg/d (up to 80 mg/d; max dose in renal failure is 40 mg/d) po; available as 2.5 mg, 5 mg, 10 mg, 20 mg, 30 mg and 40 mg tablets. Lisinopril is an orally administered long-acting angiotensin converting enzyme inhibitor. This is a very commonly used medication in medical practice and hospitals. Half-life is approximately 12 hours; absorption of Lisinopril is approximately 25%, with large intersubject variability (6% to 60%) at all doses tested (5 mg to 80 mg).	☑ Antihypertensive, vasodilatory, anti-aldosterone effect, ☑ Beneficial in CHF, ☑ Beneficial after MI, ☑ Benefits within 1 hour, peak at 6 hours, duration 24 hours; full benefit takes weeks, ☑ Concomitant administration of Lisinopril and hydrochlorothiazide further reduces blood pressure in Black and non-Black patients.	☒ Contraindicated in **pregnancy**—black box warning. Do not use during lactation. ☒ Not to be used in patients with ACEi hypersensitivity, higher risk for **life-threatening angioedema** in African-American patients, ☒ Benefit blunted by NSAIDs, ☒ Can reduce renal filtration of potassium, **lithium**—especially use caution in patients with sCr >2mg/dL. ☒ Removal of angiotensin II negative feedback on renin secretion leads to increased plasma renin activity.
Losartan: 50 mg/d (up to 100 mg/d), available as 25 mg, 50 mg and 100 mg; among the ARBs, this drug provides the additional benefit of reducing uric acid levels, which is relevant for fructose-induced urate-mediated metabolic syndrome; however, a recent clinical trial showed no differences between ramipril and losartan in lowering BP and both drugs showed a trend to improve metabolic parameters such as serum glucose, serum triglycerides, and uric acid equally.[324]	☑ Half-life is 6-9 hours with no plasma accumulation after repeated daily dosing. ☑ Food slows and reduces absorption but this is not clinically significant.	☒ Contraindicated in **pregnancy**—black box warning. Do not use during lactation. ☒ Less effective in African-American patients. ☒ Most of the anti-HTN benefits of Losartan are due to its active carboxylic acid metabolite formed via the action of cytochrome P450 2C9 and 3A4. Generally, 14% of Losartan is converted into the active metabolite; in 1% of patients, they only convert 1% of Losartan to the active metabolite and therefore the drug is inefficacious for them. ☒ Consider caution and lower doses in patients with renal disease: plasma concentrations are increased by 50 to 90% in patients with mild (creatinine clearance of 50 to 74 mL/min) or moderate (creatinine clearance 30 to 49 mL/min) renal insufficiency.

---

[324] Spinar et al; CORD Invesigators. CORD: COmparsion of Recommended Doses of ACE inhibitors and angiotensin II eceptor blockers. *Vnitr Lek*. 2009 May;55(5):481-8

Drug, starting dose, comments	Benefits	Risks
Metoprolol in extended release (Toprol-XL): 25 mg/d; available as 25 mg, 50 mg, 100 mg, 200 mg: This drug is preferred in patients with angina or MI.	☑ Benefits HTN, supraventricular tachyarrhythmia, previous MI, angina, migraine, and anxiety.	☒ Patients must not discontinue drug without tapering dose; sudden discontinuation can cause severe rebound HTN, angina, and MI. ☒ Do not use in patients with bradycardia or heart block. Fatigue, depression, sexual dysfunction, and weight gain can be caused by beta-blockers. ☒ Beta-blockers blunt the physiologic responses to hypoglycemia and are thus associated with hypoglycemic risk in diabetic patients taking glucose-lowering drugs such as insulin.
Amlodipine: 5 mg/d, or start with 2.5 mg/d if being used as a secondary drug or if patient has liver disease; available as 2.5 mg, 5 mg, 10 mg	☑ Amlodipine is indicated for HTN, chronic stable angina, vasospastic angina, and CAD if the ejection fraction is >40%. ☑ Generally safe in HTN patients with asthma, DM, angina, and PVD.	☒ Generally do not use this drug if patient has aortic stenosis, hypersensitivity, severe CAD or severe CHF. ☒ CCB are generally fourth-line drugs after thiazide diuretics, followed by either ACI/ARB and then BB. ☒ Numerous drug interactions, including barbiturates, phenytoin, rifampin, antipsychotics, amiodarone, erythromycin, fluconazole, and the related drugs sildenafil (Viagra) and tadalafil (Cialis).
Furosemide: 20 mg/d po is reasonable starting dose; may increase up to 600 mg/d as needed; available as 20 mg, 40 mg, 80 mg: Dose must be step-wise increased to find patient-specific threshold dose and frequency for individual patient, works for 6 hours (hence the name Lasix); higher doses not better than threshold dose.	☑ This is a very commonly used drug; commonly used PRN for outpatients with edema, including idiopathic edema. ☑ Used for systemic edema, pulmonary edema, CHF, hypercalcemia. ☑ This drug can be used in patients with renal insufficiency, but not with anuria or urethral obstruction	☒ This is a potent diuretic that can cause volume depletion and secondary syncope and hypoperfusion. This is a potent diuretic that can cause electrolyte depletion, including hyponatremia. Scheduled follow-up and laboratory tests for electrolytes are required. ☒ Avoid nighttime use to avoid nocturia.
Hydrochlorothiazide: Started at 12.5-25 mg/d; may use up to 50 mg/d for HTN. When used for the treatment of peripheral edema (rare), the dose is as high as 200 mg/d po qd.	☑ HCTZ is the first-line drug of choice for the routine outpatient management of chronic hypertension. Other drugs such as ACEi/ARB and BB are commonly added as second line agents after the initiation of HCTZ.	☒ HCTZ exacerbates many of the pathophysiologic components of the metabolic syndrome, such as hyperuricemia, potassium insufficiency, hyperglycemia, dyslipidemia, hypomagnesemia and magnesium insufficiency.
Spironolactone: Start HTN dose at 12.5 mg/d; available as 25 mg, 50 mg, 100 mg; dosed as high as 200 mg/d for edema and 400 mg po qd x21-28 days for the diagnosis of hyperaldosteronism.	☑ Useful as a second line or third line drug in the treatment of HTN following the use of HCTZ; also used as second line agent with Lasix. ☑ Used in the treatment of hypokalemia, hyperaldosteronism, ascities, hirsutism, CHF, and edema due to CHF, renal failure, and cirrhosis.	☒ Tumorigenic effect noted in animals suggests that spironolactone may exacerbate cancer and should therefore be used sparingly. ☒ Hyperkalemia is a real clinical concern associated with potassium-sparing diuretics such as spironolactone.

Common anti-hypertensive drugs listed in alphabetical order per class—*continued*

Drug, starting dose, comments	Benefits	Risks
Prazosin: start with 1 mg/d for the treatment of HTN; available as 1 mg, 2 mg, 5 mg; highest recommended dose for HTN is 15 mg/d.	☑ Used in the treatment of HTN, prostate enlargement (1 mg po bid).	☒ First-dose syncope and hypotension are common with prazosin.
Clonidine: start at 0.1 mg bid for HTN; max dose is 2.4 mg; available as 0.1 mg, 0.2 mg, and 0.3 mg for oral administration, also available for injection.	☑ **Useful for acute and severe HTN; not routinely used for routine chronic HTN.** Can be administered orally or intravenously for the rapid reduction of severe hypertension. ☑ Epidural administration is used in the treatment of severe pain.	☒ **High risk of rebound HTN following noncompliance or missed/skipped dose.** Taper dose over 4 days to reduce risk of rebound HTN.
Hydralazine: oral dose for moderate-severe HTN is 10-50 mg po starting with 10 mg po qid for 2-4 days then 25 mg po qid for 1 week; max dose is 300 mg po qd25-150 mg twice daily; available for oral administration 10 mg, 25 mg, 50 mg, 100 mg. For acute HTN, the parenteral dose is 10-20 mg IM or IV each 2-4 hours; switch to oral dosing as soon as possible.	☑ Monotherapy is generally only used in the treatment of pregnancy-induced HTN and moderate-severe treatment-resistant HTN. This drug is commonly used in hospitals for the treatment of pregnancy-induced HTN and pre-eclampsia.	☒ Side effects include headache due to vasodilation and drug-induced systemic lupus erythematosus (SLE). May also cause neutropenia and other blood disorders. ☒ **Warning**: Vasodilators cause reflex tachycardia that can precipitate MI and CHF.

Nutritional Treatments for Hypertension

This article was originally published in *Naturopathy Digest* in 2006
naturopathydigest.com/archives/2006/nov/vasquez.php

Introduction: Clinical problems associated with hypertension can be divided into two categories dependent upon the severity and duration of the elevated blood pressure. Mild elevations in blood pressure that are sustained over a period of many years and decades increases the risk of atherosclerosis, stroke, myocardial infarction, heart failure, and renal failure. Acute elevations in blood pressure, even if sustained for a relatively short time, can cause hypertensive encephalopathy, stroke, retinal hemorrhage, acute myocardial infarction, and acute left ventricular failure with pulmonary edema. Many different etiologies exist for hypertension, including but not limited to metabolic syndrome, hypothyroidism, renal failure, and adverse drug effects; the scope of this article is limited to uncomplicated prehypertension and Stage One Hypertension. Obviously, the goals of therapy are to bring the blood pressure down into the normal range and to prevent end-organ damage, especially to heart, brain, eyes, and kidneys.

Diagnosis: Blood pressure is assessed with a sphygmomanometer. Elevated blood pressure is a clinical finding that—if confirmed by at least two readings—leads to the diagnosis of hypertension.

Management: Guidelines for the assessment and therefore management of hypertension change periodically based on new consensus and new research data. "Prehypertension" or early hypertension begins at 120 systolic over 80 diastolic, while "Stage One hypertension" is in the range of 140/90 - 160/100. Patients beyond Stage One

Hypertension or those with a complex clinical presentation should generally be co-managed pharmaceutically (at least initially); a table describing hypertensive categories is provided below (Table 1). Doctors who choose to manage hypertension for their patients must include proper history, physical examination, laboratory assessment (e.g., chemistry/metabolic panel, urinalysis, thyroid and cardiovascular panels), and the treatment plan must include frequent follow-up (e.g., every 2-4 weeks) until the problem is resolved. If effectiveness cannot be obtained, sustained, or documented then the patient should receive both verbal and written referral to another physician, particularly an internist or cardiologist.

Table 1: Hypertension categorization and management*	
Prehypertension: >120/80	These patients are essentially normal but might take steps to lower blood pressure to a safer level.
Stage One: 140/90 - 160/100	These are perfect candidates for diet/lifestyle/integrative treatments. As with any condition: high-risk, noncompliant, and nonresponsive patients are referred for medical management.
Stage Two: 160/100 - 210/120 without symptoms and without end-organ damage (i.e., no renal damage, headache, or edema).	All integrative treatments can be used; drugs might also be used initially to reduce hypertension. Nonmedical/nonprescribing clinicians should generally refer or co-manage these patients.
Urgent: SBP ≥ 220 or DBP 125 - 129, or Stage 2 with symptoms or end-organ damage.	Immediate referral for drug treatment is appropriate.
Emergency: >220/130 is an emergency	Emergency: Intravenous medications in a hospital or urgent care clinic
* Additional considerations that affect treatment and management: Insulin resistance / pre-diabetes / metabolic syndrome: dyslipidemia / high cholesterol, obesity, inactivity, tobacco use, concomitant diseases, personal and family medical history, other chief complaints and clinical and laboratory findings.	

Nutritional treatments for hypertension: Nutritional treatments for hypertension include the following considerations, which can generally be used in combination (rather than in isolation, as studied in the research). These will be listed and discussed in order of general effectiveness (see Table 2).

1. Short-term supervised fasting: Short-term inpatient supervised fasting appears to be the most effective treatment for chronic hypertension that has ever been documented. Working closely with his multidisciplinary team, pioneering chiropractic physician Alan Goldhamer DC documented reductions in hypertension of 60/17 in patients with severe hypertension and reductions of 37/13 in patients with moderate hypertension.[325,326,327] Generally the program begins with 4-7 days of a raw vegetarian diet followed by 1-2 weeks of fasting and concluded with reintroduction of a vegetarian and health-promoting diet. Laboratory tests and professional supervision help ensure patient safety.

2. Healthy diet and exercise: Health-promoting diets such as either Paleo- and Mediterranean-style diets can lower blood pressure by as much as 17/13 according to some reports. Please see my previous articles in this magazine for description of the "supplemented Paleo-Mediterranean Diet."[328]

3. CoQ10: CoQ-10 in doses of 100-225 mg/day can lower blood pressure quite effectively, as documented in several clinical studies, some of which showed that CoQ10 is more effective and safer than the use of antihypertensive drugs.[329,330,331] Reductions in blood pressure are generally in the range of 17/12 and are dose-

[325] Goldhamer A, et al. Medically supervised water-only fasting in the treatment of hypertension. *J Manipulative Physiol Ther* 2001 Jun;24(5):335-9
[326] Goldhamer AC, et al. Medically supervised water-only fasting in the treatment of borderline hypertension. *J Altern Complement Med.* 2002 Oct;8(5):643-50
[327] Goldhamer AC. Initial cost of care results in medically supervised water-only fasting for treating high blood pressure and diabetes. *J Altern Complement Med.* 2002 Dec;8(6):696-7
[328] Vasquez A. Five-Part Nutritional Protocol that Produces Consistently Positive Results.*NutrWellness*2005 Sep
[329] "RESULTS: The mean reduction in systolic blood pressure of the CoQ-treated group was 17.8 +/- 7.3 mm Hg (mean +/- SEM). None of the patients exhibited orthostatic blood pressure changes. CONCLUSIONS: Our results suggest CoQ may be safely offered to hypertensive patients as an alternative treatment option." Burke BE, Neuenschwander R, Olson RD. Randomized, double-blind, placebo-controlled trial of coenzyme Q10 in isolated systolic hypertension. *South Med J.* 2001 Nov;94(11):1112-7
[330] "These findings indicate that treatment with coenzyme Q10 decreases blood pressure possibly by decreasing oxidative stress and insulin response in patients with known hypertension receiving conventional antihypertensive drugs." Singh RB, Niaz MA, Rastogi SS, Shukla PK, Thakur AS. Effect of hydrosoluble coenzyme Q10 on blood pressures and insulin resistance in hypertensive patients with coronary artery disease. *J Hum Hypertens.* 1999 Mar;13(3):203-8
[331] "...51% of patients came completely off of between one and three antihypertensive drugs at an average of 4.4 months after starting CoQ10." Langsjoen P, Langsjoen P, Willis R, Folkers K. Treatment of essential hypertension with coenzyme Q10. *Mol Aspects Med.* 1994;15 Suppl:S265-72

dependent. A patient who does not respond to 100 mg per day may respond very well to 200 mg per day. Since it is a fat-soluble nutrient, CoQ10 should be administered with dietary fat and/or consumed in a "pre-emulsified" form to enhance absorption which is a prerequisite for clinical effectiveness. Several trials have been reported showing enhanced absorption of CoQ10 when administered in pre-emulsified form. CoQ10 is very safe, and drug interactions are rare; caution should be used in patients taking coumadin.

4. <u>Sodium restriction</u>: Clinical responsiveness to low-sodium diets ranges from minimal to a maximal reduction in the range of 22/14 - 16/9.[332] Contraindications to low-sodium diet are uncommon (e.g., hyponatremia); low-sodium diets should generally be a component of all anti-hypertensive treatment plans.

5. <u>Vitamin D and calcium</u>: Vitamin D3 (cholecalciferol) and calcium supplementation can reduce blood pressure in hypertensive patients by approximately 13/7.[333] As I have discussed in extensive detail elsewhere, a reasonable dose of vitamin D3 for adults is in the range of 2,000 - 4,000 IU per day, and doctors new to vitamin D therapy should read my clinical monograph published in 2004 and available on-line.[334] The most important drug interaction with vitamin D is seen with hydrochlorothiazide, a commonly-used antihypertensive diuretic that promotes hypercalcemia; vitamin D therapy in patients taking hydrochlorothiazide must be implemented slowly, with professional supervision, and with weekly laboratory monitoring of serum calcium. Vitamin D probably corrects hypertension via several mechanisms, including but not limited to increased absorption of magnesium and reduction in intracellular calcium, as I described previously in this magazine.[335] Since vitamin D absorption decreases with age and in patients with intestinal disease (including dysbiosis[336]), absorption of fat-soluble vitamin D3 is enhanced when administered in pre-emulsified form.[337]

6. <u>Prescription drugs</u>: Use of the nutritional treatments described in this article can complement or replace antihypertensive drug therapy in many patients. When used singly, prescription antihypertensive drugs average a reduction in blood pressure of approximately 12/6. Initial reductions of 20/10 require combination therapy, according to a review article published in *American Family Physician* in 2003.[338]

7. <u>Exercise</u>: Moderate exercise can reduce blood pressure by approximately 7/7 in the short term. Longer-term exercise, particularly along with diet improvements and weight loss, can result in synergistic and curative benefits. Patients who have been sedentary for years and those with probable or documented cardiovascular disease should be evaluated by a physician and ECG before beginning an exercise program.

8. <u>Fish oil</u>: Fish oil supplementation had been shown to reduce blood pressure by approximately 3/2. For reasons that I have detailed elsewhere[339], fish oil should be co-administered with a source of GLA such as borage oil in order to maximize effectiveness and minimize subtle biochemical adverse effects. Importantly, fish oil is safer, less expensive, and more effective than "statin" antihypercholesterolemic drug treatment for reducing total and cardiovascular mortality.

9. <u>Food allergy elimination</u>: According to a clinical study of migraineurs published in *The Lancet*, identification and avoidance of food allergens can normalize blood pressure in hypertensive migraine patients.[340] The anti-hypertensive response to food allergy avoidance can be seen clinically even in patients who do not have migraine or other manifestations of allergy, but the more allergic symptoms that are seen and the more complete the response to allergy elimination, the more likely is a reduction in blood pressure.

[332] "The average fall in blood pressure from the highest to the lowest sodium intake was 16/9 mm Hg." MacGregor GA, Markandu ND, Sagnella GA, Singer DR, Cappuccio FP. Double-blind study of three sodium intakes and long-term effects of sodium restriction in essential hypertension. *Lancet*. 1989 Nov 25;2(8674):1244-7
[333] "A short-term supplementation with vitamin D(3) and calcium is more effective in reducing SBP than calcium alone. Inadequate vitamin D(3) and calcium intake could play a contributory role in the pathogenesis and progression of hypertension and cardiovascular disease in elderly women." Pfeifer et al. Effects of a short-term vitamin D(3) and calcium supplementation on blood pressure and parathyroid hormone levels in elderly women. *J Clin Endocrinol Metab*. 2001 Apr;86(4):1633-7
[334] Vasquez A, Manso G, Cannell J. The clinical importance of vitamin D (cholecalciferol). *Altern Ther Health Med*. 2004 Sep-Oct;10(5):28-36
[335] Vasquez A. Intracellular Hypercalcinosis. *Naturopathy Digest* 2006, September
[336] Vasquez A. Nutritional and Botanical Treatments against "Silent Infections" and Gastrointestinal Dysbiosis. *Nutritional Perspectives* 2006; January
[337] Vasquez A. Subphysiologic Doses of Vitamin D are Subtherapeutic: Comment on the Study by The Record Trial Group. *Lancet* 2005 published online May 6
[338] Magill MK, Gunning K, Saffel-Shrier S, Gay C. New developments in the management of hypertension. *Am Fam Physician*. 2003 Sep 1;68(5):853-8
[339] Vasquez A. New Insights into Fatty Acid Supplementation and Its Effect on Eicosanoid Production and Genetic Expression. *Nutritional Perspectives* 2005; January: 5-16
[340] Grant EC. Food allergies and migraine. *Lancet*. 1979 May 5;1(8123):966-9

Table 2: Anti-hypertensive effectiveness relative to standard drug treatment for outpatient chronic HTN

1. **Short-term supervised fasting**	-60/17 for severe HTN and -37/13 for moderate HTN
2. **Healthy diet and exercise**	-17/13
3. **CoQ10 100-225 mg/day**	-17/12
4. **Sodium restriction**	Reduction ranges from -16/9 up to -22/14
5. **Vitamin D and calcium**	Reductions up to -13/7 in vitamin D-deficient hypertensive patients
6. <u>Prescription drugs</u>	-12/6 Reductions of -20/10 require two-drug therapy
	"Initial combination therapy is suggested by JNC 7 for patients whose blood pressure is more than 20/10 mm Hg above their goal blood pressure." *Am Fam Physician* 2003 Sep
7. Exercise	-7/7
8. Fish oil	-3/2
9. Food allergy elimination	Variable response ranging from insignificant to curative

<u>Conclusions</u>: Many nutritional treatments for hypertension are documented in the research literature, and several of these treatments appear safer and more cost-effective than pharmaceutical antihypertensive drugs. Furthermore, the synergistic use of the nutritional and lifestyle interventions described above—e.g., supplemented Paleo-Mediterranean diet along with exercise, fish oil, vitamin D, CoQ10, and sodium restriction-results in clinical benefits that far exceed the results published in the single-intervention clinical trials that have documented the effectiveness of the individual components. The major drug interaction that one must look out for is the combination of vitamin D with hydrochlorothiazide. Switching from pharmaceutical drugs to nutrients for the management of hypertension requires diligent follow-up, informed consent, and documentation of beneficial clinical response and should be undertaken only by skilled and experienced clinicians.

Promoting Unhealthy Eating: Proatherosclerotic Recipes Endorsed by the US National Heart, Lung, and Blood Institute (NHLBI)

The following is a partial list of atherosclerosis-promoting recipes listed under the title "Stay Young at Heart: Cooking the Heart-Healthy Way"[341] advocated on the website of the NHLBI in December 2009; *horror of horrors—these recipes are still posted and advocated in 2015.* Notice the lack of nutrient density, the emphasis on simple carbohydrates, the lack of raw foods, paucity of phytonutrients, and the frequent use of baking with oil to create the effect of frying:

- <u>Stir-fried beef</u> with boiled potatoes and white rice
- <u>Beef stroganoff</u> with 6 cups of cooked macaroni pasta
- <u>Crispy oven-fried chicken</u> cooked in cornflakes and buttermilk
- <u>Classic macaroni and cheese</u>
- <u>Candied yams</u> with brown sugar, margarine, white flour, and orange juice
- <u>Oven French fries</u> (white potatoes oven-fried in vegetable oil)
- <u>White rice</u> cooked with vegetable oil and salt
- <u>Sunshine (white) rice</u> cooked with vegetable oil, orange juice, and lemon juice
- <u>Homestyle biscuits</u> made from white flour, salt, and sugar
- <u>Banana-nut bread</u> made from mashed ripe bananas, low-fat buttermilk, packed brown sugar, margarine, all-purpose white flour, egg and salt
- <u>Apricot-orange bread</u> made from dried apricots, margarine, white sugar, egg, white flour, dry milk powder, salt and orange juice
- <u>Apple coffee cake</u> made with peeled apples (please note that >90% of the antioxidants contained in apples are in the peel—thus when the peel is removed, virtually all that remains is antioxidant-poor carbohydrate), one cup of sugar, one cup of dark raisins, one-quarter cup vegetable oil, 1 egg, and two-and-a-half cups of sifted all-purpose white flour

---

[341] US National Heart, Lung, and Blood Institute (NHLBI). Stay Young at Heart: Cooking the Heart-Healthy Way. nhlbi.nih.gov/health/public/heart/other/syah/index.htm Accessed December 23, 2009. This index of recipes has been relocated to nhlbi.nih.gov/health/resources/heart/syah-html/; reviewed 2015 Nov.

- Frosted cake with 2 1/4 cups cake flour, 4 tablespoons margarine, 1 1/4 cups sugar, 4 eggs, low fat cream cheese, and 2 cups sifted confectioners' sugar!
- Tropical fruit compote with sugar
- Peach cobbler with sugar, white flour, margarine, canned peaches "packed in juice", peach nectar, and cornstarch
- Rice pudding with white rice, 3 cups of skim milk, and 2/3 cup sugar

The war is not meant to be won
"Their lives are dedicated to world conquest, but they also know that it is necessary that the war should continue everlastingly and without victory."
George Orwell in *Nineteen Eighty-four (1984)*. *Chapter 3, War is Peace*, approximately page 249

The list goes on to include many other proatherosclerotic and prodiabetic meals. Any reasonable person—*the general public has the option but healthcare professionals have the obligation*—might ask why **the US National Heart, Lung, and Blood Institute has been promoting a diet plan that is ensured to contribute to the pandemics of hypertension, obesity, and diabetes mellitus**. Actually, asking the question simply delays and allows for additional delay of the obvious solution.

Thinking Outside the (Pill) Box: Is the "Battle Against Hypertension and Diabetes" Truly Meant to be "Won" for Patients…or for the Drug Companies?

The Most Profitable "Wars" are the ones that are Fought Indefinitely and which Require Reliance on Private Industry: As with most modern sociopolitical fights, wars, and missions, a keen observer (or any high-school student who read George Orwell's classic novel *1984*) might question whether the current "**Mission: To Combat High Blood Pressure in America**"[342] is actually meant to ever be won. The US National Heart, Lung, and Blood Institute (NHLBI) invokes the language of battle, e.g., "to **mobilize** all Americans in the **fight against high blood pressure** and reduce the more than 1 million heart attacks, strokes, and kidney failure cases that it causes each year. The CDC and the NHLBI have **joined forces** to **disseminate** these materials…"[343] Ironically, the NHLBI's document entitled "Physician Fact Sheet: What Every Physician Should Know" hp2010.nhlbihin.net/mission/partner/physcian_factsheet.pdf **contains zero practical information on diet, exercise, or nutritional supplementation**. Likewise, the document under the heading "Real Possibilities for America's Health Care Providers"[344] provides nothing that a clinician or patient could use to authentically correct the common causes of HTN; it provides near-meaningless mention of "diet and exercise" accompanied by a photo of people sitting at a table with food and encourages that doctors "Support Adherence to Treatment" accompanied by a photo of a woman taking pills.

"Common Objectives" …with Drug Companies: For more than a decade, the American Heart Association has been "advised" by their "Pharmaceutical Roundtable" (PRT) comprised of **monolithic drug companies each of which must pay a least $1 million per year for each 3-year term of membership**.[345] According to the American Heart Association's website in a document last reviewed in August 2009[346], "The American Heart Association Pharmaceutical Roundtable (PRT) is a strategic coalition of 10 leading pharmaceutical companies and association volunteers and staff. It allows our association and members of the **pharmaceutical industry** to identify and pursue **common objectives** to improve cardiovascular health in the United States through research, patient education, and public and professional programs." Current (or recent) members of the American Heart Association Pharmaceutical Roundtable include:

1. AstraZeneca L.P.
2. Eli Lilly and Company
3. Bristol-Myers Squibb Company
4. GlaxoSmithKline
5. Merck/Schering-Plough Pharmaceuticals
6. Merck Pharmaceuticals
7. Novartis Pharmaceuticals Corporation
8. Pfizer, Inc.
9. Sanofi-Aventis
10. Takeda Pharmaceuticals

---

[342] National Heart, Lung, and Blood Institute (NHLBI). The Mission: To Combat High Blood Pressure in America hp2010.nhlbihin.net/mission/ Accessed December 22, 2009
[343] State Heart Disease and Stroke Prevention Program Addresses High Blood Pressure. cdc.gov/dhdsp/library/fs_state_hbp.htm Accessed December 22, 2009
[344] National Heart, Lung, and Blood Institute (NHLBI). nhlbi.nih.gov/health/prof/heart/hbp/mp/mp_health.htm Accessed December 22, 2009
[345] "Each industry participant of the PRT will sign a separate agreement with AHA that will be binding only between the AHA and that individual industry member. The agreements will commit each industry member to contribute $1,000,000 per year for three years." Letter dated March 20, 1998 from Joel I. Klein (Assistant Attorney General), US Department of Justice Antitrust Division. justice.gov/atr/public/busreview/1608.htm Accessed December 23, 2009
[346] americanheart.org/presenter.jhtml?identifier=2366 Accessed December 23, 2009

Diabetes Mellitus Type-2 & Metabolic Syndrome

Introduction:

Long ago and far away are the epochs and perspectives holding that "adult onset diabetes" resulted simply from overeating and underexcercising; we now appreciate powerful contributions from dysbiosis, mitochondrial impairment, systemic inflammation, and persistent organic pollutants (POPs) such as pesticides and plastics. The clinical phenotype of diabetes is likely changing as pollutant-induced mitochondrial dysfunction, exacerbated by gastrointestinal dysbiosis from consumption of artificial foods/sweeteners and hidden consumption of glyphosate, leads to massive preclinical and prediabetic metabolic impairment, later manifesting as insulin resistance and overt diabetes. As such, pharmacocentric treatments—ie, the drug model of treating diabetes—that focus simply and solely on reducing glucose levels are intellectually absurd and scientifically ridiculous; hyperglycemia is simply the outward manifestation—the signal, the alarm—of underlying metabolic impairment and defective cellular signaling. Outside of urgent and emergency situations, treatment of insulin resistance should be founded upon dietary improvement (e.g., carbohydrate restriction, which is clinically superior to insulin therapy), microbiome modification (e.g., especially gut flora modification, such as with berberine, which is superior to drug treatment with metformin), mitochondrial support (e.g., CoQ10 is a superior intervention for long-term management of hypertension), and pesticide/pollution avoidance and depuration. Metabolic syndrome is a clinical cluster of several components—always including hyperglycemia, dyslipidemia, abdominal obesity, and hypertension, and per more broad/inclusive criteria also encompassing inflammation and hypercoagulability—which sum to effect accelerated atherosclerosis, hence the related term cardiometabolic syndrome. Because of this, a wide range of cardiovascular risk factors are discussed in this section, with treatments for each.

Description & Pathophysiology:

- Origins of terms: The term "diabetes mellitus" is from ancient Greek, *diabetes* means "to pass through" while *mellit* refers to "honey" or "sugar." Obviously, these are references to the voluminous output of urine seen passing through untreated diabetic patients who are experiencing hyperglycemic diuresis due to the osmotic effect of excess glucose in renal filtrate.

- Introduction: Diabetes mellitus (DM) can refer to any pathological states characterized by chronic hyperglycemia. Generally, DM is divided into type-1 (DM-1), which typically begins in childhood following autoimmune destruction of pancreatic beta cells leading to insulinopenia and the resulting hyperglycemia, and type-2 (DM-2), which typically begins in adulthood as a result of an interplay of genes, poor diet, insufficient exercise, numerous vitamin and mineral deficiencies, and a myriad of metabolic malfunctions including most prominently the phenomenon of peripheral tissue insulin resistance. Thus, we could oversimplify these disorders by saying that DM-1 is a pancreatic failure of insulin output while DM-2 is a tissue failure of insulin receptivity; in both instances, hyperglycemia is the most obvious physiologic result, and hyperglycemia-induced pathophysiologic disorders are the result. Clinicians should appreciate that the insulinopenic clinical picture of DM-1 can be produced by any condition that causes destruction of pancreatic beta-cells (e.g., chronic or acute pancreatitis, iron overload and hemochromatosis [see chapter from this textbook on iron overload]) and that the clinical picture of peripheral insulin resistance can occur secondary to acromegaly, severe acute illness and excess internal production or exogenous administration of corticosteroids.

- Clinical picture of DM-2: Insulin levels are always low in DM-1, whereas in DM-2 the insulin levels typically start high (fasting hyperinsulinemia) as the pancreas produces more insulin in an appropriate physiologic response to hyperglycemia; later as DM-2 progresses, pancreatic output of insulin progressively fails, thus exacerbating the hyperglycemia. DM-2 and "the metabolic syndrome" (MetSyn, also "syndrome X") have practically become synonymous over the last few years, due to the high concordance of these two clinical entities. DM-2 can, however, exist without the full picture of the two-part (up to six-part) definition of the metabolic syndrome. Various definitions of the metabolic syndrome include at least the first 4 of the following, with increasing appreciation of the additional last two characteristics: ❶ central adiposity, abdominal obesity, ❷ hyperglycemia, ❸ dyslipidemia, ❹ hypertension, ❺ systemic inflammation, and ❻ hypercoagulability. Metabolic syndrome is more aggressive and malignant than simple diabetes mellitus because of the former's inclusion of greater degrees of dyslipidemia, oxidative stress, and systemic inflammation; thus, these patients need to be managed assertively. Because the abbreviation "MS" is synonymous with multiple sclerosis, the contraction MetSyn will be used here for expediency when discussing metabolic syndrome.

- Pathoetiology of DM-2/MetSyn: Regarding DM-2/MetSyn, a more detailed pathoetiologic list of phenomena that contribute to peripheral insulin resistance includes ❶ genetic predisposition, ❷ sedentary lifestyle, ❸ caloric excess, ❹ sarcopenia, ❺ micronutrient deficiencies (especially magnesium, cholecalciferol, chromium), ❻ metabolic perturbations due to consumption of artificial "junk foods" (e.g., fructose excess, overconsumption of *trans* fatty acids), ❼ xenobiotic exposure and accumulation with resultant activation of the aryl hydrocarbon receptor which downregulates expression of peripheral GLUT-4 glucose-insulin receptors thus leading directly to peripheral insulin resistance, and ❽ systemic inflammation, which contributes directly to insulin resistance. Chronic hyperglycemia places constant demand and therefore physiologic strain on pancreatic beta cells, leading to what has been referred to in earlier literature as "high output failure." Hyperglycemia itself is toxic to pancreatic beta-cells such that regardless of the original cause of the hyperglycemia, the final common pathway of disease progression includes impaired production of insulin, thus exacerbating the hyperglycemia. The link between diabetes and obesity is so strong that the two are increasingly merged into the single term "diabesity."[347]

Cardiovascular risk:
Inflammation, hyperglycemia, oxidant stress, dyslipidemia, hypertension, peripheral and central atherosclerosis

Infection risk:
Counterinflammation, immunocompromise, predisposition to gingival infections and skin lesions, poor tissue healing

Diabetes Mellitus type-2 & Metabolic Syndrome

Organ damage / tissue injury:
Renal failure, diabetic neuropathy, eye damage (cataracts, retinopathy), vasculopathy

Nutritional deficiencies and excesses:
Excess carbohydrate and arachidonate; deficiencies of vitamin D3, zinc, ascorbate, chromium, selenium, magnesium and numerous other vitamins, minerals, and phytonutrients; consequences include depression and infection

Venn Diagram Showing 4 Important Clinical Considerations for the Management of DM-2/MetSyn: Clinicians should consider these 4 priorities when planning a risk-management strategy for patients with DM-2/MetSyn: 1) cardiovascular risk, 2) infection risk, 3) organ damage including blindness, renal failure, and neuropathy, and 4) the underlying nutritional imbalances and dietary carbohydrate excess that underlie these pathophysiologic processes. What underlies the nutritional imbalances and carbohydrate excess?—The answer to this question will vary somewhat per patient, but clinicians should assess the psychoemotional environment that has enabled a patient to adopt the unhealthy lifestyle and mindset that allowed this situation to develop in the first place. To get to the core of these issues, integrative clinicians should appreciate concepts such as the reciprocal causality between self-esteem and self-efficacy, as well as the importance of values, self-assertiveness, self-responsibility, living purposefully and consciously (reviewed by Branden[348]) and how these core psychoemotional issues can be integrated into a program for behavior change (reviewed by Prochaska[349]).

---

[347] "Lifestyle is an expression of individual choices and their interaction with the environment and is closely associated with risks for obesity, diabetes, and cardiovascular disorders. If taken cumulatively this syndrome may be referred to as "diabesity." Mobley CC. Lifestyle interventions for diabesity. *Compend Contin Educ Dent.* 2004 Mar:207-18
[348] Branden N. *The Six Pillars of Self-Esteem.* Bantam Books, 1994
[349] Prochaska JO, Norcross JC, and DiClemente CC. *Changing for Good.* William Morrow and Company; 1994

- **Prevalence**: In the US, approximately 21 million Americans have DM with about 15 million cases diagnosed and another 6 million undiagnosed. DM-1 accounts for about 5%, with the remaining 95% due to DM-2 including MetSyn and less commonly DM secondary to drugs (e.g., exogenous corticosteroids) and diseases such as acromegaly. Costs attributed to DM are approximately $132 billion per year in direct and indirect costs.

Clinical Presentation:

- The clinical presentation is extremely variable, which is why diabetes mellitus (like hemochromatosis and syphilis) is known as a "great imitator."
- DM/MetSyn patients may be asymptomatic and "apparently healthy" or may have the following:
  - Cataracts, retinopathy, macular edema
  - Recurrent infections (most commonly presenting as gingivitis, yeast vaginitis, and skin infections)
  - Underweight with DM-1
  - Obesity (especially abdominal/visceral)
  - Peripheral neuropathy (paresthesias, burning, tingling, insensate injuries and ulcerations)
    - Slow-healing wounds
    - Dyslipidemia
    - Hypertension
    - CVD (MI, stroke)
    - PVD (peripheral vascular disease)
    - Erectile dysfunction in men
    - Menstrual disorders in women: PCOS, infertility, menstrual irregularity
  - Hyperglycemic crises: These require emergency management in a hospital/ambulance setting.
  - Diabetic ketoacidosis (DKA): Classic presentation for DM-1 characterized by the triad of ❶ **hyperglycemia,** ❷ **ketosis,** ❸ **acidosis**; 20% of DKA presentations represent new DM-1 cases. 80% of DKA presentations occur in previously diagnosed diabetics who had an acute failure of glucose control and resultant hyperglycemia due to insulin noncompliance, infection such as UTI or pneumonia, alcohol abuse, trauma or cardiopulmonary insult. The onset of DKA is typically rapid (<24h) and presents with nausea, vomiting, and abdominal pain; thus the presentation of DM DKA resembles other presentations of acute abdomen, such as pancreatitis, food poisoning, or infectious gastroenteritis. Clinical signs in addition to the triad of hyperglycemia, ketosis, and acidosis include **Kussmaul breathing** (deep labored respirations as a sign of respiratory compensation for metabolic acidosis), **fruity acetone breath, dehydration, and mental status changes**. "Paradoxical hyperkalemia" in response to acidosis may be present; acidotic patients are generally depleted of potassium, and the hyperkalemia (shift of potassium from *intra*cellular to *extra*cellular) is a buffering response to the acidosis. A "normal" potassium level in a setting of acidosis potentially portends severe hypokalemia, especially upon correction of the acidosis.
  - Hyperosmolar hyperglycemic state (HHS) or hyperosmolar hyperglycemic nonketotic coma (HHNK): Occurs with severe uncontrolled DM-2; plasma glucose exceeds 800-1,000 mg/dL but ketosis and acidosis are not present with hyperosmolar hyperglycemia. Massive glucosuria leads to osmotic diuresis and resultant severe dehydration and hyperosmolarity; the clinical presentation primarily includes severe dehydration and complications from hypovolemia as well as mental status changes including disorientation, obtundation, seizures, visual loss, paralysis and focal neurologic deficits, and coma.

Major Differential Diagnoses:

- **Corticosteroid iatrogenesis**: Assess medication history and intake.
- **Post-pancreatitis insulinopenia**: Assess for history of pancreatitis or its classic precursors (e.g., alcoholism, hypertriglyceridemia, common bile duct obstruction). Measure serum insulin and use CT imaging of pancreas as indicated.
- **Iron overload and hemochromatosis**: Assess serum ferritin and transferrin saturation in all patients with DM and MetSyn. These patients have a greater-than-average incidence of iron overload, both primary and secondary forms.
- **Acromegaly**: Clinical evaluation for classic physical manifestations; measure serum insulin-like growth factor-1 (IGF-1) as a marker for growth hormone overproduction.
- **Diabetes insipidus**: Polyuria without the hyperglycemia due to failure of secretion or reception of antidiuretic hormone (ADH, same as arginine vasopressin). Inquire about lithium use, previous head injury or other intracranial lesion. Hypernatremia may be present; careful rehydration is warranted.

Clinical Assessments:

- **History/subjective**: The classic history associated with untreated DM is either ❶ asymptomatic, ❷ the presentation of a complicating manifestation such as infection, renal failure, or tissue ischemia (e.g., stroke or MI), ❸ or the textbook presentation of polyuria, polydipsia, and hyperphagia which are all complications hyperglycemia/hyperglucosuria. Any history of recurrent yeast infections in females and balantitis in men warrants testing for DM.

- **Physical Examination/Objective**: The physical examination focuses on assessment for the presence and severity of the expected complications from the disease.

  - Body mass index, assessment of body habitus: To calculate the "Body Mass Index" simply chart height and weight to determine the BMI number. Numbers greater than 25 correlate with being "overweight" while numbers greater than 30 meet the criteria for "obesity." BMI determinations may not be reflective of disease risk for people who are pregnant, highly muscular, or for young children or the frail elderly. Waist-hip ratios can also be determined. Overweight patients need to be made acutely aware of their body weight and the use of body weight as an indicator of compliance and progress toward disease regression and health restoration. Excess weight of only a few pounds/kilograms significantly increases the risk for diabetes, so patients should be reminded that *"Every pound/kilogram counts."* Mobley wrote, "An increase in body weight of approximately 2.2 pounds (1 kg) has been shown to increase risk for diabetes by 4.5%."[350]

    Adipose tissue is biologically active, promoting systemic inflammation and "estrogen dominance", thereby promoting the development of inflammatory and malignant diseases such as psoriasis and cancers of the breast, prostate, and colon. The previous view that fat (adipose) tissue was merely serving as an inert and inactive depot for lipid/energy storage is now replaced with the view that adipose tissue is biologically-active, influencing overall health via complex mechanisms that are biochemical-inflammatory-endocrinologic and not merely mechanical (i.e., excess weight, excess mass).[351] **Excess fat tissue— especially visceral/abdominal adipose—creates a systemic proinflammatory state** evidenced most readily by the elevations in hsCRP commonly seen in patients with obesity and the metabolic syndrome.[352] Adipokines are cytokines secreted by adipose tissue and include tumor necrosis factor-alpha, interleukin-6, and leptin—a cytokine derived from fat cells that promotes inflammation and immune activation; levels are higher in obese patients and decrease after weight loss. Obese patients also appear to have "leptin resistance" with regard to the suppression of appetite by leptin. **Adipose creates excess estrogens;** concomitant hyperglycemia increases androgen production[353], and these androgens are subsequently converted to estrogens by aromatase in the adipose tissue. For example, the adrenal gland makes androstenedione, which can be converted by aromatase in adipose tissue into estrone.[354] These proinflammatory and hormonal perturbations manifest clinically as an increased risk for breast, prostate, endometrial, colon and gallbladder cancers, insulin resistance and cardiovascular disease. The combination of inflammation, reduced testosterone, and elevated estrogen is also predisposes toward the development of autoimmune/inflammatory diseases.

  - **Obesity**: Obesity is a major risk factor for cardiovascular disease, cancer, diabetes mellitus, depression, joint degeneration and pain. Obese people also commonly report difficulties with performing daily activities, and they also report higher rates of depression and social isolation than do people of normal weight. "Body Mass Index" is a clinically valuable measure of height-weight proportionality and therefore adiposity, since an excess of height-proportionate weight is more commonly due to excess adipose than to excess muscle. To calculate BMI simply chart height and weight in the table below. Numbers greater than 25 correlate with being "overweight" while numbers greater than 30 meet the criteria for "obesity." BMI

---

[350] Mobley CC. Lifestyle interventions for "diabesity": the state of the science. *Compend Contin Educ Dent.* 2004 Mar;25(3):207-8, 211-2, 214-8

[351] "The fat cell is a true endocrine cell that secretes a variety of factors, including metabolites such as lactate, fatty acids, prostaglandin derivatives and a variety of peptides, including cytokines (leptin, tumor necrosis factor, interleukin-1 and -6, adiponectin), angiotensinogen, complement D (adipsin), plasminogen activator inhibitor-1 and undoubtedly many others." Bray GA. The underlying basis for obesity: relationship to cancer. *J Nutr.* 2002 Nov;132(11 Suppl):3451S-3455S

[352] "Our results indicate a strong relationship between adipocytokines and inflammatory markers, and suggest that cytokines secreted by adipose tissue could play a role in increased inflammatory proteins secretion by the liver." Maachi M, et al. Systemic low-grade inflammation is related to both circulating and adipose tissue TNFalpha, leptin and IL-6 levels in obese women. *Int J Obes Relat Metab Disord.* 2004;28:993-7

[353] Christensen et al. Elevated levels of sex hormones and sex hormone binding globulin in male patients with insulin dependent diabetes mellitus. *Dan Med Bull.* 1997;44:547-50

[354] "Conversion of androstenedione secreted by adrenal gland into estrone by aromatase in adipose tissue stroma provides an important source of estrogen for the postmenopausal woman. This estrogen may play an important role in development of endometrial and breast cancer." Bray GA. Underlying basis for obesity. *J Nutr* 2002;3451S-3455S

determinations may not be reflective of disease risk for people who are pregnant, highly muscular, or for young children or the frail elderly. Several articles have subjugated BMI (the greatest variable of which is adiposity), under the greater importance of cardiorespiratory fitness; regardless, obesity directly encourages/causes many physical and psychosocial health problems and directly impairs cardiorespiratory fitness. Several studies have also shown that xenobiotic load is a more powerful predictor of insulin resistance than is higher adiposity/BMI. For optimal health in all dimensions, the goals remain optimization of total physical fitness, acquiring a (near-)optimal BMI, and reducing xenobiotic burden.

- ❏ Severely underweight: < 16.5
- ❏ Underweight: 16.5 - 18.4
- ❏ **Normal: 18.5 - 24.9**
- ❏ Overweight: 25 - 29.9

- ❏ Obese Class 1: 30 - 34.9
- ❏ Obese Class 2 (severe obesity): 35 - 39.9
- ❏ Obese Class 3 (morbid obesity): 40 - 47.9
- ❏ Obese Class 4 (supermorbid obesity): ≥ 48

Weight in kilograms (*derived from pounds and inches from original table below; BMI is approximate)

Height cm*	45	50	55	59	63	68	73	77	82	86	90	95	100	104	109	114
152	20	21	23	25	27	29	31	33	35	37	39	41	43	45	47	49
155	19	21	23	25	26	28	30	32	34	36	38	40	42	43	45	47
157	18	20	22	24	26	27	29	31	33	35	37	38	40	42	44	46
160	18	19	21	23	25	27	28	30	32	34	35	37	39	41	43	44
162	17	19	21	22	24	26	27	29	31	33	34	36	38	39	41	43
165	17	18	20	22	23	25	27	28	30	32	33	35	37	38	40	42
167	16	18	19	21	23	24	26	27	29	31	32	34	36	37	39	40
170	16	17	19	20	22	23	25	27	28	30	31	33	34	36	38	39
173	15	17	18	20	21	23	24	26	27	29	30	32	33	35	36	38
175	15	16	18	19	21	22	24	25	27	28	30	31	32	34	35	37
177	14	16	17	19	20	22	23	24	26	27	29	30	32	33	34	36
180	14	15	17	18	20	21	22	24	25	26	27	28	30	32	33	35
182	14	15	16	18	19	20	22	23	24	26	27	28	30	31	33	34
185	13	15	16	17	18	20	21	22	24	25	26	28	29	30	32	33
188	13	14	15	17	18	19	21	22	23	24	26	27	28	30	31	32
190	12	14	15	16	17	19	20	21	22	24	25	26	27	29	30	31
193	12	13	15	16	17	18	19	21	22	23	24	26	27	28	29	30

Weight in pounds

Height: (Ft'inch")	100	110	120	130	140	150	160	170	180	190	200	210	220	230	240	250
5'0"	20	21	23	25	27	29	31	33	35	37	39	41	43	45	47	49
5'1"	19	21	23	25	26	28	30	32	34	36	38	40	42	43	45	47
5'2"	18	20	22	24	26	27	29	31	33	35	37	38	40	42	44	46
5'3"	18	19	21	23	25	27	28	30	32	34	35	37	39	41	43	44
5'4"	17	19	21	22	24	26	27	29	31	33	34	36	38	39	41	43
5'5"	17	18	20	22	23	25	27	28	30	32	33	35	37	38	40	42
5'6"	16	18	19	21	23	24	26	27	29	31	32	34	36	37	39	40
5'7"	16	17	19	20	22	23	25	27	28	30	31	33	34	36	38	39
5'8"	15	17	18	20	21	23	24	26	27	29	30	32	33	35	36	38
5'9"	15	16	18	19	21	22	24	25	27	28	30	31	32	34	35	37
5'10"	14	16	17	19	20	22	23	24	26	27	29	30	32	33	34	36
5'11"	14	15	17	18	20	21	22	24	25	26	27	28	30	32	33	35
6'0"	14	15	16	18	19	20	22	23	24	26	27	28	30	31	33	34
6'1"	13	15	16	17	18	20	21	22	24	25	26	28	29	30	32	33
6'2"	13	14	15	17	18	19	21	22	23	24	26	27	28	30	31	32
6'3"	12	14	15	16	17	19	20	21	22	24	25	26	27	29	30	31
6'4"	12	13	15	16	17	18	19	21	22	23	24	26	27	28	29	30

- ▪ Neurologic exam: Assess baseline central and peripheral neurological status to determine history of stroke or neuropathy; assessment should include monofilament and/or vibration testing.

- **Fundoscopic eye exam**: All DM/MetSyn patients should be evaluated by an ophthalmologist. Because MetSyn is a more aggressive multisystem disorder than DM, these patients with the former should receive appropriate referral within the first year of diagnosis unless treatment is rapidly curative and compliance is high and maintained. Patients must be educated about the risks of vision loss.

- **Cardiovascular exam**: Cardiac auscultation, peripheral vascular exam, and blood pressure assessment are components of a competent clinical examination. As of August 2009, "U.S. Preventive Services Task Force (USPSTF) found insufficient evidence to recommend for or against routine screening with ECG, exercise treadmill test (ETT), or electron-beam computerized tomography (EBCT) scanning for coronary calcium for either the presence of severe coronary artery stenosis (CAS) or the prediction of CHD events in adults at increased risk for CHD events." Doppler evaluation and ankle:brachial index can be evaluated in patients with suspected PVD.

- **Foot examination**: DM patients often lose sensation in their feet; this lack of sensation can predispose them to injury, and when injury occurs it may be painless due to the anesthesia caused by the peripheral neuropathy. Add to this increased risk of infection and poor circulation and clinicians should understand why a visual and manual examination of the feet should be performed on a frequent basis. Podiatric referral and the acquisition of orthoses/orthotics and particularly well-made and properly fitting footwear should be strongly considered, especially in patients with the common combination of PDV, neuropathy, and obesity—these patients are particularly prone to foot injuries that can lead to serious complications.

- **Laboratory Assessments**: Laboratory assessments—prior to the initiation of treatment and periodically to assess the efficacy of treatment and the patient's compliance—are absolutely essential in the proper management of diabetes mellitus and the related syndromes of insulin resistance and metabolic syndrome. Renal function should be checked before the initiation of nutritional or pharmacologic treatment.

  - **Chemistry/metabolic panel**: Serum glucose, electrolytes, blood urea nitrogen, creatinine levels, and liver markers are all assessed by this battery of tests. Renal function must be assessed from "both sides" of the kidney—serum (BUN and creatinine) and urine (albumin:creatinine ratio). Keep in mind that advanced renal failure can become a contraindication to certain treatments, such as a high-potassium diet and supplementation with vitamin D, calcium, and/or magnesium.

  - **Serum glucose**: Generally this is assessed with the chemistry/metabolic panel but can be ordered separately, particularly via finger-stick blood sample. The following serum glucose levels in mg/dL are described:
    - ☺ **< 85 mg/dL**: Optimal fasting glucose; obviously symptomatic hypoglycemia would not be optimal
    - ☺ **> 85-125 mg/dL**: Impaired fasting glucose (functional), candidate for lifestyle/nutritional intervention
    - ☺ **100-125 mg/dL**: Impaired fasting glucose (medical), "prediabetes"
    - ☹ **≥ 126 mg/dL on two separate occasions**: Fasting hyperglycemia, diagnostic of diabetes mellitus
    - ☹ **≥ 200 mg/dL with nonfasting blood sample or 2 hours after of 75 g oral glucose tolerance test (GGT)**: Non-fasting severe hyperglycemia, diagnostic of DM

  - **Serum insulin (fasting)**: In patients with DM-1, insulin and C-peptide are low. In patients with DM-2, insulin levels tend to be *elevated* early in the disease due to insulin resistance and increased pancreatic output, *normal* as pancreatic function declines, and then *low(er)* after the pancreas is sufficiently "burnt out" from years of overwork in a milieu of chronic glucose toxicity. Measuring fasting serum insulin can be helpful in determining if a patient's recalcitrant hyperglycemia is due to failure to comply with treatment or failure to produce endogenous insulin—obviously these two different scenarios would need to be managed with increased compliance or exogenous insulin (or pancreatic restoration), respectively. Although the laboratory reference range can be > 24 uIU/mL as shown in the example below, clinicians should view this upper reference limit as ridiculous except when searching for insulinoma; insulin >15 uIU/mL indicates severe insulin resistance, > 10 uIU/mL is problematic, and <5 uIU/mL is optimal.

Lab results showing optimal fasting serum insulin in a 39yo physician: <5 uIU/mL (shown) is optimal

Account Number	Patient ID	Control Number	Date and Time Collected	Date Reported	Sex	Age(Y/M/D)	Date of Birth
		53023	12/18/10 11:43	12/23/10	M	39	

TESTS	RESULT	FLAG	UNITS	REFERENCE INTERVAL
Insulin	2.3		uIU/mL	0.0 - 24.9

- Glycosylated hemoglobin (Hgb-A1c): As a marker for long-term (120 days) glucose levels, Hgb-A1c is an excellent marker for assessing glucose levels and thus treatment compliance for the past month. "Healthy" Hgb-A1c is less than 6%; "at risk" Hgb-A1c is 6 to <6.5%, and an Hgb-A1c level equal to or greater than 6.5% is now considered diagnostic of DM according to criteria published in June 2009. For the treatment of DM, the goal "target" Hgb-A1c is <7%; however, pushing for this level of strict control in a population of diabetics is likely to produce a significant number of hypoglycemic events, some of which could be serious and/or result in hospitalization, and thus some clinician experts will accept 7.5% as a sufficient level of compliance and efficacy. A correlation can be found between Hgb-A1c levels and average glucose levels:

Percentage	Description	Estimated serum glucose
< 5.7	Normal:	
5.7 - 6.4	Prediabetic: Interestingly, the phrase "prediabetic" reflects the allopathic medical paradigm of the unidirectionality and unavoidability of diabetes. A more proper term could be "borderline diabetes" indicating that the patient is *not* diabetic but showing a tendency toward *insulin resistance* or *glucose intolerance*—note that either of the two latter phrases are better and more "actionable" than the pseudoprophetic phrase *prediabetic*. Unlike *insulin resistance*, the phrase *glucose intolerance* is actionable because the common-sense implication is that if a patient has a metabolic impairment to the efficient utilization and metabolism of glucose then this substance should be avoided. By popularizing the phrases insulin resistance and—even worse—*metabolic syndrome*, physicians and patients alike are distracted from the importance of reducing carbohydrate intake in the treatment of these conditions.	A1c 6% correlates with average glucose of 126 mg/dL or 7 mmol/L
> 6.5	Diabetes mellitus: Diabetes mellitus and insulin resistance are reviewed elsewhere.	A1c 6.5% correlates with average glucose of 140 mg/dL or 7.8 mmol/L
7	Goal for DM treatment: Tighter control tends to result in more hypoglycemic complications in the context of drug management	154 mg/dL or 8.6 mmol/L
7.5	Higher Hgb-A1c values (listed progressively below) indicate poor control:	169 mg/dL or 9.4 mmol/L
8		183 mg/dL or 10.1 mmol/L
8.5		197 mg/dL or 10.9 mmol/L
9		212 mg/dL or 11.8 mmol/L
9.5		226 mg/dL or 12.6 mmol/L
10		240 mg/dL or 13.4 mmol/L

- High-sensitivity C-reactive protein (hsCRP): HsCRP predicts the onset of and correlates with the severity of the systemic inflammation seen in patients with DM and MetSyn. This is an excellent objective marker (along with Hgb-A1c and body weight) to determine the effectiveness of and compliance with treatment. In a 51-year-old male patient with MetSyn and concomitant rheumatoid arthritis, the current author was able to achieve a lowering of hsCRP from 124 mg/L (normal: 1-3 mg/L) to 7.8 mg/L within about one month of multifaceted interventions as described in *Inflammation Mastery*[355]; the details of this case and the

---

[355] Vasquez A. *Integrative Rheumatology, Second Edition*. IBMRC; 2008

interventions utilized were first published in *Musculoskeletal Pain: Expanded Clinical Strategies*[356] for CME credits.

- <u>Fasting lipid profile</u>: Elevations of total Cholesterol, LDL, and triglycerides with depression of HDL is the classic pattern of dyslipidemia. Total cholesterol should be reduced to <200 mg/dl and LDL cholesterol should generally be brought to less than 100 mg/dl and is physiologically optimized—and

> **LDL levels should be <100 mg/dl and ideally <70 mg/dl**
>
> "The normal low-density lipoprotein (LDL) cholesterol range is 50 to 70 mg/dl for native hunter-gatherers, healthy human neonates, free-living primates, and other wild mammals (all of whom do not develop atherosclerosis). Randomized trial data suggest atherosclerosis progression and coronary heart disease events are minimized when LDL is lowered to <70 mg/dl."
>
> O'Keefe JH Jr, Cordain L, et al. Optimal low-density lipoprotein is 50 to 70 mg/dl: lower is better and physiologically normal. *J Am Coll Cardiol.* 2004 Jun

  consistent with a Paleo-Mediterranean diet and appropriate exercise at 50-70 mg/dl.[357]

- <u>Serum homocysteine and other cardiovascular risk factors</u>: Other cardiovascular risk factors such as homocysteine and—more controversially—lipoprotein-A might also be tested in any patient with a high risk of cardiovascular disease.

- <u>Serum ferritin (with or without transferrin saturation)</u>: DM is one of the classic presentations for hemochromatosis, which is generally considered to be one of the most common hereditary disorders in all human populations. Routine use of serum ferritin is the most reasonable and cost-effective means for diagnosing iron overload condition in symptomatic and asymptomatic patients. Elevations of ferritin (i.e., >200 mcg/L in women and >300 mcg/L in men) need to be retested along with CRP (to rule out false elevation due to excessive inflammation) before making the presumptive diagnosis of iron overload. In the absence of significant inflammation, ferritin values >200 mcg/L in women and >300 mcg/L in men indicate iron overload and the need for treatment/phlebotomy regardless of the absence of symptoms or end-stage complications.[358] Another benefit to the use of serum ferritin is the frequent detection of iron deficiency. Transferrin saturation is a good test for detecting *genetic* hemochromatosis before iron overload has occurred; values greater than 40% should be repeated *in conjunction with a measurement of serum ferritin*. As a general rule, lab tests should be performed under fasting conditions.

- <u>Thyroid assessment</u>: Among the numerous metabolic perturbations that characterize DM-2 and MetSyn, clinical and functional hypothyroidism are both quite common. Detailed thyroid assessment should include measurements of TSH, free T4, free T3, total T3, reverse T3, and anti-thyroid antibodies (anti-thyroid peroxidase and anti-thyroglobulin). TSH levels above 2 uIU/mL[359] (uIU/mL = mU/L) or 3.0 uIU/mL[360] warrant consideration for intervention as these indicate subtle thyroid dysfunction and increased risk for future thyroid disease. Progressive clinicians note the importance of the ratio of total T3 to reverse T3 (tT3:rT3 ratio) and consider the optimal range to be 10-14 with lower ratios indicating impaired formation of T3 and/or excess production of rT3.[361] Contrary to the previous view which held that rT3 was simply inactive, we now appreciate that rT3 actually impairs normal thyroid hormone metabolism thus functioning as an thyrometabolic monkeywrench or "brake" on normal metabolism. Elevated rT3 levels predict mortality among critically ill patients.[362] Aberrancies in thyroid hormone levels may reflect organic disease, psychoemotional stress, or nutritional deficiency[363], and therefore such serologic abnormalities warrant consideration of underlying problems and direct treatment when possible. If no underlying cause is apparent, then a trial of thyroid hormone(s) is reasonable in appropriately selected

---

[356] Vasquez A. *Musculoskeletal Pain: Expanded Clinical Strategies*. Institute for Functional Medicine, 2008

[357] "Randomized trial data suggest atherosclerosis progression and coronary heart disease events are minimized when LDL is lowered to <70 mg/dl. No major safety concerns have surfaced in studies that lowered LDL to this range of 50 to 70 mg/dl." O'Keefe JH Jr, Cordain L, Harris WH, Moe RM, Vogel R. Optimal low-density lipoprotein is 50 to 70 mg/dl: lower is better and physiologically normal. *J Am Coll Cardiol.* 2004 Jun 2;43(11):2142-6

[358] Barton et al. Management of hemochromatosis. Hemochromatosis Management Working Group. *Ann Intern Med.* 1998 Dec 1;129(11):932-9

[359] Weetman AP. Fortnightly review: Hypothyroidism: screening and subclinical disease. *BMJ* 1997;314: 1175

[360] American Association of Clinical Endocrinologists: "Until November 2002, doctors had relied on a normal TSH level ranging from 0.5 to 5.0 to diagnose and treat patients with a thyroid disorder who tested outside the boundaries of that range. Now AACE encourages doctors to consider treatment for patients who test outside the boundaries of a narrower margin based on a target TSH level of 0.3 to 3.04. AACE believes the new range will result in proper diagnosis for millions of Americans who suffer from a mild thyroid disorder, but have gone untreated until now." Available at aace.com/pub/tam2003/press.php on January 2004. For more current information, see "The target TSH level should be between 0.3 and 3.0 µIU/mL." American Association of Clinical Endocrinologists Medical Guidelines for Clinical Practice for the Evaluation and Treatment of Hyperthyroidism and Hypothyroidism. aace.com/pub/pdf/guidelines/hypo_hyper.pdf December 20,2005

[361] McDaniel AB. Thyroid Assessment: Controversies and Conundrums. Institute for Functional Medicine 14th International Symposium. Tucson, Arizona. May 23-26, 2007

[362] Peeters et al. Serum 3,3',5'-triiodothyronine (rT3) and 3,5,3'-triiodothyronine/rT3 are prognostic markers in critically ill patients and are associated with postmortem tissue deiodinase activities. *J Clin Endocrinol Metab.* 2005 Aug;90(8):4559-65

[363] Kelly GS. Peripheral metabolism of thyroid hormones: a review. *Altern Med Rev.* 2000 Aug;5(4):306-33

patients. Beyond stress reduction and nutritional supplementation with iodine, selenium, and zinc (as indicated per patient), correction of overt, subclinical, and functional hypothyroidism generally centers on the administration of natural or synthetic thyroid hormones in the form of T4 and T3. Correction of functional hypothyroidism (relatively reduced total T3 and increased rT3) is accomplished with either time-released or twice-daily dosing of T3 without T4 to suppress endogenous T4 conversion to T3. This allows temporary downregulation of transforming enzymes so that rT3 production is reduced and thyroid metabolism is normalized following withdrawal of T3 treatment.[364]

- <u>Serum 25-hydroxy-vitamin D</u>: Per our review by Vasquez, Manso, and Cannell[365] in 2004, we fulfilled our promise of creating a "paradigm shift" that summarized new applications for the clinical use of vitamin D beyond its application in patients with osteoporosis or malabsorption to include the mandate of empiric treatment or laboratory assessment of all patients seen in clinical practice. Daily doses generally average between 4,000-10,000 IU/d for adults, with an acceptable one-time loading dose of 100,000-300,000 IU in patients for whom it is advantageous and safe to raise serum 25-hydroxy-vitamin D levels quickly and without

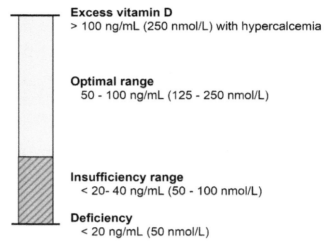

Excess vitamin D
> 100 ng/mL (250 nmol/L) with hypercalcemia

Optimal range
50 - 100 ng/mL (125 - 250 nmol/L)

Insufficiency range
< 20- 40 ng/mL (50 - 100 nmol/L)

Deficiency
< 20 ng/mL (50 nmol/L)

concern for compliance failure. The goal with vitamin D supplementation is to get serum 25-hydroxy-vitamin D levels into the optimal range, as illustrated.

- <u>Androgens and estrogens</u>: For a myriad of reasons, obese patients have adverse alterations in their sex hormones; typically "estrogens" are high in both genders, while androgens are low, particularly in males. Indeed, "Cross-sectional studies have found that between 20 and 64% of men with diabetes have hypogonadism, with higher prevalence rates found in the elderly."[366] In diabetic men, the low testosterone and high estrogens have a pathogenic role in insulin resistance; a review in 2008 by Cohen[367] concluded, "In males with increasing obesity there is increased aromatase activity, which irreversibly converts testosterone to estradiol resulting in decreased testosterone and elevated estrogen levels. Since androgens reduce the expression of ER [estrogen receptor] beta activity, **decreased testosterone levels** release the normally suppressed ER beta expression and **results in the down regulation of GLUT4 with resultant insulin resistance.**" In DM/MetSyn men with low testosterone, the exogenous/transdermal administration of testosterone is often the *wrong* solution to the problem because for many of these men the problem is not that they are not *making* enough testosterone *per se* but rather that their adipose tissue which contains the aromatase enzyme is *converting* their testosterone into estradiol. Giving these men more testosterone simply gives their adipose more substrate for converting into estrogens.

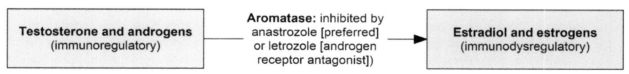

The aromatase enzyme converts androgens to estrogens: If estrogens are high and androgens are low, then estrogens can be lowered and androgens raised via inhibition of aromatase. If androgens are low and estrogens are low, then administration of androgen will raise both the androgens and the estrogens, possibly necessitating the coadministration of an aromatase inhibitor.

---

[364] "The WT3 protocol involves the use of SR-T3 taken orally by the patient every 12 hours according to a cyclic dose schedule determined by patient response. The patient is then weaned once a body temperature of 98.6 degrees F has been maintained for 3 consecutive weeks." Friedman M, Miranda-Massari JR, Gonzalez MJ. Supraphysiological cyclic dosing of sustained release T3 in order to reset low basal body temperature. *P R Health Sci J*. 2006 Mar;25(1):23-9

[365] Vasquez A, Manso G, Cannell J. The clinical importance of vitamin D (cholecalciferol). *Altern Ther Health Med*. 2004 Sep-Oct;10(5):28-36

[366] Kalyani RR, Dobs AS. Androgen deficiency, diabetes, and the metabolic syndrome in men. *Curr Opin Endocrinol Diabetes Obes*. 2007 Jun;14(3):226-34

[367] "Since androgens reduce the expression of ER beta activity, decreased testosterone levels release the normally suppressed ER beta expression and results in the down regulation of GLUT4 with resultant insulin resistance." Cohen PG. Obesity in men: the hypogonadal-estrogen receptor relationship. *Med Hypotheses*. 2008;70(2):358-60

Giving a "hypogonadal" man testosterone *without first measuring his serum estradiol level* should, in this author's opinion, be considered *mal-practice* because ❶ many of these men make sufficient testosterone but they are "rapid converters" to estradiol, ❷ giving them more testosterone raises their testosterone but can easily lead to high enough levels of estradiol to compromise sexual function, ❸ high estradiol in men appears to cause depression and fatigue, ❹ high estradiol in men appears to be a risk factor for prostate cancer. In our office, we commonly measure serum estradiol in men and administer the aromatase inhibitor anastrozole/Arimidex 1 mg (≥2-3 doses per week) to men whose estradiol level is greater than 32 picogram/mL. The Life Extension Foundation[368] advocates that the optimal serum estradiol level for a man is 10-30 picogram/mL. Clinical studies using anastrozole/Arimidex in men have shown that aromatase blockade lowers estradiol and raises testosterone[369]; generally speaking, this is exactly the result that we want. When using anastrozole/Arimidex, frequency of dosing is based on serum and clinical response. On occasion, we have seen some men who make so much endogenous testosterone→estradiol that they require both anastrozole/Arimidex *and* licorice daily in order to control their testosterone and estradiol levels. Licorice lowers testosterone[370] and thus reduces the precursor to estradiol in both men and women within about four days of oral administration. Licorice is effective for this purpose whether by standardized capsules or by tea from the cut and sifted root.

- <u>Dipstick urinalysis</u>: Begin with a urine dipstick test for overt proteinuria; results may be falsely elevated due to urinary tract infection or hematuria. Confirm positive result with repeat dipstick test within one month. Urine pH should be 7.5 to avoid chronic (diet-induced) metabolic acidosis.

- <u>Sensitive tests for occult proteinuria</u>: Urine dipstick testing is insufficiently sensitive to accurately detect minor renal damage that almost invariably affects all patients with DM and MetSyn. Urine tests for microalbuminuria include the random microalbumin-to-creatinine ratio or the timed 24-hour urine collection; these are both valid and the trend in clinical practice is away from the 24-hour urine collection toward the more convenient random microalbumin-to-creatinine ratio, with values >30 mg albumin per gram of creatinine considered positive.

- <u>Xenobiotic accumulation and toxicity; functional detoxification profiles, body burden of persistent organic pollutants (POPs)</u>: Patients with DM-2 and MetSyn have much higher-than-average levels of and diversity of toxins and xenobiotics; this literature was reviewed by Vasquez[371] in 2007 and the original article is provided at the end of this chapter. The "take home" message is that DM-2/MetSyn patients have consistent evidence of supranormal xenobiotic accumulation. Several xenobiotics stimulate the aryl hydrocarbon receptor which leads to downregulation of GLUT-4 receptors; therefore the physiologic mechanisms are clearly in place by which xenobiotic accumulation can lead directly to peripheral

> **Toxic chemical burden correlates strongly with DM-2/MetSyn**
>
> "...the expected association between obesity and diabetes was absent in people with low concentrations of persistent organic pollutants in their blood. ...the association between obesity and diabetes became stronger as the concentrations of such pollutants in the blood increased."
>
> Jones et al. Environmental pollution and diabetes. *Lancet.* 2008 Jan

insulin resistance. Recent reviews have highlighted the importance of xenobiotic accumulation over obesity as an important risk factor for diabetes.[372,373] Tests of serum, whole blood, and adipose tissue can be used to test for levels of specific xenobiotics; the current author has not found that approach particularly useful because most patients with xenobiotic accumulation and the often resultant multiple chemical sensitivity syndrome (MCS) have low-level elevations of *innumerable* xenobiotics rather than isolated elevations of

---

[368] Male Hormone Modulation Therapy, Page 4 Of 7: lef.org/protocols/prtcl-130c.shtml Accessed October 30, 2005

[369] "These data demonstrate that aromatase inhibition increases serum bioavailable and total testosterone levels to the youthful normal range in older men with mild hypogonadism." Leder et al. Effects of aromatase inhibition in elderly men with low or borderline-low serum testosterone levels. *J Clin Endocrinol Metab*. 2004 Mar;89:1174-80

[370] "The mean testosterone values decreased by 26 % after one week of treatment." Armanini D, Bonanni G, Mattarello MJ, Fiore C, Sartorato P, Palermo M. Licorice consumption and serum testosterone in healthy man. *Exp Clin Endocrinol Diabetes*. 2003 Sep;111(6):341-3

[371] Vasquez A. Chemical Exposure as a Major Contributor to the Epidemic of Diabetes Mellitus and Disorders of Insulin Resistance: From Molecular Mechanisms to Clinical Implications. *Naturopathy Digest* 2006; April.

[372] "Recent studies in populations exposed to polychlorinated biphenyls (PCBs) and chlorinated pesticides found a dose-dependent elevated risk of diabetes. An elevation in risk of diabetes in relation to levels of several POPs [persistent organic pollutants] has been demonstrated by two different groups using the National Health and Nutrition Examination Survey (NHANES), a random sampling of US citizens. The strong associations seen in quite different studies suggest the possibility that exposure to POPs could cause diabetes. One striking observation is that obese people that do not have elevated POPs are not at elevated risk of diabetes, suggesting that the POPs rather than the obesity per se is responsible for the association." Carpenter DO. Environmental contaminants as risk factors for developing diabetes. *Rev Environ Health*. 2008 Jan-Mar;23(1):59-74

[373] "...the expected association between obesity and diabetes was absent in people with low concentrations of persistent organic pollutants in their blood. ...the association between obesity and diabetes became stronger as the concentrations of such pollutants in the blood increased." Jones et al. Environmental pollution and diabetes. *Lancet*. 2008 Jan:287-8

individual xenobiotics (unless the patient had a specific overdosing exposure). Functional assessments of hepatic detoxification ability are available commercially through specialty laboratories that cater to progressive integrative clinicians; these tests can be useful either for documenting baseline, assessing response to treatment, or demonstrating to patients, colleagues, or insurers the validity of detoxification interventions. However, much of this information can be determined empirically via a thorough patient history, which specifically asks about drug intolerances, caffeine sensitivity, multiple chemical sensitivity, and to a much lesser extent known xenobiotic exposures.

- **Imaging**: From a practical clinical standpoint, clinicians may choose to provide resting/stress ECG for asymptomatic patients at high risk of CAD/CVD, especially before implementing an exercise program; the level of evidence for this recommendation is neutral.[374] Some clinicians choose to practice more defensively than others, especially if the patient's condition or demeanor indicate the need for increased caution. Patients with any CAD/CVD symptoms should receive cardiovascular evaluation. Resting and stress ECG is appropriate for screening patients at high risk for cardiovascular disease and before low-moderate risk patients begin exercise. Patients with long-standing DM/MetSyn are at high risk for cardiovascular disease, especially if they also have hypertension, dyslipidemia, any evidence of PVD, or any history of smoking. Echocardiography may be added with evidence of impaired cardiac output or ventricular hypertrophy.

- **Biopsy/Procedure**: These are generally not indicated except in special circumstances. Liver biopsies show that DM and MetSyn patients have higher-than-average rates of hepatic iron accumulation and iron overload[375,376] but iron overload can generally be determined by serologic testing with ferritin and transferrin saturation as discussed previously thus making liver biopsy unnecessary.

- **Establishing the Diagnosis**: The diagnosis of MetSyn is made by connecting the clinical constellation previously listed: ❶ central adiposity, abdominal obesity, ❷ hyperglycemia, ❸dyslipidemia, ❹ hypertension, ❺ systemic inflammation, and ❻ hypercoagulability. The diagnosis of DM-2 is made by finding a compelling clinical picture, elevated glucose levels (discussed previously and repeated in abbreviated format below) and by excluding the differential diagnoses.
    - Serum glucose: The interpretive guide below describes fasting/nonfasting glucose in units of mg/dl.
        - Fasting; diagnostic of DM: ≥126 on two separate occasions.
        - Non-fasting, diagnostic of DM: ≥ 200 with nonfasting blood sample or 2 hours after oral consumption of 75 g glucose (glucose tolerance test, GGT).

Hgb-A1c for DM diagnosis

"The diagnosis of diabetes is made if the A1C level is ≥6.5%. Diagnosis should be confirmed with a repeat A1C test unless clinical symptoms and glucose levels >200 mg/dl (>11.1 mmol/l) are present."

International Expert Committee report on the role of the A1C assay in the diagnosis of diabetes. *Diabetes Care*. 2009 Jul

---

Disease Complications: Major complications of DM and MetSyn are listed below and displayed graphically in the previous Venn diagram.

- Cardiovascular disease (CVD): MI, peripheral/visceral/cerebral/ocular vascular disease. More than 60% of nontraumatic limb amputations are due to complications from DM. Impaired circulation contributes to impaired wound healing. Hypercoagulability promotes atherosclerosis and thrombosis and resultant arterial occlusion, particularly in the coronary arteries of the heart (myocardial infarction, MI), cerebral circulation of the brain (stroke), retinal arteries of the eyes (retinal ischemia), peripheral limbs (digital necrosis), and internal organs (e.g., mesenteric ischemia, renal artery occlusion). Hypertension is highly prevalent in DM-2/MetSyn patients. Control of hypertension reduces disease-related complications by 24% while tight glucose control lowers these complications by 12%.

---

[374] "U.S. Preventive Services Task Force (USPSTF) found insufficient evidence to recommend for or against routine screening with ECG, exercise treadmill test (ETT), or electron-beam computerized tomography (EBCT) scanning for coronary calcium for either the presence of severe coronary artery stenosis (CAS) or the prediction of CHD events in adults at increased risk for CHD events." Screening for Coronary Heart Disease. Release Date: February 2004. ahrq.gov/clinic/uspstf/uspsacad.htm Accessed August 12, 2009
[375] Phelps G, Chapman I, Hall P, Braund W, Mackinnon M. Prevalence of genetic haemochromatosis among diabetic patients. *Lancet*. 1989 Jul 29;2(8657):233-4
[376] "Most of the patients (95%) had one or more of the following conditions: obesity, hyperlipidaemia, abnormal glucose metabolism, or hypertension. INTERPRETATION: We have found a new non-HLA-linked iron-overload syndrome which suggests a link between iron excess and metabolic disorders." Moirand R, Mortaji AM, Loréal O, Paillard F, Brissot P, Deugnier Y. A new syndrome of liver iron overload with normal transferrin saturation. *Lancet*. 1997 Jan 11;349(9045):95-7

- <u>Ocular diseases</u>: DM is the leading cause of blindness in adults; blindness results from cataracts (due to sorbitol accumulation and ROS production), vascular and neuropathic eye diseases. Due to the speed and severity of ocular complications of DM-2, all patients with DM-2 must be referred for ophthalmologist's evaluation upon diagnosis; follow-up exams are generally every 1-2 years.

- <u>Kidney failure, renal insufficiency</u>: Hyperglycemia is toxic to nephrons; chronic hyperglycemia eventually causes renal damage and chronic renal failure (CRF). The hypertension that is often part of the clinical picture in patients with DM/MetSyn further accelerates and exacerbates the renal disease; renal disease then becomes an additional cause of hypertension. Pharmacologic renoprotection is provided by early use of angiotensin converting enzyme (ACE) inhibitors and angiotensin receptor blockers (ARBs). Nutritional renoprotection is provided by treating the underlying cause of the syndrome and promoting its clinical resolution, as well as by CoQ10, which separately lowers blood pressure and rejuvenates nephrons, as discussed later in this chapter and in more detail in the chapter on hypertension. Assessment of renal function (detailed in Chapter 1) is mandatory in hypertensive and diabetic patients for many reasons, one of which is to screen for predisposition to hyperkalemia—which may be induced by a high-potassium diet—as discussed in a video tutorial by DrV available online: https://vimeo.com/152293616

- <u>Neuropathy</u>: Peripheral neuropathy is primarily *sensory*, predisposing to unattended injuries and proprioceptive defects that classically result in neuropathic osteoarthropathy (previously called Charcot joints). Autonomic neuropathy results in orthostatic hypotension, gastroparesis (with secondary small intestine bacterial overgrowth and tertiary malabsorption), erectile dysfunction and retrograde ejaculation.

Initial Checklist for managing DM-2/MetSyn
☑ <u>Implement "the supplemented (low-carb) Paleo-Mediterranean diet"</u> with multivitamin/multimineral, combination fatty acids, physiologic vitamin D dosage, magnesium and other nutrients as indicated
☑ <u>Blood pressure</u>: <130/85
☑ <u>Hgb-A1c</u>: <7%
☑ <u>Check renal function with serum BUN and creatinine and urine albumin:creatinine ratio</u>: Renal failure may contraindicate certain nutritional interventions and may necessitate referral to a specialist
☑ <u>LDL cholesterol</u>: <70-100 mg/dl
☑ <u>Triglycerides</u>: <100-150 mg/dl
☑ <u>HDL</u>: >40 mg/dl in men; >50 mg/dl in women
☑ <u>Serum ferritin</u>: 40-70 mcg/l
☑ <u>hsCRP</u>: 1-3 mg/L, ideal is <1
☑ <u>25(OH)vitamin D</u>: 50-100 ng/ml
☑ <u>Estradiol</u>: <30 picogram/mL in men
☑ <u>Assessments</u>: Foot exam, ophthalmology referral, ECG for patients with cardiac symptoms
☑ <u>Smoking cessation</u>
☑ <u>Low-dose aspirin for most patients >40y</u>: This recommendation has become increasingly questioned in the past few years, but is still a reasonable recommendation, especially in patients at low/normal risk for gastrointestinal bleeding and hemorrhagic stroke. "Diabetics are at high risk for atherosclerotic cardiovascular disease (ASCVD) and are considered a coronary heart disease risk equivalent. The utility of aspirin in primary prevention of ASCVD in diabetic patients has been widely studied and is still debated. Overall, the current evidence suggests a modest benefit for reduction in ASCVD events with the greatest benefit among those with higher baseline risk, but at the cost of increased risk of gastrointestinal bleeding. Diabetic patients at higher risk (with 10-year ASCVD risk >10 %) are generally recommended for aspirin therapy if bleeding risk is felt to be low. A patient-provider discussion is recommended before prescribing aspirin therapy." Desai et al. Preventing cardiovascular disease in patients with diabetes: use of aspirin for primary prevention. *Curr Cardiol Rep.* 2015 Mar

- <u>Gingival disease</u>: DM patients have an increased incidence of gum and dental disease. The relationship is bidirectional: gum disease causes systemic inflammation which exacerbates peripheral insulin resistance; hyperglycemia causes immune suppression and nutrient/antioxidant depletion which predisposes DM patients to gum disease.

- <u>Immunosuppression</u>: Most commonly presenting as gingivitis, yeast vaginitis/balantitis, and skin infections; each of these may be the presenting manifestation of DM. Clinicians must attend to each of the above clinical manifestations of DM as potential signs of DM when a new patient presents.

- <u>Hyperosmolar hyperglycemic nonketotic coma</u>: Uncontrolled DM-2 leads to extreme hyperglycemia (glucose >800-1,000 mg/dL) with resultant hyperosmolar diuresis and profound dehydration, which can result in altered mental status, stroke, or seizures.

- <u>Pregnant mothers with DM deliver babies with increased prevalence and severity of birth defects</u>: Some women may choose to delay conception until DM is resolved; risks, contraceptive options, and *most importantly* safe and effective treatments for alleviation of diabetes should be discussed with women of child-bearing potential.

Clinical Management:

- <u>Goals</u>: The goals are ❶ to address any urgent problems such as imminent MI, impending CRF, infection, electrolyte imbalance, or dehydration, ❷ assess and address anticipated complications such as CRF, CVD, dyslipidemia, retinopathy; also screen for primary causes of the clinical picture as appropriate, including iron overload, iatrogenesis (e.g., corticosteroid overdose), Cushing's disease, acromegaly, acute/chronic pancreatitis, ❸ ensure proper patient education about the nuances and curative potential of dietary and lifestyle management of uncomplicated DM-2 and the utmost importance of dietary control and overall treatment compliance—remind them that DM/MetSyn is a kidney-, heart-, limb-, vision-, and life-threatening condition, ❹ use drugs as needed to complement lifestyle and nutritional interventions, particularly for patients with complications or noncompliance; typical drugs include oral hypoglycemics, injectable insulin, aspirin, statins, antihypertensive drugs, and renoprotective drugs such as ACE-inhibitors and angiotensin receptor blockers (ARBs), ❺ practice defensively with appropriate documentation, education, co-management, and timely referral. Noncompliant patients must receive documented education, access to appropriate treatments and resources, encouragement, and co-management/referral. Clinicians should appreciate that transitioning from an unhealthy lifestyle to one compatible with health is a major challenge for many DM-2 patients; clinicians should be compassionate, patient, and diligent about documenting clinical encounters and education. Noncompliant patients put themselves at risk for devastating adverse health outcomes including blindness, death, injury, and limb amputation; likewise, noncompliant nonresponsive patients place the clinician at risk for medicolegal complications. In certain situations, clinicians may choose to provide a complete referral (i.e., call and make a confirmed appointment for the patient) to a specialist; more rarely, dangerously noncompliant patients should be appropriately referred to a specialist and then discharged from the practice by certified mail.
- <u>Patient referral, co-management and education</u>: DM and MetSyn are serious disorders that mandate thorough patient education about the disease and its treatments, and the procedures/alternatives/risks/benefits (PAR-B) for each treatment. Guidelines from the American College of Physicians[377] include the following (with slight modifications):
    1. Refer all patients for diabetes self-management education, to cover diet, glycemic management, exercise programs, and strategies to prevent complications. Review and support self-management topics at every visit.
    2. Consider referral to an endocrinologist for help in managing complex patients.
    3. Refer all patients with DM-2 to an ophthalmologist. Obtain consult to screen for diabetic eye disease at diagnosis and every 1 to 3 years, depending on risk, to reduce the risk of visual loss from diabetic retinopathy and macular edema.
    4. Consult for cardiology to perform a cardiac stress test in patients with typical/atypical cardiac symptoms and an abnormal resting ECG; consider a screening/stress cardiac stress test for those with a history of peripheral or carotid artery occlusive disease and those over age 35 with a sedentary lifestyle who plan to begin a vigorous exercise program. Exercise can induce hypoglycemia; patients are justified in starting their exercise regimen slowly so that they can adapt to the experience physiologically as well as psychologically. Patients who smoke are expediting the development of cardiovascular complications atop a condition characterized by accelerated atherosclerosis. All patients who smoke must be advised to stop smoking and this must be documented in the chart, preferably at each visit.
    5. For DM/MetSyn patients over age 40y, the benefits of a daily aspirin (75-162 mg/d) outweigh the risks for medically managed patients (common practice, yet consistently debated).

Food & Nutrition Food intake and nutritional status/supplementation always has and always will be foundational in the treatment of various forms of diabetes; carbohydrate restriction and nutritional density are the everlasting keystones of the dietary management of diabetes.

- **Low-carbohydrate Paleo-Mediterranean Diet**: The health-promoting diet of choice for the majority of people is a diet based on abundant consumption of fruits, vegetables, seeds, nuts, omega-3 and monounsaturated fatty acids, and lean sources of protein such as lean meats, fatty cold-water fish, soy and whey proteins. This diet prohibits and obviates overconsumption of chemical preservatives, artificial sweeteners, and carbohydrate-

---

[377] pier.acponline.org/physicians/public/d296/mgt.consult/d296-s9.html Accessed July 17, 2009

dominant foods such as candies, pastries, breads, potatoes, grains, and other foods with a high glycemic load and high glycemic index. This "Paleo-Mediterranean Diet" is a combination of the "Paleolithic" or "Paleo diet" and the well-known "Mediterranean diet", both of which are well described in peer-reviewed journals and the lay press. The Mediterranean diet is characterized by increased proportions of legumes, nuts, seeds, whole grain products, fruits, vegetables (including potatoes), fish and lean meats, and monounsaturated and n-3 fatty acids.[378] Consumption of this diet is consistently associated with improvements in

> **Clinical Pearl**
>
> Because inflammation is a key component of DM and MetSyn, clinicians are wise to treat DM/MetSyn as if it were an inflammatory disorder. Inflammation promotes insulin resistance, and insulin resistance promotes inflammation; both cause oxidative stress and nutritional depletion. Essentially all nutrients and dietary plans that have shown benefit in the treatment of DM/MetSyn are simultaneous inhibitors of inflammation in general and NFkB in particular, while they sensitize peripheral insulin receptors to improve glucose and serum lipid control.

insulin sensitivity and reductions in cardiovascular disease, diabetes, cancer, and all-cause mortality.[379] The Paleolithic diet detailed by collaborators Eaton[380], O'Keefe[381], and Cordain[382] is similar to the Mediterranean diet except for stronger emphasis on fruits and vegetables (preferably raw or minimally cooked), omega-3-rich lean meats, and reduced consumption of starchy foods such as potatoes and grains, the latter of which were not staples in the human diet until the last few thousand years. The current author expects that habitual consumption of this Paleo-Mediterranean Diet is immunosupportive/immunoempowering due to both ❶ increased intake of micronutrients, phytonutrients, and the alkalinizing pro-homeostatic benefits in addition to ❷ avoidance of nutrient-poor high-carbohydrate high-fat foods which are immunosuppressive and pro-inflammatory. High-carbohydrate diets deal a double-punch to the human host; first, consumption of a high-carbohydrate load causes immunosuppression, and then secondly the high-carbohydrate load promotes activation of NFkB which then promotes systemic inflammation. The Mediterranean diet has shown unparalleled safety and efficacy in the prevention of cardiovascular disease, cancer, and all-cause mortality.

- Review: Mediterranean diet and the metabolic syndrome (*Mol Nutr Food Res* 2007 Oct[383]): "Some recent studies dealing specifically with the effect of interventions on the resolution of the metabolic syndrome have demonstrated a 25% net reduction in the prevalence of the syndrome following lifestyle changes mainly based on nutritional recommendations. ... The favorable benefit/hazard ratio makes Mediterranean-style diets particularly promising to reduce the cardiovascular burden associated with the metabolic syndrome."

- Cross-sectional study: Swedish pre-school children eat too much junk food and sucrose (*Acta Paediatr* 2007 Feb[384]): An interesting finding in this study, which proved a point that integrative clinicians have been proclaiming for decades, is that obesity and nutritional deficiency can certainly co-exist. Excess caloric intake coupled with physical inactivity does not ensure

> **Clinical Insight**
>
> Question: Why do low-carbohydrate diets cause a rapid reduction/normalization in blood pressure among hypertensive patients even before significant weight loss has taken place?
>
> Answer: Because carbohydrate ingestion triggers insulin release, and insulin promotes renal retention of sodium, and therefore promotes retention of water and the development of the volume overload that is characteristic of hypertension. Low-carbohydrate diets cause a rapid reduction in serum insulin levels, and thus the endogenous trigger for sodium-water retention is abated; blood pressure then has the opportunity to normalize rapidly.

against nutritional deficiencies, despite the appearance of being "overnourished." "Eighteen percent of children were overweight/obese. ... Junk food supplied 24% of energy. Ninety-two percent had low vitamin D intake, 70% low iron and 21% low calcium intake." Astute clinicians will note that the 92% prevalence of insufficient vitamin D intake would virtually guarantee that these children will have pandemic vitamin D deficiency, since year-round sunbathing is unlikely, particularly among this group of pre-school children in Sweden.

[378] Curtis et al. Understanding the Mediterranean diet. Could this be the new "gold standard" for heart disease prevention? *Postgrad Med.* 2002 Aug;112(2):35-8, 41-5
[379] Knoops et al. Mediterranean diet, lifestyle factors, and 10-year mortality in elderly European men and women: the HALE project. *JAMA.* 2004 Sep 22;292(12):1433-9
[380] Eaton SB, Shostak M, Konner M. *The Paleolithic Prescription: A program of diet & exercise and a design for living*, New York: Harper & Row, 1988
[381] O'Keefe JH Jr, Cordain L. Cardiovascular disease resulting from a diet and lifestyle at odds with our Paleolithic genome. *Mayo Clin Proc.* 2004 Jan;79(1):101-8
[382] Cordain L. *The Paleo Diet: Lose Weight and Get Healthy by Eating the Food You Were Designed to Eat.* Indianapolis; John Wiley and Sons, 2002
[383] Esposito K, Ciotola M, Giugliano D. Mediterranean diet and the metabolic syndrome. *Mol Nutr Food Res.* 2007 Oct;51(10):1268-74
[384] Garemo M, Lenner RA, Strandvik B. Swedish pre-school children eat too much junk food and sucrose. *Acta Paediatr.* 2007 Feb;96(2):266-72

- Cross-sectional study: Micronutrient deficiency and the prevalence of mothers' overweight/obesity in Egypt (*Econ Hum Biol* 2007 Dec [385]): This study showed that micronutrient deficiency greatly increases the risk for overweight/obesity. "The ordered logit results show an overlap between micronutrient deficiency and the prevalence of mothers' overweight/obesity in Egypt. The odds of being overweight/obese are 80.8% higher for micronutrient deficient mothers than for non-deficient mothers, keeping all other variables constant." Given the firmly-established role of vitamins and minerals in basic cellular metabolism, a simple model could hold that patients with multiple micronutrient deficiencies simply do not have the enzyme cofactors to metabolize energy substrates such as lipids/adipose, and that they therefore have a biochemical predisposition toward overweight/obesity by shear virtue of not being able to metabolize energy. A second theory holds that nutritional deficiencies cause a form of *junk food pica* (note that **pica**—defined as an abnormal appetite for nonnutritive substances—is well established in relation to iron deficiency) in which nutrient-depleted patients eat more as a result of either a biochemical disturbance in the brain or a starvation-prevention instinct which is attempting to compensate for the malnutrition, or both.

  > **Clinical Pearl**
  >
  > Patients can be encouraged to aim for a "no carb" diet insofar as they are to *habitually* avoid sugar, fructose, and carb-rich grains and vegetables such as potatoes, corn, rice, squash, and the numerous variations of wheat: bread, crackers, pizza, pasta, cereals. This way, when they decide to "cheat" for occasional practical, social, or emotional reasons, this will suffice to provide some modicum of dietary carbohydrate, while generally providing the low-carb milieu that benefits glycemic control, weight loss, and blood pressure and lipid control.

- Negative effects of the standard American diet (SAD): Increase in intranuclear nuclear factor kappaB and decrease in inhibitor kappaB in mononuclear cells after a mixed meal (*Am J Clin Nutr* 2004 Apr[386]): Consumption of the standard American diet (SAD) causes oxidative stress, systemic inflammation, and activation of NFkB; clinicians must appreciate that each of these three adverse effects leads to a biochemical milieu that supports the development and perpetuation of infections, particularly viral infections. Subjects in this study consumed an egg-muffin and sausage-muffin sandwiches and 2 hash browns, which contained 81 g carbohydrate, 51 g fat, and 32 g protein "RESULTS: ROS generation by mononuclear cells and polymorphonuclear leukocytes and p47(phox) expression increased significantly. The expression of IKKalpha and IKKbeta and DNA-binding activity of NF-kappaB increased significantly, whereas IkappaBalpha expression decreased. Plasma CRP concentrations increased. The intake of 300 mL water did not induce a change in any of the above indexes. CONCLUSIONS: These data show that the intake of a mixed meal results in significant inflammatory changes characterized by a decrease in IkappaBalpha and an increase in NF-kappaB binding, plasma CRP, and the expression of IKKalpha, IKKbeta, and p47(phox) subunit. These proinflammatory changes are probably relevant to the state of chronic hypertension and obesity and to its association with atherosclerosis." Thus, some of the benefit of the Paleo-Mediterranean diet comes not only from the inherent benefits of the diet itself, but also from the avoidance of the negative effects of the SAD eating pattern that is typical in industrialized nations.

- Prospective diet-disease correlation among more than 21,000 subjects: Plasma vitamin C level, fruit and vegetable consumption, and the risk of new-onset type-2 diabetes mellitus (*Arch Intern Med* 2008 Jul[387]): This study aimed to determine whether fruit and vegetable intake and plasma vitamin C level are associated with the risk of incident type 2 diabetes by correlating fruit-vegetable intake with plasma vitamin C levels and then monitoring for development of DM-2 over the next 12 years. "RESULTS: A strong inverse association was found between plasma vitamin C level and diabetes risk. The odds ratio of diabetes in the top quintile of plasma vitamin C was 0.38 (95% confidence interval, 0.28-0.52) in a model adjusted for demographic, lifestyle, and anthropometric variables. In a similarly adjusted model, the odds ratio of diabetes in the top quintile of fruit and vegetable consumption was 0.78 (95% confidence interval, 0.60-1.00). CONCLUSIONS: **Higher plasma vitamin C level and, to a lesser degree, fruit and vegetable intake** were associated with a substantially **decreased risk of diabetes.**"

[385] Asfaw A. Micronutrient deficiency and the prevalence of mothers' overweight/obesity in Egypt. *Econ Hum Biol*. 2007 Dec;5(3):471-83
[386] Aljada A, Mohanty P, Ghanim H, Abdo T, Tripathy D, Chaudhuri A, Dandona P. Increase in intranuclear nuclear factor kappaB and decrease in inhibitor kappaB in mononuclear cells after a mixed meal: evidence for a proinflammatory effect. *Am J Clin Nutr*. 2004 Apr;79(4):682-90
[387] Harding et al. Plasma vitamin C level, fruit and vegetable consumption, and the risk of new-onset type 2 diabetes mellitus. *Arch Intern Med*. 2008 Jul 28;168(14):1493-9

- Adherence to a Mediterranean-type diet reduces the prevalence of clustered cardiovascular risk factors among 3,204 high-risk patients (*Eur J Cardiovasc Prev Rehabil* 2008 Oct[388]): "Adherence to **MeDiet [Mediterranean diet]** was inversely associated with individual risk factors and, above all, with the clustering of them. ... CONCLUSION: Following a **MeDiet** was inversely associated with the clustering of hypertension, diabetes, obesity, and hypercholesterolemia among high-risk patients."

- Pro-inflammatory effects of glucose ingestion: Glucose ingestion induces an increase in intranuclear nuclear factor kappaB, a fall in cellular inhibitor kappaB, and an increase in tumor necrosis factor alpha messenger RNA by mononuclear cells in healthy human subjects (*Metabolism* 2006 Sep[389]): Subjects in this study received glucose ingestion consistent with normal dietary habits: 300 kcal (75 g) glucose in water (300 mL). Results showed that 300 kcal of glucose causes NFkB activation, systemic inflammation, and increased expression of pro-inflammatory TNF-alpha. Clinicians should appreciate that many of the new drugs for rheumatic diseases specifically target TNF-alpha. "We conclude that glucose intake induces an immediate increase in intranuclear NF-kappaB binding, a fall in IkappaBalpha, an increase in IKKalpha, IKKbeta, IKK activity, and messenger RNA expression of TNF-alpha in MNCs (mononuclear cells) in healthy subjects. These data are consistent with **profound acute pro-inflammatory changes in MNCs after glucose intake.**"

When patients overconsume simple carbohydrates several times per day, they are inducing a clinically significant oxidative stress and pro-inflammatory state several times per day that lasts for several hours.

- Cohort study of the Mediterranean diet in elderly humans (*JAMA* 2004 Sep[390]): "Among individuals aged 70 to 90 years, **adherence to a Mediterranean diet and healthful lifestyle is associated with a more than 50% lower rate of all-causes and cause-specific mortality.**" The Mediterranean diet has shown unparalleled safety and efficacy in the prevention of cardiovascular disease, cancer, and all-cause mortality.

- Twelve-month randomized clinical trial shows that the low-carb Atkins diet is superior to other diets for weight loss (*JAMA* 2007 Mar[391]): In this 12-month randomized trial, 311 free-living, overweight/obese (body mass index, 27-40) nondiabetic, premenopausal women were randomly assigned to follow the Atkins (n = 77), Zone (n = 79), LEARN (n = 79), or Ornish (n = 76) diets. Subjects received weekly instruction for 2 months with 10-month follow-up. Body weight and laboratory parameters were measured. "RESULTS: **Weight loss was greater for women in the Atkins diet group compared with the other diet groups at 12 months,** and mean 12-month weight loss was significantly different between the Atkins and Zone diets (P<.05). Mean 12-month weight loss was

> **Diets that emphasize more protein and less carbohydrate clearly provide more metabolic and weight-loss benefits than other eating patterns, especially when combined with exercise**
>
> "Thus, a high-protein diet combined with a moderate-intensity combination aerobic and resistance training protocol **seems the ideal program** for short-term weight loss in this subject population."
>
> Meckling KA, Sherfey R. A randomized trial of a hypocaloric high-protein diet, with and without exercise, on weight loss, fitness, and markers of the Metabolic Syndrome in overweight and obese women. *Appl Physiol Nutr Metab.* 2007 Aug

> **Clinical Insight**
>
> Error: Diabetes mellitus type-2 and the metabolic syndrome are "chronic diseases" from which the patient cannot recover.
>
> Correction: Diabetes mellitus type-2 and the metabolic syndrome are conditions reflected by acute and subacute maladaptations (to nutritional deficiencies, nutrient imbalances, carbohydrate excess and possibly xenobiotic accumulation) that persist because the conditions for their perpetuation continue to exist. When these primary problems are addressed, the condition either partially abates or completely resolves, depending on the comprehensiveness of the plan, the level of compliance, and the duration/damage of the previous state. Thus, diabetes mellitus type-2 and the metabolic syndrome are not so much "chronic diseases" as they are "acute/subacute diseases that are repeated hourly and daily for many years", perhaps the rest of the patient's life, until and unless a skilled clinician and compliant patient address and correct the causes of the repetitive maladaptations.

[388] Sánchez-Taínta et al; PREDIMED group. Adherence to a Mediterranean-type diet and reduced prevalence of clustered cardiovascular risk factors in a cohort of 3,204 high-risk patients. *Eur J Cardiovasc Prev Rehabil*. 2008 Oct;15(5):589-93

[389] Aljada A, Friedman J, Ghanim H, Mohanty P, Hofmeyer D, Chaudhuri A, Dandona P. Glucose ingestion induces an increase in intranuclear nuclear factor kappaB, a fall in cellular inhibitor kappaB, and an increase in tumor necrosis factor alpha messenger RNA by mononuclear cells in healthy human subjects. *Metabolism*. 2006 Sep;55(9):1177-85

[390] Knoops et al. Mediterranean diet, lifestyle factors, and 10-year mortality in elderly European men and women: the HALE project. *JAMA*. 2004 Sep 22;292(12):1433-9

[391] Gardner CD, Kiazand A, Alhassan S, Kim S, Stafford RS, Balise RR, Kraemer HC, King AC. Comparison of the Atkins, Zone, Ornish, and LEARN diets for change in weight and related risk factors among overweight premenopausal women: the A TO Z Weight Loss Study: a randomized trial. *JAMA*. 2007 Mar 7;297(9):969-77

as follows: **Atkins, -4.7 kg**, Zone, -1.6 kg, LEARN, -2.6 kg, and Ornish, -2.2 kg. ... While questions remain about long-term effects and mechanisms, a low-carbohydrate, high-protein, high-fat diet may be considered a feasible alternative recommendation for weight loss." Clinicians should appreciate not only the exoneration of Dr Atkins, who was ostracized and harassed by groups in "conventional medicine" for his advocation of a health-promoting diet, but also that the negative associations with the *ad libitum* fat consumption are not necessarily a requirement for the success of this diet. Patients can still achieve success on a low-carb diet even if they do not overindulge in dietary lipids; what the study proves is that carbohydrate avoidance is the key to weight loss, and that avoidance of dietary fat is of lesser importance. The diet should focus on ❶ adequate consumption of high-quality protein to avoid decrements in muscle mass and immune function that are reported when patients follow a "normal" diet that is low in protein, ❷ *ad libitum* consumption of **low-carbohydrate** fruits, **vegetables, nuts, seeds**, and berries, ❸ avoidance of all dietary carbohydrate (from starchy foods such as potatoes and wheat and other grains, including rice and

Carbohydrate restriction shows therapeutic equivalence to—and therefore clinical superiority over—insulin therapy in severe diabetics
Avoidance of the following foods: 1. <u>Staple foods</u>: rice, bread, corn, spaghetti, noodle made of wheat or buckwheat, potato, sweet potato, taro and yam 2. <u>Fruits</u>: pear, apple, persimmon, mikan, orange, grapefruit, peach, grape, melon, water melon, banana, pineapple. 3. <u>Vegetables</u>: carrot, pumpkin, and autumn squash 4. <u>Confectioneries</u>: all 5. <u>Drink</u>: beverages containing sugar, glucose and fructose, and milk 6. <u>Alcohol</u>: sake, beer and wine (Distilled liquor was not restricted)
The main principle of the carbohydrate-restricted diet was to eliminate carbohydrate-rich food twice a day at breakfast and dinner, or eliminate it three times a day at breakfast, lunch and dinner. There were no other restrictions. Patients on the carbohydrate-restricted diet were permitted to eat as much protein and fat as they wanted, including saturated fat.
Haimoto et al. Effects of a low-carbohydrate diet on glycemic control in outpatients with severe type 2 diabetes. *Nutr Metab* 2009:6;21

corn) except what is found from whole-foods sources, and from the inevitable "cheating", ❹ broad-spectrum supplementation with the fatty acids ALA, GLA, EPA, and DHA along with oleic acid and the requisite polyphenolics found in olive oil, ❺ supplemental vitamin D in physiologic doses targeted to attain and maintain optimal serum levels of 25-OH-vitamin D3, and ❻ regular consumption of probiotics, either in pills or as yogurt/kefir.

- Randomized clinical trial with 100 women: Comparison of high-protein vs high-carbohydrate diet on markers of cardiovascular health in obese women (*Am J Clin Nutr* 2005 Jun[392]): Subjects were randomly assigned to 1 of 2 isocaloric 5600-kJ dietary interventions for 12 wk: either 1) a high-protein (HP) or 2) a high-carbohydrate (HC) diet. "RESULTS: ... Weight loss was 7.3 +/- 0.3 kg with both diets. Subjects with high serum triacylglycerol (>1.5 mmol/L) lost more fat mass with the HP than with the HC diet and had a greater decrease in triacylglycerol concentrations with the HP than with the HC diet. ... Fasting LDL-cholesterol, HDL-cholesterol, glucose, insulin, free fatty acid, and C-reactive protein concentrations decreased with weight loss. Serum vitamin B-12 increased 9% with the HP diet and decreased 13% with the HC diet. Folate and vitamin B-6 increased with both diets; homocysteine did not change significantly. ... CONCLUSION: An energy-restricted, high-protein, low-fat diet provides nutritional and metabolic benefits that are equal to and sometimes greater than those observed with a high-carbohydrate diet."

- Review: Metabolic effects of low glycemic index diets (*Nutr J* 2009 Jan[393]): "The currently available scientific literature shows that low glycemic-index diets acutely induce a number of favorable effects, such as a rapid weight loss, decrease of fasting glucose and insulin levels, reduction of circulating triglyceride levels and improvement of blood pressure."

- Two-year clinical trial: Weight loss with a low-carbohydrate, Mediterranean, or low-fat diet (*N Engl J Med.* 2008 Jul[394]): 322 moderately obese subjects were randomized to one of three diets: ❶ low-fat, restricted-calorie; ❷ Mediterranean, restricted-calorie; or ❸ low-carbohydrate, non–restricted-calorie. "The mean weight loss was 2.9 kg for the low-fat group, 4.4 kg for the Mediterranean-diet group, and 4.7 kg for the

[392] Noakes M, Keogh JB, Foster PR, Clifton PM. Effect of an energy-restricted, high-protein, low-fat diet relative to a conventional high-carbohydrate, low-fat diet on weight loss, body composition, nutritional status, and markers of cardiovascular health in obese women. Am J Clin Nutr. 2005 Jun;81(6):1298-306
[393] Radulian G, Rusu E, Dragomir A, Posea M. Metabolic effects of low glycemic index diets. Nutr J. 2009 Jan 29;8:5
[394] Shai I, Schwarzfuchs D, Henkin Y, et al. Weight loss with a low-carbohydrate, Mediterranean, or low-fat diet. N Engl J Med. 2008 Jul 17;359(3):229-41

low-carbohydrate group; among the 272 participants who completed the intervention, the mean weight losses were 3.3 kg, 4.6 kg, and 5.5 kg, respectively. Among the 36 subjects with diabetes, changes in fasting plasma glucose and insulin levels were more favorable among those assigned to the Mediterranean diet than among those assigned to the low-fat diet. Mediterranean and low-carbohydrate diets may be effective alternatives to low-fat diets. The more favorable effects on lipids (with the low-carbohydrate diet) and on glycemic control (with the Mediterranean diet) suggest that personal preferences and metabolic considerations might inform individualized tailoring of dietary interventions." I suggest that a *low-carb Mediterranean diet is the diet of choice because it provides the "best of both worlds"* for lipid control, weight loss, cancer prevention, mortality reduction, and the numerous other health benefits already well-established to result from habituation to the Mediterranean diet.

- Moderately low-carb diet is comparable to insulin therapy for diabetics: Effects of a low-carbohydrate diet on glycemic control in outpatients with severe type 2 diabetes (*Nutr Metab* 2009 May[395]): A 30%-carbohydrate diet was used in 33 outpatients with severe type-2 diabetes (Hgb-A1c levels of 9.0% or above). "HbA1c levels decreased sharply from a baseline of 10.9 to 7.8 at 3 months and to 7.4 at 6 months. Body mass index decreased slightly from baseline (23.8 +/- 3.3) to 6 months (23.5 +/- 3.4). … No adverse effects were observed except for mild constipation. The number of patients on sulfonylureas decreased from 7 at baseline to 2 at 6 months. No patient required inpatient care or insulin therapy. **In summary, the 30%-carbohydrate diet over 6 months led to a remarkable reduction in HbA1c levels, even among outpatients with severe type 2 diabetes, without any insulin therapy, hospital care or increase in sulfonylureas. The effectiveness of the diet may be comparable to that of insulin therapy.**"

- Randomized clinical trial: A randomized trial of a hypocaloric high-protein diet, with and without exercise, on markers of the Metabolic Syndrome in overweight and obese women (*Appl Physiol Nutr Metab* 2007 Aug[396]): This study evaluated the effects of hypocaloric diets with 3:1 and 1:1 carbohydrate-to-protein ratios, with/without exercise on physical and serologic parameters. Four groups were designated: ❶ control diet (CON), ❷ control diet with exercise (CONEx), ❸ high-protein (HP), and ❹ high-protein with exercise (HPEx)—exercise for the purpose of this study meant only three times per week (and is thus not truly representative of *exercise*, but merely of *activity*). Weight loss was as follows, with results favoring the group randomized to high-protein+exercise: -2.1 kg for the CON group, -4.0 kg in the CONEx group, -4.6 kg in the HP group, and **-7.0 kg in the HPEx.** Benefits seen in all groups were weight loss, improved body composition, decreased blood pressure, and decreased waist and hip circumference. "**A high-protein diet was superior to a low-fat, high-carbohydrate diet either alone or when combined with an aerobic/resistance-training program in promoting weight loss and nitrogen balance,** while similarly improving body composition and risk factors for the Metabolic Syndrome in overweight and obese Canadian women."

> **Nutrition-drug coordination**
>
> Clinicians must appreciate that a low-carbohydrate diet may make antihyperglycemic and antihypertensive drugs less necessary or completely unnecessary; patients need to be educated appropriately and warned of potential hypoglycemic or hypotensive complications that could occur if drug doses are not adjusted appropriately. Nutritional interventions need to be coordinated with adjustments in drug dosage so that hypoglycemic or hypotensive complications are avoided.

- Inpatient fasting as treatment for diabetes type-2 and obesity (*Am J Med* 1988 Jul[397]): "Sixty-four poorly controlled obese diabetic patients were hospitalized and placed on a precisely defined, hypocaloric diet. … **Average weight loss was 13 pounds in a mean of 23 days.** During hospitalization, the mean fasting **plasma glucose value for the group fell from 221 +/- 10 to 122 +/- 5 mg/dl.** In 45 patients (73 percent), the final fasting plasma glucose level was less than 125 mg/dl (mean: 102 +/- 2 mg/dl). Oral glucose tolerance even in those patients in whom fasting plasma glucose levels normalized was still grossly diabetic at the end of the hospital stay, deteriorating further after three days of liberalized caloric intake. In part this may have been due to decreased insulin secretory reserve as reflected by blunted plasma C-peptide response. **Forty of 42 patients who entered the study taking insulin were able to discontinue the drug within one to**

[395] Haimoto et al. Low-carbohydrate diet on glycemic control in outpatients with severe type-2 diabetes. *Nutr Metab* 2009 May:21 nutritionandmetabolism.com/content/6/1/21
[396] Meckling KA, Sherfey R. A randomized trial of a hypocaloric high-protein diet, with and without exercise, on weight loss, fitness, and markers of the Metabolic Syndrome in overweight and obese women. *Appl Physiol Nutr Metab.* 2007 Aug;32(4):743-52
[397] Bauman et al. Early and long-term effects of acute caloric deprivation in obese diabetic patients. *Am J Med.* 1988 Jul;85(1):38-46

seven days of hospitalization. After a mean follow-up period of 19 months, only 10 of 50 patients continued to maintain fasting euglycemia; five were on diet alone, and five were receiving oral hypoglycemic agents. Thirteen patients [down from 42 patients who were originally taking insulin] were receiving insulin therapy. **CONCLUSION: Diet therapy in these patients resulted in short-term improvement of glycemic control and, in the majority, normalization of fasting plasma glucose levels.** However, long-term outpatient follow-up revealed that relapse occurred in most patients." Part of the significance of this study is that it again shows the remarkable effectiveness of low-carbohydrate diet therapy for the treatment of DM-2; notice that most patients had normalization of their glucose levels, were able to discontinue insulin, and they succeeded in significant weight loss. The fact that these accomplishments were short-lived does not reflect a failure of the treatment but rather of compliance; this underscores the importance of patient support during the initiation of a low-carbohydrate diet and lifestyle.

- Clinical trial: Supplemented fasting as a large-scale outpatient program (*JAMA* 1977 Nov[398]): "Although supplemented fasting is now established as an efficient means of achieving substantial weight reduction in massively obese persons, widespread application of this treatment is contingent on its successful adaptation to a large-scale outpatient regimen. Of 519 patients treated as outpatients, 78% lost a minimum of 18.2 kg during the course of treatment. The overall rate of weight loss was 1.5 kg/wk, with females averaging 1.3 kg/wk and males, 2.1 kg/wk. The majority of patients tolerated the regimen well and were able to continue normal daily activities without experiencing any serious side effects." The importance of this study is that it showed that fasting programs can be administered safely and effectively on an outpatient basis; this does not mean that all patients will tolerate or are candidates for this treatment. Clinicians have the responsibility to select patients carefully, to screen them appropriately (e.g., ensure normal kidney function, electrolytes, and cardiac function), and to monitor them during the supervised fast with weekly or twice weekly in-office clinical assessments including blood pressure, mental status, serum electrolytes, and cardiac status assessed with auscultation and ECG.

- Outpatient diet and exercise treatment of 106 patients with massive obesity (*Arch Intern Med* 1975 Dec[399]): "This study demonstrates that massively obese persons can achieve marked weight reduction, even normalization of weight, without hospitalization, surgery, or pharmacologic intervention. Accompanying cardiovascular risk factors show great decrements concomitant with weight loss."

- **Multivitamin/multimineral supplementation**: DM/MetSyn patients generally achieved their clinical status via a lifetime of "overconsumption malnutrition." DM/MetSyn patients are at risk of nutritional deficiency because of poor dietary habits, oxidative destruction of vitamins, increased urinary losses of minerals, and—in patients with diabetes-induced autonomic neuropathy—nutrient malabsorption due to bacterial overgrowth of the small bowel due to gastroparesis or delayed intestinal transit (functional/overt hypothyroidism also contributes to the latter).

  - Review: Vitamins for chronic disease prevention in adults: clinical applications (*JAMA* 2002 Jun[400]): "Most people do not consume an optimal amount of all vitamins by diet alone. ...it appears prudent for all adults to take vitamin supplements. ... Physicians should...ensure that [patients] are taking vitamins they should..."

  - Clinical trial: Effect of a multivitamin and mineral supplement on infection and quality of life. A randomized, double-blind, placebo-controlled trial (*Ann Intern Med* 2003 Mar[401]): "A multivitamin and mineral supplement reduced the incidence of participant-reported infection and related absenteeism in a sample of participants with type 2 diabetes mellitus and a high prevalence of subclinical micronutrient deficiency."

  - Review: Contribution of selected vitamins and trace elements to immune function (*Ann Nutr Metab* 2007 Sep[402]): "Adequate intake of vitamins B(6), folate, B(12), C, E, and of selenium, zinc, copper, and iron supports a Th-1 cytokine-mediated immune response with sufficient production of proinflammatory

[398] Vertes V, Genuth SM, Hazelton IM. Supplemented fasting as a large-scale outpatient program. *JAMA*. 1977 Nov 14;238(20):2151-3
[399] Kempner et al. Treatment of massive obesity with rice/reduction diet program. Analysis of 106 patients with at least a 45-kg weight loss. *Arch Intern Med*. 1975 Dec:1575-84
[400] Fletcher RH, Fairfield KM. Vitamins for chronic disease prevention in adults: clinical applications. *JAMA*. 2002 Jun 19;287(23):3127-9
[401] Barringer et al. Effect of a multivitamin and mineral supplement on infection and quality of life. *Ann Intern Med*. 2003 Mar 4;138(5):365-71
[402] Wintergerst ES, Maggini S, Hornig DH. Contribution of selected vitamins and trace elements to immune function. *Ann Nutr Metab*. 2007;51(4):301-23

cytokines, which **maintains an effective immune response** and avoids a shift to an anti-inflammatory Th2 cell-mediated immune response and an increased risk of extracellular infections."

■ Review: Nutritional strategies to boost immunity and prevent infection in elderly individuals (*Clin Infect Dis* 2001 Dec[403]): "**Nutritional supplementation strategies can reduce this risk and reverse some of the immune dysfunction associated with advanced age.** ... The data support use of a daily multivitamin or trace-mineral supplement that includes zinc (elemental zinc, >20 mg/day) and selenium (100 microg/day), with additional vitamin E, to achieve a daily dosage of 200 mg/day."

> **Clinical Perspective**
>
> Remember that DM/MetSyn is a form of immunosuppression insofar as patients with these conditions have an increased risk for infection, poor circulation, and delayed wound healing and tissue repair. Thus, a comprehensive plan should address not only the obvious hyperglycemic, hypertensive, and pro-inflammatory issues, but also the immunocompromise that can be addressed at least partly through comprehensive nutritional supplementation.

■ Clinical trial: Effect of vitamin C on blood glucose, serum lipids & serum insulin in type 2 diabetes patients (*Indian J Med Res* 2007 Nov[404]): These authors evaluated the effect of different doses of vitamin C on blood glucose, serum lipids and serum insulin in individuals with DM-2; 84 patients with DM-2 referred to a specialty diabetic clinic in Iran were included in the study. "They received randomly either 500 mg or 1000 mg daily of vitamin C for six weeks. ... RESULTS: A significant decrease in FBS [fasting blood sugar], TG, LDL, HbA1c and serum insulin was seen in the group supplemented with 1000 mg vitamin C. The dose of 500 mg vitamin C, however, did not produce any significant change in any of the parameters studied. INTERPRETATION & CONCLUSION: Our results indicate that **daily consumption of 1000 mg supplementary vitamin C may be beneficial in decreasing blood glucose and lipids in patients with type 2 diabetes and thus reducing the risk of complications.**" To their credit, the authors of this study used a high enough dose to produce benefit. The results of 500 mg vitamin C per day are obvious—in this case, they were insignificant, and the "inefficacy of nutritional supplementation in patients with diabetes" would have made headlines in every newspaper in America, as is common when poorly conducted and underpowered trials of nutritional therapy fail.

■ Randomized double-blind placebo-controlled pilot study: High-dose thiamine therapy for patients with type 2 diabetes and microalbuminuria (*Diabetologia* 2009 Feb[405]): The authors review data showing that high-dose supplements of thiamine prevent the development of microalbuminuria in experimental diabetes. "METHODS: Type 2 diabetic patients (21 male, 19 female) with microalbuminuria were recruited at a diabetic clinic and randomized to placebo and treatment arms. Patients were given 3 x 100 mg capsules of thiamine or placebo per day for 3 months with a 2 month follow-up washout period. The primary endpoint was change in **urinary albumin excretion (UAE).** "RESULTS: **UAE was decreased in patients receiving thiamine therapy for 3 months with respect to baseline (median -17.7 mg/24 h; p < 0.001, n = 20).** There was no significant decrease in UAE in patients receiving placebo after 3 months of therapy (n = 20). UAE was significantly lower in patients who had received thiamine therapy compared with those who had received placebo (30.1 vs 35.5 mg/24 h, p < 0.01) but not at baseline. UAE continued to decrease in the 2 month washout period in both groups, but not significantly. There was no effect of thiamine treatment on glycemic control, dyslipidemia or BP. There were no adverse effects of therapy. CONCLUSIONS/INTERPRETATION: **In this pilot study, high-dose thiamine therapy produced a regression of UAE in type 2 diabetic patients with microalbuminuria. Thiamine supplements at high dose may provide improved therapy for early-stage diabetic nephropathy.**" This remarkable study disproves the medically purported "dangers" of using nutritional supplementation in patients with DM in general and DM-related renal insufficiency in particular. The mechanism of action is probably related to improved mitochondrial bioenergetics; based on this proposed mechanism of action, clinicians should readily hypothesize which other nutrient(s) would be expected to have similar clinical application—answer(s) will be provided later in this text.

---

[403] High KP. Nutritional strategies to boost immunity and prevent infection in elderly individuals. *Clin Infect Dis.* 2001 Dec 1;33(11):1892-900

[404] Afkhami-Ardekani et al. Effect of vitamin C on blood glucose, serum lipids & serum insulin in type 2 diabetes patients. *Indian J Med Res.* 2007 Nov;126(5):471-4

[405] Rabbani et al. High-dose thiamine therapy for patients with type 2 diabetes and microalbuminuria. *Diabetologia.* 2009 Feb;52(2):208-12

- Review: The potential role of thiamine (vitamin B1) in diabetic complications (*Curr Diabetes Rev* 2005 Aug[406]): Hyperglycemia causes accumulation of triose-phosphates, which are believed to contribute to the development of diabetic complications. The disposal of excess triose-phosphates via the reductive pentose-phosphate pathway relies upon the thiamine-dependent enzyme, transketolase. Correction of thiamine deficiency or supplemental thiamine has prevented diabetic complications in experimental diabetes. Given the potential clinical benefits and the paucity of adverse effects, the author concludes, "even mild thiamine deficiency in diabetes should be avoided and thiamine supplementation to high dose should be considered as adjunct nutritional therapy to prevent dyslipidemia and the development of vascular complications in clinical diabetes."

- Randomized, double-blind, controlled study: Antioxidant supplementation improves insulin sensitivity, endothelial adhesion molecules, and oxidative stress in normal-weight and overweight young adults (*Metabolism* 2009 Feb[407]): Participants (n=48) received "antioxidants" (AOX) as vitamin E 800 IU, vitamin C 500 mg, beta-carotene 10 mg or placebo for 8 weeks. The HOMA [homeostasis model assessment: a test of insulin sensitivity] values were initially higher in the overweight subjects and were lowered with AOX by week 8 (15% reduction, P = .02). Adiponectin increased in both AOX groups. (Adiponectin is a protein hormone that modulates glucose regulation and fatty acid catabolism. Adiponectin is exclusively secreted from adipose tissue, and levels of the hormone are inversely correlated with body fat percentage in adults. Adiponectin plays a protective role in the suppression of the metabolic derangements that may result in type 2 diabetes, obesity, atherosclerosis, non-alcoholic fatty liver disease (NAFLD) and the metabolic syndrome.) Furthermore, "Soluble intercellular adhesion molecule-1 and endothelial-leukocyte adhesion molecule-1 decreased in overweight AOX-treated groups by 6% and 13%, respectively (P < .05). Plasma lipid hydroperoxides were reduced by 0.31 and 0.70 nmol/mL in the normal-weight and overweight AOX-treated groups, respectively, by week 8 (P < .05)." In summary, this study showed that overweight patients have several positive and important biochemical responses to multivitamin supplementation with vitamin E 800 IU, vitamin C 500 mg, beta-carotene 10 mg for 8 weeks; integrative clinicians should appreciate the application of this protocol within a larger context that includes other nutrients as well as diet and exercise optimization.

- **Vitamin D3 (cholecalciferol, not ergocalciferol): 4,000-10,000 IU per day; for acute infections in deficient patients consider a one-time loading dose of 50,000-100,000 (up to 300,000) IU followed by a more conservative maintenance dose**: In our 2004 monograph by Vasquez, Manso, and Cannell[408], we fulfilled our promise of creating a "paradigm shift" that summarized new applications for the clinical use of vitamin D beyond its application in patients with osteoporosis or malabsorption to include the mandate of empiric treatment or laboratory assessment of all patients seen in clinical practice. Daily doses generally average between 4,000-10,000 IU/d for adults, with an acceptable one-time loading dose of 100,000-300,000 IU in patients for whom it is advantageous and safe to raise serum 25-hydroxy-vitamin D levels quickly and without concern for compliance failure; the logistical goal with vitamin D supplementation is to get serum 25-hydroxy-vitamin D levels into the optimal range, as defined in the illustration. The particular importance for using vitamin D in all diabetic patients is established by the following: ❶ DM/MetSyn patients tend to be more sedentary than the average American (who is also too sedentary), and "being sedentary" generally equates to "being indoors" where no sun exposure can occur; thus the prevalence of vitamin D deficiency is increased above the pandemic levels seen in the rest of the population. ❷ DM/MetSyn patients tend to be overweight or grossly obese, and the risk of vitamin D deficiency increases with increasing obesity/adiposity/BMI. ❸ Vitamin D levels correlate inversely with risk for heart disease, insulin resistance, renal failure, infection, cancer, and heart failure—all of these are increased in patients with DM/MetSyn. ❹ Lack of exercise that characterizes the lifestyle (or more accurately: *deathstyle*) of many patients with DM/MetSyn may also predispose a good number of these patients to osteopenia/osteoporosis; obviously vitamin D has a role in preventing this complication. ❺ Vitamin D levels correlate directly and positively with pancreatic insulin output and peripheral insulin sensitivity. ❻ DM/MetSyn patients have an increased incidence of depression, and by this time at least three separate clinical trials have shown that vitamin D has a mood-elevating and antidepressant benefit. ❼ Vitamin D can be safely

---

[406] Thornalley PJ. The potential role of thiamine (vitamin B1) in diabetic complications. *Curr Diabetes Rev.* 2005 Aug;1(3):287-98

[407] Vincent et al. Antioxidant supplementation on insulin sensitivity, endothelial adhesion molecules, oxidative stress in normal/overweight adults. *Metabolism* 2009 Feb:254-62

[408] Vasquez A, Manso G, Cannell J. The clinical importance of vitamin D (cholecalciferol). *Altern Ther Health Med.* 2004 Sep-Oct;10(5):28-36

administered to DM/MetSyn patients; patients who require more frequent monitoring of serum calcium are those with end-stage renal insufficiency and those taking hydrochlorothiazide, both of which can predispose to hypercalcemia.

- Chart review: Very high prevalence of vitamin D insufficiency in obese children and adolescents (*J Pediatr Endocrinol Metab* 2007 Jul[409]): Charts of 217 obese children were reviewed and correlated with laboratory results. **Severe vitamin D deficiency was found in 55% of obese children**, and this single nutritional **deficiency correlated with increased overweight/obesity, systolic blood pressure, and lower levels of cardioprotective HDL.** "CONCLUSION: **More than half of the obese children had vitamin D levels <20 ng/ml** with equal gender distribution. Vitamin D insufficiency was associated with increased age, BMI, and SBP, and decreased HDL-C."

Improvements in Hgb-A1c per various non-insulin treatments: ranked per safety and effectiveness, and cost-effectiveness
1. **Low-carbohydrate diet: -3.1 %***
2. **Oral magnesium supplementation: -2 %****
3. **Berberine: -1.2-2 %*****
4. Metformin: -1.5-2 %******
5. Sulfonylurea drugs: -1.5-2 %******
6. Thiazolidinedione drugs: -1.5-2 %******
*Haimoto et al. Effects of a low-carbohydrate diet on glycemic control in outpatients with severe type 2 diabetes. *Nutr Metab* 2009 ** Rodríguez-Morán et al. Oral magnesium supplementation improves insulin sensitivity and metabolic control in type 2 diabetic subjects. *Diabetes Care* 2003 Apr ***Yin et al. Efficacy of berberine in patients with type 2 diabetes mellitus. *Metabolism.* 2008 May ****Sloan PD et al [eds]. *Essentials of Family Medicine, Fifth Edition*. Lippincott Williams & Wilkins: 2008, pages 233-235

- Double-blind, parallel group, placebo-controlled randomized trial: Vitamin D improves endothelial function in patients with DM-2 and low vitamin D levels (*Diabet Med* 2008 Mar[410]): Unfortunately, this is an example of a trial that started with the wrong intervention, but was able to produce meaningful results nonetheless. The investigators used a single dose 100,000 IU vitamin D2 (they should have used vitamin D3, because it is much more effective) to see if this would improve endothelial function in patients with DM-2 and low serum 25-hydroxyvitamin D level (baseline 25-hydroxyvitamin D level was < 50 nmol/l). Significant results of this study are as follows: ❶ 49% of screened patients were vitamin D deficient. ❷ Vitamin D supplementation increased 25-hydroxyvitamin D levels by 15.3 nmol/l relative to placebo from a baseline 25-OH-vitamin D level of 38.3 nmol/l; thus the average increased to about 54 nmol/l—this is only slightly higher than the minimum of the optimal range defined and discussed previously (and again below). ❸ Vitamin D supplementation significantly improved flow mediated vasodilatation (FMD) of the brachial artery by 2.3%. ❹ **Vitamin D supplementation significantly decreased systolic blood pressure by 14 mmHg** compared with placebo; readers should note that this reduction in blood pressure is clinically meaningful and that it supports the earlier findings by Pfeifer et al[411] who found a reduction in blood pressure of approximately -13/-7 following the administration of low-dose vitamin D and calcium to elderly women.

- **Magnesium—600-1,200 mg per day or to bowel tolerance; use caution in patients predisposed to hypermagnesemia (renal failure, spironolactone):**
  - Randomized double-blind controlled trial: Oral magnesium supplementation improves insulin sensitivity and metabolic control in type 2 diabetic subjects (*Diabetes Care* 2003 Apr[412]): Oral supplementation with placebo or magnesium chloride (50 ml MgCl(2) solution containing 50 g MgCl(2) per 1,000 ml solution) was given to 63 subjects with DM-2 and hypomagnesaemia (serum magnesium levels </=0.74 mmol/l) for 16 weeks. "RESULTS: At the end of the study, **subjects who received magnesium supplementation showed significant higher serum magnesium concentration** (0.74 +/- 0.10 vs. 0.65 +/- 0.07 mmol/l, P = 0.02) and **lower HOMA-IR index** (3.8 +/- 1.1 vs. 5.0 +/- 1.3, P = 0.005), **fasting glucose levels** (8.0 +/- 2.4 vs. 10.3 +/- 2.1 mmol/l, P = 0.01), and **HbA(1c) (8.0** +/- 2.4 vs. **10.1** +/- 3.3%, P = 0.04) than control subjects. CONCLUSIONS: Oral supplementation with MgCl(2) solution restores serum magnesium levels, improving insulin sensitivity and metabolic control in type-2 diabetic patients with decreased serum magnesium levels." These results are truly remarkable considering the dramatic clinical response that these

[409] Smotkin-Tangorra et al. Prevalence of vitamin D insufficiency in obese children and adolescents. *J Pediatr Endocrinol Metab.* 2007 Jul;20(7):817-23
[410] Sugden et al. Vitamin D improves endothelial function in patients with Type 2 diabetes mellitus and low vitamin D levels. *Diabet Med.* 2008 Mar;25(3):320-5
[411] Pfeifer et al. Short-term vitamin D(3) calcium supplementation on blood pressure and parathyroid hormone levels in elderly women. *J Clin Endocrinol Metab* 2001 Apr:1633-7
[412] Rodríguez-Morán M, Guerrero-Romero F. Oral magnesium supplementation improves insulin sensitivity and metabolic control in type 2 diabetic subjects: a randomized double-blind controlled trial. *Diabetes Care.* 2003 Apr;26(4):1147-52

DM-2 patients showed to simple intervention with oral magnesium. Magnesium chloride is one of the least desirable forms of magnesium supplementation, with the citrate and malate forms being generally preferred by clinicians. The remarkable drop in Hgb-A1c levels from 10% (very poor control) to 8% (markedly improved control nearing the target of 7%) is sufficient to justify Mg supplementation in all diabetic patients (assuming result replicability).

- Randomized clinical trial: Efficacy and safety of oral magnesium supplementation in the treatment of depression in the elderly with type 2 diabetes (*Magnes Res* 2008 Dec[413]): Unfortunately, these researchers used what is generally considered to be an inferior form of magnesium supplementation—magnesium chloride—to evaluate the efficacy and safety of oral magnesium supplementation in the treatment of newly diagnosed depression in elderly hypomagnesemic patients with DM-2. Twenty-three subjects were enrolled and randomly allocated to receive either 50 mL of MgCl2 5% solution (equivalent to **450 mg of elemental magnesium**) or Imipramine 50 mg daily during 12 weeks. For inclusion criteria, hypomagnesemia was defined as serum magnesium levels < 1.8 mg/dL and depression by Yasavage and Brink score > or = 11 points; astute readers should appreciate that serum magnesium is reasonably specific but is not sensitive for magnesium deficiency. Results included the following, "At end of follow-up, there were no significant differences in the Yasavage and Brink score (11.4 +/- 3.8 and 10.9 +/- 4.3, p = 0.27) between the groups in study; whereas serum magnesium levels were significantly higher in the group with MgCl2 (2.1 +/- 0.08 mg/dL) than in the subjects with imipramine (1.5 +/- 0.07 mg/dL), p < 0.0005. **In conclusion, MgCl2 is as effective in the treatment of depressed elderly type 2 diabetics with hypomagnesemia as imipramine 50 mg daily.**" In the end, this turned out to be a remarkable study showing not only safety of oral magnesium 450 mg per day, but more importantly that magnesium is as effective as a commonly used but somewhat dangerous tricyclic antidepressant; given that the probably of *magnesium deficiency* in elderly DM-2 patients is higher than the probability of *imipramine deficiency* in these patients, correcting the underlying nutritional deficiency by the use of oral magnesium supplementation is more logical than using a tricyclic antidepressant with its numerous and serious adverse effects. Further, Mg benefits insulin sensitivity, blood pressure and other aspects of DM-2 which are not beneficially impacted by the more expensive and dangerous imipramine.

- 3-month randomized double-blind placebo-controlled trial: Oral magnesium supplementation improves insulin sensitivity in non-diabetic subjects with insulin resistance (*Diabetes Metab* 2004 Jun[414]): In this study, the researchers used oral magnesium chloride (MgCl2) 2.5 g daily in "apparently healthy" non-diabetic subjects with insulin resistance (HOMA-IR index equal or greater than 3.0) and hypomagnesemia (serum magnesium levels equal or lower than 0.74 mmol/l). Subjects were randomized to receive either, MgCl2 2.5 g daily or placebo by 3-months. "RESULTS: At baseline there were not significant anthropometric or laboratory differences between both groups. At ending of the study, magnesium-supplemented subjects significantly increased their serum magnesium levels (0.61 +/- 0.08 to 0.81 +/- 0.08 mmol/l, p<0.0001) and reduced HOMA-IR index (4.6 +/- 2.8 to 2.6 +/- 1.1, p<0.0001), whereas control subjects did not (0.62 +/- 0.08 to 0.61 +/- 0.08 mmol/l, p=0.063 and 5.2 +/- 1.9 to 5.3 +/- 2.9, p=0.087). **CONCLUSIONS: Oral magnesium supplementation improves insulin sensitivity in hypomagnesemic non-diabetic subjects.**"

- **Fatty acid supplementation with ALA (from flaxseed oil), GLA (from borage oil), EPA and DHA (from fish oil)—alone or in combination:** Fish oil supplementation is the single most effective intervention for the prevention of cardiovascular disease that has ever been consistently documented. Fish oil supplementation beneficially affects many of the physiologic phenomena that are involved in cardiovascular health and disease, including platelet adhesion, endothelial function, inflammation, serum lipids, insulin sensitivity, and mental depression; furthermore, natural-source fish oil such as cod liver oil is a notable source of cardioprotective vitamin D3, which is pandemically deficient in nearly all populations. For healthcare providers of all disciplines and pedigrees, the evidence is so strong in favor of the routine use of fish oil that—if the standards of care in healthcare truly included beneficence and nonmalfecense—failure to utilize fish oil in all patients and particularly in patients at increased risk for cardiovascular disease should be considered negligent malpractice. No other single treatment—nutritional or pharmacologic—offers the numerous benefits that fish oil

[413] Barragán-Rodríguez et al. Efficacy and safety of oral magnesium supplementation in treatment of depression in the elderly with type 2 diabetes. *Magnes Res.* 2008 Dec:218-23
[414] Guerrero-Romero et al. Oral magnesium supplementation improves insulin sensitivity in non-diabetic subjects with insulin resistance. *Diabetes Metab.* 2004 Jun;30(3):253-8

supplementation provides. Because fatty acids work in combination and synergy with other fatty acids, and because most patients have numerous fatty acid imbalances and deficiencies, fatty acid supplementation should be administered as combination fatty acid therapy that provides—at minimum—the EPA and DHA of fish oil in combination with the GLA sourced from either borage oil (most concentrated source), evening primrose oil (perhaps the best biochemical form of GLA), black currant seed oil, or hemp oil. In an earlier review[415] of this topic, I summarized the benefits of fatty acid supplementation as follows:

- ☑ N-3 alpha-linolenic acid (ALA): Increased intake of ALA appears to provide cardioprotective[416] and anti-inflammatory benefits[417,418], and ALA can help reduce the frequency and severity of migraine headaches when used as part of a comprehensive natural treatment plan that includes GLA, multivitamins, and dietary modification.[419]

- ☑ Eicosapentaenoic acid (EPA): EPA used in isolation shows benefit in lupus,[420] cancer[421], borderline personality disorder[422], mental depression[423,424,425], schizophrenia[426], and osteoporosis (when used with GLA).[427]

- ☑ Docosahexaenoic acid (DHA): Supplementation with DHA (often in the form of fish oil, which includes EPA) has been shown to benefit patients with bipolar disorder[428], Crohn's disease[429], rheumatoid arthritis[430,431,432], lupus[433], cardiovascular disease[434], psoriasis[435], and cancer.[436] DHA appears to have an "anti-stress" benefit manifested by 30% reductions in norepinephrine and improved resilience to psychoemotional stress.[437,438]

- ☑ Supplementation with EPA+DHA: This combination, naturally found in fish oil, is extremely safe and reduces all-cause mortality. [439]

- ☑ Gamma-linolenic acid (GLA): Clinical benefit associated with GLA supplementation is seen in patients with, eczema[440], breast cancer (when used with tamoxifen[441]), premenstrual syndrome[442], rheumatoid arthritis[443,444], diabetic neuropathy[445], migraine headaches (when used with ALA[446]), and respiratory distress

---

[415] Vasquez A. New Insights into Fatty Acid Supplementation and Its Effect on Eicosanoid Production and Genetic Expression. *Nutritional Perspectives* 2005; January: 5-16
[416] Hu et al. Dietary intake of alpha-linolenic acid and risk of fatal ischemic heart disease among women. *Am J Clin Nutr*. 1999 May;69(5):890-7
[417] "CONCLUSIONS: Dietary supplementation with ALA for 3 months decreases significantly CRP, SAA and IL-6 levels in dyslipidaemic patients. This anti-inflammatory effect may provide a possible additional mechanism for the beneficial effect of plant n-3 polyunsaturated fatty acids in primary and secondary prevention of coronary artery disease." Rallidis et al. Dietary alpha-linolenic acid decreases C-reactive protein, serum amyloid A and interleukin-6 in dyslipidaemic patients. *Atherosclerosis*. 2003 Apr;167(2):237-42
[418] Adam O, Wolfram G, Zollner N. Effect of alpha-linolenic acid in the human diet on linoleic acid metabolism and prostaglandin biosynthesis. *J Lipid Res*. 1986 Apr;27(4):421-6
[419] Wagner W, Nootbaar-Wagner U. Prophylactic treatment of migraine with gamma-linolenic and alpha-linolenic acids. *Cephalalgia*. 1997 Apr;17(2):127-30
[420] Duffy et al. The clinical effect of dietary supplementation with omega-3 fish oils and/or copper in systemic lupus erythematosus. *J Rheumatol*. 2004 Aug;31(8):1551-6
[421] Wigmore SJ, Barber MD, Ross JA, Tisdale MJ, Fearon KC. Effect of oral eicosapentaenoic acid on weight loss in patients with pancreatic cancer. *Nutr Cancer*. 2000;36:177-84
[422] Zanarini MC, Frankenburg FR. omega-3 Fatty acid treatment of women with borderline personality disorder. *Am J Psychiatry*. 2003 Jan;160(1):167-9
[423] Nemets et al. Addition of omega-3 fatty acid to maintenance medication treatment for recurrent unipolar depressive disorder. *Am J Psychiatry*. 2002 Mar;159(3):477-9
[424] Puri BK, Counsell SJ, Hamilton G, Richardson AJ, Horrobin DF. Eicosapentaenoic acid in treatment-resistant depression associated with symptom remission, structural brain changes and reduced neuronal phospholipid turnover. *Int J Clin Pract*. 2001 Oct;55(8):560-3
[425] Peet M, Horrobin DF. A dose-ranging study of the effects of ethyl-eicosapentaenoate in patients with ongoing depression despite apparently adequate treatment with standard drugs. *Arch Gen Psychiatry*. 2002 Oct;59(10):913-9
[426] Emsley et al. Randomized, placebo-controlled study of ethyl-eicosapentaenoic acid as supplemental treatment in schizophrenia. *Am J Psychiatry*. 2002 Sep;159(9):1596-8
[427] Kruger et al. Calcium, gamma-linolenic acid and eicosapentaenoic acid supplementation in senile osteoporosis. *Aging* (Milano). 1998 Oct;10(5):385-94
[428] Stoll et al. Omega 3 fatty acids in bipolar disorder: a preliminary double-blind, placebo-controlled trial. *Arch Gen Psychiatry*. 1999 May;56(5):407-12
[429] Belluzzi et al. Effect of an enteric-coated fish-oil preparation on relapses in Crohn's disease. *N Engl J Med*. 1996 Jun 13;334(24):1557-60
[430] Adam et al. Anti-inflammatory effects of a low arachidonic acid diet and fish oil in patients with rheumatoid arthritis. *Rheumatol Int*. 2003 Jan;23(1):27-36
[431] Lau et al. Effects of fish oil supplementation on non-steroidal anti-inflammatory drug requirement in patients with mild rheumatoid arthritis. *Br J Rheumatol*. 1993 Nov:982-9
[432] Kremer et al. Fish-oil fatty acid supplementation in active rheumatoid arthritis. A double-blinded, controlled, crossover study. *Ann Intern Med*. 1987 Apr;106(4):497-503
[433] Walton et al. Dietary fish oil and the severity of symptoms in patients with systemic lupus erythematosus. *Ann Rheum Dis*. 1991 Jul;50(7):463-6
[434] "The recent GISSI (Gruppo Italiano per lo Studio della Sopravvivenza nell'Infarto miocardico)-Prevention study of 11,324 patients showed a 45% decrease in risk of sudden cardiac death and a 20% reduction in all-cause mortality in the group taking 850 mg/d of omega-3 fatty acids." O'Keefe JH Jr, Harris WS. From Inuit to implementation: omega-3 fatty acids come of age. *Mayo Clin Proc*. 2000 Jun;75(6):607-14
[435] Bittiner SB, Tucker WF, Cartwright I, Bleehen SS. A double-blind, randomised, placebo-controlled trial of fish oil in psoriasis. *Lancet*. 1988 Feb 20;1(8582):378-80
[436] Gogos et al. Dietary omega-3 polyunsaturated fatty acids plus vitamin E restore immunodeficiency and prolong survival for severely ill patients with generalized malignancy. *Cancer*. 1998 Jan 15;82(2):395-402
[437] Hamazaki T, Itomura M, Sawazaki S, Nagao Y. Anti-stress effects of DHA. *Biofactors*. 2000;13(1-4):41-5
[438] Sawazaki S, Hamazaki T, Yazawa K, Kobayashi M. The effect of docosahexaenoic acid on plasma catecholamine concentrations and glucose tolerance during long-lasting psychological stress: a double-blind placebo-controlled study. *J Nutr Sci Vitaminol* (Tokyo). 1999 Oct;45(5):655-65
[439] "The recent GISSI (Gruppo Italiano per lo Studio della Sopravvivenza nell'Infarto miocardico)-Prevention study of 11,324 patients showed a 45% decrease in risk of sudden cardiac death and a 20% reduction in all-cause mortality in the group taking 850 mg/d of omega-3 fatty acids." O'Keefe JH Jr, Harris WS. From Inuit to implementation: omega-3 fatty acids come of age. *Mayo Clin Proc*. 2000 Jun;75(6):607-14
[440] Fiocchi et al. The efficacy and safety of gamma-linolenic acid in the treatment of infantile atopic dermatitis. *J Int Med Res*. 1994 Jan-Feb;22(1):24-32
[441] Kenny et al. Gamma linolenic acid with tamoxifen as primary therapy in breast cancer. *Int J Cancer*. 2000 Mar 1;85(5):643-8
[442] Puolakka et al. Biochemical and clinical effects of treating the premenstrual syndrome with prostaglandin synthesis precursors. *J Reprod Med*. 1985 Mar;30(3):149-53
[443] Brzeski et al. Evening primrose oil in patients with rheumatoid arthritis and side-effects of non-steroidal anti-inflammatory drugs. *Br J Rheumatol*. 1991 Oct;30(5):370-2
[444] Rothman D, DeLuca P, Zurier RB. Botanical lipids: effects on inflammation, immune responses, and rheumatoid arthritis. *Semin Arthritis Rheum*. 1995 Oct;25(2):87-96
[445] Jamal GA, Carmichael H. The effect of gamma-linolenic acid on human diabetic peripheral neuropathy. *Diabet Med*. 1990 May;7(4):319-23
[446] Wagner W, Nootbaar-Wagner U. Prophylactic treatment of migraine with gamma-linolenic and alpha-linolenic acids. *Cephalalgia*. 1997 Apr;17(2):127-30

syndrome (when used with EPA).[447] As discussed and detailed in Chapter 4, the major "biochemical risk" from using GLA is that of raising arachidonic acid levels if delta-5-desaturase is not inhibited by concomitant administration of EPA; the major "clinical risk" associated with GLA administration is that of inducing or exacerbating temporal lobe epilepsy, as noted in a few case reports and case series.

Insofar as research and statistical analyses are concerned, we have to appreciate that many of these fatty acid supplementation studies were performed by researchers who thought that olive oil was an inert placebo; no clinician or researcher in his/her right mind would make such a blunder these days—or so we might hope. The olive oil "placebo" is one of the most potent anti-inflammatory and cardioprotective interventions available; olive oil contains numerous substances with anti-cancer, cardioprotective, and anti-inflammatory benefits, including n-9 oleic acid, squalene, and the numerous polyphenolic phytonutrients. Because many of the earlier "fish oil studies" used olive oil as their control group, important benefits of fish oil were underestimated and underappreciated and thus underutilized because the "control group" (i.e., olive oil supplementation) and "treatment group" (i.e., fish oil supplementation) were both being treated with a potent anti-cancer, cardioprotective, and anti-inflammatory intervention.

- Clinical trial with very-low-dose fish oil: Effect of omega-3 fatty acids on cardiovascular risk factors in patients with type 2 diabetes mellitus and hypertriglyceridemia: an open study (*Eur Rev Med Pharmacol Sci* 2009 Jan[448]): In this group of **30 patients** with type-2 diabetes mellitus and hypertriglyceridemia, patients received two capsules of **eicosapentaenoic 465 mg and docosahexaenoic 375 mg daily** for 12 weeks. "RESULTS: Triglycerides levels and non HDL-cholesterol decreased (326 vs. 216.4 mg/dl) and (103.87 vs. 89.6 mg/dl), respectively. HDL-cholesterol levels increased (39.6 vs. 46.4 mg/dl). C-reactive protein decreased (5.98 vs. 3.9 mg/dl) and TNF-alpha levels decreased (16.24 vs. 13.3 pg/dl), without significant changes in IL-6 levels. **In conclusion, an n-3 polyunsaturated intervention improved lipid profile and inflammatory markers in patients with diabetes mellitus type 2 and hypertriglyceridemia.**" The results of this study are remarkable insofar as the dose of fish oil used was very low; generally in clinical practice we use at least 1,000 and often up to 3,000 mg per day of combined EPA and DHA; this study used only 840 mg.

- 8-week, randomized, double-blind, placebo-controlled study: Efficacy and tolerability of adding prescription omega-3 fatty acids 4 g/d to simvastatin 40 mg/d in hypertriglyceridemic patients (*Clin Ther* 2007 Jul[449]): "This study evaluated the effects on non-HDL-C and other variables of adding prescription omega-3-acid **ethyl esters** (P-OM3; Lovaza, formerly Omacor [Reliant Pharmaceuticals, Inc., Liberty Corner, New Jersey]) to stable statin therapy in patients with persistent hypertriglyceridemia. METHODS: This was a multicenter, randomized, double-blind, placebo-controlled, parallel-group study in adults who had received > or = 8 weeks of stable statin therapy and had mean fasting TG levels > or = 200 and < 500 mg/dL and mean low-density lipoprotein cholesterol levels < or = 10% above their NCEP ATP III goal. The study regimen consisted of an initial 8 weeks of open-label simvastatin 40 mg/d and dietary counseling, followed by 8 weeks of randomized treatment with double-blind P-OM3 4 g/d plus simvastatin 40 mg/d or placebo plus simvastatin 40 mg/d. The main outcome measure was the percent change in non-HDL-C from baseline to the end of treatment. RESULTS: The evaluable population included 254 patients, of whom 57.5% (146) were male and 95.7% (243) were white. The mean (SD) age of the population was 59.8 (10.4) years, and the mean weight was 92.0 (19.6) kg. At the end of treatment, the median percent change in non-HDL-C was significantly greater with P-OM3 plus simvastatin compared with placebo plus simvastatin (-9.0% vs -2.2%, respectively; P < 0.001). P-OM3 plus simvastatin was associated with **significant reductions in TG** (29.5% vs 6.3%) **and very-low-density lipoprotein cholesterol** (27.5% vs 7.2%), **a significant increase in high-density lipoprotein cholesterol (HDL-C) (3.4%** vs -1.2%), and a significant reduction in the total cholesterol:HDL-C ratio (9.6% vs 0.7%) (all, P < 0.001 vs placebo). Adverse events (AEs) reported by > or= 1% of patients in the P-OM3 group that occurred with a higher frequency than in the group that received simvastatin alone were nasopharyngitis (4 [3.3%]), upper respiratory tract infection (4 [3.3%]), diarrhea (3 [2.5%]), and dyspepsia (3 [2.5%]). There was no significant difference in the frequency of AEs [adverse

[447] Pacht ER, DeMichele SJ, Nelson JL, Hart J, Wennberg AK, Gadek JE. Enteral nutrition with eicosapentaenoic acid, gamma-linolenic acid, and antioxidants reduces alveolar inflammatory mediators and protein influx in patients with acute respiratory distress syndrome. *Crit Care Med.* 2003 Feb;31(2):491-500
[448] De Luis et al. Omega-3 fatty acids on cardiovascular risk factors in patients with type 2 diabetes mellitus and hypertriglyceridemia. *Eur Rev Med Pharmacol Sci.* 2009 Jan:51-5
[449] Davidson et al. Efficacy and tolerability of adding prescription omega-3 fatty acids 4 g/d to simvastatin 40 mg/d in hypertriglyceridemic patients. *Clin Ther.* 2007 Jul:1354-67

events] between groups. No serious AEs were considered treatment related. CONCLUSION: In these adult, mainly white patients with persistent hypertriglyceridemia, P-OM3 plus simvastatin and dietary counseling improved non-HDL-C and other lipid and lipoprotein parameters to a greater extent than simvastatin alone." Although this study was of short duration, the sample size is reasonably large (n=254) and the results are consistent with what we would have expected, namely that adding EPA+DHA supplementation would provide laboratory evidence of cardioprotection. Each 1-gram LOVAZA capsule contains 465 mg of eicosapentaenoic acid (EPA) and 375 mg of docosahexaenoic acid (DHA). Ethyl esters are the synthetic distillation product made by processing fish oil with ethanol; controversy exists about the bioavailability and biological nuances between natural fish oils with a glycerol backbone versus these semi-synthetic fish oils with an ethanol backbone.

- Meta-analysis of n-3 fatty acid supplementation in patients with DM-2: Meta-analysis of the effects of n-3 polyunsaturated fatty acids on lipoproteins and other emerging lipid cardiovascular risk markers in patients with type 2 diabetes (*Diabetologia* 2007 Aug[450]): "RESULTS: There were 23 trials on non-dietary supplementation, involving 1,075 subjects with a mean treatment duration of 8.9 weeks, with sufficient data to permit pooling. Compared with placebo, n-3 PUFA had a statistically significant effect on four outcomes, **reducing levels of (1) triacylglycerol** (18 trials, 969 subjects) by **25%**; (2) **VLDL-cholesterol** (7 trials, 238 subjects) **by 36%**; and (3) VLDL-triacylglycerol (6 trials, 178 subjects) by 39.7%; while *slightly increasing LDL* (16 trials, 565 subjects) *by 5.7%*. There were no significant effects on total cholesterol, apolipoproteins, lipid subfractions or ratios. CONCLUSIONS/INTERPRETATION: In addition to recognized triacylglycerol-lowering effects, n-3 PUFA supplementation decreases VLDL-cholesterol and VLDL-triacylglycerol, but may have an adverse effect on LDL-cholesterol. Larger and longer term clinical trials are required to conclusively establish the effect of n-3 PUFA on cardiovascular risk markers and outcomes in type 2 diabetic patients." Basically, this information reviewed the biochemical effects (rather than the clinical outcomes) of n-3 fatty acid supplementation. The fact that, per this meta-analysis, n-3 fatty acid supplementation increased LDL by 5.7% is a trend in the wrong direction, since LDL is the major target of serum lipid optimization. However, the fact that all meta-analyses that have focused on *clinical outcomes* have concluded that n-3 fatty acid supplementation reduces overall mortality (even to a greater degree than do to the highly touted and heavily advertised statin drugs) implies that clinicians should use n-3 fatty acids even at the biochemical expense of slightly elevated LDL. Furthermore, the trial by Laidlaw and Holub[451] showed that by combining n-3 fatty acids with GLA, the LDL level could be lowered by more than 11%; thus the findings from these two studies suggests that while n-3 fatty acid supplementation shows overall cardiovascular benefits at the expense of a slight increase in LDL, this biochemical adverse effect is offset by more powerful reductions in overall and cardiovascular mortality, and that even the biochemical adverse effect of raising LDL by 5% can be mitigated by combining with GLA for a total reduction in LDL of 11%. The addition of GLA would do more than lower LDL levels; it would cause additive or synergistic improvements in overall health status, given that GLA helps in a variety of clinical scenarios, such as psoriasis, eczema, and inflammatory joint pain such as rheumatoid arthritis.

- Systematic review: Effect of different antilipidemic agents and diets on mortality (*Arch Intern Med* 2005 Apr[452]): "RESULTS: A total of 97 studies met eligibility criteria, with 137,140 individuals in intervention and 138,976 individuals in control groups. Compared with control groups, **risk ratios for overall mortality** were **0.87 for statins** (95% confidence interval [CI], 0.81-0.94), **1.00 for fibrates** (95% CI, 0.91-1.11), **0.84 for resins** (95% CI, 0.66-1.08), **0.96 for niacin** (95% CI, 0.86-1.08), **0.77 for n-3 fatty acids** (95% CI, 0.63-0.94), and 0.97 for diet (95% CI, 0.91-1.04). Compared with control groups, **risk ratios for cardiac mortality** indicated benefit from statins (0.78; 95% CI, 0.72-0.84), resins (0.70; 95% CI, 0.50-0.99) and n-3 fatty acids (0.68; 95% CI, 0.52-0.90). Risk ratios for noncardiovascular mortality of any intervention indicated no association when compared with control groups, with the exception of fibrates (risk ratio, 1.13; 95% CI, 1.01-1.27).

[450] Hartweg et al. Meta-analysis of the effects of n-3 polyunsaturated fatty acids on lipoproteins and other emerging lipid cardiovascular risk markers in patients with type 2 diabetes. *Diabetologia*. 2007 Aug;50(8):1593-602
[451] Laidlaw M, Holub BJ. Effects of supplementation with fish oil-derived n-3 fatty acids and gamma-linolenic acid on circulating plasma lipids and fatty acid profiles in women. *Am J Clin Nutr*. 2003 Jan;77(1):37-42
[452] Studer et al. Effect of different antilipidemic agents and diets on mortality: a systematic review. *Arch Intern Med*. 2005 Apr 11;165(7):725-30

CONCLUSIONS: Statins and n-3 fatty acids are the most favorable lipid-lowering interventions with reduced risks of overall and cardiac mortality. Any potential reduction in cardiac mortality from fibrates is offset by an increased risk of death from noncardiovascular causes." This systematic review found that n-3 fatty acids are superior to statin drugs (and all other cholesterol-lowering cardiovascular drugs) for reducing total mortality and cardiac mortality. Clinically significant side-effects of statin drugs commonly include muscle pain and chemical hepatitis, while side effects of n-3 fatty acids such as fish oil commonly include improved mood and alleviation of depression, schizophrenia, bipolar disorder, borderline personality disorder, eczema, psoriasis, and back pain and joint pain. Even at internet prices, generic atorvastatin (same as Lipitor) at 20 mg per day for one month costs about $34 (plus fees for the office visit and follow-up laboratory and clinical monitoring), whereas one teaspoon of cod liver oil (to provide approximately 1 gram of EPA+DHA) per day for one month costs about $8 (without additional medical expenses, plus cost savings from alleviation from other conditions).

- Extrapolation of short-term effect of various fatty acid ratios on long-term cardiovascular risk: Effects of supplementation with fish oil-derived n-3 fatty acids and gamma-linolenic acid on circulating plasma lipids and fatty acid profiles in women (*Am J Clin Nutr* 2003 Jan[453]): This important study used computerized models to determine long-term cardiovascular risk based on alterations in serum lipids effected by combination fatty acid supplementation with various ratios of EPA+DHA to GLA. "DESIGN: Thirty-one women were assigned to 1 of 4 groups, equalized on the basis of their fasting triacylglycerol concentrations. They received supplements providing 4 g EPA+DHA (4:0, EPA+DHA:GLA; control group), 4 g EPA+DHA plus 1 g GLA (4:1), 2 g GLA (4:2), or 4 g GLA (4:4) daily for 28 d. Plasma lipids and fatty acids of serum phospholipids were measured on days 0 and 28. RESULTS: Plasma triacylglycerol concentrations were significantly lower on day 28 than on day 0 in the 4:0, 4:1, and 4:2 groups. **LDL cholesterol decreased significantly (by 11.3%) in the 4:2 group.** Dihomo-gamma-linolenic acid increased significantly in serum phospholipids only in the 4:2 and 4:4 groups; however, total n-3 fatty acids increased in all 4 groups. CONCLUSIONS: A mixture of **4 g EPA+DHA and 2 g GLA** favorably altered blood lipid and fatty acid profiles in healthy women. On the basis of calculated PROCAM values, the **4:2 group was estimated to have a 43% reduction in the 10-y risk of myocardial infarction**." This research shows that combination fatty acid therapy with EPA+DHA+GLA is better than EPA+DHA alone and that a 4g:2g ratio-amount is optimal. Obviously, this is an extrapolated computer model and not a long-term prospective trial, but the acute reduction in LDL of 11% is very promising; the collateral health benefits of combined EPA+DHA+GLA would be enormous if applied as widely as are the statin drugs.

- **Chromium**: Chromium has long been used in disorders of glucose metabolism: both hypoglycemia and hyperglycemia. The problem with the *medical research* in this regard is that it has generally been consistent with the *medical model* of disease, namely: the constant search for the silver bullet that can alleviate disease, without proper consideration to the use of several nutrients together, along with dietary change, and exercise and physical medicine to more accurately reflect the interventions used by integrative chiropractic and naturopathic clinicians. While we must appreciate the earlier single-intervention studies for their preliminary attempts at determining safety and efficacy of nutritional interventions, we must also appreciate what the culmination of this research has consistently shown, namely that nutrients work together synergistically and that a moderate dose of several nutrients is generally safer and more efficacious than a single dose of one nutrient, and that key metabolic pathways must be affected if clinical benefit is to be shown. Nutrients with numerous overlapping functions (especially fish oil and vitamin D) are massively more effective than single nutrients that work on only a fraction of an isolated pathway (such as chromium in the treatment of DM); simultaneously and perhaps conversely, each nutrient is necessary for optimal metabolic and immunologic function.

  - Short-term (4 weeks) placebo-controlled, double-blinded, randomized trial of chromium+biotin: The effect of chromium picolinate and biotin supplementation on glycemic control in poorly controlled patients with type 2 diabetes mellitus (*Diabetes Technol Ther* 2006 Dec[454]): Experimental studies have shown that

---

[453] Laidlaw M, Holub BJ. Effects of supplementation with fish oil-derived n-3 fatty acids and gamma-linolenic acid on circulating plasma lipids and fatty acid profiles in women. *Am J Clin Nutr.* 2003 Jan;77(1):37-42
[454] Singer et al. Effect of chromium picolinate and biotin supplementation on glycemic control in poorly controlled patients with type 2 diabetes mellitus. *Diabetes Technol Ther.* 2006 Dec;8(6):636-43

chromium picolinate together with biotin significantly enhances glucose uptake in skeletal muscle cells. This pilot study was conducted among 43 patients with DM-2 with poor glycemic control (Hgb-A1c > 7%) despite use of oral antihyperglycemic drugs. Study subjects were administered chromium 600 mcg/d (as chromium picolinate) and biotin 2 mg per day; antihyperglycemic drugs were continued during the study. "RESULTS: After 4 weeks, there was a **significantly greater reduction in the total area under the curve for glucose during the 2-h oral glucose tolerance test for the treatment group** (mean change -9.7%) compared with the placebo group (mean change +5.1%). **Significantly greater reductions were also seen in fructosamine** (P < 0.03), **triglycerides** (P < 0.02), and **triglycerides/ high-density lipoprotein cholesterol ratio** (P < 0.05) **in the treatment group**. No significant adverse events were attributed to chromium picolinate and biotin supplementation. CONCLUSIONS: … Chromium picolinate/ biotin supplementation may represent an effective adjunctive nutritional therapy to people with poorly controlled diabetes with the potential for improving lipid metabolism."

- Pilot study (n=8) of chromium in medicated HIV patients with insulin resistance: Chromium picolinate for insulin resistance in subjects with HIV disease: a pilot study (*Diabetes Obes Metab* 2008 Feb[455]): Because multidrug regimens for HIV treatment are associated with an increased incidence of insulin resistance (as much as 50%), the authors of this study used chromium picolinate (1000 mcg/day) to improve insulin sensitivity, determined with a hyperinsulinaemic-euglycaemic insulin clamp, was determined in eight HIV-positive subjects on highly active antiretroviral therapy (HAART). "RESULTS: The mean **rate of glucose disposal** during the clamp was 4.41 mg glucose/kg lean body mass (LBM)/min (range 2.67-5.50), which increased to 6.51 mg/kg LBM/min (range 3.19-12.78, p = .03), an **increase of 25% after 8 weeks of treatment with chromium picolinate**. There were no significant changes in blood parameters, HIV viral burden or CD4+ lymphocytes with chromium picolinate treatment. Two subjects experienced abnormalities of liver function during the study.

> **Chromium (picolinate) can modulate appetite in depressed overweight patients who crave carbohydrates**
>
> "While these findings require replication in a prospective trial, they suggest that CrPic may be beneficial for patients with atypical depression who are also high carbohydrate cravers."
>
> Docherty et al. A double-blind, placebo-controlled, exploratory trial of chromium picolinate in atypical depression: effect on carbohydrate craving. *J Psychiatr Pract*. 2005 Sep

Another subject experienced an elevation in blood urea nitrogen. CONCLUSIONS: The study shows that **chromium picolinate therapy improves insulin resistance in some HIV-positive subjects, but with some concerns about safety in this population.**" These findings are of interest for several reasons: ❶ While the dose used in this study is higher than what has been used in most studies (generally 200 mcg), the 1,000 mcg dose is consistent with what clinicians might use in clinical practice. ❷ These results, even though based on a very small number of patients, suggests that clinicians should use a smaller dose or use careful patient selection or frequent laboratory surveillance when using high-dose chromium in patients with HIV who are taking HAART. ❸ The lack of placebo/control group makes impossible the attribution of adverse effects to chromium, but nonetheless, clinicians should use caution when using high-dose chromium in this patient population based on these results.

- Double-blind, placebo-controlled, multicenter, 8-week replication study: Chromium picolinate in overweight patients with atypical depression: effect on carbohydrate craving (*J Psychiatr Pract* 2005 Sep[456]): The authors report that in a pre-publication small pilot trial, patients with atypical depression demonstrated significant positive therapeutic response to chromium picolinate. These 113 overweight (average BMI = 29.7) adult outpatients with atypical depression were randomized 2:1 to receive chromium 600 mcg/d (as chromium picolinate (CrPic)) or placebo. Patients were assessed with the 29-item Hamilton Depression Rating Scale (HAM-D-29) and the Clinical Global Impressions Improvement Scale (CGI-I). "RESULTS: … There was no significant difference between the CrPic and placebo groups in both the ITT [intention to treat] and evaluable populations on the primary efficacy measures, with both groups showing significant improvement from baseline on total HAM-D-29 scores during the course of treatment (p < 0.0001). However, in the evaluable population, **the CrPic group showed significant improvements from**

---

[455] Feiner et al. Chromium picolinate for insulin resistance in subjects with HIV disease: a pilot study. *Diabetes Obes Metab*. 2008 Feb;10(2):151-8
[456] Docherty et al. A trial of chromium picolinate in atypical depression: effect on carbohydrate craving. *J Psychiatr Pract*. 2005 Sep;11(5):302-14

baseline compared with the placebo group on 4 HAM-D-29 items: appetite increase, increased eating, carbohydrate craving, and diurnal variation of feelings. A supplemental analysis of data from the subset of 41 patients in the ITT population with high carbohydrate craving (26 CrPic, 15 placebo; mean BMI = 31.1) showed that **the CrPic patients had significantly greater response on total HAM-D-29 scores** than the placebo group (65% vs. 33%; p < 0.05) as well as **significantly greater improvements on the following HAM-D-29 items: appetite increase, increased eating, carbohydrate craving, and genital symptoms (e.g., level of libido)**. Chromium treatment was well-tolerated. CONCLUSIONS: In a population of adults with atypical depression, most of whom were overweight or obese, CrPic produced improvement on the following HAM-D-29 items: appetite increase, increased eating, carbohydrate craving, and diurnal variation of feelings. In a subpopulation of patients with high carbohydrate craving, overall HAM-D-29 scores improved significantly in patients treated with CrPic compared with placebo. **The results of this study suggest that the main effect of chromium was on carbohydrate craving and appetite regulation in depressed patients and that 600 mcg of elemental chromium may be beneficial for patients with atypical depression who also have severe carbohydrate craving.** Further studies are needed to evaluate chromium in depressed patients specifically selected for symptoms of increased appetite and carbohydrate craving as well as to determine whether a higher dose of chromium would have an effect on mood." Interpretation of this study may be a little confusing to clinicians unfamiliar with the clinical spectrum of depression, especially when combined with an overweight BMI. On the one hand, we would like to see overweight depressed patients eat less if we are more focused on their weight; on the other hand, since lack of appetite is one of the defining characteristics of depression, the fact that some of these patients actually began to eat more can be interpreted as a reflection of an antidepressant effect. Further the observation that patients with severe carbohydrate craving actually began to eat less shows that, overall, chromium supplementation in depressed+overweight patients might be expected to have a homeostatic effect: following chromium supplementation, patients with anorexia begin to eat more, while patients with food cravings begin to eat less.

- ▪ Review: Chromium and polyphenols from cinnamon improve insulin sensitivity (*Proc Nutr Soc* 2008 Feb[457]): "The signs of Cr deficiency are similar to those for the metabolic syndrome and supplemental Cr has been shown to improve all these signs in human subjects. In a double-blind placebo-controlled study it has been demonstrated that glucose, insulin, cholesterol and HbA1c are all improved in patients with type 2 diabetes following Cr supplementation."

- **Cinnamon**: Cinnamon supplementation/consumption has shown benefit in the treatment of DM.
  - ▪ Small placebo-controlled study of the impact of cinnamon on glycemic control in healthy patients: Changes in glucose tolerance and insulin sensitivity following 2 weeks of daily cinnamon ingestion in healthy humans (*Eur J Appl Physiol* 2009 Apr[458]): Eight male volunteers underwent two 14-day interventions involving cinnamon 3g/d or placebo supplementation. "Oral glucose tolerance tests (OGTT) were performed on days 0, 1, 14, 16, 18, and 20. Cinnamon ingestion reduced the glucose response to OGTT on day 1 (-13.1 +/- 6.3% vs. day 0; P < 0.05) and day 14 (-5.5 +/- 8.1% vs. day 0; P = 0.09). Cinnamon ingestion also reduced insulin responses to OGTT on day 14 (-27.1 +/- 6.2% vs. day 0; P < 0.05), as well as improving insulin sensitivity on day 14 (vs. day 0; P < 0.05)." This small study shows that orally administered cinnamon 3g/d improves the response of OGTT in healthy humans.
  - ▪ Review: Chromium and polyphenols from cinnamon improve insulin sensitivity (*Proc Nutr Soc* 2008 Feb[459]): "It has also been shown that cinnamon polyphenols improve insulin sensitivity in in vitro, animal and human studies. Cinnamon reduces mean fasting serum glucose (18-29%), TAG (23-30%), total cholesterol (12-26%) and LDL-cholesterol (7-27%) in subjects with type 2 diabetes after 40 d of daily consumption of 1-6 g cinnamon. Subjects with the metabolic syndrome who consume an aqueous extract of cinnamon have been shown to have improved fasting blood glucose, systolic blood pressure, percentage body fat and increased lean body mass compared with the placebo group. Studies utilizing an aqueous extract of cinnamon, high in type A polyphenols, have also demonstrated improvements in fasting glucose, glucose

---

[457] Anderson RA. Chromium and polyphenols from cinnamon improve insulin sensitivity. *Proc Nutr Soc.* 2008 Feb;67(1):48-53
[458] Solomon et al. Glucose tolerance and insulin sensitivity following 2 weeks of daily cinnamon ingestion in healthy humans. *Eur J Appl Physiol.* 2009 Apr;105(6):969-76
[459] Anderson RA. Chromium and polyphenols from cinnamon improve insulin sensitivity. *Proc Nutr Soc.* 2008 Feb;67(1):48-53

tolerance and insulin sensitivity in women with insulin resistance associated with the polycystic ovary syndrome."

- **Systematic review of the safety and efficacy of common and cassia cinnamon bark: From type 2 diabetes to antioxidant activity** (*Can J Physiol Pharmacol* 2007 Sep[460]): Common cinnamon (*Cinnamomum verum, C. zeylanicum*) and cassia cinnamon (*C. aromaticum*) are well known for their centuries-old use as spices and flavoring agents. Regarding cinnamon's applications in DM-2, "Two of 3 randomized clinical trials on type 2 diabetes provided strong scientific evidence that cassia cinnamon demonstrates a therapeutic effect in reducing fasting blood glucose by 10.3%-29%; the third clinical trial did not observe this effect. Cassia cinnamon, however, did not have an effect at lowering glycosylated hemoglobin (HbA1c). One randomized clinical trial reported that cassia cinnamon lowered total cholesterol, low-density lipoprotein cholesterol, and triglycerides; the other 2 trials, however, did not observe this effect."

- **Vanadium**: Vanadium is probably the most controversial nutrient purported to have benefit in the treatment of DM. At current, the lack of documented benefit and the narrow therapeutic window precludes its routine clinical utilization.

  - **Systematic review: Vanadium oral supplements for glycemic control in type 2 diabetes mellitus** (*QJM* 2008 May[461]): Using reasonable criteria for study inclusion (controlled human trials of vanadium vs. placebo in adults with type 2 diabetes of minimum 2 months duration, and a minimum of 10 subjects per arm) the authors found 151 studies, but none met the inclusion criteria. Using weaker criteria, the authors found five studies: "These demonstrated significant treatment-effects, but due to poor study quality, must be interpreted with caution. Treatment with vanadium often results in gastrointestinal side-effects." Appropriately, the authors concluded, "There is no rigorous evidence that oral vanadium supplementation improves glycemic control in type 2 diabetes. The routine use of vanadium for this purpose cannot be recommended. A large-scale randomized controlled trial is needed to address this clinical question."

Infections, Microbiome | Diabetes patients are at increased risk for various types of overt infections and are thus candidates for supportive immunonutrition, such as with glutamine, zinc, and vitamin D3. Beyond the obvious, we now appreciate that diabetes patients have dysbiosis of the mouth, gut, and skin; see overall protocol in Chapter 4, Section 2—a few highlights will be provided here. Berberine has emerged as a superior intervention in DM2, with euglycemic benefits safely mediated via several mechanisms, including that of modulating the gut microbiome; the clinical efficacy of berberine is similar to that of metformin, thus giving berberine clinical superiority due to its low cost, wide availability, collateral benefits, and excellent safety.

- **Berberine: 200-500 mg twice-thrice daily for dyslipidemia**: Most naturopathic physicians would probably and appropriately first think of its antimicrobial benefits when first asked about the clinical benefits of berberine; indeed berberine has been used for thousands of years to help the body's immune system clear infections, particularly gastrointestinal infections such as due to *Giardia lamblia*. More recently, clinical trials have allowed us to expand the clinical applications of this popular botanical extract to the treatment of dyslipidemia. Berberine appears to have a beneficial impact on negative serum lipid profiles by promoting increased production of LDL cholesterol receptors.

  - **Review and trials: Berberine is a novel cholesterol-lowering drug working through a unique mechanism distinct from statins** (*Nat Med* 2004 Dec[462]): Oral administration of berberine 500 mg orally twice daily for 3 months in 32 hypercholesterolemic patients reduced serum cholesterol by 29%, triglycerides by 35% and LDL-cholesterol by 25%. In an animal study, treatment with berberine in hyperlipidemic hamsters reduced serum cholesterol by 40% and LDL-cholesterol by 42%, with a 3.5-fold increase in hepatic LDL-receptor mRNA and a 2.6-fold increase in hepatic LDL-receptor protein. In vitro studies showed that berberine upregulates LDLR expression through a post-transcriptional mechanism that stabilizes the mRNA. The authors concluded, "These findings show [berberine] as a new hypolipidemic drug with a mechanism of action different from that of statin drugs."

[460] Dugoua et al. From type 2 diabetes to antioxidant activity: a systematic review of the safety and efficacy of cinnamon bark. *Can J Physiol Pharmacol*. 2007 Sep;85(9):837-47
[461] Smith DM, Pickering RM, Lewith GT. A systematic review of vanadium oral supplements for glycaemic control in type 2 diabetes mellitus. *QJM*. 2008 May;101(5):351-8
[462] Kong et al. Berberine is a novel cholesterol-lowering drug working through a unique mechanism distinct from statins. *Nat Med*. 2004 Dec;10(12):1344-51

- Randomized clinical trial: Treatment of type 2 diabetes and dyslipidemia with the natural plant alkaloid berberine (*J Clin Endocrinol Metab* 2008 Jul[463]): 116 patients with DM-2 and dyslipidemia were randomly allocated to receive berberine (1.0 g daily) and the placebo for 3 months. Results showed that berberine reduced fasting and postload plasma glucose from 7.0 to 5.6 and from 12.0 to 8.9 mm/liter, HbA1c from 7.5% to 6.6%, triglyceride from 2.51 to 1.61 mm/liter, total cholesterol from 5.31 to 4.35 mm/liter, and low-density lipoprotein-cholesterol from 3.23 to 2.55 mm/liter, with all parameters differing from placebo significantly. Only 5 patients had mild to moderate constipation as the adverse effect in the berberine group. "CONCLUSIONS: Berberine is effective and safe in the treatment of type 2 diabetes and dyslipidemia."

- Animal study and human clinical trial: Combination of simvastatin with berberine improves the lipid-lowering efficacy (*Metabolism* 2008 Aug[464]): Animal studies confirmed that berberine alone was nearly as effective as simvastatin in normalizing lipids, but that the combination of berberine+simvastatin was significantly more effective than either treatment alone. The mechanism of action appears to be stabilization of the low-density lipoprotein receptor (LDLR) messenger RNA. In a human clinical trial, the therapeutic efficacy of the berberine+simvastatin was then evaluated in 63 hypercholesterolemic patients; the combination showed an improved lipid-lowering effect with 31.8% reduction of serum LDL cholesterol with similar efficacies observed in the reduction of total cholesterol as and triglyceride levels. The authors concluded, "Our results display the rationale, effectiveness, and safety of the combination therapy for hyperlipidemia using BBR and SIMVA. It could be a new regimen for hypercholesterolemia."

Nutritional Immunomodulation Obese and diabetic patients tend to demonstrate an excess of inflammation generally and Th-17 dominance in particular. Given such, these patients are candidates for the nutritional immunomodulation protocol detailed in Chapter 4, Section 3.

Dysmetabolism & Dysfunctional Mitochondria Clearly, the vast majority of diabetic patients—like their euglycemic counterparts—show overwhelming evidence of increased body burden of pesticides and other persistent organic pollutants. High levels of chemical accumulation correlate more strongly with hyperglycemia than does obesity, per many studies; likewise, population-wide trends in diabetes incidence are wisely attributed to population-wide exposure to pollutants, rather than simple "lack of willpower" with regard to individual choices in diet and exercise. Indeed, reducing the global burden/prevalence of diabetes will require individual nations and the global community as a whole to implement effective controls against polluting their inhabitants; governments must implement stronger controls against reckless and rampant corporate polluting. As stated plainly by the article and specific example provided by Lee[465], "I do not believe the diabetes epidemic in China occurred because Chinese people were lazy when they were achieving huge economic growth during the period of 2000–2010. They did not live a luxurious life either. They were not even obese when they became diabetic. The mean body mass index of Chinese diabetic patients reported in the 2010 survey was 23.7, and waist circumference was 80.2 cm. ... My Chinese friends should read the very compelling review by Lee et al. showing that various persistent organic pollutants (POPs) are associated with obesity and diabetes. My fellow diabetologists would agree that, rather than a few individual POPs, background exposure to POP mixtures, including organochlorine pesticides and polychlorinated biphenyls, might increase diabetes. All those POPs might enter our body through foods, water and air." Readers are encouraged to review the two interviews by Drs Lee and Vasquez in *International Journal of Human Nutrition and Functional Medicine* (2015, Spring Edition), available freely online: IntJHumNutrFunctMed.org.[466]

- **Carbohydrate avoidance/reduction, fasting**: The major causes of secondary dysmetabolism are 1) carbohydrate excess, 2) nutritional deficiencies, 3) microbial effects, and 4) xenobiotic effects. As such, each must be addressed as noted in the respective sections of Chapter 4. In the case of diabesity, fasting, low-carbohydrate diets, and exercise all serve to "burn" excess saturated fats and ceramide which otherwise

[463] Zhang et al. Treatment of type 2 diabetes and dyslipidemia with the natural plant alkaloid berberine. *J Clin Endocrinol Metab.* 2008 Jul;93(7):2559-65
[464] Kong et al. Combination of simvastatin with berberine improves the lipid-lowering efficacy. *Metabolism.* 2008 Aug;57(8):1029-37
[465] Lee HK. Success of 2013-2020 World Health Organization action plan to control non-communicable diseases would require pollutants control. *J Diabetes Investig.* 2014 Nov;5(6):621-2
[466] Vasquez A. "Dr Hong Lee's Personal and Educational Path: The New Field of Mitochondrial Toxicology and Its Clinical Relevance to Endocrine Disruption and Meaningful Control of the Diabetes Epidemic" and "Dr Vasquez's Personal and Educational Path, the 2015 CAM Summit, and Mitochondrial Medicine as the Conversational and Conceptual Hub for Interconnecting Nutrition, Lifestyle, Microbes, and Political Pollution—Beyond Nutritional Myopia into Social Contextualization." *International Journal of Human Nutrition and Functional Medicine* 2015 Spring http://intjhumnutrfunctmed.org/

promote inflammation and mitochondrial impairment. Again, sugar-induced production of dysmetabolic and proinflammatory fatty acids leads to metabolic impairment (e.g., mitochondrial dysfunction via ceramide accumulation[467]) and inflammation, including hypothalamic inflammation that drives nonsatiation and overconsumption.[468] Rather than seeking to always "add something good", clinicians should emphasize "taking away the harmful substances that are causing disease", especially toxins—microbial, xenobiotic, metabolic.

- **Coenzyme Q-10 (CoQ10)**: CoQ10 is an endogenous antioxidant, NFkB inhibitor, favorable immune modulator, and essential component of several steps in the electron transport chain. CoQ10 has shown benefit in hypertensive patients, patients with dyslipidemia, and in patients with renal failure, but as of 2009 the current author is not aware of any studies showing positive benefit of CoQ10 on indexes of glycemic control in patients with DM/MetSyn; CoQ10 may still be used in these patients for cardioprotective, renoprotective, and anti-dyslipidemic benefits.

  - Double-blind crossover study: Coenzyme Q10 improves endothelial dysfunction in statin-treated type 2 diabetic patients (*Diabetes Care* 2009 May[469]): The authors investigated whether oral CoQ10 supplementation (200 mg/d) improves endothelial dysfunction in statin-treated type-2 diabetic patients (n=23). "RESULTS: Compared with placebo, CoQ(10) supplementation increased brachial artery FMD [flow-mediated dilatation] by 1.0%, but did not alter NMD [nitrate-mediated dilatation]. CoQ10 supplementation also did not alter plasma F(2)-isoprostane or urinary 20-HETE levels. CONCLUSIONS: **CoQ10 supplementation improved endothelial dysfunction in statin-treated type 2 diabetic patients**, possibly by altering local vascular oxidative stress."

  - Letter to the editor: Lackluster effect of coenzyme Q10 on microcirculatory endothelial function of subjects with type-2 diabetes mellitus (*Atherosclerosis* 2008 Feb[470]): This trial used 200 mg per day of CoQ10 for 12 weeks in medicated patients with DM-2 and found a serologic response to supplementation (increased CoQ10 levels by 3x over baseline) but no significant benefit to CoQ10 supplementation in this group (treatment n=40; placebo n=40). Furthermore, although CoQ10 levels increased, the metabolism of CoQ10 was impaired in these DM-2 patients in the absence of dietary modification; in this regard the authors write, "CoQ10 supplementation without reducing the burden of other metabolic derangements (e.g. hyperglycemia) could not alter the distribution of ubiquinol/ubiquinone favorably." The authors suggest that a higher dose such as 300 mg per day might have shown benefit, as documented in other trials, and surmise, "In conclusion, oral CoQ10 supplementation can replete the plasma concentration without altering its ubiquinol/ubiquinone composition. This intervention was, however, ineffective in improving microcirculatory endothelial function in subjects with T2DM."

  - Clinical trial with water-soluble CoQ10: Effect of hydrosoluble coenzyme Q10 on blood pressures and insulin resistance in hypertensive patients with coronary artery disease (*J Hum Hypertens* 1999 Mar[471]): In this randomized, double-blind trial, placebo-controlled trial among patients receiving antihypertensive medication and with coronary artery disease (n=59: 30 in treatment group, 29 in placebo group), patients received oral coenzyme Q10 (60 mg twice daily) for 8 weeks. In the coenzyme Q10 group, **beneficial reductions were noted in systolic and diastolic blood pressures (average 168/106 reduced to 152/97 [-16/-9]), heart rate, waist–hip ratio, fasting and 2-h plasma insulin and glucose levels, triglyceride levels and angina; CoQ10 supplementation also effected a net increase in HDL-cholesterol.** The authors concluded, "These findings indicate that treatment with coenzyme Q10 decreases blood pressure possibly by decreasing oxidative stress and insulin response in patients with known hypertension receiving conventional antihypertensive drugs."

- **Lipoic acid (thioctic acid)—oral doses range from 600 mg to 1,800 mg per day in divided doses**: Lipoic acid is produced endogenously as well as consumed in foods; it has been referred to as "the universal antioxidant"

[467] Chavez JA, Summers SA. A ceramide-centric view of insulin resistance. *Cell Metab.* 2012 May 2;15(5):585-94
[468] Milanski et al. Saturated fatty acids produce an inflammatory response predominantly through the activation of TLR4 signaling in hypothalamus: implications for the pathogenesis of obesity. *J Neurosci.* 2009 Jan 14;29(2):359-70
[469] Hamilton SJ, Chew GT, Watts GF. Coenzyme Q10 improves endothelial dysfunction in statin-treated type 2 diabetic patients. *Diabetes Care.* 2009 May;32(5):810-2
[470] Lim et al. The effect of coenzyme Q10 on microcirculatory endothelial function of subjects with type 2 diabetes mellitus. *Atherosclerosis.* 2008 Feb;196(2):966-9
[471] Singh RB, Niaz MA, Rastogi SS, Shukla PK, Thakur AS. Effect of hydrosoluble coenzyme Q10 on blood pressures and insulin resistance in hypertensive patients with coronary artery disease. *J Hum Hypertens.* 1999 Mar;13(3):203-8

because it is both water-soluble and fat-soluble. In addition to its antioxidant roles, lipoic acid is also a potent inhibitor of NFkB, and as such has broad applications, including the treatment of viral infections. Lipoic acid is an essential component of the pyruvate dehydrogenase complex, which is the intermediate pathway between glycolysis and the Kreb's cycle. When used in supplemental doses, lipoate should always be used in a comprehensive plan that includes a high-potency broad-spectrum multivitamin and multimineral. With regard to DM-2, lipoate has been mostly studied in the treatment of diabetic polyneuropathy; however, clinicians should not lose sight of its broad anti-oxidant benefits that extend beyond this single application. Nor should diabetic neuropathy be taken lightly as it represents a major health problem; it is responsible for increased mortality as well as substantial morbidity and impaired quality of life. The most important treatment for DM-neuropathy is control of blood glucose levels; specific treatments such as lipoate play a secondary but very important role.

- Literature review: Alpha-lipoic acid in the treatment of diabetic polyneuropathy in Germany: current evidence from clinical trials (*Exp Clin Endocrinol Diabetes* 1999[472]): The authors review at least 15 clinical trials, which, as a group, have shown beneficial effects of lipoic/thioctic acid on either "neuropathic symptoms and deficits due to polyneuropathy or reduced heart rate variability resulting from cardiac autonomic neuropathy." Studies reporting positive results have used at least 600 mg per day. The authors enumerate the following findings:
  1. "Short-term treatment for 3 weeks using 600 mg of thioctic acid i.v. per day appears to reduce the chief symptoms of diabetic polyneuropathy. A 3-week pilot study of 1800 mg per day given orally indicates that the therapeutic effect may be independent of the route of administration, but this needs to be confirmed in a larger sample size.
  2. The effect on symptoms is accompanied by an improvement of neuropathic deficits.
  3. **Oral treatment for 4-7 months tends to reduce neuropathic deficits and improves cardiac autonomic neuropathy**.
  4. Preliminary data over 2 years indicate possible long-term improvement in motor and sensory nerve conduction in the lower limbs.
  5. Clinical and postmarketing surveillance studies have revealed a highly favorable safety profile of the drug."

- Critical review: Thioctic acid for patients with symptomatic diabetic polyneuropathy (*Treat Endocrinol* 2004[473]): The author reviews evidence that oxidative stress resulting from enhanced free-radical formation and/or defects in antioxidant defense is implicated in the pathogenesis of diabetic neuropathy; if this is true, then control of endogenous oxidant production such as through improved glycemic control as well as the administration of supplemental/exogenous antioxidants would appear to be the obvious and reasonable therapeutic interventions. Supporting this oxidative-neuropathic link is the observation that superoxide anion and peroxynitrite production are increased in diabetic patients in relation to the severity of polyneuropathy. **The author also discusses a meta-analysis that included the largest sample of diabetic patients (n = 1258) ever to have been treated with a single drug or class of drugs to reduce neuropathic symptoms, and confirmed the favorable effects of thioctic acid based on the highest level of evidence (Class Ia: evidence from meta-analyses of randomized, controlled trials).** The author enumerates the following conclusions:
  1. Short-term treatment for 3 weeks using intravenous thioctic acid 600 mg/day reduces the chief symptoms of diabetic polyneuropathy to a clinically meaningful degree;
  2. This effect on neuropathic symptoms is accompanied by an improvement of neuropathic deficits, suggesting potential for the drug to favorably influence underlying neuropathy;
  3. Oral treatment for 4-7 months tends to reduce neuropathic deficits and improve cardiac autonomic neuropathy;
  4. Clinical and postmarketing surveillance studies have revealed a highly favorable safety profile of the drug."

---

[472] Ziegler et al. Alpha-lipoic acid in the treatment of diabetic polyneuropathy in Germany: current evidence from clinical trials. *Exp Clin Endocrinol Diabetes*. 1999;107:421-30
[473] Ziegler D. Thioctic acid for patients with symptomatic diabetic polyneuropathy: a critical review. *Treat Endocrinol*. 2004;3(3):173-89

- Controlled, randomized, open-label study: Alpha-lipoic acid in the treatment of autonomic diabetic neuropathy (*Rom J Intern Med* 2004[474]): In this study, 46 patients with type-1 diabetes and different forms of autonomic neuropathy (mean duration of diabetes 16.8 years) were treated with alpha-lipoic acid 600 mg/d intravenously (IV or iv) for 10 days; thereafter they received 600 mg/d orally for 50 days. The control group consisted of 29 type-1 diabetic patients with autonomic diabetic neuropathy. "RESULTS: **There was a significant improvement** after treatment in the score for severity of cardiovascular autonomic neuropathy--from 6.43 +/- 0.9 to 4.24 +/- 1.8 (p<0.001), while in the control group it worsened from 6.18 +/- 1.3 to 6.52 +/- 0.9 (p>0.1). We found improvement in the Valsalva maneuver after treatment - from 1.05 +/- 0.04 to 1.13 +/- 0.08 (p<0.001); in the deep-breathing test -from 3.4 +/- 2.8 to 10.4 +/- 5.7 (p<0.001); and in the lying-to-standing test--from 0.99 +/- 0.01 to 1.01 +/- 0.02 (p>0.1), while **in the control group there was no improvement**. … We found improvement in diabetic enteropathy in six patients; in the complaints of dizziness, instability upon standing in six patients; in neuropathic edema of the lower extremities in four patients and in erectile dysfunction in four patients after treatment, while in the control group no change was reported in the symptoms and signs of autonomic neuropathy by the end of the follow-up period. There were changes in the laboratory parameters of oxidative stress after therapy--**total serum antioxidant capacity increased** from 20.42 +/- 1.8 to 22.96 +/- 2.3 microgH2O2/ml/min (p<0.05), **serum SOD activity** - from 269.8 +/- 31.1 to 319.8 +/- 29.IU/l (p=0.02) and **erythrocyte SOD**--from 0.89 +/- 0.10 to 1.11 +/- 0.09 U/gHb (p=0.04). CONCLUSION: Our results demonstrate that alpha-lipoic acid (Thiogamma) appears to be an effective drug in the treatment of the different forms of autonomic diabetic neuropathy."
- Multicenter clinical trial: The role of alpha-lipoic acid in diabetic polyneuropathy treatment (*Bosn J Basic Med Sci.* 2008 Nov[475]): These researchers investigated the effect of alpha-lipoic acid on the symptoms of diabetic neuropathy by administering lipoate 600 mg intravenously for 3 weeks, followed by 3 months of oral lipoate 300-600 mg/d. The 100 patients in this study had either DM-1 (n=16) or DM-2 (n=80) with 4 patients not classified; average age was 61y, and average duration of disease was 11y. 69 patients were taking insulin and 31 were treated with oral hypoglycemics; average duration of polyneuropathic symptoms was 3y. The authors reported the following results, "**Significant statistic differences in improvement** were recorded (P>0,05) according to Fridman's test for repeated measurements compared to initial findings in assessments: **sensory symptoms of polyneuropathy, pain sensations as polyneuropathy symptoms, total score of polyneuropathy symptoms, subjective assessment of patients, subjective findings of physicians**, and significant differences were not found (P>0,05) in autonomous and motoric neuropathy. Based on the conducted study, we have concluded that the application of **alpha-lipoic acid during 3 months has helped to decrease the symptoms of diabetic neuropathy** and in only one case out of 100 included patients there was no subjective improvement after drug application." Thus, in summary, these authors loaded patients with intravenous administration of lipoate for 3 weeks, then followed with oral administration for 3 months; **they report that 99 out of 100 patients had a positive response** in the reduction of the severity of diabetic polyneuropathy.
- **Acetyl-L-carnitine 500-1,000 mg three times daily between meals for diabetic neuropathy**:
  - Review: Acetyl-L-carnitine in the treatment of diabetic peripheral neuropathy (*Ann Pharmacother* 2008 Nov[476]): These authors review data from two large clinical trials (n=1679) using acetyl-L-carnitine (ALC) in the treatment of diabetic peripheral neuropathy (DPN). Results showed, "Subjects who received at least 2 g daily of ALC showed decreases in pain scores. One study showed improvements in electrophysiologic factors such as nerve conduction velocities, while the other did not. Patients who had neuropathic pain reported reductions in pain using a visual analog scale. Nerve regeneration was documented in one trial. The supplement was well tolerated. A proprietary form of ALC was used in both studies. CONCLUSIONS: Data on treatment of DPN with ALC support its use. It should be recommended to patients early in the disease process to provide maximal benefit."

[474] Tankova et al. Alpha-lipoic acid in the treatment of autonomic diabetic neuropathy (controlled, randomized, open-label study). *Rom J Intern Med*. 2004;42(2):457-64
[475] Bureković A, Terzić M, Alajbegović S, Vukojević Z, Hadzić N. The role of alpha-lipoic acid in diabetic polyneuropathy treatment. *Bosn J Basic Med Sci*. 2008 Nov;8:341-5
[476] Evans JD, Jacobs TF, Evans EW. Role of acetyl-L-carnitine in the treatment of diabetic peripheral neuropathy. *Ann Pharmacother*. 2008 Nov;42(11):1686-91

- Acetyl-L-carnitine improves pain, nerve regeneration, and vibratory perception in patients with chronic diabetic neuropathy: an analysis of two randomized placebo-controlled trials (*Diabetes Care* 2005 Jan[477]): "CONCLUSIONS: These studies demonstrate that ALC treatment is efficacious in alleviating symptoms, particularly pain, and improves nerve fiber regeneration and vibration perception in patients with established diabetic neuropathy."

Style of Living Diabetes must be approached in its totality—socially, politically, emotionally, physically, nutritionally, etc.

- **Sleep**: Sleep deprivation causes systemic inflammation that promotes insulin resistance and the development of DM-2. Patients should be encouraged to practice good "sleep hygiene" by allowing sufficient time for quality sleep; some patients will need to reduce caffeine intake appropriately. Assessment for sleep apnea by history or polysomnography should be employed.

- **Psychological support, group support, and individual counseling**: The development of obesity requires years of under-exercising, overeating, allowing/denying progressive decrements in physical and (generally) social and psychological functioning. These cannot be reversed by a purely nutritional or medical approach. Patients must be willing to receive counseling, feedback, support, and to actively participate in psychological counseling *with a competent therapist* who holds the patient accountable to homework, behavioral change, the achievement of goals, and the integration (or more often *creation*) of important life goals which can pull the patient forward into a positive future via a health-promoting lifestyle. A healthy lifestyle is the means by which patients attain, maintain, and protect an optimized health status which helps them achieve their overall life goals; patients with no goals and without high standards for the expectations of their life experience will readily fall into the pattern of noncompliance and failure that have made obese, DM-2, and MetSyn patients notoriously hard to help and deal with clinically.
  - Review: A comprehensive psychological approach to obesity (*Psychiatr Med* 1983 Sep[478]): "The management of obesity must be a joint venture between psychiatry and medicine. ... Many obese patients lack a fundamental knowledge of nutrition, exercise, and health. In addition, most are poorly socialized and require assistance in learning assertiveness and other interpersonal skills. A behaviorally oriented component is very effective in providing these skills."

- **Specific therapeutic and management considerations for specific aspects of the DM/MetSyn interconnected matrix**: The previous sections have reviewed therapeutics considered by this author to be most poignant in the routine management of DM, particularly DM-2 and MetSyn. The single most important treatment is the low-carbohydrate supplemented Paleo-Mediterranean diet; this is simply a low-carbohydrate version of "the supplemented Paleo-Mediterranean diet" which I described in *Integrative Orthopedics* (2004), *Integrative Rheumatology* (2006), *Musculoskeletal Pain: Expanded Clinical Strategies* (2008) and originally in *Nutritional Wellness* in 2005.[479] In the section that follows, I provide a problem-based itemization of various therapeutics worthy of consideration when specific problems need to be targeted within a context of overall diabetes management. These are "reasonable" considerations based on clinical experience generally with but sometimes without high-quality peer-reviewed trials.
  - **Cardiovascular risk**: Hypertension and hyperglycemia both lead to accelerated atherosclerosis; the combination of hypertension with hyperglycemia is additive/synergistic, hence the term "accelerated atherosclerosis" to describe the cardiometabolic syndrome. Clinicians must address whole-body physiology while also addressing various individualized facets and nuances per patient.
    - Clinical patient assessment with resting/stress ECG, consider adding echocardiography: These are considerations per patient; guidelines do not recommend these for all patients as benefit has not been demonstrated unless clinically indicated.
    - Hyperglycemia, oxidative stress, hypercoagulability: Assess and address with tests and interventions detailed above, especially low-carb supplemented Paleo-Mediterranean diet; add low-dose aspirin for most DM patients over age 40y.

---

[477] Sima et al. Acetyl-L-carnitine improves pain, nerve regeneration, and vibratory perception in patients with chronic diabetic neuropathy. *Diabetes Care.* 2005 Jan;28(1):89-94

[478] Fawzy FI, Pasnau RO, Wellisch DK, Ellsworth RG, Dornfeld L, Maxwell M. A comprehensive psychological approach to obesity. *Psychiatr Med.* 1983 Sep;1(3):257-73

[479] Vasquez A. A Five-Part Nutritional Protocol that Produces Consistently Positive Results. *Nutritional Wellness* 2005 Sept

- o **Optimize glycemic control**: Use additional chromium, biotin, grapeseed extract, cinnamon, and *Gymnema* as necessary.
- o **Co-manage or refer unresponsive or noncompliant patients**: The clinician's technical goal is the objective documentation of a positive serologic (e.g., glucose, Hgb-A1c, lipids, CRP) and clinical (e.g., blood pressure, weight loss) response to treatment within not more than 2-3 months' time from the initiation of treatment. If such documentation cannot be made due to treatment failure or patient noncompliance, or if documentable positive responses are not occurring quickly enough and the patient remains at an unacceptable level of risk, the patient should be co-managed with pharmaceutical drugs (especially statins) until the diet and lifestyle interventions have taken effect. Clinicians must be aware of the politics and medicolegal consequences, especially if a state medical board is involved: A patient who dies while taking statins and antihypertensive polypharmacy will be considered "well managed" while a patient who dies despite the prescription of an evidence-based nutritional protocol will likely be considered "mismanaged." The topic being debated is not research or patient care; rather, the issue is "standard of care" which is defined by what doctors and specialists are doing in the community (and nationally). Standard-of-care issues are decided by majority rule; when most cardiologists and internists rely solely on drugs for the treatment of diet-induced disease, the drug treatment is the standard of care, regardless of research showing that nutritional interventions are superior or equivalent. When in doubt, refer or co-manage.

- **Hypercholesterolemia and dyslipidemia**: Assess with serum testing; strongly consider the following interventions.
  - o **Low-carb supplemented Paleo-Mediterranean diet**: Best single intervention for reducing cardiovascular and total mortality; fish oil, vitamin D, and Mg supplementation make the intervention particularly more powerful.
  - o **Berberine 500 mg once or twice or thrice daily**: Most studies have been short-term in the range of about 3 months when using the 1,000 mg per day dose; long-term safety of berberine 1,000 mg/d has not been established.
  - o **Policosanol 10-20 mg/d**: Policosanol appears efficacious for some patients, despite some controversy in the research literature, with some studies showing statin-like results and others showing no benefit. The most effective policosanol comes from sugar cane (not bee's wax) and is standardized for the octacosanol content Early in my (DrV) clinical practice, I recall witnessing the reduction of 100 mg/dL (from 280 mg/dL to 180 mg/dL) within one month simply by use of dietary carbohydrate restriction plus policosanol.
  - o **Niacin 500 mg 2-4 times per day**: Very effective for raising HDL, but the uncomfortable skin flushing sensation limits its tolerability; pretreatment with aspirin can help mitigate this benign adverse effect. Plain niacin is the product of choice for serum lipid modification; other forms such as niacinamide and inositol hexaniacinate are much less effective in this regard. Niacin, like EFAs when given in excessive doses, may worsen glycemic control.

- **Diabetic neuropathy**:
  - o **Biotin 10-20 mg/d**: Clinicians should recall from their training in basic/clinical nutrition that biotin is essentially nontoxic; toxicity of biotin has not been reported in patients receiving daily doses of up to 200 mg orally and up to 20 mg intravenously for the treatment of biotin-responsive inborn errors of metabolism and acquired biotin deficiency.[480]
  - o **Gamma linolenic acid**: 500-1,000 mg/d: Preferably administered with food
  - o **Lipoic acid 400 mg 2-4 times daily**.
  - o **Acetyl-L-carnitine 500 mg 2-6 times daily**.
  - o **B vitamins especially vitamin B12 and thiamine**: Oral B-12 given 2,000-4,000 mcg daily as hydroxocobalamin (or the methyl- or adenosyl- forms); about half that dose if given intramuscularly. Thiamine is available in water-soluble and fat-soluble forms and can be given orally 50-300 mg per day.

---

[480] Ames BN, et al. High-dose vitamin therapy stimulates variant enzymes with decreased coenzyme binding affinity (increased K(m)). *Am J Clin Nutr*. 2002 Apr;75(4):616-58

- o Capsaicin cream: Applied topically for pain relief only, 2-4 times per day. The burning sensation abates with continued use. Avoid contact with eyes and mucus membranes.
- **Diabetic retinopathy**: Emphasize blood pressure control, glycemic control, lipid control, and antioxidants especially zinc, selenium, and phytonutrients from bilberry (e.g., standardized to >25% anthocyanosides given 240-600 mg/day) and other flavonoids (e.g., quercetin) and proanthocyanidins. **Referral to an ophthalmologist is absolutely mandatory for all DM and MetSyn patients.**
- **Nephropathy and renal failure**: These patients are best co-managed by an internist, nephrologist, or excellent family medicine doctor; the legal ramifications and consent and compliance issues, along with preparation for hemodialysis or transplant need to be addressed quickly in preparation for the expenses and procedures likely to come.
  - o Adjust the diet to avoid excess potassium, magnesium, or protein: Adjust the diet and use serum testing as indicated.
  - o High-dose (300 mg per day) thiamine therapy for patients with type-2 diabetes and microalbuminuria: "METHODS: Type 2 diabetic patients (21 male, 19 female) with microalbuminuria were recruited at a diabetic clinic and randomized to placebo and treatment arms. Patients were given 3 x 100 mg capsules of thiamine or placebo per day for 3 months with a 2 month follow-up washout period. The primary endpoint was change in urinary albumin excretion (UAE). "RESULTS: UAE was decreased in patients receiving thiamine therapy for 3 months with respect to baseline (median -17.7 mg/24 h; $p < 0.001$, n = 20). There was no significant decrease in UAE in patients receiving placebo after 3 months of therapy (n = 20). UAE was significantly lower in patients who had received thiamine therapy compared with those who had received placebo (30.1 vs 35.5 mg/24 h, $p < 0.01$) but not at baseline. UAE continued to decrease in the 2 month washout period in both groups, but not significantly. There was no effect of thiamine treatment on glycemic control, dyslipidemia or BP. There were no adverse effects of therapy. CONCLUSIONS/INTERPRETATION: In this pilot study, high-dose thiamine therapy produced a regression of UAE in type 2 diabetic patients with microalbuminuria. Thiamine supplements at high dose may provide improved therapy for early-stage diabetic nephropathy."[481]
  - o CoQ10 200-300 mg/day with food: CoQ10 is one of the most effective treatments for reversing renal failure according to Singh et al.[482,483]
  - o Other nephroprotective nutrients: Selenium and silymarin have also shown nephroprotective benefits in humans treated with nephrotoxic anti-cancer chemotherapy.
- **Hypertension**: See Hypertension section for details and interventions beyond those mentioned in this chapter.
- **Infection risk**: See chapter on Viral Infections, revisit treatments and management strategies throughout this chapter while focusing on:
  - o Foot care: Examine the feet at nearly every visit.
  - o Dental/mouth care: DM and MetSyn patients should receive dental care at least annually. Encourage use of antimicrobial mouthwashes, regular brushing, and frequent sterilization/replacement of toothbrushes.
  - o Treat all infections aggressively: From pneumonia to sinus and ear infections to boils, treat all infected DM patients aggressively and with in-office follow-up within 48-72 hours.
- **Impaired pancreatic function**: Beta-cell failure is the hallmark of DM-1 and—as previously mentioned—it also occurs in DM-2 after the disease has progressed for many years (previously termed "high output failure"). In patients with pancreatic failure due to acute/chronic pancreatitis—such as seen due to hypertriglyceridemia, alcoholism, or (rarely) major abdominal trauma—a clinician might aspire to promote regeneration/protection of remaining pancreatic beta-cells. The following therapeutics might be considered; although they have more experimental/animal research support than support from clinical trials in humans.

[481] Rabbani et al. High-dose thiamine therapy for patients with type 2 diabetes and microalbuminuria. *Diabetologia.* 2009 Feb;52(2):208-12
[482] Singh et al. Randomized, double-blind placebo-controlled trial of coenzyme Q10 in chronic renal failure: discovery of a new role. *J Nutr Environ Med* 2000;10:281-8
[483] Singh et al. Randomized, Double-blind, Placebo-controlled Trial of Coenzyme Q10 in Patients with Endstage Renal Failure. *J Nutr Environ Med* 2003; 13 (1): 13–22

- o Niacinamide 2-3 g/d in divided doses: Niacinamide has shown the ability to protect pancreatic beta-cells in several studies in animal models of DM-1. A reasonable daily dose of 2,000 mg should be divided into several smaller doses, such as 500 mg 4 times daily, or 250 mg 8 times daily. As with plain niacin, hepatitis from niacinamide can occur, but this is exceedingly rare; clinicians should monitor liver enzymes before starting treatment, at about 2-4 weeks after starting treatment, again at 3-6 months. Nausea or abdominal pain should prompt appropriate follow-up and testing of serum AST and ALT; patients should be educated appropriately.
- o Gymnema (*Gymnema sylvestre*): Gymnema appears to have some benefit in selected patients. Clinicians might have to try more than one brand/manufacturer in order to find a product that works for a particular patient; in my own clinical experience with difficult-to-control DM-2, I found that some products were inefficacious, while another provided clear benefit by reducing glucose levels. Admittedly, some of the research on Gymnema is not entirely clear; hence my reservation of this intervention as a last resort. The typical therapeutic dose of a standardized extract, standardized to contain 24% gymnemic acids, is 400-600 mg/d, with some preference for dosing with meals.[484]
  - □ Systematic review: Use of Gymnema sylvestre for diabetes mellitus (*J Altern Complement Med* 2007 Nov[485]): "Given that *G. sylvestre* targets several of the etiological factors connected with diabetes, including chronic inflammation, obesity, enzymatic defects, and pancreatic beta-cell function, and no single oral hypoglycemic drug presently exerts such a diverse range of effects, suggests that *gymnema* may be useful in the management of diabetes and the prevention of associated pathological changes. However, as this systematic review shows, the clinical efficacy of *gymnema* has only been supported by a small number of nonrandomized, open-label trials."
  - □ Clinical trial: Antidiabetic effect of a leaf extract from Gymnema sylvestre in non-insulin-dependent diabetes mellitus patients (*J Ethnopharmacol* 1990 Oct [486]): "The effectiveness of GS4, an extract from the leaves of Gymnema sylvestre, in controlling hyperglycemia was investigated in 22 Type 2 diabetic patients on conventional oral anti-hyperglycemic agents. GS4 (400 mg/day) was administered for 18-20 months as a supplement to the conventional oral drugs. During GS4 supplementation, the **patients showed a significant reduction in blood glucose, glycosylated hemoglobin and glycosylated plasma proteins, and conventional drug dosage could be decreased.** Five of the 22 diabetic patients were able to discontinue their conventional drug and maintain their blood glucose homeostasis with GS4 alone. These data suggest that the beta cells may be regenerated/repaired in Type 2 diabetic patients on GS4 supplementation. This is supported by the appearance of raised insulin levels in the serum of patients after GS4 supplementation."
- **Elevated homocysteine (hyperhomocysteinaemia, hyperhomocysteinuria):** Reasonable doses are listed; clinicians will have to combine and "dose to effect" per patient. All of these treatments are well-accepted as safe and generally effective.
  - o Folinic acid or methylfolate 5 mg/d: Use in combination with other vitamins, especially vitamin B12, in the form of hydroxocobalamin, adenosylcobalamin, or methylcobalamin—cyanocobalamin is obviously to be avoided because of its clinically relevant content of cyanide.
  - o Vitamin B12 >2,000 mcg per day: Use in the form of hydroxocobalamin, adenosylcobalamin, or methylcobalamin—cyanocobalamin is to be avoided because of its clinically relevant content of cyanide.
  - o Vitamin B6, pyridoxine 50-250 mg/d: The phosphorylated form (P5P) can also be used; when the HCL form is used, additional attention must be given to magnesium status/supplementation and urinary alkalinization.
  - o Riboflavin 20-400 mg/d: Small doses of 2 mg/d have been shown to significantly reduce homocysteine levels, and doses of 400 mg/d are common and well-tolerated in the treatment of migraine.

---

[484] [No authors listed] Gymnema sylvestre. *Altern Med Rev.* 1999 Feb;4(1):46-7
[485] Leach MJ. Gymnema sylvestre for diabetes mellitus: a systematic review. *J Altern Complement Med.* 2007 Nov;13(9):977-83
[486] Baskaran et al. Antidiabetic effect of a leaf extract from Gymnema sylvestre in non-insulin-dependent diabetes mellitus patients. *J Ethnopharmacol.* 1990 Oct;30(3):295-300

- o **NAC 600 mg per day and upward to 500-1,500 mg thrice daily**: Doses of NAC 4,800 mg/d have been used with success and safety in the treatment of SLE. NAC binds directly to homocysteine to form a NAC-homocysteine conjugate that is excreted in the urine.
- o **Thyroid optimization**: Hypothyroidism causes elevated homocysteine and promotes insulin resistance[487] and should be treated appropriately per Chapter 1.
- o **Avoidance of homocysteine-elevating factors**: High coffee intake (>5 cups per day), ethanol, tobacco smoking, and medications/treatments (such as methotrexate, metformin, niacin and fibrate drugs); fish oil can raise homocysteine levels in some patients. Metformin is well-known to cause malabsorption of vitamin B12 and to thereby exacerbate "diabetic neuropathy" and promote depression and dementia/psychosis.
- o **Choline, phosphatidylcholine, lecithin (approximately 2.6 g choline/d)**: Each TBS (tablespoon, approximately 15 mL) of lecithin contains 275 mg of choline; thus, if the goal is to get to 2.6 g choline, one would need to use 10 TBS (150 mL) per day of granulated lecithin.
- o **Betaine, trimethylglycine 6–12 g/day**: Effects are weak/modest; likely more relevant for patients taking drugs such as metformin and fibrates that promote loss of betaine in urine.

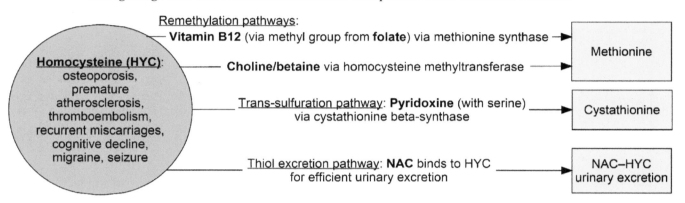

Lowering homocysteine (HYC) via nutritional supplementation: Folate gives methyl group to cobalamin (vitamin B12) to convert HYC via methionine synthase to methionine; choline/betaine can remethylate homocysteine via homocysteine methyltransferase to form methionine. Pyridoxine promotes conversion of HYC via cystathionine beta-synthase to cystathionine. The amino acid N-acetyl-cysteine (NAC) binds to HYC for efficient renal excretion of NAC-HYC.[488]

Endocrine Imbalances Obese/diabetic patients generally have hyperinsulinemia (previously reviewed in this chapter); excesses of estrogen and cortisol with deficiencies of DHEA, testosterone, and thyroid are expected—see Chapter 4, Section 6 for review of assessments and interventions.

Xenobiotic Exposure and Detoxification Detoxification must be optimized, as reviewed in Chapter 4, Section 7.

Drug Treatments The three classes of oral drugs and the injectable insulin can be remembered by the mnemonic "MIST" for metformin, insulin, sulfonylureas, and thiazolidinediones. The sequence of medicalization is generally as follows: ❶ provide cursory and nonspecific diet and lifestyle advice, ❷ start with metformin, increase dose as necessary until maximized at 2,500 mg/d, ❸ add sulfonylurea, ❹ add thiazolidinedione, ❺ discontinue sulfonylurea and add injectable insulin when the previous measures have "failed."

> **Xenobiotic-induced mitochondrial dysfunction is what leads to xenobiotic-induced HTN and diabetes**
>
> Pesticides and other pollutants commonly induce mitochondrial dysfunction, thereby contributing to insulin resistance and vasoconstriction, both of which promote HTN and DM.

[487] Yang N et al. Novel Clinical Evidence of an Association between Homocysteine and Insulin Resistance in Patients with Hypothyroidism or Subclinical Hypothyroidism. *PLoS One*. 2015 May 4;10(5):e0125922

[488] "NAC intravenous administration induces an efficient and rapid reduction of plasma thiols, particularly of Hcy; our data support the hypothesis that NAC displaces thiols from their binding protein sites and forms, in excess of plasma NAC, mixed disulphides (NAC-Hcy) with a high renal clearance." Ventura et al. N-Acetyl-cysteine reduces homocysteine plasma levels after single intravenous administration by increasing thiols urinary excretion. *Pharmacol Res*. 1999 Oct;40(4):345-50

Drug treatment of diabetes mellitus

Drugs	Clinical considerations
• <u>Metformin</u>: Promoted as initial pharmacologic management due to benefits (reduction of HgbA1c by 2% max; reduction in mortality) and safety (less hypoglycemia); reduces hepatic gluconeogenesis and increases peripheral insulin sensitivity with additional benefits for lipids, blood pressure, and (hyper)coagulation. Berberine is safer and more effective than metformin per a 3-month equivalent-dose 500mg TID study (Yin et al, *Metabolism* 2008 May)	• <u>Renal excretion of metformin</u> prohibits use in patients with renal insufficiency; relative contraindications are serum creatinine >1.5 in men or >1.4 in women (per what we learned in medical school/training) • <u>Adverse GI effects</u>: anorexia, N/V/D; may be transient. • <u>Hypoglycemia</u> is more likely with fasting exercise, alcohol, and concomitant use of other hypoglycemic treatments. • <u>Lactic acidosis</u>: Occurs 3-5 cases per 100,000 patient-years. Increased risk with hepatic or renal insufficiency/compromise, also older age, diuretics, radiographic contrast, dehydration, diarrhea, vomiting, hepatic insufficiency, alcoholism. Metformin should be avoided 48 hours before and after radiographic contrast. • <u>Contraindicated with pregnancy & lactation</u> • <u>Start at 500 mg with dinner</u>, titrating upward weekly as needed with a max dose of 2,500 mg/d in divided doses with food. Extended-release preparations are conveniently administered once daily.
• <u>Sulfonylurea drugs—glyburide, glipizide, glimepiride</u>: Stimulate pancreatic insulin production and improve peripheral insulin sensitivity.	• <u>Start with low dose with breakfast, titrate upward weekly PRN</u> • **Hypoglycemia is the biggest risk** occurring in 1% of patients per year; reduce dose when fasting. Sulfonylurea "gli-ide" drugs should be discontinued when rapid-acting insulins are added, ie, when moving from "basal only" to "basal-bolus." • **Glipizide**: Shortest half-life and thus the least hypoglycemia
• <u>Thiazolidinedione drugs—pioglitazone and rosiglitazone</u>: Improve peripheral insulin sensitivity; reduction of HgbA1c by 1.5% max; with reductions in Trigs, increases in LDL and HDL.	• <u>"-glitazones" are extensively metabolized in the liver and are thus contraindicated with liver disease</u> • <u>Liver monitoring</u> by measurement of ALT and AST should occur before treatment and every 2 months for the first year of treatment • <u>Exacerbation of heart failure</u>: Contraindicated in Class 3-4 CHF
• <u>Insulin</u>: Pancreatic beta-cells constantly produce insulin (basal) accentuated by increased production postprandially (bolus). Pharmacologic insulins function as endogenous insulin but vary in their cellular bioavailability and thus onset and duration of action. Patients with type-1 DM require frequent insulin injections with each meal or must use a continuous infusion pump.	• <u>Initial starting dose of insulin</u>: 0.1 units/kg, or divide the fasting glucose level in mg/dL by 18. • <u>Basal insulin is given at bedtime</u>, with the dose adjusted every 3 days; the nighttime basal insulin dose is increased by 2 units every 3 days for as long as the mean fasting glucose level is greater than 100 mg/dl. The long-acting insulins NPH and Glargine (insulin analog) are equally efficacious but Glargine produces less hypoglycemia. "Basal" insulin is given as one nighttime injection of NPH or Glargine. • <u>Basal-bolus therapy is introduced when oral+basal treatments are insufficient</u>: Generally this is a 70/30 combination of rapid and intermediate acting insulins administered twice daily before meals; the original nighttime basal dose of a long-acting insulin is replaced by two doses of 70/30 rapid/intermediate doses administered before breakfast and dinner.
• <u>Inhibitors of dipeptidyl peptidase 4</u>: DPP-4 inhibitors, such as sitagliptin/Januvia	• This relatively new class of drugs provide an antidiabetic effect by increasing pancreatic output of insulin and reducing hepatic gluconeogenesis. In contrast to other agents, sitagliptin/Januvia is reported to cause less weight gain (a side-effect of insulin) and less hypoglycemia (a problem with insulin and the sulfonylurea drugs). • The botanical medicine berberine inhibits DPP-4, which at least partly explains its anti-hyperglycemic activities.[489]

---

[489] "Our findings suggest that DPP IV inhibition is, at least, one of the mechanisms that explain the anti-hyperglycemic activity of berberine." Al-Masri et al. Inhibition of dipeptidyl peptidase IV (DPP IV) is one of the mechanisms explaining the hypoglycemic effect of berberine. *J Enzyme Inhib Med Chem*. 2009 Oct;24(5):1061-6

Chemical Exposure as a Major Contributor to the Epidemic of Diabetes Mellitus and Disorders of Insulin Resistance: From Molecular Mechanisms to Clinical Implications

This article was originally published in *Naturopathy Digest* in 2007
naturopathydigest.com/archives/2007/apr/diabetes.php

Introduction: Evidence has been consistently accumulating over the past few years implicating chemical exposure as a plausible and important cause of insulin resistance and diabetes mellitus. In this article, I will survey current literature and explain the causes, mechanisms, and clinical implications of the toxin-diabetes link, and I will expand some of my previous work on chemical exposure and clinical detoxification methods[490] as specifically related to the genesis and treatment of diabetes. By the time they finish reading this article, chiropractic and naturopathic doctors should appreciate the role of chemical exposure in the genesis and perpetuation of insulin resistance, understand the mechanisms of chemical accumulation and detoxification, and have an awareness of some of the methods used to alleviate and prevent chemical-induced disease.

Chemical Exposure and Type-2 Diabetes in Humans: Numerous animal models have irrefutably established the ability of specific chemicals and toxic metals to destroy pancreatic beta-cells and thus reduce insulin production to such an extent that hyperglycemia and diabetes result; these models establish that toxin exposure can result in a form of type-1 "low insulin" diabetes. However, the largest burden of hyperglycemic diabetes (distinguished from diabetes insipidus) in industrialized nations is associated not with insufficiency of insulin as in type-1 diabetes but rather with the hallmark findings of excess insulin, peripheral insulin resistance, and associated clinical presentations that include overweight/obesity, hypertension, hyperglycemia and dyslipidemia. The current dominant paradigm of type-2 diabetes and its synonyms and closely related conditions including insulin resistance, adult-onset diabetes, metabolic syndrome, and syndrome X is that the condition results from excess caloric intake and an insufficiency of exercise in patients with one or more genetic predispositions. Medical treatment generally consists of inadequate dietary-lifestyle advice and the use of one or more prescription drugs. However, the diet-exercise-gene-drug model of diabetes is clearly incomplete; other factors, including micronutrient status (particularly vitamin D, cholecalciferol[491]) and hormonal milieu also clearly influence adiposity and insulin receptor sensitivity. Exposure to and accumulation of toxic chemicals, either from occupational exposure or chronic background exposure to these chemicals which pervade our environment appears to be a hitherto underappreciated factor influencing insulin receptor sensitivity and the risk and prevalence of diabetes mellitus; a sampling of primary research is provided in the following section.

In 1997, Henriksen et al[492] showed that military veterans exposed to dioxin showed increased prevalence of glucose abnormalities, insulin abnormalities, and diabetes prevalence and faster development of diabetes compared to veterans of the same era who had lower levels of dioxin in their blood. In 1999, Calvert et al[493] showed that among workers occupationally exposed to a highly toxic form of dioxin, those with the highest blood levels of dioxin showed higher average levels of blood glucose. In 2000, Longnecker and Michalek[494] showed that among 1,197 veterans Air Force Veterans with no history of chemical exposure and normal serum levels of dioxins, patients with higher levels of dioxins showed an increased prevalence of diabetes. In 2003, Fierens et al[495] reported that diabetic patients showed significantly increased serum levels of dioxins, coplanar PCBs, and 12 PCB markers compared to unaffected control patients, and the level of chemical accumulation in diabetics was very significant; diabetic patients showed a 62% higher level of PCB toxins than healthy patients, and higher levels of toxins were associated with a higher risk of diabetes in a dose-dependent manner. In 2006, Fujiyoshi et al[496] showed that higher levels of dioxin correlated with higher levels of systemic inflammation (as measured by NFkB activity, which I have reviewed elsewhere[497]) and higher levels of blood glucose and increased risk of clinical diabetes; the results of this

---

[490] Vasquez A. "Detoxification: Clinical Relevance and Interventional Strategies for Adjunctive Treatment and Preventive Healthcare" in AFMCP: Applying Functional Medicine in Clinical Practice hosted by the Institute for Functional Medicine. Tampa, Florida November 2004 and Seattle, Washington March 2005. See Chapter 4.7 for review.

[491] Vasquez A, et al. The clinical importance of vitamin D (cholecalciferol). *Altern Ther Health Med.* 2004 Sep-Oct;10(5):28-36

[492] Henriksen GL, Ketchum NS, Michalek JE, Swaby JA. Serum dioxin and diabetes mellitus in veterans of Operation Ranch Hand. *Epidemiology.* 1997 May;8(3):252-8

[493] Calvert GM, Sweeney MH, Deddens J, Wall DK. Evaluation of diabetes mellitus, serum glucose, and thyroid function among United States workers exposed to 2,3,7,8-tetrachlorodibenzo-p-dioxin. *Occup Environ Med.* 1999 Apr;56(4):270-6. While the findings of this study are significant, the strength of the relationship between chemical exposure and insulin resistance was probably underestimated due to the researchers' focus on the specific dioxin subfraction 2,3,7,8-tetrachlorodibenzo-p-dioxin.

[494] Longnecker et al. Serum dioxin level in relation to diabetes mellitus among Air Force veterans with background levels of exposure. *Epidemiology.* 2000 Jan;11(1):44-8

[495] Fierens et al. Dioxin/polychlorinated biphenyl body burden, diabetes and endometriosis. *Biomarkers.* 2003 Nov-Dec;8(6):529-34

[496] Fujiyoshi et al. Molecular epidemiologic evidence for diabetogenic effects of dioxin exposure in US Air force veterans. *Environ Health Perspect.* 2006 Nov;114(11):1677-83

[497] Vasquez A. Nutritional and Botanical Inhibition of NF-kappaB, the Major Intracellular Amplifier of the Inflammatory Cascade. *Nutritional Perspectives* 2005;July: 5-12

study are particularly alarming because serum levels of toxins that correlated with increased risk of insulin resistance were comparable to levels found in the general population and which are generally considered "normal", assuming that chemical exposure and accumulation could ever be considered normal. **This research shows that background "every day" environmental exposure to dioxins and other chemical increases the risk of diabetes and insulin resistance even among patients with no occupational or accidental acute exposure to these chemicals.** Also in 2006, Vasiliu et al[498] showed that women with higher levels of polychlorinated biphenyls showed increased risk of diabetes. Further in 2006, Lee et al[499] showed a "striking dose-response relations between serum concentrations of six selected POPs [persistent organic pollutants] and the prevalence of diabetes" among a sample of more than 2,000 American citizens; note that this study is unique in that it analyzed a group of chemicals rather than a single or a small number of chemicals as performed in most of the previous studies. In 2007, Lee et al[500] published a follow-up study which again showed a clinically significant correlation between body burden of toxic chemicals and the incidence of insulin resistance and risk of diabetes.

Given the strong and consistent link between diabetes and the accumulation of toxic chemicals, two causal possibilities exist: either chemical accumulation causes diabetes, or diabetes causes chemical accumulation. While the former is more likely, the latter would not exclude clinicians and patients from the need to take action on this data because of the inherent risks associated with chemical accumulation. Toxic chemicals such as the ones associated with diabetes in the aforementioned studies are the same chemicals associated with induction of Parkinson's disease, and current evidence does indeed show increased risk of Parkinson's disease among diabetic patients.

Molecular Mechanisms of Xenobiotic Diabetogenesis: Toxic chemicals (xenobiotics) can cause insulin resistance and clinical diabetes mellitus by several different mechanisms. The aryl hydrocarbon receptor (hereafter: hydrocarbon receptor) is generally viewed as the molecular mechanism by which dioxin-like chemicals exert their adverse biological actions.[501] Stated simply, a leading hypothesis suggests that dioxin-like chemicals stimulate the hydrocarbon receptor to suppress glucohomeostatic activity of PPAR-gamma (peroxisome proliferator activated receptor gamma). PPAR-gamma is an intranuclear receptor that powerfully modulates insulin sensitivity and glucose utilization; indeed PPAR-gamma is the main target of the drug class of thiazolidinediones (TZDs) which are used in diabetes mellitus and other disorders of insulin resistance.[502] PPAR-gamma activation promotes insulin sensitivity and thus has a clear anti-diabetic effect by increasing the number of GLUT-4 receptors on the surface of muscle and adipose cells. Conversely, inhibition of PPAR-gamma (by toxin activation of the hydrocarbon receptor) causes a reduction in the number of GLUT-4 transporters which are required to move glucose from the serum into the intracellular space of muscle and adipose tissue. **Thus, the molecular mechanism and biologic plausibility by which toxic chemicals can lead to insulin resistance is clearly and firmly established based on in vitro studies, animal experiments, and the consistent data reported in humans.** Furthermore, secondary effects such as the estrogen-like action of many toxic chemicals may further complicate and exacerbate the diabetogenic effect of these toxins via upregulation of adipose accumulation. Increased adiposity from whatever cause correlates with increased serum levels of estrogens because adipose tissue expresses the aromatase enzyme which converts androgens into estrogens. Furthermore, adipose tissue is pro-inflammatory via the elaboration of cytokines (adipokines) which induce systemic inflammation and downregulate insulin sensitivity by decreasing the number of insulin receptors in adipose and muscle cell membranes. Many of the toxic chemicals that correlate with increased risk for diabetes have been shown in other studies to adversely affect thyroid function, directly leading to clinical and subclinical hypothyroidism and the resultant reduction in metabolic rate and propensity for weight gain and increased adiposity. Once established, the hyperglycemia of diabetes results in increase urinary excretion of nutrients such as magnesium, which is essential for peripheral insulin sensitivity and hepatic detoxification of xenobiotics; thus diabetes-induced magnesium deficiency can impair xenobiotic detoxification and thus contribute

---

[498] Vasiliu et al. Polybrominated biphenyls, polychlorinated biphenyls, body weight, and incidence of adult-onset diabetes mellitus. *Epidemiology.* 2006;17(4):352-9.

[499] Lee DH, Lee IK, Song K, Steffes M, Toscano W, Baker BA, Jacobs DR Jr. A strong dose-response relation between serum concentrations of persistent organic pollutants and diabetes: results from the National Health and Examination Survey 1999-2002. *Diabetes Care.* 2006 Jul;29(7):1638-44

[500] Lee et al. Association between serum concentrations of persistent organic pollutants and insulin resistance among nondiabetic adults. *Diabetes Care.* 2007 Mar;30(3):622-8

[501] Remillard RB, Bunce NJ. Linking dioxins to diabetes: epidemiology and biologic plausibility. *Environ Health Perspect.* 2002 Sep;110(9):853-8

[502] "PPAR-gamma is the main target of the drug class of thiazolidinediones (TZDs), used in diabetes mellitus and other diseases that feature insulin resistance." en.wikipedia.org/wiki/PPAR Accessed March 11, 2007

to an exacerbation of chemical accumulation. Lastly, some clinicians have proposed that increased adiposity may be a defensive means by which the body attempts to protect itself from chemical exposure, since increased fat stores will serve to dissipate and dilute absorbed chemicals and thus lessen their toxic effects. Anecdotal reports of rapid and effective weight loss have been observed in some patients following the implementation of clinical detoxification procedures, such as those outlined by the current author (Chapter 4, *Inflammation Mastery*) and detailed by others, notably Walter Crinnion ND as cited below.

Diabetes Treatment by Routine Methods—Unintentional Detoxification: I propose here that some of the commonly used methods for treating diabetes actually derive their benefits at least in part from their ability to enhance excretion of toxic chemicals. Exercise increases lipolysis which liberates fat-stored xenobiotics from adipose tissue, resulting in higher serum levels of toxins which thus increases urinary excretion of these toxins. Furthermore, the hyperventilation induced by exercise promotes respiratory alkalosis and the resultant alkalinization of the urine increases excretion of weakly acidic poisons. Relatedly, increased intake of fruits and vegetables promotes systemic and urinary alkalinization and thereby facilitates urinary excretion of poisons. Given evidence that systemic inflammation (in human studies of endotoxinemia) suppresses hepatic detoxification of xenobiotics, then the glucohomeostatic benefits of exercise, phytonutrient-rich diets, vitamin D3, fatty acid supplementation, and lipoic acid may be derived in part from the ability of these interventions to reduce systemic inflammation and thus facilitate (via derepression) xenobiotic biotransformation. The fiber of fruits and vegetables binds to chemicals which have undergone detoxification/biotransformation and which have been excreted in the bile; high-fiber diets reduce the recycling of toxins excreted into the gut. Magnesium supplementation improves insulin sensitivity, enables hepatic detoxification, and promotes urinary alkalinization. Fruits, vegetables, fiber, exercise, and magnesium supplementation all promote increased frequency of bowel movements to reduce enterohepatic recycling of (de)conjugated toxins. "Statin" cholesterol-lowering drugs (designed to inhibit the HMG-CoA reductase enzyme) activate the pregnane X receptor which upregulates xenobiotic detoxification and results enhanced toxin excretion. Cholestyramine, a drug that binds cholesterol in the gut and that is used in the treatment of diabetic hypercholesterolemia, also binds toxic chemicals excreted in the gut and can be used as effective therapy in patients with chronic chemical poisoning.[503] Therefore, the anti-diabetic, hypocholesterolemic, and insulin-sensitizing clinical effects of many commonly employed therapeutics may result directly and in part from the enhanced elimination of xenobiotics; this is a hitherto unappreciated mechanism of action for these treatments.

Diabetes Treatment by Detoxification—Proposal for Large-Scale Clinical Trials: Given the strength and direction of the research (sampled above) indicating that xenobiotic exposure and chemical accumulation is a major contributor to the epidemic of type-2 diabetes mellitus and other disorders of insulin resistance, all of us as researchers, clinicians, and healthcare consumers are potentially on the verge of a major paradigm shift in regard to our view of these disorders and their clinical management. If chemical exposure and accumulation contributes to insulin resistance, then healthcare professionals will have ethical and professional obligations to address these underlying problems in their patients who present with insulin resistance. Detoxification protocols, rather than endless and additive drug prescriptions to suppress the symptoms of the problem, could become the standard of care if such protocols are shown safe and effective for restoring glucohomeostasis. However, given the ubiquitous nature of xenobiotic exposure and the numeric infinity and methodological complexity of measuring levels of xenobiotics in individual patients, doctors and patients alike will be fighting an uphill battle against the constant onslaught of toxins, and both groups will have to start with an understanding of the body's inherent detoxification processes and the means by which these defense mechanisms can be supported in their respective roles. Given that we already have molecular mechanisms, animal research, and human data linking xenobiotic exposure to the genesis and perpetuation of insulin resistance, the only piece of the diabetes-xenobiotic puzzle that is missing is a large-scale clinical trial of effective therapeutic detoxification in patients with diabetes. If such a trial were to be skillfully designed and successfully implemented and was able to demonstrate amelioration of insulin resistance by interventions that are—to the extent possible—specific to the detoxification process (rather than directed toward

---

[503] "Cholestyramine offers a practical means for detoxification of persons exposed to chlordecone and possibly to other lipophilic toxins." Cohn WJ, Boylan JJ, Blanke RV, Fariss MW, Howell JR, Guzelian PS. Treatment of chlordecone (Kepone) toxicity with cholestyramine. Results of a controlled clinical trial. *N Engl J Med*. 1978 Feb 2;298(5):243-8

enhancement of insulin sensitivity), then an authentic breakthrough in the management of the rising pandemic of diabetes mellitus would have been achieved. Further, such a breakthrough would open the door to other trials in xenobiotic-associated diseases, particularly Parkinson's disease, autism[504], and many of the systemic autoimmune diseases such as systemic lupus erythematosus. In order to design and implement such trials, clinician researchers must start from an understanding of the biochemical and physiologic means by which detoxification occurs and the means by which such process can be supported and expedited to effect rapid elimination of toxins, and an overview of important concepts will be provided in the following section. Citations to research will be limited here due to space restrictions; excellent reviews of this subject include the works of Liska[505] and Crinnion.[506] What follows here is an excerpt from my previous work in the role of therapeutic detoxification in the treatment of musculoskeletal inflammation; see Chapter 4 of *Inflammation Mastery 4th Edition* for the complete list of references to the following paragraph.

Biochemistry and Physiology of Detoxification—Rationale for Clinical Therapeutics: Studies using blood tests and tissue samples from Americans across the nation have consistently shown that **all** Americans have toxic chemical **accumulation** whether or not they work in chemical factories or are exposed at home or work.[507,508] We cannot escape from the chemical consequences of living in a world with tens of thousands of synthetic chemicals. According to limited analyses, the average American has accumulated at least 18 different chemicals[509], and analyses that are more detailed show that even more chemicals and metals have been accumulated.[510] Common sources of these chemicals include pesticides, synthetic fertilizers, herbicides, fungicides, industrial pollution, car exhaust, solvents, paints, perfumes, plastic food/drink containers, non-stick cookware, Styrofoam, trichloroethylene from dry cleaning, rubber, carpet, plastics, glues, propellants, petroleum fuels such as gasoline, detergents, and other "cleaners." Clinical consequences of chemical toxicity are diverse, can affect nearly every organ system, and may be predicted to some extent by the pattern of chemical exposure since some chemicals have characteristic sequelae. Most of these chemicals are fat-soluble and can readily enter the body via respiratory, gastrointestinal, and transdermal routes. Once in the bloodstream, chemicals are either detoxified (inactivated and/or solubilized) by the liver and then excreted via urine or bile, or to a lesser extent exhaled from the lungs or excreted via sweat. Chemicals which are not excreted from the body are stored in the tissues, particularly lipid-rich organs such as the liver, adipose, and brain. Molecular turnover and recycling (particularly lipolysis) liberates fat-stored xenobiotics for another opportunity for either detoxification or additional toxicity. The main route for detoxification is the liver, which hydrosolublizes xenobiotics via oxidation ("phase one") and conjugation ("phase two"). Generally speaking, oxidation reactions are dependent on the cytochrome P-450 system, which can be inhibited by various drugs (e.g., ketoconazole, erythromycin, ritonavir, cimetidine, omeprazole, ethanol), foods such as ethanol and grapefruit juice, bacterial endotoxin from bacterial overgrowth of the bowel, and/or by genetic defects known as single nucleotide polymorphisms ("SNiPs") which reduce xenobiotic clearance. Similarly, conjugation reactions can be inhibited by a low-vegetable diet, SNiPs, and insufficiencies of conjugation moieties such as glutathione, glycine, glutamine, taurine, ornithine, sulfur, and methyl groups. If oxidation is too slow, then xenobiotics are insufficiently detoxicated and insufficiently processed for conjugation, leading to xenobiotic accumulation. If oxidation is too fast *relative to conjugation*, then reactive intermediates are formed which are commonly more toxic than the original xenobiotic. Optimally oxidized and conjugated xenobiotics are excreted in the urine or expelled in the bile. Supranormal hydration and urinary alkalinization enhance renal clearance of weakly acidic xenobiotics and drugs, whereas dehydration and urinary acidity impair toxin excretion, generally speaking. Conjugated toxins expelled in the bile can be deconjugated by bacteria so that the toxin is reabsorbed, a

[504] Vasquez A. "Chapter 10: Organ System Function and Underlying Mechanisms: The Interconnected Web." In Jones DS (Editor-in-Chief). *Textbook of Functional Medicine*. Institute for Functional Medicine, 2005. Vasquez A. Web-like Interconnections of Physiological Factors. *Integrative Med* 2006 April: 32-37 ichnfm.academia.edu/AlexVasquez
[505] Liska DJ. The detoxification enzyme systems. *Altern Med Rev*. 1998 Jun;3(3):187-98
[506] Crinnion WJ. Results of a decade of naturopathic treatment for environmental illnesses. *J Naturopathic Med* 1994;17:21-27. Crinnion WJ. Human burden of environmental toxins and their common health effects. *Altern Med Rev*. 2000 Feb:52-63; Crinnion WJ. Health effects of ubiquitous airborne solvent exposure. *Altern Med Rev* 2000 Apr:133-43
[507] "The average concentration of 2,3,7,8-tetrachlorodibenzo-p-dioxin in the adipose tissue of the US population was 5.38 pg/g, increasing from 1.98 pg/g in children under 14 years of age to 9.40 pg/g in adults over 45." Orban JE, Stanley JS, Schwemberger JG, Remmers JC. Dioxins and dibenzofurans in adipose tissue of the general US population and selected subpopulations. *Am J Public Health* 1994;84(3):439-45
[508] "Although the use of HCB as a fungicide has virtually been eliminated, detectable levels of HCB are still found in nearly all people in the USA." Robinson PE, Leczynski BA, Kutz FW, Remmers JC. An evaluation of hexachlorobenzene body-burden levels in the general population of the USA. *IARC Sci Publ* 1986;(77):183-92
[509] Schafer et al. Chemical Trespass: Pesticides in Our Bodies and Corporate Accountability. Pesticide Action Network North America. May 2004 panna.org/ on August 1, 2004
[510] Body Burden: The Pollution in People. ewg.org/issues/siteindex/issues.php?issueid=5004 Accessed February 6, 2006

phenomenon commonly referred to as "enterohepatic recycling" or "enterohepatic recirculation." Such recirculation is obviously less likely if gastrointestinal status and diet have been optimized to minimize the presence of deconjugating bacteria and to maximize fiber intake and laxation for the adsorption and expulsion of intraluminal toxins. Therapeutic colonics and enemas can be employed to stimulate bile flow from the liver[511,512] and to remove bile-secreted toxins from the gut before deconjugation and re-absorption occur. Bile formation and expulsion are further stimulated by botanical medicines such as beets, ginger, curcumin/turmeric[513], *Picrorhiza*, milk thistle, *Andrographis paniculata,* and *Boerhaavia diffusa*. Respiratory exhalation of toxins is enhanced by deep breathing and exercise, and hyperventilation promotes respiratory alkalosis which elevates urine pH and promotes excretion of weakly acidic drugs and xenobiotics as previously mentioned. Dermal excretion of toxins via sweat and expedited lipolysis are stimulated via low-temperature saunas and regular aerobic exercise. Xenobiotic oxidation can be promoted (cautiously) by reducing endotoxins from the gut and by the use of botanicals such as *Hypericum perforatum* which induce several isoforms of cytochrome P-450 via activation of the pregane X receptor. Xenobiotic conjugation is likewise promoted via nutrigenomic induction stimulated by cruciferous vegetables and their derivatives such as indole-3-carbinol (I3C) and dimethylindolylemethane (DIM). The plant-based diet is employed to provide fiber for bowel cleansing and the urinary alkalinization that is necessary for optimal urinary excretion of toxins, the majority of which are weak acids and are thus excreted more efficiently in alkaline urine. Sodium bicarbonate can also be used to induce urinary alkalinization. The diet must contain high-quality protein and can be supplemented with amino acids to support amino acid and glutathione conjugation. Serum, urine, and adipose samples can be analyzed to determine the intensity and diversity of chemical accumulation. For most patients, their chemical accumulation is so diverse that they may not display abnormally high levels of a specific chemical; their clinical manifestations are rather a manifestation of a wide plethora of different chemicals, which individually may be only modestly increased. Detoxification characteristics can be assessed from genotypic and phenotypic perspectives using appropriate laboratory tests. Phenotype can be assessed by serum and urine measurements of post-challenge detoxification of benzoate, caffeine, acetylsalicylic acid, and acetaminophen. Amino acid status can be

> **Xenobiotic-induced HTN and DM**
>
> Pesticides and other pollutants commonly induce mitochondrial dysfunction, thereby contributing to insulin resistance (impaired insulin secretion and reception) and vasoconstriction (via ROS-induced endothelial dysfunction), which promote HTN and DM.

quantified and qualified via serum or urine amino acid analysis. Stool testing assesses digestion, absorption, and microflora status. Clinical implementation of therapeutic detoxification follows a screening physical examination and basic laboratory assessment (minimally including CBC, metabolic panel, and urinalysis). Stool testing for dysbiosis is always reasonable when working with patients with fatigue and/or autoimmunity[514]; however, this and the other detoxification-related tests can often be deferred and/or used selectively. The Paleo-Mediterranean diet provides ample high-quality protein, alkalinization, fiber, and phytonutrients to which may be added supplements of protein, amino acids (especially NAC, glycine, and glutamine), and vitamins and minerals. Antioxidant teas and fresh fruit and vegetable juices are consumed to increase frequency of urination and promote urinary alkalinization due primarily to the content of potassium citrate. Exercise and low-temperature saunas promote sweating and xenobiotic-mobilizing lipolysis. Bile flow is further stimulated by consumption of beets, ginger, curcumin/turmeric, *Picrorhiza*, milk thistle, *Andrographis paniculata* and *Boerhaavia diffusa*. These interventions work in concert to enhance xenobiotic removal and cleanse the tissues of accumulated toxins. Intervention can be acute or periodic, but must be maintained for the long-term in order to resist the re-accumulation that is destined to result from the chemical onslaught that is inescapable in our polluted world.

Conclusion: Clinicians should now have an appreciation of the emerging research that links chemical accumulation to the development of diabetes. The molecular mechanisms have been explained, and the basic science and clinical research has been reviewed. Lastly, major considerations for the design and implementation of therapeutic detoxification programs have been presented. Formal clinical trials must be pursued, while individual clinicians explore the use of detoxification in their diabetic patients.

---

[511] Garbat, AL, Jacobi, HG. Secretion of bile in response to rectal installations. *Arch Intern Med* 1929; 44: 455-462

[512] "Caffeine enemas cause dilation of bile ducts, which facilitates excretion of toxic cancer breakdown products by the liver and dialysis of toxic products from blood across the colonic wall. The therapy must be used as an integrated whole." Gerson M. The cure of advanced cancer by diet therapy. *Physiol Chem Phys.* 1978;10(5):449-64

[513] "On the basis of the present findings, it appears that curcumin induces contraction of the human gall-bladder." Rasyid A, Lelo A. The effect of curcumin and placebo on human gall-bladder function: an ultrasound study. *Aliment Pharmacol Ther.* 1999 Feb;13(2):245-9

[514] Vasquez A. Nutritional and Botanical Treatments against "Silent Infections" and Gastrointestinal Dysbiosis. *Nutr Perspect* 2006; Jan. ichnfm.academia.edu/AlexVasquez

Migraine, Cluster and Other Headaches

Introduction:

This section focuses on migraine headaches in their classic and prototypic manifestations, originating primarily from the additive/synergistic combination of glial activation (and the related neurogenic inflammation and neuroinflammation) and mitochondrial dysfunction; understood as such, migraine and its closely related variant cluster headache can reasonably and very accurately be categorized within my model of metabolic inflammation— the manifestation of inflammation strongly associated with or caused by metabolic impairment, most generally noted in causal/contributory association with mitochondrial dysfunction. Per the origination of this work in my clinical textbooks (*Integrative Orthopedics*, 2004, 2007, 2012) and clinical monographs (*Musculoskeletal Pain*, 2008), this section includes clinical evaluation and differential diagnosis.

Description/pathophysiology:

- **Introduction**: Headaches are a common symptom-based diagnosis with a wide variety of underlying causes ranging from commonplace and benign (e.g., muscle tension headache) to catastrophic (e.g., meningitis or stroke). This section deals only with the pathophysiology and amelioration of routine benign headaches (migraine, cluster, allergic, tension, and cervicogenic); emphasis is placed on migraine headaches as the prototype for these disorders. Once serious pathological causes of headache have been excluded, the headache can be treated with symptom-suppressing drugs (which have associated risks and expenses without collateral benefits) or by biological/nutritional/natural interventions that address the underlying causative mechanisms and thereby improve overall health.

- **Social and medical significance**: Headaches and migraine—while seemingly insignificant compared to life-threatening diseases such as cancer and autoimmune diseases—account for huge losses in quality of life and productivity. Headache is a diagnosis based on the patient's subjective report of pain *in* (deep) or *on* (superficial) the head. The potential causes are numerous, ranging from benign muscle tension to life-threatening intracranial hemorrhage or meningitis. Of important note: migraine headache patients have increased risk for neurologic and cardiovascular diseases[1,2]; simply treating the *pain* of migraine does not address the underlying biochemical, physiologic, and inflammatory disturbances whereas nutritional and anti-inflammatory interventions hold great potential for both *alleviation of pain* and *improvement of overall health* via correction of the underlying pathophysiology.

- **Mechanism of pain sensation in headache**: The final common pathway for "primary" headaches (e.g., migraine and cluster headaches) is currently reported to be neurogenic/brain inflammation: inflammatory mediators from the brain generally and nerves specifically activate trigeminal (cranial nerve V) neurons to produce both vasoconstriction and the sensation of pain.[3]

- **A contemporary integrated model of migraine**: The task of intellectuals is the creation of cohesion, integration, and understanding; as such, one of the first tasks in the conversation on migraine is to define and characterize the disorder. Effective treatment, excepting blind luck, must be based on a comprehensive and cohesive understanding of the disorder in its *essential* totality. The major

---

Dysfunction precedes disease; understanding precedes efficacy

The best model of any disease is one that incorporates all of the major known facts into a cohesive and sequential understanding, predicting and being supported by efficacious treatments that are known to address the abnormal physiology—the dysfunction that precedes and causes the disease. The intellectual error of previous models of migraine is that they had no specific starting point, other than to attribute the genesis to "genetic traits and environmental triggers." As such, these earlier descriptions "started from the middle" and simply explained ongoing pathophysiology. By failing to start at the beginning, these earlier models likewise based their treatment on the downstream effects rather than on the treatment of the original cause of the disease. As such, the medical treatments based on this faulty model were necessarily ineffective. Here, I present a complete model, facilitating both understanding and treatment of various headache types.

---

[1] "Depression [adjusted OR = 2.12] and migraine [adjusted OR = 3.65] were more commonly recorded before the diagnosis of dementia in the DLB group." Fereshtehnejad et al. Comorbidity profile in dementia with Lewy bodies versus Alzheimer's disease. *Alzheimers Res Ther.* 2014 Oct 6;6(5-8):65

[2] "The migraine cohort had a higher prevalence of diabetes, hypertension, coronary artery disease, head injury and depression at baseline (p < 0.0001). After adjusting the covariates, migraine patients had a 1.33-fold higher risk of developing dementia [hazard ratio (HR) 1.33]. The sex-specific incidence rate of dementia was higher in men than in women in both cohorts, with an HR of 1.09 for men compared to women. Kaplan-Meier analysis shows that the cumulative incidence of dementia was 1.48% greater in the migraine cohort than in the nonmigraine cohort. This study shows that migraines are associated with a future higher risk of dementia after adjusting for comorbidities. Specifically, the association between migraine and dementia is greater in young adults than in older adults." Chuang et al. Migraine and risk of dementia. *Neuroepidemiology.* 2013;41:139-45

[3] Tierney ML. McPhee SJ, Papadakis MA (eds). *Current Medical Diagnosis and Treatment 2006, 45ᵗʰ Edition*. New York: Lange Medical Books; 2006, pages 31-33

themes from experimental studies and clinical trials have to be integrated and reconciled so that the best model of the disorder emerges triumphantly above the trivia of anecdote and the dogma of pharmaceutical profiteering. Beyond, in addition to, and in support of clinical efficacy, we need a grand unified theory (GUT) that helps us perceive the disease and prioritize the treatments; otherwise, a disarticulated understanding will perpetuate the disarrayed medical management and dependency that we currently observe in migraine and headache management. Each of the following components are sequentially ordered, starting with the first most important primary cause: mitochondrial dysfunction. Importantly, given that—as Thoreau noted in _Civil Disobedience_ (1849, p. 26)—"We love eloquence for its own sake, and not for any truth which it may utter", we cannot be satisfied with a clear explanation; the explanation has to have high merit in the real world, being proven by the safety and efficacy of the treatments that it advocates. This standard reveals the falsity of the medical model of both migraine and fibromyalgia, since both the models are selectively incomplete in order to justify drug treatment, and the interventions are unnecessarily hazardous and inadequately efficacious.

1. <u>Mitochondrial impairment is the origin of migraine and cluster headache</u>: Patients with migraine (and cluster headache) have very clear and consistent defects in mitochondrial performance, leading to cellular energy/ATP deficiency, excess production of free radicals (reactive oxygen species—ROS, which promote cellular damage and inflammation). Patients with migraine are often deficient in coenzyme Q-10 (CoQ10), and this causes mitochondrial dysfunction and reduced antioxidant protection against the harmful and pro-inflammatory effects of ROS. Nutritional treatments, such as riboflavin and CoQ10, which support mitochondrial function are consistently the safest and most effective anti-migraine treatments available, thereby proving the mitochondrial origin of migraine. Defects in cellular energy/ATP production cause neurons to be more unstable, resulting in excessive activation, resulting in pain sensation and sensitization. Mitochondrial dysfunction always promotes inflammation, at the very least by increasing formation of free radicals and the liberation of free ATP via leaky mitochondrial membranes; these molecules are perceived by cellular receptors as danger signals, thereby triggering the nonspecific alarm response of inflammation. The metabolic impairment likely contributes to vasodilation, as arteries dilate to bring more oxygen to support metabolic demand (in physiology, this is termed "reactive hyperemia").

   Increasingly over the past several years, the model of microglial activation along with mitochondrial dysfunction is gaining strength and due popularity; this model helps explain many divergent aspects of migraine and provides unification of previously fragmented models and disconnected facts. One of the strongest primary drivers of migraine is mitochondrial dysfunction, which shows a severity-response relationship and is maternally inheritable. Mitochondrial dysfunction is sufficient to promote (micro)glial activation, and the two then form a vicious cycle, ultimately promoting neocortical excitation and the resultant pain sensitization, thereby again promoting continuance and reinforcement of this vicious cycle. By analogy, the brains of these patients are "physiologically fragile" with a constant smoldering sterile inflammation; the brain is either constantly smoldering (e.g., chronic neuroinflammation) or actively "on fire" (e.g., migraine attack).

2. <u>Sustained glial activation results from mitochondrial dysfunction and causes brain inflammation and hyperexcitation</u>: Glial cells are the "glue"—the interconnecting cells—of the brain comprised chiefly of microglia and astrocytes. Microglia (the immune cells of the brain) are sensitive to ROS and inflammatory signals, and become "activated" (microglial activation) in response to peripheral inflammation (including obesity, trauma, infection and vaccination) and central "within the nervous system" events such as trauma and stress. When microglia become activated, they signal the astrocytes (cells that physically and chemically support neurons) to change behavior by providing _less protective support_ to brain neurons and _causing more stimulation_ of these same neurons; more stimulation with less protection causes the neurons to become "sensitized" and hyperresponsive and eventually promotes the "burn-out" of these neurons. The combinations of more excitation, more inflammation, less energy/ATP and less protection is called "excitotoxicity" (neuronal injury by overstimulation) and eventually leads to neurodegeneration, damage to neurons, brain structures, and the brain as a whole. Stated again and differently: microglia cells in the brain receive inflammatory stimuli and then trigger astrocytes to increase stimulation of neurons via the excitatory neurotransmitter glutamate, which activates a receptor called the NMDA receptor (NMDAr, detailed later); in this manner, inflammatory signals are converted into altered levels of neurotransmitters

(especially glutamate, also quinolinic acid [QUIN], a metabolite of tryptophan produced during conditions of inflammation, discussed later) which stimulate neurons to perceive more pain. Excessive stimulation of neurons feeds-back into causing more microglial activation, resulting in a vicious cycle.

3. <u>Brain inflammation, neuroinflammation, neurogenic inflammation all result from glial activation and promote additional brain inflammation</u>: Nerve cells become inflamed in response to any insult; this is called **neuroinflammation**, and it promotes various neurologic and psychiatric disorders, such as pain and depression (e.g., the components of **sickness behavior**), respectively. The neurons themselves can also release inflammatory mediators; this is called **neurogenic inflammation** because the inflammation is coming from the nerve cells while also affecting those same nerve cells. When **brain inflammation** is triggered, it affects all of the major cells types of the brain and becomes a self-reinforcing cycle, sometimes called "**brain on fire**."[4] Inflammation in the brain has many consequences; for example, ❶ inflamed neurons release neuropeptides and inflammatory mediators that activate endothelial cells (thereby causing vasoconstriction) and promote additional inflammation, and ❷ activation of mast cells and platelets causes these cells to secrete inflammatory/vasoactive amines, arachidonate metabolites (such as prostaglandins, leukotrienes, isoprostanes); these substances promote additional inflammation and also promote constriction of blood vessels. Remarkably, the brain inflammation and metabolic impairment seen in migraine known as **cortical spreading depression** triggers release of the inflammation-associated and tissue-destructive enzyme matrix metalloproteinase (MMP), which causes leakiness of the blood-brain barrier (BBB), leading to brain edema and enhanced uptake of inflammatory molecules from the blood.[5]

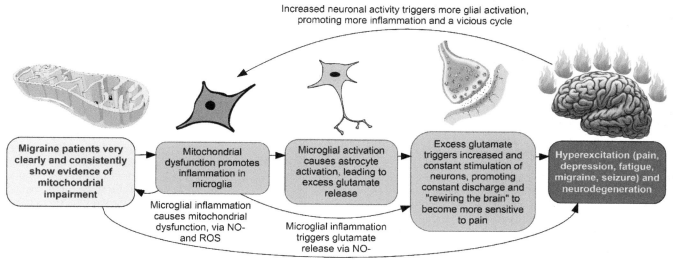

Increased neuronal activity triggers more glial activation, promoting more inflammation and a vicious cycle

| Migraine patients very clearly and consistently show evidence of mitochondrial impairment | Mitochondrial dysfunction promotes inflammation in microglia | Microglial activation causes astrocyte activation, leading to excess glutamate release | Excess glutamate triggers increased and constant stimulation of neurons, promoting constant discharge and "rewiring the brain" to become more sensitive to pain | Hyperexcitation (pain, depression, fatigue, migraine, seizure) and neurodegeneration |

Microglial inflammation causes mitochondrial dysfunction, via NO- and ROS

Microglial inflammation triggers glutamate release via NO-

Mitochondrial impairment causes neurons to be more vulnerable to normal activity and makes these neurons more sensitive to minor insults and stressors such as sound/light stimulation, hormonal fluctuations, emotional stress. The combination of mitochondrial dysfunction with excess excitation is particularly devastating to neurons, leading to neuron death: neurodegeneration.

<u>Foundational model of migraine</u>: ❶ Migraine patients very clearly and consistently show evidence of mitochondrial impairment: This genotropic mitochondrial dysfunction can be due to different factors, including 1) defects in CoQ10 synthesis, 2) defects in the citric acid cycle, and 3) defects in the function of the electron transport chain (ETC). The majority of these problems can be partly/largely circumvented by use of nutritional interventions. ❷ Mitochondrial dysfunction promotes inflammation in microglia: Sterile inflammation promoted by excess free radicals produced by dysfunctional mitochondria promote microglial activation. Microglial inflammation causes mitochondrial dysfunction via NO- (nitric oxide, causes impairment of Complex #4 in the electron transport chain[ETC], leading to reduced cellular energy/ATP production), ROS (reactive oxygen species, free radicals), and perhaps directly via inflammatory cytokines thereby creating a vicious cycle. ❸ Microglial activation causes astrocyte activation, leading to excess glutamate release. ❹ Excess glutamate triggers increased and constant stimulation of neurons, promoting constant discharge and "rewiring the brain" to become more sensitive to pain. ❺ Hyperexcitation promotes pain, depression, fatigue, seizure, migraine and neurodegeneration. The combination of mitochondrial dysfunction with excess excitation is particularly devastating to neurons, leading to neuron death: neurodegeneration. Image of brain by IsaacMao per Flickr.com via creativecommons.org/licenses/by/2.0. See educational videos and updates at www.inflammationmastery.com/pain

---

[4] Cohen G. The brain on fire? *Ann Neurol.* 1994 Sep;36(3):333-4
[5] Moskowitz MA. Genes, proteases, cortical spreading depression and migraine: impact on pathophysiology and treatment. *Funct Neurol.* 2007 Jul-Sep;22(3):133-6

Brain neuron excitation

- Glutamate/NMDA receptors are activated by glutamate, QUIN and homocysteine
- Reduced mitochondrial performance impairs homeodynamics in response to excessive NMDAr stimulation
- Free radicals from mitochondria, neurons, and glia promote molecular and cellular damage thereby triggering inflammation and metabolic collapse of neurons
- Excess intracellular calcium triggers inflammation
- Hyperexcitation promotes pain, pain sensitization, and neurodegeneration

Mitochondrial dysfunction

- Increases in oxidant production promote progressive inflammation and metabolic collapse
- Promotes inflammation in all affected cells
- Depletes antioxidant nutrients such as CoQ10, thereby leading to additional vulnerability, inflammation, and mitochondrial dysfunction
- Makes neurons vulnerable/fragile to excessive activation (eg, lowered depolarization threshold) due to oxidant damage and increased intracellular calcium
- Mitochondrial ROS cause mitochondrial damage, which increases ROS production in a vicious cycle

Central sensitization, cortical spreading depression, metabolic collapse

Image © by Dr Alex Vasquez, ICHNFM.ORG

Microglial activation, astrocyte activation

- Increased oxidant production promotes progressive inflammation and metabolic collapse
- NO- causes mitochondrial dysfunction at ETC #4 and triggers glutamate release to activate NMDAr
- Inflammatory response creates QUIN to activate NMDAr
- Inflammation promotes leaky blood-brain barrier and additional inflammation, edema

The vicious cycles of migraine, free radical production/damage, "metabolic collapse" and cortical spreading depression: Illustration of the interconnecting cycles that promote persistent and additive/synergistic brain inflammation, neuron dysfunction, stemming from primary mitochondrial dysfunction. Integrated models of migraine are now available, providing better understanding, more effective treatment, and less medical dependency. This model of *brain hypersensitivity induced by mitochondrial dysfunction* helps explain why migraine patients 1) are vulnerable to otherwise innocuous stimuli such as hormonal fluctuations and changes in weather, 2) respond poorly to drug treatments, which generally fail to address these components sufficiently, and 3) respond brilliantly to nutritional interventions that support mitochondrial function and reduce inflammation. Independently from my own models of migraine (described and illustrated in this section), Malkov et al[6] proved the merit of the model I have illustrated by showing that "Reactive oxygen species initiate metabolic collapse" in brain neurons, and that this free radical damage that tripartitely damages neurons, glia, and mitochondria is a major cause of cortical spreading depression. See educational videos and updates at www.inflammationmastery.com/pain

4. <u>Mitochondrial dysfunction and glial activation combine to cause altered brain neuron function—brain destabilization, metabolic fragility; in its entirety, this three-part combination of mitochondrial dysfunction, glial inflammation, and neuronal dysfunction is called cortical spreading depression (CSD)</u>: Neurons are simultaneously hyperactive due to (NMDA) neurotransmitter receptor activation and also hyporesponsive due to the mitochondrial impairment; this "physiologic confusion" contributes to the altered brain function seen in migraine, especially migraine with aura. In migraine, the brain is "destabilized" (per Moskowitz[7]), leading to what I call "metabolic fragility" or "brain fragility" that makes migraine patients more sensitive to changes in diet, climate, hormones, stress and sleep. These combinations of ❶ metabolic/mitochondrial impairment with ❷ increased/altered brain activity (e.g., specifically mediated by glutamate at the NMDA

Mitochondrial dysfunction is a key component of migraine
"In migraine, the degree of the mitochondrial impairment ... is related to the severity of the clinical phenotype."
Lodi et al. *J Neurol Sci.* 1997 Feb

---

[6] Malkov et al. Reactive oxygen species initiate a metabolic collapse in hippocampal slices: potential trigger of cortical spreading depression. *J Cereb Blood Flow Metab.* 2014 Sep;34(9):1540-9

[7] Moskowitz MA. Genes, proteases, cortical spreading depression and migraine: impact on pathophysiology and treatment. *Funct Neurol.* 2007 Jul-Sep;22(3):133-6

receptor) and ❸ glial/neuronal/brain inflammation is what creates the wave of abnormal brain function—cortical spreading depression—that typifies migraine and which promotes its exacerbation; cortical spreading depression (CSD) leads to elaboration of the inflammatory and destructive enzyme MMP9 which causes leakiness of the BBB and subsequent brain edema (secondary to protein and water entry into the brain) and increased brain entry of substances from the blood, such as peripherally derived proinflammatory cytokines.[8,9] Brain edema in migraine is associated with and likely contributes to reduced brain perfusion (ie, reduced blood flow).[10] Very importantly, enhanced glutaminergic neurotransmission is itself sufficient to induce cortical spreading depression in experimental models. In an insightful article published in 2014 that supports the model that I have proposed, Malkov et al[11] showed that cortical spreading depression is caused by elaboration of reactive oxygen species (ROS, free radicals) and that these initiate "metabolic collapse" in brain cells.

> **All of these components are interconnected and thus the terms and components become (ultimately/practically) conceptually synonymous**
>
> Since microglial activation causes astrocyte activation, these terms can be summarized as glial activation. Microglial activation triggers formation of QUIN, which along with glutamate from astrocyte activation, causes stimulation of the NMDA receptor, promoting excitation of neurons. Since glial activation causes neuronal excitation, we can generally state that glial activation is synonymous with hyperexcitation of neurons, which segues into excitotoxic death of neurons and neurodegeneration. Persistent and prolonged hyperexcitation of neurons causes these neurons to strengthen their connections with each other, leading to facilitated pain perception, called central sensitization, as noted in **migraine, fibromyalgia**, and **complex regional pain syndrome**. Microglial activation—via release of nitric oxide (NO-) —causes mitochondrial dysfunction and additional glutamate release, causing the combination of metabolic impairment (e.g., reduced ATP formation) and increased metabolic demand, because activation of the NMDA receptor by glutamate and QUIN imposes increased metabolic demand on the neuron cells as they must control the resulting influx of calcium, which if not controlled will promote additional inflammation, impairment, and neuronal cell death.

5. Pain route—the covering of the brain is sensitive to metabolic and inflammatory changes within the brain, and interprets the inflammatory substances as pain signals: The trigeminal nerve (cranial nerve V, #5) receives transmissions from nerve endings surrounding the blood vessels of the membrane surrounding the brain (pia mater) and inside of the skull (dura mater). Recall as previously discussed and cited that the blood-brain barrier becomes more permeable when the brain is inflamed, thereby promoting passage/diffusion of inflammatory mediators from the brain to nearby neurons that receive noxious stimuli and convert the reception of those substances into nerve impulses received and interpreted as pain signals (nociception). While sensory innervation of the supratentorial dura mater membrane is via small meningeal branches of the trigeminal nerve, the innervation for the infratentorial dura mater is via upper cervical nerves, thereby establishing a bidirectional relationship between neck pain (and other subconscious neurologic inputs) and intracranial stimuli and structures.

6. Pain sensitization: As more pain signals are received, the brain facilitates the reception of these messages and thereby becomes more sensitive to the reception of pain; this is called central sensitization, and is greatly facilitated by brain inflammation and mitochondrial impairment.

7. Blood vessel dilation and constriction, and the role of serotonin-1D receptors: Metabolic impairment can trigger vasodilation, while inflammatory mediators promote vasoconstriction; both vasodilation and vasoconstriction have been noted in migraine.

8. Nuances in the contribution of various factors leads to different clinical presentations (e.g., migraine headaches vs cluster headaches); however, in the main primary headache conditions—migraine and cluster—the main themes of mitochondrial dysfunction and brain inflammation dominate the causal pathophysiology and therefore guide treatment: The model presented and used here is that cluster headache is simply a variant of migraine headache, with secondary rather than primary causes of the

---

[8] Moskowitz MA. Genes, proteases, cortical spreading depression and migraine: impact on pathophysiology and treatment. *Funct Neurol*. 2007 Jul-Sep;22(3):133-6

[9] Wilson CJ, Finch CE, Cohen HJ. Cytokines and cognition--the case for a head-to-toe inflammatory paradigm. *J Am Geriatr Soc*. 2002 Dec;50(12):2041-56

[10] For evidence of brain edema (with associated hypoperfusion) in patients with migraine: Kim et al. Recurrent steroid-responsive cerebral vasogenic edema in status migrainosus and persistent aura. *Cephalalgia*. 2015 Jul;35:728-34. See also: Bereczki et al. Cortical spreading edema in persistent visual migraine aura. *Headache*. 2008 Sep;48:1226-9

[11] Malkov et al. Reactive oxygen species initiate a metabolic collapse in hippocampal slices: cortical spreading depression. *J Cereb Blood Flow Metab*. 2014 Sep;34(9):1540-9

underlying mitochondrial dysfunction, and with a greater contribution by psychoemotional stress, muscle tension, and nutritional deficiencies. Mitochondrial dysfunction is seen in both migraine and cluster headache.[12] Nutritional deficiencies (e.g., folic acid) and excesses of systemic inflammation and serum homocysteine are noted in various types of headache, in both adult and pediatric populations.[13]

- Pathophysiology—from past to current models: The sensation of headache pain results from activation and sensitization of sensory trigeminal pain neurons that service intracranial blood vessels and meninges. For many years, the debate focused on whether *vasculogenic* or *neurogenic* influences predominated; most if not all headaches appear to involve *both* of these main components, thus allowing for the consensus that headaches have a *neurovascular* component. That said, the weight of evidence increasingly shifted to support the *neurological* origin—from within the brain and neurons (rather than the blood vessels)—of headaches in general and migraines in particular. "Brain-initiated events" such as cortical spreading depression—a wave of electrical and metabolic disturbance that sweeps across the brain surface, making the brain tissue physiologically unstable, and thus more fragile and vulnerable to various insults—culminate in the release of pain-inducing nociceptive substances including hydrogen ions and arachidonate metabolites, which irritate trigeminovascular sensory neurons surrounding pial vessels.[14,15]

Both dilation and constriction of arteries has been noted in migraine. Dilation of arteries may be an early compensatory response to impaired cellular energy/ATP production as mitochondrial dysfunction progresses from mild to more severe as vicious cycles exacerbate an ever-present primary defect; vasodilation in response to impaired energy/ATP production is well known in physiology as "reactive hyperemia." As mitochondrial

Brain sensitization to pain: 4 main components
1. Pain signals: Defects in cellular energy/ATP production cause neurons to be more unstable, resulting in excessive activation, resulting in pain sensation and sensitization. Mitochondrial dysfunction always promotes inflammation, at the very least by increasing formation of free radicals, which are perceived by cellular receptors as danger signals. The metabolic impairment likely contributes to vasodilation, as arteries dilate to bring more oxygen to support metabolic demand (in physiology, this is termed "reactive hyperemia").
2. Brain inflammation: Microglia and astrocytes in the brain transform inflammatory signals into altered levels of neurotransmitters which further activate neurons.
3. Mitochondrial dysfunction: Nerve cells become inflamed in response to any insult; this is called **neuroinflammation**, and it promotes various neurologic and psychiatric disorders. The neurons themselves can also release inflammatory mediators; this is called **neurogenic inflammation** because the inflammation is coming from the nerve cells. When **brain inflammation** is triggered, it affects all of the major cell types of the brain and becomes a self-reinforcing cycle that has been called **brain on fire**. Released neuropeptides activate endothelial cells, mast cells, and platelets to then increase extracellular levels of amines, arachidonate metabolites, peptides, and ions; these substances promote additional inflammation and also promote constriction of blood vessels.
4. Free radicals, reactive oxygen species (ROS): "We show that ROS accumulation...is capable of triggering an abrupt metabolic collapse (MC) that reproduces most features of cortical spreading depression (CSD). This suggests that oxidative stress may be the primary cause of CSD and not just its consequence. In pathological conditions, the failure to neutralize ROS during the excessive ROS surge and/or deficiency of the neuronal antioxidant system may result in the MC and subsequent ignition of CSD. Indeed, our in vivo results show that when the oxidative stress-induced ROS accumulation is suppressed by an exogenous antioxidant, CSD occurrence is strongly reduced."*

*Malkov et al. Reactive oxygen species initiate a metabolic collapse: potential trigger of cortical spreading depression. *J Cereb Blood Flow Metab.* 2014 Sep

function deteriorates before and during a migraine attack, it segues from a metabolic problem to an inflammatory problem, and the consequences of mitochondrial dysfunction (e.g., ROS, inflammation, failure of calcium homeostasis) plus brain neuron dysfunction due to excessive excitation (e.g., ROS, inflammation, failure of calcium homeostasis) lead to vasoconstriction specifically via increased intracellular calcium in

---

[12] "The maximum rate of mitochondrial ATP production (Qmax), calculated from the rate of post-exercise PCr recovery and the end-exercise [ADP], was low in cluster headache patients as well as in migraine patients except MwoA. In migraine the degree of the mitochondrial impairment, that apparently is associated with a reduced glycolytic flux, is related to the severity of the clinical phenotype." Lodi et al. Quantitative analysis of skeletal muscle bioenergetics and proton efflux in migraine and cluster headache. *J Neurol Sci.* 1997 Feb 27;146(1):73-80

[13] "Mean values for body mass index, C-reactive protein, and homocysteine were higher in children with than without headaches, and more children with headaches were in the highest quintile of risk for these factors. Serum and red blood cell folate levels were lower in children with headache. More children with headache were in the highest quintile of risk for 3 or more of these factors. Several important risk factors for long-term vascular morbidity cluster in children and adolescents with severe or recurrent headache or migraine. Further study and screening of children with headaches may permit improved preventive management." Nelson et al. Headache and biomarkers predictive of vascular disease in a representative sample of US children. *Arch Pediatr Adolesc Med.* 2010 Apr;164(4):358-62

[14] Moskowitz MA. Pathophysiology of headache—past and present. *Headache.* 2007 Apr;47 Suppl 1:S58-63

[15] Moskowitz MA. Genes, proteases, cortical spreading depression and migraine: impact on pathophysiology and treatment. *Funct Neurol.* 2007 Jul-Sep;22(3):133-6

astrocytes and inflammation-triggered phospholipase-A2-catalized formation of vasoconstrictive prostaglandins, specifically prostaglandin E2 (PGE2) and F2-alpha (PGF2), which are also elaborated from endometrial tissue, thereby supporting the biochemical basis of menstrual migraine.[16]

Neurogenic inflammation (in this conversation, the release of neuropeptides from trigeminal nerve [cranial nerve V] neurons to local blood vessels and meninges) is also important and contributes to a vicious cycle of pain and inflammation.[17] Elevated intracellular calcium levels that trigger inflammatory pathways can be promoted by arachidonate, secondary hyperparathyroidism due to vitamin D deficiency, a relative insufficiency of magnesium, and also by mitochondrial impairment. Mast cell degranulation releases inflammatory mediators such as serotonin, prostaglandin I-2, and histamine, which induce local inflammation and activation of meningeal nociceptors[18,19] and might serve as a pathophysiological link between emotional stress or allergen exposure and headache (i.e., the link between environmental stressors and headache pain). Mast cells can also be activated by neuropeptides that originate from neurons in the brain parenchyma/tissue. Further substantiating the role of local inflammation in migraine is the finding of increased activity of nuclear transcription factor-kappa B (NFkB) in jugular blood of migraine patients during migraine episode[20]; NFkB is an important mediator of inflammation through its ability to enhance transcription of genes that encode for inflammatory mediators.[21] This model provides for the often observed continuum between external and biopsychosocial factors such as exposure to bright lights, hypoglycemia, stress, anxiety, allergen exposure, and hormonal fluctuations with the triggering of new or recurrent headaches. An appreciation for the intraneuronal genesis of headaches such as migraines sharpens our focus on events occurring *within the neuronal cell*, particularly impaired mitochondrial bioenergetics, increased intraneuronal calcium, and the elaboration of inflammatory mediators derived from omega-6 (n6) polyunsaturated fatty acids. With the realization of mitochondrial and eicosanoid contributions to headache, clinicians can intervene with nutritional intervention and fatty acid supplementation to enhance mitochondrial function and modulate eicosanoid production, respectively. Failure to appreciate these underlying pathophysiological mechanisms forces clinicians and patients to rely on pharmacological symptom suppression while the underlying processes remain unaddressed.

The historically documented failure of migraine treatments has arisen largely from the incomplete model of the disease upon which those treatments are founded. Without raw luck, a treatment based on an erroneous or incomplete model has no chance of providing *major*—let alone *optimal*—benefit. Any listing of medical treatments for migraine reveals a catalog of chaos: bits and pieces of incomplete and inconsistent models and the resulting therapy—ie, drugs—which address a small fraction of the problem and therefore have to be overpowered in effect to compensate for their minor significance; hence the low efficacy and high risk of adverse effects.

Important for the perpetuation of any ongoing disease are the vicious cycles that are initiated and maintained; skilled clinicians focus on breaking these vicious cycles because failure to do so allows the disease condition to re-initiate and perpetuate, even after limited therapeutic efficacy of incomplete treatment. I might introduce the concept of "double-stranded" or "triple-stranded" (etc) therapies that simultaneously break multiple vicious cycles, in contrast to treatments such as with drugs which focus only on a single molecule or a single pathway, ie, single-stranded therapy. In this metaphor, the "strands" are biochemical and physiologic pathways; the more that we can optimize the maximum number of pathways, the greater our opportunities for restoring and enjoying optimal health.

A 2015 review discussing fibromyalgia (FM) and complex regional pain syndrome (CRPS) focused on "neurogenic neuroinflammation", the essential definition/concept of which is that that neuronal activity in general and its inflammatory effects in particular can become autonomous and self-perpetuating; neuroinflammation could be initiated externally so-to-speak by stress or trauma and then become a vicious

[16] Shaik MM, Gan SH. Vitamin supplementation as possible prophylactic treatment against migraine with aura and menstrual migraine. *Biomed Res Int.* 2015;2015:469529
[17] Tierney ML. McPhee SJ, Papadakis MA (eds). *Current Medical Diagnosis and Treatment 2006, 45th Edition*. New York: Lange Medical Books; 2006, pages 31-33
[18] Levy D, Burstein R, Kainz V, Jakubowski M, Strassman AM. Mast cell degranulation activates a pain pathway underlying migraine headache. *Pain.* 2007 Jul;130(1-2):166-76
[19] Zhang XC, et al. Sensitization and activation of intracranial meningeal nociceptors by mast cell mediators. *J Pharmacol Exp Ther.* 2007 Aug;322(2):806-12
[20] Sarchielli et al. NF-kappaB activity and iNOS expression in monocytes from internal jugular blood of migraine without aura during attacks. *Cephalalgia.* 2006 Sep; 1071-9
[21] Tak PP, Firestein GS. NF-kappaB: a key role in inflammatory diseases. *J Clin Invest.* 2001 Jan;107(1):7-11

cycle within the nervous system promoting chronic pain and neurodegeneration.[22] The existence of neurogenic neuroinflammation is physiologically *likely* and becomes *probable* within dysfunctional and predisposed (i.e., "primed") metabolic and physiologic systems; such "priming factors" clearly include a pro-inflammatory diet, nutrient deficiencies (especially of vitamin B6, magnesium, vitamin D, and CoQ10), mitochondrial dysfunction, and dysbiosis. Hence, the treatment of persistently painful and inflammatory disorders—including but not limited to migraine, recurrent headaches, fibromyalgia and CRPS—needs to focus on the treatment of factors which continue to sustain these disease processes.

- The importance of glutamate and the NMDA receptor in headache, migraine, and chronic pain syndromes: The excitatory neurotransmitter glutamate stimulates neurons by binding to the NMDA (N-methyl-D-aspartate) receptor (NMDAr). As shown in the diagram, excitatory glutamate (which promotes pain, seizure, migraine, anxiety and depression) can be converted into inhibitory GABA (gamma-amino butyric acid, which has an inhibitory, relaxing effect on neurons and the brain as a whole) via the enzyme glutamic acid decarboxylase, which is dependent upon and also dose-dependently stimulated by the vitamin pyridoxine (vitamin B6). Stimulation of the NMDA receptor by glutamate and other receptor activators such as QUIN (quinolinic acid, a "dysfunctional metabolite" of the amino acid L-tryptophan which is formed in response to inflammation and which causes additional inflammation, oxidative damage, and neurotoxicity) causes calcium to enter into the stimulated neuron cells to trigger activation or "firing" of the neuron. A moderate amount of NMDAr stimulation is a normal part of learning and the formation of memories—normal and healthy neurologic function; however, too much NMDAr stimulation causes overstimulation (excitotoxicity) of neurons thereby promoting pain, depression, anxiety, migraine, seizure/epilepsy, and neurodegeneration. Magnesium and zinc partly block the NMDAr calcium channel to reduce/modulate calcium entry into neurons; in this way, magnesium and zinc might be thought of as "softening the effect" of NMDAr activation. The safety and efficacy of supplemental pyridoxine (vitamin B6) in reducing glutamate levels—and thus reducing excessive stimulation of the NMDAr by glutamate—necessitates its inclusion in the treatment of any and all chronic pain disorders, especially migraine and fibromyalgia. Pyridoxine does more than simply lower glutamate levels, as pyridoxine also helps to lower homocysteine (HYC) levels. Glutamate and HYC are both amino acids that activate the NMDAr and mGluR[23]—the metabotropic glutamate receptor (detailed shortly). Generally, higher homocysteine levels correlate with fatigue and pain in patients with fibromyalgia and chronic fatigue syndrome, and with headache pain and increased cardiovascular disease risk in patients with migraine.[24]

- In the treatment of pain—including headaches and fibromyalgia—reducing the effects of glutamate-mediated neurotransmission and cellular effects is of very high importance: Glutamate is an amino acid with many functions, including serving as a precursor to the antioxidant glutathione (GSH), serving as a precursor to alpha-keto-glutarate (a substrate for energy production in the Krebs/citrate cycle in mitochondria) and serving as an excitatory neurotransmitter. Our concern in this conversation is with glutamate's role as a stimulator of neurotransmission in the peripheral and central nervous system; while some minimal glutaminergic stimulation is normal and necessary, excess glutaminergic neurotransmission very clearly promotes anxiety, depression, fibromyalgia pain, myofascial pain and myofascial trigger points, migraine and headaches, seizures and epilepsy; in the extreme, excess glutamate in the brain causes over-excitation of neurons leading to cell death—neurodegeneration—and either mild or massive, acute or chronic, brain damage. In the following image and subsequent descriptors, I provide an accurate and yet simplified overview of important concepts, but I will state plainly here what everyone needs to know about this section: Because glutaminergic neurotransmission promotes pain/anxiety/depression/neurodegeneration, our therapeutic goals are to 1) reduce glutamate levels with vitamin B6 and by avoiding/treating microglial activation (ie, "brain inflammation"), 2) reduce glutamate-triggered influx of calcium with zinc and magnesium, also vitamin D, alkalinization (increased consumption of base-forming foods, such as fruits and vegetables which contain citrate which is converted to bicarbonate to promote alkalinization, one effect of which is to promote magnesium retention, thereby alleviating pain[25]), omega-3 fatty acids such as from fish oil, 3) reduce the effects

[22] Littlejohn G. Neurogenic neuroinflammation in fibromyalgia and complex regional pain syndrome. *Nat Rev Rheumatol.* 2015 Nov;11(11):639-48
[23] Abushik et al. NMDA and mGluR5 in calcium mobilization and neurotoxicity of homocysteine in trigeminal/cortical neurons and glial cells. *J Neurochem.* 2014 Apr; 264-74
[24] "Mean homocysteine plasma levels - as well as the proportion of subjects with hyperhomocysteinaemia - were significantly higher in patients with MA than in healthy controls." Moschiano et al. Homocysteine plasma levels in patients with migraine with aura. *Neurol Sci.* 2008 May;29 Suppl 1:S173-5
[25] Vormann et al. Supplementation with alkaline minerals reduces symptoms in patients with chronic low back pain. *J Trace Elem Med Biol.* 2001;15(2-3):179-83

of glutamate/NMDA receptor activation by counterbalancing with benzodiazepine/GABA receptor activation by promoting conversion of glutamate to GABA and perhaps also by using niacinamide and botanicals that act as ligands for the GABA receptor. Because much of this information is both important and a bit complicated, I will create some teaching videos on this material and make them available per the following internet link/redirect: www.inflammationmastery.com/pain

Glutamate is increased by dietary MSG, deficiencies of B6 and Mg, glial activation, genotropic enzyme defects

Other agonists (eg, QUIN, homocysteine) and co-agonists

Glutamate (neuroexcitatory)

Glutamic acid decarboxylase requires P5P, the active form of vitamin B6

GABA (neuroinhibitory)

Other agonists (eg, niacinamide, ethanol, several botanicals)

NMDA-type glutamate receptor

Zn

Mg

GABA receptor

Calcium entry following activation of glutamate receptor: excitatory/stimulatory effect

Chloride entry following activation of GABA receptor: inhibitory effect

NMDA receptors are located in the brain, spinal cord, and peripheral tissues, including nerves, muscles and skin

Neuron cell membrane

Glutamate-activated calcium channel

Excess dietary arachidonate and insufficient EPA increases intracellular calcium

Mild hyperparathyroidism (most commonly due to vitamin D3 insufficiency)

Excess intracellular calcium: relative to magnesium, secondary to true magnesium deficiency or mild chronic metabolic acidosis with resultant loss of intracellular magnesium

Increased/excess intracellular calcium; nerve depolarization activation of intracellular pathways

GABA receptor activation increases intracellular chloride which has inhibitory, calming, relaxing, analgesic effects

Glutamate receptors in the brain: Neurocortical excitation, promotion of inflammation (neuroinflammation), promotion of mitochondrial dysfunction, apoptosis/neurodegeneration

Glutamate receptors in the periphery: Glutamate receptors (including NMDAr) are located throughout the body; increased glutamate signaling promotes neurogenic inflammation, peripheral pain sensitization, muscle contraction

Central sensitization, increased pain sensitivity (hyperalgesia), depression and anxiety, migraine and seizure

Muscle contraction/hypertonicity, myofascial trigger points (MFTP), muscle cramps, hypertension due to increased peripheral resistance

Clinically relevant conceptual illustration of the NMDA-type glutamate receptor (NMDAr), its activation, effects, and nutritional modulation: The image above provides a conceptually accurate and clinically applicable model of glutamate reception and the effects thereof; categorized details are provided below, listed from top to bottom of the image and also prioritized to clinical relevance (top) and additional details and context (bottom). See instructional videos at ICHNFM.ORG.

Image caption—continued from previous page:

- Various types of glutamate receptors in the central nervous system and periphery share the common themes of promoting pain and inflammation: Glutamate receptors are described in two broad categories; **ionotropic glutamate receptors—iGluR**—(divided into three groups: AMPA, NMDA and kainate receptors) transpose ions such as sodium and calcium upon activation and thus can be considered mostly involved with propagation of nerve impulses, while **metabotropic glutamate receptors—mGluR**—(also with several subtypes, such as mGluR5) lead more to activation of intracellular pathways with results dependent on the cell type but generally consistent with some type of cellular activation and/or inflammation.

- Glutamate reception, with the NMDA receptor (NMDAr) as the prototype receptor: Many types and subtypes of glutamate receptors exist, and the specific subtype NMDA is very clearly the most discussed for its relevance in both chronic pain disorders and neurodegenerative diseases. The NMDA receptor is activated by glutamate, QUIN (quinolinic acid, a metabolite of tryptophan made in inflammatory conditions, discussed in more detail in the section on fibromyalgia), aspartate, homocysteine and other substances which act as agonists/activators or required co-activators/co-agonists (e.g., D-serine, glycine). Different forms of the NMDA receptor exist in the central and peripheral nervous systems, each with slightly different characteristics and sensitivity to agonists and requirement for co-agonists; thus, the image presented here is a generalized version that is conceptually accurate (rather than all-inclusive; for more details see reviews[26]) and clinically relevant. Although we have traditionally thought of glutamate/NMDA receptors as existing separately (ie, on different cell types) from the GABA/benzodiazepine receptors, that fact remains true (ie, some cells are clearly dominated by one receptor type over others) while we are also increasingly appreciating that glutamate/NMDA receptors can coexist with GABA/benzodiazepine receptors on the same cell and that these receptors are interactive, not simply oppositional, and occasionally behave/interact in paradoxical and age-specific manners.[27,28]

- Homocysteine (HYC), a toxic intermediate of amino acid metabolism, activates glutamate receptors, thereby promoting pain, headache/migraine/seizure: Glutamate is the prototypic excitatory neurotransmitter, activating a wide range of ionotropic glutamate receptors (including the NMDA receptor) and metabotropic glutamate receptors (mGluR) which are present throughout the central and peripheral nervous systems and all of which are generally involved in (enhanced) pain processing. We have exacting clarity that both NMDA receptors and mGluR5 are activated by homocysteine with resultant calcium influx just as with glutamate-mediated activation of these same receptors; Abushik et al[29] published in 2014, "Thus, elevation of intracellular calcium (Ca2) by HCY in neurons is mediated by NMDA and mGluR5 receptors while SGC are activated through the mGluR5 subtype. Long-term neurotoxic effects in peripheral and central neurons involved both receptor types. Our data suggest glutamatergic mechanisms of HCY-induced sensitization and apoptosis of trigeminal nociceptors." This is of very high clinical importance, because we gain the mechanistic insight that lowering of homocysteine levels (technique detailed later) will reduce the total stimulation of these glutamate receptors in the brain, spinal cord, and periphery to reduce the pain and fatigue of migraine, fibromyalgia, and other pain conditions.

- Glutamate promotes pain and inflammation; therefore, reducing levels of glutamate or reducing the effects of its reception are important therapeutic goals, especially in the treatment of pain, anxiety/depression, migraine, and seizure/epilepsy: Glutamate levels are increased by microglial inflammation and the subsequent astrocyte activation[30]; therefore, reducing inflammation generally and "brain inflammation" specifically is an important therapeutic goal. Reducing inflammation must always focus on the trigger of the inflammation, most commonly microbial (e.g., gastrointestinal dysbiosis[31]) and/or metabolic (e.g., excess sugar and "junk/fast food" in the diet[32], vitamin D deficiency, lack of phytonutrients due to insufficient intake of fruits and vegetables, insufficient omega-3 fatty acids from fish oil, etc). Glutamate is excitatory to neurons, promoting pain, depression, migraine, seizure and neurodegeneration; glutamate is readily converted by the enzyme glutamic acid decarboxylase to GABA—gamma-amino-butyric acid—which has opposing effects to those of glutamate.

- Modulation of calcium entry/accumulation following NMDA receptor activation: Following NMDAr activation, sodium (Na) enters to propagate nerve impulses, and calcium (Ca) enters and promotes intracellular signaling, including the promotion of pain and inflammatory pathways. Intracellular calcium is a famous "second messenger" responsible for physiologic processes such as the pancreatic release of insulin; however, excess intracellular calcium triggers the activation of pathways that can promote pain, migraine and hypertension, hence the well-established use of calcium-channel blocking (CCB) drugs to treat migraine and hypertension. Calcium entry following glutamate stimulation of the NMDA receptor is reduced or "modulated" by both zinc and magnesium, both of which "adhere" to the NMDA receptor to reduce calcium influx; in fact, magnesium is often described as a "cork" or "plug" of the NMDA receptor. Magnesium (Mg) can also be thought of as competing for space with calcium or otherwise blocking some of the effects of intracellular calcium; as such, Mg reduces the effect of glutamate receptor stimulation. Excess intracellular calcium also challenges or stresses the capacity of mitochondria, while magnesium supports mitochondrial function. Intracellular calcium promotes muscle contraction, important in hypertension (due to systemic constriction of arteries/arterioles) and myofascial trigger points (MFTP, an important cause of and contributor to pain in migraine and fibromyalgia), while magnesium promotes muscle relaxation, arterial dilation, and pain relief. Thus, we would expect—and indeed we see clinically—that magnesium supplementation (typically 600 mg per day for adults) provides many of its benefits by offsetting the adverse effects of glutaminergic stimulation and excess intracellular calcium, while also supporting mitochondrial function. Many of the factors that contribute

[26] Vyklicky et al. Structure, function, and pharmacology of NMDA receptor channels. *Physiol Res.* 2014;63 Suppl 1:S191-203

[27] Ben-Ari et al. GABAA, NMDA and AMPA receptors: a developmentally regulated 'ménage à trois'. *Trends Neurosci.* 1997 Nov;20(11):523-9

[28] Ben-Ari Y. Excitatory actions of gaba during development: the nature of the nurture. *Nat Rev Neurosci.* 2002 Sep;3(9):728-39

[29] Abushik et al. The role of NMDA and mGluR5 receptors in calcium mobilization and neurotoxicity of homocysteine in trigeminal and cortical neurons and glial cells. *J Neurochem.* 2014 Apr;129(2):264-74

[30] Béchade C, Cantaut-Belarif Y, Bessis A. Microglial control of neuronal activity. *Front Cell Neurosci.* 2013 Mar 28;7:32

[31] Vasquez A. Nutritional and Botanical Treatments against "Silent Infections" and Gastrointestinal Dysbiosis. *Nutr Perspectives* 2006. Translating Microbiome (Microbiota) and Dysbiosis Research into Clinical Practice. *Int J Hum Nutr Funct Med* 2015 https://ichnfm.academia.edu/AlexVasquez

[32] Aljada et al. Increase in intranuclear nuclear factor kappaB and decrease in inhibitor kappaB in mononuclear cells after a mixed meal: proinflammatory effect. *Am J Clin Nutr.* 2004 Apr;79(4):682-90. Mohanty et al. Glucose challenge stimulates reactive oxygen species (ROS) generation by leucocytes. *J Clin Endocrinol Metab.* 2000 Aug;85(8):2970-3

to excess intracellular calcium—vitamin D deficiency, magnesium deficiency, an acidic acid-base balance, excess omega-6 arachidonic acid relative to omega-3 fatty acids—are easily treated with vitamin D supplementation, magnesium supplementation, promotion of systemic alkalinization, and omega-3 fatty acid supplementation, respectively; proof-of-principle is demonstrated by the observation that each of these interventions provides analgesic, antihypertensive, and other clinical benefits.[33]

- <u>Stimulation of the GABA/benzodiazepine receptor</u>: GABA reception at the GABA receptor—a large multicomponent receptor that also receives benzodiazepine and barbiturate drugs—promotes analgesia, euphoria, relaxation and antiseizure benefits. GABA receptors are also activated by the niacinamide form of vitamin B3 as well as by alcohol/ethanol in beer, wine, and liquors. Botanical medicines that have proven clinical benefit via—at least in large part—their activation of the GABA/benzodiazepine receptor include *Matricaria recutita* (Chamomile), *Melissa officinalis* (lemon balm), *Passiflora incarnata* (passionflower), *Piper methysticum* (kava), *Scutellaria lateriflora* (skullcap), *Valeriana species* (valerian), *Withania somnifera* (ashwagandha).[34]

- <u>Conversion of glutamate to GABA, the importance of vitamin B6 in neuroprotection and pain alleviation</u>: Conversion of glutamate to GABA via glutamic acid decarboxylase requires vitamin B6 (pyridoxine), and the speed/efficiency of this conversion is generally proportionate to the provision of B6. Giving more vitamin B6 results in lower glutamate levels and therefore less activation of the glutamate receptor, thereby providing anti-pain, anti-depression, and anti-seizure benefits. As such, what is obvious is that supplementation with vitamin B6 clearly has an essential role in the treatment of pain, depression, migraine, and seizure; all patients affected by such disorders should receive high-potency vitamin B6 supplementation, at least as a therapeutic trial if not as a default component of therapy. Very importantly, vitamin B6 alleviates pain and the excess brain activity seen with migraine and seizure by means other than serving as a cofactor for glutamic acid decarboxylase; vitamin B6 also provides analgesic and antiinflammatory benefits in peripheral tissues/nerves, in the spinal cord, in the deep brain structures of the brain such as the pain-relaying thalamus, as well as in the neurocortex.

- <u>Activation of the glutamate receptor, especially the NMDA receptor, in the nervous system results in stimulation/depolarization of neurons and the promotion of new connections, promoting memory/learning as well as pain</u>: Activation of the NMDA receptor allows sodium (Na) and calcium (Ca) to enter the cell; entry of Na promotes depolarization of the nerve membrane to allow propagation of the nerve impulse, sometimes called nerve "firing." Entry of Ca following glutamate receptor activation triggers intracellular events, some of which are beneficial for processes such as learning and memory, while others—especially if intracellular calcium levels are too high for too long—are harmful and promote inflammatory responses and mitochondrial stress. While we have typically thought of glutamate receptors and the classic NMDA receptor as existing in the brain and neocortex, we now share the clarity that NMDA receptors exist throughout the nervous system including the spinal cord and peripheral nerves. Activation of NMDAr is important for learning and memory and is also important for the generation of excessive neuronal/brain activity that is seen in seizure/epilepsy, chronic pain, and overactivation of neurons that leads to neuron/brain damage—neuroexcitation, neurodegeneration, and neuroexcitatory neuronal death.

- <u>Activation of the glutamate receptor in peripheral tissues (outside of the nervous system) is not well understood, but again mostly correlates with pain and inflammation</u>: Beyond the NMDA receptor and beyond the nervous system, other types of glutamate receptors are active throughout the body. Given that most tissues and cells are innervated by the nervous system, the distinction between glutaminergic effect via the nervous system and the direct effect on the cells is a bit challenging; however, one of the most important themes observed in the research and science literature is that elevated levels of glutamate in the periphery are clearly and causatively associated with increased pain sensation and to a lesser extent with adverse physiologic changes. For example, activation of mGluR5 in skin is seen with inflammatory and irritating/itchy/pruritic skin disorders, and blockade of the receptor is therapeutic; this same subtype mGluR5 also participates in hypersensitivity to pain in inflammatory diseases.[35] Elevated levels of glutamate are seen in malignant diseases (ie, cancer) and appear to suppress immune function; blockade of iGluR reduces cancer invasiveness. Overall, the associations with excessive glutamate signaling are pain and inflammation; when glutamate is injected into muscles, the result is increased intensity of pain and enlargement of the receptive field (ie, spreading of pain, increased area of heightened sensitivity).[36] Therefore, treatments to reduce glutamate levels (especially vitamin B6) and to reduce the effect of glutamate-triggered increases in intracellular calcium (e.g., magnesium and vitamin D) are expected to reduce glutamate-triggered pain and inflammation.

- <u>Conclusion of this image caption with a few more details and bit of redundancy</u>: Conversion of glutamate to GABA requires vitamin B6 and provides analgesic and "calming" benefits to brain and muscles. Neuroexcitatory glutamate is converted to neuroinhibitory GABA by the enzyme glutamic acid decarboxylase, which—as firmly established in the disease pyridoxine-dependent/responsive epilepsy—shows very clear dose-responsiveness in its ability to reduce glutamate levels in response to high-dose vitamin B6 supplementation. Magnesium and zinc (and perhaps copper) retard the passage of calcium through this channel, thereby mitigating some of the effects of NMDAr activation. Quenching NO- (for example with the hydroxocobalamin form of vitamin B12), which would otherwise trigger glutamate release, and dousing glial activation (for example, with anti-inflammatory nutrients such as vitamin D3 and EPA and DHA from fish oil) which otherwise promotes elaboration of glutamate and QUIN are important considerations not included in this illustration. Glycine is generally considered a necessary co-activator of the NMDAr; but given that glycine is ubiquitous and mostly invariable, it is not immediately malleable and therefore not considered of high relevance as a clinical therapeutic target.

---

[33] Vasquez A. Intracellular Hypercalcinosis. *Naturopathy Digest* 2006 naturopathydigest.com/archives/2006/sep/vasquez.php. Included at the end of this section/chapter.
[34] Sarris et al. Plant-based medicines for anxiety disorders, part 2: a review of clinical studies with supporting preclinical evidence. *CNS Drugs*. 2013 Apr;27(4):301-19
[35] Julio-Pieper et al. Exciting times beyond the brain: metabotropic glutamate receptors in peripheral and non-neural tissues. *Pharmacol Rev*. 2011 Mar;63(1):35-58
[36] Wang et al. Spatial pain propagation over time following painful glutamate activation of latent myofascial trigger points in humans. *J Pain*. 2012 Jun;13(6):537-45

Clinical presentations:

- **Headache—general considerations**: Head pain, with a wide range of differential diagnoses and possible causes and contributions, ranging from simple "stress" and so-called "reactive hypoglycemia" to life-threatening causes such as stroke, aneurysm, tumor, meningitis. Especially for new headaches or acute-onset headaches, concomitant subjective complaints (e.g., lethargy, sleepiness, mood/cognitive changes, changed vision) and/or objective presentations (e.g., fever, skin rash, galactorrhea, or neurologic deficits) indicate the need for additional evaluation to exclude important intracranial lesions such as pituitary adenoma, meningitis, tumor, or subdural hematoma. Since the trigeminal sensory pathway is activated in any condition associated with brain inflammation, relief of headache with analgesic medications does not exclude serious underlying disease such as hemorrhage or meningitis.

- **Migraine**: Periodic headache characterized by unilateral distribution, commonly with a pulsatile sensation; severity ranges from moderate to severe and disabling; commonly begin in adolescence; commonly with a maternal inheritance, consistent with inheritance of mitochondrial DNA from the mother; twice as common in women (5-25%) as in men (2-10%); typical duration of migraine "attack" is 4-72 hours. 80% of migraine is "common migraine" or "migraine without aura." Photophobia and phonophobia (excessive sensitivity to light and sound, respectively) are common, as is nausea, sometimes leading to vomiting. Patients with migraine show a consistent pattern of different—additive and synergistic—mitochondrial defects affecting various locations in the pathway of substrate conversion to cellular energy/ATP: ❶ enzymatic impairment of citrate synthase—the first enzyme in the Krebs cycle, ❷ impaired function of complexes #1-4 of the electron transport chain, ❸ deficiency of coenzyme Q-10 due to insufficient endogenous production, thereby promoting failure of performance of the electron transport chain as well as reduced antioxidant and antiinflammatory defense, and ❹ magnesium deficiency—noted in all headache types—which leads to impairment of complex #5 (ATP synthase) of the electron transport chain, and also leading to increased intracellular calcium influx following activation of the NMDA receptor, leading to increased metabolic demand in neurons.

- **Migraine with aura**: Migraine with aura is characterized by focal neurologic symptoms/deficits; the localization of the neurologic involvement has traditionally been attributed to regional brain vasospasm, leading to reduced blood flow and compromised neuron/brain function in the affected areas. Migraine with aura may present with any combination of the following: blurred/altered vision including scotoma (the perception of "flashing lights"), vertigo/dizziness, hallucinations such as hearing nonreal sounds or seeing nonreal images. Some patients experience the aura as hyper/hypo-activity, depression, food cravings, yawning, mood changes. More than 50% of migraine patients report significant impairment in life tasks and personal relationships as a result.

- **Cluster headache**: Cluster headache (CH) affects predominantly middle-aged men. Although the "pathophysiology is unclear" according to *Current Medical Diagnosis and Treatment 2014*, triggering of trigeminal pain sensation and vasoconstriction are clearly involved, identically to migraine. CH patients generally lack a family history of headache or migraine. CH manifests with episodes of severe unilateral periorbital pain, generally with one or more of the following: ipsilateral nasal congestion, rhinorrhea (runny nose), lacrimation (tearing), redness of the eye, and Horner syndrome (ptosis/drooping of the eyelid, meiosis/constriction of the pupil, and anhidrosis—reduced sweating on the affected side). CH attacks may occur daily (especially nightly) for several weeks, and patients often feel restless and agitated. CH attacks typically last 15 minutes - 3 hours and occur in clusters for weeks or months, then remit. Triggers include alcohol, stress, glare, or specific foods. The prototypic CH patient is a stressed male entrepreneur who smokes, with varying levels of alcohol intake. Mechanistically, stress promotes muscle tension especially in the neck; ethanol/alcohol and tobacco smoke's cyanide are both mitochondrial toxins, and the prototypical stressed male entrepreneur is not eating sufficient fruits and vegetables to maintain urinary alkalinization and sufficient magnesium intake/retention. The facts that CH patients generally ❶ have no family history of the disorder, ❷ have a characteristic lifestyle pattern known to promote mitochondrial impairment, and ❸ respond acutely to oxygen therapy (obviously a form of mitochondrial support, since the primary function of oxygen in the human body is to drain hydrogen protons from the intramembrane space via the formation of ATP and water), support the contention that these patients have a *secondary* lifestyle-generated mitochondrial impairment leading to their headaches, via the aforementioned glial activation and resultant brain inflammation and the remainder of the pain-inducing cascade of events.

Major differential diagnoses: The differential diagnosis of headache by history, examination, and laboratory and imaging assessments should be familiar to clinicians. In particular, the neurological examination should include psychoemotional assessment, as well as cranial nerve and fundoscopic examination, and any new headache symptoms, even in a patient with a history of headaches, must receive due diligence on the part of the clinician.

- Cervical spondylosis: Cervical spine dysfunction and arthropathy can cause and contribute to head pain and headaches; confer with history and examination.
- Cluster headache: Presents with intense unilateral periorbital pain often associated with ipsilateral nasal congestion, rhinorrhea, lacrimation, eye redness, and transient/chronic Horner's syndrome; more common in men, especially in smokers; exacerbated by alcohol; tend to recur at the same time each day/night.
- Cough headache: Severe transient headache triggered by coughing, straining, sneezing, or laughing; patients with recurrent complaints need to be evaluated with a complete neurologic examination and are candidates for CT/MRI since 10% of patients with persistent cough headache have an intracranial lesion.[37]
- Dental or occlusive disorders: Mouth examination, history, oral/dental exam.
- Depression: Check for history consistent with depression: apathy, recent stressful life events.
- Drug side-effect: Check each drug to see if side-effects correlate with clinical complaints.
- Food allergy: Evaluate with elimination/challenge, history; consider blood tests for recalcitrant cases.
- Head injury: Evaluate with history and examination.
- Hyperparathyroidism: Begin by assessing serum calcium.
- Hypertension: Assess blood pressure; although most patients with hypertension do not have headaches, and most patients with headaches do not have hypertension, acute exacerbations of hypertension commonly precipitate headache. Assess for papilledema and hyperreflexia.
- Hyperthyroidism: Weight loss, tremor; assess TSH (generally low) and free T4 (always high).
- Hypothyroidism: Assess TSH (typically elevated), free T4 (generally low), free T3 (may be low or normal), anti-TPO antibodies (seen with autoimmune hypothyroidism: Hashimoto's disease); effective treatment with thyroid hormone alleviates most headaches in hypothyroid-headache patients.[38]
- HIV infection: Patients with HIV are at increased risk for infections, including intracranial infections, particularly toxoplasmosis; intracranial lymphoma is also more common in HIV-positive patients.
- Intracranial aneurysm: May present with throbbing pain; assessed with contrast angiography. In one large international study with 1449 patients[39], the risk of rupture was less than 1% per year, whereas complications from surgery were seen in approximately 14%. A Japanese study[40] found that 95% of patients had a favorable outcome with surgery, implying that 5% had an unfavorable outcome, which is still greater than the risk of rupture, being less than 1% per year for untreated aneurysms reported previously.[41] A more recent study also suggested that the risks of treatment might exceed the risk of spontaneous rupture.[42] Thus the clinical management of intracranial aneurysms must be determined per patient, neuroanatomic location, available techniques/technology, current research, and experience of the neurosurgeon.
- Iron deficiency: Iron is necessary for function of the mitochondrial electron transport chain as well as for formation of the neurotransmitters dopamine and serotonin, both of which can be said to have an analgesic effect. As such, iron deficiency can promote headaches in general and migraine in particular; iron deficiency might also contribute to the clinical presentation of fibromyalgia.[43] Optimal iron status correlates with serum ferritin values of 40-70 ng/ml; rarely, a person with what can be described as a defect in the blood-brain barrier transport of iron into the brain will need to have a serum ferritin value of 120 ng/ml in order to promote entry of iron into the brain.

[37] Tierney ML. McPhee SJ, Papadakis MA (eds). *Current Medical Diagnosis and Treatment 2002, 41st Edition*. New York: Lange; 2002. Page 999-1005

[38] "Thirty-one patients with hypothyroidism of 102 (30%) presented with headache 1-2 months after the first symptoms of hypothyroidism. The headache was slight, nonpulsatile, continuous, bilateral, and salicylate responsive and disappeared with thyroid hormone therapy." Moreau et al. Headache in hypothyroidism. *Cephalalgia* 1998 Dec:687-9

[39] International UIA Investigators. Unruptured intracranial aneurysms—risk of rupture and risks of surgical intervention. *N Engl J Med* 1998 Dec 10;339(24):1725-33

[40] Orz et al. Risks of surgery for patients with unruptured intracranial aneurysms. *Surg Neurol* 2000 Jan;53(1):21-7; discussion 27-9

[41] International UIA Investigators. Unruptured intracranial aneurysms—risk of rupture and risks of surgical intervention. *N Engl J Med* 1998 Dec 10;339(24):1725-33

[42] Risks associated with spontaneous rupture "were often equaled or exceeded by the risks associated with surgical or endovascular repair of comparable lesions." Wiebers DO, et al. Unruptured intracranial aneurysms: natural history, clinical outcome, and risks of surgical and endovascular treatment. *Lancet*. 2003 Jul 12; 362(9378): 103-10

[43] "The mean serum ferritin levels in the fibromyalgia and control groups were 27.3 and 43.8 ng/ml, respectively, and the difference was statistically significant. Binary multiple logistic regression analysis with age, body mass index, smoking status and vitamin B12, as well as folic acid and ferritin levels showed that having a serum ferritin level <50 ng/ml caused a 6.5-fold increased risk for FMS." Ortancil et al. Association between serum ferritin level and fibromyalgia syndrome. *Eur J Clin Nutr*. 2010 Mar;64(3):308-12

- Iron overload, with or without genetic hemochromatosis: For reasons reviewed in Chapter 1 and per my previous reviews[44], all patients must be tested for iron overload. Iron overload causes headaches; iron depletion can relieve headaches.[45,46] Optimal iron status correlates with serum ferritin values of 40-70 ng/ml.

- Magnesium deficiency: Magnesium deficiency is common in industrialized nations[47,48,49,50] and can be assessed clinically (e.g., response to supplementation) or with laboratory tests (e.g., intracellular magnesium). Associated findings common with magnesium deficiency are muscle cramps, bruxism, constipation, and cravings of sweets/candies and especially chocolate.

- Meningitis: Evaluate fundoscopic examination, skin rash, fever, CBC, CRP; immediate transport to emergency department if meningitis is suspected.

- Migraine: Classic presentation includes periodicity, unilaterality, with prodrome, photophobia, nausea, vomiting, visual changes, and positive family history and onset in early teens or adulthood; a large percentage of migraine patients do not have the classic presentation. Migraine can be associated with transient neurologic deficits: numbness, aphasia, clumsiness, and weakness.

- Muscle tension and tension headaches: Assessed with palpation/provocation of cervical/cranial musculature; worse with stress and generally worse at the end of the workday; generally responsive to manual therapies, stress reduction, stretching of affected musculature, and magnesium supplementation.

- Myofascial trigger points: Palpation/provocation of cervical/cranial musculature; treat with post-isometric stretching, ergonomic improvements, and the supplemented Paleo-Mediterranean diet[51] with an emphasis on supplementation with vitamin D, calcium, and magnesium.

- Ocular disorders: Assess with history (e.g., recent change in prescription, new glasses or contacts), and neurologic, eye, and fundoscopic examination; consider diabetes mellitus, multiple sclerosis, and glaucoma and test or refer appropriately.

- Preeclampsia: Headache in a pregnant woman may indicate preeclampsia; assess for hypertension, edema, and proteinuria; emergency or urgent obstetrical referral will be indicated in most cases.

- Pheochromocytoma: Common presentation is periodic headache concurrent with exacerbations of hypertension, sweats, and tachycardia/palpitations.

- Sinusitis or sinus infection: History, fever, pain with palpation of sinuses, nasal discharge; test CBC and CRP; consider radiographic or CT imaging.

- Temporal arteritis (TA), giant cell arteritis (GCA), polymyalgia rheumatica (PMR): History of diffuse head/shoulder pain and jaw claudication generally with systemic complaints of myalgia and fatigue in a patient over 50 years of age; if suspected, must assess CRP/ESR and palpation of artery. **Remember that temporal arteritis can result in blindness; any visual change in a patient with TA/PMR should be considered a medical emergency.** "Loss of vision is the most feared manifestation and occurs quite commonly."[52]

- Temporomandibular joint (TMJ) dysfunction: Assess with examination, history, oral/dental exam, pain worse with chewing (DDX temporal arteritis); notably associated with excess interstitial glutamate.

- Tumor other intracranial lesion: One-third of brain tumor patients present with headache[53], typically worse upon waking and worse with exertion. Assess with neurologic exam/imaging as indicated.

---

[44] See Chapter 1 of either *Inflammation Mastery* / *Functional Inflammmology* (2014 or later) for the most complete reviews, including assessment, management, and radiographic presentations. See also: Vasquez A. Musculoskeletal disorders and iron overload disease: comment on the American College of Rheumatology guidelines for the initial evaluation of the adult patient with acute musculoskeletal symptoms. [Letter] *Arthritis & Rheumatism* 1996; 39:1767-8. Vasquez A. High body iron stores. *Nutr Perspect* 1994 October
[45] In a study involving more than 51,000 patients: "Phenotypic hemochromatosis and the C282Y/C282Y genotype were both associated with an 80% increase in headache prevalence evident only among women. The reason for this association is unclear, but one may speculate that iron overload alters the threshold for triggering a headache by disturbing neuronal function." Hagen K, et al. High headache prevalence among women with hemochromatosis. *Ann Neurol* 2002;51(6):786-9
[46] "...the temporary improvement of headache from depletion of iron stores may indicate a causal relation, possibly mediated by iron deposits in pain-modulating centres in the brainstem." Stovner et al. Hereditary haemochromatosis in two cousins with cluster headache. *Cephalalgia* 2002 May;22(4):317-9
[47] "The American diet is low in magnesium, and with modern water systems, very little is ingested in the drinking water." Innerarity S. Hypomagnesemia in acute and chronic illness. *Crit Care Nurs Q*. 2000 Aug;23(2):1-19
[48] "Altogether 43% of 113 trauma patients had low magnesium levels compared to 30% of noninjured cohorts." Frankel et al. Hypomagnesemia in trauma patients. *World J Surg*. 1999 Sep;23(9):966-9
[49] "There was a 20% overall prevalence of hypomagnesemia among this predominantly female, African American population." Fox et al. An investigation of hypomagnesemia among ambulatory urban African Americans. *J Fam Pract*. 1999 Aug;48(8):636-9
[50] "Suboptimal levels were detected in 33.7 per cent of the population under study. These data clearly demonstrate that the Mg supply of the German population needs increased attention." Schimatschek HF, Rempis R. Prevalence of hypomagnesemia in an unselected German population of 16,000 individuals. *Magnes Res*. 2001 Dec;14(4):283-90
[51] Vasquez A. A Five-Part Nutritional Protocol that Produces Consistently Positive Results. *Nutritional Wellness* 2005Sept.
[52] Tierney ML. McPhee SJ, Papadakis MA (eds). *Current Medical Diagnosis and Treatment 2002, 41st Edition*. New York: Lange; 2002, page 999-1005
[53] Tierney ML. McPhee SJ, Papadakis MA (eds). *Current Medical Diagnosis and Treatment 2002, 41st Edition*. New York: Lange; 2002, page 999-1005

Clinical assessment:

- **History/subjective:**
  - Subacute or chronic/periodic head pain: Most likely benign if course is not progressive and if no neurologic deficits and other findings are present.
  - Acute headache: Recent onset of severe headache in a previously healthy patient suggests intracranial lesion or meningitis.[54] Approximately 1% of patients with acute headache who present to emergency departments will have a life-threatening disorder.[55]
- **Physical examination/objective:**
  - Neurologic examination should be performed on all patients with a recent onset of new headaches or a change from their previous headache. The finding of any mental abnormality or neurologic deficit indicates immediate need for further evaluation: brain CT/MRI and/or emergency department referral.[56]
  - Muscle strength and reflexes
  - Fundoscopic examination for papilledema
  - Cranial nerve examination
  - Blood pressure
  - Spinal and cervical musculature assessment for joint dysfunction and myofascial trigger points[57]
  - Signs for meningeal irritation:

> **Spinal and myofascial assessment**
>
> "Because treating myofascial problems may be the only way to offer complete relief from certain types of headache, clinicians must learn to diagnose and manage trigger points in neck, shoulder, and head muscles."
>
> Davidoff RA. *Cephalalgia.* 1998 Sep

  - - Nuchal rigidity (previously referred to as Soto-Hall maneuver): Patient supine on examining table; doctor gently-yet-assertively forces patient's neck into flexion: positive sign for meningeal irritation is undue pain or resistance. This test must not be performed in patients who may have atlantoaxial instability or cervical spine fracture.
    - Kernig sign: Patient supine with hip flexed, slowly extend knee; positive sign: pain in posterior thigh with or without flexion of opposite knee.
    - Brudzinski sign: Bilateral hip flexion following forced cervical flexion when the patient is supine.
- **Imaging & laboratory assessments:**
  - Imaging: Rarely required except to assess for or exclude intracranial pathology or cervical spondylosis. Importantly, **new onset of headache in an elderly patient or a patient with HIV warrants neuroimaging** *even if the neurologic examination is normal.*[58]
  - Lumbar puncture for CSF analysis: This procedure assesses for infection and subarachnoid hemorrhage and must not be performed unwittingly in patients with increased intracranial hypertension/papilledema.
  - Laboratory evaluation is generally routine and includes the following:
    - 25-OH-vitamin D (serum): Should be between 50-100 ng/mL. All patients with pain need to be assessed for vitamin D deficiency and/or supplemented with 2,000 IU/d (children) or at least 4,000 IU/d (adults).[59]
    - CBC: Assess for anemia and evidence of infection.
    - Chemistry panel: Screening for diabetes, hypercalcemia/electrolytes, liver and kidney function.
    - CRP: Helps to exclude an infectious or inflammatory etiology.
    - Ferritin: Should be 40-70 and certainly less than 120 mcg/L for most people. Assessment for iron overload is indicated in African Americans[60,61], white men over age 30 years[62], patients with peripheral

[54] "The onset of severe headache in a previously well patient is more likely than chronic headache to relate to an intracranial disorder such as subarachnoid hemorrhage or meningitis." Tierney ML. McPhee SJ, Papadakis MA (eds). *Current Medical Diagnosis and Treatment 2002, 41ˢᵗ Edition*. New York: Lange Medical Books; 2002, page 999

[55] Tierney ML. McPhee SJ, Papadakis MA (eds). *Current Medical Diagnosis and Treatment 2006, 45ᵗʰ Edition*. New York: Lange Medical Books; 2006, pages 31-33

[56] Tierney ML. McPhee SJ, Papadakis MA (eds). *Current Medical Diagnosis and Treatment 2006, 45ᵗʰ Edition*. New York: Lange Medical Books; 2006, pages 31-33

[57] Davidoff RA. Trigger points and myofascial pain: toward understanding how they affect headaches. *Cephalalgia.* 1998 Sep;18(7):436-48

[58] Tierney ML. McPhee SJ, Papadakis MA (eds). *Current Medical Diagnosis and Treatment 2006, 45ᵗʰ Edition*. New York: Lange Medical Books; 2006, pages 31-33

[59] Vasquez et al. Clinical Importance of Vitamin D: Paradigm Shift for All Healthcare Providers. *Altern Ther Health Med* 2004; 10: 28-37 ichnfm.academia.edu/

[60] Barton JC, Edwards CQ, Bertoli LF, Shroyer TW, Hudson SL. Iron overload in African Americans. *Am J Med.* 1995 Dec;99(6):616-23

[61] Wurapa RK, Gordeuk VR, Brittenham GM, Khiyami A, Schechter GP, Edwards CQ. Primary iron overload in African Americans. *Am J Med.* 1996;101(1):9-18

[62] Baer DM, et al. Hemochromatosis screening in asymptomatic ambulatory men 30 years of age and older. *Am J Med.* 1995 May;98(5):464-8

arthropathy[63], diabetics[64] and is advisable in children[65], women[66], young adults[67] and the general population.[68] Iron overload causes headaches.[69,70]

- Homocysteine (serum): Optimal level is below 7 micromoles/liter in blood/serum; all patients with pain disorders—including but not limited to migraine/headaches, fibromyalgia and CRPS—should be tested for elevated homocysteine. Importantly, we need to appreciate that the most "pathologic" increases in homocysteine occur in the fluid around the brain—the cerebrospinal fluid (CSF) which is typically not subject to laboratory assessment due to the pain, risk, technical needs and skill involved in the procedure.[71]
  - Thyroid assessment: Especially in patients with classic manifestations of hypothyroidism: fatigue, depression, cold hands and feet, dry skin, constipation, and delayed Achilles return.[72] See Chapter 1.
  - Food allergy testing: May be helpful when elimination-and-challenge procedures are nonproductive and when other therapeutic measures have failed. I personally (DrV) think food allergy testing is overused and that addressing mucosal barrier defects and phenotype immunomodulation (Chapter 4, Section 3) is more important than laboratory testing for food allergies.
- Establishing the diagnosis:
  - Headache is considered a diagnosis based on the patient's subjective report of head pain. However, the headache is always secondary to some other cause of pain, which is the true diagnosis. A clinical or empirical process of elimination must consider common and dangerous causes of head pain, including meningitis, temporal arteritis, sinus infections, cervicogenic pain, intracranial lesions such as brain tumors, hypertension, drug side-effects, and food intolerances.
  - **Serious causes of head pain must be considered with each recurrence, as a patient with a long-term history of benign headaches may contract meningitis or develop hypertension as a new or additive cause of his/her headaches.**

Complications:
- Pain, nausea/vomiting/diarrhea, secondary inability to engage in work, play, and other daily activities.
- Cost and adverse effects of drugs.
- Complications may arise if an underlying cause (e.g., tumor, meningitis, hemorrhage) is undiagnosed.

Clinical management:
- A complete patient history and the above-mentioned lab tests and a physical examination with neurologic assessment will exclude most of the lethal differential diagnoses, allowing the provisional assessment of "benign headache" or "migraine headache" to be established. New onset of headaches or a progressive headache disorder always requires investigation. Refer to neurologist if clinical outcome is unsatisfactory or if complications become evident. For benign headaches including migraine, standard medical treatment is targeted at the alleviation of symptoms. To this end, analgesics and anti-inflammatory drugs such as acetaminophen, aspirin, ibuprofen, naproxen, and ketoprofen are the medical mainstays. Antidepressant drugs ranging from amitriptyline to fluoxetine also might be used for both migraine and tension headaches. Other drugs used for migraine include beta-adrenergic blockers such as propanolol, calcium-channel antagonists such as verapamil, anticonvulsants such as gabapentin and topiramate, and serotonin-modulating drugs such as methysergide and sumatriptan, as well as monoamine oxidase inhibitors and angiotensin-2 receptor blockers. Treatments unique to cluster headaches include inhaled oxygen, lithium carbonate, and prednisone.

[63] Olynyk J, Hall P, Ahern M, KwiatekR, MackinnonM. Screening for hemochromatosis in a rheumatology clinic. *Aust NZ J Med* 1994; 24: 22-5
[64] Phelps G, Chapman I, Hall P, Braund W, Mackinnon M. Prevalence of genetic haemochromatosis among diabetic patients. *Lancet* 1989; 2: 233-4
[65] Kaikov Y, et al. Primary hemochromatosis in children: report of three newly diagnosed cases and review of the pediatric literature. *Pediatrics* 1992; 90: 37-42
[66] Edwards CQ, Kushner JP. Screening for hemochromatosis. *N Engl J Med* 1993; 328: 1616-20
[67] Gushusrt TP, Triest WE. Diagnosis and management of precirrhotic hemochromatosis. *W Virginia Med J* 1990; 86: 91-5
[68] Balan V, Baldus W, Fairbanks V, et al. Screening for hemochromatosis: a cost-effectiveness study based on 12, 258 patients. *Gastroenterology* 1994; 107: 453-9
[69] Hagen K, Stovner LJ, Asberg A, et al. High headache prevalence among women with hemochromatosis: the Nord-Trondelag health study. *Ann Neurol* 2002 Jun;51(6):786-9
[70] Stovner LJ, Hagen K, Waage A, Bjerve KS. Hereditary haemochromatosis in two cousins with cluster headache. *Cephalalgia* 2002 May;22(4):317-9
[71] "The concentration of free HC did not differ significantly from normal controls, but the total HC concentration was significantly higher in MOA and MWA patients (41% increase in MOA and 376% increase in MWA). These findings suggest that an increase of total HC concentration in the brain is commonly seen in migraine patient and is particularly pronounced in MWA sufferers." Isobe C, Terayama Y. A remarkable increase in total homocysteine concentrations in the CSF of migraine patients with aura. *Headache*. 2010 Nov;50(10):1561-9
[72] DeQowin RL. *DeQowin and DeQowin's Diagnostic Examination. Sixth Edition*. New York, McGraw-Hill; 1994, page 900

Migraine patients may become dependent on prescription narcotic drugs, which carry inherent risks of dependence and abuse. Topiramate (Topomax®) is one of the most commonly used pharmaceutical drugs for the treatment of migraine, and a brief description of its efficacy and expense is warranted in order to provide clinical perspective. A recent clinical trial in a leading headache journal concluded that topiramate "resulted in statistically significant improvements" and that the drug is "safe and generally well tolerated"[73]; these statements would appear to support clinical use of the drug. However, more than 10% of patients stopped using the drug due to adverse

> **Patients with migraine headaches—noted in 50% of patients with fibromyalgia and some patients with hypertension—often have food allergies/sensitivities/intolerances**
>
> "The commonest foods causing reactions were wheat (78%), orange (65%), eggs (45%), tea and coffee (40% each), chocolate and milk (37%) each), beef (35%), and corn, cane sugar, and yeast (33% each). When an average of ten common foods were avoided there was a dramatic fall in the number of headaches per month, 85% of patients becoming headache-free."
>
> Grant EC. Food allergies and migraine. *Lancet*. 1979 May

effects, and the statistically significant benefit largely consisted of a reduction in headache days by 1.5 days per 91 days of treatment compared to placebo. The out-of-pocket cost for 3 months of this drug treatment (not including physician fees, recommended laboratory monitoring, and management of adverse effects) is in the range of $400 to $600. Thus, for a yearly cost of approximately $2000, the total reduction in headache days over placebo would be approximately 6 days per year. This study was funded by the company that makes the drug, and 11 of the 13 authors received funding, employment, or direct payment from Ortho-McNeil Neurologics, Inc. Therapeutic trials are implemented to address the underlying problem(s); natural treatments may be superior to drug treatments especially when used in combination.[74]

- <u>Medical standard for migraine—symptomatic relief</u>: "Management of migraine consists of avoidance of any precipitating factors, together with prophylactic or symptomatic pharmacologic treatment if necessary."[75] The goals of medical management are to reduce pain and other manifestations of migraine such as nausea and aura; this symptom-based approach ignores—conceptually and therapeutically—nearly all of the underlying biochemical and nutritional components of the illness, thereby providing minimal/modest benefit while fostering drug-dependency; additional medical goals are to reduce use of high-cost higher-risk emergency "rescue" drugs as well as the utilization of urgent/emergency medical services.

- <u>Treatments (all benign headaches)</u>: Standard medical treatment for headaches is expensive and fraught with adverse effects, drug dependence, and suboptimal efficacy. Further, such symptom-suppressive treatment fails to address the causative food intolerances, nutritional deficiencies, and mitochondrial defects that are common in headache patients and migraineurs. Following the exclusion of serious underlying disease, headache patients should be counseled on allergen identification (free and highly efficacious) and should receive nutritional supplementation with combination fatty acids (e.g., ALA, GLA, EPA, DHA) and therapeutic doses of vitamins and minerals, particularly riboflavin, vitamin D3, and magnesium. CoQ10, 5-HTP, melatonin, spinal manipulation, post-isometric stretching, and the other treatments listed above can be used in combination as appropriate per patient to optimize the therapeutic response.

| Food & Nutrition | The foundational diet is the 5pSPMD as described previously; this "Paleo template"—a diet of fruits, vegetables, nuts, seeds, berries, and lean sources of protein (thereby excluding grains in general and gluten-containing grains in particular)—immediately helps patients increase potassium and magnesium intake specifically and increase nutritional density and systemic alkalinization generally while reducing intake of sodium chloride, common allergens and triggers such as wheat/gluten and milk/dairy, and chemicals such as MSG and aspartame. Patients should—generally speaking—base the diet on "fruits, vegetables, nuts, seeds, and berries with adequate protein intake." Grains that contain the most inflammatory and allergenic form of gluten are rye, barley, and wheat; these foods should be avoided due to their pro-inflammatory properties, their ability to promote gastrointestinal

---

[73] Silberstein SD, et al. Efficacy and safety of topiramate for the treatment of chronic migraine. *Headache*. 2007 Feb;47(2):170-80

[74] Vasquez A. Interventions need to be consistent with osteopathic philosophy. *J Am Osteopath Assoc*. 2006 Sep;106(9):528-9 jaoa.org/cgi/content/full/106/9/528

[75] Tierney ML. McPhee SJ, Papadakis MA (eds). <u>*Current Medical Diagnosis and Treatment 2002, 41st Edition*</u>. New York: Lange; 2002. Page 999-1005

dysbiosis generally and small intestine bacterial overgrowth (SIBO) in particular, and their promotion of gastrointestinal damage, release of zonulin and—in some patients—promotion of systemic inflammation and brain inflammation, both leading to pain while also likely promoting neurodegeneration.[76] The ability of gluten-containing grains to trigger brain inflammation (triggering migraine and other headaches) and autoimmune brain conditions (mimicking multiple sclerosis [MS] and amyotrophic lateral sclerosis [ALS]) has been well proven for decades and is irrefutable; a gluten-free diet is curative.[77,78,79] Beyond custom, convenience, and the government subsidies that make "junk foods"—many of

---

Dr Vasquez's Five-part Nutrition Protocol: The "Supplemented Paleo-Mediterranean Diet" (SPMD)

1. **Diet: Emphasize fruits, vegetables, nuts, seeds, berries, and lean sources of protein** (fish, grass-fed lamb/beef). Make modifications for patient-specific food allergies and sensitivities; this is especially important for patients with known allergy-related conditions such as migraine headaches. Patients with kidney disease should use caution when consuming a potassium-rich diet. Vasquez A. Revisiting the Five-Part Nutritional Wellness Protocol: The Supplemented Paleo-Mediterranean Diet. *Nutritional Perspectives* 2011 Jan

2. **Multivitamin and multimineral supplement**: Nutrient deficiencies are common and are easily treated with nutritional supplementation. Fletcher and Fairfield. Vitamins for chronic disease prevention in adults. *JAMA* 2002 Jun

3. **Vitamin D dosed at 2,000-10,000 IU per day**: The adult requirement for vitamin D3 is approximately 4,000 IU per day; some patients may achieve optimal blood levels with lower doses, but generally daily doses of 4,000-10,000 IU are necessary. Vasquez A et al. The Clinical Importance of Vitamin D. *Alternative Therapies in Health and Medicine* 2004 Sep

4. **Combination fatty acid supplementation**: A combination of flax oil, borage oil, and fish oil provides the health-promoting fatty acids (ALA, GLA, EPA, DHA). Patients should consume organic virgin olive oil liberally with foods. Vasquez A. New Insights into Fatty Acid Supplementation and Its Effect on Eicosanoid Production and Genetic Expression. *Nutritional Perspectives* 2005; Jan

5. **Probiotics**: Health-promoting bacteria can be consumed in the form of powders, pills, and fermented foods such as yogurt and kefir.

For a video review of this foundational diet and introduction to the functional inflammology protocol, see Dr Vasquez "Functional Inflammology Protocol, part 1" from the 2013 International Conference on Human Nutrition and Functional Medicine (ICHNFM.ORG): https://vimeo.com/100089988 Password: "DrVprotocol_volume1"

---

which contain gluten and other inflammatory dietary components—inexpensive and widely available, no legitimate medical or nutritional reason exists for the consumption of gluten-containing foods; the myth that "whole grain foods promote health" is a lie foisted on an ignorant public and an equally uninformed population of nutritionally ignorant medical professionals.[80]

- Food allergy elimination (*Lancet* 1979 May): Mitochondrial dysfunction promotes inflammation, including allergic inflammation; as a result of mitochondrial dysfunction, elevated glutamate levels, and microglial activation, headache patients in general and migraine patients in particular are more sensitive to triggers (e.g., emotional, environmental, hormonal, nutritional) that might otherwise not cause problems. Food allergy is among the most common causes/triggers of headaches[81,82], particularly migraine headaches, particularly those that do not respond to drug treatments.[83,84] In the important study by Grant[85], the following foods were identified as the most common headache triggers: wheat (78%), orange (65%), eggs (45%), tea and coffee (40% each), chocolate and milk (37% each), beef (35%), corn, cane sugar, and yeast (33% each); when an average of 10 triggering foods were avoided, patients experienced a "dramatic fall in the number of headaches per month, 85% of patients becoming headache-free." Food allergen identification via the *elimination and challenge technique*[86] is accurate and inexpensive, and problem-causing foods are then eliminated from the diet.

---

[76] Daulatzai MA. Non-celiac gluten sensitivity triggers gut dysbiosis, neuroinflammation, gut-brain axis dysfunction, and vulnerability for dementia. *CNS Neurol Disord Drug Targets*. 2015;14(1):110-31

[77] Finsterer J, Leutmezer F. Celiac disease with cerebral and peripheral nerve involvement mimicking multiple sclerosis. *J Med Life*. 2014 Sep 15;7(3):440-4

[78] "The authors describe 10 patients with gluten sensitivity and abnormal MRI. All experienced episodic headache, six had unsteadiness, and four had gait ataxia. MRI abnormalities varied from confluent areas of high signal throughout the white matter to foci of high signal scattered in both hemispheres. Symptomatic response to gluten-free diet was seen in nine patients." Hadjivassiliou et al. Headache and CNS white matter abnormalities associated with gluten sensitivity. *Neurology*. 2001 Feb 13;56(3):385-8

[79] "CD is an autoimmune-mediated disorder of the gastrointestinal tract. Initial symptom presentation is variable and can include neurologic manifestations that may comprise ataxia, neuropathy, dizziness, epilepsy, and cortical calcifications rather than gastrointestinal-hindering diagnosis and management. We present a case of a young man with progressive neurologic symptoms and brain MR imaging findings worrisome for ALS. During the diagnostic work-up, endomysium antibodies were discovered, and CD was confirmed by upper gastrointestinal endoscopy with duodenal biopsies. MR imaging findings suggestive of ALS improved after gluten-free diet institution." Brown et al. White matter lesions suggestive of amyotrophic lateral sclerosis attributed to celiac disease. *AJNR Am J Neuroradiol*. 2010 May;31(5):880-1

[80] Adams et al. Nutrition education in U.S. medical schools: latest update of a national survey. *Acad Med*. 2010 Sep;85(9):1537-42

[81] Egger J, Carter CM, Wilson J, Turner MW, Soothill JF. Is migraine food allergy? A double-blind controlled trial of oligoantigenic diet treatment. *Lancet* 1983 Oct ;2:865-9

[82] Monro J, Brostoff J, Carini C, Zilkha K. Food allergy in migraine. Study of dietary exclusion and RAST. *Lancet* 1980 Jul 5;2(8184):1-4

[83] Monro J, Carini C, Brostoff J. Migraine is a food-allergic disease. *Lancet* 1984 Sep 29;2(8405):719-21

[84] Finn R, Cohen HN. "Food allergy": Fact or Fiction? *Lancet* 1978 Feb 25;1(8061):426-8

[85] Grant EC. Food allergies and migraine. *Lancet* 1979 May 5;1(8123):966-9

[86] "Elimination diets can be both a diagnostic tool and a therapeutic intervention for people with a suspected food sensitivity or allergy." Denton C. The elimination/challenge diet. *Minn Med*. 2012 Dec;95(12):43-4. The classic book on the topic of the elimination and challenge technique is William G. Crook MD's *Detecting Your Hidden Allergies* or *Tracking Down Hidden Food Allergy*. Professional Books; 2 edition (June 1980).

- <u>Gluten-free diet alleviates migraine and fibromyalgia in a significant proportion of affected patients (*Rheumatol Int*. 2014)</u>: "The level of widespread chronic pain improved dramatically for all patients; for 15 patients, chronic widespread pain was no longer present, indicating remission of FM. Fifteen patients returned to work or normal life. In three patients who had been previously treated in pain units with opioids, these drugs were discontinued. Fatigue, gastrointestinal symptoms, migraine, and depression also improved together with pain. … For some patients, the clinical improvement after starting the gluten-free diet was striking and observed after only a few months; for other patients, improvement was very slow and was gradually observed over many months of follow-up."

- <u>Avoidance of food additives</u>: Red wine, aged cheeses, sardines, sausage, bacon, and monosodium glutamate (MSG)-containing foods are common triggers for headache and migraine in susceptible patients and should therefore be avoided or at least trialed, ie, avoided and reintroduced to observe for any reduction and recurrence, respectively, of headache or other inflammatory manifestations. Most of these foods contain tyramine, nitrites, or other neuroexcitatory or vasoactive substances, in addition to components (allergens) to which migraine patients tend to be immunologically sensitized. MSG consumption can trigger headache, nausea, and increased blood pressure in apparently normal healthy people.[87] Sulfites in red wine are also noted to trigger migraine and headache in some patients; many wines are available on the market now which contain no detectable sulfites. Sulfites trigger migraine by directly triggering the release of inflammatory mediators and by impairing mitochondrial function; sulfite inhibits the enzyme glutamate dehydrogenase in its conversion of glutamate into alpha-keto-glutarate thereby blocking substrate/fuel entry into the Krebs/citrate cycle (leading to a 50% reduction in cellular energy/ATP production in an experimental study using rat brain cells[88]) while perhaps also leaving excess glutamate present for NMDAr activation—note here again, as previously mentioned, that the combination of mitochondrial dysfunction with glutamate-mediated NMDAr activation is particularly lethal for neurons because the mitochondrial dysfunction starves the neurons of energy/ATP and mitochondria-mediated calcium homeostasis at the exact moment when these same neurons are overstimulated.

- <u>Fish oil supplying 3,000 mg of eicosapentaenoic acid (n3 EPA) and docosahexaenoic acid (n3 DHA) per day, with additional 400 IU mixed tocopherols</u>: Fish oil has been shown to reduce the frequency, duration, and intensity of migraine headaches[89] and the effectiveness of fish oil may be mediated via alterations in cytokine production.[90] More specifically per current research, we appreciate that EPA and especially DHA alleviate glial activation, thereby reducing excessive glutamate-driven pain-inducing excitatory neurotransmission.

- <u>Gamma-linolenic acid (n6 GLA, from plants such as borage and hemp) and alpha-linolenic acid (n3 ALA, notably from flaxseed oil)</u>: Supplementation with GLA and ALA—along with the use of a multivitamin and multimineral supplement and avoidance of dietary arachidonic acid—has been shown to significantly reduce the intensity, frequency, and duration of migraine headaches.[91] Exacerbation of temporal lobe epilepsy (TLE) with GLA combined with n6 linoleic acid has been reported; this exacerbation can be problematic or diagnostically useful (e.g., temporary exacerbation of TLE aids in the differential from schizophrenia).[92] Relatedly and importantly, Al-Khamees et al[93] reported a case of previously well 41-year-old female (i.e., 41yoF) who developed temporal lobe status epilepticus following one week of 1.5-3 g/d borage oil; the amount of GLA and LA and any contaminants in the product were not determined but serum fatty acid analysis showed elevations of GLA 345 microg/g of blood (control 191 microg/g), and LA 259 microg/g of blood (control 165 microg/g). Migraine patients could reasonably limit GLA intake to not more than 500 mg/d; other treatments within this protocol such as vitamin D, pyridoxine, and magnesium have established anti-seizure benefits.

---

[87] "A statistically significant increase in systolic and diastolic blood pressures after MSG administration was observed, as well as a significantly higher frequency of reports of nausea and headache in the MSG group. No robust effect of MSG on muscle sensitivity was found." Shimada et al. Differential effects of repetitive oral administration of monosodium glutamate on interstitial glutamate concentration and muscle pain sensitivity. *Nutrition*. 2015 Feb;31(2):315-23

[88] Zhang et al. A mechanism of sulfite neurotoxicity: direct inhibition of glutamate dehydrogenase. *J Biol Chem*. 2004 Oct 8;279(41):43035-45

[89] "In fact, results of this preliminary study suggest that both fish oil and olive oil may be beneficial in the treatment of recurrent migraines in adolescents." Harel et al. Supplementation with omega-3 polyunsaturated fatty acids in the management of recurrent migraines in adolescents. *J Adolesc Health* 2002 Aug;31(2):154-61

[90] Smith RS. The cytokine theory of headache. *Med Hypotheses* 1992 Oct;39(2):168-74

[91] "In 129 patients available for study, 86% experienced reduction in severity, frequency and duration of migraine attacks, 22% became free of migraine and more than 90% had reduced nausea and vomiting." Wagner et al. Prophylactic treatment of migraine with gamma-linolenic and alpha-linolenic acids. *Cephalalgia*. 1997 Apr;17(2):127-30

[92] Vaddadi KS. The use of gamma-linolenic acid and linoleic acid to differentiate between temporal lobe epilepsy and schizophrenia. *Prostaglandins Med*. 1981 Apr;6(4):375-9

[93] Al-Khamees et al. Status epilepticus associated with borage oil ingestion. *J Med Toxicol*. 2011 Jun;7(2):154-7

Generally, the minimal dose of GLA for systemic anti-inflammatory effect is 500 mg/d; doses up to 2-4 grams per day have been used with safety and efficacy in other inflammatory/metabolic disorders such as cancer, asthma, psoriasis, and rheumatoid arthritis.

- Magnesium supplementation to bowel tolerance (generally with additional pyridoxine): Magnesium deficiency is common, affecting approximately 30% of different populations in various industrialized nations.[94,95,96,97] Regardless of headache etiology or classification, magnesium deficiency is more common in headache patients than in headache-free controls. Magnesium deficiency directly contributes to headache by at least 4 mechanisms: (1) facilitating brain cortex hyperexcitability and hypesthesia due to a reduction in the partial blockade of N-methyl-D-aspartate (NMDA) neurotransmitter receptor sites by magnesium[98], (2) impairing cellular energy production, specifically at the level of mitochondrial electron chain complex #5, the ATP synthase enzyme, (3) promoting vasoconstriction, and (4) promoting increased muscle tension, with the latter 2 mechanisms caused in part by impaired energy production, as well as altered intracellular calcium-to-magnesium ratios. Conversely, adequate magnesium nurture and use of magnesium supplementation help prevent headaches by modulation of NMDA receptor sensitivity and support of energy production, vasorelaxation, and myorelaxation. Not only is magnesium deficiency common in female patients with menstrual migraine[99] and in patients with post-traumatic headaches[100], but magnesium supplementation is justified in headache patients based on the findings of "disturbances in magnesium ion homeostasis" which appear to contribute to brain cortex hyperexcitability.[101] **Except when contraindicated due to renal failure or drug interaction, magnesium supplementation is safe, effective, and reasonable for essentially all patients with headache.**[102,103,104,105,106] Intravenous magnesium (sulfate) is more effective than drug therapy with dexamethasone/metoclopramide for the treatment of acute migraine headaches.[107] A reasonable clinical approach is to 1) evaluate patient with history, physical examination, and screening laboratory tests to exclude contraindications such as renal insufficiency (assess with BUN, creatinine, and urinalysis), 2) assess for possible drug interactions, and then 3) begin the patient with 200 mg elemental magnesium (citrate or malate) with the dose increased by 200 mg every 1-2 days until bowel tolerance is reached. Reduce dose if excessively loose stools or diarrhea occur. When high-dose magnesium supplementation is used in patients with renal insufficiency or drugs that predispose to hypermagnesemia, cautious professional supervision is warranted, with periodic measurement of serum or ionized magnesium. Efficacy of magnesium supplementation is enhanced with concomitant pyridoxine supplementation (e.g., 100-250 mg per day with food) and with an alkalinizing Paleo-Mediterranean Diet as described in Chapter 2. The Paleo-Mediterranean Diet can promote alkalinization[108] which facilitates systemic mineral and magnesium

> **Clinical Pearl**
>
> The importance of alkalinization for the renal retention and intracellular uptake of magnesium can hardly be overemphasized; so-called failure of magnesium therapy is generally due to failure to attain systemic alkalinization, without which magnesium is both hyperexcreted in the urine and "underabsorbed" into the intracellular space. As discussed in this context, systemic pH can be assessed by measuring urine pH, which should range from 7.5 up to approximately 8.5.

[94] Innerarity S. Hypomagnesemia in acute and chronic illness. *Crit Care Nurs Q*. 2000 Aug;23(2):1-19

[95] Frankel H, Haskell R, Lee SY, Miller D, Rotondo M, Schwab CW. Hypomagnesemia in trauma patients. *World J Surg*. 1999 Sep;23(9):966-9

[96] Fox CH, Ramsoomair D, Mahoney MC, et al. An investigation of hypomagnesemia among ambulatory urban African Americans. *J Fam Pract*. 1999 Aug;48(8):636-9

[97] Schimatschek HF, Rempis R. Prevalence of hypomagnesemia in an unselected German population of 16,000 individuals. *Magnes Res*. 2001 Dec;14(4):283-90

[98] Boska et al. Contrasts in cortical magnesium, phospholipid and energy metabolism between migraine syndromes. *Neurology* 2002 Apr 23;58(8):1227-33

[99] "CONCLUSIONS: The high incidence of IMg2+ deficiency and the elevated ICa2+/IMg2+ ratio during menstrual migraine confirm previous suggestions of a possible role for magnesium deficiency in the development of menstrual migraine." Mauskop A, Altura BT, Altura BM. Serum ionized magnesium levels and serum ionized calcium/ionized magnesium ratios in women with menstrual migraine. *Headache* 2002 Apr;42(4):242-8

[100] "Abnormalities in serum IMg(2+) concentrations and ICa(2+)/IMg(2+) ratios were found in children with post-traumatic headaches, but total magnesium levels were normal." Marcus JC, Altura BT, Altura BM. Serum ionized magnesium in post-traumatic headaches. *J Pediatr* 2001 Sep;139(3):459-62

[101] "...disturbances in magnesium ion homeostasis may contribute to brain cortex hyperexcitability and the pathogenesis of migraine syndromes associated with neurologic symptoms." Boska et al. Contrasts in cortical magnesium, phospholipid and energy metabolism between migraine syndromes. *Neurology* 2002 Apr 23;58(8):1227-33

[102] Mazzotta G, Sarchielli P, Alberti A, Gallai V. Intracellular Mg++ concentration and electromyographical ischemic test in juvenile headache. *Cephalalgia* 1999 Nov;19(9):802-9

[103] Mishima K, et al. Platelet ionized magnesium, cyclic AMP, and cyclic GMP levels in migraine and tension-type headache. *Headache* 1997 Oct;37(9):561-4

[104] "After a prospective baseline period of 4 weeks they received oral 600 mg (24 mmol) magnesium (trimagnesium dicitrate) daily for 12 weeks or placebo... High-dose oral magnesium appears to be effective in migraine prophylaxis." Peikert et al. Prophylaxis of migraine with oral magnesium. *Cephalalgia* 1996 Jun;16(4):257-63

[105] Mauskop A, Altura BT, Cracco RQ, Altura BM. Intravenous magnesium sulfate rapidly alleviates headaches of various types. *Headache* 1996 Mar;36(3):154-60

[106] Wang et al. Oral magnesium oxide prophylaxis of frequent migrainous headache in children: a randomized, double-blind, placebo-controlled trial. *Headache*. 2003;43:601-610

[107] "We gave dexamethasone/metoclopramide to one group and magnesium sulfate to the other group, and evaluated pain severity at 20 min and at 1- and 2-h intervals after infusion. ... According to the results, magnesium sulfate was a more effective and fast-acting medication compared to a combination of dexamethasone/metoclopramide for the treatment of acute migraine headaches." Shahrami et al. Comparison of therapeutic effects of magnesium sulfate vs. dexamethasone/metoclopramide on alleviating acute migraine headache. *J Emerg Med*. 2015 Jan;48(1):69-76

[108] Sebastian et al. Estimation of the net acid load of the diet of ancestral preagricultural Homo sapiens and their hominid ancestors. *Am J Clin Nutr* 2002;76:1308-16

retention[109,110] and increases intracellular magnesium levels; alkalinization and increased intracellular magnesium levels are associated with reductions in low-back pain according to a clinical trial.[111] **Magnesium may decrease the absorption or effectiveness of several drugs**, including: Azithromycin (Zithromax), Cimetidine (Tagamet), Ciprofloxacin (Ciloxan, Cipro), Doxycycline (Atridox, Doryx, Doxy, Monodox, Periostat, Vibramycin), Famotidine (Mylanta-AR, Pepcid, Pepcid AC), Hydroxychloroquine (Plaquenil), Levofloxacin (Levaquin), Nitrofurantoin (Furadantin, Macrobid, Macrodantin), Nizatidine (Axid, Axid AR), Ofloxacin (Floxin, Ocuflox), Tetracycline (Achromycin, Sumycin, Helidac), and Warfarin (Coumadin). Misoprostol (Cytotec, Arthrotec) with magnesium may result in diarrhea. **Spironolactone (Aldactone, Aldactazide) or Amiloride (Midamor, Moduretic) may cause hypermagnesemia.**

- Oral magnesium for migraine prophylaxis. (*J Pak Med Assoc.* 2013 Feb[112]): "In this clinical trial study, effects of 500 mg/day oral magnesium oxide for migraine prophylaxis and serum magnesium concentration in 77 migrainous adults (case=33, control=44) aged 34.10±9.61 years, were assessed. Significant reduction in migraines, migraine days, headache severity and migraine index in both the groups compared with baseline, were observed. In magnesium oxide group compared with control group, 50% or greater reduction in migraines (P<0.01) and headache severity (P<0.05) were significant. ... Magnesium supplementation increased significantly (P<0.001) serum magnesium concentration while in control group no difference was seen. Considering that oral oxide magnesium supplementation resulted in positive outcomes in decreasing frequency and severity of migraine seizures without leaving any serious side effects, it seems that magnesium oxide supplementation associated with the routine treatments may be effective especially in patients with low level of serum magnesium."

- Vitamin C, ascorbate: Ascorbate promotes mitochondrial function at cytochrome c, between complexes 3 and 4. My personal hypothesis is that ascorbate provides analgesic benefits via enhancement of central dopaminergic mechanisms and via its ability to lower histamine levels[113] thereby potentially alleviating neurogenic inflammation.[114] Appreciating its safety and efficacy in treating CRPS, migraine, neuropathic and postsurgical pain[115,116], I think all patients with pain should receive ascorbate 2-6 grams daily in divided doses.

- Hydroxocobalamin (hydroxo-vitamin-B12, OH-B12): Hydroxocobalamin is a nitric oxide (NO-) scavenger and appears to benefit the majority of patients with migraine headaches; this study used OH-B12 1 mg/d via aqueous intranasal administration to obviate the need for parenteral administration.[117] If the route of administration is unimportant, then high-dose oral supplementation with 2,000-6,000 mcg/d may prove to be just as effective, according to comparable research using cyanocobalamin.[118] NO- promotes migraine by two mechanisms—induction of mitochondrial dysfunction and promotion of glutamate release—which function synergistically to promote pain amplification, central sensitization as discussed in great detail in the following section on fibromyalgia. Therefore, hydroxocobalamin's effectiveness in migraine is mediated by NO- scavenging is simultaneously mitoprotective (protective of mitochondria) and neuroprotective (protective of neurons).

NO- scavenging with hydroxocobalamin
"Drugs which directly counteract nitric oxide (NO), such as endothelial receptor blockers, NO-synthase inhibitors, and NO-scavengers, may be effective in the acute treatment of migraine, but are also likely to be effective in migraine prophylaxis. ...This is the first prospective, open study indicating that intranasal hydroxocobalamin may have a prophylactic effect in migraine."
van der Kuy et al. Hydroxocobalamin, a nitric oxide scavenger, in the prophylaxis of migraine. *Cephalalgia.* 2002 Sep

---

[109] Sebastian et al. Improved mineral balance and skeletal metabolism in postmenopausal women treated with potassium bicarbonate. *N Engl J Med.* 1994;330(25):1776-81
[110] Tucker et al. Potassium, magnesium, and fruit and vegetable intakes are associated with greater bone mineral density in elderly men and women. *Am J Clin Nutr.* 1999;69(4):727-36
[111] "The results show that a disturbed acid-base balance may contribute to the symptoms of low back pain. The simple and safe addition of an alkaline multimineral preparate was able to reduce the pain symptoms in these patients with chronic low back pain." Vormann J, Worlitschek M,Goedecke T,Silver B. Supplementation with alkaline minerals reduces symptoms in patients with chronic low back pain. *J Trace Elem Med Biol.* 2001;15(2-3):179-83
[112] Talebi M, Goldust M. Oral magnesium; migraine prophylaxis. *J Pak Med Assoc.* 2013 Feb;63(2):286
[113] Johnston CS, Martin LJ, Cai X. Antihistamine effect of supplemental ascorbic acid and neutrophil chemotaxis. *J Am Coll Nutr.* 1992 Apr;11(2):172-6
[114] Rosa AC, Fantozzi R. The role of histamine in neurogenic inflammation. *Br J Pharmacol.* 2013 Sep;170(1):38-45
[115] Hasanzadeh Kiabi et al. Can vitamin C be used as an adjuvant for managing postoperative pain? A short literature review. *Korean J Pain.* 2013 Apr;26(2):209-10
[116] Mohseni M. Use of vitamin C as placebo in anesthesiology. *Anesth Pain Med.* 2013 Winter;2(3):141
[117] van der Kuy PH, et al. Hydroxocobalamin, a nitric oxide scavenger, in the prophylaxis of migraine: an open, pilot study. *Cephalalgia.*2002; 22:513 –519
[118] "In cobalamin deficiency, 2 mg of cyanocobalamin administered orally on a daily basis was as effective as 1 mg administered intramuscularly on a monthly basis and may be superior." Kuzminski et al. Effective treatment of cobalamin deficiency with oral cobalamin. *Blood* 1998 Aug 15;92(4):1191-8 bloodjournal.org/cgi/content/full/92/4/1191

- Folic acid in the form of folinic acid or methylfolate ("5-methyltetrahydrofolate" or "5-MTHF"): Most nutrition-knowledgeable doctors do not use "folic acid" in the form of folic acid due to concerns about increased free radical generation and possible increased risk of cellular damage and malignant disease; we still use the term "folic acid" but nowadays this is—in practice—meant to imply the use of either folinic acid or methylfolate, two forms of folic acid that are considered safer, if not also more effective. Strictly speaking, "folic acid" refers to the synthetic form of the vitamin, whereas "folate" refers to derivatives of tetrahydrofolate that are found in food, especially leafy green vegetables, of which most people do not consume a sufficient amount. Some people develop antibodies against the folic acid transporter (cerebral folate receptor autoantibodies) that facilitates entry of folate into the brain, and they must receive either folinic acid or methylfolate to avoid neurologic devastation due to cerebral folate deficiency, wherein blood/serum levels of folate are normal but the brain (on the other side of the "wall" formed by the blood-brain barrier) is starved for this nutrient.[119] Folic acid from diet and/or supplementation serves many roles and thereby provides numerous benefits, largely centered on the provision of single-carbon methyl groups for metabolic processes (e.g., homocysteine metabolism) and DNA methylation, which regulates/suppresses gene transcription and thereby reduces risk of cancer and viral activation (e.g., cervical cancer following exposure to the human papilloma virus [HPV][120]). In this conversation, we are primarily concerned with optimizing folate intake to optimize "neurologic function" (i.e., generally speaking: normalization of homocysteine-mediated NMDAr activation in the brain, spinal cord and periphery) by reducing homocysteine levels because elevated homocysteine levels will cause excessive pain/fatigue/depression due to activation of the NMDA-receptor, mostly in the brain but also in the periphery. The most important nutrients for reducing homocysteine are folate (vitamin B9), pyridoxine (vitamin B6), cobalamin (vitamin B12) and the amino acid N-acetyl-cysteine (NAC); some people have a defect in their ability to convert folate into its active form via the enzyme methylenetetrahydrofolate reductase (MTHFR) and therefore need more nutritional supplementation to push this sluggish pathway to metabolic completion and reduce/normalize homocysteine levels. Diagrams illustrating these pathways tend to be repulsively complex, immemorably curvaceous, and/or incomplete and thereby clinically valueless; the illustration below is perhaps the most simple for efficient understanding of the means by which nutritional supplementation lowers homocysteine levels.

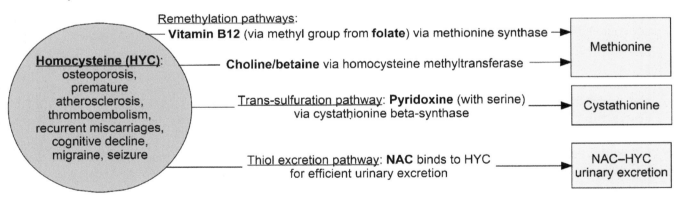

Lowering homocysteine (HYC) via nutritional supplementation: Folate gives methyl group to cobalamin (vitamin B12) to convert HYC via methionine synthase to methionine; choline/betaine can remethylate homocysteine via homocysteine methyltransferase to form methionine. Pyridoxine promotes conversion of HYC via cystathionine beta-synthase to cystathionine. The amino acid N-acetyl-cysteine (NAC) binds to HYC for efficient renal excretion of NAC-HYC.[121]

Increased consumption of folate from diet and/or supplements can alleviate depression, fatigue, and pain and is therefore recommended for all "pain patients", including those with migraine, fibromyalgia, and chronic fatigue syndrome. Adult doses of folate 1-5 mg (1,000-5,000 mcg) per day are reasonable and should be

[119] Gordon N. Cerebral folate deficiency. *Dev Med Child Neurol.* 2009 Mar;51(3):180-2

[120] Piyathilake et al. Indian women with higher serum concentrations of folate and vitamin B12 are significantly less likely to be infected with carcinogenic or high-risk (HR) types of human papillomaviruses (HPVs). *Int J Womens Health.* 2010 Aug 9;2:7-12

[121] "NAC intravenous administration induces an efficient and rapid reduction of plasma thiols, particularly of Hcy; our data support the hypothesis that NAC displaces thiols from their binding protein sites and forms, in excess of plasma NAC, mixed disulphides (NAC-Hcy) with a high renal clearance." Ventura et al. N-Acetyl-cysteine reduces homocysteine plasma levels after single intravenous administration by increasing thiols urinary excretion. *Pharmacol Res.* 1999 Oct;40(4):345-50

coadministered with a roughly equal amount of vitamin B12. Anti-seizure drugs (especially phenytoin, carbamazepine, barbiturates[122]), some of which are used in the treatment of migraine and chronic pain, are notorious for causing folate deficiency and homocysteine elevation[123]; obviously, the drugs would paradoxically promote pain and seizure if folate deficiency develops—coadministration of folate with anti-seizure drugs should be supervised by the prescribing physician.

- Vitamin supplementation to lower homocysteine levels alleviates migraine. (*Pharmacogenet Genomics*. 2009 Jun[124]): "This was a randomized, double-blind placebo, controlled trial of 6 months of daily vitamin supplementation (i.e. 2 mg of folic acid, 25 mg vitamin B6, and 400 microg of vitamin B12) in 52 patients diagnosed with migraine with aura. Vitamin supplementation reduced homocysteine by 39% (approximately 4 mumol/l) compared with baseline, a reduction that was greater than placebo (P=0.001). Vitamin supplementation also reduced the prevalence of migraine disability from 60% at baseline to 30% after 6 months, whereas no reduction was observed for the placebo group. Headache frequency and pain severity were also reduced, whereas there was no reduction in the placebo group. In this patient group the treatment effect on both homocysteine levels and migraine disability was associated with MTHFRC677T genotype whereby carriers of the C allele experienced a greater response compared with TT genotypes."

- Higher levels of dietary folate intake reduce migraine disability and frequency. (*Headache*. 2015 Feb[125]): "A significant inverse relation was observed between dietary folate equivalent and (folic acid) FA consumption and migraine frequency. It was also observed that in individuals with the CC genotype for the methylenetetrahydrofolate reductase (MTHFR) C677T variant, migraine frequency was significantly linked to FA consumption. The results from this study indicate that folate intake in the form of FA may influence migraine frequency in female MA sufferers."

• Pyridoxine (vitamin B6) 50-250 mg/d taken with food and aided by concomitant supplementation with magnesium and riboflavin: Pyridoxine promotes the conversion, via glutamic acid decarboxylase, of neuroexcitatory glutamate into neuroinhibitory GABA, as previously discussed and diagrammed. Pyridoxine also lowers levels of homocysteine, which functions as does glutamate in excitation of the NMDA receptor; thus, pyridoxine protects brain neuron cells from excess stimulation by lowering both glutamate and homocysteine. Experimental and clinical data are both very clear that B6 has analgesic and anti-seizure benefits that are independent from its support of glutamic acid decarboxylase's conversion of glutamate to GABA; pyridoxine functions both peripherally and centrally, with those central locations including the spinal cord, deep brain structures such as the thalamus (where it inhibits neuron firing), and cortex.[126] The conversion of pyridoxine to its intermediate form pyridoxine-5-phosphate requires magnesium (Mg), as expected with phosphorylation reactions; further, magnesium modulates/reduces calcium entry following NMDAr activation, and thus magnesium has a dual effect in reducing excess NMDAr activation. Conversion of pyridoxine-5-phosphate to the fully activated form pyridoxal-5-phosphate (P5P or PLP) requires an oxidase enzyme which requires riboflavin (vitamin B2); thus, as expected, some patients respond to B6 supplementation optimally/only when B2 is coadministered.[127] Not surprisingly, some patients respond better—or exclusively— to administration of the active P5P when pyridoxine previously failed to provide efficacy[128]; thus, what should be obvious by now is that pyridoxine therapy cannot be considered inefficacious until B2, and Mg have been used concomitantly with it and/or until P5P has been used. Furthermore, pyridoxine doses for adults should be in the range of 50-250 (up to 500) mg/d while determining the proper dosage (ie, response to treatment); multiyear use of extremely high doses, e.g., 2,000 mg/d, can cause sensory nerve damage (dorsal root

---

[122] Morrell MJ. Folic Acid and Epilepsy. *Epilepsy Curr*. 2002 Mar;2(2):31-34

[123] "Patients who consume antiepileptic drugs are susceptible to high levels of homocysteine and low levels of folate in the blood." Paknahad et al. Effects of Common Anti-epileptic Drugs on the Serum Levels of Homocysteine and Folic Acid. *Int J Prev Med*. 2012 Mar;3(Suppl 1):S186-90

[124] Lea et al. Effects of vitamin supplementation and MTHFR (C677T) genotype on homocysteine-lowering and migraine disability. *Pharmacogenet Genomics*. 2009 Jun:422-8

[125] Menon et al. Effects of dietary folate intake on migraine disability and frequency. *Headache*. 2015 Feb;55(2):301-9

[126] Zimmerman M, Bartoszyk GD, Bonke D, et al. Antinociceptive properties of pyridoxine. Neurophysiological and behavioral findings. *Ann N Y Acad Sci*. 1990;585:219-30

[127] Folkers et al. Enzymology of the response of the carpal tunnel syndrome to riboflavin and to combined riboflavin and pyridoxine. *Proc Natl Acad Sci*. 1984 Nov;81(22):7076-8

[128] "We present a female infant with seizures responsive to pyridoxal phosphate but that are resistant to pyridoxine. ... It is suggested that in addition to glutamic acid decarboxylase abnormality, the path from the absorption, transportation, phosphorylation, and oxidation of pyridoxine to pyridoxal phosphate in this patient might be defective. It should be considered whether pyridoxal phosphate can be the drug of choice instead of pyridoxine in treating patients suspected of pyridoxine-dependent epilepsy to reduce failure rate and further delay in seizure control." Kuo MF, Wang HS. Pyridoxal phosphate-responsive epilepsy with resistance to pyridoxine. *Pediatr Neurol*. 2002 Feb;26(2):146-7

ganglionopathy[129]) but this is not a concern when P5P is used (because P5P is considered nontoxic relative to pyridoxine[130]) lower doses are used for shorter periods of time, especially with professional supervision and a modicum of awareness and common sense. Studies using B6 in the treatment of premenstrual syndrome have used doses of 50-500 mg/d; however, regarding dosing, we all need to appreciate the differences between clinical trials (short-term studies with close supervision), use of B6 in epilepsy (high doses are warranted to prevent death and brain damage), and long-term unsupervised use (more likely—although still generally unlikely—to result in adverse effects). Of additional note regarding dosing is the observation that pyridoxine is commonly administered in doses 5-10 mg/kg/d for infants (up to 50 mg/kg/d of P5P[131]) and of 100-500 mg/d for children and adults with the seizure disorder "pyridoxine-dependent epilepsy" (of note: to correct the unfortunate error in the naming of this condition, the name should have been "pyridoxine-responsive epilepsy" or "epilepsy of pyridoxine dependency"). Patients with B6-dependent epilepsy have a gene defect that causes accumulation of a natural substance that blocks the function of P5P; this coenzyme inhibition is overpowered via daily megadosing of B6.[132]

- Effects of pyridoxine supplementation on severity, frequency and duration of migraine attacks in migraine patients with aura. (*Iran J Neurol*. 2015 Apr[133]): "This double-blind randomized clinical trial study was conducted on 66 patients with migraine with aura (MA)... Patients were randomly allocated to receive either pyridoxine supplements (80 mg pyridoxine per day) or placebo.... Pyridoxine supplementation led to a significant decrease in headache severity, attacks duration, and HDR (headache diary results) compared with placebo, but was not effective on the frequency of migraine attacks. CONCLUSION: Pyridoxine supplementation in patients with MA was effective on headache severity, attacks duration and HDR, but did not affect the frequency of migraine attacks."

- Antiseizure benefit of pyridoxine administration in an infant with normal blood levels of pyridoxine and deficient brain levels of GABA (*Neuropediatrics*. 1992 Oct[134]): "In an infant with typical pyridoxine-dependent seizures, CSF GABA level, was determined before treatment with pyridoxine. Before onset of treatment, level of GABA in CSF was highly lowered (16 pmol/ml), pyridoxine level in serum was within normal range. Immediately after application of 80 mg pyridoxine fits stopped and the EEG was without seizure activity. The data substantiate previous findings in brain tissue from a patient with pyridoxine-dependent seizures. They are proof of a disturbed GABA metabolism in pyridoxine dependent seizures."

- Pyridoxine deficiency is extremely common in adult patients with severe epilepsy. (*Epilepsy Behav*. 2015 Nov[135]): "An 8-year-old girl treated at our facility for superrefractory status epilepticus was found to have a low pyridoxine level at 5microg/L. After starting pyridoxine supplementation, improvement in the EEG for a 24-hour period was seen. ... All but six [of 81] patients admitted for status epilepticus [SE] had low normal or undetectable pyridoxine levels. A selective pyridoxine deficiency was seen in 94% of patients with status epilepticus (compared to 39.4% in the outpatients) which leads us to believe that there is a relationship between status epilepticus and pyridoxine levels." Very clearly, all seizure/epilepsy patients must be tested for vitamin B6 deficiency and/or treated empirically with pyridoxine; relatedly and very importantly, several anti-seizure medications cause deficiency of folic acid and/or vitamin D—deficiency of either can promote seizure. Thus, testing for serum pyridoxine, homocysteine, and 25-OH-vitamin D should be mandatory in all seizure/epilepsy patients; empiric nutritional treatment is safe and provides collateral benefits.

- Pyridoxine lowers serum/blood glutamate levels (*Am J Clin Nutr* 1992 Apr[136]): "Initially, the plasma PLP concentration of the subjects was 45 ± 2 nmol/L ... and after 7 d of oral supplementation with 27 mg PN-HC1 it reached 377 nmol/L. This represented an 8.5-fold increase from the initial concentration (P < 0.0001).

[129] Baxter P. Pyridoxine-dependent seizures: a clinical and biochemical conundrum. *Biochim Biophys Acta*. 2003 Apr 11;1647(1-2):36-41

[130] Lewis PJ. Pain in the hand and wrist. Pyridoxine supplements may help patients with carpal tunnel syndrome. *BMJ*. 1995 Jun 10;310(6993):1534

[131] Wang HS et al. Pyridoxal phosphate is better than pyridoxine for controlling idiopathic intractable epilepsy. Arch Dis Child. 2005 May;90(5):512-5

[132] The gene defect leads to reduced activity of antiquitin which would leads to accumulation of L-alpha-aminoadipic semialdehyde (L-AASA) and its reciprocal L-alpha-piperideine 6-carboxylate (P6C), the latter of which inhibits P5P. Mills et al. Genotypic and phenotypic spectrum of pyridoxine-dependent epilepsy (ALDH7A1 deficiency). *Brain*. 2010 Jul;133(Pt 7):2148-59

[133] Sadeghi et al. Effects of pyridoxine supplementation on severity, frequency and duration of migraine attacks in migraine patients with aura. *Iran J Neurol*. 2015 Apr 4;14:74-80

[134] Kurlemann et al. Disturbance of GABA metabolism in pyridoxine-dependent seizures. *Neuropediatrics*. 1992 Oct;23(5):257-9

[135] Dave et al. Pyridoxine deficiency in adult patients with status epilepticus. Epilepsy Behav. 2015 Nov;52(Pt A):154-8

[136] Kang-Yoon SA, Kirksey A. Relation of short-term pyridoxine-HCl supplementation to plasma vitamin B-6 vitamers and amino acid concentrations in young women. *Am J Clin Nutr*. 1992 Apr;55(4):865-72

PLP concentration remained essentially unchanged as long as PN supplementation was continued; after 14 d of vitamin supplementation the plasma PLP concentration was 429 ± 16 nmol/L. The increase in plasma PLP concentrations of individuals ranged from 400% to 1400% after supplementation. The concentration of plasma glutamic acid decreased 31% in the supplemented group after 7d of supplementation and 47% after 14 d of supplementation compared with the unsupplemented group." This very important study shows that supplementation with 27mg per day of synthetic pyridoxine hydrochloride raised blood levels of the pyridoxine and the active phosphorylated form P5P—pyridoxal-5-phosphate. Important for patients with migraine, chronic pain and seizures is the fact that serum glutamate levels were reduced by 31%. The authors somewhat erroneously describe 27 mg as a "large oral dose"; most nutritional doctors comfortably and frequently use doses of 50 to 250 to 500 mg per day of pyridoxine. Also noteworthy is that 2 of 10 of the patients showed moderate elevations—not reductions—in serum glutamate. Magnesium (typical adult dose is 600 mg/d) should always be supplemented when vitamin B6 is used. Also of high importance is the fact that—although this study showed clear safety and effectiveness for lowering blood levels of glutamate—levels of glutamate that surround the brain in the CSF were not measured.

- <u>Vitamin administration improves the analgesic efficacy of pharmacotherapy with diclofenac following knee surgery</u> (*Drug Res* 2013 Jun[137]): "Forty eight patients programmed to total knee arthroplasty with a pain level =7 in a 1-10 cm visual analogue scale were allocated to receive a single intramuscular injection of sodium diclofenac (75 mg) alone or combined with thiamine (100 mg), pyridoxine (100 mg) and cyanocobalamin (5 mg), and the pain level was evaluated during 12 h post-injection. Diclofenac+B vitamins mixture showed a superior analgesic effect during the assessed period and also a better assessment of the pain relief perception by patients than diclofenac alone."

- <u>Pyridoxine (vitamin B6) alleviates neuropsychiatric aspects of premenstrual syndrome</u> (*J R Coll Gen Pract.* 1989 Sep[138]): "A randomized double-blind crossover trial was conducted to study the effects of pyridoxine (vitamin B6) at a dose of 50 mg per day on symptoms characteristic of the premenstrual syndrome. ...In these women a significant beneficial effect (P less than 0.05) of pyridoxine was observed on emotional type symptoms (depression, irritability and tiredness)."

- <u>Vitamin D3 (cholecalciferol)</u>: All patients with persistent pain must be tested for non-optimal vitamin D status and empirically treated with vitamin D3 to optimize serum vitamin D.[139,140] Failure to assess and correct vitamin D deficiency and implement effective correction in patients with persistent pain is medical-professional negligence; the data is very clear on the induction of chronic and often debilitating pain by vitamin D deficiency and the merits of vitamin D supplementation in alleviating pain. Several case reports have documented the effectiveness of vitamin D supplementation in the treatment and prevention of migraine.[141,142] Vitamin D is

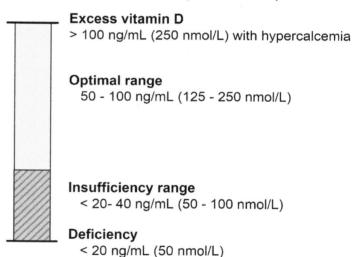

Excess vitamin D
> 100 ng/mL (250 nmol/L) with hypercalcemia

Optimal range
50 - 100 ng/mL (125 - 250 nmol/L)

Insufficiency range
< 20- 40 ng/mL (50 - 100 nmol/L)

Deficiency
< 20 ng/mL (50 nmol/L)

Image © 2004-2015 by Vasquez A in "**Functional Inflammology, volume 1**" published 2014 and "**Inflammation Mastery, 4th Edition**" published 2015. See InflammationMastery.com/reprints for Dr Vasquez's original paper Vasquez et al. The clinical importance of vitamin D (cholecalciferol): a paradigm shift with implications for all healthcare providers. *Altern Ther.Health Med.* 2004 Sep-Oct

---

[137] Magaña-Villa et al. B-vitamin mixture improves the analgesic effect of diclofenac in patients with osteoarthritis: a double blind study. *Drug Res.* 2013 Jun;63(6):289-92

[138] Doll H, Brown S, Thurston A, Vessey M. Pyridoxine (vitamin B6) and the premenstrual syndrome: a randomized crossover trial. *J R Coll Gen Pract.* 1989 Sep;39(326):364-8

[139] Moore D, Wahl R, Levy P. Hypovitaminosis D presenting as diffuse myalgia in a 22-year-old woman: a case report. *J Emerg Med.* 2014 Jun;46(6):e155-8

[140] "The findings suggest a role of low vitamin D levels for heightened central sensitivity, particularly augmented pain processing upon mechanical stimulation in chronic pain patients." von Känel et al. Vitamin D and central hypersensitivity in patients with chronic pain. *Pain Med.* 2014 Sep;15(9):1609-18

[141] "Therapeutic replacement with vitamin D and calcium resulted in a dramatic reduction in the frequency and duration of their migraine headaches." Thys-Jacobs S. Alleviation of migraines with therapeutic vitamin D and calcium. *Headache.* 1994 Nov-Dec;34(10):590-2

[142] "These observations suggest that vitamin D and calcium therapy should be considered in the treatment of migraine headaches." Thys-Jacobs S. Vitamin D and calcium in menstrual migraine. *Headache.* 1994 Oct;34(9):544-6

anti-inflammatory (including reductions in glial activation) and immunomodulatory[143] and also modulates vascular tone by reducing intracellular hypercalcinosis.[144] Reasonable replacement doses are 2,000 IU per day for children and 4,000 IU per day for adults; monitoring serum calcium ensures safety. Optimal vitamin D status correlates with serum 25(OH)D levels of 50-100 ng/mL, or 125-250 nmol/L—see our review article for more details[145]; levels greater than 100 ng/mL are unnecessary and increase the risk of hypercalcemia.

- 5-Hydroxytryptophan (5-HTP)—typical dose is 50-300 mg per day in divided doses: 5-Hydroxytryptophan (5-HTP) is a natural constituent of the human body and is also found in some plants and is thus available as a nutritional supplement. Altered serotonin metabolism has been observed in headache patients, and this observation serves to support the use of selective serotonin reuptake inhibitors (SSRIs) in headache patients, while supplementation with 5-HTP increases serotonin levels naturally. Among various types of headache, migraine would be expected to show the best response to 5-HTP because the conversion of serotonin to melatonin would extend the benefits of serotonin-mediated analgesia to include the protection of mitochondrial function, an important benefit of melatonin.

> **Tryptophan/serotonin insufficiency & glial activation: common in migraine, chronic pain, and fibromyalgia**
>
> "The recently shown **high prevalence of migraine in the population of fibromyalgia sufferers**, suggests a common ground shared by fibromyalgia and migraine. Migraine has been demonstrated to be characterized by a defect in the serotonergic and adrenergic systems. A parallel dramatic failure of serotonergic systems and a defect of adrenergic transmission have been evidenced to affect fibromyalgia sufferers, too."
>
> Nicolodi M, Sicuteri F. Fibromyalgia and migraine, two faces of the same mechanism. Serotonin as the common clue. *Adv Exp Med Biol*. 1996;398:373-9

Conversion of serotonin to melatonin occurs in non-migraine headaches but is of lesser therapeutic importance since these disorders (cluster headaches excepted) are not associated directly with mitochondrial dysfunction. 5-HTP has a better safety and efficacy profile than does the drug methysergide in the treatment of migraine according to a study of 124 adults and children with migraine.[146]

- Vitamin E supplementation with mixed tocopherols 400-1,200 IU/d: As noted previously, free radicals and prostaglandins contribute to migraine pathophysiology; both are reduced by administration of supplemental doses of vitamin E.[147] Vitamin E—known chemically as tocopherol—is present in several forms, arguably the most important of which is the gamma form; most nutritionally competent clinicians generally recommend that vitamin E supplementation contain approximately 40% gamma tocopherol. Another form of vitamin E with more specificity for enhancing/protecting mitochondrial function is known as tocopherol succinate; a combination of various tocopherols is reasonable and is likely to produce enhanced therapeutic efficacy. Isoprostanes are lipid-derrived mediators produced in direct proportion to free radical burden; isoprostanes directly trigger pain and their production is inhibited by antioxidant protection, especially with vitamin E.

  - Vitamin E for the treatment of menstrual migraine. (*Med Sci Monit.* 2009 Jan[148]): "During a placebo-controlled double-blinded trial, 72 women with menstrual migraine received placebo (identical in appearance to vitamin E) daily for five days, two days before to three days after menstruation for two cycles followed by a one-month wash-out and one vitamin E softgel (400 IU) daily for five days in the next two cycles. ... There were statistically significant differences in the pain severity and functional disability scales between the placebo and the vitamin E treatments. Vitamin E effect was also superior to placebo regarding photophobia, phonophobia, and nausea. CONCLUSIONS: Vitamin E is effective in relieving symptoms due to menstrual migraine."

- Combination nutritional supplementation: Patients with migraine show multiple abnormalities in metabolism, inflammation, and oxidative stress; as expected therefore, multi-nutrient supplementation shows benefits via numerous mechanisms.

[143] Timms et al. Circulating MMP9, vitamin D and variation in the TIMP-1 response with VDR genotype. *QJM*. 2002 Dec;95(12):787-96
[144] Vasquez A. Intracellular Hypercalcinosis. *Naturopathy Digest* 2006 September naturopathydigest.com/archives/2006/sep/vasquez.php
[145] Vasquez et al. The Clinical Importance of Vitamin D (Cholecalciferol). *Alternative Therapies in Health Med* 2004; 10: 28-37. ichnfm.academia.edu/AlexVasquez
[146] "The most beneficial effect of 5-HTP appears to be felt with regard to the intensity and duration rather than the frequency of the attacks... These results suggest that 5-HTP could be a treatment of choice in the prophylaxis of migraine." Titus et al. 5-Hydroxytryptophan versus methysergide in prophylaxis of migraine. *Eur Neurol*.1986; 25:327-329
[147] Shaik MM, Gan SH. Vitamin supplementation as possible prophylactic treatment against migraine with aura and menstrual migraine. *Biomed Res Int*. 2015;2015:469529
[148] Ziaei S, Kazemnejad A, Sedighi A. The effect of vitamin E on the treatment of menstrual migraine. *Med Sci Monit*. 2009 Jan;15(1):CR16-9

- <u>Alleviation of migraine symptoms with a supplement containing riboflavin, magnesium, Q10, and other nutrients. (*J Headache Pain.* 2015 Dec[149])</u>: "130 adult migraineurs (age 18 - 65 years) with ≥ three migraine attacks per month were randomized into two treatment groups: dietary supplementation or placebo in a double-blind fashion." The product contained "400 mg riboflavin (vitamin B2), 600 mg magnesium, 150 mg coenzyme Q10 along with a multivitamin/trace elements combination per 4 capsules. The amount of additional multivitamin/trace elements per 4 capsules is as follows: 750 mcg vitamin A, 200 mg vitamin C, 134 mg, vitamin E, 5 mg thiamin, 20 mg niacin, 5 mg vitamin B6, 6 mcg vitamin B12, 400 mcg folic acid, 5 mcg vitamin D, 10 mg pantothenic acid, 165 mcg biotin, 0.8 mg iron, 5 mg zinc, 2 mg manganese, 0.5 mg copper, 30 mcg chromium, 60 mcg molybdenum, 50 mcg selenium, 5 mg bioflavonoids." "Migraine days per month declined from 6.2 days during the baseline period to 4.4 days at the end of the treatment with the supplement and from 6.2.days to 5.2 days in the placebo group. The intensity of migraine pain was significantly reduced in the supplement group compared to placebo. The sum score of the HIT-6 questionnaire was reduced by 4.8 points from 61.9 to 57.1 compared to 2 points in the placebo-group. The evaluation of efficacy by the patient was better in the supplementation group compared to placebo."

- <u>Use of a pine bark extract and antioxidant vitamin combination product as therapy for migraine refractory to pharmacologic medication. (*Headache.* 2006 May[150])</u>: "Twelve patients with a long-term history of migraine with and without aura who had failed to respond to multiple treatments with beta-blockers, antidepressants, anticonvulsants, and 5-hydroxytryptamine receptor agonists were selected for the study. They were treated with 10 capsules of an antioxidant formulation of 120 mg pine bark extract, 60 mg vitamin C, and 30 IU vitamin E in each capsule daily for 3 months. ... There was a significant mean improvement in migraine disability assessment (MIDAS) score of 50.6% for the 3-month treatment period compared with the 3 months prior to baseline. The treatment was also associated with significant reductions in number of headache days and headache severity score. Mean number of headache days was reduced from 44.4 days at baseline to 26.0 days after 3 months' therapy and mean headache severity was reduced from 7.5 of 10 to 5.5. CONCLUSION: These data suggest that the antioxidant therapy used in this study may be beneficial in the treatment of migraine possibly reducing headache frequency and severity."

| Infections & Dysbiosis | Patients with migraine have a higher-than-average prevalence of gastric infection with *H. pylori*, and significant symptomatic improvement is obtained following eradication of *H pylori* in these patients, according to two studies[151,152] and refuted by two others.[153,154] As usual, gastrointestinal dysbiosis should be assessed and corrected on a *per patient* (rather than *per disease*) basis—see Chapter 4 of *Integrative Rheumatology / Functional Inflammology* for details and interventions. For patients with recalcitrant headaches (and for those seeking comprehensive whole-patient health care), assessment of digestion, absorption, and gastrointestinal microecology is a reasonable component of evaluation that can help guide treatment. Although *Helicobacter pylori* is a common inhabitant of the human gastrointestinal tract (found in more than 50% of Americans over age 50), immunologic responses to the organism can range from nonreactive on one end of the spectrum to diverse diseases like chronic gastritis, chronic urticaria, autoimmune thrombocytopenia, or reactive arthritis on the more severe and systemic end of the spectrum. Thus, the host-microbe relationship is of greater significance than the identity and microbiological characteristics of the microbe. As a Gram-negative bacterium that produces endotoxin (LPS), the obvious means by which *H pylori* can contribute to migraine is via LTR-4 mediated systemic inflammation and microglial activation.

---

[149] Gaul et al. Improvement of migraine symptoms with a proprietary supplement containing riboflavin, magnesium and Q10: a randomized, placebo-controlled, double-blind, multicenter trial. *J Headache Pain.* 2015 Dec;16:516

[150] Chayasirisobhon S. Use of a pine bark extract and antioxidant vitamin combination product as therapy for migraine in patients refractory to pharmacologic medication. *Headache.* 2006 May;46(5):788-93

[151] "H. pylori is common in subjects with migraine. Bacterium eradication causes a significant decrease in attacks of migraine. The reduction of vasoactive substances produced during infection may be the pathogenetic mechanism underlying the phenomenon." Gasbarrini et al. Beneficial effects of Helicobacter pylori eradication on migraine. *Hepatogastroenterology.* 1998 May-Jun;45(21):765-70

[152] "Helicobacter pylori should be examined in migranous patients and eradication of the infection may be helpful for the treatment of the disease." Tunca et al. Is Helicobacter pylori infection a risk factor for migraine? A case-control study. *Acta Neurol Belg.* 2004 Dec;104(4):161-4

[153] "Our study suggests that chronic Helicobacter pylori infection is not more frequent in patients with migraine than in controls and that infection does not modify clinical features of the disease." Pinessi et al. Chronic Helicobacter pylori infection and migraine: a case-control study. *Headache.* 2000 Nov-Dec;40(10):836-9

[154] "In conclusion, our results do not support any specific correlation between Hp infection and migraine." Ciancarelli et al. Helicobacter pylori infection and migraine. *Cephalalgia.* 2002 Apr;22(3):222-5

Nutritional Immunomodulation Migraine is most essentially viewed as a combination of mitochondrial dysfunction and glial activation—those two primary components are fundamental, consistent, and explanatory of nearly all other permutations— resulting in physiologic fragility and sensitivity toward (intolerance of) otherwise minor "subclinical" or "subsymptomatic" stressors such as dietary, hormonal, and environmental stressors. With regard to immunohyperresponsiveness—specifically in this case the glial activation, treatments to reduce neuroinflammation should be implemented, such as vitamin D, anti-inflammatory polyphenolics, resveratrol, the n3 fatty acids EPA and DHA, etc. For patients with overt systemic inflammation, allergy, and/or autoimmunity, a more comprehensive antiinflammatory protocol can and should be implemented, especially 1) identifying and removing the inflammatory triggers, and 2) promoting immunotolerance with the complete nutritional immunomodulation protocol outlined in Chapter 4, Section 3. Elevated homocysteine can promote microglial activation, and reducing homocysteine levels with nutritional supplementation is indicated for hyperhomocysteinemic migraineurs as described in protocol component #5: *Style of Living and Special Considerations*.

Dysmetabolism & Mitochondrial Dysfunction We must appreciate that migraine is a multifaceted phenomenon with neuroemotional, structural, allergic-immunologic-inflammatory, and mitochondrial components. With regard to the latter, we can understand migraine from the perspective of defects in the mitochondrial electron transport chain (ETC), namely **NADH-dehydrogenase**, **citrate synthase** and **cytochrome-c-oxidase**; defects in **NADH-cytochrome-c-reductase** appear to be specific to migraine with aura.[155] Thus, not surprisingly, nutrients which are intimately involved with these steps of the ETC have shown impressive efficacy in the treatment and prevention of migraine via the Le Chatelier principle which states—from the perspective of orthomolecular nutrition—that metabolic defects can be compensated for by the administration of supraphysiologic quantities of nutrients to push defective pathways toward completion; this is a main component of Linus Pauling's orthomolecular concept[156] (ie, that using the right molecules in the right amounts can optimize health by optimizing biochemistry and metabolism, as most recently and authoritatively reviewed by his colleague Bruce Ames in a masterful review.[157] In the case of migraine, we are bypassing or compensating for defects in mitochondrial function by supplying supraphysiologic doses of the nutrients involved in those pathways with the end result being enhancement/restoration/normalization/optimization of

> **The evidence of mitochondrial dysfunction in migraine is strong, consistent and irrefutable**
>
> 1. <u>Biochemical evidence</u>: High intracellular calcium, excessive production of free radicals, low activity of superoxide dismutase, activation of cytochrome-c oxidase and nitric oxide, high levels of lactate and pyruvate, and low ratios of phosphocreatine-inorganic phosphate and "deficient oxidative phosphorylation, which ultimately causes energy failure in neurons and astrocytes, thus triggering migraine mechanisms, including spreading depression."
> 2. <u>Cellular, histologic evidence</u>: Muscle biopsy shows ragged red fibers, accumulation of giant mitochondria with paracrystalline inclusions
> 3. <u>Genetic evidence</u>: Various mitochondrial DNA polymorphisms/mutations have been demonstrated
> 4. <u>Therapeutic evidence</u>: "Several agents that have a positive effect on mitochondrial metabolism have shown to be effective in the treatment of migraines. The agents include riboflavin (B2), coenzyme Q10, magnesium, niacin, carnitine, topiramate, and lipoic acid."
>
> Yorns WR Jr, Hardison HH. Mitochondrial dysfunction in migraine. *Semin Pediatr Neurol*. 2013 Sep;20:188-93

mitochondrial function. In the world of nutritional medicine, we would probably not be familiar with these concepts were it not for the independent and synergistic works of Roger Williams, Linus Pauling, Jeff Bland, and Bruce Ames; to these men do we owe gratitude for our understanding of this phenomenon and its clinical application. Furthermore however, we must also appreciate that nutrients have numerous functions and *affect* and *effect* numerous (not singular) pathways and processes, such that a "mitochondrial nutrient" may exert its action via a *non-mitochondrial* effect, as mentioned per nutrient in the itemized section that follows:

- CoQ10—100-400 mg per day: CoQ10 supplementation significantly reduces migraine headache frequency, duration, and intensity.[158] As shown in the diagram below, CoQ10 shuttles electrons from Complex 1 to Complex 2, and from "Complex 2" to Complex 3. Thus, CoQ10 supplementation helps to bypass defects in the electron transport chain (ETC) of mitochondria to promote, preserve, and protect optimal cellular energy/ATP

---

[155] "NADH-dehydrogenase, citrate synthase and cytochrome-c-oxidase activities in both patient groups were significantly lower than in controls, while NADH-cytochrome-c-reductase activity was reduced in migraine with aura." Sangiorgi et al. Abnormal platelet mitochondrial function in migraine with and without aura. *Cephalalgia* 1994 Feb; 21-3

[156] Pauling L. Orthomolecular psychiatry. Varying concentrations of substances normally present in human body may control mental disease. *Science*. 1968 Apr 19;160:265-71

[157] Ames et al. High-dose vitamin therapy stimulates variant enzymes with decreased coenzyme binding affinity (increased K(m)). *Am J Clin Nutr*. 2002 Apr;75(4):616-58

[158] Rozen et al. Open label trial of coenzyme Q10 as a migraine preventive. *Cephalalgia* 2002;22(2):137-41

production. Furthermore, research by Folkers et al[159] strongly suggests that CoQ10 has an anti-allergy and immunomodulatory role; thus the anti-migraine benefits of CoQ10 may be mediated via immunomodulation in addition to enhancement of mitochondrial function.

- Riboflavin (vitamin B2)—50-400 mg per day: Flavin adenine dinucleotide (FAD) is required at Complex 2 of the ETC. High-dose vitamin B2 shows "high efficacy, excellent tolerability, and low cost" in the prevention of migraine headaches.[160] The standard dose for riboflavin in the treatment of migraine is 400 mg taken orally each morning; identical or lower doses can be used in children and/or when riboflavin is used with other nutrients such as CoQ10, magnesium, etc. Riboflavin is safe and effective for long-term use in children and adults[161]; riboflavin is also effective in the long-term treatment of the migraine variant condition known as cyclic vomiting syndrome (CVS) in children.[162] So-called "B vitamins" such as riboflavin—as with zinc and iron— should always be taken with food to avoid the nausea that commonly occurs when vitamins are taken on an empty stomach; other vitamins such as vitamins A, D, and E are generally well tolerated on an empty stomach.
  - Riboflavin prophylaxis in pediatric and adolescent migraine. (*J Headache Pain*. 2009 Oct[163]): "This retrospective study reports on our experience of using riboflavin for migraine prophylaxis in 41 pediatric and adolescent patients, who received 200 or 400 mg/day single oral dose of riboflavin for 3, 4 or 6 months. ... In conclusion, riboflavin seems to be a well-tolerated, effective, and low-cost prophylactic treatment in children and adolescents suffering from migraine."

- Acetyl-L-Carnitine—1,000-2,000 mg taken twice daily between meals: The amino acid L-carnitine is necessary for fatty acid transport into the mitochondria for oxidative metabolism and energy production. Deficiency of or metabolic inability to use carnitine can precipitate or perpetuate migraine headaches, which can be alleviated by carnitine supplementation.[164] As a natural component of the human diet, carnitine has a wide safety margin, and supplemental doses of 2-4 g/d are commonly used; acetyl-L-carnitine is generally the preferred form. Carnitine and acetyl-carnitine provide best benefit when combined with other nutrients, especially CoQ10, magnesium, and lipoic acid. A study in 2015 using 3 grams per day of acetyl-carnitine as monotherapy showed no benefit in the treatment of migraine[165]; one possibility is that 3 grams per day of acetyl-carnitine as monotherapy is an excessive dose. A study using magnesium 500 mg/d and/or carnitine 500 mg/d showed benefit in all groups.[166]

- Lipoic acid—300 mg twice-thrice daily: Lipoic (thiotic) acid is an essential component of the pyruvate dehydrogenase complex, is a potent antioxidant, and it also inhibits NFkB-mediated inflammation. A placebo-controlled clinical trial showed benefit of lipoic acid (600 mg/d) supplementation in migraine patients.[167]

- Melatonin—5-20 mg at night: As mentioned previously, melatonin is a potent protector of mitochondrial function, which has been demonstrated in experimental models of mitochondrial inhibition by bacterial endotoxin. As a powerful antioxidant, melatonin scavenges oxygen and nitrogen-based reactants generated in mitochondria and thereby limits the loss of the intramitochondrial glutathione; this prevents mitochondrial protein and DNA damage. Melatonin increases the activity of Complexes 1 and 4 of the ETC, promoting mitochondrial ATP synthesis under various physiological/experimental conditions.[168]

- Niacin, including inositol hexaniacinate and niacinamide—dose varies per type used: High-dose niacin alleviates migraine headaches and headaches of various etiologies, whether administered orally,

[159] Ye CQ, Folkers K, et al. A modified determination of coenzyme Q10 in human blood and CoQ10 blood levels in diverse patients with allergies. *Biofactors*. 1988 Dec;1:303-6
[160] Schoenen J, Jacquy J, Lenaerts M. Effectiveness of high-dose riboflavin in migraine prophylaxis. A randomized controlled trial. *Neurology* 1998;50(2):466-70
[161] Sherwood M, Goldman RD. Effectiveness of riboflavin in pediatric migraine prevention. *Can Fam Physician*. 2014 Mar;60(3):244-6
[162] "They received prophylactic monotherapy with riboflavin for at least 12 months. Excellent response and tolerability was observed." Martinez-Esteve Melnikova et al. Riboflavin in cyclic vomiting syndrome: efficacy in three children. *Eur J Pediatr*. 2015 Jul 31. [Epub ahead of print]
[163] Condò et al. Riboflavin prophylaxis in pediatric and adolescent migraine. *J Headache Pain*. 2009 Oct;10(5):361-5
[164] Kabbouche et al. Carnitine palmityltransferase II (CPT2) deficiency and migraine headache: two case reports. *Headache*. 2003 May;43(5):490-5
[165] "After a four-week run-in-phase, 72 participants were randomized to receive either placebo or 3 g acetyl-l-carnitine for 12 weeks. ...In this triple-blind crossover study no differences were found in headache outcomes between acetyl-l-carnitine and placebo. Our results do not provide evidence of benefit for efficacy of acetyl-l-carnitine as prophylactic treatment for migraine." Hagen et al. Acetyl-l-carnitine versus placebo for migraine prophylaxis: A randomized, triple-blind, crossover study. *Cephalalgia*. 2015 Oct;35(11):987-95
[166] "In this clinical trial, 133 migrainous patients were randomly assigned into three intervention groups: magnesium oxide (500 mg/day), L-carnitine (500 mg/day), and Mg-L-carnitine (500 mg/day magnesium and 500 mg/day L-carnitine), and a control group. .. Oral supplementation with magnesium oxide and L-carnitine and concurrent supplementation of Mg-L-carnitine besides routine treatments could be effective in migraine prophylaxis; however, larger trials are needed to confirm these preliminary findings." Tarighat Esfanjani et al. The effects of magnesium, L-carnitine, and concurrent magnesium-L-carnitine supplementation in migraine prophylaxis. *Biol Trace Elem Res*. 2012 Dec;150(1-3):42-8
[167] Magis D, Ambrosini A, et al. A randomized double-blind placebo-controlled trial of thioctic acid in migraine prophylaxis. *Headache*. 2007 Jan;47(1):52-7
[168] León J, Acuña-Castroviejo D, Escames G, Tan DX, Reiter RJ. Melatonin mitigates mitochondrial malfunction. *J Pineal Res*. 2005 Jan;38(1):1-9

intramuscularly, or intravenously; niacin can also be used to halt acute migraine attacks.[169,170] Niacinamide adenine dinucleotide (NADH) is an essential component of the first stage (Complex 1) of the ETC, a step that is commonly defective in migraine patients. High-dose niacin facilitates this step and thus enhances energy production. Another anti-migraine benefit of high-dose niacin is its sparing effect on tryptophan, allowing its conversion to serotonin. Niacin also has a vasodilating action and may thereby address the vasculogenic component of headache. Efficacious oral doses of niacin can range from 300 to 1500 mg/d; lower doses are used for children. High-dose niacin, particularly in time-released tablets, presents some risk for hepatic damage, and thus safer forms of niacin such as plain niacin, slow-release niacin (e.g., Niaspan®), and inositol hexaniacinate are preferred; niacinamide and NADH might also be efficacious but neither has vasodilating actions provided by the other forms of niacin. Doses of niacin exceeding 500 to 1000 mg/d are probably unnecessary in headache patients if other treatments such as coenzyme Q10 (CoQ10), vitamin D, and fatty acids are being used; before implementing high-dose niacin, patients should be selected, informed, and monitored appropriately.

- Oxygen: One-hundred percent oxygen delivered by facial mask at 8 L/min for 10 minutes can help abort an attack of cluster headache. Oxygen is the required electron and proton acceptor of the mitochondrial electron transport chain (ETC) for ATP production; thus, supraphysiologic oxygen, like supraphysiologic doses of mitochondria-specific nutrients, generally improves mitochondrial energy (ATP) production. The model of pain sensitization in so-called "chronic pain syndromes"—specifically migraine, cluster headache, fibromyalgia, myofascial pain syndrome and complex regional pain syndrome (CRPS)—that I have developed includes a tripartite vicious cycle of mitochondrial dysfunction, glial activation, and neuronal hyperexcitation, all of which promote brain inflammation, central sensitization, and perpetuation and amplification of pain. Strong support for this model comes from both its biochemical and physiologic rationale as well as the efficacy of corresponding treatments that address each of the main components: mitochondrial dysfunction, glial activation, neuronal hyperexcitation, brain inflammation.

  Appreciation of the efficacy of oxygen therapy—whether as normobaric (more available and affordable) or hyperbaric (more effective and more expensive; hyperbaric oxygen therapy [HBOT])—in various pain states invites us to revisit the naturopathic profession's hierarchy of therapeutics. Symptomatic therapy clearly has a role in patient care but, in order to avoid repeated use of urgent/emergency care and the creation of unnecessary medical dependency, repeated acute care or even "maintenance therapy" should never replace treatment of the underlying cause(s). Patients need to receive treatment aimed at the underlying pathophysiology so that health is optimized and patients are moved toward better general well-being and disease-specific health. Oxygen therapy is abortive of pain and shows some contribution to breaking the vicious cycles of mitochondrial impairment (immediate treatment of headaches, current-prospective treatment of fibromyalgia and CRPS) but this therapy does not address the other aspects of mitochondrial dysfunction (e.g., CoQ10 deficiency) and does not address the cause (e.g., small intestine bacterial overgrowth [SIBO] in fibromyalgia) and therefore should remain as supplemental, abortive/acute, and adjunctive therapy not as the foundation of therapy. Obviously, hyperbaric therapy makes more money for doctors/clinics and—(except/including) when patients buy their own home hyperbaric units—will therefore receive more press and more endorsement than therapies that are curative and empowering (ie, autonomous, without medical dependence). Given that most patients with persistent inflammation and pain are antioxidant deficient and therefore at increased risk for oxygen toxicity (including subclinical damage), antioxidant repletion should occur prior to oxygen therapy; the idea of administering supraphysiologic doses of oxygen to pull more protons and electrons through an *already damaged* and *pro-inflammatory* and *ROS-generating* electron transport chain is not meritorious, although some will defend it—weakly—on the theoretic basis of hormesis.

  - High-flow oxygen therapy for all types of headache (*Am J Emerg Med* 2012 Nov[171]): "We performed a prospective, randomized, double-blinded, placebo-controlled trial of patients presenting to the ED with a chief complaint of headache. The patients were randomized to receive either 100% oxygen via nonrebreather mask at 15 L/min or the placebo treatment of room air via nonrebreather mask for 15 minutes in total. ... A total of 204 patients agreed to participate in the study and were randomized to the oxygen

[169] Velling DA, Dodick DW, Muir JJ. Sustained-release niacin for prevention of migraine headache. *Mayo Clin Proc.* 2003 Jun;78(6):770-1
[170] Prousky J, Seely D. The treatment of migraines and tension-type headaches with intravenous and oral niacin (nicotinic acid). *Nutr J.* 2005 Jan 26;4:3
[171] Ozkurt et al. Efficacy of high-flow oxygen therapy in all types of headache: a prospective, randomized, placebo-controlled trial. *Am J Emerg Med.* 2012 Nov;30(9):1760-4

(102 patients) and placebo (102 patients) groups. Patient headache types included tension (47%), migraine (27%), undifferentiated (25%), and cluster (1%). Patients who received oxygen therapy reported significant improvement in visual analog scale scores at all points when compared with placebo: 22 mm vs 11 mm at 15 minutes, 29 mm vs 13 mm at 30 minutes, and 55 mm vs 45 mm at 60 minutes. ... In addition to its role in the treatment of cluster headache, high-flow oxygen therapy may provide an effective treatment of all types of headaches in the ED setting.

- <u>Oxygen (normobaric/hyperbaric) for migraine</u> (*Headache* 1995 Apr[172]): "The purpose of this study was to compare the effects of hyperbaric oxygen and normobaric oxygen in migraine. Twenty migraineurs were divided randomly into two groups and studied in a hyperbaric chamber during a typical headache attack. ... One group received 100% oxygen at 1 atmosphere of pressure (normobaric) while the other received 100% oxygen at 2 atmospheres of pressure (hyperbaric). One of the 10 patients in the normobaric group achieved significant relief of headache symptoms, while 9 of 10 in the hyperbaric group found relief. Based on a chi-square test, this difference is significant at the P < .005 level. Those patients who did not find significant relief from normobaric oxygen were given hyperbaric oxygen as above. All nine found significant relief. The results suggest that hyperbaric (but not normobaric) oxygen may be useful in the abortive management of migraine headache. Possibilities for the mechanism of this effect, in addition to vasoconstriction, include an increase in the rate of energy-producing and neurotransmitter-related metabolic reactions in the brain which require molecular oxygen."

- <u>Hyperbaric oxygen in the treatment of migraine with aura.</u> (*Headache* 1998 Feb[173]): "Female subjects with confirmed migraine were randomly assigned to begin with either the control (100% oxygen, no pressure) or hyperbaric treatment (100% oxygen, pressure). ... Results suggest that hyperbaric oxygen treatment reduces migraine headache pain…"

- <u>Minimal prophylactic/preventive effect of hyperbaric oxygen therapy on migraine.</u> (*Cephalalgia* 2004 Aug[174]): Not surprisingly, this study found that prophylactic administration of oxygen was generally inefficacious in reducing future migraine attacks; while patients with migraine always have a basal level of mitochondrial dysfunction, oxygen administration does not prevent future attacks. Oxygen is of main value in the treatment of active migraine (and other headache) attacks.

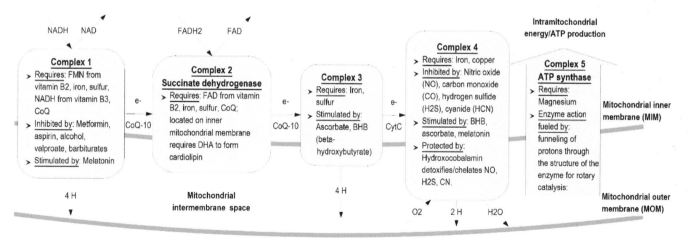

Mitochondrial ETC: Schematic diagram of the electron transport chain, function of which is wholly dependent upon niacin, riboflavin, CoQ10, iron, copper, and—to a lesser extent—vitamin C. Beyond showing where nutrients function in the ETC, this diagram also shows where drugs inhibit ETC function while endogenous substances such as melatonin and beta-hydroxybutyrate stimulate the ETC at complexes 1 and 4 (melatonin) and 3 and 4 (BHB), respectively. For thorough reviews of mitochondrial nutrition and mitochondrial medicine, see vimeo.com/ondemand/mitochondrialmedicine.

---

[172] Myers DE, Myers RA. A preliminary report on hyperbaric oxygen in the relief of migraine headache. *Headache*. 1995 Apr;35(4):197-9

[173] Wilson et al. Hyperbaric oxygen in the treatment of migraine with aura. *Headache*. 1998 Feb;38(2):112-5

[174] Eftedal et al. A randomized, double blind study of the prophylactic effect of hyperbaric oxygen therapy on migraine. *Cephalalgia*. 2004 Aug:639-44

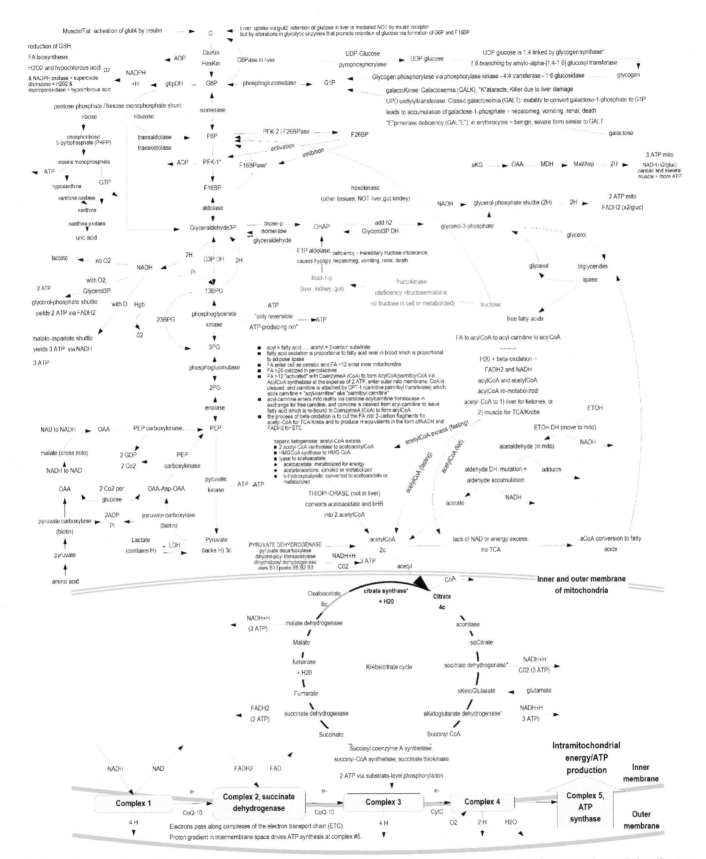

Schematic overview of glycolytic pathways, pyruvate dehydrogenase complex, the Krebs/citrate cycle, and the electron transport chain: Items in bold/red are those which are commonly defective in patients with migraine headaches (and fibromyalgia)—consult your biochemistry text as needed for details and definitions. Note from DrV: The origin of this diagram is from my first year of medical school, during which I created this diagram for my study notes and could recite it from memory.

Style of Living, Special Considerations, Surgical & Somatic/Spinal Treatments

- <u>Style of living—lifestyle optimization</u>: Patients with cluster headaches show a greater percentage of increased work-related stress, self-employment, tobacco smoking, and alcohol use or abuse. These concerns should be addressed per patient as indicated. Lifestyle factors such the standard American diet, overconsumption of caffeine and alcohol, and use of tobacco can result in mitochondrial impairment through various mechanisms, not the least of which are nutrient (especially magnesium) deficiency and accumulation of cyanide (from tobacco smoke), a known mitochondrial poison.

- <u>Self-knowledge—psychological exploration of emotional tension</u>: If someone has chronic "tension headaches" then the question becomes *"Why does this person have chronic tension?"* Generally, the answer is a combination of magnesium deficiency along with some underlying emotional issue(s). If someone feels compelled to maintain a static posture all day without taking a necessary and healthful break to stretch and relax, this suggests that they are over-focusing on their work at the expense of taking care of their body and health—this is not a sign of health, and it suggests an underlying compulsion or dissociation. Patients with cluster headaches show a greater percentage of increased work-related stress, self-employment, tobacco smoking and alcohol use and abuse.[175] Address as indicated.

> **Osteopathic treatment should include manual musculoskeletal medicine and nutritional interventions**
>
> "In contrast to the description of the osteopathic medical profession by the American Osteopathic Association, namely, "doctors of osteopathic medicine, or D.O.s, apply the philosophy of treating the whole person to the prevention, diagnosis and treatment of illness, disease and injury," [the authors of the article in question] essentially reviewed only pharmacologic treatment. ... It is hoped that future reviews in this journal can include a more balanced survey of the literature, inclusive of non-pharmacologic and "holistic" interventions that are consistent with osteopathic philosophy."
>
> **Vasquez A**. Interventions Need to be Consistent with Osteopathic Philosophy. [Letter] *JAOA: Journal of the American Osteopathic Association* 2006 Sep
> http://jaoa.org/cgi/content/full/106/9/528

- <u>Stress reduction, relaxation and biofeedback</u>: Biofeedback is proven effective in the prevention of chronic headaches, including pediatric migraine.[176,177] Relaxation and stress management are more effective than drug treatment with metoprolol for pediatric migraine.[178]

- <u>Somatic treatments—cervical myofascial trigger points</u>: Check the upper cervical spine musculature (especially suboccipital muscles and sternocleidomastoid) for the characteristic manifestations of myofascial trigger points (MFTP, see Chapter 3): palpable nodule, twitch response, and elicitation of referred pain with deep palpation/provocation. Myofascial trigger points are much more common in patients with migraine[179] than in non-headache controls, and they are an important cervicogenic contribution to chronic headaches.[180,181] If located, the MFTP can be effectively treated with in-office/at-home post-isometric stretching and exercises.[182]

> **Post-isometric stretching is of high value in the treatment of cervical MFTP that contribute to headache**
>
> If deep palpation of the upper cervical musculature produces referred pain to the head or face, then you know the patient has MFTP, and you can then treat them with at-home and in-office stretching and exercises. Generally their "chronic pain" will be greatly reduced within 3-10 days. Better results will be obtained with alkalinization and concomitant supplementation with magnesium, vitamin D, and fish oil.

- <u>Somatic treatments—spinal manipulation</u>: Myofascial, arthrogenic, and dyskinetic contributions to headache are significant, and these cervicogenic problems can be addressed with manual spinal and myofascial manipulation. Spinal manipulation can help alleviate headaches with efficacy comparable to commonly used

[175] Manzoni GC. Cluster headache and lifestyle: remarks on a population of 374 male patients. *Cephalalgia* 1999 Mar;19(2):88-94

[176] Scharff L, Marcus DA, Masek BJ. A controlled study of minimal-contact thermal biofeedback treatment in children with migraine. *J Pediatr Psychol*.2002; 27:109 –119

[177] "Feedback training was accompanied by significant reduction of cortical excitability. This was probably responsible for the clinical efficacy of the training; a significant reduction of days with migraine and other headache parameters was observed." Siniatchkin et al. Self-regulation of slow cortical potentials in children with migraine: an exploratory study. *Appl Psychophysiol Biofeedback*.2000; 25:13 –32

[178] "The overall results of the study showed that relaxation training combined with stress management training was significantly more effective in reducing the headache index than treatment with the betablocker metoprolol." Sartory et al. A comparison of psychological and pharmacological treatment of pediatric migraine. *BehavResTher*1998;36:1155-1170

[179] "Trigger points were found in 92 (93.9%) migraineurs and in nine (29%) controls (P < 0.0001). The number of individual migraine trigger points varied from zero to 14, and was found to be related to both the frequency of migraine attacks, and the duration of the disease." Calandre et al. Trigger point evaluation in migraine patients: an indication of peripheral sensitization linked to migraine predisposition? *Eur J Neurol*. 2006 Mar;13(3):244-9

[180] "Myofascial trigger points can refer pain to the head and face in the cervical region, thus contributing to cervicogenic headache." Borg-Stein J. Cervical myofascial pain and headache. *Curr Pain Headache Rep*. 2002 Aug;6(4):324-30

[181] "Because treating myofascial problems may be the only way to offer complete relief from certain types of headache, clinicians must learn to diagnose and manage trigger points in neck, shoulder, and head muscles." Davidoff RA. Trigger points and myofascial pain: toward understanding how they affect headaches. *Cephalalgia*. 1998 Sep;18(7):436-48

[182] Lewit K, Simons DG. Myofascial pain: relief by post-isometric relaxation. *Arch Phys Med Rehabil* 1984 Aug;65(8):452-6. This is a classic "must read" article.

first-line prophylactic prescription medications. [183,184,185,186] Spinal manipulation should be performed only by professionals with graduate and postgraduate training in relevant spinal biomechanics, patient assessment, and manipulative technique. [187,188,189,190]

- <u>Somatic treatments—acupuncture</u>: Acupuncture is effective symptomatic treatment for migraine and tension headaches, with cost-effectiveness comparable to standard medical treatment. [191,192,193] Acupuncture is known to affect regional blood flow, and the neurophysiological mechanisms involved include increased release of endogenous analgesics such as endomorphin-1, beta-endorphin, enkephalin, and serotonin [194] In a head-to-head study of acupuncture versus drug treatment with metoprolol, "2 of 59 patients randomized to acupuncture withdrew prematurely from the study compared to 18 of 55 randomized to metoprolol … The proportion of responders was 61% for acupuncture and 49% for metoprolol. Both physicians and patients reported fewer adverse effects in the acupuncture group." [195] While pain relief is an important benefit, it should not be the primary goal in treatment if an underlying physiological or biochemical disturbance (including nutritional deficiencies or imbalances) can be corrected.

- <u>Somatic treatment—exercise</u>: When people have pain, they are disinclined to move and exercise; however, lack of movement and exercise promotes the continuation of pain via several mechanisms including allowing the formation of myofascial adhesions and contractions, "untraining" of vestibulocerebellar circuits that are necessary for neuromuscular coordination, which is important for reducing musculoskeletal microtrauma that results from uncoordinated/dyscoordinated movements. Exercise and movement are necessary for maintaining myofascial elasticity; all three of these (exercise, movement/stretching, elasticity) support flow of blood, nutrients, oxygen, interstitial fluid, lymph throughout tissues to maintain cellular metabolism and remove wastes and inflammatory mediators. Movement also reduces pain directly via proprioceptive/sensory inhibition of nociception; stated simply: *movement sensation blocks pain reception*.

  - <u>Intensive dynamic training for females with chronic neck/shoulder pain. (*Clin Rehabil*. 1998 Jun[196])</u>: In a clinical research study with 77 women who suffered from chronic neck and shoulder pain, women who performed their exercises **three times per week for 5 sets of 20 repetitions** had better results than those who performed their exercises three times per week for 1 set of 20 repetitions. *More exercise gives better results—faster and more complete relief of pain.*

- <u>Special supplementation for hyperhomocysteinaemia/hyperhomocysteinuria</u>: Reasonable doses are listed; clinicians will have to combine and "dose to effect" per patient. All of these treatments are well-accepted as safe and generally effective. Homocysteine contributes to the increased cardiovascular and stroke risk seen in patients with migraine, while also contributing directly to neuroinflammation and NMDA receptor activation resulting in—identically as with glutamate—increased intracellular calcium and neurotoxicity. [197]

  - <u>Folinic acid or methylfolate 2-5 mg/d</u>: Use in combination with other vitamins, especially vitamin B12, in the form of hydroxocobalamin, adenosylcobalamin, or methylcobalamin—cyanocobalamin is obviously to be avoided because of its clinically relevant content of cyanide.

  - <u>Vitamin B12 >2,000 mcg per day orally, or 1-2 mg per week by injection</u>: Use in the form of hydroxocobalamin, adenosylcobalamin, or methylcobalamin—cyanocobalamin is obviously to be avoided because of its clinically relevant content of cyanide.

[183] Bronfort et al. Efficacy of spinal manipulation for chronic headache: a systematic review. *J Manipulative Physiol Ther* 2001 Sep;24(7):457-66

[184] Tuchin PJ, Pollard H, Bonello R. A randomized controlled trial of chiropractic spinal manipulative therapy for migraine. *J Manipulative Physiol Ther.* 2000 Feb;23(2):91-5

[185] "SMT appears to have a better effect than massage for cervicogenic headache. It also appears that SMT has an effect comparable to commonly used first-line prophylactic prescription medications for tension-type headache and migraine headache." Bronfort et al. Efficacy of spinal manipulation for chronic headache: a systematic review. *J Manipulative Physiol Ther* 2001 Sep;24(7):457-66

[186] "The average response of the treatment group (n = 83) showed statistically significant improvement in migraine frequency (P < .005), duration (P < .01), disability, and medication use..." Tuchin et al. A randomized controlled trial of chiropractic spinal manipulative therapy for migraine. *J Manipulative Physiol Ther.* 2000 Feb;23(2):91-5

[187] Kirk CR, Lawrence DJ, Valvo NL. *States Manual of Spinal, Pelvic, and Extravertebral Technics. Second Edition.* Lombard, Illinois: National College of Chiropractic; 1985

[188] Kimberly PE. *Outline of Osteopathic Manipulative Procedures. The Kimberly Manual 2006.* Kirksville College of Osteopathic Medicine. Walsworth Publishing

[189] Bergmann TF, Peterson DH, Lawrence DJ. *Chiropractic Technique.* New York; Churchill Livingstone: 1993

[190] Gatterman MI. *Chiropractic Management of Spine Related Disorders.* Baltimore; Williams and Wilkins: 1990

[191] Endres et al. Acupuncture for tension-type headache. *J Headache Pain.* 2007 Oct; 8(5): 306–314

[192] Vickers et al. Acupuncture of chronic headache disorders in primary care: randomised controlled trial and economic analysis. *Health Technol Assess.* 2004 Nov;8(48):iii, 1-35

[193] Wonderling D, et al. Cost effectiveness analysis of a randomised trial of acupuncture for chronic headache in primary care. *BMJ.* 2004 Mar 27;328(7442):747

[194] Cabyoglu MT, Ergene N, Tan U. The mechanism of acupuncture and clinical applications. *Int J Neurosci.* 2006 Feb;116(2):115-25

[195] Streng et al. Effectiveness and tolerability of acupuncture compared with metoprolol in migraine prophylaxis. *Headache.* 2006 Nov-Dec;46(10):1492-502

[196] "... pain scores were only significantly improved in the intensive group at 12 months follow-up." Randlov et al. Intensive dynamic training for females with chronic neck/shoulder pain. *Clin Rehabil.* 1998 Jun:200-10

[197] Abushik et al. The role of NMDA and mGluR5 receptors in calcium mobilization and neurotoxicity of homocysteine in trigeminal and cortical neurons and glial cells. *J Neurochem.* 2014 Apr;129(2):264-74

- <u>Vitamin B6, pyridoxine 50-250 mg/d</u>: The phosphorylated form (P5P) can also be used; when the HCL form is used, additional attention must be given to magnesium status/supplementation and urinary alkalinization.
- <u>Riboflavin 20-400 mg/d</u>: Small doses of 2 mg/d have been shown to significantly reduce homocysteine levels, and doses of 400 mg/d are common and well-tolerated in the treatment of migraine.
- <u>Thyroid optimization</u>: Hypothyroidism causes elevated homocysteine and promotes insulin resistance[198] and should be treated appropriately per Chapter 1.
- <u>NAC 600 mg per day and upward to 500-1,500 mg thrice daily</u>: Doses of NAC 4,800 mg/d have been used with success and safety in the treatment of SLE.
- <u>Avoidance of homocysteine-elevating factors</u>: High coffee intake (>5 cups per day), ethanol, tobacco smoking, and medications/treatments (such as methotrexate, metformin, niacin and fibrate drugs); fish oil can raise homocysteine levels in some patients. Metformin is well-known to cause malabsorption of vitamin B12 and to thereby exacerbate "diabetic neuropathy" and promote depression and dementia/psychosis.
- <u>Choline, phosphatidylcholine, lecithin (approximately 2.6 g choline/d)</u>: Each TBS (tablespoon, approximately 15 mL) of lecithin contains 275 mg of choline; thus, if the goal is to get to 2.6 g choline, one would need to use 10 TBS (150 mL) per day of granulated lecithin.
- <u>Betaine, trimethylglycine 6–12 g/day</u>: Effects are weak/modest; likely more relevant for patients taking drugs such as metformin and fibrates that promote loss of betaine in urine.

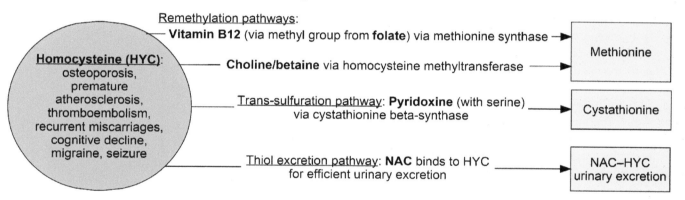

Lowering homocysteine (HYC) via nutritional supplementation: Folate gives methyl group to cobalamin (vitamin B12) to convert HYC via methionine synthase to methionine; choline/betaine can remethylate homocysteine via homocysteine methyltransferase to form methionine. Pyridoxine promotes conversion of HYC via cystathionine beta-synthase to cystathionine. The amino acid N-acetyl-cysteine (NAC) binds to HYC for efficient renal excretion of NAC-HYC.[199]

- <u>Special supplementation—Feverfew (*Tanacetum parthenium*) as monotherapy or with ginger, willow</u>: Results of numerous studies support the use of feverfew for the safe and cost-effective treatment and prevention of migraine headaches. Feverfew has several mechanisms of action including antithrombosis and inhibition of NFkB. Feverfew products are generally concentrated to 0.2% to 0.7% parthenolide, and a reasonable starting dose is 250 mcg/d of parthenolide; lower doses can be used within a context of multicomponent treatment. Feverfew can be used alone, with other nutrients, or with other botanical medicines. The combination of ginger and feverfew has shown efficacy for halting incipient migraine attacks when started within 2 hours of pain onset.[200] Similarly, the combination of feverfew and willow extract was shown to be remarkably safe and effective in preventing and reducing migraine.[201]

[198] Yang N et al. Novel Clinical Evidence of an Association between Homocysteine and Insulin Resistance in Patients with Hypothyroidism or Subclinical Hypothyroidism. *PLoS One.* 2015 May 4;10(5):e0125922
[199] "NAC intravenous administration induces an efficient and rapid reduction of plasma thiols, particularly of Hcy; our data support the hypothesis that NAC displaces thiols from their binding protein sites and forms, in excess of plasma NAC, mixed disulphides (NAC-Hcy) with an high renal clearance." Ventura et al. N-Acetyl-cysteine reduces homocysteine plasma levels after single intravenous administration by increasing thiols urinary excretion. *Pharmacol Res.* 1999 Oct;40(4):345-50
[200] Cady RK, Schreiber CP, Beach ME, Hart CC. Gelstat Migraine (sublingually administered feverfew and ginger compound) for acute treatment of migraine when administered during the mild pain phase. *Med Sci Monit.* 2005 Sep;11(9):PI65-9
[201] Shrivastava R, Pechadre JC, John GW. Tanacetum parthenium and Salix alba (Mig-RL) combination in migraine prophylaxis. *Clin Drug Investig.* 2006;26(5):287-96

- <u>Special supplementation—Butterbur (*Petasites hybridus*)</u>: Butterbur/*Petasites* has consistently shown excellent efficacy in the prophylaxis of migraine, with frequency reductions of ~60%.[202,203] Adult doses used in clinical trials have been variantly described per product as "two capsules 25 mg BID" for a total of 100 mg and "Petasites extract 75 mg bid, Petasites extract 50 mg bid" with the higher doses showing greater efficacy. Anderson et al[204] noted that antimigraine and anti-allergy benefits are mediated via sesquiterpene esters of petasin and furanopetasin which reduce leukotriene biosynthesis, inhibit cyclooxygenase (COX-1 and COX-2), ameliorate activation of p38 mitogen–activated protein kinase stress signaling, and reduce NFkB activation in rat microglial cells; partial blockade of calcium channels has also been noted. Rare (< 0.01%) cases of liver damage (acute hepatitis) and liver failure have been reported; Anderson et al (op cit) per their comparative *in vitro* studies recommend limiting the petasin content (<17%) to improve the hepatobiliary safety profile. Differently, Utterback et al[205] attributed the hepatotoxicity to pyrrolizidine alkaloids (PAs) and stated that products should be virtually PA-free, with less than 0.08 ppm PA; their review concluded that butterbur is safe for antimigraine treatment in children (>6yo) and adults. Contraindications include hypersensitivity/allergy to butterbur or any of the related Asteraceae plants: ragweed, marigolds, daisies, and chrysanthemums.
- <u>Special supplementation—botanical medicines with anti-inflammatory and/or GABA agonist effects</u>: Numerous botanical medicines have proven anti-inflammatory and analgesic benefits. *Zingiber officinale* (ginger) demonstrates multiple antiinflammatory mechanisms and is commonly consumed as food, juice and as a nutritional supplement in the form of pills/powder. Components of ginger reduce production of the leukotriene LTB4 by inhibiting 5-lipoxygenase and reduce production of the prostaglandin PG-E2 by inhibiting cyclooxygenase.[206,207] With its dual reduction in the formation of inflammation-promoting prostaglandins and leukotrienes, ginger has been shown to safely reduce musculoskeletal pain in general[208,209] and to provide relief from osteoarthritis of the knees and migraine headaches.[210] The traditional Chinese herbal medicine *Scutellaria baicalensis* contains, among other active phytochemicals, baicalein, which is anti-inflammatory, neuroprotective, and protective/therapeutic against persistent pain and neuroinflammation[211]; baicalein, oroxylin A, and skullcapflavone II bind the benzodiazepine site of GABA-A receptors with a Ki value of 13.1, 14.6 and 0.36 micromol/L, respectively.[212] Since Ki value increases with decreasing affinity (ie, the lower the value, the stronger the ligand-receptor interaction), we note that skullcapflavone has more GABA receptor affinity than does the more "famous" baicalein. Botanical medicines that have proven clinical benefit via—at least in large part—their activation of the GABA/benzodiazepine receptor include *Matricaria recutita* (Chamomile), *Melissa officinalis* (lemon balm), *Passiflora incarnata* (passionflower), *Piper methysticum* (kava), *Scutellaria lateriflora* (skullcap), *Valeriana species* (valerian), and *Withania somnifera* (ashwagandha).[213]
- <u>Special supplementation—intranasal capsaicin</u>: Capsaicin is the "hot" spicy component of hot chili peppers; when applied to the skin or mucus membranes, it damages pain-sensing nerves and thereby reduces the sensation of pain after an initial exacerbation of pain. Intranasal capsaicin (300 mcg/100 microliters) is remarkably well studied in the treatment and prevention of cluster headaches, beginning with the first report published by Sicuteri et al[214] in 1989. Treatment of active cluster headache with intranasal capsaicin (compared

[202] Grossmann M, Schmidramsl H. An extract of Petasites hybridus is effective in the prophylaxis of migraine. *Int J Clin Pharmacol Ther.* 2000 Sep;38(9):430-5. See also Grossman W, Schmidramsl H. An extract of Petasites hybridus is effective in the prophylaxis of migraine. *Altern Med Rev.* 2001 Jun;6(3):303-10
[203] Lipton et al. Petasites hybridus root (butterbur) is an effective preventive treatment for migraine. *Neurology.* 2004 Dec 28;63(12):2240-4
[204] Anderson et al. Toxicogenomics applied to cultures of human hepatocytes enabled an identification of novel petasites hybridus extracts for the treatment of migraine with improved hepatobiliary safety. *Toxicol Sci.* 2009 Dec;112(2):507-20
[205] Utterback et al. Butterbur extract: prophylactic treatment for childhood migraines. *Complement Ther Clin Pract.* 2014 Feb;20(1):61-4
[206] Kiuchi et al. Inhibition of prostaglandin and leukotriene biosynthesis by gingerols and diarylheptanoids. *Chem Pharm Bull* (Tokyo) 1992 Feb;40(2):387-91
[207] Tjendraputra et al. Effect of ginger constituents and synthetic analogues on cyclooxygenase-2 enzyme in intact cells. *Bioorg Chem* 2001 Jun;29(3):156-63
[208] Srivastava KC, Mustafa T. Ginger (Zingiber officinale) in rheumatism and musculoskeletal disorders. *Med Hypotheses.* 1992 Dec;39(4):342-8
[209] Srivastava KC, Mustafa T. Ginger (Zingiber officinale) and rheumatic disorders. *Med Hypotheses.* 1989 May;29(1):25-8
[210] "It is proposed that administration of ginger may exert abortive and prophylactic effects in migraine headache without any side-effects." Mustafa T, Srivastava KC. Ginger (Zingiber officinale) in migraine headache. *J Ethnopharmacol.* 1990 Jul;29(3):267-73
[211] "Baicalein (BE), isolated from the traditional Chinese herbal medicine Scutellaria baicalensis Georgi (or Huang Qin), has been demonstrated to have anti-inflammatory and neuroprotective effects. ...Intrathecal and oral administration of BE at different doses could alleviate the mechanical allodynia in CIBP rats. Intrathecal 100 µg BE could inhibit the production of IL-6 and TNF-α in the spinal cord of CIBP rats. ...The analgesic effect of BE may be associated with the inhibition of the expression of the inflammatory cytokines IL-6 and TNF-α and through the activation of p-p38 and p-JNK MAPK signals in the spinal cord." Hu et al. The Analgesic and Antineuroinflammatory Effect of Baicalein in Cancer-Induced Bone Pain. *Evid Based Complement Alternat Med.* 2015;2015:973524
[212] "A benzodiazepine binding assay directed separation led to the identification of 3 flavones baicalein (1), oroxylin A (2), and skullcapflavone II (3) from the water extract of Scutellaria baicalensis root. Compounds 1, 2, and 3 interacted with the benzodiazepine binding site of GABAA receptors with a Ki value of 13.1, 14.6 and 0.36 micromol/L, respectively." Liao et al. Benzodiazepine binding site-interactive flavones from Scutellaria baicalensis root. *Planta Med.* 1998 Aug;64(6):571-2
[213] Sarris et al. Plant-based medicines for anxiety disorders, part 2: a review of clinical studies with supporting preclinical evidence. *CNS Drugs.* 2013 Apr;27(4):301-19
[214] Sicuteri et al. Beneficial effect of capsaicin application to the nasal mucosa in cluster headache. *Clin J Pain.* 1989;5(1):49-53

with placebo) reduced severity after 7 days of treatment.[215] In a small controlled clinical trial, patients stated that intranasal capsaicin alleviated chronic migraine suffering by 50% to 80%.[216] Burning pain, sneezing, and increased nasal secretions induced by topical capsaicin application are intense for the first few applications but decrease over time, generally within a week or so; clinical benefits generally begin on the eighth day of consecutive treatment. Episodic cluster headache patients appear to benefit more than do chronic cluster headache patients. Cluster headaches are typically unilateral, and capsaicin should be applied to the nostril on the same side as the head pain.[217]

- Surgical closure of patent foramen ovale: While the prevalence of patent foramen ovale in the general adult population is approximately 20% to 30%, patients with migraine—especially migraine with aura—show a higher prevalence (55–65%) of this physiological cardiopulmonary shunt. Surgical closure of a patent foramen ovale can provide relief from headache in many migraine patients.[218,219] If the cardiopulmonary shunt is severe enough to result in reduced blood oxygenation, it can exacerbate the already reduced energy production caused by the aforementioned mitochondrial dysfunction. More likely, bypassing the lungs results in failure of pulmonary degradation of proinflammatory mediators. The lungs inactivate proinflammatory mediators such as prostaglandins E1, E2, and F2-alpha, all of the leukotrienes, and norepinephrine (30% reduction). Thus, surgical closure of the patent foramen ovale stops inflammatory mediators from bypassing the lungs and may provide a systemic anti-inflammatory benefit that reduces migraine severity.

| Endocrine Imbalances | All hormones have either pro-inflammatory or anti-inflammatory effects. As such, patients with pain and inflammation are candidates for complete hormonal evaluation, as reviewed in Chapter 4, Section 5. Melatonin's utility in migraine—as in fibromyalgia—is more likely related to its antioxidant and mitochondrial-supportive effects than to a true "hormonal" effect. Thyroid status must be optimized in all migraine patients.

- Melatonin—3-20 mg at night: Melatonin is a hormone made in the pineal gland from the neurotransmitter serotonin which is derived from the amino acid tryptophan and 5-hydroxytryptophan. Melatonin levels are low in patients with migraine and cluster headache. According to case reports and studies with small numbers of patients, 10 mg of melatonin taken at night relieves cluster headaches in approximately 50% of patients, with results beginning 3 to 5 days after the start of treatment and continuing for the duration of treatment.[220,221] Clinical trials using melatonin in migraine patients have shown consistently positive results, with a significant number of patients becoming completely migraine-free.[222] Melatonin is generally administered at night in doses ranging from 3 to 10 mg, although studies in cancer patients have safely used doses as high as 20 to 40 mg and have shown antitumor and pro-survival benefits. Melatonin has antioxidant and immunomodulatory actions in addition to its ability to preserve mitochondrial function, which is particularly relevant to migraine and cluster headaches. According to small studies and case reports with small numbers of patients, 10 mg of melatonin taken at night relieves cluster headaches in approximately 50% of patients.[223,224]

- Testosterone: Testosterone has antiinflammatory/immunomodulatory actions, and as such has clinical utility in migraine, cluster headache, rheumatoid arthritis, and fibromyalgia via reduction/modulation of peripheral inflammation and the brain inflammation and microglial activation that promote central sensitization to pain. In this study[225], following subcutaneous testosterone implant, "Improvement in headache severity was noted by 92% of patients and the mean level of improvement was statistically significant (3.3 on a 5 point scale). ... Seventy-four percent of patients reported a headache severity score of '0' (none) on testosterone implant therapy

[215] Marks et al. A double-blind placebo-controlled trial of intranasal capsaicin for cluster headache. *Cephalalgia*. 1993 Apr;13(2):114-6
[216] Fusco et al. Repeated intranasal capsaicin applications to treat chronic migraine. *Br J Anaesth*. 2003 Jun;90(6):812
[217] Fusco et al. Preventative effect of repeated nasal applications of capsaicin in cluster headache. *Pain*. 1994 Dec;59(3):321-5
[218] Rigatelli et al. Primary patent foramen ovale closure to relieve severe migraine. *Ann Intern Med*. 2006 Mar 21;144(6):458-60
[219] Dubiel et al. Migraine Headache Relief after Percutaneous Transcatheter Closure of Interatrial Communications. *J Interv Cardiol*. 2007 Dec 18; [Epub ahead of print]
[220] Leone et al. Melatonin versus placebo in the prophylaxis of cluster headache: a double-blind pilot study with parallel groups. *Cephalalgia* 1996 Nov;16(7):494-6
[221] "Melatonin levels have been found to be decreased in cluster headache patients. ... We report two chronic cluster headache patients who had both daytime and nocturnal attacks that were alleviated with melatonin." Peres MF, Rozen TD. Melatonin in the preventive treatment of chronic cluster headache. *Cephalalgia*. 2001 Dec;21(10):993-5
[222] Vogler et al. Role of melatonin in the pathophysiology of migraine: implications for treatment. *CNS Drugs*. 2006;20(5):343-50
[223] "Five of the 10 treated patients were responders whose attack frequency declined 3-5 days after treatment, and they experienced no further attacks until melatonin was discontinued." Leone et al. Melatonin versus placebo in the prophylaxis of cluster headache: a double-blind pilot study with parallel groups. *Cephalalgia* 1996 Nov;16(7):494-6
[224] "Melatonin levels have been found to be decreased in cluster headache patients. ... We report two chronic cluster headache patients who had both daytime and nocturnal attacks that were alleviated with melatonin." Peres MF, Rozen TD. Melatonin in the preventive treatment of chronic cluster headache. *Cephalalgia*. 2001 Dec;21(10):993-5
[225] Glaser et al. Testosterone pellet implants and migraine headaches: a pilot study. *Maturitas*. 2012 Apr;71(4):385-8

for the 3-month treatment period. Continuous testosterone was effective therapy in reducing the severity of migraine headaches in both pre- and post-menopausal women." In another study, "Seven male and 2 female patients, seen between July 2004 and February 2005, and between the ages of 32 and 56, are reported with histories of treatment resistant cluster headaches accompanied by borderline low or low serum testosterone levels. The patients failed to respond to individually tailored medical regimens, including melatonin doses of 12 mg a day or higher, high flow oxygen, maximally tolerated verapamil, antiepileptic agents, and parenteral serotonin agonists. Seven of the 9 patients met 2004 International Classification for the Diagnosis of Headache criteria for chronic cluster headaches; the other 2 patients had episodic cluster headaches of several months duration. After neurological and physical examination all patients had laboratory investigations including fasting lipid panel, PSA (where indicated), LH, FSH, and testosterone levels (both free and total). All 9 patients demonstrated either abnormally low or low, normal testosterone levels. After supplementation with either pure testosterone in 5 of 7 male patients or combination testosterone/estrogen therapy in both female patients, the patients achieved cluster headache freedom for the first 24 hours. Four male chronic cluster patients, all with abnormally low testosterone levels, achieved remission."[226]

Xenobiotic Accumulation/Detoxification Persistent organic pollutants promote inflammation generally and mitochondrial dysfunction specifically. Treat as described throughout this text and as reviewed in Chapter 2 and also in Chapter 4, Section 7.

---

[226] Stillman MJ. Testosterone replacement therapy for treatment refractory cluster headache. *Headache*. 2006 Jun;46(6):925-33

Fibromyalgia (FM, FMS, FMD) &
Complex Regional Pain Syndrome (CRPS)

Introduction:

Fibromyalgia (FM)—also referred to as fibromyalgia syndrome (FMS) but more properly referred to as fibromyalgia disease (FMD)—is an organic clinical entity that has remained enigmatic to the medical profession despite the consistent publication of research that delineates its cause and its effective treatments. This chapter summarizes clinical assessments, treatments, and essential background information that—when properly applied—should provide empowering knowledge for clinicians and for the patients suffering with this condition. For any disease, we as scientists and clinicians must establish a model of the disease so that we can start with *some shared idea about the disease itself* and have some common language and understanding so that we can engage in meaningful conversations and valuable research. The model of FM that I have been the first and only clinician researcher to construct (starting in 2008) is that FM starts from small intestine bacterial overgrowth, and that the absorbed microbial molecules lead to the pain-amplifying central sensitization and fatigue-inducing mitochondrial dysfunction that clearly characterize this condition; variations of and deviations from the classic model of any disease will undoubtedly be encountered, but they can always be traced back to this classic model.

Fibromyalgia is uniquely exemplary in its clouded diagnostic criteria and etiology; I argue in this review and the associated videos and related articles that the diagnostic criteria for FM have been intentionally clouded and deconstructed via influence of drug companies that want the FM label to be applied to as many patients as possible for the longest duration possible and that the etiology and very nature of the disorder has been clouded and hijacked by medical/science writers who are heavily paid by drug companies that sell the FDA-approved drugs for fibromyalgia and which directly profit from a population of confused doctors and helpless patients which create a multi-billion dollar international drug/medical market.

After considerable literature review and personal deliberation, I have decided to include information about complex regional pain syndrome (CRPS) in this section that is otherwise exclusive to fibromyalgia. At the time of this writing, I am impressed that these are two variants of essentially the same pathophysiology, just as migraine and cluster headaches are variants on the same theme. With all due respect for the differences and distinctions between these conditions, I appreciate that their pathophysiologic similarities are of greater importance for understanding and treating both disorders. Both FM and CRPS share 1) central sensitization, 2) peripheral sensitization, 3) neuroinflammation, 4) neurogenic inflammation, 5) increased glutaminergic/NMDA-mediated central and peripheral neurotransmission, 6) mitochondrial dysfunction, 7) increased intestinal permeability, and 8) gastrointestinal dysbiosis. Relative to my study of migraine and fibromyalgia which has a history of publications over many years, I have only recently begun to study CRPS, but my impression is that it is a spinal cord (SC)-specific regional activation of glia and neurons and failure of regional neuroinhibition; somewhat analogous to a spinal cord migraine/seizure or at least the spinal cord variant of fibromyalgia. I agree with Littlejohn[227] that both FM and CRPS have a component of neurogenic inflammation; I think the role of neurogenic inflammation in CRPS is stronger than it is in FM, also—perhaps obviously—more focal, limited to a region of spinal cord segments. While the pathophysiologic similarities among FM and CRPS suggest that effective nutritional therapeutics for FM will be at least partly efficacious for CRPS, we generally do not have such proof due to lack of studies in CRPS; however, the risk:benefit ratio of these highly safe and frequently efficacious interventions clearly favors empiric implementation followed by monitoring of therapeutic response in a condition notorious for its debilitating severity and therapeutic recalcitrance.

Introduction and Clinical Presentation

- <u>Overview</u>: Fibromyalgia (FM) is commonly described as an "idiopathic" (of unknown origin) syndrome principally characterized by widespread body pain and numerous myofascial tender points at specific locations. FM is most common in women 20-50 years of age, and the condition often presents with associated complaints of fatigue, headaches, subjective numbness, altered sleep patterns, and gastrointestinal disturbances. FM in children and adolescents presents similarly to FM in adults except for the comparatively higher prevalence of sleep disturbance and the finding of fewer tender points in children.[228] Until recently,

---

[227] Littlejohn G. Neurogenic neuroinflammation in fibromyalgia and complex regional pain syndrome. *Nat Rev Rheumatol.* 2015 Nov;11(11):639-48. At the time this citation is added in 2015 Dec, I (DrV) had recently submitted a reply to *Nat Rev Rheumatol*; my reply will be posted at ichnfm.academia.edu/AlexVasquez as soon as possible.

[228] Siegel DM, Janeway D, Baum J. Fibromyalgia syndrome in children and adolescents: clinical features at presentation and status at follow-up. *Pediatrics* 1998;101:377-82

fibromyalgia was considered a *diagnosis of exclusion* after infection, autoimmunity, or other primary causes of widespread pain were excluded by clinical and laboratory assessment. However, current criteria base the diagnosis on positive findings of chronic, widespread musculoskeletal pain in characteristic locations; these criteria will be described below. Fibromyalgia shares several clinical, demographic, and pathologic features with chronic fatigue syndrome (CFS) and irritable bowel syndrome (IBS); the reason for these overlaps is not generally understood by most clinicians and researchers but will be made plain in this writing.

- The common medical view—scientifically inaccurate, financially leveraged: The prevailing medical view, expressed by most medical doctors and the authors of widely cited articles, is that fibromyalgia is idiopathic—*of unknown origin*—with strong neuropsychogenic (*neuro*=nerves and brain, *psyche*=mind, *genic*=origin) influences (in other words, "It's all in your head.") and that, since the underlying causes of the condition have not been identified, the best therapeutic approach is symptom suppression via perpetual pharmacotherapy with adjunctive use of psychotherapy and limited exercise.[229,230,231] This prevailing medical view is unscientific (not based on science) and counterscientific (ignores and contradicts published and validated research), unethical (fails to provide effective treatment when such treatment is available; condemns patients to medicalization and suffering), and commercially leveraged (diagnostic criteria revision and many review articles discussing treatment are sponsored by drug companies; medical profession benefits financially by having many long-term drug-dependent patients).

- Fibromyalgia—in its original "1990-based" description—is a disease, not a syndrome: The term *syndrome* connotes that a cluster of symptoms is of a nonorganic, psychogenic, or idiopathic nature, whereas *disease* validates the organic and pathophysiological nature of an illness. This author advocates the use of *disease* rather than *syndrome* when describing fibromyalgia in appreciation of the real, organic, biochemical, and histopathological (*histo*=cells and tissues, *pathological*=disease) findings which clearly indicate that fibromyalgia is a specific disease entity and not simply a psychogenic or enigmatic cluster of symptoms. If fibromyalgia is a real, organic clinical entity (as will be documented here), then the appropriate designation is *fibromyalgia disease* (FMD) rather than *fibromyalgia syndrome* (FMS). For consistency and clarity within this section, the general term "fibromyalgia" will be used. Relatedly, the term "irritable bowel syndrome" (IBS) is also a misnomer that confuses professionals as well as the general public into thinking that the condition does not have identified causes and (nonpharmaceutical) treatments; despite promulgations to the contrary, the cause of IBS is well-known[232], and effective treatment is readily available. When in 2010 the American College of Rheumatology (ACR) mistakenly allowed the diagnostic criteria for FM to be hijacked to leverage more drug sales—facilitate the making of the diagnosis, broaden the number of people affected, and impair the "cure" of and escape from the disease—the legitimate meaning of the diagnosis of course became less specific and much broader and therefore less meaningful. Per the original diagnostic criteria published in 1990, fibromyalgia is a legitimate functional disease and should be described and labeled as such; per the ridiculous diagnostic criteria published in 2010, fibromyalgia is a symptom cluster of aches, pains, and other signs and symptoms that can accompany virtually any other disease. Classic legitimate "FM" or "FMD" is what is described in this section (per the 1990 criteria), not simply the pain and symptom cluster (FMS) per the 2010 criteria. The idea that any and all patients with widespread pain should qualify for a diagnosis of fibromyalgia is ludicrous, and the 2010 ACR criteria for fibromyalgia are an obfuscating disservice to patients, doctors, and researchers while only benefiting the drug companies that can now sell their expensive and ineffective drugs *more quickly* to a *larger audience* for a *longer duration*. Patients develop true *primary* FM/FMD per the description that follows; patients can develop "fibromyalgia-like syndrome" or "fibromyalgia syndrome"—ie, FMS—by many means, including head injury or major trauma—these cases are more legitimately titled *secondary* hyperalgesic/allodynic central sensitization and/or myofascial pain syndromes.

- Prevalence, symptoms, and clinical findings: Fibromyalgia is one of the most common chronic pain conditions, affecting an estimated 10 million people in the U.S. and an estimated 3-6% of people world-wide.[233]

[229] Chakrabarty S, Zoorob R. Fibromyalgia. *Am Fam Physician*. 2007 Jul 15;76(2):247-54
[230] Tierney ML. McPhee SJ, Papadakis MA (eds). *Current Medical Diagnosis and Treatment 2006, 45th Edition*. New York: Lange Medical Books, pages 820-821
[231] Simms RW. Nonarticular soft tissue disorders. In Andreoli TE, Carpenter CCJ, Griggs RC, Benjamin IJ (eds). *Cecil Essentials of Medicine. 7th Edition*. Elsevier 2007:851-2
[232] Lin HC. Small intestinal bacterial overgrowth: a framework for understanding irritable bowel syndrome. *JAMA*. 2004 Aug 18;292(7):852-8
[233] "Fibromyalgia is one of the most common chronic pain conditions. The disorder affects an estimated 10 million people in the U.S. and an estimated 3-6% of the world population." National Fibromyalgia Association. fmaware.org/PageServera6cc.html?pagename=fibromyalgia_affected Accessed Sept 2012.

Approximately 10% of affected patients have severe symptoms resulting in partial or total disability. Affected patients report chronic aches, pains, and stiffness with a proclivity for localization near the neck, shoulders, low back, and hips. Pain and fatigue are typically exacerbated following physical exertion or psychological stress. Associated manifestations include fatigue, sleep disorders (including insomnia, unrefreshing sleep, and objective abnormalities such as an increase in stage 1 sleep, a reduction in delta sleep, and alpha-delta sleep anomaly), subjective numbness, headaches, and gastrointestinal disturbances consistent with a clinical diagnosis of irritable bowel syndrome (IBS). Clinical findings shared between FM and IBS include abdominal pain and discomfort, changed frequency of stool, diarrhea and/or constipation, abdominal bloating/distention/gas and flatulence, dyspepsia/heartburn, headaches especially migraine-type headaches), fatigue, myalgias, restless leg syndrome, anxiety, and depression. The **high prevalence (>50%) of migraine-type headaches in FM patients** suggests an underlying pathogenesis shared between cephalgia (*ceph*=head, *algia*=pain) and widespread myalgia (*myo*=muscle, *algia*=pain); one of the established and most likely causative abnormalities shared between migraine and FM is impaired mitochondrial function, which will be explained in greater detail later in this publication. Cognitive symptoms such as "brain fog" ("fibro-fog") and difficulty with memory and word retrieval, as well as **environmental intolerance (EI) and multiple chemical sensitivity (MCS)**, are seen in both FM and CFS[234]; again, this overlap of shared symptoms suggests a common etiopathogenesis (*etio*=cause, *patho*=disease, *genesis*=initiation). Routine physical examination and laboratory findings are generally normal, with the exception the physical examination finding of fibromyalgia tender points (described and diagrammed below in the section on Diagnosis per the 1990 diagnostic criteria).

Objective "organic" (ie, real) abnormalities in fibromyalgia dispel the myth that the condition is psychogenic

1. Histologic and functional abnormalities in muscle tissue: Disorganization of actin filaments, accumulation of lipofuscin bodies consistent with premature muscle aging, increased DNA fragmentation, and focal areas of chronic muscle contraction, reduced perfusion of muscle tissue during exercise (i.e., reduced blood flow to muscles).

2. Mitochondrial defects: Accumulation of glycogen (muscle sugar) and lipid (fat) indicate that intracellular energy production is impaired and that the cells are unable to efficiently convert fuel sources into energy in the form of ATP, adenosine triphosphate, which is the basic fuel source for cellular metabolism. Also noted are significant reductions in the number of mitochondria, reduced activity of important enzymes such as 3-hydroxy-CoA dehydrogenase, citrate synthase, and cytochrome oxidase. Nutritional deficiencies, such as CoQ-10 deficiency, promote mitochondrial dysfunction, thus leading to mitochondrial destruction (mitophagy) which ultimately results in reduced numbers of mitochondria and perpetuates and aggravates muscle fatigue, pain, and neurocognitive dysfunction (i.e., brain fog, difficulty thinking, depression).

3. Oxidative stress: Increased oxidative stress results from mitochondrial dysfunction and nutrient depletion.

4. Neuroendocrine abnormalities: Hypothalamic-pituitary-adrenal (HPA) disturbance indicates impaired function of the brain and endocrine system.

5. Elevated brain glutamate, homocysteine, and interlukin-8: See in FM, also CFS and CRPS.

6. Low-grade immune activation: Increased cytokine production indicates a pro-inflammatory state.

7. Bacterial overgrowth in the intestines: FM patients have excess/overgrowth of bacteria in their intestines, referred to as SIBO (small intestine bacterial overgrowth); CRPS patients have an abnormal pattern of microbial growth.

8. Increased intestinal permeability, "leaky gut": Generally this indicates a gastrointestinal disorder, including but not limited to microbial imbalance (dysbiosis) or overt infection. Leaky gut is seen in both FM and CRPS.

9. High prevalence of vitamin D deficiency: Common in the general population but more common in patients with chronic pain; vitamin D deficiency causes chronic pain, depression/anxiety, and low-grade inflammation—all of these problems are seen in patients with fibromyalgia.

10. Low blood levels of L-tryptophan: FM patients have low levels of the amino acid tryptophan in their blood, despite adequate dietary intake. The most likely explanation for the deficiency of tryptophan is destruction of tryptophan by bacterial enzyme action. Several intestinal bacteria produce the enzyme tryptophanase, which destroys the amino acid tryptophan. Bacterial overgrowth results in more tryptophanase, resulting in tryptophan deficiency. Deficiency of tryptophan results in deficiencies of the hormones serotonin and melatonin, which result in anxiety, depression, food/sugar cravings, unrestful sleep, and mitochondrial dysfunction, since deficiency of melatonin causes reduced mitochondrial energy-production efficiency.

---

[234] Brown MM, Jason LA. Functioning in individuals with chronic fatigue syndrome: increased impairment with co-occurring multiple chemical sensitivity and fibromyalgia. *Dyn Med.* 2007 May 31;6:6 dynamic-med.com/content/6/1/6

Pathophysiology of Pain and Mitochondrial Dysfunction in Fibromyalgia

- Patients with FM demonstrate multiple biochemical abnormalities, centering on mitochondrial dysfunction, oxidative stress, and increased pain perception: Ultrastructural and biochemical abnormalities appear to be more pathologically significant and clinically relevant than the noted histological changes in skeletal muscle biopsy samples. Importantly, **the biochemical abnormalities** *are the cause* **of the histologic/tissue abnormalities.** Numerous **mitochondrial enzyme defects are seen**, including reduced activity of 3-hydroxy-CoA dehydrogenase, citrate synthase, and cytochrome oxidase. Levels of free magnesium are reduced by 31%, and levels of complexed ATP-magnesium are reduced by 12% in muscle from FM patients compared with levels seen in healthy controls; these biochemical and bioenergetic defects contribute to rapid-onset fatigue and muscle pain. From a neurophysiological perspective, *magnesium deficiency* can promote hypersensitivity to pain due to a reduction in the partial blockade of N-methyl-D-aspartate (NMDA) neurotransmitter receptor sites.[235] Reduced perfusion of muscle tissue during exercise results in relative tissue hypoxia, reduced muscle healing after the microtrauma of exercise, and promotion of muscle soreness due to accumulation of L-lactate (lactic acid).[236] **Increased oxidative stress** is also seen in FM patients,[237] providing additional objective evidence of the systemic, organic, and non-psychogenic nature of the illness. Evidence of hypothalamic-pituitary-adrenal disturbance and **increased cytokine production (particularly interleukin-8, which promotes sympathetic pain, and interleukin-6, which induces hyperalgesia [increased perception of pain], fatigue, and depression**[238]) further characterize the systemic and organic nature of this condition and are well documented in the research literature. **The majority of fibromyalgia patients demonstrate laboratory evidence of bacterial overgrowth in the small bowel**[239], and the details and important implications of this will be discussed below. **Vitamin D deficiency**—a recognized cause of chronic widespread pain as well as depression, muscle fatigue, and chronic low-grade inflammation—is also common in fibromyalgia patients.[240,241] FM patients have **significantly elevated blood levels of pentosidine**, which is an advanced glycation end-product (AGE) and marker of oxidative stress and glycosylation (sugar-protein binding); AGEs promote chronic inflammation and nociceptive sensitization leading to chronic pain.[242] Another AGE very similar to pentosidine, **carboxy-methyl-lysine (CML) is found in higher levels in the blood and muscle of FM patients**[243]; both pentosidine and CML cause expedited "muscle aging" and promote chronic pain and inflammation. These objective abnormalities of biochemical, histological, nutritional, and microbiological/gastrointestinal status force clinicians to appreciate the valid and organic nature of fibromyalgia. As previously stated, this evidence refutes promulgations espoused within standard allopathic/pharmaceutical medicine that fibromyalgia is an idiopathic condition warranting lifelong medicalization with expensive and potentially hazardous analgesic and antidepressant drugs; the focus on drug treatment to mask/suppress the pain of fibromyalgia detours doctors and patients away from focusing on the legitimate and validated causes of fibromyalgia and physiology-based (rather than pharmacology-based) means for alleviating the suffering and pain that these patients experience. CRPS patients also show evidence of biochemical and metabolic abnormalities, including increased oxidative stress and impaired mitochondrial function.[244]

  - Chronic widespread pain: increased glutamate and lactate concentrations in the trapezius muscle and plasma. (*Clin J Pain*. 2014 May[245]): "Chronic widespread pain (CWP), including fibromyalgia syndrome (FM), is associated with prominent negative consequences. CWP has been associated with alterations in

[235] Park JH, Niermann KJ, Olsen N. Evidence for metabolic abnormalities in the muscles of patients with fibromyalgia. *Curr Rheumatol Rep*. 2000 Apr;2(2):131-40

[236] Elvin et al. Decreased muscle blood flow in fibromyalgia patients during standardised muscle exercise. *Eur J Pain*. 2006 Feb;10(2):137-44

[237] Altindag O, Celik H. Total antioxidant capacity and the severity of the pain in patients with fibromyalgia. *Redox Rep*. 2006;11(3):131-5

[238] Wallace DJ, Linker-Israeli M, Hallegua D, et al. Cytokines play an aetiopathogenic role in fibromyalgia. *Rheumatology* (Oxford). 2001 Jul;40(7):743-9

[239] Pimentel et al. A link between irritable bowel syndrome and fibromyalgia may be related to findings on lactulose breath testing. *Ann Rheum Dis*. 2004 Apr;63(4):450-2

[240] Huisman AM, White KP, Algra A, et al. Vitamin D levels in women with systemic lupus erythematosus and fibromyalgia. *J Rheumatol*. 2001 Nov;28(11):2535-9

[241] Armstrong DJ, Meenagh GK, Bickle I, et al. Vitamin D deficiency is associated with anxiety and depression in fibromyalgia. *Clin Rheumatol*. 2007 Apr;26(4):551-4

[242] Hein G, Franke S. Are advanced glycation end-product-modified proteins of pathogenetic importance in fibromyalgia? *Rheumatology* (Oxford). 2002 Oct;41(10):1163-7

[243] "In the interstitial connective tissue of fibromyalgic muscles we found a more intensive staining of the AGE CML, activated NF-kappaB, and also higher CML levels in the serum of these patients compared to the controls. RAGE was only present in FM muscle." Rüster M, Franke S, Späth M, Pongratz DE, Stein G, Hein GE. Detection of elevated N epsilon-carboxymethyllysine levels in muscular tissue and in serum of patients with fibromyalgia. *Scand J Rheumatol*. 2005 Nov-Dec;34(6):460-3

[244] "Recent evidence demonstrates that oxidative stress is associated with clinical symptoms in patients with CRPS-I. ... This review summarises the effect of oxidative stress and mitochondrial dysfunction in the pathogenesis of CRPS." Taha R, Blaise GA. Update on the pathogenesis of complex regional pain syndrome: role of oxidative stress. *Can J Anaesth*. 2012 Sep;59(9):875-81

[245] Gerdle et al. Chronic widespread pain: increased glutamate and lactate concentrations in the trapezius muscle and plasma. *Clin J Pain*. 2014 May;30(5):409-20. See also "Significantly higher interstitial concentrations of pyruvate and lactate were found in patients with fibromyalgia- syndrome. The multivariate regression analyses of group membership and pressure pain thresholds of the trapezius confirmed the importance of pyruvate and lactate." Gerdle et al. Increased interstitial concentrations of pyruvate and lactate in the trapezius muscle of patients with fibromyalgia: a microdialysis study. *J Rehabil Med*. 2010 Jul;42(7):679-87

the central processing of nociception. ...CWP patients had significantly increased interstitial muscle and plasma concentrations of lactate and glutamate. No significant differences existed in blood flow between CWP and CON [controls]. The interstitial concentrations-but not the plasma levels-of glutamate and lactate correlated significantly with aspects of pain such as pressure pain thresholds of the trapezius and tibialis anterior and the mean pain intensity in CWP but not in CON." Elevated lactate correlates with and suggests the presence of impaired energy/ATP production, consistent with mitochondrial dysfunction, while elevated glutamate levels is expected to promote enhanced pain reception, given that glutamate is the classic excitatory neurotransmitter (activator of glutamate receptors in general and the NMDA receptor in particular). The combination of elevated lactate (e.g., muscle impairment leading to muscle pain) and elevated glutamate (e.g., enhanced sensitivity to pain) is the perfect recipe and explanation for muscle-generated pain with enhanced sensitivity to pain that might otherwise be well tolerated. In addition to lactate and glutamate, patients with chronic muscle pain also show tissue-specific elevations of pyruvate (again indicating impaired energy/ATP production in muscles, leading to easy fatigability and increased achiness/pain) and elevated serotonin[246]; although we generally think of serotonin as having a relaxing and analgesic effect in the *central* nervous system, serotonin in the *periphery* appears to promote pain perception and sensitization while also promoting inflammation.[247]

- <u>Patients with FM demonstrate abnormalities in muscle tissue and mitochondrial function</u>: Muscle biopsies from patients with fibromyalgia show numerous histological, ultrastructural, and biochemical abnormalities, including defects in mitochondrial structure and function, reduced numbers of capillaries in skeletal muscle (leading to reduced blood supply to muscles), thickened capillary endothelium (thicker vessel walls), and ragged red fibers consistent with the development of **mitochondrial myopathy** (*myo*=muscle, *pathos*=disease). The histological finding of "rubber-band morphology" with reticular threads connecting neighboring cells in muscle biopsies of FM patients is associated with prolonged contractions in adjacent/neighboring muscle fibers; these abnormalities result in and perpetuate a low-energy state within myocytes (*myo*=muscle, *cytes*=cells).[248] Other studies have shown disorganization of actin filaments, accumulation of lipofuscin (cellular debris) consistent with premature muscle aging, accumulation of glycogen and lipid accumulation consistent with **mitochondrial impairment**, increased DNA fragmentation, **significant reductions in the number of mitochondria**, and focal areas of chronic muscle contraction.[249] These histological abnormalities are important and establish the fact that **fibromyalgia is a *disease of metabolic dysfunction*** rather than an *emotional disorder of psychogenic origin*; therefore, attributing the pain and fatigue of fibromyalgia to a mental-psychological cause or a central nervous system disorder such as central sensitization is unscientific and illogical. Patients with CRPS also show evidence of impaired oxygen diffusion and mitochondrial impairment[250], and Tan et al[251] specifically noted that mitochondrial ETC "complex II activity in the CRPS I patients was significantly lower."

---

[246] "Several studies clearly showed elevated levels of serotonin, glutamate, lactate, and pyruvate in localized chronic myalgias and may be potential biomarkers." Gerdle et al. Chronic musculoskeletal pain: review of mechanisms and biochemical biomarkers as assessed by the microdialysis technique. *J Pain Res.* 2014 Jun 12;7:313-26
[247] "5-HT, acting in combination with other inflammatory mediators, may ectopically excite and sensitize afferent nerve fibers, thus contributing to peripheral sensitization and hyperalgesia in inflammation and nerve injury." Sommer C. Serotonin in pain and analgesia in the periphery. *Mol Neurobiol.* 2004 Oct:117-25. See also: "5-HT sensitizes afferent nerve fibers, thus contributing to hyperalgesia in inflammation and nerve injury." Sommer C. Is serotonin hyperalgesic or analgesic? *Curr Pain Headache Rep.* 2006 Apr; 101-6
[248] Olsen NJ, Park JH. Skeletal muscle abnormalities in patients with fibromyalgia. *Am J Med Sci.* 1998 Jun;315(6):351-8
[249] Sprott H, Salemi S, Gay RE, et al. Increased DNA fragmentation and ultrastructural changes in fibromyalgic muscle fibres. *Ann Rheum Dis.* 2004 Mar;63(3):245-51
[250] "The mean venous oxygen saturation (S(v)O(2)) value (94.3% ± 4.0%) of the affected limb was significantly higher than S(v)O(2) values found in healthy subjects (77.5% ± 9.8%) pointing to a severely decreased oxygen diffusion or utilization within the affected limb. ... Ultrastructural investigations of soleus skeletal muscle capillaries revealed thickened endothelial cells and thickened basement membranes. Muscle capillary densities were decreased in comparison with literature data. High venous oxygen saturation levels were partially explained by impaired diffusion of oxygen due to thickened basement membrane and decreased capillary density. ...The abnormal skeletal muscle findings points to severe disuse but only partially explain the impaired diffusion of oxygen; mitochondrial dysfunction seems a likely explanation in addition." Tan et al. Impaired oxygen utilization in skeletal muscle of CRPS I patients. *J Surg Res.* 2012 Mar;173(1):145-52
[251] "We observed that mitochondria obtained from CRPS I muscle tissue displayed reduced mitochondrial ATP production and substrate oxidation rates in comparison to control muscle tissue. Moreover, we observed reactive oxygen species evoked damage to mitochondrial proteins and reduced MnSOD levels." Tan et al. Mitochondrial dysfunction in muscle tissue of complex regional pain syndrome type I patients. *Eur J Pain.* 2011 Aug;15(7):708-15

CONTROL

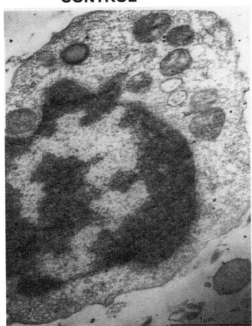

PATIENT

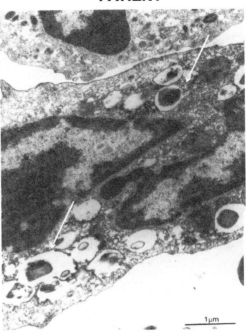

Blood cells in FM patients show mitochondrial destruction (mitophagy), smaller size and lower number of mitochondria: Structure of blood mononuclear cells (BMCs, cells of the immune system) from FM patients. The healthy/control BMCs show mitochondria with a normal structure. Autophagosomes (indicated by arrows), where mitochondria are destroyed (the process of mitophagy [*mito*=mitochondria, *phagy*=consumption], are noted in the BMCs of patients with FM. [Bar = 1 micrometer]. This open-access image is respectfully attributed to the brilliant research published by these researchers Cordero MD, De Miguel M, Moreno Fernández AM, Carmona López IM, Garrido Maraver J, Cotán D, Gómez Izquierdo L, Bonal P, Campa F, Bullon P, Navas P, Sánchez Alcázar JA. Mitochondrial dysfunction and mitophagy activation in blood mononuclear cells of fibromyalgia patients. *Arthritis Res Ther.* 2010;12(1):R17 arthritis-research.com/content/12/1/R17

Mitophagy: The body's inherent mechanism for the destruction of dysfunctional mitochondria

Concept: Autophagic destruction of mitochondria is termed "mitophagy" and is the body's inherent mechanism for eliminating superfluous or dysfunctional mitochondria; this generally has a protective and life-sustaining effect. However, in the case of fibromyalgia wherein the mitochondrial dysfunction is persistent, prolonged mitophagy contributes to failure of adequate energy production and thereby contributes to clinical manifestations of fatigue, dyscognition, and impaired exercise/activity performance. Further, the consistent documentation of significant mitophagy in patients with fibromyalgia proves the biological/organic/real/pathophysiologic character of the illness and refutes the pharmacocentric paradigm which holds that the condition is of psychogenic or neurologic origin and thus to be treated with so-called "antidepressants" and/or analgesic drugs, respectively.

- "The removal of damaged mitochondria that could contribute to cellular dysfunction or death is achieved through process of mitochondrial autophagy, i.e. mitophagy." Novak I. *Antioxid Redox Signal.* 2011
- "Mitochondrial number and health are regulated by mitophagy, a process by which excessive or damaged mitochondria are subjected to autophagic degradation." Rambold. *Cell Cycle.* 2011
- **"Autophagy can be beneficial for the cells by eliminating dysfunctional mitochondria, but massive autophagy can promote cell injury and may contribute to the pathophysiology of FM."** Cordero. *Arthritis Res Ther.* 2010

- <u>Pain in fibromyalgia originates peripherally and is amplified centrally</u>: The pain of fibromyalgia originates from the muscles[252] secondary to stimulation by oxidative and inflammatory mediators and is excessively amplified in the brain and spinal cord; another possible peripheral contribution to pain inputs is degeneration of nerve fibers in the skin.[253] To risk redundancy for clarity: **FM pain originates *peripherally* in the muscles**

---

[252] "Results of these studies suggest that FM pain is associated with widespread primary and secondary cutaneous hyperalgesia, which are dynamically maintained by tonic impulse input from deep tissues and likely by brain-to-spinal cord facilitation. Enhanced somatic pains are accompanied by mechanical hyperalgesia and allodynia in FM patients as compared with healthy controls. FM pain is likely to be at least partially maintained by peripheral impulse input from deep tissues. This conclusion is supported by results of several studies showing that injection of local anesthetics into painful muscles normalizes somatic hyperalgesia in FM patients." Staud R. Is it all central sensitization? Role of peripheral tissue nociception in chronic musculoskeletal pain. *Curr Rheumatol Rep.* 2010 Dec;12(6):448-54
[253] "The study's instruments comprised the Michigan Neuropathy Screening Instrument (MNSI), the Utah Early Neuropathy Scale (UENS), distal-leg neurodiagnostic skin biopsies, plus autonomic-function testing (AFT). We found that 41% of skin biopsies from subjects with fibromyalgia vs 3% of biopsies from control subjects were diagnostic for small-fiber polyneuropathy (SFPN), and MNSI and UENS scores were higher in patients with fibromyalgia than in control subjects (all $P \leq 0.001$). Abnormal AFTs were equally prevalent, suggesting that fibromyalgia-associated SFPN is primarily somatic. Blood tests from subjects with fibromyalgia and SFPN-diagnostic skin biopsies provided insights into causes. All glucose tolerance tests were normal, but 8 subjects had dysimmune markers, 2 had hepatitis C serologies, and 1 family had apparent genetic causality. These

(and likely in the skin as well, at least in some patients) and is amplified *centrally* in the spinal cord and brain. Following reception and amplification of the original muscular pain, the peripheral "receptive field" grows both in size and intensity/hypersensitivity to include the skin, so that various skin inputs are perceived as pain; the two main types of dysfunctional pain sensitivity/sensations are allodynia (reception of nonpainful stimuli as pain) and hyperalgesia (extended duration and increased intensity of pain).

- <u>Enhanced central pain processing of fibromyalgia patients is maintained by muscle afferent input</u> (*Pain.* 2009 Sep[254]): "Lidocaine injections increased local pain thresholds and decreased remote secondary heat hyperalgesia in FM patients, emphasizing the important role of peripheral impulse input in maintaining central sensitization in this chronic pain syndrome; similar to other persistent pain conditions such as irritable bowel syndrome and complex regional pain syndrome."

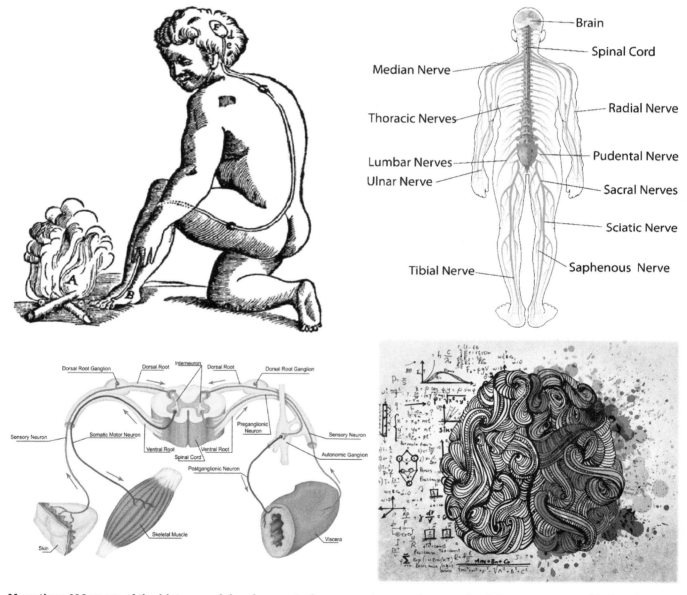

More than 400 years of the history and development of neuroanatomy and neurophysiology represented in four images: These four images in sequence represent the history and development of the fields of neuroanatomy and neurophysiology, ❶ starting with the drawing by Descartes in the 1600s, ❷ the tracing of nerves throughout the body, ❸ what might be called the

findings suggest that some patients with chronic pain labeled as fibromyalgia have unrecognized SFPN, a distinct disease that can be tested for objectively and sometimes treated definitively." Oaklander et al. Objective evidence that small-fiber polyneuropathy underlies some illnesses currently labeled as fibromyalgia. *Pain.* 2013 Nov;154(11):2310-6
[254] Staud et al. Enhanced central pain processing of fibromyalgia patients is maintained by muscle afferent input. *Pain.* 2009 Sep;145(1-2):96-104

start of the "functional neurology revolution" with the work of Melzack and Wall in 1965, and ❹ culminating with today's understanding of neurophysiology and neuropathophysiology as highly dynamic and interactive processes, far advanced from the simple models of sequential reception, perception, and interpretation.

1. ***Image upper left—Peripheral reception and central perception of pain as simple linear connectivity***: The famous historical image from Rene Descartes (French polymath, 1596-1650) was an important beginning in society's understanding that pain had a neurophysiologic basis; in this model, pain sensations were received peripherally, transmitted by nerves to the brain where they were perceived and acted upon (e.g., reflexive withdrawal from painful stimuli).

2. ***Image upper right—Nervous system as simple anatomic connectivity***: Advances in anatomy and neuroanatomy later provided more details about neurologic pathways and synapses (connections between nerves), but the overall model remained very mechanical, resembling electric circuitry (e.g., wiring) transmitting signals which were simply received in the brain for interpretation. Important within this obvious, simple, and overly simplistic model of neuroanatomy is the facile assumption of "stimulus-response specificity"—the idea that specific sensory receptors receive only one type of sensory input such as temperature or light touch or vibration; what we appreciate instead is that receptors, nerves, and their connections within the spinal cord, brainstem, and brain can communicate a wide range of sensory inputs in ways that commonly defy anatomic expectations. As stated by Wall[255], "Obviously anatomy does not predict physiology." Wall goes on to dismantle "the specificity theory" with the observations that "nociceptors become sensitized by prolonged or repeated noxious stimulation so that their threshold drops and they are excited by normally innocuous stimuli" and "one should be cautious in attributing one and only one function to a particular cell …the degree of convergence is under control of other afferents and descending systems and is also dependent on the activity of segmental interneurons."

3. ***Image lower left—Interconnections of nerves allows for "spill over" of sensory inputs and dynamic changes in perception, including amplification and misinterpretation***: Research published by Melzack and Wall[256] in 1965 is commonly credited with revolutionizing our view of pain processing by changing the paradigm from a static model of linear connectivity (e.g., sensory receptors to peripheral nerve to spinal cord to the brain) to one of dynamic interconnectivity, with interactive interconnections and opportunities for inhibition, amplification and misinterpretation at nearly every level. The perception of pain is neither simple, nor solely anatomy-based, nor static; it is a dynamic process reflecting the sum total interplay of peripheral reception (e.g., modifiable by inflammation), nerve transmission (e.g., modifiable by nutritional status and glutamate levels), reception and "intermixing" (e.g., pre-synaptic inhibition/facilitation, post-synaptic inhibition/facilitation) in the spinal cord, brain stem, subcortical structures such as the thalamus, and the "conscious" brain cortex. Furthermore and very importantly, we know that sensory nerves and sensory nerve endings do much more than simply receive information; in addition to sensing various types of stimuli through various types of sensors in nerve endings, sensory nerves directly influence the peripheral environment by releasing inflammatory mediators via a process called "neurogenic inflammation." Neurogenic (*neuro*—nerve, *genic*—generated, originating) inflammation again forces us to expand our perception of the nervous system and its components; in neurogenic inflammation, stimulated sensory nerves respond to painful stimuli by releasing inflammatory mediators into the self-same environment, thereby adding an inflammatory component to whatever is perceived as pain-inducing. One can think of this as providing a survival advantage in the short-term, as the inflammatory response generated by the release of these pro-inflammatory mediators released by nerves will serve to prepare the area for infiltration by immune cells to remove and repair damage and repel any infectious agents that might have entered with the injury. However, when chronically sustained in so-called "chronic diseases", neurogenic inflammation contributes to tissue injury, as we see in complex regional pain syndrome (CRPS). Indeed, CRPS might be considered a prototype of the effects of neurogenic inflammation. In a review published in 2015, Littlejohn[257] writes, "Neurogenic inflammation—comprising tissue swelling, vasomotor changes and marked allodynia—also contributes substantially to the clinical features of CRPS."; he goes on to mention the clinical sequelae that have a strong or dominant origination from neurogenic inflammation, including bone marrow edema, osteopenia, visceral pain, hyperalgesia (increased intensity and duration of pain sensitivity), allodynia (misperception of sensory input as pain), abnormal hair and nail growth (including absence of same), rashes, sweating, vasodilation (causing heat and redness), vasoconstriction (causing cold and blueness), skin ulceration and fibrosis of skin and joints. Littlejohn goes on to describe how neurogenic inflammation can promote itself, as nerve-released inflammatory mediators cause tissue damage that leads to pain, the self-same sensory nerves respond to the self-generated pain by causing more neurogenic inflammation; the proper term for this concept and phenomenon is "*neurogenic* neurogenic inflammation" or "neurogenic inflammation-induced neurogenic inflammation", a vicious cycle. I (DrV[258]) disagree with Littlejohn that this vicious cycle is at the core of fibromyalgia, although I agree that it could and likely does play a contributing part. Lastly and also included in the review by Littlejohn, the idea of "neurogenic neuroinflammation" likely has merit based on our current understanding of neuropathophysiology; especially in the spinal cord and brain, neuronal activity triggers microglial inflammation, which thereby inflames the nearby nerves for a vicious cycle of neurogenic neuroinflammation. This neurogenic neuroinflammation is almost certain to play a major role in CRPS, importantly but to a lesser degree in FM (chronic) and migraine (periodic). In the context of the brain and spinal cord,

---

[255] Wall PD. The gate control theory of pain mechanisms. A re-examination and re-statement. *Brain*. 1978 Mar;101(1):1-18

[256] Melzack R, Wall PD. Pain mechanisms: a new theory. *Science*. 1965 Nov 19;150(3699):971–979

[257] Littlejohn G. Neurogenic neuroinflammation in fibromyalgia and complex regional pain syndrome. *Nat Rev Rheumatol*. 2015 Nov;11(11):639-48

[258] At the time this citation is added in 2015 Dec, I (DrV) had recently submitted a reply to the article by Littlejohn (Neurogenic neuroinflammation in fibromyalgia and complex regional pain syndrome. *Nat Rev Rheumatol*. 2015 Nov) pointing out some of the bitemporal hemianopsia of the aforecited article; my reply will be published either by *Nat Rev Rheumatol* or elsewhere and will be posted at ichnfm.academia.edu/AlexVasquez as soon as possible. In reply to the previously cited article, Cordeo —a preeminent researcher in the field of fibromyalgia's mitochondrial dysfunction and its remediation by the vitamin-like substance coenzyme Q10 (CoQ10)—noted that neurogenic neuroinflammation includes activation of the NLRP3 inflammasome, which he suggests could be a therapeutic target (e.g., by CoQ10). "Interestingly, inflammasome activation in the CNS primarily occurs in microglia and macrophages. Microglia have been highly studied as key contributors to pathological and chronic pain mechanisms, and are involved in hyperalgesia and allodynia in both fibromyalgia and chronic fatigue syndrome, as well as pain in CRPS. Microglial inflammasome activation promotes the recruitment of peripheral innate immune cells (macrophages) and adaptive immune cells (T cells and B cells), as well as further activating nearby glial cells." Cordero MD. The inflammasome in fibromyalgia and CRPS: a microglial hypothesis? *Nat Rev Rheumatol*. 2015 Nov;11(11):630. See also Cordero MD et al. NLRP3 inflammasome is activated in fibromyalgia: the effect of coenzyme Q10. *Antioxid Redox Signal*. 2014 Mar 10;20(8):1169-80

neurogenic neuroinflammation contains an important pro-inflammatory contributor that is phenotypically ready to perceive, amplify, and exacerbate neuroinflammation caused by increased neuroactivity—the microglial cells; thus, neurogenic (in this context, including the microglia and astrocytes as components of the brain and spinal cord) neuroinflammation would be expected to participate in seizure disorders and vaccine-induced encephalomyelitis.

4. ***Image lower right*—The nervous system (represented by artistic brain image) is now appreciated as dynamic and interactive receiver and processor of sensory information**: In modern times, pain processing is appreciated as a dynamic, complex, and interactive process at every level, from ❶ peripheral reception of stimuli (e.g., in the skin or muscles), to the ❷ spinal cord, to the ❸ brainstem, to the ❹ subcortical structures especially the thalamus, to the ❺ cortex. Generally appreciated is that much "spill-over", "misinterpretation", inhibition and amplification" can occur in the spinal cord, brainstem, and structures of the brain, so that the initial perception of pain—in the muscles for example in the case of FM—is amplified at multiple levels and "spills over" to be perceived as skin pain, resulting in allodynia (misinterpretation of light touch as pain) and hyperalgesia (pain perception is amplified in intensity and duration). The brain is constantly adapting to input; for example the brain forms neuron-neuron connections in various patterns to produce memory. When the brain is constantly receiving messages of pain, the brain "rewires" the neuron-neuron interconnections to increase pain processing—what might be called a "pain memory"—in a way that facilitates the perception of pain, leading to enhanced pain perception, e.g., more pain felt by the patient.

Diagnosis

- Clinical criteria—description and contrast of the 1990 criteria and the 2010 criteria: Per guidelines published in 1990 by the American College of Rheumatology (ACR), a diagnosis of fibromyalgia can be made in a patient with inexplicable, widespread myofascial pain of at least 3 months' duration; *inexplicable* denotes normalcy of routine laboratory and physical examination findings and failure to find an alternate explanation or diagnosis, while *widespread* denotes bilateral pain above and below the waist not attributable to trauma or rheumatic disease and with pain at 11 of 18 classic tender point locations (see illustration below).

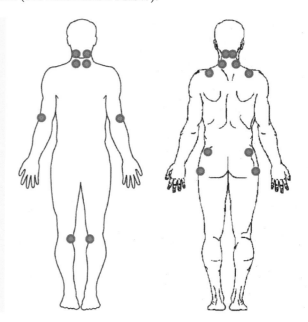

Illustration of the 9 paired locations of FM tender points:
Pain, on digital palpation, must be present in at least 11 of the following 18 tender point sites:
1. Occiput: at the suboccipital muscle insertions.
2. Low cervical: at the anterior aspects of the intertransverse spaces at C5-C7.
3. Trapezius: at the midpoint of the upper border.
4. Supraspinatus: at origins, above the scapula spine near the medial border.
5. Second rib: upper lateral to the second costochondral junction.
6. Lateral epicondyle: 2 cm distal to the epicondyles.
7. Gluteal: in upper outer quadrants of buttocks in anterior fold of muscle.
8. Greater trochanter: posterior to the trochanteric prominence.
9. Knee: at the medial fat pad proximal to the joint line.

Per 1990 ACR guidelines, the diagnosis of FM is supported when at least 11 out of 18 of these locations are painful. Digital palpation should be performed with an approximate force of 4 kg (9 lbs). A tender point has to be painful at palpation, not just "tender."[259]

FM tender points are assessed bilaterally at 9 paired sites: (sub)occiput (below the head at the neckline), low cervical spine (lower neck), trapezius and supraspinatus (two of the shoulder muscles), second rib (anterior, near costosternal [rib-breastbone] junction), lateral epicondyle, gluteal region, greater trochanter, and medial fat pad of the knees. Tender points are provoked by the clinician's application of approximately 9 pounds of fingertip pressure, which is sufficient to cause blanching of the clinician's nail bed. The tender points of fibromyalgia are distinguished from myofascial trigger points (MFTP, described by Travell[260]) and strain-counterstrain tender points (described in the osteopathic literature by Jones[261]). Pain must have been consistent

[259] The American College of Rheumatology 1990 Criteria for the Classification of Fibromyalgia. nfra.net/Diagnost.htm Accessed Nov 2011
[260] Simons DG, Travell JG, Simons LS. *Travell & Simons' Myofascial Pain and Dysfunction. The Trigger Point Manual*. Baltimore: Lippincott Williams & Wilkins; 1999
[261] Jones L, Kusunose R, Goering E. *Jones Strain-Counterstrain*. Carlsbad, Jones Strain Counterstrain Incorporated, 1995. [ISBN 0964513544]

for at least three months and must not be attributable to another (obvious) cause. In contrast to MFTP, which are located toward the center of the muscle fiber and which refer pain and show spontaneous electrocontractile activity[262], tender points of fibromyalgia are located near the tendinous insertions of muscle to bone and cause local pain only, without pain referral or contractile activity.

The new 2010 ACR guidelines for the diagnosis and assessment of FM[263] are significantly different from the 1990 guidelines. These new guidelines are mostly illogical and appear to have been structured to broaden the definition of fibromyalgia, to allow patients and nonphysicians to make the diagnosis, and generally to increase the patient population available for a diagnosis of fibromyalgia, thereby increasing the sales of drugs. Very curiously, the authors state that one of their objectives was to create criteria that "do not require a tender point examination"; at first, this seems odd and clinically inconsistent considering that the tender point examination ❶ takes only about 60 seconds to perform, ❷ is noninvasive, ❸ was previously the standard by which the diagnosis was made, and ❹ is reasonable and responsible—physical examination of patients with pain is a reasonable standard of care. Oddly, the authors of the new guidelines note several "important problems" with the 1990 ACR criteria, such as "Patients who improved or whose symptoms and tender points decreased could fail to satisfy the ACR 1990 classification definition" and "there was little variation in symptoms among fibromyalgia patients." Clinicians should note that these so-called "problems" *are not problems at all* because patients who improve and thus no longer meet diagnostic criteria should not be considered to have an active disease/diagnosis, and that high-quality clinical criteria should indeed result in the specific definition of clinical disorder and thus in a well-defined cohort of patients; correcting these "problems" results in patients being diagnosed for longer periods of time (more *long-term* patients) and also results in more patients being diagnosed with fibromyalgia (more *total* patients). Perhaps even more curious is the fact that development of these new guidelines was sponsored by Lilly Research Laboratories—the front page of the article states "these criteria were developed with support from the study sponsor, Lilly Research Laboratories", which is the "research" section of Eli Lilly and Company, one of the world's largest drug companies and the manufacturer of duloxetine/Cymbalta® which is one of the only drugs approved by the US Food and Drug Administration (FDA) for the treatment of fibromyalgia.[264] Among patients labeled with fibromyalgia, the new criteria increase the percentage of patients diagnosable by criteria from 75% to 88%; whether the motivation to expand the patient population diagnosed with fibromyalgia is altruistic or financially motivated is subject to debate. The new criteria rely on a summation of two tallies—"widespread pain index" (WPI) and "symptom severity" (SS, parts 1 and 2)—with the diagnosis being supported by either **"WPI >7 and SS >5"** or **"WPI 3–6 and SS >9"**.

A descriptive video of the distinctions between the 1990 and 2010 diagnostic criteria is available for free from www.InflammationMastery.com/pain.

[262] Hubbard DR, Berkoff GM. Myofascial trigger points show spontaneous needle EMG activity. *Spine*. 1993 Oct 1;18(13):1803-7
[263] Wolfe F, et al. The ACR preliminary diagnostic criteria for fibromyalgia and measurement of symptom severity. *Arthritis Care Res*. 2010;62(5):600-10
[264] lilly.com/research/Pages/research.aspx and newsroom.lilly.com/ReleaseDetail.cfm?releaseid=316740 Accessed January 2012

Widespread pain index (WPI): Each positive location receives one point (max = 19)

1. Shoulder girdle, left	7. Hip (buttock/trochanter), left	13. Jaw, left
2. Shoulder girdle, right	8. Hip (buttock/trochanter), right	14. Jaw, right
3. Upper arm, left	9. Upper leg, left	15. Chest (sternum area)
4. Upper arm, right	10. Upper leg, right	16. Abdomen
5. Lower arm, left	11. Lower leg, left	17. Neck
6. Lower arm, right	12. Lower leg, right	18. Upper back
		19. Lower back

Symptom severity (SS)—part 1: Each of these three problems is quantified with the following scale (max = 9):
  0 none: no problem **1 mild**: intermittent or mild problems
  2 moderate: often present, considerable problems **3 severe**: continuous, life-disturbing problems

0 1 2 3 Fatigue	0 1 2 3 Waking unrefreshed	0 1 2 3 Cognitive symptoms

---

Symptom severity (SS)—part 2: The clinician considers the patient's "somatic symptoms in general" (listed below) and applies the following scale (max = 3):
  0 no symptoms 1 few symptoms
  2 a moderate number of symptoms 3 a great deal of symptoms

0 1 2 3 muscle pain	0 1 2 3 itching
0 1 2 3 irritable bowel syndrome	0 1 2 3 wheezing
0 1 2 3 fatigue/tiredness	0 1 2 3 Raynaud's phenomenon
0 1 2 3 thinking or remembering problems	0 1 2 3 hives/welts
0 1 2 3 muscle weakness	0 1 2 3 ringing in ears
0 1 2 3 headache	0 1 2 3 vomiting
0 1 2 3 pain/cramps in the abdomen	0 1 2 3 heartburn
0 1 2 3 numbness/tingling	0 1 2 3 oral ulcers
0 1 2 3 dizziness	0 1 2 3 loss of/change in taste
0 1 2 3 insomnia	0 1 2 3 seizures
0 1 2 3 depression	0 1 2 3 dry eyes
0 1 2 3 constipation	0 1 2 3 shortness of breath
0 1 2 3 pain in the upper abdomen	0 1 2 3 loss of appetite
0 1 2 3 nausea	0 1 2 3 skin rash
0 1 2 3 nervousness	0 1 2 3 sun sensitivity
0 1 2 3 chest pain	0 1 2 3 hearing difficulties
0 1 2 3 blurred vision	0 1 2 3 easy bruising
0 1 2 3 fever	0 1 2 3 hair loss
0 1 2 3 diarrhea	0 1 2 3 frequent urination
0 1 2 3 dry mouth	0 1 2 3 painful urination
	0 1 2 3 bladder spasms

Tally points from above; patients may be diagnosed with FM if **"WPI >7 and SS >5"** or **"WPI 3-6 and SS >9"**.
WPI = _____
SS1 + SS2 = _____

2010 Fibromyalgia diagnostic criteria—summary, chart for clinical use, discussion: Per the 2010 diagnostic criteria[265], patients may be diagnosed with fibromyalgia if "WPI >7 and SS >5" or "WPI 3–6 and SS >9". Of note, these new criteria reflect a major departure from the former criteria published and codified in 1990; of additional note, publication of these new criteria received sponsorship from a drug company which has an FDA-approved drug for this condition—this represents a massive conflict of interest, full manifestation of which would have the same for-profit entity influencing the criteria used by doctors for the diagnosis and then providing (i.e., selling for profit) one of the only approved drug treatment options. I have discussed these conundrums in video format at Vimeo.com/ICHNFM and Vimeo.com/DrVasquez.

- Clinical profile and findings on common laboratory tests: New-onset fibromyalgia is unlikely over age 50, and the condition never causes fever, significant weight loss, or other objective signs of acute or subacute illness. Hypothyroidism is common and can produce widespread myofascial pain along with depression and other complaints, resulting in a clinical picture that closely resembles FM; thus, a complete thyroid evaluation (detailed later) is essential during the initial evaluation of any fibromyalgia-like condition. Common rheumatic

---

[265] Wolfe F, et al. The ACR preliminary diagnostic criteria for fibromyalgia and measurement of symptom severity. *Arthritis Care Res.* 2010;62(5):600-10

conditions such as rheumatoid arthritis (RA) and systemic lupus erythematosus (SLE) are excluded by the lack of other clinical manifestations (e.g., joint pain and swelling) and the lack of positive laboratory findings such as anti-cyclic citrullinated protein (CCP) antibodies and antinuclear antibodies (ANA), respectively. C-reactive protein (CRP) and erythrocyte sedimentation rate (ESR) are normal in FM patients; abnormalities with these or other common laboratory assessments suggest inflammatory disease, infection, or other concomitant illness. Hypophosphatemia (a low level of the electrolyte phosphate in the blood) can cause bone pain and muscle weakness; this condition is easily excluded by demonstration of normal serum phosphate level.

Standard Medical Treatment for Fibromyalgia

- Overview: Mild exercise, "patient education", and the use of pain-relieving drugs are mainstays of standard medical treatment delivered by most allopathic medical doctors (MDs), and osteopathic medical doctors (DOs) may add manual musculoskeletal treatments to enhance the benefits of drugs.[266] These interventions are only partially effective and offer no hope of actually curing the disease; thus, medical treatment relegates patients to a future of drug dependency, potential adverse effects (some of which can be fatal), and therapeutic inefficacy insofar as none of these treatments addresses the underlying cause of the disorder.

  - Amitriptyline: For many years, the most widely used drug for symptomatic treatment of fibromyalgia was amitriptyline (a tricyclic antidepressant), which has been used "off label"—without approval from the FDA—for this application. In the treatment of FM, the drug has low efficacy and high potential for adverse effects; up to 20% of patients suffer from weight gain, constipation, orthostatic hypotension, and/or agitation as a side-effect of the drug. Only 25% to 30% of fibromyalgia patients experience clinically significant improvement with amitriptyline.[267] According to recent research in rats, administration of amitriptyline causes deficiency of CoQ10, impaired mitochondrial function, reduced ATP/energy production, and increased oxidative stress and free radical damage[268]; all of these drug-induced problems (discussed in detail later in this paper) are expected to worsen the pain and suffering experienced by FM patients. Thus, the use of amitriptyline cannot be considered to be consistent with the practice of good medicine due to its low efficacy and unacceptable risks for adverse effects.

  - Pregabalin: In 2007, the United States Food and Drug Administration (US FDA) approved pregabalin (Lyrica® sold/marketed by Pfizer) for symptomatic treatment of fibromyalgia[269]; however, because the drug does not address the primary cause(s) of the disease, patients must continue treatment indefinitely. Adverse effects of pregabalin include

Suicide and depression risk warning for pregabalin/Lyrica from the US FDA
"Antiepileptic drugs (AEDs), including Lyrica, increase the risk of suicidal thoughts or behavior in patients taking these drugs for any indication. Patients treated with any AED for any indication should be monitored for the emergence or worsening of depression, suicidal thoughts or behavior, and/or any unusual changes in mood or behavior."
fda.gov/Safety/MedWatch/SafetyInformation/Safety-RelatedDrugLabelingChanges/ucm154524.htm

    dizziness, sleepiness, blurred vision, weight gain, dry mouth, swelling of hands and feet, impairment of motor function, and problems with concentration and attention. Pregabalin when given at the recommended dose of 150-225 mg twice per day for fibromyalgia costs $94-190 per month (pricing in 2013).

  - Duloxetine: In 2008, the FDA announced duloxetine (Cymbalta® sold/marketed by Lilly) as the second approved drug for the treatment of fibromyalgia. Ironically, many physicians consider any "approved" drug to have scientific substantiation; however, in the case of duloxetine (as well as pregabalin) the exact mechanism of action is unknown[270] although duloxetine appears to inhibit reuptake of norepinephrine and serotonin, thereby increasing the action of these neurotransmitters in the synaptic cleft. Adverse effects from duloxetine include nausea, dry mouth, sleepiness, constipation, decreased appetite, and increased

[266] Gamber RG, Shores JH, Russo DP, Jimenez C, Rubin BR. Osteopathic manipulative treatment in conjunction with medication relieves pain associated with fibromyalgia syndrome: results of a randomized clinical pilot project. *J Am Osteopath Assoc.* 2002 Jun;102(6):321-5 jaoa.org/content/102/6/321.full.pdf

[267] Leventhal LJ. Management of fibromyalgia. *Ann Intern Med.* 1999 Dec 7;131(11):850-8

[268] "Amitriptyline is a tricyclic antidepressant commonly prescribed for the treatment of several neuropathic and inflammatory illnesses. We have already reported that amitriptyline has cytotoxic effect in human cell cultures, increasing oxidative stress, and decreasing growth rate and mitochondrial activity." Bautista-Ferrufino MR, Cordero MD, Sánchez-Alcázar JA, et al. Amitriptyline induces coenzyme Q deficiency and oxidative damage in mouse lung and liver. *Toxicol Lett.* 2011 Jul 4;204(1):32-7

[269] FDA Approves First Drug for Treating Fibromyalgia. fda.gov/bbs/topics/NEWS/2007/NEW01656.html

[270] "exact mechanism of action unknown; inhibits norepinephrine and serotonin reuptake" https://online.epocrates.com; "Both Lyrica and Cymbalta reduce pain and improve function in people with fibromyalgia. While those with fibromyalgia have been shown to experience pain differently from other people, the mechanism by which these drugs produce their effects is unknown. fda.gov/ForConsumers/ConsumerUpdates/ucm107802.htm. Accessed January 2012

sweating; **duloxetine can also increase the risk of suicidal thinking and behavior and for this reason the drug carries a black box warning on the container.** Duloxetine can cause serious and fatal adverse effects including the following: worsening depression and suicidality, serotonin syndrome, neuroleptic malignant syndrome, seizures, and Stevens-Johnson syndrome. Duloxetine given at the recommended dose of 60 mg per day for FM costs $170 per month (pricing in 2013).

Suicide and depression risk warning for duloxetine/Cymbalta
"WARNING: Suicidality and Antidepressant Drugs: Antidepressants increased the risk compared to placebo of suicidal thinking and behavior (suicidality) in children, adolescents, and young adults in short-term studies of major depressive disorder (MDD) and other psychiatric disorders. Anyone considering the use of Cymbalta or any other antidepressant in a child, adolescent, or young adult must balance this risk with the clinical need. Short-term studies did not show an increase in the risk of suicidality with antidepressants compared to placebo in adults beyond age 24; there was a reduction in risk with antidepressants compared to placebo in adults aged 65 and older. Depression and certain other psychiatric disorders are themselves associated with increases in the risk of suicide. Patients of all ages who are started on antidepressant therapy should be monitored appropriately and observed closely for clinical worsening, suicidality, or unusual changes in behavior. Families and caregivers should be advised of the need for close observation and communication with the prescriber. Cymbalta is not approved for use in pediatric patients."
pi.lilly.com/us/cymbalta-pi.pdf

- <u>Milnacipran</u>: Approved for the treatment of FM by the US FDA in 2009, milnacipran (Savella® sold/marketed by Forest Pharmaceuticals) inhibits norepinephrine and serotonin reuptake, i.e., it potentiates (increases the effect of) the neurotransmitters norepinephrine and serotonin, both of which decrease the experience of pain and elevate mood. Of course, other non-drug treatments (such as nutrients and dietary optimization) can have the same effect, but most medical doctors have no training in nondrug

Suicide and depression risk warning for milnacipran/Savella
"Savella is a selective serotonin and norepinephrine reuptake inhibitor (SNRI), similar to some drugs used for the treatment of depression and other psychiatric disorders. Antidepressants increased the risk compared to placebo of suicidal thinking and behavior (suicidality) in children, adolescents, and young adults in short-term studies of major depressive disorder (MDD) and other psychiatric disorders."
frx.com/pi/Savella_pi.pdf, linked as "Full Prescribing Information" from savella.com/important-risk-information.aspx

treatments[271,272,273,274] and thus habitually turn to drugs as the one-and-only answer to the patients' problems[275], especially when these are sanctified by FDA/government approval. Nondrug treatments that enhance serotonergic and noradrenergic neurotransmission include exercise, relaxation, massage, and nutritional supplementation with omega-3 fatty acids (as found in fish oil), nutritional supplementation in general and vitamin D supplementation in particular. Adverse effects associated with use of milnacipran include seizures, suicidality, depression, worsening hypomania/mania, Stevens-Johnson syndrome (which is a medical emergency that can be fatal), serotonin syndrome, neuroleptic malignant syndrome, hypertensive (elevated blood pressure) crisis, tachycardia (rapid heart rate), hyponatremia (low sodium in the blood, which can occasionally result in permanent brain damage), abnormal bleeding (due to abnormal platelet function), glaucoma, and liver toxicity.[276] Treatment of fibromyalgia is the only FDA-approved use of this medication, which when used at the recommended dose of 50 mg twice daily costs $144 per month (pricing in April 2013).

- <u>Cyclobenzaprine, Tramadol, and acetaminophen</u>: Cyclobenzaprine (a muscle-relaxing drug), Tramadol (a non-typical opioid, centrally-acting narcotic analgesic) and acetaminophen (centrally acting analgesic),

---

[271] "Internal medicine interns' perceive nutrition counseling as a priority, but lack the confidence and knowledge to effectively provide adequate nutrition education." Vetter ML, Herring SJ, Sood M, Shah NR, Kalet AL. What do resident physicians know about nutrition? An evaluation of attitudes, self-perceived proficiency and knowledge. *J Am Coll Nutr*. 2008 Apr;27(2):287-98 ncbi.nlm.nih.gov/pmc/articles/PMC2779722/

[272] "The amount of nutrition education that medical students receive continues to be inadequate." Adams KM, Kohlmeier M, Zeisel SH. Nutrition education in U.S. medical schools: latest update of a national survey. *Acad Med*. 2010 Sep;85(9):1537-42

[273] "Scientific advances on the relationship of dietary substances to the cellular mechanisms of disease occur with regularity and frequency. Yet, despite the prevalence of nutritional disorders in clinical medicine and increasing scientific evidence on the significance of dietary modification to disease prevention, present day practitioners of medicine are typically untrained in the relationship of diet to health and disease." Halsted CH. The relevance of clinical nutrition education and role models to the practice of medicine. *Eur J Clin Nutr*. 1999 May;53 Suppl 2:S29-34

[274] Vasquez A. Interventions need to be consistent with osteopathic philosophy. *J Am Osteopath Assoc*. 2006 Sep;106(9):528-9 jaoa.org/content/106/9/528.full.pdf

[275] Ely et al. Analysis of questions asked by family doctors regarding patient care. *BMJ*. 1999 Aug 7;319(7206):358-61 ncbi.nlm.nih.gov/pmc/articles/PMC28191/

[276] https://online.epocrates.com/noFrame/showPage.do?method=drugs&MonographId=4950 Accessed April 2012.

show low efficacy and have little research supporting their use in the treatment of FM; these drugs also carry important risks for adverse effects, and they do not favorably alter the course of the disease over the long-term.[277] Per recent information from the American College of Rheumatology (ACR), treatment of FM with opioid drugs "may cause greater pain sensitivity or make pain persist."[278]

- Exercise: Low-intensity aerobic exercise may initially exacerbate symptoms but can result in very modest mental and physical improvement. Exercise alone cannot cure FM.

- Cognitive-behavioral therapy (CBT): Cognitive-behavioral therapy helps patients deal with and adapt to the impact of the illness. Therapy alone cannot cure FM.

- Patient (mis)education in standard medicine: "Patient education" from a *medical* perspective generally means telling patients that ❶ they will probably have the condition forever, ❷ they will not immediately die from it, ❸ they need to take it seriously (i.e., comply with medical treatment), and ❹ they need to rely on drugs for alleviation of symptoms since no cause of the condition is known and therefore no direct treatment is available. From the medical perspective, these communications are considered "helpful" and "reassuring"; however, part of the effect that is created is **dependency** ("You need these drugs from me."), **passivity** ("There's nothing you can do about this, so don't even try to think for yourself or seek 'alternative' treatments."), and **co-victimization** ("We are both victims of our ignorance; I am in this with you in that we are both blind and dependent on drug management."). In the examples that follow, I will review and summarize patient educational materials from major medical groups; for efficiency, I will use quotes followed by my comments in *italics*:

- Press release from the American Pain Society "Fibromyalgia Has Central Nervous System Origins", written by an author heavily funded by drug companies[279]:
  - "Fibromyalgia is the second most common rheumatic disorder behind osteoarthritis and, though still widely misunderstood, is now considered to be a lifelong central nervous system disorder, which is responsible for amplified pain that shoots through the body in those who suffer from it." — *This lunacy does not require additional refutation: the American Pain Society clearly affiliates with drug companies and wants to promote drug sales and use of their specialty organization; for this, they need to foster the illusion that FM begins in the brain, has no cure, and needs to be treated with drugs for the duration of patients' lives.*

- "Patient Education" from the American College of Rheumatology, Rheumatology.org[280]:
  - "Though there is no cure, medications can relieve symptoms." — *This is a commonly used statement within the medical community from doctors to patients to create passivity and drug/medical dependency.*
  - "There likely are certain genes that can make people more prone to getting fibromyalgia and the other health problems that can occur with it. Genes alone, though, do not cause fibromyalgia." — *These are common statements in the medical community, basically summed as "We don't know what we are doing but your only hope is to depend on us."*
  - "For the person with fibromyalgia, it is as though the "volume control" is turned up too high in the brain's pain processing centers." — *This promotes the concept of "primary central sensitization" (i.e., the brain has defied normal physiology and has somehow [without known cause, by itself] become too sensitive to pain); this "blame the brain" concept is used to leverage drug sales for pain-relieving and anti-depressant drugs as I have recently reviewed in video:* youtube.com/watch?v=41opevN87qs
  - "There is no cure for fibromyalgia. However, symptoms can be treated with both medication and non-drug treatments." — *This is the standard "party line" for the medical profession, whose chief goal is not to cure diseases but rather to drug them indefinitely, thereby creating a perpetual audience for their services and prescriptions. Honorable mention (more accurately: dishonorable mention) is generally given to "lifestyle modification" but is generally done so in a way that provides vague advice for ineffective interventions, thereby **creating the illusion of options** while undercutting any potential for these "options" to actually work.*
  - Non-drug treatments reviewed: relaxation, deep breathing, meditation, sleep, avoidance of nicotine and caffeine, exercise including such miniscule revelations as "take the stairs instead of the elevator, or park further [sic] away from the store", and "education" from other medical and special interest groups. — *These*

[277] Goldenberg DL, Burckhardt C, Crofford L. Management of fibromyalgia syndrome. *JAMA*. 2004 Nov 17;292(19):2388-95
[278] rheumatology.org/practice/clinical/patients/diseases_and_conditions/fibromyalgia.asp Accessed April 2012
[279] Fibromyalgia Has Central Nervous System Origins. americanpainsociety.org/about-us/press-room/fibromyalgia-clauw May 16, 2015
[280] rheumatology.org/practice/clinical/patients/diseases_and_conditions/fibromyalgia.asp Accessed March 31, 2012

> *are all essentially worthless suggestions, but they are effective distractions for patients and doctors so that effective treatments are marginalized and drug/medical dependency is fostered.*

- □ Prescription drugs are given the primary emphasis in the treatment section.—*Whether drugs are effective or not, the medical profession relies on drugs for its societal position and will therefore reflexively advocate them.*

- ▪ <u>Patient education from American Academy of Family Physicians, FamilyDoctor.org[281]</u>:
  - □ "…your muscles and organs are not being damaged."—*This is false/inaccurate information. Several primary research studies have demonstrated consistently pathologic and biochemical abnormalities in muscle tissue from patients with fibromyalgia; this research has been published in widely available peer-reviewed medical journals. While the muscle damage in FM is not gross or overt myopathy, stating that no damage is occurring is not histologically accurate and supports the drug-friendly model that FM is idiopathic and (neuro)psychiatric.*
  - □ "This condition is not life-threatening, but it is chronic (ongoing). Although there is no cure,…"—*This is false information because obviously the condition is curable; the statement as it reads produces patient passivity and drug-dependency, which is exactly what the medical profession and the drug industry want.*
  - □ "There isn't currently a cure for fibromyalgia. Your care will focus on helping you minimize the impact of fibromyalgia on your life and treating your symptoms. Your doctor can prescribe medicine to help with your pain,… The treatment recommendations your doctor makes won't do any good unless you follow them."—*Again, false information promoting passivity and drug-dependency. This is basically drug propaganda, encouraging passivity and compliance on the parts of doctors and patients alike.*
  - □ Weak recommendations under the guise of "taking an active role in your healthcare" include 1) maintaining a healthy outlook, 2) support groups, 3) **"take medicines exactly as prescribed"**, 4) moderate exercise, 5) stress management, 6) "establish healthy sleep habits", 7) make a routine daily schedule, 8) "make healthy lifestyle choices." —*Most of these recommendations are blatantly passive, vague, and ineffective while fostering drug-dependency.*

The most common pattern in medical books and articles: components of the medical paradigm
1. <u>Diseases are describable yet incomprehensible</u>: The condition generally is described as a complex interplay of genetic factors with numerous environmental factors; generally little or no intellectually worthwhile effort is made to understand these environmental factors, so the ultimate view that medical physicians are taught is the disease is not understood and that drug therapy is the best available treatment.
2. <u>Nearly always the disease is described as chronic and incurable</u>: Even if a cure is known and published in available peer-reviewed research, most medical books and articles conclude that the causes are unknown and that palliative drug treatment is therefore warranted.
3. <u>Characteristics and diagnostic criteria are reviewed</u>: The medical profession is very good at defining and diagnosing problems, but the reliance on drugs often detours from the more effective nondrug treatments. The idea that every disease needs a drug is absurd, but this very same idea is embraced as the axiom of medicine and indeed as proof of its insight and resourcefulness.
4. <u>Drug treatments are emphasized</u>: Drug benefits are inflated and adverse effects are minimized if mentioned at all. Many review articles published in clinical journals are authored by consultants to the drug industry who profit from the sale of the drugs used to treat the condition about which they write; the general conclusion of these articles is that "Medical research is making considerable advances in our understanding of Disease X, which results from a complex interplay of genetic and environmental factors. The appropriate treatment for Disease X is Drug X, then Drug X2…along with generally meaningless lifestyle advice.
5. <u>Nondrug treatments are marginalized</u>: Brief mention is made of diet and lifestyle and other non-drug treatments, but the information is nonspecific, very general, and almost always diluted to the point of inefficacy.
6. <u>Authentic integrative/functional medicine approaches are essentially never mentioned</u>: Generally, the only nondrug treatments that are mentioned are weak or are mentioned so casually that no effective action can be implemented.
7. <u>Hope for the future is always placed back in the hands of "more research" and "drug development"</u>: Often some mention of "hope for the future" is made, generally in the guise of "medical research" and "drug development"; all the while, safe and effective non-drug treatment approaches that go far beyond diet and lifestyle are virtually never mentioned.
Most medical students start medical school in their early 20s, when they are notably young and impressionable, with practically zero life experience other than creating the perfect medical school application (ie, high scores plus some foray into volunteer work to appear socially concerned), and eager to "be a doctor." Medical training is typically 7 years—4 years of school followed by 3 years of hospital-based residency training—during which students and residents are stressed, sleep-deprived, hazed, and fearful of expulsion for any minor infraction. Medical training induces a trance-like state, with several features of Stockholm syndrome, wherein doctors become accustomed in their early training to memorize, pathologize, and conform to expectations. They are eager to do the things that define a doctor's authority and privilege—write prescriptions or recommend procedures/surgery; nutrition—a "nonmedical" treatment that is considered "alternative"—is for "quacks" (nonscientists, nonrationalists, especially those who could not enter a "real" medical school) and dieticians (hierarchically inferior to doctors). With the time pressure (2-7 minutes per patient) and formulary restrictions (zero outpatient nutritional options) of hospital/clinic-based training/practice, practically no *conscientious* medical student/clinician would consider deviation from well ingrained (and intellectually inbred) *expectations*.

---

[281] American Academy of Family Physicians. familydoctor.org/familydoctor/en/diseases-conditions/fibromyalgia.html Accessed March 31, 2012

Functional/Naturopathic Considerations, Assessments, and Interventions

- Foundational perspectives: Two fundamental premises of are: (1) ~~chronic~~ sustained *diseases* are manifestations of ~~chronic~~ sustained *dysfunctions,* and (2) dysfunction can result from a wide range of interconnected genotropic (gene-influenced), metabolic, nutritional, microbial, inflammatory, toxic, environmental, and psychological and social influences. **Many of these dysfunctions lie outside the narrow, pathology-based, pharmacocentric (drug-centered) view of standard allopathic medicine.** The functional/naturopathic medicine approach to each individual fibromyalgia patient is based firstly on the presumption that the condition has an underlying primary cause (or several interconnected causes) and that the cause(s) can be identified and addressed—in this manner, the clinical approach is one of positive psychoepistimology (ie, affirmative that we can understand this situation), rather than pathodefetism (ie, "we can't understand this disease") resulting pharmacodependency. The cause(s) may be manifold and multifaceted and may differ among patients with the same diagnostic label. This approach includes the diagnostic and therapeutic considerations of standard medicine but extends far beyond these in assessment, treatment, and understanding. Clinicians should appreciate that as a diagnostic label, fibromyalgia is commonly applied to any patient with chronic, widespread pain and that the current trend to limit diagnostic evaluation in such patients will clearly result in failure to identify and address readily diagnosable and treatable problems that can result in a clinical picture that resembles FM. Clinicians must consider chronic infections (such as with hepatitis C virus, *Borrelia burgdorferi* [the bacteria strongly associated with Lyme disease], *Chlamydia/Chlamydophila pneumoniae,* and the protozoan parasite *Babesia,* which is also associated with Lyme disease and co-infection with *Borrelia burgdorferi*), cancerous conditions such as multiple myeloma and lymphoma, and autoimmune/rheumatic diseases such as polymyositis and polymyalgia rheumatica. A few of the other more exemplary conditions to consider in patients with widespread pain are vitamin D deficiency, hypothyroidism, iron overload, and chronic exposure to and accumulation of xenobiotics—perhaps most importantly mercury and lead.

Common differential diagnoses—conditions that can mimic (or contribute to) fibromyalgia

- Vitamin D deficiency: A clinical picture nearly identical to fibromyalgia—chronic widespread pain, mental depression/anxiety, headaches, low-grade systemic inflammation—can result from vitamin D deficiency.[282] Fibromyalgia patients are commonly deficient in vitamin D, and indeed, **vitamin D deficiency—with its attendant pain, anxiety/depression, and normal lab values on routine laboratory testing—is often misdiagnosed as fibromyalgia,** as reported by Holick.[283] Increased severity of the deficiency correlates with worsening depression and anxiety in these patients.[284] Correction of vitamin D deficiency by administration of vitamin D3 (cholecalciferol) in doses of 5,000-10,000 IU (international units) per day for several months has resulted in a dramatic alleviation of pain; such intervention among patients with low back pain has resulted in cure rates greater than 95%.[285] Other studies with vitamin D3 using doses 400-4,000 IU/day have shown that vitamin D3 supplementation for the correction of vitamin D deficiency alleviates depression and enhances sense of well-being. Vitamin D3 supplementation—or adequate endogenous production from ultraviolet light exposure (approximately 10-30 minutes per day of full-body exposure at midday, near the equator)—to meet physiological requirements of approximately 4,000 IU/day is safe and results in numerous major health benefits.[286,287,288] The only risk associated with vitamin D supplementation is hypercalcemia—too much calcium in the blood, mostly as a result of increased gastrointestinal absorption of calcium; hypercalcemia can cause abdominal pain, bone pain, fatigue, constipation, abnormal heart rhythm (arrhythmia), kidney stones, increased thirst and urination [additional details[289]]. Hypercalcemia caused solely by vitamin D3 supplementation is extremely rare; vitamin D supplementation in the range of 2,000 – 10,000 IU per day for

---

[282] Plotnikoff GA, Quigley JM. Prevalence of severe hypovitaminosis D in patients with persistent, nonspecific musculoskeletal pain. *Mayo Clin Proc.* 2003;78(12):1463-70

[283] Holick MF. Vitamin D: importance in the prevention of cancers, type 1 diabetes, heart disease, and osteoporosis. *Am J Clin Nutr.* 2004 Mar;79(3):362-71

[284] Armstrong DJ, et al. Vitamin D deficiency is associated with anxiety and depression in fibromyalgia. *Clin Rheumatol.* 2007 Apr;26(4):551-4

[285] Al Faraj S, Al Mutairi K. Vitamin D deficiency and chronic low back pain in Saudi Arabia. *Spine.* 2003;28:177-9

[286] Holick MF. Vitamin D: importance in the prevention of cancers, type 1 diabetes, heart disease, and osteoporosis. *Am J Clin Nutr.* 2004 Mar;79(3):362-71

[287] Vieth R. Vitamin D supplementation, 25-hydroxyvitamin D concentrations, and safety. *Am J Clin Nutr.* 1999 May;69(5):842-56

[288] Zittermann A. Vitamin D in preventive medicine: are we ignoring the evidence? *Br J Nutr.* 2003 May;89(5):552-72

[289] Mild hypercalcemia is not necessarily a problem by itself and must be evaluated within the patient's clinical context. When blood levels of calcium (normal range: 8.7-10.4 mg/dL) reach approximately 12.0 mg/dL, patients will start to develop symptoms; with levels of 14 mg/dL or higher, the patient is generally experiencing symptoms and complications and is in need of treatment (initially with administration of intravenous fluids and a loop diuretic such as furosemide).

adults is remarkably safe.[290,291] The main drug-nutrient interaction of relevance to vitamin D supplementation is with the drug hydrochlorothiazide, which is a diuretic drug used for the treatment of high blood pressure; this drug causes calcium retention by the kidney and when combined with vitamin D supplementation may lead to high levels of calcium in the blood (hypercalcemia). *Note from Dr Vasquez: I have only seen this occur one time in my clinical practice in a hypertensive patient taking hydrochlorothiazide who was vitamin D deficient; vitamin D supplementation at 2,000 IU/d caused a mild hypercalcemia within 10 days which was treated simply by discontinuing the vitamin D supplementation (also note that discontinuation of appropriate nutritional supplementation in favor of continuing a symptom-suppressing drug is generally not my preference but in this particular situation it was the best choice).* A group of conditions called granulomatous diseases—which can include lymphoma, sarcoidosis, and Crohn's disease—increase the risk for hypercalcemia; caution and more frequent laboratory monitoring must be employed when using physiological doses of vitamin D3 in patients with these conditions. Diagnosis of vitamin D3 deficiency is simple and is based upon measurement of serum 25-hydroxy vitamin D3 (25[OH]D) levels. Supplementation effectiveness and safety are monitored by measuring 25(OH)D levels and serum calcium, respectively. The two goals with supplementation of vitamin D3 are ❶ safety—avoidance of hypercalcemia or any calcium-related complications, and ❷ efficacy—serum 25[OH]D levels should enter into the optimal range of 50 – 100 ng/mL (125 - 250 nmol/L).

- Functional/metabolic hypothyroidism: Insufficient levels of thyroid hormone lead to an associated clinical condition called hypothyroidism (*hypo*=low, *thyroidism*=thyroid condition). Both mild and overt hypothyroidism are well known in the rheumatology literature as causes of diffuse body pain. As a cause of diffuse muscle pain, mild-moderate hypothyroidism can mimic fibromyalgia; more severe cases of hypothyroidism cause "hypothyroid myopathy" which typically manifests as polymyositis-like disease with proximal muscle weakness and an increased serum level of the enzyme creatine kinase, indicating muscle damage. In its most extreme, hypothyroid myopathy presents as muscle enlargement (pseudohypertrophy); in adults, this condition is called Hoffmann syndrome while in children it is known as Kocher-Debré-Sémélaigne syndrome.[292] Hypothyroidism is well known to cause depression and low-grade systemic inflammation; these are two findings

Thyroid hormone production and metabolism
 - TSH—thyroid stimulating hormone: Hormone secreted from the anterior pituitary gland to stimulate T4 and T3 production from the thyroid gland. - T4: The inactive form of thyroid hormone, accounting for about 80% of thyroid gland output. Oddly and contrary to physiology, doctors have been trained to use this inactive form of the hormone despite known problems in conversion to the active T3 form described immediately below. - T3: The active form of thyroid hormone produced from conversion of T4, accounts for about 20% of thyroid gland output. This is the form of thyroid hormone that is most important, because it is active and ready to stimulate metabolic processes; of note, the brain is unable to convert T4 to T3 and thus when patients are deficient in thyroid hormone and substituted with T4 only, they commonly have suboptimal improvement, especially for brain-specific issues of depression and fatigue. - rT3—reverse T3: During times of stress and also as a result of some drugs, T4 is preferentially converted to rT3, which is inactive and may actually impair the utilization of active T3. In some people, especially after a period of severe emotional stress, their thyroid hormone metabolism becomes skewed toward rT3 production, perhaps as an adaptive mechanism to conserve energy. However, increased rT3 production results in impaired thyroid hormone function and thereby promotes a clinical picture of hypothyroidism even when gland function is adequate; the problem is the hormone's peripheral metabolism, not its production from the gland.

common in FM. Another related problem commonly seen with both FM and hypothyroidism is IBS and small intestinal bacterial overgrowth (SIBO); hypothyroidism causes a slowing of intestinal motility, promoting stasis in the gastrointestinal tract which leads to an overgrowth of bacteria.[293] Detailed thyroid assessment should include measurements of thyroid stimulating hormone (TSH), free T4, free T3, total T3, reverse T3 (rT3), and antithyroid peroxidase (anti-TPO) and antithyroglobulin antibodies. Management of hypothyroidism is detailed in Chapter 1 of *Inflammation Mastery* / *Functional Inflammology* (2014 and later editions).

---

[290] Vieth R. Vitamin D supplementation, 25-hydroxyvitamin D concentrations, and safety. *Am J Clin Nutr.* 1999 May;69(5):842-56
[291] Vasquez et al. Clinical Importance of Vitamin D: Paradigm Shift for All Healthcare Providers. *Altern Ther Health Med* 2004; 10: 28-37 ichnfm.academia.edu/AlexVasquez
[292] Kedlaya D. Hypothyroid Myopathy. emedicine.medscape.com/article/313915-overview Accessed April 2012
[293] Lauritano EC, Bilotta AL, Gabrielli M, et al. Association between hypothyroidism and small intestinal bacterial overgrowth. *J Clin Endocrinol Metab.* 2007 Nov;92(11):4180-4

- Occult infections, especially with _Mycoplasma_ species and _Chlamydia/Chlamydophila pneumoniae_: Clinicians are increasingly appreciating the role of occult intracellular infections in the genesis and/or perpetuation of chronic health problems, including some previously perplexing problems such as chronic fatigue syndrome (CFS), inflammatory arthritis, and multiple sclerosis (MS). For chronic _Chlamydophila_ (previously _Chlamydia_) _pneumoniae_ infection, testing for serum levels of antibodies is useful followed by treatment with antibacterial drugs such as azithromycin and nutritional supplements such as N-acetyl-cysteine (NAC) in appropriately selected patients; for chronic _Mycoplasma_ infections, because of the various subspecies involved, polymerase chain reaction (PCR) testing appears to be preferred followed by treatment with doxycycline in adults.

  - Review: _Mycoplasma_ blood infection in chronic fatigue and **fibromyalgia** syndromes (_Rheum Int_ 2003 Sep[294]): The author notes that "**Chronic fatigue syndrome (CFS) and fibromyalgia syndrome (FMS)** are characterized by a lack of consistent laboratory and clinical abnormalities. Although they are distinguishable as separate syndromes based on established criteria, a great number of patients are diagnosed with both." He goes on to say, "In studies using **polymerase chain reaction [PCR] methods, mycoplasma blood infection has been detected in about 50% of patients with CFS and/or FMS**, including patients with Gulf War illnesses and symptoms that overlap with one or both syndromes. **Such infection is detected in only about 10% of healthy individuals**, significantly less than in patients. Most patients with CFS/FMS who have mycoplasma infection appear to recover and reach their pre-illness state after **long-term antibiotic therapy with doxycycline**, and the infection cannot be detected after recovery. … It is not clear whether mycoplasmas are associated with CFS/FMS as causal agents, cofactors, or opportunistic infections in patients with immune disturbances."

  - Clinical investigation: High prevalence of Mycoplasmal infections in symptomatic (chronic fatigue syndrome) family members of _Mycoplasma_-positive Gulf War illness patients (_Journal of Chronic Fatigue Syndrome_ 2003[295]): The authors state, "…a relatively common finding in Gulf War Illness patients is a bacterial infection due to _Mycoplasma_ species, we examined military families (149 patients: 42 veterans, 40 spouses, 32 other relatives and 35 children with at least one family complaint of illness) selected from a **group of 110 veterans with Gulf War Illness who tested positive (~41%) for at least one of four _Mycoplasma_ species**: _M. fermentans, M. hominis, M. pneumoniae_ or _M. genitalium_. Consistent with previous results, over 80% of Gulf War Illness patients who were positive for blood mycoplasmal infections had **only one _Mycoplasma_ species, in particular _M. fermentans_** (Odds ratio = 17.9, P <0.001). In healthy control subjects the incidence of mycoplasmal infection was ~8.5% and none were found to have multiple mycoplasmal species."

  - Clinical investigation: Prevalence of antibodies to _Chlamydophila pneumoniae_ in persons without clinical evidence of respiratory infection (_Journal of Clinical Pathology_ 2002 May[296]): The authors note that "Because there is as yet no standardization of serological criteria for persistent infection, we considered antibody titers of > 1/20 in the IgA fraction, together with **IgG titers of 1/64 to 1/256, to be indicative of persistent infection**." This article supports clinical experience and post-graduate presentations[297] showing that in persons with fatigue and various other chronic health disorders characterized by pain and inflammation (such as chronic inflammatory arthritis[298] or spine[299] inflammation), the finding of IgG antibody levels >1:64 suggests that the patient has a persistent _Chlamydophila pneumoniae_ infection which may be alleviated by the administration of—for example—the antibiotic **azithromycin** (adult dose 250 mg every other day due to the drug's long half-life, given for several weeks or months until symptoms are resolved and/or antibody

---

[294] Endresen GK. Mycoplasma blood infection in chronic fatigue and fibromyalgia syndromes. _Rheumatol Int_. 2003 Sep;23(5):211-5

[295] Nicolson GL, Nasralla MY, Nicolson NL. High prevalence of Mycoplasmal infections in symptomatic (chronic fatigue syndrome) family members of _Mycoplasma_-positive Gulf War illness patients. _Journal of Chronic Fatigue Syndrome_ 2003; 11(2): 21-36 immed.org/GulfWarIllness/10.01.11update/GWIfamilyJCFS_.pdf

[296] Ben-Yaakov et al. Prevalence of antibodies to Chlamydia pneumoniae in an Israeli population without clinical evidence of respiratory infection. _J Clin Pathol_. 2002 May;55(5):355-8 jcp.bmj.com/content/55/5/355.long

[297] Stratton C. The Role of Chlamydophila in Autoimmune Disease. 2011 International Symposium. "The Challenge of Emerging Infections in the 21st Century: Terrain, Tolerance, and Susceptibility" hosted by Institute for Functional Medicine in Seattle, Washington in May 2011

[298] "This study was a 9-month, prospective, double-blind, triple-placebo trial assessing a 6-month course of combination antibiotics as a treatment for Chlamydia-induced ReA. Groups received 1) doxycycline and rifampin plus placebo instead of azithromycin; 2) azithromycin and rifampin plus placebo instead of doxycycline; or 3) placebos instead of azithromycin, doxycycline, and rifampin. … These data suggest that a 6-month course of combination antibiotics is an effective treatment for chronic Chlamydia-induced ReA." Carter JD, Espinoza LR, Inman RD, et al. Combination antibiotics as a treatment for chronic Chlamydia-induced reactive arthritis: a double-blind, placebo-controlled, prospective trial. _Arthritis Rheum_. 2010 May;62(5):1298-307

[299] "The frequency of Chlamydia-positive ST samples, as determined by PCR, was found to be significantly higher in patients with uSpA than in patients with OA. Our results suggest that in many patients with uSpA, chlamydial infection, which is often occult, may be the cause." Carter et al. Chlamydiae as etiologic agents in chronic undifferentiated spondylarthritis. _Arthritis Rheum_. 2009 May;60(5):1311-6

titers are normalized) and **N-acetyl-cysteine** (NAC: 500-1,200 mg 1-3 times per day by mouth between meals). Positive antibody titers (levels) are common because the infection itself is common *as a transient condition*; the issue here is the determination of which patients have a *chronic* and *persistent* low-grade infection. The finding of an elevated antibody titer—that is a level greater than 1:64—indicates the need to consider long-term antimicrobial intervention.

Chlamydia pneumoniae IgG	**>1:256**	**High**	Neg:<1:16
Chlamydia pneumoniae IgM	<1:10		Neg:<1:10

Elevated titers to *Chlamydia/Chlamydophila pneumoniae* suggesting chronic persistent infection in a 40yo male physician *without pulmonary symptoms* but with a positive history of chronic sinus congestion and low-grade fatigue—improvement with azithromycin and NAC: This patient experienced years of severe psychologic and physiologic stress during a doctorate program and then had an acute upper respiratory illness onset in September 2010 while working in hospital emergency rooms and urgent care clinics; recurrent bouts of upper respiratory illness—attributed to viral infections—persisted for five months until February 2011. By the summer of 2011, the patient was relatively asymptomatic except for persistent sinus congestion and low-grade fatigue. No pulmonary symptoms such as shortness of breath were ever present. Following detection of the elevated antibody titer, the patient started on azithromycin and NAC, which resulted in a short-term (12-hour) exacerbation of symptoms followed by complete and sustained resolution of sinus congestion and improved energy levels and exercise endurance.

- Hemochromatosis and iron overload: Genetic hemochromatosis is a common iron-accumulation disease that causes chronic persistent musculoskeletal pain, even while most routine laboratory tests are normal; thus, the clinical presentation of iron overload may be confused with that of fibromyalgia—both are common conditions commonly presenting with inexplicable (i.e., normal values of routine laboratory tests) nontraumatic musculoskeletal pain. Hemochromatosis is one of the most common hereditary disorders among Caucasians, with a homozygote (two of the same genes, results in more severe disease) frequency of approximately 1 in 200 to 250 persons and a heterozygote (only one affected gene, less severe disease) frequency of approximately 1 in 7 persons. Various other hereditary iron overload disorders affect all races, with the highest prevalence in persons of African descent (as high as 1 in 80 according to some small studies among hospitalized African-American patients).[300,301] Eighty percent of hemochromatosis patients have chronic musculoskeletal pain, which is commonly the earliest or only presenting complaint.[302] In contrast to the clinical presentation of FM, the musculoskeletal manifestations of iron overload are classically arthritic (i.e., in the joints) rather than muscular, with the joints of the hands, wrists, hips, and knees most commonly affected. However, due to the widespread distribution of pain and the normalcy of routine laboratory results, iron overload can mimic fibromyalgia. Given the high population prevalence of iron overload and the high frequency with which it presents with musculoskeletal manifestations, all patients with chronic, nontraumatic musculoskeletal pain must be tested for iron overload. Serum ferritin, which can be used alone or with transferrin saturation, is the best single laboratory test; confirmed results greater than 200 mcg/L in women and 300 mcg/L in men necessitate treatment with diagnostic and therapeutic phlebotomy (frequent "blood donation" is the most effective treatment for chronic iron overload).[303]

- Iron deficiency: Iron is necessary for function of the mitochondrial electron transport chain as well as for formation of the neurotransmitters dopamine and serotonin, both of which can be said to have an analgesic effect. As such, iron deficiency can promote headaches in general and migraine in particular; iron deficiency might also contribute to the clinical presentation of fibromyalgia.[304] Per my previous extensive reviews of the

[300] Wurapa RK, Gordeuk VR, Brittenham GM, Khiyami A, Schechter GP, Edwards CQ. Primary iron overload in African Americans. *Am J Med*. 1996 Jul;101(1):9-18
[301] Barton JC, Edwards CQ, Bertoli LF, Shroyer TW, Hudson SL. Iron overload in African Americans. *Am J Med*. 1995 Dec;99(6):616-23
[302] Vasquez A. Musculoskeletal disorders and iron overload disease: comment on the American College of Rheumatology guidelines for the initial evaluation of the adult patient with acute musculoskeletal symptoms. *Arthritis Rheum*. 1996 Oct;39(10):1767-8 Ichnfm.academia.edu/AlexVasquez
[303] Barton JC, McDonnell SM, Adams PC, et al. Management of hemochromatosis. Hemochromatosis Management Working Group. *Ann Intern Med*. 1998 Dec 1;129(11):932-9
[304] "The mean serum ferritin levels in the fibromyalgia and control groups were 27.3 and 43.8 ng/ml, respectively, and the difference was statistically significant. Binary multiple logistic regression analysis with age, body mass index, smoking status and vitamin B12, as well as folic acid and ferritin levels showed that having a serum ferritin level <50 ng/ml caused a 6.5-fold increased risk for FMS." Ortancil et al. Association between serum ferritin level and fibromyalgia syndrome. *Eur J Clin Nutr*. 2010 Mar;64(3):308-12

literature on the topics of iron overload and iron deficiency[305], optimal iron status correlates with serum ferritin values of 40-70 ng/ml. Rarely, a person with what can be described as a defect in the blood-brain barrier transport of iron into the brain will need to have a serum ferritin value of 120 ng/ml in order to promote entry of iron into the brain.

- Accumulation of xenobiotics (including mercury and lead): Xenobiotic (foreign chemical) accumulation may occasionally cause widespread pain resembling fibromyalgia, and xenobiotic detoxification (depuration) can alleviate pain in affected patients. Toxic chemical and toxic metal accumulation is common in humans worldwide and has been well-documented in Americans. Eight percent (8%) of American women of childbearing age have sufficiently high levels of mercury in their blood to increase the risk of health problems such as neurological damage in their

> **Potential benefits of reducing the body burden of mercury in patients with chronic pain and fatigue**
>
> "We suggest that **metal-driven inflammation** may affect the hypothalamic-pituitary-adrenal axis (HPA axis) and indirectly trigger psychosomatic multisymptoms characterizing **chronic fatigue syndrome, fibromyalgia**, and other diseases of unknown etiology."
>
> Sterzl et al. Mercury and nickel allergy: risk factors in fatigue and autoimmunity. *Neuro Endocrinol Lett.* 1999

children.[306] Americans in general show alarmingly high concentrations and combinations of neurotoxic (nerve-damaging), carcinogenic (cancer-causing), diabetogenic (diabetes-causing), and immunotoxic (immune-poisoning) xenobiotics/toxins.[307] Adverse effects of toxic chemicals (e.g., pesticides, herbicides, solvents, plastics, formaldehyde, petroleum byproducts) and heavy metals (especially lead and mercury) are well described throughout the biomedical literature and have been clinically reviewed by Crinnion.[308,309,310,311] Among toxins with the ability to produce chronic muscle pain, mercury may deserve special recognition given its ubiquitous distribution in the human population and the scientific evidence detailing its numerous adverse effects.[312,313] Whether by metabolic, neurological, or endocrinologic means, occult mercury toxicity may manifest as a syndrome of widespread muscle pain that resembles fibromyalgia.[314] Acrodynia is a subacute peripheral pain syndrome due to mercury toxicity classically seen in children.[315] Acute mercury intoxication can result in severe skeletal muscle damage (rhabdomyolysis).[316] Mercury in organic and inorganic forms interferes with acetylcholine reception and several crucial aspects of the sarcoplasmic reticulum, including calcium-magnesium-ATPase and calcium transport; these adverse effects establish a molecular basis for a *mercurial myopathy* (mercury-induced muscle disease).[317,318] The toxicity of mercury is greatly increased by simultaneous accumulation of lead, elevated levels of which are also common in the U.S. population. Demonstration of high mercury and lead levels in urine following administration of a chelating agent such as dimercaptosuccinic acid (DMSA) can be used to diagnose chronic mercury or lead overload, and orally administered DMSA is also used for treatment.[319,320,321,322] Failure to preadminister a chelating agent prior to measurement of urine mercury renders the test insensitive for chronic accumulation and can thus give the false impression that mercury is not contributory to fibromyalgia, as concluded by Kotter et al.[323] Orally administered selenium, phytochelatins (metal-binding peptides from plants[324]), a high-fiber diet, and potassium citrate can be used to augment mercury excretion.

---

[305] See Chapter 1 of either *Inflammation Mastery* / *Functional Inflammology* (2014 or later) for the most complete reviews, including assessment, management, and radiographic presentations. See also: Vasquez A. Musculoskeletal disorders and iron overload disease. [Letter] *Arthritis & Rheumatism* 1996; 39:1767-8. Vasquez A. High body iron stores: causes, effects, diagnosis, and treatment. *Nutritional Perspectives* 1994 October

[306] "However, approximately 8% of women had concentrations higher than US Environmental Protection Agency's recommended reference dose (5.8 µg/L), below which exposures are considered to be without adverse effects." Schober et al. Blood mercury levels in US children and women of childbearing age,1999-2000. *JAMA* 2003;289:1667-74

[307] Kristin et al. Chemical Trespass. Pesticide Action Network North America. Available at panna.org. See also: Body Burden: The Pollution in People. ewg.org/ 2006 Feb

[308] Crinnion WJ. Environmental medicine, part 1: the human burden of environmental toxins and their common health effects. *Altern Med Rev.* 2000 Feb;5(1):52-63

[309] Crinnion WJ. Environmental medicine, part 2: health effects of and protection from ubiquitous airborne solvent exposure. *Altern Med Rev.* 2000 Apr;5(2):133-43

[310] Crinnion WJ. Environmental medicine, part 3: long-term effects of chronic low-dose mercury exposure. *Altern Med Rev.* 2000 Jun;5(3):209-23

[311] Crinnion WJ. Environmental medicine, part 4: pesticides - biologically persistent and ubiquitous toxins. *Altern Med Rev.* 2000 Oct;5(5):432-47

[312] Elemental Mercury Vapor Poisoning -- North Carolina, 1988. cdc.gov/mmwr/preview/mmwrhtml/00001499.htm

[313] Shih H, Gartner JC Jr. Weight loss, hypertension, weakness, and limb pain in an 11-year-old boy. *J Pediatr.* 2001 Apr;138(4):566-9

[314] Sterzl I, Prochazkova J, Hrda P, et al. Mercury and nickel allergy: risk factors in fatigue and autoimmunity. *Neuro Endocrinol Lett.* 1999;20:221-8

[315] Padlewska KK. Acrodynia. Last Updated: February 15, 2007 eMedicine emedicine.com/derm/topic592.htm Accessed October 25, 2007

[316] Chugh KS, Singhal PC, Uberoi HS. Rhabdomyolysis and renal failure in acute mercuric chloride poisoning. *Med J Aust.* 1978 Jul 29;2(3):125-6

[317] Chiu VC, Mouring D, Haynes DH. Action of mercurials on the active and passive transport properties of sarcoplasmic reticulum. *J Bioenerg Biomembr.* 1983 Feb;15(1):13-25

[318] Shamoo AE, Maclennan DH, Elderfrawi ME. Differential effects of mercurial compounds on excitable tissues. *Chem Biol Interact.* 1976 Jan;12(1):41-52

[319] Kalra V, et al. Succimer in Symptomatic Lead Poisoning. *Indian Pediatrics* 2002; 39:580-585 indianpediatrics.net/june2002/june-580-585.htm

[320] Bradstreet et al. Case-control study of mercury burden in children with autistic spectrum disorders. *J Am Physicians Surgeons* 2003; 8: 76-79 jpands.org/vol8no3/geier.pdf

[321] Forman et al. A cluster of pediatric metallic mercury exposure cases treated with meso-2,3-dimercaptosuccinic acid (DMSA). *Environ Health Perspect.* 2000 Jun;108(6):575-7

[322] Miller AL. Dimercaptosuccinic acid (DMSA), a non-toxic, water-soluble treatment for heavy metal toxicity. *Altern Med Rev.* 1998 Jun;3(3):199-207

[323] Kotter I, Durk H, Saal JG, et al. Mercury exposure from dental amalgam fillings in the etiology of primary fibromyalgia. *J Rheumatol.* 1995;22:2194-5

[324] Cobbett CS. Phytochelatins and their roles in heavy metal detoxification. *Plant Physiol.* 2000;123:825-32 plantphysiol.org/content/123/3/825

- **Case report: Therapeutic detoxification to reduce the body burden of lead and mercury in a woman diagnosed with FM leads to complete relief of FM symptoms**: This 54-year-old athletic female with healthy diet, lifestyle, and supportive relationship presented with chronic diffuse musculoskeletal pain. Health history was significant for decades of environmental illness/intolerance (EI) and multiple chemical sensitivity (MCS). Family history was positive for maternal temporal (giant cell) arteritis. Physical examination revealed numerous tender points consistent with FM. Stool analysis was unremarkable and unsupportive of either identifiable infection or nonspecific bacterial overgrowth. Laboratory investigations revealed normal results for hsCRP (high-sensitivity c-reactive protein), CK (creatine kinase, a marker of muscle damage), ANA (anti-nuclear antibodies, elevated in many autoimmune diseases such as lupus/SLE), vitamin D, calcium, phosphorus, and comprehensive thyroid evaluation. The patient was then (defensively) referred to an excellent osteopathic medical internist who diagnosed the patient with fibromyalgia. The patient was unsatisfied with the diagnosis of FM and returned to the current author, who then performed urine heavy metal testing provoked with 10 mg per kilogram of dimercaptosuccinic acid (DMSA). Results revealed the highest levels of lead and mercury encountered in the author's practice at that time. As in the accompanying lab results, lead levels were 6x above the reference range and mercury levels were 7x above the reference range. The patient was commenced on DMSA 10 mg/kg/d three days "on" and 4 days "off" (cyclic dosing is used to avoid toxicity in general and bone marrow toxicity [neutropenia] in particular), selenium 800 mcg/d to promote excretion of toxic metals and to support renal and antioxidant protection, vegetable juices to provide potassium and citrate for urinary alkalinization and enhanced excretion of xenobiotics[325], and a proprietary phytochelatin (metal-binding peptides from plants) concentrate to bind toxic metals in the gut and thereby promote their fecal excretion by blocking enterohepatic recycling/recirculation. DMSA chelation is approved by the US Food and Drug Administration (FDA) for the treatment of lead toxicity in children.[326] The use of DMSA for children and adults is supported by peer-reviewed literature.[327,328,329,330,331] After approximately 8 months of treatment, the patient was completely free of pain, and the clinical improvement was associated with a reduction in both lead and mercury of approximately 50% as demonstrated by follow-up laboratory testing. This case was published in peer-reviewed literature for continuing medical education (CME) for physicians.[332]

Date Completed: **10/22/2005**

Lead	30	<	5
Mercury	21	<	3

Date Completed: **6/30/2006**

Lead	15	<	5
Mercury	8.2	<	4

Marked accumulation of lead and mercury in a patient diagnosed with FM—complete elimination of pain and stiffness following identification and reduction in the body burden of lead and mercury: 54yo woman presents with nontraumatic widespread pain consistent with a diagnosis of fibromyalgia; the diagnosis of FM is confirmed by two clinicians. All laboratory test results were normal except for urine toxic metal testing which showed 6x elevations of lead and 7x elevations of mercury. Treatment (DMSA, citrate, selenium, and phytochelatins per above) for 8 months effected safe reductions in body burden of lead and mercury and alleviation of all pain.

---

[325] Crinnion WJ. Environmental medicine, part3:long-term effects of chronic low-dose mercury exposure. *Altern Med Rev* 2000 Jun;5:209-23

[326] "The Food and Drug Administration has recently licensed the drug DMSA (succimer) for reduction of blood lead levels >/= 45 micrograms/dl. This decision was based on the demonstrated ability of DMSA to reduce blood lead levels. An advantage of this drug is that it can be given orally." Goyer RA, Cherian MG, Jones MM, Reigart JR. Role of chelating agents for prevention, intervention, and treatment of exposures to toxic metals. *Environ Health Perspect.* 1995 Nov;103(11):1048-52

[327] Bradstreet et al. A case-control study of mercury burden in children with autistic spectrum disorders. *Journal of American Physicians and Surgeons* 2003; 8: 76-79

[328] Crinnion WJ. Environmental medicine, part three: long-term effects of chronic low-dose mercury exposure. *Altern Med Rev.* 2000 Jun;5(3):209-23

[329] Forman et al. A cluster of pediatric metallic mercury exposure cases treated with meso-2,3-dimercaptosuccinic acid (DMSA). *Environ Health Perspect.* 2000 Jun;108(6):575-7

[330] Miller AL. Dimercaptosuccinic acid (DMSA), a non-toxic, water-soluble treatment for heavy metal toxicity. *Altern Med Rev.* 1998 Jun;3(3):199-207

[331] DMSA. *Altern Med Rev.* 2000 Jun;5(3):264-7 thorne.com/altmedrev/.fulltext/5/3/264.pdf

[332] Vasquez A. *Musculoskeletal Pain: Expanded Clinical Strategies*. Institute for Functional Medicine. 2008

> **Small intestine bacterial overgrowth (SIBO) is the primary cause of and most logical explanation for FM; all other characteristics of the disease can be understood by understanding the protean effects of SIBO.**

In the restructuring of this work in 2015 from its previous versions, I am—based on a more confident description of FM that moves from hypothesis to assertion—choosing to organize the pathophysiologic descriptions, upon which are based the therapeutic interventions, in the following four categories, each with their respective evidence:

1. The primary cause of fibromyalgia is SIBO—small intestinal bacterial overgrowth.
2. As a result of SIBO, fibromyalgia patients suffer somatic/body fatigue from mitochondrial dysfunction.
3. As a result of SIBO, fibromyalgia patients suffer increased sensitivity to pain due to heightened sensitivity of the brain and spinal cord—central sensitization—as well as from peripheral sensitization and impaired muscle function due to the previously established mitochondrial dysfunction.
4. All other biochemical and pathophysiologic abnormalities seen in fibromyalgia are explained from SIBO.

The primary focus of this section—establishing that SIBO is the cause of FM—is the provision of a cohesive and coherent explanation of FM; examples of treatments will be provided in this section on pathophysiology because the efficacy of treatments substantiates and helps prove the model that I have developed. Following these proofs substantiating this pathophysiologic model, a separate section detailing treatments will be provided. Allowing some repetition of citations used in the establishment of the pathophysiologic model, in the section on therapeutics I will review treatments using the format of my FINDSEX ® acronym to maintain consistency with my treatment protocols. Several diagrams will be provided, each providing novelty, emphasis, and repetition.

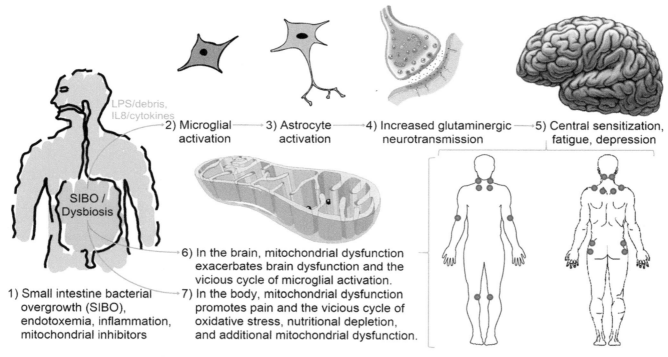

LPS/debris, IL8/cytokines

2) Microglial activation → 3) Astrocyte activation → 4) Increased glutaminergic neurotransmission → 5) Central sensitization, fatigue, depression

SIBO / Dysbiosis

1) Small intestine bacterial overgrowth (SIBO), endotoxemia, inflammation, mitochondrial inhibitors

6) In the brain, mitochondrial dysfunction exacerbates brain dysfunction and the vicious cycle of microglial activation.

7) In the body, mitochondrial dysfunction promotes pain and the vicious cycle of oxidative stress, nutritional depletion, and additional mitochondrial dysfunction.

A simple integrated model of fibromyalgia, emphasizing dysbiosis-induced glial activation and mitochondrial dysfunction—first published in *Nutritional Perspectives* 2015 Oct: Small intestine bacterial overgrowth (SIBO) elaborates endotoxin/lipopolysaccharide (LPS) with other inflammogens and mitochondrial inhibitors (including D-lactate and hydrogen sulfide [H2S]). Microglial activation can be triggered directly by LPS or indirectly by peripheral and central cytokines (especially IL-8), and it then triggers astrocyte activation and results in increased glutaminergic neurotransmission, which promotes central sensitization and the resulting depression, central fatigue, and pain sensitivity. In the brain, mitochondrial dysfunction exacerbates brain dysfunction and the vicious cycle of microglial activation. In the body, mitochondrial dysfunction promotes pain and the vicious cycles of oxidative stress, nutritional depletion, and additional mitochondrial dysfunction. Vitamin D deficiency, common in many conditions of persistent pain, exacerbates central pain by allowing increased microglial activation while also contributing to peripherally-sourced pain from muscle (myalgia) and bone (osteomalacia). Illustration by Vasquez; image of brain by IsaacMao per Flickr.com via creativecommons.org/licenses/by/2.0. See educational videos and updates at www.inflammationmastery.com/pain

❶ <u>**Primary Cause of FM—SIBO:**</u> **The primary cause of fibromyalgia is small intestinal bacterial overgrowth.** Small intestine bacterial overgrowth (SIBO)—also referred to as "intestinal bacterial overgrowth" or simply "bacterial overgrowth"—provides the single best model for explaining the clinical and pathophysiological manifestations of fibromyalgia. Although commonly underappreciated by many clinicians, SIBO is common in clinical practice, affecting for example approximately 40% of patients with rheumatoid arthritis, 84% of patients with IBS, and 90% to 100% of patients with fibromyalgia. **In a study of 42 fibromyalgia patients, all 42 FM patients showed laboratory evidence of SIBO, and the severity of the intestinal bacterial overgrowth correlated positively with the severity of the fibromyalgia,** thus indicating the plausibility of a causal relationship.[333] The links between fibromyalgia and IBS are also strong; **most IBS patients meet strict diagnostic criteria for fibromyalgia, and most fibromyalgia patients meet strict criteria for IBS.** Lubrano et al[334] showed that fibromyalgia severity correlated with IBS severity among patients who met strict diagnostic criteria for both conditions. The high degree of overlap between these two diagnostic labels suggests that these conditions are two variations of a common pathophysiological process—SIBO.[335] SIBO causes altered bowel function, immune activation, and visceral hypersensitivity, and it is the best causative explanation for the clinical and pathophysiological manifestations of IBS; for more details and citations, see the excellent review by Lin published in *Journal of the American Medical Association* in 2004.[336] IBS is characterized by *visceral* hyperalgesia (hypersensitivity to pain), just as fibromyalgia is characterized by *skeletal muscle* hyperalgesia. Given that strong evidence indicates that IBS is caused by SIBO and that IBS and fibromyalgia are variations of the same pathophysiological process, then fibromyalgia may therefore be caused by SIBO. However, these links and interconnections require substantiation, as provided throughout this section.

Bacterial LPS and other antigens absorbed from the intestine during SIBO contribute to a subclinical inflammatory state that results in pain hypersensitivity and increased cytokine release, both of which are characteristics of fibromyalgia. In animal models and in human research studies, exposure to bacterial endotoxin/LPS has been shown to increase the brain's sensitivity to and perception of pain. Immune-mediated and inflammation-mediated pathways that promote pain sensitivity and pain perception include ❶ increased production of nitric oxide with ❷ increased production of prostaglandins and cytokines, resulting in ❸ the sensitization of peripheral and/or central neurons to pain perception/transmission. In support of this concept, Lin[337] wrote in 2004, **"The immune response to bacterial antigen in SIBO provides a framework for understanding the hypersensitivity in both fibromyalgia and IBS."** A later paper by Othmanm, Agüero, and Lin[338] in 2008 stated, "...a recent animal study demonstrated that exposure to endotoxin increased the production of prostaglandins and simultaneously decreased nitrous oxide production, resulting in inflammatory hyperalgesia" and "These observations suggest that SIBO is a common feature in both [IBS and FM] disorders and that altered gut microbiota in SIBO may play a role in the induction of somatic or visceral hypersensitivity, with affected patients meeting the diagnostic criteria for IBS, fibromyalgia or both disorders."

Gut bacteria also affect CNS/brain neurotransmission via vagal stimulation. According to a 2014 review by Galland, "Intrinsic primary afferent neurons (IPANs) are cellular targets of neuroactive bacteria and transmit microbial messages to the brain via the vagus nerve. Live bacteria may not be needed for these effects; in the case of *B. fragilis*, a lipid-free polysaccharide is both necessary and sufficient for IPAN activation. ... Gut bacteria influence reactivity of the HPA axis and the induction and maintenance of nREM sleep. They may influence mood, pain sensitivity and normal brain development."[339]

- <u>Fibromyalgia is tightly correlated with irritable bowel syndrome, a condition caused by small intestine bacterial overgrowth</u>: Fibromyalgia and IBS are strongly convergent, and the evidence indicates that IBS is caused largely or completely by SIBO; again, for more details and citations, see the brilliant article by Lin, cited previously. Small intestine bacterial overgrowth is highly prevalent in fibromyalgia. Several studies have

---

[333] Pimentel et al. A link between irritable bowel syndrome and fibromyalgia may be related to findings on lactulose breath testing. *Ann Rheum Dis.* 2004 Apr;63(4):450-2
[334] Lubrano E, et al. Fibromyalgia in patients with irritable bowel syndrome. An association with the severity of the intestinal disorder. *Int J Colorectal Dis.* 2001 Aug;16(4):211-5
[335] Veale et al. Primary fibromyalgia and the irritable bowel syndrome: different expressions of a common pathogenetic process. *Br J Rheumatol.* 1991 Jun;30(3):220-2
[336] Lin HC. Small intestinal bacterial overgrowth: a framework for understanding irritable bowel syndrome. *JAMA.* 2004 Aug 18;292(7):852-8
[337] Lin HC. Small intestinal bacterial overgrowth: a framework for understanding irritable bowel syndrome. *JAMA.* 2004 Aug 18;292(7):852-8
[338] Othman M, Agüero R, Lin HC. Alterations in intestinal microbial flora and human disease. *Curr Opin Gastroenterol.* 2008 Jan;24(1):11-6
[339] Galland L. The gut microbiome and the brain. *J Med Food.* 2014 Dec;17(12):1261-72

shown that 90% to 100% of fibromyalgia patients have evidence of SIBO; such a strong correlation and the dose-response relationship imply causality and must be integrated into any science-based model of fibromyalgia.

- □ <u>Clinical study: Patients with FM have evidence of frequent and severe bacterial overgrowth in the intestines</u> (<u>*Annals of the Rheumatic Diseases* 2004 Apr[340]</u>): The **breath hydrogen test** is used for the detection of SIBO and involves orally administering a carbohydrate (such as lactulose, a source of sugar for bacteria) which is converted to hydrogen through bacterial fermentation; the exhaled hydrogen in the breath is measured as an indirect quantification of the amount of bacteria in the intestines. In this study, 20% of "healthy" control patients were found to have intestinal bacterial overgrowth via an abnormal hydrogen breath test compared with 93/111 (84%) subjects with IBS and **42/42 (100%) with fibromyalgia**. Subjects with fibromyalgia had higher hydrogen production (indicating more severe SIBO), peak hydrogen, and area under the curve than subjects with IBS. **The degree of somatic pain in fibromyalgia correlates significantly with the hydrogen level seen on the breath test**.

- • <u>Small intestine bacterial overgrowth leads to systemic absorption of toxins that impair brain/nerve and muscle/mitochondrial function</u>: SIBO is associated with overproduction and absorption of bacterial cellular debris (e.g., lipopolysaccharide [LPS], bacterial DNA, peptidoglycans, teichoic acid, exotoxins) and antimetabolites—substances which are directly toxic to cellular energy/ATP production and muscle and nerve function—such as D-lactic acid, tyramine, tartaric acid, hydrogen sulfide. Intestinal gram-negative bacteria produce endotoxin (also known as lipopolysaccharide, LPS), which impairs skeletal muscle energy/ATP production (by stimulating skeletal muscle sodium-potassium-ATPase). Endotoxin also raises blood lactate (indicating impaired cellular energy production) under aerobic conditions in humans.[341] **Thus, via direct and indirect effects on cellular metabolism, chronic low-dose bacterial LPS/endotoxin exposure can result in impaired muscle metabolism and reduced ATP synthesis via impairment of mitochondrial function.** Intestinal bacteria also produce D-lactate, a well-known metabolic toxin in humans; SIBO often results in variable levels of D-lactate acidosis, severe cases of which can progress from fatigue and malaise to encephalopathy (e.g., confusion, ataxia, slurred speech, altered mental status) and death.[342] Supporting the proposal that bacterial overgrowth with D-lactate-producing bacteria is a contributor to the chronic fatigue syndromes including fibromyalgia is an excellent study published in 2009 showing that **patients with chronic fatigue syndrome have intestinal overgrowth of bacteria that produce the cellular toxin D-lactate**; specifically the research showed that these chronic fatigue patients have **a 7-fold increase in D-lactate producing *Enterococcus* and 1,100-fold increase in D-lactate producing *Streptococcus*.** Energy/ATP underproduction and lactate overproduction cause muscle fatigue and muscle pain. An additional cellular toxin produced by intestinal bacteria is hydrogen sulfide (H2S), which causes DNA damage[343] (noted previously to be increased in fibromyalgia patients) and which impairs cellular energy production, a finding relevant to *but not necessarily limited to* the pathogenesis of ulcerative colitis.[344,345] Bacteria and yeast in the intestines produce H2S, which can bind to the mitochondrial enzyme cytochrome c oxidase (part of Complex IV of the electron transport chain), thereby impairing oxidative phosphorylation and ATP production; this may partly explain the association of gastrointestinal dysbiosis and small intestine bacterial overgrowth (SIBO) with conditions such as chronic fatigue syndrome (CFS) and fibromyalgia.[346] Given that sulfur-containing molecules such as sulfite and hydrogen sulfide bind to vitamin B12[347,348], we should reasonably expect that patients with excess exposure to H2S from the gastrointestinal tract would have an increased prevalence of vitamin B12 deficiency, and indeed this has been documented; vitamin B12 deficiency in CFS and FM patients promotes fatigue and brain dysfunction via the effects of vitamin B12 deficiency directly (ie, vitamin B12 deficiency is well known to cause

---

[340] Pimentel et al. A link between irritable bowel syndrome and fibromyalgia may be related to findings on lactulose breath testing. *Ann Rheum Dis.* 2004 Apr;63(4):450-2

[341] Bundgaard et al. Endotoxemia stimulates skeletal muscle Na+-K+-ATPase and raises blood lactate under aerobic conditions in humans. *Am J Physiol Heart Circ Physiol.* 2003 Mar;284(3):H1028-34

[342] Vella A, Farrugia G. D-lactic acidosis: pathologic consequence of saprophytism. *Mayo Clin Proc.* 1998 May;73(5):451-6

[343] Attene-Ramos MS, Wagner ED, Gaskins HR, Plewa MJ. Hydrogen sulfide induces direct radical-associated DNA damage. *Mol Cancer Res.* 2007 May;5(5):455-9

[344] Magee et al. Contribution of dietary protein to sulfide production in large intestine: in vitro and controlled feeding study in humans. *Am J Clin Nutr.* 2000 Dec;72(6):1488-94

[345] Babidge W, Millard S, Roediger W. Sulfides impair short chain fatty acid beta-oxidation at acyl-CoA dehydrogenase level in colonocytes. *Mol Cell Biochem.* 1998 Apr:117-24

[346] Lemle MD. Hypothesis: chronic fatigue syndrome is caused by dysregulation of hydrogen sulfide metabolism. *Med Hypotheses.* 2009 Jan;72(1):108-9

[347] Añíbarro et al. Asthma with sulfite intolerance in children: a blocking study with cyanocobalamin. *J Allergy Clin Immunol.* 1992 Jul;90(1):103-9

[348] Fujita et al. A fatal case of acute hydrogen sulfide poisoning caused by hydrogen sulfide: hydroxocobalamin therapy for acute hydrogen sulfide poisoning. *J Anal Toxicol.* 2011 Mar;35(2):119-23

nerve damage and brain damage) and indirectly via impaired metabolism of homocysteine, which then triggers pain sensitivity and accelerated neurodegeneration via activation of NMDA receptors in the brain.[349]

- Experimental study: Effect of *E. coli* endotoxin on mitochondrial form and function (*Annals of Surgery* 1971 Dec[350]): Authors of this paper show that treatment of normal rat liver mitochondria with *E. coli* endotoxin results in mitochondrial impairment. They note previous research showing that animal exposure to *E. coli* endotoxin causes inhibition of mitochondrial respiration and uncoupling of oxidative phosphorylation. Near their conclusion, the authors write, "Thus we have evidence to show that topical ***E. coli* endotoxin has pathologic effects on both membrane integrity and internal mechanochemical systems of isolated mitochondria.**" Readers should appreciate that *E. coli* is a common inhabitant of the gastrointestinal tract of humans and that its population is quantitatively increased during states of bacterial overgrowth of the small bowel, as is commonly seen in most patients with fibromyalgia. More recently, research has shown that impairment of mitochondrial function (noted in patients with fibromyalgia) can lead to destruction of mitochondria by a process termed "mitophagy" (noted in patients with fibromyalgia); over time, loss of mitochondria via mitophagy leads to reduced numbers of mitochondria in muscle and other tissues (noted in patients with fibromyalgia) and contributes to the fatigue and other symptoms which characterize FM.

- Clinical study: Increased D-lactic acid intestinal bacteria in patients with chronic fatigue syndrome (*In Vivo* 2009 Jul-Aug[351]): The authors of this 2009 study state in the summary of their research, "Patients with chronic fatigue syndrome (CFS) are affected by symptoms of cognitive dysfunction and neurological impairment, the cause of which has yet to be elucidated. However, these symptoms are strikingly similar to those of patients presented with D-lactic acidosis. A significant increase of Gram-positive facultative anaerobic fecal microorganisms in 108 CFS patients as compared to 177 control subjects is presented in this report. The viable count of D-lactic acid producing *Enterococcus* and *Streptococcus* spp. in the fecal samples from the CFS group (3.5 x 10(7) cfu [colony forming units]/L and 9.8 x 10(7) cfu/L respectively) were significantly higher than those for the control group (5.0 x 10(6) cfu/L and 8.9 x 10(4) cfu/L respectively). [**Note: This is approximately a 7x increase in D-lactate producing *Enterococcus* and 1,100x increase in D-lactate producing *Streptococcus*.**] Analysis of exometabolic profiles of *Enterococcus faecalis* and *Streptococcus sanguinis*, representatives of *Enterococcus* and *Streptococcus* spp. respectively, by NMR and HPLC showed that these organisms produced significantly more lactic acid from (13)C-labeled glucose, than the Gram negative *Escherichia coli*. Further, **both *E. faecalis* and *S. sanguinis* secrete more D-lactic acid than *E. coli*.** This study suggests a probable link between intestinal colonization of Gram-positive facultative anaerobic D-lactic acid bacteria and symptom expressions in a subgroup of patients with CFS. Given the fact that **this might explain not only neurocognitive dysfunction in CFS patients but**

> **Patients with "chronic fatigue syndrome" and the associated neurologic dysfunction and muscle dysfunction have intestinal overgrowth of bacteria that produce D-lactic acid, a known neurotoxin and metabolic poison**
>
> In 2007 and 2008, the current author (AV) wrote and published *Musculoskeletal Pain: Expanded Clinical Strategies** with the Institute for Functional Medicine; this chapter on fibromyalgia is derived and updated from that work. In that publication, I reviewed evidence that fibromyalgia—at that time considered mysterious, idiopathic, chronic, relentless, and treatable only by pain-relieving drugs—was most likely caused by small intestine bacterial overgrowth (SIBO) and the resultant absorption of metabolic toxins and immunogenic debris. This perspective has been supported by numerous publications, particularly the article published by Sheedy et al** in 2009, which showed for the first time that patients with chronic fatigue syndrome—a condition tightly correlated with and which often overlaps with fibromyalgia—have SIBO with various bacteria that are high-output producers of D-lactic acid, a known neurotoxin and metabolic poison which potentially contributes to many of the main clinical, biochemical, and histologic manifestations of FM, namely mental fatigue and dyscognition (difficulty thinking), muscle fatigue and pain, biochemical evidence of mitochondrial impairment, and histologic evidence of mitochondrial myopathy.
>
> *Vasquez A. *Musculoskeletal Pain*. Institute for Functional Medicine, 2008. **Sheedy, et al. Increased d-lactic acid intestinal bacteria in patients with chronic fatigue syndrome. *In Vivo*. 2009 Jul

---

[349] Regland et al. Increased concentrations of homocysteine in the cerebrospinal fluid in patients with fibromyalgia and chronic fatigue syndrome. *Scand J Rheumatol.* 1997;26(4):301-7

[350] White et al. Effect of E. coli endotoxin on mitochondrial form and function. *Ann Surg.* 1971 Dec;174(6):983-90

[351] Sheedy JR, Wettenhall RE, Scanlon D, et al. Increased d-lactic acid intestinal bacteria in patients with chronic fatigue syndrome. *In Vivo.* 2009 Jul-Aug;23(4):621-8

also **mitochondrial dysfunction, these findings may have important clinical implications.**" A note of personal experience: the current author (Dr Vasquez) had one event of severe headache and dyscognition following consumption of a prebiotic (FOS) supplement during my 6-year bout with a CFS-related condition; from this experience, I furthered my understanding of dysbiosis and continued to do so *via personal experience* for the following 10 years. Of further note, based on my personal experience and review of the biomedical literature, I proposed in the CME monograph *Musculoskeletal Pain: Expanded Clinical Strategies* (Institute for Functional Medicine, 2008) that D-lactic acidosis was one of the pathophysiologic mechanisms by which microbial overgrowth of the intestines causes fibromyalgia; I was therefore gratified to see this article—published in 2009, nearly 2 years after I had proposed this mechanism—verifying my hypothesis.

- <u>Commensal microbiota are necessary for the development of inflammatory pain</u> (*Proc Natl Acad Sci.* 2008 Feb[352]): In this remarkably insightful article, the authors introduce their work by stating, "The sensation of pain can be enhanced by acute or chronic inflammation", and that in their experimental model using germ-free and "conventional" (colonized) mice, they "show that inflammatory hypernociception induced by carrageenan, lipopolysaccharide, TNF-alpha, IL-1beta, and the chemokine CXCL1 was reduced in germ-free mice" while hypernociception induced by prostaglandins and dopamine was not altered by the presence/absence of bacteria. However, "reposition of the microbiota" or systemic administration of LPS essentially restored the pain and inflammation that was absent in germ-free mice, which also produced more IL-10, which—via experiments using anti-IL-10 antibody—proved to mediate both anti-inflammation and anti-nociception. The authors concluded that, "Therefore, these results show that contact with commensal microbiota is necessary for mice to develop inflammatory hypernociception. … Therefore, these results show that contact with commensal microbiota [or LPS] is necessary for mice to develop inflammatory hypernociception possibly in a TLR-dependent manner. "

- <u>Low-dose LPS 'priming' of muscle provides an animal model of persistent elevated mechanical sensitivity for the study of chronic pain</u> (*Eur J Pain* 2011 Aug[353]): In this experiment using intramuscular hypertonic saline with either high or low doses of LPS, the authors found that low-dose LPS exacerbated long-term pain, while high-dose LPS caused the expected acute inflammatory response but did not promote development of chronic pain; the authors speculate that the low dose of LPS "primed" inflammatory and neurologic pathways for the persistence of pain perception while the higher dose may have invoked counter-inflammatory mechanisms ("larger-dose of LPS in this experiment may have provoked a protective effect such as invoking negative feedback loops") that failed to promote the development of central sensitization. By showing that low-level locally-administered systemically-circulated LPS could promote the development of chronic pain, these authors have supported a model consistent with an integrated model of fibromyalgia, in which SIBO/LPS can explain the entirety of this common condition.

---

[352] Amaral et al. Commensal microbiota is fundamental for the development of inflammatory pain. *Proc Natl Acad Sci U S A.* 2008 Feb 12;105(6):2193-7
[353] Yamaguchi et al. Low rather than high dose lipopolysaccharide 'priming' of muscle provides an animal model of persistent elevated mechanical sensitivity for the study of chronic pain. *Eur J Pain.* 2011 Aug;15(7):724-31

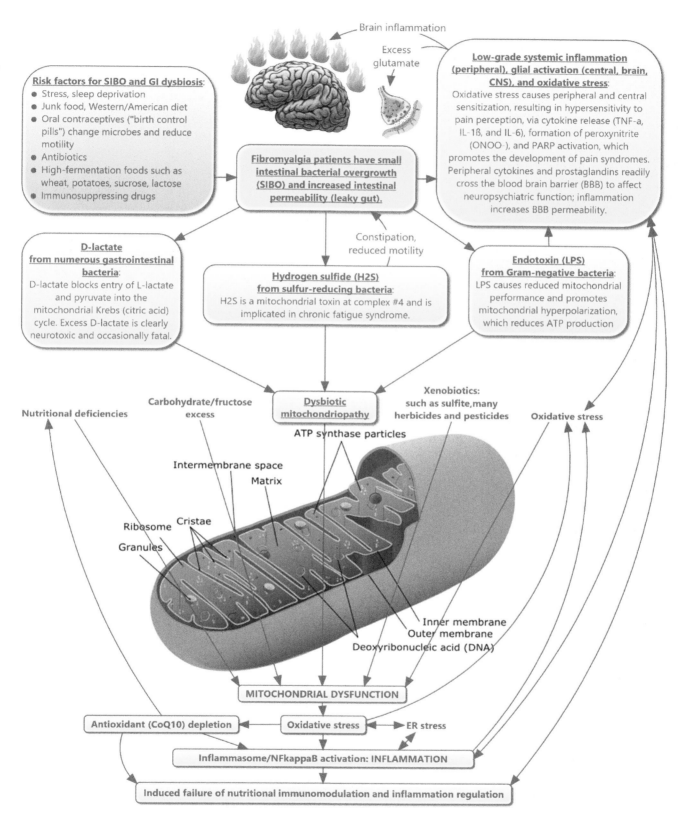

Brain inflammation

Excess glutamate

Risk factors for SIBO and GI dysbiosis:
- Stress, sleep deprivation
- Junk food, Western/American diet
- Oral contraceptives ("birth control pills") change microbes and reduce motility
- Antibiotics
- High-fermentation foods such as wheat, potatoes, sucrose, lactose
- Immunosuppressing drugs

Fibromyalgia patients have small intestinal bacterial overgrowth (SIBO) and increased intestinal permeability (leaky gut).

Low-grade systemic inflammation (peripheral), glial activation (central, brain, CNS), and oxidative stress:
Oxidative stress causes peripheral and central sensitization, resulting in hypersensitivity to pain perception, via cytokine release (TNF-a, IL-1ß, and IL-6), formation of peroxynitrite (ONOO-), and PARP activation, which promotes the development of pain syndromes. Peripheral cytokines and prostaglandins readily cross the blood brain barrier (BBB) to affect neuropsychiatric function; inflammation increases BBB permeability.

D-lactate from numerous gastrointestinal bacteria:
D-lactate blocks entry of L-lactate and pyruvate into the mitochondrial Krebs (citric acid) cycle. Excess D-lactate is clearly neurotoxic and occasionally fatal.

Constipation, reduced motility

Hydrogen sulfide (H2S) from sulfur-reducing bacteria:
H2S is a mitochondrial toxin at complex #4 and is implicated in chronic fatigue syndrome.

Endotoxin (LPS) from Gram-negative bacteria:
LPS causes reduced mitochondrial performance and promotes mitochondrial hyperpolarization, which reduces ATP production

Nutritional deficiencies

Carbohydrate/fructose excess

Dysbiotic mitochondriopathy

Xenobiotics: such as sulfite, many herbicides and pesticides

Oxidative stress

ATP synthase particles

Intermembrane space

Matrix

Ribosome

Cristae

Granules

Inner membrane

Outer membrane

Deoxyribonucleic acid (DNA)

MITOCHONDRIAL DYSFUNCTION

Antioxidant (CoQ10) depletion ◄── **Oxidative stress** ◄──► **ER stress**

Inflammasome/NFkappaB activation: INFLAMMATION

Induced failure of nutritional immunomodulation and inflammation regulation

Fibromyalgia is a unique combination of SIBO-induced mitochondrial impairment with SIBO-induced glial activation: The synergistic combination of mitochondrial impairment (clearly evidenced in FM) with glial activation and the resulting central sensitization (clearly evidenced in FM) produces the clinical pattern of fibromyalgia. Image copyright © 2016 by Dr Alex Vasquez, all rights reserved and enforced. Image of brain by IsaacMao per Flickr.com via creativecommons.org/licenses/by/2.0.

❷ **Secondary Cause of FM (part 1)—Mitochondrial Dysfunction: Fibromyalgia patients suffer somatic/body and central/brain fatigue from mitochondrial dysfunction as a result of SIBO.**

The evidence is clear to the point of being irrefutable that FM patients have mitochondrial impairment; given the critical role of mitochondria in somatic and cerebral function, this mitochondrial impairment (dysmitochondriosis) alone would be sufficient to explain virtually all manifestations of FM. Dysmitochondriosis is evident biochemically and histologically, thus obviously accounting for—or at least contributing to—the muscle/somatic pain and fatigue; what makes the situation in FM unique is the coupling of mitochondrial impairment with central nervous system inflammation, ie, brain inflammation, glial activation, and central sensitization. Glial activation is exacerbated by mitochondrial dysfunction, because—at least in part—the hyperglutaminergic neurotransmission induced by microglial-astrocyte activation puts heavier demands on energy/ATP production to maintain neuronal homeostasis, for maintaining the increased metabolic activity in general and for maintaining intracellular calcium homeostasis in particular. The excess glutaminergic neurotransmission contributes to additional glial activation and mitochondrial impairment, thereby forming a reinforced vicious cycle. Mitochondrial dysfunction causes excess ROS production and resultant depletion of multifunctional nutrients/chemicals such as CoQ10, which again feeds back to promote additional mitochondrial impairment and reduction in antioxidant defenses, leading to altered and consequential ROS signaling and the perpetuation of inflammation (e.g., inflammasome activation), mitochondrial impairment, and glial activation. Clinicians and researchers need to appreciate that because of their pathophysiologic connections and consequences, microglial activation leads to astrocyte activation which leads to excessive glutaminergic (hyperglutaminergic) neurotransmission and the brain/neocortical hyperexcitation that promotes the manifestations of depression (and other components of sickness behavior) and pain via central sensitization; as such these terms become interconnected and largely interchangeable when discussed in their totality of effect.

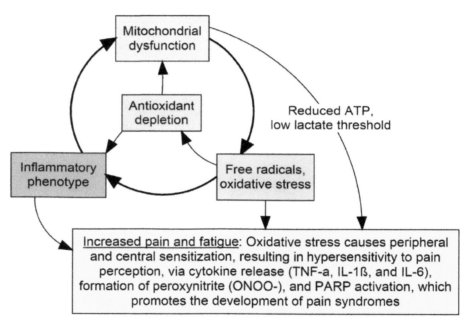

Mitochondrial dysfunction promotes central sensitization via oxidative stress and cytokine release: Mitochondrial dysfunction increases free radical production, which promotes "neurologic hypersensitivity" to pain, i.e., the pain in fibromyalgia is not simply due to muscle fatigue due to mitochondrial dysfunction although that is clearly a major component. The mitochondrial dysfunction also promotes central sensitization, which should be treated directly via alleviating the mitochondrial dysfunction and the causative dysbiosis, in addition to patient-specific factors.

Mitochondrial dysfunction

Antioxidant depletion

Reduced ATP, low lactate threshold

Inflammatory phenotype

Free radicals, oxidative stress

Increased pain and fatigue: Oxidative stress causes peripheral and central sensitization, resulting in hypersensitivity to pain perception, via cytokine release (TNF-a, IL-1ß, and IL-6), formation of peroxynitrite (ONOO-), and PARP activation, which promotes the development of pain syndromes

- Antimetabolites—microbial products that directly and indirectly impair mitochondrial performance: Yeast and bacteria can produce certain molecules which *jam up, monkey wrench*, or otherwise interfere with normal human cellular metabolism. The best example is **D-lactic acid**, which impairs human metabolic pathways that are designed to work with the "human" form of this metabolite—the levo isomer—L-lactic acid. Commonly resulting in headache, fatigue, depression, and sometimes death, D-lactic acidosis is extensively well documented in the medical research literature and commonly occurs in association with bacterial overgrowth of the intestine, particularly following intestinal bypass surgery.[354] Other antimetabolites produced from

---

[354] "D-Lactic acidosis is a potentially fatal clinical condition seen in patients with a short small intestine and an intact colon. Excessive production of D-lactate by abnormal bowel flora overwhelms normal metabolism of D-lactate and leads to an accumulation of this enantiomer in the blood." Vella A, Farrugia G. D-lactic acidosis: pathologic consequence of saprophytism. *Mayo Clin Proc.* 1998 May;73(5):451-6

(intestinal) microbes which are associated with human disease and dysfunction include **ammonia, tryptamine, tyramine, octopamine, mercaptates, aldehydes, alcohol (ethanol), tartaric acid, indolepropionic acid, indoleacetic acid, skatole, indole, putrescine,** and **cadaverine**. Many of these metabolites are seen in higher amounts in patients with migraine, depression, weakness, confusion, schizophrenia, agitation, hepatic encephalopathy, chronic arthritis and rheumatoid arthritis. **Gut-derived neurotoxins** from bacteria and yeast may contribute to autistic symptomatology[355,356], and case reports have consistently demonstrated that excess absorption of bacterial metabolites can alter behavior in humans and result in acute

D-lactate triad: SIBO, CHO, and IP—bacterial overgrowth, carbohydrate, and increased permeability; the solutions are to reduce SIBO, reduce/modify CHO, heal gut, promote motility
"D-lactate is usually produced in excess when small bowel resection allows delivery of a high carbohydrate load to the colon. Elevation of D-lactate in plasma may also occur after other types of abdominal surgery, as a result of increased intestinal permeability and bacterial translocation across the intestinal mucosal barrier. Nonsurgical causes of intestinal hyperpermeability also increase absorption of D-lactate from the intestinal lumen." Galland L. *J Med Food*. 2014 Dec

neurocognitive decline and behavioral abnormalities in children.[357] **Hydrogen sulfide (H2S)**, produced by intestinal bacteria such as *Citrobacter freundii*[358], is a mitochondrial poison[359] and is strongly associated with disease activity in ulcerative colitis.[360] Degradation of tryptophan by bacterial tryptophanase predisposes the host to a "functional tryptophan deficiency" and may result in insufficiency of serotonin which would contribute to hyperalgesia, depression, impaired adrenal responsiveness[361] ("hypoadrenalism"), and insomnia; **indole** and **skatole**, which are gut-derived bacterial degradation products of tryptophan, produce an inflammatory arthritis identical to rheumatoid arthritis in animal models.[362,363]

▪ Increased D-lactic acid intestinal bacteria in chronic fatigue syndrome (*In Vivo* 2009 Jul[364]): The authors report finding a **significant increase of Gram-positive facultative anaerobic fecal microorganisms** in 108 CFS patients as compared to 177 control subjects. Specifically, they report, "The viable count of D-lactic acid producing *Enterococcus* and *Streptococcus* spp. in the fecal samples from the CFS group (3.5 x 10(7) cfu/L and 9.8 x 10(7) cfu/L respectively) were significantly higher than those for the control group (5.0 x 10(6) cfu/L and 8.9 x 10(4) cfu/L respectively). **Readers should note that this is approximately a 10-fold increase in *Enterococcus* and a >1,000-fold increase in *Streptococcus* in the CFS group compared with the control group. These Gram-positive bacteria produced not only more lactic acid in general but specifically they produced more of the dextro isomer D-lactic acid** than the Gram negative *Escherichia coli*. The authors correctly conclude that these findings "might explain not only neurocognitive dysfunction in CFS patients but also mitochondrial dysfunction, these findings may have important clinical implications."

▪ Short bowel syndrome and D-lactic acidosis (*Arch Dis Child* 1980 Oct[365]): The three-sentence abstract of this case report reads, "Metabolic acidosis in a 3-year-old child with short bowel syndrome led to the discovery of massive D-lactic aciduria. After normalization of the intestinal bacterial flora, D-lactate disappeared together with the acidosis. Dysbacteriosis with excessive production of D-lactate by intestinal bacteria (unidentified) and subsequent absorption explains this unusual cause of metabolic acidosis." Note the use

---

[355] Sandler RH, Finegold SM, Bolte ER, et al. Short-term benefit from oral vancomycin treatment of regressive-onset autism. *J Child Neurol*. 2000 Jul;15(7):429-35

[356] Shaw et al. Increased urinary excretion of analogs of Krebs cycle metabolites and arabinose in two brothers with autistic features. *Clin Chem* 1995;41(8Pt1):1094-104

[357] "The neurological features consisted of a depressed conscious state, confusion, aggressive behaviour, slurred speech and ataxia. The organic acid profile of urine demonstrated increased amounts of lactic, 3-hydroxypropionic, 3-hydroxyisobutyric, 2-hydroxyisocaproic, phenyllactic, 4-hydroxyphenylactic and 4-hydroxyphenyllactic acids. Of the lactic acid 99% was D-lactic acid." Haan et al. Severe illness caused by products of bacterial metabolism in child with short gut. *Eur J Pediatr*. 1985;144:63-5

[358] Lennette EH (editor in chief). *Manual of Clinical Microbiology, Fourth Edition*. Washington DC; American Society for Microbiology: 1985, page 269. See also web.indstate.edu/thcme/micro/GI/general/sld038.htm Accessed 10/27/2005

[359] "Treatment of H2S poisoning may benefit from interventions aimed at minimizing ROS-induced damage and reducing mitochondrial damage." Eghbal MA, Pennefather PS, O'Brien PJ. H2S cytotoxicity mechanism involves reactive oxygen species formation and mitochondrial depolarisation. *Toxicology*. 2004 Oct 15;203(1-3):69-76

[360] "CONCLUSIONS: Metabolic effects of sodium hydrogen sulfide on butyrate oxidation along the length of the colon closely mirror metabolic abnormalities observed in active ulcerative colitis, and increased production of sulfide in ulcerative colitis suggests that the action of mercaptides may be involved in the genesis of ulcerative colitis." Roediger WE, et al. Reducing sulfur compounds of the colon impair colonocyte nutrition: implications for ulcerative colitis. *Gastroenterology* 1993 Mar;104:802-9

[361] "This hypothesis is supported by the findings in chronic MS patients of a significantly diminished adrenal cortisol reactivity to insulin-induced hypoglycemia which is considered a stress response mediated through the 5-HT system. Consequently, since patients with MS exhibit an abnormal response to stress it follows that increased tryptophan availability through dietary supplementation would diminish their vulnerability to psychological stress." Sandyk R. Tryptophan availability and the susceptibility to stress in multiple sclerosis: a hypothesis. *Int J Neurosci*. 1996 Jul;86(1-2):47-53

[362] Nakoneczna I, Forbes JC, Rogers KS. The arthritogenic effect of indole, skatole and other tryptophan metabolites in rabbits. *Am J Pathol*. 1969 Dec;57(3):523-38

[363] Rogers KS, Forbes JC, Nakoneczna I. Arthritogenic properties of lipophilic, aryl molecules. *Proc Soc Exp Biol Med*. 1969 Jun;131(2):670-2

[364] Sheedy JR, et al. Increased d-lactic acid intestinal bacteria in patients with chronic fatigue syndrome. *In Vivo*. 2009 Jul-Aug;23(4):621-8

[365] Schoorel EP, Giesberts MA, Blom W, van Gelderen HH. D-Lactic acidosis in a boy with short bowel syndrome. *Arch Dis Child*. 1980 Oct;55(10):810-2

of "dysbacteriosis" which is more commonly abbreviated to "dysbiosis", with the latter being more accurate in its nonspecificity since the disease-producing microbes may be from several different kingdoms and thus not exclusive to bacteria. The young boy in this case report underwent bowel resection secondary to multiple congenital malformations and complications from infection, i.e., mesenteric thrombosis tertiary to dehydration secondary to infectious diarrhea. After several episodes of neurocognitive dysfunction including weakness and dyspnea, the child was eventually diagnosed with multiple nutritional deficiencies, malabsorption, and lactic acidosis secondary to intestinal overgrowth of Gram-positive D-lactate-producing bacteria and an insufficiency of Gram-negative bacteria. The child was treated only with probiotic supplementation—no antibiotics were given—and D-lactate levels fell quickly within 4 days and were virtually undetectable by day 11. Thus, probiotic therapy alone may be sufficient treatment for some cases of D-lactic acidosis, particularly when an "insufficiency dysbiosis" of beneficial bacteria and a relative or absolute "overgrowth dysbiosis" of harmful bacteria coexist.

❸ **Secondary Cause of FM (part 2)—Central Sensitization: As a result of SIBO, fibromyalgia patients suffer increased sensitivity to pain due to heightened sensitivity of the brain and spinal cord—as well as from peripheral sensitization and impaired muscle function due to the previously established mitochondrial dysfunction. In other words, inflammation induced by microbial debris promotes sensitization to pain.**

- The *existence* of central sensitization in fibromyalgia—real and generally accepted: Central sensitization—the increased perception of "pain" from otherwise nonpainful stimuli—is a well-accepted component of fibromyalgia; in fact, some authors and medical societies have claimed that sensitization of the brain and spinal cord is indeed the sole cause of fibromyalgia. The emphasis on *central* is to specify that the sensitization is localized in the *central* nervous system (comprised only of the brain and spinal cord) and not in the *peripheral* nervous system—the peripheral nerves (e.g., in the arms and legs) nor in their receptors (e.g., in skin, muscles, and other tissues). Again, the consensus is that central sensitization is present in fibromyalgia, that these patients have heightened sensitivity to pain and the perception of pain from stimuli that would not otherwise be painful to "normal" persons whom do not have fibromyalgia.

- The *origin* of central sensitization—an issue of the highest importance in the treatment of fibromyalgia: What is needed in the conversation on central sensitization is not debating is *presence* but rather an understanding of its *cause*, or purported lack of cause. In medicine, when we say that a condition is "primary" we are saying that conceptually the condition has *no known cause*, that it is *idiopathic*, that the primary origin is *inherent* within the disease condition itself; to say that something is *primary* is to say that it itself is the origin of the disease process. In contrast, when we describe a

> **Dysbiosis—SIBO and LPS—alter brain function, neurotransmission, to promote pain, fatigue, depression**
>
> "Structural bacterial components such as **lipopolysaccharides** provide low-grade tonic stimulation of the innate immune system. Excessive stimulation due to bacterial **dysbiosis, small intestinal bacterial overgrowth**, or increased intestinal permeability may produce systemic and/or central nervous system inflammation."
>
> Galland L. *J Med Food.* 2014 Dec

condition or aspect of disease as *secondary*, we are saying that it is due to a preceding primary problem, that it follows some other event, that it is second in line in the disease process. Likewise, we can say that a problem that occurs *causally* (not simply *chronologically*) after a secondary problem is a tertiary problem, and so on. If two events happen at the same time but one event does not cause the other, then the events are *associated* (somehow related) or *concomitant* (occurring at the same time).

- Example—distinguishing *primary*, from *secondary*, from *tertiary*, from *associated*: If a person has an automobile or sporting accident (the *primary* event) and suffers a painful injury, we would say that the injury is *secondary* to trauma, and that any resulting psychological distress would be *secondary* to the pain and impairment from the injury, or *tertiary* to the primary trauma. If the psychological distress were due to the accident itself (e.g., distressing memories of what occurred), then the psychological distress would be *secondary* to experiencing the event of the accident itself, independent from or complicated by any pain or impairment. If the patient also had a skin disease that existed previously, we would say that the patient has a *concomitant* skin disease but that it is unrelated to the accident or the injury, unless perhaps the patient intentionally injured himself/herself as a result of the skin disease (for example in a suicide attempt or some other form of self-harm secondary to the primary illness).

In the conversation on central sensitization in fibromyalgia, the distinction between *primary* and *secondary* is of the highest importance. If we say that central sensitization in fibromyalgia is *primary*, we are saying that the problem originates in the brain and spinal cord, and that the appropriate treatments are therefore those that target the brain and spinal cord, such as pain-relieving drugs; other treatments might be useful, but they are of secondary importance to directly influencing the *primary* problem in the brain and spinal cord. For ethical and professional reasons, doctorate-level physicians are obligated to address the primary cause of disease whenever possible; this is a matter of acumen and beneficence because failing to address the primary cause of the problem when possible firstly allows the primary disease to fester and develop and progress while secondly leaving the patient dependent upon—enslaved to—symptom alleviation.

- o Example—distinguishing *professional* and *ethical* behavior (e.g., treating the primary problem) from *unprofessional/irresponsible/unethical* behavior (e.g., failing to treat the primary problem, promoting dependency and exposing the patient to excess risk and expense, etc) among physicians: If a patient sits on a nail but cannot see the nail and then reports to the physician's office with a complaint of pain, the physician is professionally obligated to assess the situation by providing treatment of the primary problem—in this case, by removing the nail. The cause of the pain is the embedded nail, removing the nail will shortly alleviate the pain (assuming no infection or other complication). But let's say that an unethical physician is paid by a drug company to sell analgesic drugs, and the physician neglects his/her professional responsibility and his/her ethical responsibility to the patient; this physician fails to address the primary problem (the painful nail) and instead prescribes a dangerous drug to partly alleviate the pain at a cost of $200 and the doctor also receives a cash "gift" of $50 from the drug company for having promoted the sale of the drug. Because the doctor failed to address the *primary* problem (the painful nail) and only addressed the *secondary* problem (the pain), the doctor has failed to provide professional and ethical care, and this is further complicated by the physician's nondisclosed conflict of interest and receipt of a cash reward for having ordered the patient to spend $200 on a drug that he/she did not need. What is worse, the patient might be injured from the drug, or might eventually develop and infection because of the ongoing nature of the embedded nail. The doctor has created dependency (e.g., return visits and fees for more prescriptions) and income (e.g., from office fees and from payments by the drug company) while failing to treat the primary cause of the patient's problem.

If we say that pain and central sensitization in fibromyalgia are *primary*—without identifiable cause—then we have to treat symptomatically by suppressing/targeting the pain itself; this is reasonable, but increasingly unlikely as science advances and we better understand the nature and causes of diseases. If we say that pain and central sensitization in fibromyalgia are *secondary*—caused by a primary problem—then we are professionally and ethically obligated to address the primary cause of the pain. If physicians and medical groups say that pain and central sensitization in fibromyalgia are *primary* when in fact the research has made clear the cause of and treatment for the pain, then these physicians and medical groups—possibly to advance their own importance in society and income from drug companies—are behaving unprofessionally and unethically and unscientifically by cheating their patients of the opportunity for cure and putting these patients at risk for complications from the primary disease, at risk for adverse drug effects including injury and death, and burdening patients and the healthcare system with the costs of thousands of dollars individually and billions of dollars collectively/systematically by frauding the nature of the illness and its treatment. There it is; that is the defining line between *ethical* and *professional* behavior and *unethical* and *unprofessional* behavior, whether by individual physicians affecting the lives of hundreds of patients or by medical organizations affecting millions of patients for billions of dollars. If fibromyalgia has a legitimate cause, then doctors have an obligation to treat the cause of the problem rather than profit by unnecessary clinical patronage (coerced by pain, made necessary by the "necessary" need for repeated assessments and prescription refills). Relatedly, medical organizations that fraud the practice of medicine by distributing false information and promoting inefficacious treatment protocols that culminate in nontreatment of the primary disorder, the unnecessary use of dangerous treatments that harm patients, and unnecessary expenses to healthcare systems in the billions of dollars would be culpable for same.

- <u>Describing central sensitization in fibromyalgia as "primary" is unscientific, magical thinking that promotes drug dependency, drug sales, and physician dependency</u>: This promulgation, based on the selective ignoring of a vast and readily integrated body of scientific body of information, harms patients and costs healthcare systems billions of dollars.
- <u>Describing central sensitization in fibromyalgia as "secondary" is scientific, logical thinking</u>: This affirmation, based on the integration of a large body of scientific information, benefits patients, empowers doctors, and saves healthcare systems billions of dollars.

Given that the existence of central sensitization in animal and human models of pain, and that its presence is reasonably well established in human patients with fibromyalgia, the main question(s) to address are ❶ What is the cause of the central sensitization?, ❷ How can the cause be effectively treated?, ❸ Only if no cause can be found are we then allowed to ask, "What treatments—natural or pharmaceutical—are appropriate for the direct treatment of central sensitization?" Anytime that doctors and policymakers are discussing treatments, we have to consider 1) cost, availability, distributive justice, 2) effectiveness, 3) cost-effectiveness ratio, 4) safety, contraindications, adverse effects, and 5) drug-drug and drug-nutrient interactions; in shorthand, we can think of the risk:benefit ratio as a summation of these considerations, wherein "risk" is everything negative and "benefit" is everything positive. Except perhaps in Emergency Medicine and Urgent Care, doctors for the most part are trained to ignore the cause of problems and to just prescribe the "appropriate" drug for each diagnosis[366]; this is why medical care for nonacute/chronic/persistent diseases is so abysmal—because doctors have been trained to turn off their investigative brains, to recite the *idiopathic dogma*[367] that "chronic diseases are a complex interplay genes and environment, and while we don't yet know the exact cause, we can give you medicines that will help", to focus on molecules rather than context and cause, and to basically just practice as MDs—medicine dispensers. Exacerbating the problem are the medical/science writers and the medical organizations (e.g., specialists organizations in pain, rheumatology, and general medicine) that are paid hundreds of thousands and millions of dollars, respectively, to selectively ignore *causal* data and emphasize the *drug-selling* data.

In the following sections, I will establish that ❶ central sensitization in fibromyalgia is caused by microbial debris and secondary metabolic and inflammatory effects, that ❷ rational treatment of microbe-induced pain and inflammation must focus on 1) the eradication/modulation of the inflammatory microbial load, 2) the restoration of barrier defenses (e.g., the defensive lining of the skin and the gut wall) to reduce absorption of and exposure to microbial molecules (enhancing elimination of already-absorbed microbial toxins is a possibility, but is of lesser importance and is mentioned in some of my other writings), and ❸ treatments to directly address the inflammatory pain and central sensitization.

---

[366] Ely JW, Osheroff JA, Ebell MH, et al. Analysis of questions asked by family doctors regarding patient care. *BMJ*. 1999 Aug 7;319(7206):358-61
[367] Vasquez A. Twilight of the Idiopathic Era and the Dawn of New Possibilities in Health and Healthcare. *Naturopathy Digest* 2006 Mar naturopathydigest.com/archives/2006/mar/idiopathic.php. See also: Ely et al. Analysis of questions asked by family doctors regarding patient care. *BMJ*. 1999 Aug:358-61

Central sensitization in fibromyalgia is caused by microbial debris and secondary metabolic and inflammatory effects: My main thesis is stated immediately above, that central sensitization in fibromyalgia is caused by microbial debris and the secondary metabolic and inflammatory effects. I think this is easily demonstrated in graphic form, and so I will use the following image and its caption do most of the explaining, then I will follow the caption with a bit more discussion before concluding this section with a few notes and comments on research.

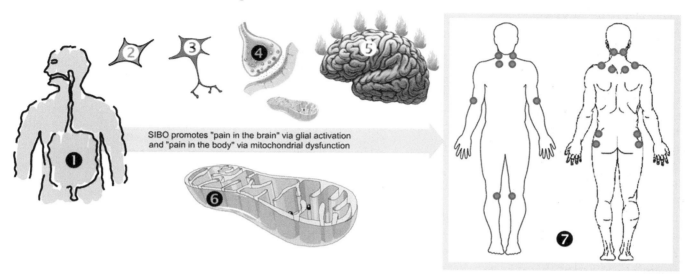

SIBO promotes "pain in the brain" via glial activation and "pain in the body" via mitochondrial dysfunction

SIBO promotes glial activation and mitochondrial impairment which are the major causes of fibromyalgia syndrome: *From gut to "brain pain"*: ❶ Small intestine bacterial overgrowth (SIBO) leads to intestinal absorption and systemic distribution of low levels of bacterial endotoxin (endotoxemia) and other ***inflamm**ation-**gen**erating* molecules (inflammogens); this results in low-grade inflammation (including release of cytokines, prostaglandins and other inflammatory mediators and oxidants).[368] Microbial inflammogens cause systemic inflammation, and cytokines and prostaglandins produced peripherally (ie, outside of the central nervous system [CNS], which is the brain and spinal cord) can readily traverse the blood-brain barrier (BBB) and enter the CNS to promote glial activation—brain inflammation.[369] Some of these microbial inflammogens may be able to bypass the BBB directly, when the BBB becomes permeable/leaky following induction of systemic inflammation. SIBO can also elaborate mitochondrial inhibitors such as endotoxin (lipopolysaccharide, LPS)[370], hydrogen sulfide (H2S)[371], and D-lactate.[372] In the brain, mitochondrial dysfunction exacerbates brain dysfunction and the vicious cycle of microglial activation.[373] ❷ Microglia are immune cells in the brain that respond to cytokines, prostaglandins, and microbial inflammogens; when microglia become stimulated or "activated" by inflammatory triggers/signals, the microglia signal/activate/irritate the nearby ❸ astrocytes, which are cells in the brain that respond by causing an increase in neuron-to-neuron communication (neurotransmission) via the neurotransmitter glutamate, which is stimulatory to neurons.[374] ❹ While glutamate is necessary in small and regulated amounts, higher levels of glutamate promote central sensitization, pain amplification, "brain fatigue", depression and anxiety; when very elevated, glutamate can promote migraine headaches, seizures and epilepsy.[375] ❺ High levels of glutamate cause excitation of brain neurons, and this increased activity leads to increased production of free radicals, which cause additional local inflammation and mitochondrial dysfunction within the brain, leading back to microglial activation for a vicious cycle. The brain is now in a "positive feedback loop" which promotes additional pain/fatigue/depression independently from ongoing stimulation from the original trigger. As you can see from this description, microglial activation causes astrocyte activation in a close relationship; since microglia—the brain's immune cells—and astrocytes—the brain's supportive or helper or "nurse" cells—are both categorized as glial cells (glia = glue = the mass of cells that creates the supporting structure for the neurons of the brain), you can see that *microglial activation* and *astrocyte activation* and *glial activation* are extensions of each other and can be used somewhat interchangeably. Excess or prolonged microglial activation promotes neurodegeneration via hyperexcitation of neurons, basically causing them to "burn out" in a process

[368] Patel et al. Human experimental endotoxemia in modeling pathophysiology, genomics, and therapeutics of innate immunity in complex cardiometabolic diseases. *Arterioscler Thromb Vasc Biol* 2015 Mar:525-34. Ferguson et al. Omega-3 PUFA supplementation response to endotoxemia in healthy volunteers. *Mol Nutr Food Res* 2014 Mar;601-13

[369] Wilson CJ, Finch CE, Cohen HJ. Cytokines and cognition--the case for a head-to-toe inflammatory paradigm. *J Am Geriatr Soc*. 2002 Dec;50(12):2041-56

[370] Scirocco et al. Exposure of Toll-like receptors 4 to bacterial lipopolysaccharide (LPS) impairs human colonic smooth muscle cell function. *J Cell Physiol*. 2010 May; 442-50

[371] Lemle MD. Hypothesis: chronic fatigue syndrome is caused by dysregulation of hydrogen sulfide metabolism. *Med Hypotheses*. 2009 Jan;72(1):108-9

[372] Sheedy et al. Increased d-lactic Acid intestinal bacteria in patients with chronic fatigue syndrome. *In Vivo*. 2009 Jul-Aug;23(4):621-8

[373] Nguyen et al. A new vicious cycle involving glutamate excitotoxicity, oxidative stress and mitochondrial dynamics. *Cell Death Dis*. 2011 Dec 8;2:e240

[374] Béchade C, Cantaut-Belarif Y, Bessis A. Microglial control of neuronal activity. *Front Cell Neurosci*. 2013 Mar 28;7:32

[375] Devinsky O, Vezzani A, Najjar S, De Lanerolle NC, Rogawski MA. Glia and epilepsy: excitability and inflammation. *Trends Neurosci*. 2013 Mar;36(3):174-84

that has been described as "brain on fire."[376] The exception to this occurs after a period of particularly protracted microglial activation, which can cause damage or "burn out" of the astrocytes, too; this "astrocyte degeneration" leads to neurodegeneration when the astrocytes become impaired and cannot perform their supportive and "nursing" functions to the neurons. ❺ *From gut to "body pain and fatigue"*: SIBO can also elaborate mitochondrial inhibitors such as endotoxin (lipopolysaccharide, LPS), hydrogen sulfide (H2S), and D-lactate, as previously stated and cited. In the body, mitochondrial dysfunction promotes pain and the vicious cycle of oxidative stress, nutritional depletion, and additional mitochondrial dysfunction. Mitochondrial dysfunction in muscle leads to the cellular/cytologic and histologic/tissue changes that are typical and well-documented in cell and muscle samples of patients with fibromyalgia.[377] These peripheral (e.g., non-brain) changes in muscle also prove beyond any doubt that fibromyalgia is not a "brain disease" or solely a "disorder of pain processing." ❻ **Thus, fibromyalgia can be easily explained/understood as SIBO-induced central sensitization and mitochondrial dysfunction, resulting in pain and fatigue**; all other abnormalities in FM can be traced back to these key problems. Image of brain by IsaacMao per Flickr.com via creativecommons.org/licenses/by/2.0. See educational videos and updates at www.inflammationmastery.com/pain

Central sensitization (enhanced and autonomous pain hypersensitivity) seen in FM can be caused by bacterial LPS: Somewhat independent from the immune/inflammation-mediated hyperalgesia induced by LPS is the hyperalgesia mediated by central nervous system responses. The central sensitization seen with fibromyalgia[378] might be explained as being caused by intestinally-derived bacterial toxins. **Bacterial LPS/endotoxin promotes central sensitization via (microglia-driven astrocyte-induced glutamate-mediated) activation of NMDA receptors and by inducing hyperalgesia (elevated pain perception) and anti-analgesia (reduced response to pain inhibition).**[379] Accumulated evidence suggests that fibromyalgia may be a disorder of somatic hypersensitivity induced by bacterial toxins derived from quantitative excess or qualitative abnormalities in gut bacteria.[380]

> **Exposure to the bacterial endotoxin lipopolysaccharide (LPS) causes increased sensitivity to painful stimuli (hyperalgesia) and a reduction in opioid analgesia (anti-analgesia)**
>
> "Intraperitoneal injection of toxins, such as the bacterial endotoxin lipopolysaccharide (LPS), is associated with a well-characterized increase in sensitivity to painful stimuli (hyperalgesia) and a longer-lasting reduction in opioid analgesia (anti-analgesia) when pain sensitivity returns to basal levels."
>
> Johnston et al. Inhibition of morphine analgesia by LPS. *Behav Brain Res* 2005 Jan

Gut dysbiosis—generally speaking—can promote syndromes of pain, fatigue and depression via systemic inflammation (triggered directly by microbial molecules), immune activation via increased intestinal permeability, and increased glutaminergic neurotransmission via glial activation—microglial activation followed by astrocyte activation. As the name implies, central sensitization describes a condition of heightened perception of / responsiveness to sensory stimuli, particularly pain. In an authoritative review by Woolf[381] in 2011, the following introduction provides both definition and description, "Nociceptor inputs can trigger a prolonged but reversible increase in the excitability and synaptic efficacy of neurons in central nociceptive pathways, the phenomenon of central sensitization. Central sensitization manifests as pain hypersensitivity, particularly dynamic tactile allodynia, secondary punctate or pressure hyperalgesia, aftersensations, and enhanced temporal summation." Woolf goes on to note that central sensitization (CS) can be elicited in humans by diverse experimental noxious stimuli to skin, muscles or viscera, and that CS "results in secondary changes in brain activity that can be detected by electrophysiological or imaging techniques." Clinical conditions in which CS plays a role include fibromyalgia, osteoarthritis, headache, temporomandibular joint disorders, chronic musculoskeletal pain, dental pain, neuropathic pain, visceral pain hypersensitivity disorders (such as irritable bowel syndrome, IBS), and post-surgical/traumatic pain. In essence, anything that causes pain (e.g., injury) or contributes to increased pain perception (e.g., sleep deprivation, magnesium deficiency, vitamin D deficiency) can contribute to central sensitization simply by virtue of neuronal plasticity, which makes repeatedly activated pathways—in this case the perception of and response to pain—become more permanent via synaptogenesis, e.g., pain chronification via activity/repetition-dependent synaptic plasticity. In experimental models, bacterial LPS has been shown to promote central sensitization via activation of microglial release of extracellular ATP which in turn triggers astrocytes to

---

[376] Cohen G. The brain on fire? *Ann Neurol.* 1994 Sep;36(3):333-4

[377] Cordero et al. Mitochondrial dysfunction and mitophagy activation in blood mononuclear cells of fibromyalgia patients: implications in the pathogenesis of the disease. *Arthritis Res Ther.* 2010;12(1):R17. Olsen NJ, Park JH. Skeletal muscle abnormalities in patients with fibromyalgia. *Am J Med Sci.* 1998 Jun;315(6):351-8

[378] Meeus et al. Central sensitization: biopsychosocial explanation for chronic widespread pain in patients with fibromyalgia and chronic fatigue syndrome. *Clin Rheumatol.* 2007 Apr;26(4):465-73

[379] Johnston IN, Westbrook RF. Inhibition of morphine analgesia by LPS: role of opioid and NMDA receptors and spinal glia. *Behav Brain Res.* 2005;156(1):75-83

[380] Othman M, Agüero R, Lin HC. Alterations in intestinal microbial flora and human disease. *Curr Opin Gastroenterol.* 2008 Jan;24(1):11-6

[381] Woolf CJ. Central sensitization: implications for the diagnosis and treatment of pain. *Pain.* 2011 Mar;152(3 Suppl):S2-15

promote glutaminergic neurotransmission, thereby increasing neurocortical hyperexcitability and promoting pain, depression, central fatigue, and migraine/seizure. As paraphrased here and noted in the diagram from Béchade et al[382], LPS stimulates microglia to externalize the DAMP extracellular ATP, recruiting astrocytes to release glutamate leading to increased excitatory transmission via a glutamate, the major excitatory neurotransmitter. Clinicians should appreciate that LPS is a prototype agonist but certainly not the only "environmental factor" capable of triggering hyperglutaminergic neurotransmission (excess glutamate activating the glutamate-sensitive NMDA receptors) or what might be called glutamate-mediated hypertransmission (normal levels of glutamate triggering a hypersensitive receptor, or a hypersensitive or "loaded" or "primed" intracellular cascade). The clinical correlates of this model are relevant for chronic pain, depression, central fatigue, neurodegeneration, post-traumatic pain, post-traumatic stress disorder (PTSD), epilepsy and migraine. LPS is one of many "noxious stimuli" that can trigger microglia activation for eventual hyperglutaminergic neurocortical hyperexcitability and excitotoxicity; other factors include trauma and inflammatory cytokines and prostaglandins. LPS, other microbial immunogens, and other inflammatory triggers need not originate in the gut, as many long-term/chronic "dysbiotic-like" infections are localized within the brain and central nervous system, such as HSV[383], *Chlamydia pneumoniae*[384], and "algal" chlorovirus ATCV-1[385]; neuropathologic infections, antigens and neurotoxins such as the aluminum used in vaccines/immunizations as an adjuvant can be trafficked from the periphery into the brain by the immune system.[386] This author's perspective is that gut-derived microbial signals do indeed evoke central sensitization, most likely via direct CNS entry (via a "leaky" blood-brain barrier; perhaps trafficked by immunocytes), but at the very least indirectly by peripheral immune activation and the systemic proinflammatory state characterized by increased production of cytokines and prostaglandins which readily cross the blood-brain barrier to produce microglial activation and the subsequent hyperexcitation, excitotoxicity, and sickness behavior—including fatigue, depression, sensitivity. Microglial activation promotes neuronal hyperexcitation/excitotoxicity, and the reverse is also true: neuronal (hyper)activity promotes microglial activation; thereby forming a vicious cycle. Additionally, factors such as heightened glutamate/NMDA receptor sensitivity, depleted antioxidant defenses and specific nutrient deficiencies (e.g., pyridoxine, magnesium, zinc, vitamin D, n3 fatty acids), mitochondrial impairment, and an pro-inflammatory microenvironment combine additively/synergistically to promote the progressively accelerated pace of reciprocal microglial activation and neuronal hyperexcitation/excitotoxicity noted in several neurodegenerative states. This could be complicated by gut *Clostridia* production of 3-3-hydroxyphenyl-3-hydroxypropionic acid (HPHPA) and p-cresol causing neurotransmitter imbalance—elevated dopamine and reduced norepinephrine.

Defining and describing what is meant by "brain inflammation" relative to central sensitization in pain syndromes: Encephalitis (*enceph*—brain, *itis*—inflammation) classically refers to acute brain inflammation resultant from brain infection, such as a viral infection, e.g., herpes encephalitis. However, we now appreciate more subtle forms of chronic/persistent brain inflammation—metabolic-immunologic inflammation—in neurologic and psychiatric conditions such as chronic pain, autism, Parkinson's and Alzheimer's DZs, as well as chronic depression and schizophrenia. As such, we can reasonably expand the use of the term *encephalitis* beyond the acute and infectious to include the chronic and metabolic, ie

---

Glial activation = brain inflammation = promotion of central sensitization = pain hypersensitivity and other manifestations of sickness behavior

Typical manifestations of brain inflammation and sickness behavior include:
- Reduced physical activity, inertia
- Reduced food intake
- Reduced social interaction
- Reduced sexual behavior
- Reduced mood, depression
- Impaired memory
- Heightened sensitivity to pain

Maier SF, Watkins LR. Consequences of the Inflamed Brain. *Report on Progress 2012, University of Colorado at Boulder. Dana Alliance* 2012 Aug

---

[382] Béchade C, Cantaut-Belarif Y, Bessis A. Microglial control of neuronal activity. *Front Cell Neurosci.* 2013 Mar 28;7:32

[383] Ball et al. Intracerebral propagation of Alzheimer's disease: strengthening evidence of a herpes simplex virus etiology. *Alzheimers Dement.* 2013 Mar;9(2):169-75

[384] Hammond et al. Immunohistological detection of Chlamydia pneumoniae in the Alzheimer's disease brain. *BMC Neurosci.* 2010 Sep 23;11:121

[385] Yolken et al. Chlorovirus ATCV-1 is part human oropharyngeal virome associated changes in cognitive functions in humans and mice. *Proc Natl Acad Sci* 2014 Nov:16106-11

[386] "We previously showed that poorly biodegradable aluminum-coated particles injected into muscle are promptly phagocytosed in muscle and the draining lymph nodes, and can disseminate within phagocytic cells throughout the body and slowly accumulate in brain." Gherardi et al. Biopersistence and brain translocation of aluminum adjuvants of vaccines. *Front Neurol* 2015 Feb;6:4. See also: "Detection of Al(III) in tissues indicated presence of aluminum in the nervous tissue of experimental animals." Luján et al. Autoimmune/autoinflammatory syndrome induced by adjuvants (ASIA syndrome) in commercial sheep. *Immunol Res* 2013 Jul:317-24

chronic/persistent metabolic-immunologic brain inflammation. Not all brain inflammation leads to central sensitization, but all central sensitization has a (neuro)inflammatory component. If we say "central sensitization", then we are a bit lost, because we are describing too many things at once (e.g., pain, emotions, MRI changes, early experiences, neurotransmitters...); as such, overuse of the term central sensitization can lead us astray or leave us unclear and therefore easily manipulated. If we say "brain inflammation" then we can reasonably appreciate a process that is: 1) causal—only so many things cause brain inflammation, so we can organize a plan of discovery and treatment, and 2) limited—we appreciate that most inflammatory disorders and responses should resolve. Any inflammatory trigger will be expected to trigger brain inflammation; while insults to the brain are obvious, peripheral cytokines and immunocytes can cross the blood brain barrier (BBB) to trigger inflammation in the brain, even when the problem started in the periphery. If you know that "the brain has an immune system", and that when the brain's immune system triggers inflammation—whether via central/brain insult or peripheral/body inflammation—that the result is neuroinflammation, pain, depression, and expedited neurodegeneration, then you can appreciate the intermixing of systemic inflammation with brain inflammation, with microglial activation and the resultant changes in neurotransmission that lead to pain sensitivity and changes in mood/affect called "sickness behavior." In this work, I show that fibromyalgia is a unique combination of dysbiosis-induced glial activation and mitochondrial impairment; both of these components need to be treated effectively and at the same time in order to alleviate the brain inflammation—unique—in fibromyalgia. "Glial activation with mitochondrial impairment" is different from and worse than glial activation or mitochondrial impairment by itself; the combination of the two together exacerbates both while also causing a vicious cycle that promotes ongoing pain, fatigue, and emotional/psychiatric changes.

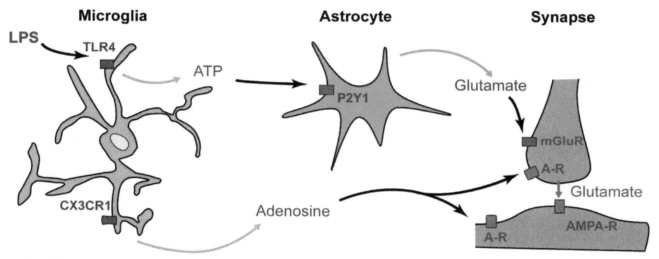

Microglial LPS reception leads to (extracellular) ATP elaboration, which stimulates astrocytes to produce glutamate, which increases glutaminergic neurotransmission: "Upon LPS stimulation, microglia rapidly produce ATP, which recruits astrocytes. Astrocytes subsequently release glutamate, and this leads to increased excitatory transmission via a metabotropic glutamate receptor-dependent mechanism." Illustration and quote from: Béchade C, Cantaut-Belarif Y, Bessis A. Microglial control of neuronal activity. *Front Cell Neurosci*. 2013 Mar 28;7:32[387]

Verified in animal models and likely contributory to clinical pain syndromes such as fibromyalgia is the observation that bacterial endotoxin/LPS can also contribute to central sensitization. This concept is introduced here and will be further substantiated in a following section on clinical pain syndromes and more so in separate writings, whether specific to fibromyalgia[388] or general to rheumatology.[389] The basic pathophysiology is quite simple and linear, as depicted below and itemized with citations thereafter.

Bacterial LPS ➔ microglial activation ➔ astrocyte hyperglutaminogenesis ➔ neurocortical hyperexcitation ➔ pain

[387] Béchade C, Cantaut-Belarif Y, Bessis A. Microglial control of neuronal activity. *Front Cell Neurosci*. 2013 Mar 28;7:32 doi: 10.3389/fncel.2013.00032 journal.frontiersin.org/article/10.3389/fncel.2013.00032/abstract. Copyright © 2013 Béchade, Cantaut-Belarif and Bessis. *Front Cell Neurosci* is an open-access journal distributed under terms of Creative Commons Attribution License, which permits use/distribution/reproduction in other forums, provided original authors/source are credited.
[388] Vasquez A. *Fibromyalgia in a Nutshell: A Safe and Effective Functional Medicine Strategy*. 2012, and later versions.
[389] Vasquez A. *Functional Medicine Rheumatology v3.5*. 2014, and later versions.

However, the correlation of serum LPS (or its indirect marker, anti-LPS antibodies) with increased intestinal permeability provides another interpretation, wherein serum LPS activity is simply a correlate with increased IP which promotes pain via nonspecific and non-LPS mechanisms, as shown in the following sequence:

SIBO/LPS-induced mucosal damage ➔ absorption of gut-derived immunogens and toxins ➔ microglial activation ➔ astrocyte-mediated hyperglutaminogenesis ➔
neurocortical hyperexcitation ➔ pain/depression/fatigue and associated low-grade immune activation

- Endotoxemia induces visceral hypersensitivity and altered pain evaluation in healthy humans (*Pain.* 2012 Apr[390]): "...transient systemic immune activation results in decreased visceral sensory and pain thresholds and altered subjective pain ratings."
- LPS-induced hyperalgesia in healthy humans (*Brain Behav Immun* 2014 Oct[391]): "Our results revealed widespread increases in musculoskeletal pain sensitivity in response to a moderate dose of LPS (0.8 ng/kg), which correlate both with changes in IL-6 and negative mood."
- Widespread hyperalgesia in adolescents with symptoms of irritable bowel syndrome (*J Pain.* 2014 Sep[392]): "We examined pain sensitivity in 961 adolescents from the general population (mean age 16.1 years), including pain threshold and tolerance measurements of heat (forearm) and pressure pain (fingernail and shoulder) and cold pressor tolerance (hand). ... Our results indicate that adolescents in the general population with IBS symptoms, like adults, have widespread hyperalgesia. ... Our results suggest that central pain sensitization mechanisms in IBS may contribute to triggering and maintaining chronic pain symptoms."

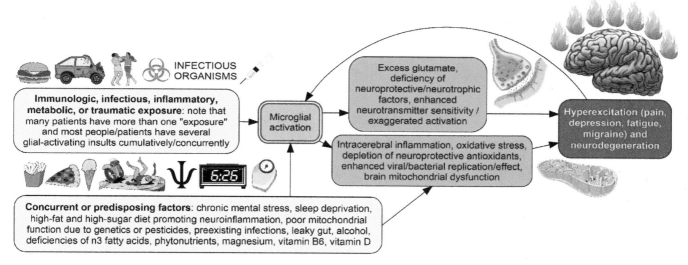

Numerous insults—immunologic, inflammatory, infectious, metabolic, traumatic, toxins—can "team up" or act individually to incite glial activation: Very importantly, glial activation can remain in an activated state promoting neurotransmitter imbalance, hyperexcitation, and neurodegeneration for several years after a single biochemical, infectious, or physical assault. High-fat foods, physical trauma from sports and accidents, psychological and mental stress, sleep deprivation, and the metabolic stress of hyperglycemia, insulin resistance, and obesity all contribute to brain inflammation—also called "the brain on fire" per Cohen, *Annals of Neurology* 1994—to promote pain, depression, migraine/seizure, and neurodegeneration. Images and descriptions above © 2015-2015 by Dr Vasquez except for image of brain by IsaacMao per Flickr.com via creativecommons.org/licenses/by/2.0. See educational videos and updates at www.inflammationmastery.com/pain

Proof of accelerated neurodegeneration in fibromyalgia: The model I have presented—dysbiosis-induced glial activation and mitochondrial dysfunction leading to both pain sensitivity and accelerated neurodegeneration—is supported by research showing accelerated brain aging and loss of gray matter (neuron cell bodies) in patients with fibromyalgia. As such, I consider my model of fibromyalgia to be very complete and consistent.

[390] Benson et al. Acute experimental endotoxemia induces visceral hypersensitivity and altered pain evaluation in healthy humans. *Pain.* 2012 Apr;153(4):794-9
[391] Wegner et al. Inflammation-induced hyperalgesia: timing, dosage, and negative affect on somatic pain in human endotoxemia. *Brain Behav Immun.* 2014 Oct;41:46-54
[392] Stabell et al. Widespread hyperalgesia in adolescents with symptoms of irritable bowel syndrome: results from a large population-based study. *J Pain.* 2014 Sep;15(9):898-906

- Accelerated brain gray matter loss and premature aging of the brain in fibromyalgia patients (*J Neurosci* 2007 Apr[393]): "In this study, we investigate anatomical changes in the brain associated with fibromyalgia. Using voxel-based morphometric analysis of magnetic resonance brain images, we examined the brains of 10 female fibromyalgia patients and 10 healthy controls. We found that fibromyalgia patients had significantly less total gray matter volume and showed a 3.3 times greater age-associated decrease in gray matter than healthy controls. The longer the individuals had had fibromyalgia, the greater the gray matter loss, with each year of fibromyalgia being equivalent to 9.5 times the loss in normal aging. In addition, fibromyalgia patients demonstrated significantly less gray matter density than healthy controls in several brain regions, including the cingulate, insular and medial frontal cortices, and parahippocampal gyri. The neuroanatomical changes that we see in fibromyalgia patients contribute additional evidence of CNS involvement in fibromyalgia. In particular, fibromyalgia appears to be associated with an acceleration of age-related changes in the very substance of the brain."

Additional comments and perspectives on central sensitization—integrating the model of SIBO-induced central sensitization via glial activation and other mechanisms

We appreciate that FM contains the aspect of central sensitization and the associated pain amplification; our intellectual task is to understand the most likely origin or—alternatively—to ascribe the central sensitization

> **Follow the pathophysiologic trail from bacterial exposures to IL-8 to brain inflammation and central sensitization**
>
> Various microbial exposures are known to cause elevations in IL-8, elevated CSF levels of which are characteristic of and perhaps unique to fibromyalgia, a condition causatively associated with intestinal bacterial overgrowth. The best summation of data at this point reads that the brain inflammation of fibromyalgia pain is triggered by microbial exposure. The alternate hypothesis that all of these pathophysiologic characteristics are unrelated is illogical and subintellectually immeritous.

to a magical/idiopathic origination. My contention is that microbial exposure leads to pain amplification via central sensitization in fibromyalgia; the means by which this can occur are both direct/primary causality and indirect/secondary, etc. Most of these were summarized in the above image and caption; in the sections that follow I will review some additional and also new information and show how it further supports this model.

- Systemic inflammation causes suppression of brain noradrenergic signaling (experimental study; *Science* 1983 Aug[394]) and is likely to contribute to fatigue, depression, pain sensitivity, and a heightened stress response: This experimental study shows that systemic inflammation leads to reduction in norepinephrine signaling in the (rat) brain. This would be expected to lead to fatigue, depression, and pain sensitivity. Secondarily, lack of adrenergic stimulation of the central alpha-2 receptor would be expected to stimulate the sympathetic nervous system; we note that bacterial overgrowth of the intestines (SIBO) causes enhanced sympathetic activity that is noted in patients with IBS which is closely related to fibromyalgia.[395] Low-grade systemic inflammation is known to be a component of FM, and generally speaking the molecules in or near the human body that are most likely to trigger inflammation are of microbial origin. Patients with IBS and FM are both known to have small intestine bacterial overgrowth. **In sum, we can reasonably opine that SIBO in FM and IBS leads to low-grade inflammation which leads to suppression of brain noradrenergic signaling, leading directly to fatigue and depression while likely also contributing to a heightened stress/sympathetic response; all of these components are noted in patients with IBS/FM.**
- FM patients have elevated CSF levels of IL-8 (*J Neuroimmunol* 2012 Jan[396] and *J Neuroimmunol* 2015 Mar[397]): Kadetoff et al did good work in 2012 when they were the first to find that patients with FM showed elevated levels of the inflammatory cytokine IL-8 in the cerebrospinal fluid (CSF) of patients with FM; research suggests that IL-8 promotes central sensitization via brain inflammation, and again this is consistent with FM. Although these authors note that "The release of pro-inflammatory cytokines/chemokines (including IL-8), by glia cells

---

[393] Kuchinad et a. Accelerated brain gray matter loss in fibromyalgia patients: premature aging of the brain? *J Neurosci.* (2007 Apr 11;27(15):4004-7

[394] "We report here that the immune response elicits a decrease in NA synthesis in the hypothalamus and that soluble products of activated immunological cells induce a decrease in NA content in the hypothalamus." Besedovsky et al. The immune response evokes changes in brain noradrenergic neurons. *Science.* 1983 Aug 5;221(4610):564-6

[395] Lin HC. Small intestinal bacterial overgrowth: a framework for understanding irritable bowel syndrome. *JAMA.* 2004 Aug 18;292(7):852-8

[396] "To our knowledge, this is the first study assessing intrathecal concentrations of pro-inflammatory substances in fibromyalgia. We report elevated cerebrospinal fluid and serum concentrations of interleukin-8, but not interleukin-1beta, in FM patients." Kadetoff D, Lampa J, Westman M, Andersson M, Kosek E. Evidence of central inflammation in fibromyalgia-increased cerebrospinal fluid interleukin-8 levels. *J Neuroimmunol.* 2012 Jan;242:33-8

[397] Kosek E, Altawil R, Kadetoff D, et al. Evidence of different mediators of central inflammation in dysfunctional and inflammatory pain--interleukin-8 in fibromyalgia and interleukin-1 β in rheumatoid arthritis. *J Neuroimmunol.* 2015 Mar 15;280:49-55

can be triggered by stress, immune activation and afferent nociceptive input [pain]", they ultimately pin the blame on pain by concluding in their abstract that their findings are "in accordance with FM symptoms being mediated by sympathetic activity...and supports the hypothesis of glia cell activation in response to pain mechanisms." The error these authors make is when they prematurely and without citation ascribe the elevation of IL-8 to pain and sympathetic activation in FM. The authors are thereby stating in essence that pain causes stress which causes more pain; they completely failed to both 1) substantiate this claim, and/or to 2) consider alternate hypotheses. Their attribution of the sympathetic activation to pain appears premature at best; they provide no substantiation for this claim, and it appears to have been promulgated and accepted simply because it is convenient and in accord with the prevailing drug-funded model of fibromyalgia which states that, in fibromyalgia, pain/stress causes pain/stress via a vicious cycle of glial activation (central sensitization, brain inflammation). In 2015, this same team of researchers replicated their 2012 finding of elevated IL-8 in FM; however they exacerbated their error of attribution by stating that their findings are—citing the work of Clauw—"in line with the proposal to regard FM as a sympathetically mediated pain syndrome." I believe that these authors are inappropriately connecting their finding of elevated IL-8 in FM with elevated sympathetic activity and pain in FM, and then concluding conveniently and hastily that these are the only variables worth considering and that therefore these must cause each other; they give zero consideration to the fact that these FM patients have SIBO[398] and that microbial molecules and intestinal inflammation can cause elevations in IL-8. So while we can reasonably accept that IL-8 is elevated in FM and may contribute to pain sensitization via brain inflammation and central sensitization, ascribing the elevation of IL-8 to the same pain that it promotes is circular thinking which in this case is also faulty thinking without consideration and exclusion of the obvious microbial overload noted in these patients with FM. Their citation to Clauw is particularly questionable since Clauw has been heavily funded by drug companies and consistently cheerleads the idea that FM is a primary disorder of the brain that needs—in accord with his sources of funding—perpetual drug treatment.[399] While stress and pain may lead to elevations in IL-8, an inflammatory cytokine that appears to promote central pain sensitization, stress and pain alone are less likely to be the primary contributors to the central sensitization in FM than are microbial and mitochondrial contributors, especially in combination. If stress and pain were sufficient to cause central sensitization, then virtually all medical students/residents (and working single mothers, persons living in war zones, persons living in prison and in conditions of gross social inequality, etc) and all competitive athletes would have central sensitization and FM; thus the general lack of population-wide correlation argues against the stress/pain model of *IL-8 induced central sensitization* in FM. Furthermore and even more clearly, the stress/pain model of pain sensitization in FM absolutely fails to account for the mitochondrial and other molecular abnormalities. In contrast, SIBO and microbial exposure is the perfect explanation of/for central sensitization in FM.

- <u>Elevations in IL-8 can be triggered by various bacterial exposures</u>: In an experimental cell culture model, exposure to the Gram-negative bacterium *Pseudomonas aeruginosa* was shown to increase production of IL-8.[400] Similarly, exposure to protein from the Gram-negative bacterium *Streptococcus pyogenes* also triggered expression of IL-8.[401]

- <u>Elevations in IL-8 correlate with gastrointestinal infection with *Blastocystis* in patients with IBS, known to be correlated with FM</u> (*PLoS One* 2015 Sep[402]): "Among 109 (IBS n = 35 and non-IBS n = 74) adults, direct stool

---

[398] Pimentel et al. A link between irritable bowel syndrome and fibromyalgia may be related to findings on lactulose breath testing. *Ann Rheum Dis.* 2004 Apr;63(4):450-2

[399] American Pain Society. Fibromyalgia Has Central Nervous System Origins. May 16, 2015. americanpainsociety.org/about-us/press-room/fibromyalgia-clauw and "Dr Clauw has received grants/research support from Pfizer and Forest Laboratories. He is a consultant and a member of the advisory boards for Pfizer, Eli Lilly and Company, Forest Laboratories, Cypress Biosciences, Pierre Fabre Pharmaceuticals, UCB, and AstraZeneca. Dr Arnold has received grants/research support from Eli Lilly and Company, Pfizer, Cypress Biosciences, Wyeth Pharmaceuticals, Boehringer Ingelheim, Allergan, and Forest Laboratories. She is a consultant for Eli Lilly and Company, Pfizer, Cypress Biosciences, Wyeth Pharmaceuticals, Boehringer Ingelheim, Forest Laboratories, Allergan, Takeda, UCB, Theravance, AstraZeneca, and sanofi-aventis. Dr McCarberg has received honoraria from Cephalon, Eli Lilly and Company, Endo Pharmaceuticals, Forest Laboratories, Merck & Co, Pfizer, and Purdue Pharma. The FibroCollaborative group was sponsored by Pfizer." "Editorial support was provided by Gayle Scott, PharmD, of UBC Scientific Solutions and funded by Pfizer." Clauw DJ, Arnold LM, McCarberg BH; FibroCollaborative. The science of fibromyalgia. *Mayo Clin Proc.* 2011 Sep;86(9):907-11

[400] "Thus, IL-8 mRNA expression was prolonged after P. aeruginosa stimulation in CF epithelial cells, and this sustained IL-8 expression may contribute to the excessive inflammatory response in CF." Joseph T, Look D, Ferkol T. NF-kappaB activation and sustained IL-8 gene expression in primary cultures of cystic fibrosis airway epithelial cells stimulated with Pseudomonas aeruginosa. *Am J Physiol Lung Cell Mol Physiol.* 2005 Mar;288(3):L471-9

[401] "Our results showed that following exposure to SPE B or G308S, the levels of IL-8 protein and mRNA were increased and the increase was inhibited by the addition of anti-Fas antibody, suggesting that the increased production of IL-8 by SPE B is mediated through Fas receptor." Chang CW, Wu SY, Chuang WJ, Lin YS, Wu JJ, Liu CC, Tsai PJ, Lin MT. The IL-8 production by Streptococcal pyrogenic exotoxin B. *Exp Biol Med* (Maywood). 2009 Nov;234(11):1316-26

[402] Ragavan et al. Blastocystis sp. in Irritable Bowel Syndrome (IBS) - Detection in Stool Aspirates during Colonoscopy. *PLoS One.* 2015 Sep 16;10(9):e0121173

examination and culture of colonic aspirates were initially negative for *Blastocystis*. However, PCR analysis detected *Blastocystis* in 6 (17%) IBS and 4 (5.5%) non-IBS patients. In the six positive IBS patients by PCR method, subtype 3 was shown to be the most predominant (3/6: 50%) followed by subtype 4 (2/6; 33.3%) and subtype 5 (1/6; 16.6%). IL-8 levels were significantly elevated in the IBS Blasto group and IBS group (p<0.05) compared to non-IBS and non-IBS Blasto group. … Meanwhile, the IL-5 levels were significantly higher in IBS Blasto group (p<0.05) compared to non-IBS and non-IBS Blasto group. This study implicates that detecting Blastocystis by PCR method using colonic aspirate samples during colonoscopy, suggests that this may be a better method for sample collection due to the parasite's irregular shedding in Blastocystis-infected stools. Patients with IBS infected with parasite showed an increase in the interleukin levels demonstrate that *Blastocystis* does have an effect in the immune system." Additionally, *Blastocystis* is known to cause intestinal damage and to thereby increase intestinal permeability[403], and fibromyalgia patients are also noted to have increased intestinal permeability[404]; the possibility exists that *Blastocystis* induces increased IL-8 via intestinal mucosal damage which leads to increased absorption of microbial debris/inflammogens rather than directly, although an additive and synergistic mechanism/effect is more likely.

- Elevations in IL-8 are seen in patients with IBS, known to be triggered by SIBO and causatively dose-dependently correlated with FM (*Am J Gastroenterol.* 2010 Oct[405]): If my model is correct that the elevated IL-8 in FM is caused by the SIBO and not by the FM itself, then we should see elevated in IL-8 in patients with IBS, which is caused by SIBO. In a study with more than 120 human subjects, results showed that patients with IBS/SIBO have increased plasma levels of IL-6 and IL-8. Note that this study used blood/plasma/serum testing rather than cerebrospinal fluid (CSF) as in the previously reviewed studies; IL-8 levels in blood and CSF tend to correlate, as demonstrated in FM patients who typically have elevations in both locations (ie, peripherally and centrally).

- Bacterial overgrowth in ulcerative colitis patients correlates with increased inflammatory mediator production, including IL-8 (*J Crohns Colitis.* 2014 Aug[406]): Among patients with ulcerative colitis, SIBO is common and correlates with reduced intestinal motility and increased production of inflammatory mediators: "observed that there was a significant correlation between SIBO with IL-6, IL-8, TNF-α, and IL-10, LPO and GSH."

- Small intestinal bacterial overgrowth association with TLR4 expression and IL-8 (*Dig Dis Sci.* 2011 May[407]): SIBO was more common in nonalcoholic steatohepatitis (NASH) patients than control subjects (77% v 31.25%) and only IL-8 levels were significantly higher in patients than control and correlated positively with TLR-4 expression. "NASH patients have a higher prevalence of small intestinal bacterial overgrowth which is associated with enhanced expression of TLR-4 and release of IL-8. SIBO may have an important role in NASH through interactions with TLR-4 and induction of the pro-inflammatory cytokine, IL-8."

Microbe-induced brain inflammation without brain infection and without high fever, vasculitis or autoimmunity
Viral infections
• Measles
• Mumps
• Rubella
• Influenza A and B
• Herpes simplex
• Epstein-Barr virus
• Varicella
• Vaccinia
Bacterial infections
• Mycoplasma pneumoniae
• Chlamydia
• Legionella
• Streptococcus
• Campylobacter
• Shigella
Immunizations*
• Rabies
• DPT—Diphtheria, pertussis tetanus
• Smallpox
• Measles
• Japanese B encephalitis
• Influenza

*Of important note, vaccinations commonly contain numerous adjuvants, toxic metals such as mercury and aluminum, highly allergenic antibiotics and cell culture components including egg, aborted human cells, and monkey kidney cells; as such, the inflammatory encephalitis that results cannot be ascribed solely to the microbial component of the vaccination.

cdc.gov/vaccines/pubs/pinkbook/ downloads/appendices/B/ excipient-table-2.pdf
Accessed 2015 Nov

---

[403] "The IP was found to have increased in patients with protozoan infections compared with control patients (7.20+/-5.52 vs. 4.47+/-0.65%, P=0.0017). The IP values were 9.91+/- 10.05% in Giardia intestinalis group, 6.81+/-2.25% in Blastocystis hominis group, 5.78+/-2.84% in Entamoeba coli group. In comparison with the control group, the IP was significantly higher in G. intestinalis and B. hominis patients (P=0.0025, P=0.00037, respectively), but not in E. coli patients. In conclusion, the IP increases in patients with G. intestinalis and B. hominis but not with E. coli infection. This finding supports the view that IP increases during the course of protozoan infections which cause damage to the intestinal wall while non-pathogenic protozoan infections have no effect on IP. The increase in IP in patients with B. hominis brings forth the idea that B. hominis can be a pathogenic protozoan." Dagci H, Ustun S, Taner MS, Ersoz G, Karacasu F, Budak S. Protozoon infections and intestinal permeability. *Acta Trop.* 2002 Jan;81(1):1-5
[404] Goebel et al. Altered intestinal permeability in patients with primary fibromyalgia and in patients with complex regional pain syndrome. *Rheumatology* 2008 Aug;47(8):1223-7
[405] Scully et al. Plasma cytokine profiles in females with irritable bowel syndrome and extra-intestinal co-morbidity. *Am J Gastroenterol.* 2010 Oct;105(10):2235-43
[406] Rana et al. Relationship of cytokines, oxidative stress and GI motility with bacterial overgrowth in ulcerative colitis patients. *J Crohns Colitis.* 2014 Aug;8(8):859-65
[407] Shanab et al. Small intestinal bacterial overgrowth in nonalcoholic steatohepatitis: toll-like receptor 4 and plasma levels of interleukin 8. *Dig Dis Sci.* 2011 May;1524-34

Stress/pain is an insufficient explanation for the origination of FM: While stress and pain may lead to elevations in IL-8, an inflammatory cytokine that appears to promote central pain sensitization, stress and pain alone are less likely to be the primary contributors to the central sensitization in FM than are microbial and mitochondrial contributors, especially in combination. If stress and pain were sufficient to cause central sensitization, then virtually all medical students/residents (and working single mothers, persons living in war zones, etc) and all competitive athletes would have central sensitization and FM; thus the general lack of population-wide correlation argues against the stress/pain model of IL8-induction of central sensitization in FM. Furthermore and even more clearly, the stress/pain model of pain sensitization in FM absolutely fails to account for the mitochondrial and other molecular abnormalities. In contrast, **SIBO and microbial exposure is the perfect explanation of/for FM.**

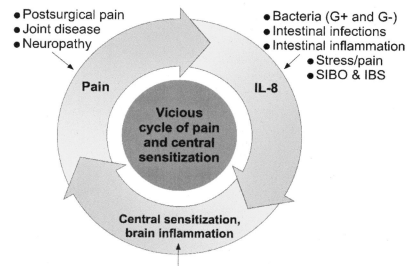

- Postsurgical pain
- Joint disease
- Neuropathy

- Bacteria (G+ and G-)
- Intestinal infections
- Intestinal inflammation
  - Stress/pain
  - SIBO & IBS

Pain — IL-8

Vicious cycle of pain and central sensitization

Central sensitization, brain inflammation

- Microbial inflammogens and systemic inflammation
- Deficiencies of anti-inflammatory nutrients, such as vitamin D, n3FA and phytochemicals
- Mitochondrial dysfunction, per migraine (primary) and fibromyalgia (secondary)

In sum, the data clearly show that microbial exposure in general and bacterial overgrowth of the small intestine in particular trigger increased IL-8 production. While elevated IL-8 is not specific to a particular disease per se, it is consistently elevated in patients with small intestine bacterial overgrowth, regardless of disease association. Many conditions causatively related to SIBO are noted to have elevated IL-8 levels, and we should reasonably attribute the elevated IL-8 levels in fibromyalgia to bacterial exposure, especially given the exceptionally high and dose-dependent correlation of SIBO with FM. IL-8 promotes pain sensitization, and the hyperalgesic effects of IL-8 are mediated in part by activation of beta-adrenergic receptors[408], chronic/sustained activation of which would be expected to promote depression, anxiety, and fatigue in addition to pain. IL-8 promotes activation of the sympathetic nervous system via beta-adrenergic receptors, and activation of the sympathetic nervous system via beta-adrenergic receptors feeds back to cause additional IL-8 production, thereby promoting a vicious cycle; my contention is that microbial debris is the initiating factor in this cycle, and that exposure to microbial inflammogens from SIBO is both more powerful (microbial debris is clearly pro-inflammatory, and LPS in particular is the most potent inflammogen known to science) and more durable (24/7 for months and years) than any "stress response." As such, the microbial inflammatory load is the more reasonable recipient of the burden of physiologic guilt than is the "stress level" of these patients. Stress is transient, and highly stressed people (e.g., medical students and residents, air traffic controllers, etc) do not show an undue burden of pain and mitochondrial impairment as do patients with an excessive total microbial load, specifically—as previously shown per literature review—SIBO. Thus having established that SIBO is sufficient to induce brain inflammation, I will now review more severe cases of what might be considered true gastrointestinal infection as a cause of severe brain inflammation; I am moving from the *mild and functional* to the truly *infectious and pathologic* to further exemplify this model.

- Gastrointestinal infection/dysbiosis as a cause of severe brain inflammation: criteria and review: We might reasonably expect that if *comparatively/relatively mild* cases of dysbiosis and SIBO can cause *mild* brain inflammation, then cases may have been reported wherein *more severe* gastrointestinal infections have led to *more severe* brain inflammation (ie, encephalitis and encephalomyelitis), and indeed such cases are impressively

---

408 Kosek E, Altawil R, Kadetoff D, et al. Evidence of different mediators of central inflammation in dysfunctional and inflammatory pain--interleukin-8 in fibromyalgia and interleukin-1 β in rheumatoid arthritis. *J Neuroimmunol*. 2015 Mar 15;280:49-55. Kadetoff D, Lampa J, Westman M, Andersson M, Kosek E. Evidence of central inflammation in fibromyalgia-increased cerebrospinal fluid interleukin-8 levels. *J Neuroimmunol*. 2012 Jan;242:33-8

abundant. The most important distinction is that of what is being discussed here, specifically brain inflammation induced by gastrointestinal-specific microbes, their inflammatory debris, and the resulting inflammatory response within the brain, *versus* an infection that originated in the gut and then spread to the brain, or an infection that induced sepsis and systemic complications that resulted in altered cognition. Accordingly, viral infections which can easily penetrate the brain are selected against (e.g., essentially omitted) in this discussion; emphasis here is on *bacterial infections* with *no evidence of direct brain/meningeal infection* in *otherwise healthy people* resulting in severe brain inflammation via "indirect" inflammatory effects. Inflammatory bowel disease (IBD) is known to be causatively/contributively associated with gut dysbiosis; IBD patients can develop brain inflammation and brain/CNS antibody-mediated autoimmunity[409], apparently triggered by the gut dysbiosis, but such cases are excluded from the discussion below for the sake of clarity in establishing a more pure causative connection between gut dysbiosis and brain inflammation *mediated via cytokines* and *microglial activation* in *otherwise healthy people*. Likewise, cases of infection-induced encephalitis wherein high fever or vasculitis were present are likewise excluded. As I have discussed and presented recently in 2015[410], dysbiosis-induced disease is generally effected via multiple mechanisms, one of which is the inflammatory-cytokine response, which in this conversation would "spill from the periphery into the brain" to cause microglial activation and the resulting brain inflammation—encephalitis.

- o Acute disseminated encephalomyelitis (ADEM) secondary to transient gastroenteritis in an otherwise healthy adult (*Case Rep Neurol Med.* 2015 Jun[411]): "A 62-year-old man presented with encephalopathy and rapid neurological decline following a gastrointestinal illness. A brain MRI revealed extensive supratentorial white matter hyperintensities consistent with ADEM and thus he was started on high dose intravenous methylprednisolone. He underwent a brain biopsy showing widespread white matter inflammation secondary to demyelination. At discharge, his neurological exam had significantly improved with continued steroid treatment and four months later, he was able to perform his ADLs."

- o Acute disseminated encephalomyelitis with Campylobacter gastroenteritis (*J Neurol Neurosurg Psychiatry* 2004 May[412]): "We report a case of acute disseminated encephalomyelitis (ADEM) temporally associated with Campylobacter gastroenteritis in a previously fit man. ... Two days after admission (day 16 of illness), his family reported a change in his personality and he complained of slurring of speech, intermittent diplopia, and difficulty in walking. Examination revealed mild dysarthria, left sided facial weakness, mild left pyramidal limb weakness, and decreased sensation in the left leg. Tendon reflexes were brisk but plantar responses were flexor. His gait was ataxic. ... In the majority of cases, the condition develops after systemic viral infections most commonly measles, mumps, rubella, influenza A and B, herpes simplex, Epstein-Barr virus, varicella, and vaccinia. It has also been reported following bacterial infections with Mycoplasma pneumoniae, Chlamydia, Legionella, and Streptococcus, or following immunizations for rabies, diphtheria/tetanus/pertussis, smallpox, measles and Japanese B encephalitis."

- o Bickerstaff's brainstem encephalitis related to Campylobacter jejuni gastroenteritis (*J Clin Pathol.* 2007 Oct[413]): "Here we report a case of BBE following a gastrointestinal infection with Campylobacter jejuni. The patient presented with acute onset of confusion and ophthalmoplegia. The cerebrospinal fluid (CSF) showed lymphocytic pleocytosis and raised protein. This acute presentation was preceded by an episode of Campylobacter-related diarrhea as confirmed by high titers of Campylobacter-specific IgM antibodies."

- o Acute encephalopathy preceding Shigella infection (*Isr Med Assoc J.* 2001 May[414]): This is a case of a 3yo girl with encephalitis which preceded mild mucus diarrhea which lead to the discovery of *Shigella sonnei*. Thus, this case is doubly unique for 1) the fact that the encephalopathy *preceded* any gastrointestinal manifestations, and 2) the gastrointestinal manifestations were impressively *mild*.

[409] Yamamoto et al. Bickerstaff's brainstem encephalitis associated with ulcerative colitis. *BMJ Case Rep.* 2012 Sep 21;2012
[410] The presentations to which I make reference here are specifically video presentations 1-3 wherein I describe the molecular mechanisms of dysbiosis-induced disease in our CE/CME program hosted at http://www.nutritionandfunctionalmedicine.org/lms/ and derived from the printed monograph *Human Microbiome and Dysbiosis in Clinical Disease*. International College of Human Nutrition and Functional Medicine 2015
[411] Mahdi et al. A Case of Acute Disseminated Encephalomyelitis in a Middle-Aged Adult. *Case Rep Neurol Med.* 2015;2015:601706
[412] Orr et al. Acute disseminated encephalomyelitis temporally associated with Campylobacter gastroenteritis. *J Neurol Neurosurg Psychiatry.* 2004 May;75(5):792-3
[413] Hussain et al. Bickerstaff's brainstem encephalitis related to Campylobacter jejuni gastroenteritis. *J Clin Pathol.* 2007 Oct;60(10):1161-2
[414] Somech R, Leitner Y, Spirer Z. Acute encephalopathy preceding Shigella infection. *Isr Med Assoc J.* 2001 May;3(5):384-5

Means by which inflammatory cytokines in the periphery (body) can result in inflammation in the brain
1. Cytokines enter the brain where the blood–brain barrier (BBB) is weak or non-existent (i.e. circumventricular organs).
2. Cytokines are transported into the brain by selective uptake systems (transporters), thus bypassing BBB.
3. Cytokines may act directly or indirectly on peripheral nerves that can send afferent signals to the brain.
4. Cytokines can act on peripheral tissues, inducing the secretion of molecules whose ability to penetrate the brain is not limited by the barrier. A major target appears to be endothelial cells, which bear receptors for IL-1 and endotoxin.
5. Cytokines can be synthesized by immune cells that infiltrate the brain.
6. Cytokines and the resultant increased ROS production can also impair mitochondrial function; impaired mitochondrial function in the periphery/body drains antioxidants (such as glutathione) and nutritive substances (such as CoQ10, tocopherols, and lipoic acid) that are important for the maintenance of cellular function and homeodynamics. Thereby, peripheral inflammation and mitochondrial impairment becomes a "sink" for draining nutrients and protectants while also becoming a "faucet" for inflammatory mediators, molecular debris and alarm signals. Increased production of glutamate, QUIN, and NO- fuel NMDAr activation and mitochondrial dysfunction. (DrV)
7. Cytokines may be transported in a retrograde manner from the periphery, via axonal mechanisms.
8. Cytokines may be transported in a retrograde manner from the periphery, via axonal mechanisms. (Zhang, An)
Contents 1-5 of this table are fully credited to Dunn AJ. Effects of cytokines and infections on brain neurochemistry. *Clin Neurosci Res.* 2006 Aug;6(1-2):52-68. Zhang JM, An J. Cytokines, inflammation, and pain. *Int Anesthesiol Clin.* 2007 Spring;45(2):27-37

Beyond glutamate in microbe-triggered brain inflammation: alterations in tryptophan, serotonin and additional triggering of NMDA receptors for more brain/pain activation and less inhibition

- Introduction to altered intracerebral tryptophan metabolism: Microbial, psychological, and inflammatory stressors cause elevations in IFN-g and TNF-a; "IFN-g induces the enzyme indoleamine 2,3-dioxygenase (IDO, found in immune cells such as macrophages and dendritic cells), which causes reduction in tryptophan availability, leading to a reduction in serotonin synthesis in the brain."[415] Paraphrasing the brilliantly excellent 2015 review by Jo, Zhang, Emrich, and Dietrich[416]: Following induction, IDO catabolizes/converts tryptophan into kynurenine (KYN), is converted to kynurenic acid (KA) or quinolinic acid (QUIN); "KA and QUIN have contrasting roles influencing the glutamatergic system, the first acting as antagonist and the latter as agonist of the glutamate N-methyl-D-aspartate receptor (NMDAr). Microglia are the main producers of QUIN in the brain, whereas astrocytes are the CNS-key cells involved in KA synthesis. This is explained by the fact that microglia express kynurenine 3-monooxygenase (KMO), the rate-limiting enzyme in the production of QUIN. Conversely, astrocytes exclusively express kynurenine aminotransferases, which are essential in the conversion of KYN to KA." Thus, in relevant summary, glial activation in the brain leads to cerebral tryptophan depletion, thereby depleting this important precursor of serotonin and melatonin while also leading to additional NMDAr agonism via QUIN. As such we are able to advance our understanding of this utmost-important pathophysiology that is occurring in the brain following/during inflammatory events/exposures, as illustrated and additionally detailed in the caption.

---

[415] Hurley LL, Tizabi Y. Neuroinflammation, neurodegeneration, and depression. *Neurotox Res.* 2013 Feb;23(2):131-44

[416] Jo WK, Zhang Y, Emrich HM, Dietrich DE. Glia in the cytokine-mediated onset of depression: fine tuning the immune response. *Front Cell Neurosci.* 2015 Jul 10;9:268

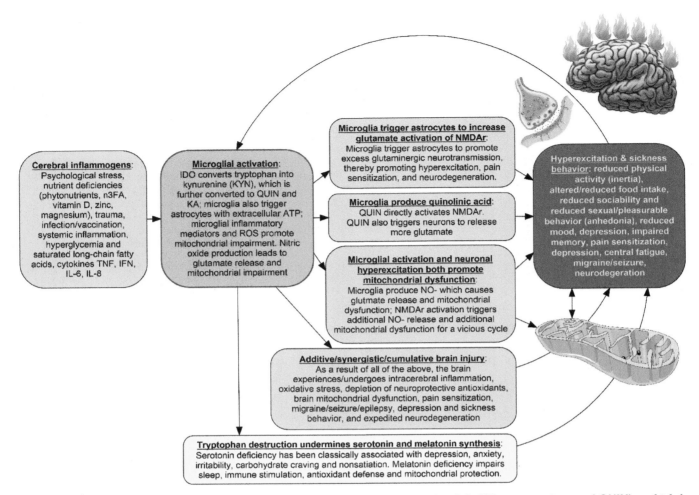

Cerebral inflammogens:
Psychological stress, nutrient deficiencies (phytonutrients, n3FA, vitamin D, zinc, magnesium), trauma, infection/vaccination, systemic inflammation, hyperglycemia and saturated long-chain fatty acids, cytokines TNF, IFN, IL-6, IL-8

Microglial activation:
IDO converts tryptophan into kynurenine (KYN), which is further converted to QUIN and KA; microglia also trigger astrocytes with extracellular ATP; microglial inflammatory mediators and ROS promote mitochondrial impairment. Nitric oxide production leads to glutamate release and mitochondrial impairment

Microglia trigger astrocytes to increase glutamate activation of NMDAr:
Microglia trigger astrocytes to promote excess glutaminergic neurotransmission, thereby promoting hyperexcitation, pain sensitization, and neurodegeneration.

Microglia produce quinolinic acid:
QUIN directly activates NMDAr. QUIN also triggers neurons to release more glutamate

Microglial activation and neuronal hyperexcitation both promote mitochondrial dysfunction:
Microglia produce NO- which causes glutmate release and mitochondrial dysfunction; NMDAr activation triggers additional NO- release and additional mitochondrial dysfunction for a vicious cycle

Hyperexcitation & sickness behavior: reduced physical activity (inertia), altered/reduced food intake, reduced sociability and reduced sexual/pleasurable behavior (anhedonia), reduced mood, depression, impaired memory, pain sensitization, depression, central fatigue, migraine/seizure, neurodegeration

Additive/synergistic/cumulative brain injury:
As a result of all of the above, the brain experiences/undergoes intracerebral inflammation, oxidative stress, depletion of neuroprotective antioxidants, brain mitochondrial dysfunction, pain sensitization, migraine/seizure/epilepsy, depression and sickness behavior, and expedited neurodegeneration

Tryptophan destruction undermines serotonin and melatonin synthesis:
Serotonin deficiency has been classically associated with depression, anxiety, irritability, carbohydrate craving and nonsatiation. Melatonin deficiency impairs sleep, immune stimulation, antioxidant defense and mitochondrial protection.

Brain inflammation leads directly to triple enhancement of NMDAr activation (via NO-, astrocytes, and QUIN) and triple impairment of mitochondrial function (via NO-, ROS, and inflammatory barrage): Details and citations provided in the following caption. Images above by DrV. Image of brain by IsaacMao per Flickr.com via creativecommons.org/licenses/by/2.0. See educational videos and updates at www.inflammationmastery.com/pain.

- **Cerebral inflammation can be triggered by any indirect or direct insult**, including psychological stress, nutrient deficiencies (phytonutrients, n3FA, vitamin D, zinc, magnesium), trauma, infection/vaccination, systemic inflammation, hyperglycemia and saturated long-chain fatty acids, cytokines TNF, IFN, IL-6, IL-8. We need to change the way that we appreciate inflammation: we have traditionally/historically/conveniently/simplistically thought of inflammation as needing a trigger and occurring in response to that trigger; while that remains largely but not absolutely true, we need to appreciate that inflammation—especially metabolic inflammation—occurs as a manifestation of cellular dysfunction in general and mitochondrial dysfunction in particular and as such can be initiated by nutritional deficiency, including phytonutrient deficiency. For example, the fact that nutritional supplementation in physiologic subpharmacologic doses provides an antiinflammatory benefit (e.g., multivitamin/mineral[417] and vitamin D3[418]) is proof that the preexisting nutritional deficiency—even though slight and subclinical—was itself the cause of the inflammatory response. We have crystalline clarity now that peripheral inflammation leads to central/brain inflammation, whether from trauma, infection, or vaccination[419,420,421] and as such we can reasonably state—and should accept as true—that any significant inflammatory/immunologic response in the periphery is going to cause/promote central/brain inflammation and the resulting hyperexcitation, pain sensitization, and sickness behavior. Important in this conversation is that while the model of "microglial activation = astrocyte activation = neuroinflammation / central sensitization / sickness behavior" is generally accurate, this same model is actually quite nuanced and contains different variations, leading to different clinical phenotypes. Data is giving shape to the idea that different cytokines have different effects on brain cellular components, leading to different phenotypic manifestations. Taking a single example, we note the recent 2015 report showing that beta amyloid induced IL-8 mediated microglial activation, and that the resulting astrocytic activation is mediated by a different (nonIL-8) pathway; also noted is the 2015 report showing

[417] Church TS, Earnest CP, Wood KA, Kampert JB. Reduction of C-reactive protein levels through use of a multivitamin. *Am J Med.* 2003 Dec 15;115(9):702-7

[418] Timms et al. Circulating MMP9, vitamin D and variation in the TIMP-1 response with VDR genotype. *QJM.* 2002 Dec;95(12):787-96

[419] Wright CE et al. Acute inflammation and negative mood: mediation by cytokine activation. *Brain Behav Immun.* 2005 Jul;19(4):345-50

[420] Harrison NA et al. Inflammation causes mood changes through alterations in subgenual cingulate activity and mesolimbic connectivity. *Biol Psychiatry.* 2009 Sep:407-14

[421] Wilson CJ, Finch CE, Cohen HJ. Cytokines and cognition—the case for a head-to-toe inflammatory paradigm. *J Am Geriatr Soc.* 2002 Dec;50(12):2041-56

that central/brain neuroinflammation in RA is mediated by IL-1 while that in FM is mediated by IL-8. As such, we should speak of neuroinflammations and glial activations in the plural rather than singular forms.

- **Microglial activation drains tryptophan** by triggering IDO conversion of tryptophan into kynurenine (KYN), which is further converted to QUIN and KA.[422] Tryptophan destruction undermines serotonin and melatonin synthesis: Serotonin deficiency has been classically associated with depression, anxiety, irritability, carbohydrate craving and nonsatiation. Melatonin deficiency impairs sleep, immune stimulation, antioxidant defense and mitochondrial protection.

- **Microglia trigger astrocytes to increase glutamate activation of NMDAr**: Microglia trigger astrocytes with extracellular ATP. Microglial activation triggers astrocytes to promote excess glutaminergic neurotransmission[423], thereby promoting hyperexcitation, pain sensitization, and neurodegeneration.

- **Microglial activation and increased nitric oxide (NO-) production leads to glutamate release and mitochondrial impairment**. Microglial inflammatory mediators and ROS promote mitochondrial impairment. Readers should appreciate the implications of this vicious cycle, where in "fire in the brain" can readily burn out of control; in context with other information in this section, this understanding helps explain, for example, how immunologic triggers in the periphery such as vaccination/immunization can cause devastating brain injury, basically leading to "metabolic-inflammatory meltdown of the brain" as seen in the most horrific of vaccination responses—vaccination encephalopathy/encephalitis.[424,425] Encephalitis can also result from gastrointestinal infection. [426]

- **Microglia produce quinolinic acid (QUIN) to activate NMDAr: Microglia produce QUIN which activates NMDAr while QUIN also triggers neurons to release more glutamate, thereby leading to additional contribution to NMDAr activation.**[427] Astrocytes can produce the NMDAr agonist kynurenic acid (KA); however, in settings of glial activation, NMDAr activation clearly predominates.

- **Microglial activation and neuronal hyperexcitation both promote mitochondrial dysfunction.**[428] Microglia produce (or induce astrocytic production of*) NO- which causes glutamate release and mitochondrial dysfunction; NMDAr activation triggers additional NO- release and additional mitochondrial dysfunction for a vicious cycle. Neuronal excitation and microglial activation both promote mitochondrial dysfunction; this is physiologically disastrous because neurons need optimized mitochondrial performance generally and especially when faced with increased/dysregulated demand. Very important here is the appreciation that mitochondrial dysfunction is itself pro-inflammatory (via ROS and DAMP/PAMP receptor activation by mitochondrial fragments), thereby adding to the vicious cycle. Further, mitochondrial dysfunction triggers excess release of inflammatory cytokines from a wide range of cell types; the range of cell types showing increased pro-inflammatory cytokine release following induction of mitochondrial impairment is so wide that possibly all cells (in this conversation, including microglia and neurons) are involved/affected. *Kim and Nagai[429] noted that human microglia do not produce NO- and that NO- production in the human brain glia originates chiefly from astrocytes; still, in the context of an intact brain, we might summarize that the microglia induce NO- production by triggering astrocytes, even if human microglia—distinguished from other animal models—cannot directly produce NO-.

- **Additive/synergistic/cumulative brain injury manifesting generally and chronically as increased brain fragility**: As a result of all of the above, the brain experiences/undergoes intracerebral inflammation, oxidative stress, depletion of neuroprotective antioxidants, enhanced viral/bacterial replication/effect, brain mitochondrial dysfunction, pain sensitization, migraine/seizure/epilepsy, depression and sickness behavior, and expedited neurodegeneration. Since many of these metabolic impairments are both common and silent, these lead to the promotion of neurodegeneration and "brain fragility" (or per Morley and Seneff: "diminished brain resilience syndrome"[430]) wherein the brain is supranormally vulnerable to other insults, such as trauma, dietary insult, glyphosate/pesticide exposure, infections and vaccinations.

<u>**As clinicians, pragmatists, and intellectuals, we are obligated to employ the available data**</u>: We already have sufficient evidence for this model, and clinicians should move forward and implement this model in clinical practice; use of this model is considerably more attractive than ascribing the associated conditions to spontaneous generation and condemning the associated patients to eternal medicalization. For ethical and logistical reasons, we will probably never have "perfect proof" of this model, because such would require induction of disease in healthy people, and this would be clearly risky and unethical and would therefore never be approved by any competent IRB (institutional review board, tasked with approving research investigations). What we might call *perfect proof* of this would have to be established by *prospective* studies showing that ❶ administration of a sufficient total microbial load (TML)—specifically SIBO in the case of FM—causes central sensitization as assessed by some reliable

[422] Jo WK, Zhang Y, Emrich HM, Dietrich DE. Glia in the cytokine-mediated onset of depression: fine tuning the immune response. *Front Cell Neurosci.* 2015 Jul 10;9:268
[423] Béchade C, Cantaut-Belarif Y, Bessis A. Microglial control of neuronal activity. *Front Cell Neurosci.* 2013 Mar 28;7:32
[424] Alicino et al. Acute disseminated encephalomyelitis with severe neurological outcomes following virosomal seasonal influenza vaccine. *Hum Vaccin Immunother.* 2014;10(7):1969-73
[425] Lee et al. An adverse event following 2009 H1N1 influenza vaccination: a case of acute disseminated encephalomyelitis. *Korean J Pediatr.* 2011 Oct;54(10):422-4
[426] Mahdi N, Abdelmalik PA, Curtis M, Bar B. A Case of Acute Disseminated Encephalomyelitis in a Middle-Aged Adult. *Case Rep Neurol Med.* 2015;2015:601706
[427] Jo WK, Zhang Y, Emrich HM, Dietrich DE. Glia in the cytokine-mediated onset of depression: fine tuning the immune response. *Front Cell Neurosci.* 2015 Jul 10;9:268
[428] Brown GC, Bal-Price A. Inflammatory neurodegeneration mediated by nitric oxide, glutamate, and mitochondria. *Mol Neurobiol.* 2003 Jun;27(3):325-55
[429] Kim SU Nagai A. Microglia as immune effectors of the central nervous system: Expression of cytokines and chemokines. *Clin Experiment Neuroimmunol.* 2010 May; 1: 61–69
[430] Morley WA, Seneff S. Diminished brain resilience syndrome: A modern day neurological pathology of increased susceptibility to mild brain trauma, concussion, and downstream neurodegeneration. *Surg Neurol Int.* 2014 Jun ; 5: 97

technology such as functional magnetic resonance imaging (fMRI) of the brain or evidence of inflammatory changes within the cerebrospinal fluid (CSF). A prospective trial of this nature would almost certainly be considered unethical and would be almost impossible to perform, either technically (how would the microbial load be delivered safely, effectively, and *temporarily* without risk of long-term harm?) and the related near-impossibility of being passed/approved by a responsible research IRB. **Natural life provides this trial via the observation that people who naturally develop small intestine bacterial overgrowth and other forms of gastrointestinal dysbiosis frequently develop syndromes of central sensitization such as irritable bowel syndrome, fibromyalgia, and complex regional pain syndrome[431]; prospective experimental studies have shown that animals exposed to microbial inflammogens indeed develop central sensitization.** Secondarily and of lesser importance, we would also want prospective evidence that ❷ the above-mentioned microbe-induced central sensitization can be alleviated by removal of the inflammatory microbial load. Ideally, we would look for *direct* evidence of alleviation of central sensitization, again by looking at the brain and its surrounding fluid for functional/molecular evidence of normalization, but without the ideal situation, we could look for *indirect* evidence of alleviation of central sensitization by looking for alleviation of pain. **Clinical studies with humans have already shown that removing the excessive microbial load—specifically SIBO in the case of FM—alleviates the clinical manifestations of central sensitization, namely excessive pain, fatigue, and other physical and mental manifestations of the illness.** Supportively, we can appreciate data showing that ❸ mitochondrial dysfunction (mitodysfunction) and systemic inflammation in general promote central sensitization, and thereby the alleviation of either mitodysfunction or inflammation by alleviating the TML/SIBO would be expected to alleviate central sensitization. In a world of imperfect research, incomplete data, and the vast majority of doctors/researchers having had zero training in nutrition, mitochondrial optimization and treatments for dysbiosis, let us look at the support for this thesis while emphasizing the importance of incorporating the available data while recalling that absence of evidence (ie, the studies have not been performed) is neither evidence of refutation (ie, no evidence refutes the thesis) nor evidence of absence (ie, we have an abundance of supporting data, even if we are currently and perhaps always will be lacking a perfect prospective study of microbe-induced central sensitization followed by relief of same via antimicrobial/antidysbiotic interventions).

The medicomonetary reality: The goal of most research is not cure of disease, but translation of biology into drug sales: In order to further understand the nature, goals, and constraints of "biomedical research", one first needs to have some *insights into the obvious*: namely, that the general goal of *biomedical* research is to understand enough of nature and biology so that a drug can be developed to address the condition being studied. This is the *translation* of biology into the practice of medicine, and generally this culminates in the development and sales of drugs. Of note, these drugs generally do not cure

---

Basic science research and the practice of medicine are shaped by powerful financial interests

"A clinician who is unaware of the political forces that shape healthcare policy and research is analogous to a captain of an oceangoing ship not knowing how to use a compass, sextant, or coastline map. Medical science and healthcare policy are influenced by a myriad of powerful private interests motivated by their own goals, at times different from the stated goal of medicine, which purports to hold paramount the patient's welfare. Scientific objectivity and the guiding ethical principles of informed consent, beneficence, autonomy, and non-malfeasance are subject to different interpretations depending on the lens through which a dilemma is viewed. This gives rise to a disarrayed tug-of-war between factions and private interests, with paradigmatic victory often being awarded to those with the best marketing campaigns and political influence while less importance is given to safety, efficacy, and the economic burden to consumers. To be ignorant of such considerations is to be blind to the nature of research, policy, and our own biased inclinations for and against particular paradigms, assessments, and interventions. Research articles and sources of authority must be approached with an artist's delicacy and with a willingness to consider new information that may contradict deeply rooted beliefs."

Vasquez A. *Musculoskeletal Pain: Expanded Clinical Strategies*. Institute for Functional Medicine, 2008

---

the disease nor solve the problems, but rather alleviate select and occasionally irrelevant biochemical or clinical indexes of the disease to show "improvement" and therefore justify regulatory "approval" and therefore empower drug sales. Consciously or unconsciously, this is how the system operates, and this is how people within the system generally think; in medical research centers—ie, medical research centers are almost always affiliated with hospitals or medical schools—generally everyone within these systems is a devotee of the medical paradigm, which generally holds that diseases are *idiopathic* and *need to be treated with drugs*, generally multiple drugs (polypharmacy) for

---

[431] Reichenberger et al. Establishing a relationship between bacteria in the human gut and complex regional pain syndrome. *Brain Behav Immun.* 2013 Mar;29:62-9

indefinite periods of time. The lifeblood of biomedical research centers is funding, and this is generally tied to the expectation of "advancing the practice of medicine" which by definition means using—and therefore developing for sale—more drugs. (Drugs are tangible, and drugs are profitable; drugs keep doctors employed, and they keep so-called healthcare centers [e.g., clinics and hospitals] open and profitable because patients are obligated to seek consultations and constantly renew their prescriptions—the profitability and repeat business are guaranteed when patients are told, "You have a disease that is not understood, and this disease will kill or harm you unless you take and continue to take these drugs." Drugs also maintain our power-over paradigm[432],

> **Paradigms—goals, components, needs and fears—are created to support the prevailing power structures**
>
> 248   PUBLIC OPINION
>
> consciously what facts, in what setting, in what guise he shall permit the public to know.
>
> 4
>
> That the manufacture of consent is capable of great refinements no one, I think, denies. The process by which public opinions arise is certainly no less intricate than it has appeared in these pages, and the opportunities for manipulation open to anyone who understands the process are plain enough.
>
> Lippmann W. *Public Opinion*. Harcourt & Brace, 1922

which holds that our worldview is centered on the feeling that we have *power over our problems* [rather than accepting them as they are and working with them as they are], and again we tend to seek this through concrete and obvious and simple-minded means because these are the means that have immediate appeal.) Any basic science or medical researcher who finds that a disease can be cured and the problem solved by a simple treatment will at best be the *Hero of the Day* before being forgotten (and—quite often—later fired); the doctor or researcher who finds that a drug *might* help a problem and who thereafter receives speaking opportunities at national and international medical society meetings (always directly or indirectly funded by drug companies) and who receives several hundred thousand dollars in research grants (always directly or indirectly funded by drug companies and/or the private interests tied to them) will be remembered and championed.

Limited thought—systematic addictions to searching for parts without appreciating the whole, and to disregarding the obvious as simple and therefore without merit: Within the medical paradigm is the belief that diseases are complex and serious and that therefore the treatments must be complex and serious; ironically, drug therapy is actually based on simplistic thinking evidenced by the fact that drugs almost always work on only *one single* pathway/process while complex chronic/persistent diseases are always *multifaceted*. When diseases are indeed simple or at least understandable, they must be made to appear complex and enigmatic by the confusion of research and the perpetual reenactment of ignoring previous research and starting from zero. In this manner, researchers can apply for grants using the words and phrases "new" and "innovative" and "translational" and "advancing medical science to advance patient care" and thus fall into the line of *common thought*—drug production, drug sales, medical dependency to which we are all indoctrinated and accustomed—which makes these ideas and phrases easily acceptable. A doctor or researcher who advances the idea that a disease can be treated by simple means runs the risk of appearing himself/herself as *simple* rather than *insightful*. Collectively as a society, we have created illusions of complexity on many facets of life, ranging from poverty to diabetes to perpetual war; each of these— like the majority of illnesses that bind patients and busy/occupy healthcare systems—can be understood and managed effectively, but not if we allow ourselves to be convinced that they are complex and not if we allow the profiteers to hold the reigns of conversation and intervention. I state that biomedical researchers by virtue of the society in which they live and the environments in which they work are inclined to state and perhaps believe (ie, honestly accept as their own perception) that fibromyalgia is complex, not understood, and ultimately only treatable with drugs—that is the "prescribed" line of medical thinking; we get that paradigm of thought hammered into us via reading, exams, and sleep deprivation in medical school, and medical school courses are the initial training ground for both doctors and their biomedical research colleagues (e.g., many PhD students have to take medical school courses if the PhD program is housed within a university system that contains a medical school). Thus, virtually everyone in "medicine" whether as a physician or researcher is indoctrinated with the *idiopathic-*

---

[432] Largent C, Breton D. *The Paradigm Conspiracy: Why Our Social Systems Violate Human Potential*. Hazelden, 1998

polypharmacy model. Finally, we must also appreciate the profiteering bias manifested by medical journals—who profit from sales of drug-friendly articles when drug companies pay for associated advertising and for article reprints[433]—and magazines/newspapers/websites/television that also receive more advertising money when they publish drug-friendly articles and news. In this way, research and news is inherently biased toward publishing drug-friendly articles and news.

Private control over public paradigms: Notably in the United States—the country that most strongly influences international healthcare, science, and policy—the largest media outlets for news, science, and television are owned by a small handful of multicorporation conglomerates that are interconnected—either directly, paradigmatically, or financially—with drug companies; indeed, each facet of health and healthcare in American society—including medical education itself[434] and the lack of labeling of GMO foods and the horrific failure to regulate the pesticide industry's contamination of food, air, and water[435,436]—is strongly influenced by lobbying and money from drug companies and private business interests.[437]

Denial of the obvious, especially that which is natural and immediate: Western culture has been largely built on the denial of the present moment and denial of what is natural, hence our fascination with anything new, "modern", "sophisticated", and laboratory-clean. As such, our treatment paradigms tend to avoid the *actionable* and *clear* and *natural* in favor of the passive (e.g., drugs), squeaky-clean (e.g., drugs), and the future (e.g., idiopathic now, but we are supposed to wait for future developments while postponing action and thought and in the meanwhile resign our consciousness to "the powers that be" which are supposed to make the decisions for us by their "virtue" of divine insight). Given that Western culture in its entirety is based on denial of now, natural, and actionable (except when stirred to war)—and any look at our generally passive, listless, and deferent society will confirm this—we should not be surprised that our medical paradigm is largely the same, characterized by passive drugs and passive medical care, apathy in personal thought and action (including medical professionals themselves who are taught

[433] Smith R. Medical Journals Are an Extension of the Marketing Arm of Pharmaceutical Companies. *PLoS Med.* 2005 May; 2(5): e138
[434] Drug-company influence on medical education in USA. *Lancet.* 2000 Sep 2;356(9232):781
[435] Bøhn T, Cuhra M, Traavik T, Sanden M, Fagan J, Primicerio R. Compositional differences in soybeans on the market: glyphosate accumulates in Roundup Ready GM soybeans. *Food Chem.* 2014 Jun 15;153:207-1 sciencedirect.com/science/article/pii/S0308814613019201
[436] Majewski MS, Coupe RH, Foreman WT, Capel PD. Pesticides in Mississippi air and rain: a comparison between 1995 and 2007. *Environ Toxicol Chem.* 2014 Jun;33:1283-93
[437] For anyone paying attention to America's political scene, especially since 1980, this statement will be self-evident and abundantly buttressed by the observance of national events that favor small numbers of rich and therefore powerful private and business interests over the interests of the American people and the overall welfare of the nation.

While some would reasonably argue that American society has always been a populist façade run amuck by a puppeteering financial elite, the population-wide data is very clear that the financial balance of the nation was essentially "inverted" in the 1980s during a time when—a fact that nobody can refute—the stated policy of the government was specifically to give more money, more power, and less responsibility to the rich at the expense of the rest of the nation; this was called "trickle-down economics" and was sold to the public via the illusion that by making the rich more rich the wealth of the nation would eventually "trickle down" to the financially lower segments of society and everyone would bathe in the wealth of the nation via the generosity and altruism of the financial elite. Obviously, this did not occur; along with the government's deregulation of industry and the demolition of public power generally and unions in particular, deceptively termed "free trade agreements" shipped American jobs overseas to nations with comparatively zero worker and environmental protections to the benefit of multinational corporations. As shown in the image from President Obama's 2015 State of the Union address, the largest section of the American population—the bottom 90%—now have access to but a small piece of the American national pie, while the top 1% own nearly 70% of the country's resources. As a result, rich individuals and companies gained even more power while the citizens saw their interests ignored; finally in 2014, the obvious was published: America no longer functioned as a democracy by and for the people but rather as an oligarchy, with the government controlled by private interests controlling policies ranging from public health to education and public transportation. Studies and press are listed below:

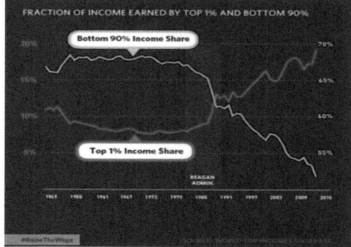

1. US is an oligarchy, not a democracy. bbc.com/news/blogs-echochambers-27074746
2. America is an oligarchy, not a democracy or republic, university study finds. washingtontimes.com/news/2014/apr/21/americas-oligarchy-not-democracy-or-republic-unive/
3. The US is an oligarchy, study concludes: "Report by researchers from Princeton and Northwestern universities suggests that US political system serves special interest organisations, instead of voters." telegraph.co.uk/news/worldnews/northamerica/usa/10769041/The-US-is-an-oligarchy-study-concludes.html
4. Is the USDA Silencing Scientists? theatlantic.com/science/archive/2015/11/is-the-usda-silencing-scientists/413803/
5. One Nation, Under Monsanto. counterpunch.org/2013/02/26/one-nation-under-monsanto Of special note, this article is written by Paul Craig Roberts PhD (Economics), a former Assistant Secretary of the US Treasury and Associate Editor of the *Wall Street Journal*.

not to think but rather to defer to authority and guidelines while they focus on diagnoses and drugs[438]). In Western medicine, natural treatments whether diets or vitamins are constantly attacked and obfuscated, despite their self-evident value and importance; meanwhile, drugs in general and vaccines in particular are sacrosanct, despite their generally artificial importance, indebting/bankrupting expenses, and adverse effects that often exceed their benefit.

❹ All other biochemical and pathophysiologic abnormalities seen in fibromyalgia can likewise be explained from the primary SIBO.

- **Restless leg syndrome and fibromyalgia commonly co-exist, and restless leg syndrome can be alleviated by eradication of SIBO:** Restless leg syndrome (RLS) occurs in approximately 30% of FM patients and can be effectively treated by addressing SIBO with a combination of antibiotics (drugs or botanical medicines that eradicate bacteria) and probiotics (products containing beneficial bacteria, which help restore "microbial balance" in the gastrointestinal tract).[439]

- **SIBO commonly causes nutrient malabsorption and thus predisposes to subclinical selective malnutrition, specifically micronutrient deficiency:** SIBO causes nutrient malabsorption[440] and can thereby contribute to the vitamin D and magnesium deficiencies that promote pain and mitochondrial dysfunction, respectively, and which are common in fibromyalgia. Intestinal bacterial overgrowth causes nutrient malabsorption via intestinal inflammation and villus atrophy (anatomic impairment) and impairment of digestion, specifically the enzymatic degradation of mucosal peptidases and disaccharidases by bacterial proteases (biochemical impairment). As reported by McEvoy and colleagues[441], bacterial contamination [overgrowth] of the small intestine is an important cause of occult malabsorption and malnutrition, especially in the elderly.

- **SIBO can be triggered or exacerbated by emotional stress:** SIBO can be triggered in humans by reduced mucosal immunity following stressful life events, and this helps explain the link between psychoemotional stress and the SIBO-related conditions IBS and FM. Chronic mental-emotional stress causes reduced production of the antibody secretory IgA (sIgA) which is the primary line of defense against bacteria and other microorganisms in the gastrointestinal tract; thus, mental-emotional stress can reduce intestinal immunity and thereby promote SIBO. Further, stress in humans triggers enhanced microbial pathogenicity via microbial endocrinology.

- **Oxidative stress triggers exaggerated pain perception—hyperalgesia (hypersensitivity to pain) and allodynia (perception of pain from normal stimuli):** Patients with fibromyalgia show evidence of increased free radical (oxidant) production and reduced antioxidant defenses. Increased oxidative stress can be caused by immune activation and mitochondrial dysfunction; immune activation and mitochondrial dysfunction also promote oxidative stress and depletion of antioxidants, resulting in a vicious cycle, as illustrated. In the excellent review by Cordero et al[442], the authors note that recent studies have shown that oxidative stress causes peripheral and central sensitization and alters nerve sensitivity to pain (nociception), resulting in hyperalgesia—hypersensitivity to normal stimuli. The free radical (oxidant) superoxide promotes the development of pain through direct peripheral sensitization and the release of various cytokines (such as TNF-α, IL-1β, and IL-6), the formation of peroxynitrite (ONOO-), and PARP activation. PARP—poly-ADP-ribose-polymerase—is a nuclear enzyme activated by superoxide/peroxynitrite radicals; activation of PARP promotes the development of pain syndromes, including the components of small sensory fiber neuropathy, thermal and mechanical hyperalgesia, tactile allodynia, and exaggerated pain behavior in animal models of diabetic neuropathy.[443,444]

- **Low plasma levels of L-tryptophan seen in fibromyalgia patients can be caused by degradation of dietary tryptophan by the bacterial enzyme tryptophanase:** Patients with fibromyalgia have low blood levels of the amino acid L-tryptophan[445], which is used in the body to make serotonin (important for mood maintenance,

[438] Ely et al. Analysis of questions asked by family doctors regarding patient care. *BMJ.* 1999 Aug 7;319(7206):358-61 ncbi.nlm.nih.gov/pmc/articles/PMC28191/
[439] Weinstock et al. Restless Legs Syndrome in Patients with Irritable Bowel Syndrome: Response to Small Intestinal Bacterial Overgrowth Therapy. *Dig Dis Sci* 2007 May:1252-6
[440] Elphick HL, Elphick DA, Sanders DS. Small bowel bacterial overgrowth. An underrecognized cause of malnutrition in older adults. Geriatrics. 2006 Sep;61(9):21-6
[441] McEvoy et al. Bacterial contamination of the small intestine is an important cause of occult malabsorption in the elderly. *Br Med J* 1983 Sep 17;287(6395):789-93
[442] Cordero MD, et al. Mitochondrial dysfunction and mitophagy activation in blood mononuclear cells of fibromyalgia patients. *Arthritis Res Ther.* 2010;12(1):R17
[443] Wang ZQ, Porreca F, Cuzzocrea S et al. A newly identified role for superoxide in inflammatory pain. *J Pharmacol Exp Ther.* 2004 Jun;309(3):869-78
[444] Ilnytska O, et al. Poly(ADP-ribose) polymerase inhibition alleviates experimental diabetic sensory neuropathy. *Diabetes* 2006 Jun;55:1686-94
[445] "Plasma-free tryptophan is inversely related to the severity of subjective pain in 8 patients who fulfilled criteria for a variety of non-articular rheumatism, the "fibrositis syndrome". The observation is consistent with animal and human studies suggesting a relationship between reduced brain serotonin metabolism and pain reactivity." Moldofsky H, Warsh JJ. Plasma tryptophan and musculoskeletal pain in non-articular rheumatism ("fibrositis syndrome"). *Pain.* 1978 Jun;5(1):65-71

pain alleviation, and appetite control) and melatonin (important for normal sleep, support of mitochondrial function [stimulant of ETC complexes #1 and #4], and antioxidant protection, given that melatonin is one of the most powerful antioxidants). Bacteria such as *Escherichia coli*, *Proteus vulgaris*, and *Bacteroides* produce the enzyme tryptophanase[446], which destroys L-tryptophan in the gut before it is absorbed from ingested foods; thus, generalized bacterial overgrowth of the small intestine could reasonably be expected to exacerbate this phenomenon. In patients with fibromyalgia, higher tryptophan levels correlate positively with serotonin levels and with less pain and better sleep, while lower tryptophan levels are associated with sleep impairment, reduced serotonin levels, and higher levels of substance P, a neurotransmitter that promotes inflammation and pain perception.[447] Fibromyalgia patients produce 31% less melatonin than do healthy controls, and "this may contribute to impaired sleep at night, fatigue during the day, and changed pain perception."[448] Thus, a likely sequence of events is that, for example, a period of stressful life events can cause impair gastrointestinal immunity leading to intestinal bacterial overgrowth, which itself causes tryptophan degradation via elaboration of bacterial tryptophanase, causing tryptophan deficiency and resultant deficiencies of serotonin (leading to pain, depression, anxiety, and food/carbohydrate craving) and melatonin (leading to sleep disturbance, impaired antioxidant defense and mitochondrial function, and impaired immune responsiveness). Enhanced degradation of tryptophan can also be effected by the liver via enhanced activation of the enzyme tryptophan pyrrolase (tryptophan 2,3-dioxygenase, TDO) in response to "stress" and increased cortisol and by immune cells such as macrophages and dendritic cells via the enzyme indoleamine 2,3-dioxygenase (IDO) which is upregulated via the Th1-type cytokine interferon-gamma (IFNg).[449] Pregnancy induces accelerated tryptophan degradation; however, for the focus of this conversation we note that most FM patients are not pregnant and thus the likely causes of tryptophan deficiency in FM patients, who show evidence of SIBO, stress, and inflammation are ❶ intraluminal bacterial tryptophanase, ❷ hepatic tryptophan pyrrolase, and ❸ immune/inflammatory 2,3-dioxygenase.

- <u>The therapies that help fibromyalgia share mechanisms of action consistent with the model presented here</u>: As will be reviewed below under *Therapeutic Interventions*, essentially all of the most successful therapies for fibromyalgia have effects on intestinal flora, muscle perfusion/contractility, or mitochondrial bioenergetics (biological production of cellular energy/ATP). This is true for vegetarian diets (which favorably alter gut flora and improve antioxidant defenses), supplementation with tryptophan/melatonin (which preserve mitochondrial function during bacterial LPS/endotoxin exposure), physical treatments such as acupuncture (which improves tissue perfusion), and the use of nutrients such as magnesium, acetyl-L-carnitine, D-ribose, creatine, and coenzyme Q-10—all of which support or improve mitochondrial function.

Overall and when integrated together, the research literature provides compelling evidence linking intestinal bacterial overgrowth with the genesis and perpetuation of fibromyalgia. Chronic low-dose exposure to bacterial debris such as lipopolysaccharide/endotoxin and metabolic toxins such as hydrogen sulfide and D-lactic acid from SIBO is a plausible cause of impaired cellular energy production that results in chronic, widespread muscle fatigue and soreness and which may culminate in the clinical presentation of fibromyalgia. The individual components of this model have been substantiated by mechanistic studies in animals and/or research studies in humans. CFS also shares many epidemiological and clinical similarities with FM, and a similar pathophysiology is therefore highly probable.

A consistent report from many CFS and fibromyalgia patients is that of environmental intolerance (EI) and multiple chemical sensitivity (MCS), often grouped together as EI-MCS; these are complex disorders that the medical profession has failed to appreciate and which are characterized by adverse physiological responses to ambient levels of toxic chemicals and other environmental exposures. EI-MCS can be plausibly explained by SIBO because bacterial LPS/endotoxin impairs hepatic cytochrome P450 detoxification enzymes, resulting in reduced

[446] Demoss RD, Moser K. Tryptophanase in Diverse Bacterial Species. *Journal of Bacteriology* 1969; 98: 167-171
[447] "A strong negative correlation between SP and 5-HIAA as well as between SP and TRP could be demonstrated. High serum concentrations of 5-HIAA and TRP showed a significant relation to low pain scores. Moreover, 5-HIAA was strongly related to good quality of sleep, while SP was related to sleep disturbance." Schwarz et al. Relationship of substance P, 5-hydroxyindole acetic acid and tryptophan in serum of fibromyalgia patients. *Neurosci Lett*. 1999 Jan 15;259(3):196-8
[448] "The FMS patients had a 31% lower MT secretion than healthy subjects during the hours of darkness... Patients with fibromyalgic syndrome have a lower melatonin secretion during the hours of darkness than healthy subjects. This may contribute to impaired sleep at night, fatigue during the day, and changed pain perception." Wikner J, Hirsch U, Wetterberg L, Röjdmark S. Fibromyalgia syndrome associated with decreased nocturnal melatonin secretion. *Clin Endocrinol* (Oxf). 1998 Aug;49:179-83
[449] Schröcksnadel K, Wirleitner B, Winkler C, Fuchs D. Monitoring tryptophan metabolism in chronic immune activation. *Clin Chim Acta*. 2006 Feb;364(1-2):82-90

drug metabolism and impaired clearance of xenobiotics/toxins.[450] Accumulation of xenobiotics in CFS patients[451] might therefore be explained in part by LPS-induced inhibition of xenobiotic clearance secondary to SIBO. Further, the metabolic and immunologic effects of LPS can also account for the immune activation, neurological dysfunction, and musculoskeletal complaints noted in patients with CFS, IBS, and FM. A simplified yet accurate model of fibromyalgia which accounts for the major clinical and objective abnormalities seen with this condition is presented in the diagram that follows. Following the exclusion of diagnosable and treatable conditions that can contribute to or mimic fibromyalgia, and by using an integrated model, clinicians can design treatment plans based on the previously reviewed pathogenesis and on the therapeutic considerations detailed in the following section.

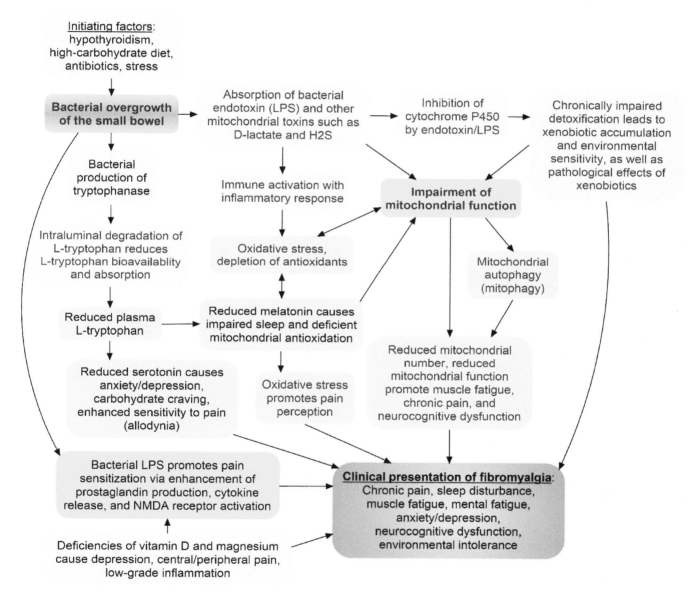

How small intestine bacterial overgrowth (SIBO) causes fibromyalgia: Bacterial overgrowth of the small bowel leads to chronic low-grade tryptophan insufficiency resulting in reduced endogenous production of serotonin (important for positive mood and relief from anxiety pain) and of melatonin (important for restful sleep and protection of mitochondria from oxidative stress). Bacterial mitochondrial toxins such as endotoxin, H2S, D-lactate cause impaired mitochondrial energy production, which leads to mitophagy, muscle fatigue, pain, and cognitive impairment. See educational videos and updates at www.inflammationmastery.com/pain

---

[450] Shedlofsky et al. Endotoxin administration to humans inhibits hepatic cytochrome P450-mediated drug metabolism. *J Clin Invest*. 1994 Dec;94(6):2209-14
[451] Dunstan et al. A preliminary investigation of chlorinated hydrocarbons and chronic fatigue syndrome. *Med J Aust*. 1995 Sep 18;163(6):294-7

<u>Introduction to Therapeutic Approach</u>: Rational treatment of microbe-induced pain and inflammation as seen in FM must focus on the eradication/modulation of the inflammatory microbial load as well as on the restoration of barrier defenses (e.g., the defensive lining of the skin and the gut wall) to reduce absorption of and exposure to microbial molecules (enhancing elimination of already-absorbed microbial toxins is a possibility, but is of lesser importance and is mentioned in some of my other writings). Enhancement of mitochondrial dysfunction and glial activation (brain inflammation) should also be pursued.

This section begins with a review of evidence showing important gut involvement in FM, CFS/SEID, and CRPS—all of which are variants on the same themes of microbe-induced microglial activation and mitochondrial dysfunction, as depicted in the following image, showing the relative contribution and combination of dysbiosis-induced mitochondrial impairment and brain inflammation (e.g., glial activation and central sensitization).

Complex regional pain syndrome: severe sensitization, often localized

Fibromyalgia: moderate-severe sensitization combined with mitochondrial dysfunction

Chronic fatigue syndrome (SEID): mitochondrial dysfunction predominates over sensitization

Irritable bowel syndrome: mild general sensitization, gastrointestinal symptoms predominate

Dysbiotic neurotoxicity / mitochondriopathy

Dysbiotic encephalitis / pain

<u>Microbe-induced mitochondriopathy/neurotoxicity and brain inflammation—a schematic diagram of relative contributions and combinations</u>: In CFS/SEID, microbial induction of mitochondrial dysfunction and (D-lactate) neurotoxicity predominate, whereas fibromyalgia is a unique combination of both microbial mitochondriopathy with central sensitization. In IBS, central sensitization is potent, along with a more disruptive gut microbiome leading to bloating and constipation/diarrhea; meanwhile in CRPS, a neuroinflammatory dysbiosis clearly dominates the clinical picture.

- <u>Patients with chronic fatigue syndrome (SEID), fibromyalgia (FM), and complex regional pain syndrome (CRPS) show evidence of increased intestinal permeability, leading to increased absorption of antigens, immunogens, inflammogens, and mitochondrial inhibitors (etc)</u>: Finally and most importantly, **antimicrobial therapy alleviates FM (and IBS) symptoms in direct proportion to the success of bacterial overgrowth eradication**, thus adding strong direct evidence in support of SIBO as a main cause of FM.[452,453] Recent clinical trials have shown that treatment of the fibromyalgia-related conditions IBS and SIBO by use of the nonabsorbed oral antibiotic rifaximin results in significant diminution of IBS-SIBO symptomatology with benefits lasting after the discontinuation of therapy.[454,455]

  - <u>Increased intestinal permeability (IP) in patients with primary fibromyalgia (FM) and in patients with complex regional pain syndrome (CRPS) (*Rheumatology* 2008 Aug[456])</u>: Authors of this study used well-established tests of mucosal permeability for gastroduodenal permeability (sucrose) and small intestinal permeability (lactulose and mannitol, as discussed in Chapter 1) to find that both FM and CRPS patients

[452] Wallace DJ, Hallegua DS. Fibromyalgia: the gastrointestinal link. *Curr Pain Headache Rep.*2004 Oct;8(5):364-8
[453] Pimentel et al. Improvement of symptoms by eradication of small intestinal overgrowth in FM: a double-blind study. [Abstract] *Arthritis Rheum* 1999, 42:S343
[454] Pimentel et al. The effect of a nonabsorbed oral antibiotic (rifaximin) on the symptoms of the irritable bowel syndrome. *Ann Intern Med.* 2006 Oct 17;145(8):557-63
[455] Sharara et al. A randomized double-blind placebo-controlled trial of rifaximin in patients with abdominal bloating and flatulence. *Am J Gastroenterol.* 2006 Feb;101(2):326-33
[456] Goebel et al. Altered intestinal permeability in patients with primary fibromyalgia and in patients with complex regional pain syndrome. *Rheumatology* 2008 Aug;47(8):1223-7

show increased burden of intestinal involvement; they write, "Patients with FM had a significantly higher IP than healthy volunteers. Indeed, both FM and CRPS groups had significantly higher IP values than healthy volunteers for both gastroduodenal permeability and small bowel permeability. The difference in gastroduodenal permeability between the two patient groups did not reach significance. Gastroduodenal permeability, as measured with the sucrose test, was increased in 13 patients with FM (32.5%) and in six patients with CRPS (35.3%) and in one healthy volunteer. The small bowel permeability index [using lactulose and mannitol] was increased in 15 patients with FM (37.5%), three patients with CRPS (17.6%) and in none of the volunteers." A wonderful addition to / extension of this work would have been the measurement of serum LPS levels, but this was not performed in the current study and has not been performed as of early 2015—noted and summarized immediately below is one study (Maes et al, *J Affect Disord* 2007 Apr) that measured antibodies to LPS (not LPS directly) in patients with CFS—chronic fatigue syndrome. Notably, increased IP in FM did not correlate with GI symptoms; however increased IP did correlate with serologic positivity against *Helicobacter pylori, Yersinia enterocolitica* and *Campylobacter jejuni.*

- **Increased serum IgA and IgM against LPS of enterobacteria in chronic fatigue syndrome (CFS) shows involvement of gram-negative enterobacteria and increased gut-intestinal permeability in the etiology of CFS** (*J Affect Disord* 2007 Apr[457]): These investigators measured IgA and IgM to LPS of the enterobacteria *Hafnia alvei, Pseudomonas aeruginosa, Morganella morganii, Proteus mirabilis, Pseudomonas putida, Citrobacter koseri,* and *Klebsiella pneumoniae* and "found that the prevalences and median values for serum IgA against the LPS of enterobacteria are significantly greater in patients with CFS than in normal volunteers and patients with partial CFS. Serum IgA levels were significantly correlated to the severity of illness, as measured by the FibroFatigue scale and to symptoms, such as irritable bowel, muscular tension, fatigue, concentration difficulties, and failing memory. The results show that enterobacteria are involved in the etiology of CFS and that an increased gut-intestinal permeability has caused an immune response to the LPS of gram-negative enterobacteria."

- **Gut inflammation in chronic fatigue syndrome.** (*Nutr Metab* 2010 Oct[458]): "Many CFS patients complain of gut dysfunction. In fact, patients with CFS are more likely to report a previous diagnosis of irritable bowel syndrome (IBS), a common functional disorder of the gut, and experience IBS-related symptoms. Recently, evidence for interactions between the intestinal microbiota, mucosal barrier function, and the immune system have been shown to play a role in the disorder's pathogenesis. Studies examining the microecology of the gastrointestinal (GI) tract have identified specific microorganisms whose presence appears related to disease; in CFS, a role for altered intestinal microbiota in the pathogenesis of the disease has recently been suggested. Mucosal barrier dysfunction promoting bacterial translocation has also been observed. ...For example, the administration of probiotics could alter the gut microbiota, improve mucosal barrier function, decrease pro-inflammatory cytokines, and have the potential to positively influence mood in patients where both emotional symptoms and inflammatory immune signals are elevated. Probiotics also have the potential to improve gut motility, which is dysfunctional in many CFS patients."

- **Altered intestinal microbiota and organic acids may be the origin of symptoms in irritable bowel syndrome.** (*Neurogastroenterol Motil.* 2010 May[459]): "Irritable bowel syndrome patients showed significantly higher counts of Veillonella and Lactobacillus than controls. They also expressed significantly higher levels of acetic acid, propionic acid, and total organic acids than controls. The quantity of bowel gas was not significantly different between controls and IBS patients. Finally, IBS patients with high acetic acid or propionic acid levels presented with significantly worse GI symptoms, QOL and negative emotions than those with low acetic acid or propionic acid levels or controls."

- **Intestinal permeability and hypersensitivity in the irritable bowel syndrome.** (*Pain* 2009 Nov[460]): "Here we demonstrate that diarrhea-predominant IBS (D-IBS) patients display increased intestinal permeability. We

[457] Maes et al. Increased serum IgA and IgM against LPS of enterobacteria in chronic fatigue syndrome (CFS): indication for the involvement of gram-negative enterobacteria in the etiology of CFS and for the presence of an increased gut-intestinal permeability. *J Affect Disord* 2007 Apr, 99:237–240
[458] Lakhan SE, Kirchgessner A. Gut inflammation in chronic fatigue syndrome. *Nutr Metab* (Lond). 2010 Oct 12;7:79
[459] Tana et al. Altered profiles of intestinal microbiota and organic acids may be the origin of symptoms in irritable bowel syndrome. *Neurogastroenterol Motil.* 2010 May;22(5):512-9, e114-5
[460] Zhou Q, Zhang B, Verne GN. Intestinal membrane permeability and hypersensitivity in the irritable bowel syndrome. *Pain.* 2009 Nov;146(1-2):41-6

have also found that increased intestinal membrane permeability is associated with visceral and thermal hypersensitivity in this subset of D-IBS patients. We evaluated 54 D-IBS patients and 22 controls for intestinal membrane permeability using the lactulose/mannitol method. ... We also evaluated the mean mechanical visual analogue scale (M-VAS) pain rating to nociceptive thermal and visceral stimulation in all subjects. ... Approximately 39% of diarrhea-predominant IBS patients had increased intestinal membrane permeability as measured by the lactulose/mannitol ratio. These IBS patients also demonstrated higher M-VAS pain intensity reading scale. Interestingly, the IBS patients with hypersensitivity and increased intestinal permeability had a higher Functional Bowel Disorder Severity Index (FBDSI) score (100.8 + or - 5.4) than IBS patients with normal membrane permeability and sensitivity (51.6 + or - 12.7) and controls (6.1 + or - 5.6) (p<0.001). A subset of D-IBS patients had increased intestinal membrane permeability that was associated with an increased FBDSI score and increased hypersensitivity to visceral and thermal nociceptive pain stimuli. Thus, increased intestinal membrane permeability in D-IBS patients may lead to more severe IBS symptoms and hypersensitivity to somatic and visceral stimuli."

- Antimicrobial/antibiotic treatment alleviates fibromyalgia in most FM patients, just as it also alleviates gastrointestinal symptoms in patients with irritable bowel syndrome (IBS): Finally and most importantly, **antimicrobial therapy alleviates FM (and IBS) symptoms in direct proportion to the success of bacterial overgrowth eradication**, thus adding strong direct evidence in support of SIBO as a main cause of FM.[461,462] Recent clinical trials have shown that treatment of the fibromyalgia-related conditions IBS and SIBO by use of the nonabsorbed oral antibiotic rifaximin results in significant diminution of IBS-SIBO symptomatology with benefits lasting after the discontinuation of therapy.[463,464]

  - Clinical trial: Rifaximin therapy for patients with irritable bowel syndrome without constipation (*New England Journal of Medicine* 2011 Jan[465]): Authors of this study evaluated rifaximin, a minimally absorbed antibiotic, as treatment for IBS. Subjects were given rifaximin at a dose of 550 mg or placebo, three times daily for 2 weeks and were followed for 10 weeks thereafter. "Significantly more patients in the rifaximin group than in the placebo group had adequate relief of global IBS symptoms during the first 4 weeks after treatment (40.8% vs. 31.2%). Similarly, more patients in the rifaximin group than in the placebo group had adequate relief of bloating (39.5% vs. 28.7%). In addition, significantly more patients in the rifaximin group had a response to treatment as assessed by daily ratings of IBS symptoms, bloating, abdominal pain, and stool consistency. The incidence of adverse events was similar in the two groups." Thus, among patients who had IBS without constipation, treatment with rifaximin for 2 weeks provided significant relief of IBS symptoms, bloating, abdominal pain, and loose or watery stools. *Comments by Dr Vasquez: Shortcomings of the intervention used in this IBS-rifaximin study include ❶ failure to use long-term treatment, which is often necessary in the treatment of chronic SIBO, ❷ failure to co-administer an antifungal agent to avert fungal growth in the intestines which commonly occurs as a result of antimicrobial/antibacterial drug treatment, ❸ failure to administer probiotics to re-establish beneficial flora, and ❹ failure to implement dietary modification to sustain the beneficial eradication of excess bacteria—allowing patients to continue their unhealthy diets and lifestyles is the most assured way to ensure that the condition (SIBO-IBS) will return.*

  - Review of clinical trials: Rifaximin as treatment for SIBO and IBS (*Expert Opinion on Investigational Drugs* 2009 Mar[466]): A recognized expert in the treatment of SIBO-related conditions, Dr Pimentel writes, "**Rifaximin is a broad-range, gastrointestinal-specific antibiotic that demonstrates no clinically relevant bacterial resistance**. Therefore, rifaximin may be useful in the treatment of gastrointestinal disorders associated with altered bacterial flora, including irritable bowel syndrome (IBS) and small intestinal bacterial overgrowth (SIBO)." He also notes regarding the use of rifaximin in the treatment of IBS, "Rifaximin improved global symptoms in 33 - 92% of patients and eradicated SIBO in up to 84% of patients with IBS, with results sustained up to 10 weeks post-treatment. Rifaximin caused a lower number of

[461] Wallace DJ, Hallegua DS. Fibromyalgia: the gastrointestinal link. *Curr Pain Headache Rep.* 2004 Oct;8(5):364-8
[462] Pimentel et al. Improvement of symptoms by eradication of small intestinal overgrowth in FM: a double-blind study. [Abstract] *Arthritis Rheum* 1999, 42:S343
[463] Pimentel et al. The effect of a nonabsorbed oral antibiotic (rifaximin) on the symptoms of the irritable bowel syndrome. *Ann Intern Med.* 2006 Oct 17;145(8):557-63
[464] Sharara et al. A randomized double-blind placebo-controlled trial of rifaximin in patients with abdominal bloating and flatulence. *Am J Gastroenterol.* 2006 Feb;101(2):326-33
[465] Pimentel M, Lembo A, Chey WD, et al. Rifaximin therapy for patients with irritable bowel syndrome without constipation. *N Engl J Med.* 2011 Jan 6;364(1):22-32
[466] Pimentel M. Review of rifaximin as treatment for SIBO and IBS. *Expert Opin Investig Drugs.* 2009 Mar;18(3):349-58

adverse events compared with metronidazole or levofloxacin and may have a more favorable adverse event profile than systemic antibiotics, without clinically relevant antibiotic resistance."

- <u>Results of two clinical trials of antibiotics in the treatment of fibromyalgia (*Current Pain and Headache Reports* 2004 Oct[467])</u>: This article discusses the results of two experiments using antibiotics in the treatment of FM: ❶ 96 patients with SIBO diagnosed by lactulose hydrogen breath testing (LHBT) were offered antibiotic treatment for the reduction of gastrointestinal bacteria; 25 of the 96 patients returned for a follow-up LHBT. Neomycin was the most commonly used antibiotic. Eleven of the 25 patients achieved complete transient eradication of SIBO after antibiotic treatment and experienced better improvement in more of their FM symptom scores when compared with the patients who did not achieve complete eradication. This indicates that **a direct relationship exists between the presence of SIBO and intestinal and extraintestinal symptoms in fibromyalgia, and that FM can be alleviated by effective antimicrobial/antibiotic treatment.** ❷ In this double-blind trial of eradication of SIBO in fibromyalgia, 46 patients fulfilling the established criteria for FM were tested for SIBO using LHBT. Forty-two of the 46 patients (91.3%) were positive for SIBO and were randomized to receive placebo or 500 mg of liquid neomycin (a minimally-absorbed gastrointestinal-specific antibiotic drug) twice daily for 10 days. Only six of the 20 patients (30%) in the neomycin group achieved eradication (indicating inefficacy of treatment); thus, no statistically significant difference between groups was available for analysis. Thereafter, 28 patients in the double-blind study testing positive for SIBO went on to receive open-label antibiotic treatment to eradicate SIBO, and this time 17 of the 28 patients (60.7%) achieved eradication of SIBO. When these 23 patients were compared with the 15 patients who failed to eradicate or did not undergo open-label treatment, significant improvement attributable to antibiotic treatment in the FM scores was detected. **Results show that eradication of bacterial overgrowth results in a clinically significant alleviation of FM symptoms.**

Most experienced functional medicine clinicians generally and naturopathic physicians specifically—collectively these are the clinicians with the most experience in the assessment and treatment of various forms of dysbiosis—will agree that ultimate correction of dysbiosis is no easy task. Many aspects must be addressed simultaneously, and these will be detailed in the section on *Therapeutics and Clinical Interventions*. For the here and now, I will simply outline some of the more common and important considerations, in no particular order because order implies importance, which implies effectiveness, which is dependent on the patient's response:

1. <u>Dietary optimization</u>: The diet must be diverse, varied, and plant-based in order to optimize microbial diversity and reduce intake of carbohydrates in general and simple carbohydrates in particular.
2. <u>Probiotic therapy</u>: Administering probiotics to patients who have SIBO can be effective or can cause exacerbations; patients might need to wait until other aspects are optimized before adding "good bacteria."
3. <u>Antimicrobial therapy</u>: Botanicals such as berberine, oregano oil, and others are safe and highly efficacious.
4. <u>Stimulation/normalization of peristalsis</u>: Magnesium and ascorbate can be used to promote laxation; optimization of thyroid function/status is of utmost importance. Exercise, water, relaxation, fiber are important.
5. <u>Systemic health optimization, stress reduction, sleep optimization</u>: Fatty acid intake (e.g., n3 fatty acids) and mitochondrial function need to be optimized in order to optimize gut flora. Stress promotes dysbiosis and microbial virulence; sleep deprivation impairs mitochondria, redox balance, hormones, and immunity.

In this space before diving into *Therapeutics and Clinical Interventions*, I'll briefly mention three concepts that are interrelated. ❶ Microbial identity and location are irrelevant, given that most of the adverse physiologic effects seen can be mediated by a wide range of Gram-negative bacteria; their identities and locations are irrelevant as long as they produce sufficient LPS. The only aspect that is almost entirely dependent on localization to the gut is the production of the mitochondrial neurotoxins H2S and D-lactate. ❷ Any combination of glial activation and mitochondrial dysfunction would be sufficient to induce the fibromyalgia phenotype; the agents most likely to accomplish both are pesticides and corporate toxins such as glyphosate, widely sprayed internationally and pervasive in the American food, air, and water supply. ❸ The variations in microbial combinations and total load, individual patient fragilities and vulnerabilities, nutritional status and xenobiotic permutations give rise to the nuances and variations in clinical presentations and therapeutic responses. However, the model presented

---

[467] Wallace DJ, Hallegua DS. Fibromyalgia: the gastrointestinal link. *Curr Pain Headache Rep.* 2004 Oct;8(5):364-8

throughout this section is an accurate description of the most important and common pathoetiologic considerations and clinical interventions; once these core considerations are addressed, others can be addressed with greater specific and overall efficacy.

Therapeutics and Clinical Interventions

- Overview: Treatments for FM should be ❶ science-based and should ❷ directly address the cause(s) of the disorder; treatments should be ❹ safe (generally) and ❺ effective and ❻ without potential for serious adverse effects. Drug treatment of FM does not meet these criteria; the integrative, nutritional, and functional medicine approaches outlined below can—when properly employed by a skilled clinician—address the cause(s) of FM in a way that is scientific, direct, safe, effective, and well tolerated by essentially all patients. **Treatments for FM must emphasize eradication of SIBO, prevention of SIBO recurrence, the restoration/establishment of optimal nutritional status, and specific support for optimal mitochondrial function; anything less than this will fail to be effective.** Clinical interventions for the treatment of SIBO include dietary carbohydrate restriction, normalization of slow gastrointestinal transit time (e.g., correction of hypothyroidism), selective use of probiotic supplements to normalize intestinal flora, support of mucosal immunity (with nutrients such as vitamin A, zinc, and L-glutamine), and eradication of bacterial overgrowth with drugs (such as ciprofloxacin, rifaximin, amoxicillin/Augmentin[468], metronidazole) and/or natural products (such as berberine[469], *Artemisia annua*, peppermint oil[470], and emulsified time-released oil of oregano[471])—each of these have been reviewed in greater detail elsewhere by this author.[472] Failure of any monotherapeutic approach to immediately resolve the clinical manifestations of FM can explained by the secondary metabolic, immune, and neurophysiological effects that have generally persisted over periods ranging from years to decades for most patients; in other words, the treatment program must be multifaceted in order to address the numerous major problems that cause FM, and the treatment plan must also be sustained long enough to correct the abnormal physiologic patterns that have been established by the body's response/adaptation to the disease process. The treatment program (examples provided) must be complete in order to facilitate correction of systemic oxidative damage (broad-spectrum antioxidant support), resultant nutritional deficiencies (diet optimization, vitamin and mineral supplementation), immune sensitization and induction of proinflammatory cycles (anti-inflammatory nutrition), alterations in neurotransmission and membrane receptor function (amino acid and fatty acid supplementation), and the inflammation-induced disturbances in pain reception and hypothalamic-pituitary-endocrine function (assess/correct hormonal imbalances; supplement with n-3 fatty acids and olive oil to reduce hypothalamic inflammation[473], etc.). Further, patients treated for SIBO who do not positively change their diets and lifestyles (which probably promoted the genesis and perpetuation of the disease-causing SIBO in the first place) are subject to continual recurrence until such changes are implemented and faithfully maintained.

FOOD & NUTRITION As with many rheumatologic/painful/inflammatory conditions with a strong component of gastrointestinal dysbiosis, the single best diet is a vegan or pesco-vegetarian diet free of gluten and most grains (judicious use of brown rice excepted); clearly the diet must emphasize vegetable intake and avoidance of fermentable substrate to induce quantitative reductions and qualitative improvements in microbial populations and metabolic activity. Beyond the gut, the benefits of minimized carbohydrate intake include weight loss (generally beneficial in this patient population), alleviation of physiologic and psychologic dependence on carbohydrate (over)consumption, and increased endogenous production of beta-hydroxy-butyrate which stimulates the terminal complexes of the mitochondrial electron transport chain while also promoting histone acetylation (via inhibition of histone deacetylase) for enhanced DNA transcription resulting in what has been referred to as a rejuvenative phenotype. My foundational diet-nutritional program—the 5-part "supplemented Paleo-Mediterranean Diet"—can easily be modified to pesco-vegetarian or lacto-pesco-vegetarian variants to

[468] Malik BA, Xie YY, Wine E, Huynh HQ. Diagnosis and pharmacological management of small intestinal bacterial overgrowth in children with intestinal failure. *Can J Gastroenterol.* 2011 Jan;25(1):41-5. This is a remarkable article and probably one of the most brilliant articles on the treatment of SIBO with drugs.
[469] [No authors listed] Berberine. *Altern Med Rev.* 2000 Apr;5(2):175-7
[470] "A case report of a patient with SIBO who showed marked subjective improvement in IBS-like symptoms and significant reductions in hydrogen production after treatment with ECPO is presented. While further investigation is necessary, results in this case suggest one of mechanisms by which ECPO improves IBS symptoms is antimicrobial activity in small intestine." Logan et al. Treatment of small intestinal bacterial overgrowth with enteric-coated peppermint oil: a case report. *Altern Med Rev.* 2002 Oct;7(5):410-7
[471] Force M, Sparks WS, Ronzio RA. Inhibition of enteric parasites by emulsified oil of oregano in vivo. *Phytother Res.* 2000 May;14(3):213-4
[472] Vasquez A. Nutritional and Botanical Treatments against "Silent Infections" and Gastrointestinal Dysbiosis. *Nutr Perspect* 2006; Jan: 5-21 ichnfm.academia.edu/AlexVasquez
[473] Milanski et al. Saturated fatty acids produce inflammatory response predominantly through activation of TLR4 signaling in hypothalamus. *J Neurosci.* 2009 Jan;29(2):359-70

enhance high-quality protein intake while continuing to emphasize vegetable, nut, and seed intake to maximize fiber and micronutrient intake. In particular, whey protein isolate is attractive in this patient population due to the high content of tryptophan (to correct the common tryptophan deficiency), the glutathione precursors (to alleviate oxidative stress and enhance mitochondrial function), immunoglobulins (to support mucosal defenses against bacterial overgrowth), and growth factors including whey's insulotrophic effect to promote anabolism with resultant improvements in muscle function and gut mucosal integrity. Systemic alkalinization supported by plant-based potassium citrate promotes xenobiotic excretion (reduction in total load of persistent organic pollutants and toxic metals such as lead and mercury) and endogenous production of endorphins (enhanced mood, pain relief). The increased intake of vitamins (including physiologic doses of vitamin D3), minerals, ALA, GLA, EPA, DHA, and probiotics all synergize to alleviate SIBO, oxidative stress, pain and inflammation while also promoting optimal immune and mitochondrial functions. Allergy identification and avoidance is easily achieved via the very practical and no-cost elimination-and-challenge technique. In particular for patients with fibromyalgia, magnesium intake is increased via consumption of dark green vegetables and nutritional supplements while magnesium absorption is promoted by optimized vitamin D status while renal retention of magnesium is promoted with urinary alkalinization. The consistent and pathologic secondary tryptophan deficiency is foremost corrected by eradicating the causative SIBO and the resultant intraintestinal bacterial tryptophanase-catalyzed degradation of ingested tryptophan and via dietary supplementation with L-tryptophan, 5-hydroxytryptophan, and/or whey protein isolate.

> **Dr Vasquez's summary of the medical indication for gluten-containing grains/foods**
>
> The only medical indication for the consumption of gluten-containing grains is prevention/treatment of acute starvation, assuming no other food is available.

- Diet optimization with the five-part "supplemented Paleo-Mediterranean Diet" (*Nutr Perspect* 2011 Jan[474]): The "supplemented Paleo-Mediterranean Diet" (SPMD)—the 5-part nutritional wellness protocol—as described in most of my textbooks in "chapter 2" and also in my articles available on-line at ichnfm.academia.edu/AlexVasquez should be implemented for most FM patients; exceptions to this general rule might include patients with renal insufficiency due to the risk for potassium excess (hyperkalemia [Note 475]). Because any patient might have an allergy or intolerance to any food (even a healthy food like citrus fruit, chicken or eggs), patients and doctors must be aware of the potential for food allergies and will therefore have to customize the Paleo-Mediterranean diet *for each individual patient* to exclude foods to which the patient might be allergic or sensitive/intolerant. Otherwise, this 5-part nutrition protocol is based on ❶ vegetables, nuts, seeds, (berries, fruits, and juices generally have to be avoided during treatment for SIBO due to the high content of sugars and—with juice—the rapid passage through the gastrointestinal tract) and lean sources of protein, ❷ high-potency multivitamin and multimineral supplementation, ❸ physiologic doses of vitamin D3 to optimize blood levels of vitamin D3 (measured as 25-OH-vitamin D), ❹ combination fatty acid supplementation (with flax oil [for ALA], fish oil [for EPA and DHA], and borage oil [for GLA] with oleic acid from olive oil incorporated into the diet), and ❺ probiotics—foods or supplements that contain living bacteria with beneficial qualities. The diet should emphasize strict avoidance of grains in general and gluten-containing grains *especially wheat* in particular. This diet is essential for the provision of sufficient protein, fiber, phytonutrients, and alkalinization—potassium citrate is most concentrated in vegetables and helps the body maintain proper acid-alkaline balance.[476] The diet should be low in carbohydrates to reduce fermentable substrate to intestinal bacteria. The most important books for patients to read in support of this diet are *The Paleo Diet* by Dr Loren Cordain and *Breaking the Vicious Cycle* by Elaine Gottschall.

---

[474] Vasquez A. Revisiting the Five-Part Nutritional Wellness Protocol: Supplemented Paleo-Mediterranean Diet. *Nutr Perspect* 2011 Jan Ichnfm.academia.edu/AlexVasquez

[475] Because the kidneys are responsible for excreting potassium, reduced kidney function (kidney failure, renal insufficiency) implies that the kidneys may not be able to perform the function of excreting potassium; thus, consumption of a potassium-rich diet could contribute to a dangerous situation of excess potassium in the blood known as hyperkalemia (*hyper*=too much, *kal*=potassium, *emia*=blood disorder). For patients with renal insufficiency, consumption of an otherwise health-promoting diet rich in fruits and vegetables might cause a problem if potassium accumulates in the blood due to impaired excretion. Blood tests can assess renal function as well as the blood potassium level. This is one example of why a clinician/doctor should be employed by patients before implementing diet modification and nutritional supplementation.

[476] "The modern Western-type diet is deficient in fruits and vegetables and contains excessive animal products, generating the accumulation of non-metabolizable anions and a lifespan state of overlooked metabolic acidosis, whose magnitude increases progressively with aging due to the physiological decline in kidney function." Adeva MM, Souto G. Diet-induced metabolic acidosis. *Clin Nutr*. 2011 Aug;30(4):416-21

- Vegetarian diet: Fibromyalgia syndrome improved using a mostly raw vegetarian diet (*BMC Complementary and Alternative Medicine* 2001 Sep[477]): Diets high in fruits, vegetables, nuts, berries, and seeds provide ample fiber to promote laxation and can be useful as adjunctive treatment for gastrointestinal dysbiosis in general and SIBO in particular (i.e., *quantitative* reduction in GI dysbiosis). Perhaps more importantly, plant-based diets result in *qualitative* benefits by changing microbial behavior and reducing production of irritants, toxins, and bacterial metabolites, including the mitochondrial poisons D-lactate and hydrogen sulfide. Fibromyalgia patients who consume a mostly vegetarian diet have experienced significant improvements in function and reductions in FM symptomatology. Poorly designed dietary interventions that allow abundant intake of whole-grain bread, pasta, rice, and fruit juice[478] would be expected to fail because such high-carbohydrate diets feed intestinal bacteria with an abundance of substrate and would therefore be expected to sustain or exacerbate SIBO. Another advantage to a plant-based mostly-raw diet is the avoidance of dietary advanced glycation end-products (AGEs) which are inflammation-promoting chemical combinations of proteins with sugars, which can be consumed in the diet (e.g., baked deserts) or formed endogenously/internally as a result of oxidative stress and elevated blood sugar levels (e.g., diabetes mellitus). As discussed previously, FM patients show higher levels of AGEs in blood cells and muscle tissue; AGEs promote chronic pain and inflammation[479], and therefore dietary and nutritional strategies that reduce AGE intake and/or AGE formation are 1) without risk, and 2) likely to provide manifold health benefits, including but not limited to reductions in pain and inflammation.

Dr Vasquez's Nutrition Protocol: The 5-part "Supplemented Paleo-Mediterranean Diet" (5pSPMD or SMPD)

1. **Diet: Emphasize fruits, vegetables, nuts, seeds, berries, and lean sources of protein** (fish, grass-fed lamb/beef). Minimize fruit intake due to higher sugar content while treating SIBO; the goal is to deprive the bacteria and yeast in the intestines of their preferred food source (carbohydrates, sugars). Make modifications for patient-specific food allergies and sensitivities; this is especially important for patients with known allergy-related conditions such as migraine headaches. Patients with kidney disease should use caution when consuming a potassium-rich diet. Vasquez A. Revisiting the Five-Part Nutritional Wellness Protocol: The Supplemented Paleo-Mediterranean Diet. *Nutritional Perspectives* 2011 Jan

2. **Multivitamin and multimineral supplement**: Nutrient deficiencies are common and are easily treated with nutritional supplementation. Fletcher and Fairfield. Vitamins for chronic disease prevention in adults. *JAMA* 2002 Jun

3. **Vitamin D dosed at 2,000-10,000 IU per day**: The adult requirement for vitamin D3 is approximately 4,000 IU per day; some patients may achieve optimal blood levels with lower doses, but generally daily doses of 4,000-10,000 IU are necessary. Vasquez et al. Clinical Importance of Vitamin D. *Alternative Therapies in Health and Medicine* 2004 Sep

4. **Combination fatty acid supplementation**: A combination of flax oil, borage oil, and fish oil provides the health-promoting fatty acids (ALA, GLA, EPA, DHA). Patients should consume organic virgin olive oil liberally with foods. Vasquez A. New Insights into Fatty Acid Supplementation and Its Effect on Eicosanoid Production and Genetic Expression. *Nutritional Perspectives* 2005; Jan

5. **Probiotics**: Health-promoting bacteria can be consumed in the form of powders, pills, and fermented foods such as yogurt, kefir, pickles and sauerkraut.

For a video review of this foundational diet and introduction to the functional inflammology protocol, see Dr Vasquez "Functional Inflammology Protocol, part 1: Introduction and Foundational Diet" from the 2013 International Conference on Human Nutrition and Functional Medicine: https://vimeo.com/100089988 Password: "DrVprotocol_volume1"

- Vitamin B12 in the form of hydroxo-/methyl-/adenosyl-cobalamin, should be administered to all FM and CFS patients to alleviate pain, glial inflammation, accelerated neurodegeneration; reasonable doses are at least 2,000 mcg per day orally and/or 2,000 mcg per week by subcutaneous/intramuscular injection: Given that sulfur-containing molecules such as sulfite and hydrogen sulfide bind to vitamin B12[480,481], we should reasonably expect that patients with excess exposure to H2S from the gastrointestinal tract would have an increased prevalence of vitamin B12 deficiency, and indeed this has been documented; vitamin B12 deficiency in CFS and FM patients promotes fatigue and brain dysfunction via the effects of vitamin B12 deficiency directly (ie, vitamin B12 deficiency is well known to cause nerve damage and brain damage) and indirectly via impaired

[477] Donaldson et al. Fibromyalgia syndrome improved using a mostly raw vegetarian diet. *BMC Complement Altern Med.* 2001;1:7 biomedcentral.com/1472-6882/1/7

[478] Michalsen et al. Mediterranean diet or extended fasting's influence on changing the intestinal microflora, immunoglobulin A secretion and clinical outcome in patients with rheumatoid arthritis and fibromyalgia: an observational study. *BMC Complement Altern Med.* 2005 Dec 22;5:22

[479] "In the interstitial connective tissue of fibromyalgic muscles we found a more intensive staining of the AGE CML, activated NF-kappaB, and also higher CML levels in the serum of these patients compared to the controls. RAGE was only present in FM muscle." Rüster et al. Detection of elevated N epsilon-carboxymethyllysine levels in muscular tissue and in serum of patients with fibromyalgia. *Scand J Rheumatol.* 2005 Nov-Dec;34(6):460-3

[480] Añíbarro et al. Asthma with sulfite intolerance in children: a blocking study with cyanocobalamin. *J Allergy Clin Immunol.* 1992 Jul;90(1):103-9

[481] Fujita et al. A fatal case of acute hydrogen sulfide poisoning caused by hydrogen sulfide: hydroxocobalamin therapy for acute H2S poisoning. *J Anal Toxicol.* 2011 Mar:119-23

metabolism of homocysteine, which then triggers pain sensitivity and accelerated neurodegeneration via activation of NMDA receptors in the brain.

- ▪ Patients with FM and CFS have decreased vitamin B12 and increased homocysteine in the fluid surrounding the brain while blood test results are generally normal. (*Scand J Rheumatol.* 1997[482]): "Twelve outpatients, all women, who fulfilled the criteria for both fibromyalgia and chronic fatigue syndrome were rated on 15 items of the Comprehensive Psychopathological Rating Scale (CPRS-15). ... Blood laboratory levels were generally normal. The most obvious finding was that, in all the patients, the homocysteine (HCY) levels were increased in the cerebrospinal fluid (CSF). There was a significant positive correlation between CSF-HCY levels and fatigability, and the levels of CSF-B12 correlated significantly with the item of fatigability and with CPRS-15. The correlations between vitamin B12 and clinical variables of the CPRS-scale in this study indicate that low CSF-B12 values are of clinical importance. Vitamin B12 deficiency causes a deficient remethylation of HCY and is therefore probably contributing to the increased homocysteine levels found in our patient group. We conclude that increased homocysteine levels in the central nervous system characterize patients fulfilling the criteria for both fibromyalgia and chronic fatigue syndrome."

- • Folic acid in the form of folinic acid or methylfolate ("5-methyltetrahydrofolate" or "5-MTHF"): Most nutrition-knowledgeable doctors do not use "folic acid" in the form of folic acid due to concerns about increased free radical generation and possible increased risk of cellular damage and malignant disease; we still use the term "folic acid" but nowadays this is—in practice—meant to imply the use of either folinic acid or methylfolate, two forms of folic acid that are considered safer, if not also more effective. Strictly speaking, "folic acid" refers to the synthetic form of the vitamin, whereas "folate" refers to derivatives of tetrahydrofolate that are found in food, especially leafy green vegetables, of which most people do not consume a sufficient amount. Some people develop antibodies against the folic acid transporter (cerebral folate receptor autoantibodies) that facilitates entry of folate into the brain, and they must receive either folinic acid or methylfolate to avoid neurologic devastation due to cerebral folate deficiency, wherein blood/serum levels of folate are normal but the brain (on the other side of the "wall" formed by the blood-brain barrier) is starved for this nutrient.[483] Folic acid from diet and/or supplementation serves many roles and thereby provides numerous benefits, largely centered on the provision of single-carbon methyl groups for metabolic processes (e.g., homocysteine metabolism) and DNA methylation, which regulates/suppresses gene transcription and thereby reduces risk of cancer and viral activation (e.g., cervical cancer following exposure to the human papilloma virus [HPV][484]). In this conversation, we are primarily concerned with optimizing folate intake to optimize "neurologic function" (i.e., generally speaking: normalization of homocysteine-mediated NMDAr activation in the brain, spinal cord and periphery) by reducing homocysteine levels because elevated homocysteine levels will cause excessive pain/fatigue/depression due to activation of the NMDA-receptor, mostly in the brain but also in the periphery. The most important nutrients for reducing homocysteine are folate (vitamin B9), pyridoxine (vitamin B6), cobalamin (vitamin B12) and the amino acid N-acetyl-cysteine (NAC); some people have a defect in their ability to convert folate into its active form via the enzyme methylenetetrahydrofolate reductase (MTHFR) and therefore need more nutritional supplementation to push this sluggish pathway to metabolic completion and reduce/normalize homocysteine levels. Increased consumption of folate from diet and/or supplements can alleviate depression, fatigue, and pain and is therefore recommended for all "pain patients", including those with migraine, fibromyalgia, and chronic fatigue syndrome. Adult doses of folate 1-5 mg (1,000-5,000 mcg) per day are reasonable and should be coadministered with a roughly equal amount of vitamin B12. Anti-seizure drugs (especially phenytoin, carbamazepine, barbiturates[485]), some of which are used in the treatment of

---

[482] Regland et al. Increased concentrations of homocysteine in the cerebrospinal fluid in patients with fibromyalgia and chronic fatigue syndrome. *Scand J Rheumatol.* 1997;26(4):301-7

[483] Gordon N. Cerebral folate deficiency. *Dev Med Child Neurol.* 2009 Mar;51(3):180-2

[484] Piyathilake et al. Indian women with higher serum concentrations of folate and vitamin B12 are significantly less likely to be infected with carcinogenic or high-risk (HR) types of human papillomaviruses (HPVs). *Int J Womens Health.* 2010 Aug 9;2:7-12

[485] Morrell MJ. Folic Acid and Epilepsy. *Epilepsy Curr.* 2002 Mar;2(2):31-34

migraine and chronic pain, are notorious for causing folate deficiency and homocysteine elevation[486]; obviously, the drugs would paradoxically promote pain and seizure if folate deficiency develops—coadministration of folate with anti-seizure drugs should be supervised by the prescribing physician. Diagrams illustrating these pathways tend to be repulsively complex, immemorably curvaceous, or incomplete and thereby unusable; the illustration below is perhaps the most simple for efficient understanding of the means by which nutritional supplementation lowers homocysteine levels.

- **Positive response to vitamin B12 and folic acid in myalgic encephalomyelitis and fibromyalgia (*PLoS One*. 2015 Apr[487]):** "The individual doses of B12 and folic acid, as well as the form of B12 used (i.e. hydroxocobalamin or methylcobalamin), had been due to individual decisions made by the five doctors in interplay with their patients – to a large extent following common sense in a process of trial and error – and limited by the patient's desire and the doctor's permission. It was a general experience that the patients deteriorated when returning to oral treatment, or when the injection interval was prolonged. After such a dose-finding period, they continued injective B12 therapy and learned how to self-administer the injections. In Sweden, the common form of B12 injective substrate has for more than forty years been hydroxocobalamin, provided in 1 mL ampoules with 1 mg/mL. By the end of last century, also methylcobalamin became available, in 2 mL ampoules with 5 mg/mL; i.e. an ampoule of methylcobalamin contains ten times more cobalamin than an ampoule of hydroxocobalamin. Folate in pharmacological doses is available by using tablets of folic acid (1 mg or 5 mg). ... Frequent injections of high-concentrated vitamin B12, combined with an individual daily dose of oral folic acid, may provide blood saturations high enough to be a remedy for good and safe relief in a subgroup of patients with ME/FM. Moreover, we suspect a counteracting interference between B12/folic acid and certain opioid analgesics and other drugs which have to be demethylated as part of their metabolism. Furthermore, it is important to be alert on co-existing thyroid dysfunction."

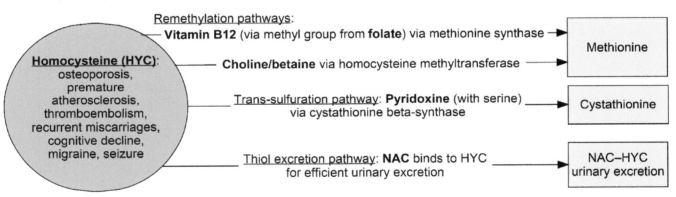

Lowering homocysteine (HYC) via nutritional supplementation: Folate gives methyl group to cobalamin (vitamin B12) to convert HYC via methionine synthase to methionine; choline/betaine can remethylate homocysteine via homocysteine methyltransferase to form methionine. Pyridoxine promotes conversion of HYC via cystathionine beta-synthase to cystathionine. The amino acid N-acetyl-cysteine (NAC) binds to HYC for efficient renal excretion of NAC-HYC.[488]

- **Tryptophan and 5-hydroxytryptophan (5-HTP):** Tryptophan is an amino acid found in many foods and is essential for human health and survival. Tryptophan is available as a nutritional supplement only by a doctor's prescription; it is available over-the-counter in a nonprescription supplement in the form of 5-hydroxytryptophan (5-HTP), which is commonly sourced from the seeds of *Griffonia simplicifolia*, a woody climbing shrub native to West and Central Africa. Tryptophan is the precursor to the neurotransmitter serotonin, which has antidepressant, anti-anxiety, and analgesic properties. Patients with FM are known to have low blood levels (i.e., functional nutritional insufficiency) of tryptophan, and the severity of the deficiency

[486] "Patients who consume antiepileptic drugs are susceptible to high levels of homocysteine and low levels of folate in the blood." Paknahad et al. Effects of Common Anti-epileptic Drugs on the Serum Levels of Homocysteine and Folic Acid. *Int J Prev Med*. 2012 Mar;3(Suppl 1):S186-90
[487] Regland et al. Response to vitamin B12 and folic acid in myalgic encephalomyelitis and fibromyalgia. *PLoS One*. 2015 Apr 22;10(4):e0124648
[488] "NAC intravenous administration induces an efficient and rapid reduction of plasma thiols, particularly of Hcy; our data support the hypothesis that NAC displaces thiols from their binding protein sites and forms, in excess of plasma NAC, mixed disulphides (NAC-Hcy) with an high renal clearance." Ventura et al. N-Acetyl-cysteine reduces homocysteine plasma levels after single intravenous administration by increasing thiols urinary excretion. *Pharmacol Res*. 1999 Oct;40(4):345-50

correlates with the severity of pain.[489,490,491] Blood levels of serotonin are often below normal in FM patients.[492] The accepted *medical-pharmacological* use of selective serotonin reuptake inhibitors (SSRI) drugs to treat the pain, depression, and anxiety associated with FM supports the use of 5-HTP to raise serotonin levels *naturally* by correcting the underlying nutritional insufficiency. As an over-the-counter nutritional supplement, the 5-hydroxylated form of tryptophan (5-HTP) has been used clinically and in numerous research studies. **Supplementation with 5-HTP has been shown to significantly alleviate symptoms of fibromyalgia.**[493] Commonly used doses range from 50 to 300 mg/d, with larger doses divided throughout the day. If tryptophan rather than 5-HTP is used, results are improved when taken on an empty stomach with carbohydrate (such as honey or fruit juice) to induce insulin secretion, which preferentially promotes uptake of tryptophan into the brain. Deficiency of either magnesium or vitamin B6 impairs conversion of 5-HTP into serotonin, and therefore the interventional program must ensure nutritional supra-sufficiency.

- Primary fibromyalgia syndrome and 5-hydroxy-L-tryptophan: a 90-day open study (*Journal of Internal Medicine Research* 1992 Apr[494]): An open 90-day study in 50 fibromyalgia patients showed significant improvement in all measured parameters (number of tender points, anxiety, pain intensity, quality of sleep, fatigue) after treatment with 5-HTP; global clinical improvement assessed by the patient and the investigator indicated a "good" or "fair" response in nearly 50% of the patients during the treatment period.

- Double-blind study of 5-hydroxytryptophan versus placebo in the treatment of primary fibromyalgia syndrome (*Journal of Internal Medicine Research* 1990 May-Jun[495]): A double-blind, placebo-controlled study using 5-HTP in 50 fibromyalgia patients showed significant improvement in all measured parameters, with only mild and transient side effects. *Note by DrV: Again, the common dose range for 5-HTP is 50 to 300 mg per day with doses greater than 100 mg generally best divided throughout the day (e.g., 50 mg thrice per day). I generally recommend starting with 50-100 mg about one hour before bedtime, then adding incremental additions of 50 mg throughout the day for a maximum daily dose of 300 mg. Effectiveness is increased with additional supplementation with magnesium, vitamin B6 (pyridoxine), and the fatty acids found in fish oil (EPA and DHA).*

- Magnesium: Magnesium deficiency is epidemic in industrialized societies due to insufficient dietary intake (e.g., from mineral water and leafy green vegetables) and concomitant metabolic-urinary acidosis, which increases urinary magnesium loss.[496,497] Additional causes of magnesium deficiency in fibromyalgia patients include vitamin D deficiency, malabsorption due to SIBO, and the stress of chronic illness. Magnesium deficiency exacerbates the symptoms of fibromyalgia by contributing to impairment of energy/ATP production in skeletal muscle, increased muscle tone and spasms (hypomagnesemic tetany), and anxiety and increased pain sensitivity—hyperalgesia via NMDA receptor overstimulation and neurocortical hyperexcitability. Magnesium deficiency also promotes constipation and intestinal stasis, which exacerbates SIBO. Magnesium supplementation (600 mg or to bowel tolerance to a limit of 1,500 mg in divided doses [bowel tolerance is defined as the dose—commonly of magnesium or vitamin C—that produces slightly loose stools due to the osmotic laxative effect]) should be used routinely in fibromyalgia patients; the primary cautions with magnesium use are renal insufficiency and the use of magnesium-sparing drugs such as the diuretic drug spironolactone. Modest benefits demonstrated in clinical trials with magnesium and malic acid[498] can easily be exceeded with concomitant interventions to address vitamin D deficiency, SIBO, and mitochondrial dysfunction.

- Vitamin C, ascorbate: Textbooks[499] and recent metaanalyses[500,501] consistently advocate use of ascorbic acid (ascorbate) 500-1,500 mg/d x50 days for the prevention of CRPS following trauma or surgery, especially to/of

[489] Moldofsky H, Warsh JJ. Plasma tryptophan and musculoskeletal pain in non-articular rheumatism ("fibrositis syndrome"). *Pain*. 1978 Jun;5(1):65-71
[490] Yunus MB, Dailey JW, Aldag JC, Masi AT, Jobe PC. Plasma tryptophan and other amino acids in primary fibromyalgia: a controlled study. *J Rheumatol*. 1992 Jan;19(1):90-4
[491] Russell IJ, Michalek JE, Vipraio GA, Fletcher EM, Wall K. Serum amino acids in fibrositis/fibromyalgia syndrome. *J Rheumatol* Suppl. 1989 Nov;19:158-63
[492] Wolfe F, Russell IJ, Vipraio G, Ross K, Anderson J. Serotonin levels, pain threshold, and fibromyalgia symptoms in the general population. *J Rheumatol*. 1997;24(3):555-9
[493] Caruso I, et al. Double-blind study of 5-hydroxytryptophan versus placebo in the treatment of primary fibromyalgia syndrome. *J Int Med Res*. 1990 May-Jun;18(3):201-9
[494] Sarzi Puttini P, Caruso I. Primary fibromyalgia syndrome and 5-hydroxy-L-tryptophan: a 90-day open study. *J Int Med Res*. 1992 Apr;20(2):182-9
[495] Caruso I et al. Double-blind study of 5-hydroxytryptophan versus placebo in the treatment of primary fibromyalgia syndrome. *J Int Med Res*. 1990 May-Jun;18(3):201-9
[496] Cordain L, et al. Origins and evolution of the Western diet: health implications for the 21st century. *Am J Clin Nutr*. 2005 Feb;81(2):341-54
[497] Rylander R, Remer T, Berkemeyer S, Vormann J. Acid-base status affects renal magnesium losses in healthy, elderly persons. *J Nutr*. 2006 Sep;136(9):2374-7
[498] Russell et al. Treatment of fibromyalgia syndrome with Super Malic: randomized, double blind, placebo controlled, crossover pilot study. *J Rheumatol*. 1995 May;22(5):953-8
[499] Papadakis, Maxine; McPhee, Stephen J.; Rabow, Michael W. *Current Medical Diagnosis and Treatment 2014*. McGraw-Hill Education.
[500] Shibuya et al. Efficacy and safety of high-dose vitamin C on complex regional pain syndrome in extremity trauma and surgery. *J Foot Ankle Surg*. 2013 Jan-Feb;52(1):62-6
[501] Meena et al. Role of vitamin C in prevention of complex regional pain syndrome after distal radius fractures. *Eur J Orthop Surg Traumatol*. 2015 May;25(4):637-41

the upper or lower limb. Mechanisms of action include the antioxidant effect[502] (thereby protecting the microvasculature following trauma) and the healing effect (promotion of bone and connective tissue repair, via hydroxyproline). Ascorbate also promotes mitochondrial function at cytochrome c, between complexes 3 and 4. My personal hypothesis is that ascorbate provides analgesic benefits via enhancement of central dopaminergic mechanisms and—via its ability to lower histamine levels (38% reduction following oral administration of ascorbate 2g/d)[503]—alleviation of neurogenic inflammation's vicious cycle, within which histamine plays a major role.[504] Appreciating its safety and efficacy in treating neuropathic, postsurgical, and migraine pain[505,506], I think all patients with pain should receive ascorbate 2-6 grams daily in divided doses. Two potential contraindications to vitamin C supplementation are iron overload and renal insufficiency.

- **S-adenosylmethionine (SAMe)**: Studies using oral or intravenous administration of the nutritional supplement SAMe have reported conflicting results; however, the overall trend seems to indicate that SAMe (800 mg/d orally) is safe and beneficial in the treatment of fibromyalgia.[507] SAMe helps maintain mitochondrial function by preserving glutathione, and its contribution of methyl groups is important for the regulation of gene expression and neurotransmitter synthesis. *Comment: I do not regularly use this supplement, and I would only use it as a last resort if nothing else had worked or if a particular patient had a specific indication for this supplement.*

INFECTIONS & DYSBIOSIS As reviewed in a previous section, fibromyalgia patients have a remarkably high prevalence of occult SIBO, the severity of which directly correlates with the severity of FM symptomatology and the eradication of which directly correlates with alleviation of FM. SIBO is the single primary pathoetiologic mechanism that explains each and every abnormality seen in this condition; the response of fibromyalgia patients to gastrointestinal-specific nonabsorbable antimicrobial treatments such as rifaximin provides diagnostic proof of effective treatment of the causative SIBO. Jejunal aspiration is expensive, inconvenient, cumbersome, invasive, and not completely sensitive, while breath hydrogen and methane testing is also cumbersome and relatively expensive (especially when compared to making a clinical diagnosis and confirmatory treatment) and is likewise not completely reliable. Post-prandial gas and bloating is a reliable clinical indicator of SIBO, and empiric treatment of SIBO with a low-carbohydrate diet (LCD) and antimicrobial agents that results in clinical improvement (which may include alleviation of musculoskeletal pain, improved cognition, alleviation of fatigue, and—especially in elderly patients—alleviation of malabsorption and malnutrition) confirms the diagnosis. Stated more plainly, effective implementation of LCD with antimicrobial treatment is both diagnostic and therapeutic; this allows the diagnosis to be made efficiently and with high specificity, (sensitivity depends upon efficacy) and bypassing expensive/insensitive/nontherapeutic/cumbersome diagnostic methods expedites physicians' efficacy and patients' relief in a manner that is safe and cost-effective, especially when compared to perpetual nontherapeutic symptomatic polypharmacy.

- **Low-carbohydrate diet, specific-carbohydrate diet**: Patients can follow a diet that emphasizes consumption of low-carbohydrate vegetables, nuts, and seeds and excludes grains (especially wheat, which is very highly fermentable), starches from foods such as potatoes, and disaccharides such as lactose and sucrose; most of the characteristics of a competent low-carbohydrate diet can be achieved within a "Paleo diet" such as described and popularized by Cordain. Alternatively or additionally, patients can follow the specific-carbohydrate diet described and popularized by Gottschall.
- **Probiotics**: Probiotics are beneficial bacteria that can be consumed in foods or as nutritional supplements to populate the gut, particularly following antibiotic use or long-term dietary neglect. In addition to their availability in capsules and powders, probiotics are widely consumed in the form of yogurt, kefir, and other cultured foods, and they have an excellent record of safety. Probiotic supplements are available in different strengths (quantity), potencies (viability), and combinations of bacteria (diversity). Some probiotics also contain fermentable carbohydrates (prebiotics) such as fructooligosaccharides (FOS) and inulin, which are substrates to nourish the beneficial bacteria. From a practical clinical perspective, the clinician can choose probiotic foods and supplements and instruct the patient to use these on an ongoing, periodic, or rotational basis. Probiotics

---

[502] Kapoor S. Vitamin C and its emerging role in pain management: beneficial effects in pain conditions besides post herpetic neuralgia. *Korean J Pain*. 2012 Jul;25(3):200-1
[503] Johnston CS, Martin LJ, Cai X. Antihistamine effect of supplemental ascorbic acid and neutrophil chemotaxis. *J Am Coll Nutr*. 1992 Apr;11(2):172-6
[504] Rosa AC, Fantozzi R. The role of histamine in neurogenic inflammation. *Br J Pharmacol*. 2013 Sep;170(1):38-45
[505] Hasanzadeh Kiabi et al. Can vitamin C be used as an adjuvant for managing postoperative pain? A short literature review. *Korean J Pain*. 2013 Apr;26(2):209-10
[506] Mohseni M. Use of vitamin C as placebo in anesthesiology. *Anesth Pain Med*. 2013 Winter;2(3):141
[507] Leventhal LJ. Management of fibromyalgia. *Ann Intern Med*. 1999 Dec 7;131(11):850-8

(i.e., bacteria only) may have a therapeutic advantage over prebiotics or synbiotics (probiotics+prebiotics) when treating SIBO because the fermentable carbohydrate in prebiotics and synbiotics may exacerbate the preexisting bacterial overgrowth by providing already overpopulated bacteria with additional substrate. The benefits of probiotic supplementation have been demonstrated in patients with IBS, rotavirus infection, eczema and increased intestinal permeability, and SIBO associated with renal failure. To date, no studies using probiotics in the treatment of fibromyalgia have been published.

- **Antimicrobial agents**: Antimicrobial agents can be categorized as either natural or pharmaceutical, and as absorbable and systemic or nonabsorbable and gastrointestinal-specific. These can be used empirically, as such treatment for suspected SIBO is well documented in the peer-reviewed clinical medicine literature; however, clinicians must always consider risk-to-benefit ratios especially when using the pharmaceutical antimicrobials which can induce systemic adverse effects (e.g., drug allergy or Stevens-Johnson syndrome or quinolone tendonopathy) or gastrointestinal adverse effects (e.g., nonspecific diarrhea, yeast overgrowth, *Clostridium difficile* diarrhea). Clinicians must always determine the proper choice and dose of therapeutic agents per patient. Two of the best and most important articles on the subject of SIBO are "Lin HC. Small intestinal bacterial overgrowth: a framework for understanding irritable bowel syndrome. *JAMA* 2004 Aug" (concepts and system-wide pathophysiology) and "Malik et al. Diagnosis and pharmacological management of small intestinal bacterial overgrowth in children with intestinal failure. *Can J Gastroenterol* 2011 Jan" (excellent sections on clinical diagnosis and pharmacologic management emphasizing rotational implementation of gut-specific antimicrobials). I prefer to use natural antimicrobial agents continuously for an extended period of time either alone or in conjunction with pharmaceutical antibacterial drugs, which I tend to use on a rotating basis of 7-14 days. Occasionally I will use a short course of an antiparasitic drug such as metronidazole or tinidazole, and I nearly always implement an extended course of antifungal treatment—either oregano oil or nystatin as nonabsorbable agents—punctuated by fluconazole/Diflucan if I suspect treatment resistant gastrointestinal yeast or any dermatologic or sinorespiratory yeast. Clinicians should appreciate that *yeast* colonization of the intestines promotes *bacterial* colonization of the intestines via—for example—elaboration by *Candida albicans* of a sIgA-protease and gliotoxin, an appreciated immunosuppressant. The following list emphasizes the antimicrobial agents I most commonly utilize, always in conjunction with nutritional supplementation (to restore immune function and mucosal defenses) and reduction in dietary carbohydrate intake (to reduce fermentable substrate and thereby "starve the microbes"). Although some dosage and duration suggestions are provided, the clinical reality is that patients need to be treated with *"dose and duration to effect"* or *"titrate to effect"*—meaning that the milligram dose per day and the duration of treatment can and should be customized per the patient's response to treatment. Combination therapy (i.e., more than one treatment at a time), prolonged therapy (treatment of chronic [poly]dysbiosis generally requires longer duration of treatment than does treatment of acute monomicrobial infections), and periodic/punctual treatment (for exacerbations and recurrences).

  - <u>Clinical support favoring "open label" empiric antimicrobial treatment of SIBO in patients with fibromyalgia</u> (*Current Pain and Headache Reports* 2004 Oct[508]): This article discusses the results of two experiments using antibiotics in the treatment of FM: ❶ 96 patients with SIBO diagnosed by lactulose hydrogen breath testing (LHBT) were offered **antibiotic treatment** for the reduction of gastrointestinal bacteria; 25 of the 96 patients returned for a follow-up LHBT. **Neomycin** was the most commonly used antibiotic. Eleven of the 25 patients achieved complete transient eradication of SIBO after antibiotic treatment and experienced better improvement in more of their FM symptom scores when compared with the patients who did not achieve complete eradication. This indicates that a direct relationship exists between the presence of SIBO and intestinal and extraintestinal symptoms in fibromyalgia, and that FM can be alleviated by effective antimicrobial/antibiotic treatment. ❷ In this double-blind trial of eradication of SIBO in fibromyalgia, 46 patients fulfilling the established criteria for FM were tested for SIBO using LHBT. Forty-two of the 46 patients (91.3%) were positive for SIBO and were randomized to receive placebo or 500 mg of **liquid neomycin** (a minimally-absorbed gastrointestinal-specific antibiotic drug) twice daily

---

[508] Wallace DJ, Hallegua DS. Fibromyalgia: the gastrointestinal link. *Curr Pain Headache Rep.* 2004 Oct;8(5):364-8

for 10 days. Only six of the 20 patients (30%) in the neomycin group achieved eradication (indicating inefficacy of treatment); thus, no statistically significant difference between groups was available for analysis. Thereafter, 28 patients in the double-blind study testing positive for SIBO went on to receive **open-label antibiotic treatment** to eradicate SIBO, and this time 17 of the 28 patients (60.7%) achieved eradication of SIBO. When these 23 patients were compared with the 15 patients who failed to eradicate or did not undergo open-label treatment, significant improvement attributable to antibiotic treatment in the FM scores was detected. Results suggest that eradication of bacterial overgrowth results in a statistically and clinically significant alleviation of FM symptoms.

- Nonprescription antimicrobial agents—examples: Most of the agents listed below have their primary or exclusive area of effectiveness within the lumen of the gastrointestinal tract. These agents are generally broad-spectrum and nonspecific, which is perfectly appropriate when treating nonspecific SIBO.
- Prescription-restricted antimicrobial agents—examples: In this section specific for the SIBO of fibromyalgia, nonabsorbable agents (rifaximin, vancomycin, nystatin) are appropriate; agents with systemic absorption (Augmentin and fluconazole) are listed here due to their high efficacy and frequent clinical utilization.
    - Rifaximin/Xifaxan: Rifaximin (gut-specific antibacterial drug) should not be confused with rifampin (systemic antibacterial drug, often used in the treatment of mycobacterium infections such as tuberculosis but also used for other bacterial infections); remember to "get your **facts/fax** right by using ri**fax**imin/Xi**fax**an" while you "use ri**famp**in **to amp**lify the effectiveness of systemic antibiotics in the treatment of chronic infections but it also **amps up** cytochrome p450 and adverse drug effects."
    - Vancomycin orally administered: Clinicians should consider this non/poorly-absorbed antibiotic which is effective against Gram-positive bacteria. Human studies have shown effectiveness in the treatment of IBS, constipation, and primary sclerosing cholangitis. In one particularly remarkable case of a patient with rheumatoid arthritis, I prescribed 125mg/d with great success with the intention to target Gram-positive Th17-inducing segmented filamentous bacteria.
    - Augmentin 1-2g BID: This combination of amoxicillin and clavulanate shows efficacy against more than 90% of gastrointestinal bacteria which contribute to SIBO.
    - Nystatin 500,000 units BID-TID PO duration as needed (e.g., 1-6 months empirically or with any use of antibacterial drugs: Nystatin is a safe nonabsorbable gentle and commonly effective antifungal agent originally derived from a natural source of soil microorganisms. Its lack of significant intestinal absorption reduces the incidence of adverse effects while also prohibiting systemic antifungal effectiveness, except for reducing the total microbial load (TML) by reducing gastrointestinal fungal

---

A practical summary of SIBO: small intestine bacterial overgrowth

1. <u>Definition</u>: Generalized nonspecific overpopulation of bacteria (commonly with other microbes such as yeast) in the small intestine (and large intestine, too).
2. <u>Frequency</u>: Very common in clinical practice and the general population.
3. <u>Primary symptoms</u>: Gas and bloating, especially after carbohydrate consumption; may also have constipation and/or diarrhea.
4. <u>Secondary symptoms</u>: Fatigue, muscle aches, difficulty with concentration and cognition ("brain fog"), nutritional deficiencies due to malabsorption, immune activation due to absorption of microbial debris and metabolites, muscle pain due to dysbiotic mitochondriopathy and LPS- and cytokine-induced central sensitization.
5. <u>Diagnosis</u>: ❶ Based on the symptoms above, ❷ jejunal aspiration is the gold standard but is expensive, cumbersome, and potentially hazardous, ❸ measurement of fermentation products (hydrogen and methane) in breath following consumption of a carbohydrate such as glucose, sucrose, or lactulose; the amount of "gas" produced is proportional to the bacterial population, ❹ may find elevated short chain fatty acids (SCFA) in stool or elevated folate in blood, but not all cases of SIBO produce high levels of SCFA or folate, ❺ clinical response to low-carbohydrate diet and/or antibiotic drugs or antimicrobial herbs. The current author (AV) uses #1 in conjunction with #5 most commonly.
6. <u>Treatments</u>: Low-carbohydrate diet with antibiotic drugs (e.g., Xifaxan/Rifaximin (200 or 550 mg each) 400-550 mg tid po [1,200-1,650 mg daily] for 10-30 days) or antimicrobial herbs (e.g., time-released emulsified oregano oil 600 mg daily for 4-6 weeks, and/or berberine 400-1,500 mg daily for 4-12 weeks). Restoration of normal flora with probiotics, plant-based dietary diversity and authentically fermented foods.

population. Nystatin is safe for long-term use, is inexpensive, and should generally be used anytime that antibiotic/antibacterial drugs are employed.

- ▫ <u>Fluconazole/Diflucan 100-150-200 mg every other day for 4-5 doses over 8-10 days</u>: The long half-life of 30 hours allows discontinuous alternate-day dosing without loss of efficacy for most routine outpatient applications. This drug is absorbed systemically with excellent tissue penetration for the delivery of multifocal antifungal effectiveness (e.g., alleviation of sinus and genitourinary fungal infections/colonization)

NUTRITIONAL IMMUNOMODULATION My use of the term and technique "nutritional immunomodulation" refers to a specific protocol designed to induce epigenetic modifications in undifferentiated Th-0 cells for their preferential promotion into the T-regulatory (Treg) FOXp3+ phenotype while shifting immune (im)balance away from the proinflammatory Th-1, Th-2, and Th-17 phenotypes. The primary components of this protocol can be safely implemented in essentially any and all patients without adverse effect; these fundamental components include low-carbohydrate plant-based diet to promote a systemic anti-inflammatory state, vitamin D3, combination fatty acid supplementation for n-3 fatty acids and GLA, probiotics (note that the first four components of the protocol are already represented in the foundational five-part nutritional protocol), vitamin A, lipoic acid, green tea, and a low-sodium diet. More assertive antidysbiotic interventions to promote healthy microbial balance in the gastrointestinal lumen may include botanical/nutritional/pharmacologic antimicrobial interventions, with some preferential utilization of orally administered vancomycin based on research supporting its effectiveness against segmented filamentous bacteria which are specific inducers of the Th-17 phenotype. Since fibromyalgia in its pure form is not directly due to an immune imbalance in the way considered here, this component of the functional inflammology protocol is not specifically relevant; however, for the many patients with concomitant diagnoses of fibromyalgia with another systemic/inflammatory/autoimmune disease (such as diabetes mellitus, rheumatoid arthritis, multiple sclerosis, or psoriasis) then of course this nutritional immunomodulation protocol should be implemented.

DYSFUNCTIONAL MITOCHONDRIA The basic view that mitochondria are the "powerhouses" of the cell responsible for the formation of cellular energy in the form of ATP is what most people learn in high school biology, and little if any additional knowledge is added to medical physicians' appreciation of the diversity of mitchondria's biologic roles in medical school. Lack of appreciation of the importance of the role of mitochondrial in general and mitochondrial dysfunction in particular in health and disease has left a huge blind spot in the therapeutic vision of most clinicians; by failing to appreciate and correct mitochondrial dysfunction, clinicians have missed a valuable component to the treatment plans of many and probably most of their patients. In addition to the well-known role that mitochondria have in the formation of energy/ATP, mitochondria also play major roles in pancreatic insulin secretion, peripheral insulin reception, microbial surveillance, and maintenance of inflammatory balance, insofar as mitochondrial dysfunction clearly contributes to a pro-diabetic and insulin-insulin resistant state, as well as enhanced pro-inflammatory responsiveness to microbial (including viral) stimuli. Fibromyalgia is clearly identified with mitochondrial dysfunction, and while the secondary mitochondrial dysfunction is one of the major causes of fibromyalgic muscle pain and fatigue, the mitochondrial dysfunction does not itself cause fibromyalgia, the primary cause of which is SIBO. Thus, SIBO's generation of LPS, D-lactate, and other mitochondrial toxins is the primary/direct cause of the mitochondrial dysfunction; effective treatment must emphasize SIBO eradication and mitochondrial resuscitation. We can compartmentalize major components of mitochondrial structure and function into these three main components: ❶ citric acid cycle, ❷ electron transport chain, ❸ and the structural integrity of the inner and outer mitochondrial membranes. The main area of clinical importance can be discussed within a conversation of the electron transport chain (ETC) since this is fed by the citric acid cycle and is structurally interwoven into the inner mitochondrial membrane and fully dependent upon the nonpermeability of the outer mitochondrial membrane for the maintenance of the electromechanical proton gradient. Primary treatment must always be directed at the primary cause of any disease—not its secondary complications; in the case of FM, the SIBO must always be treated. Among mitochondria-specific treatments for fibromyalgia, supplementation with CoQ10, melatonin, and acetyl-carnitine (preferably with lipoic acid) are the best studied and most efficacious.

- Coenzyme Q10 (CoQ10): An endogenous antioxidant, vitamin-like substance, and essential component of the mitochondrial electron transport chain, oral supplementation with CoQ10 has been used therapeutically in numerous studies for the successful treatment of migraine, heart failure, hypertension, and renal failure. Additional data have shown immunomodulatory roles for CoQ10, and many clinicians employ it as adjunctive treatment for viral infections, cancer, and allergies.[509,510] The electron transport chain is the terminal step in mitochondrial energy/ATP production; as readers can see in the following diagram, each step or "complex" of the electron transport chain requires nutrients, without which energy/ATP production will be impaired, and provision of which (via supplementation) will generally enhance mitochondrial energy/ATP production. Per Cordero et al[511] in 2012, **CoQ10 levels are 40% lower in blood cells of patients with FM compared with levels in healthy persons**, and reduced levels of CoQ10 correlate with markers associated with expedited destruction of mitochondria (mitophagy).
  - Clinical investigation: Mitochondrial dysfunction and mitophagy activation in blood mononuclear cells of fibromyalgia patients (*Arthritis Research Therapy* 2010 Jan[512]): The authors studied 2 male and 18 female FM patients and 10 healthy controls. They evaluated mitochondrial function in blood mononuclear cells from FM patients measuring CoQ10 levels with high-performance liquid chromatography (HPLC) and measuring mitochondrial membrane potential with flow cytometry. Oxidative stress was determined by measuring mitochondrial superoxide production and lipid peroxidation in blood mononuclear cells and plasma from FM patients. Autophagy activation was evaluated in blood mononuclear cells; mitophagy was confirmed by measuring citrate synthase activity and electron microscopy examination of blood mononuclear cells. The authors **found reduced levels of CoQ10, decreased mitochondrial membrane potential, increased levels of mitochondrial superoxide in blood mononuclear cells (indicating increased oxidative stress and reduced antioxidant defense)**, and increased levels of lipid peroxidation in both blood mononuclear cells and plasma from FM patients. Importantly, the authors note that "mitochondrial dysfunction was also associated with increased expression of autophagic genes and the elimination of dysfunctional mitochondria with mitophagy." *What this means in practical terms is that the biochemical aberrations that cause mitochondrial dysfunction lead to destruction of mitochondria via "mitophagy" which literally means "mitochondrial consumption", a process by which dysfunctional mitochondria are eliminated by degradative processes.*
  - Case series of FM patients treated with CoQ10 (*Mitochondrion* 2011 Jul[513]): The authors note that CoQ10 is an essential electron carrier in the mitochondrial respiratory chain and a strong antioxidant and that **low CoQ10 levels have been detected in patients with FM**. The authors found that "**FM patients with CoQ10 deficiency showed a statistically significant reduction in symptoms after CoQ10 treatment during 9 months (300 mg/day)**. Determination of deficiency and consequent supplementation in FM may result in clinical improvement." *This is a small but important study documenting 1) that CoQ10 deficiency is common in FM patients, and 2) that CoQ10 supplementation alleviates the clinical manifestations/symptoms of FM, consistent with the integrated model of FM presented in this book, which includes the components of nutrient deficiency and mitochondrial dysfunction. Although standardized blood testing for CoQ10 levels is widely available, testing for and documentation of CoQ10 deficiency is not necessary before the use of CoQ10 supplementation.*
  - Clinical trial using a combination of *Ginkgo biloba* and CoQ10 (*Journal of Internal Medicine Research* 2002 Mar[514]): In an open trial of 23 fibromyalgia patients, the combination of 200 mg CoQ10 and 200 mg *Ginkgo biloba* (for a total dose of 48 mg flavone glycosides and 12 mg terpene lactones) daily for 84 days was shown to provide clinical benefit in 64% of patients. CoQ10 is often deficient in FM patients, and this deficiency both *causes* and *results from* mitochondrial dysfunction; stated differently, CoQ10 depletion and mitochondrial dysfunction form a vicious cycle, a relationship of reciprocal causality. *Ginkgo biloba* extract is an extensively researched botanical medicine with a long history of safe and effective clinical use for various conditions, especially those associated with reduced blood flow and impaired mitochondrial

[509] Gaby AR. The role of Coenzyme Q10 in clinical medicine: Part 1. *Altern Med Rev* 1996;1:11-17
[510] Gaby AR. The role of Coenzyme Q10 in clinical medicine: Part 2. *Altern Med Rev* 1996;1:168-175
[511] Cordero MD, De Miguel M, Moreno Fernández AM, et al. Mitochondrial dysfunction and mitophagy activation in blood mononuclear cells of fibromyalgia patients: implications in the pathogenesis of the disease. *Arthritis Res Ther*. 2010;12(1):R17
[512] Cordero et al. Mitochondrial dysfunction and mitophagy activation in blood mononuclear cells of fibromyalgia patients. *Arthritis Res Ther*. 2010;12(1):R17
[513] Cordero MD et al. Coenzyme Q(10): a novel therapeutic approach for Fibromyalgia? case series with 5 patients. *Mitochondrion*. 2011 Jul;11(4):623-5
[514] Lister. Open, pilot study to evaluate potential benefits of coenzyme Q10 combined with Ginkgo biloba extract in fibromyalgia syndrome. *J Int Med Res* 2002 Mar-Apr;30:195-9

function. *Ginkgo biloba* is a botanical/herbal medicine with a long history of human use; the three most important physiologic effects of *Ginkgo biloba* are ❶ vasodilation—improves blood circulation (which is often compromised in FM patients), ❷ improves mitochondrial function and ATP/energy production, and ❸ antioxidant benefits—quenches/absorbs free radicals, which are oxygen-containing molecules that cause damage to cell structures and body tissues. Given these therapeutic benefits, *Ginkgo* would appear to be a reasonable therapeutic agent to address the secondary pathophysiology in fibromyalgia. *Ginkgo biloba* products are generally standardized for the content of flavone glycosides (approximately 24%) and terpene lactones (approximately 6%) with adult doses ranging from 60-240 mg/d and generally 120 mg/d. *Comment by Dr Vasquez: Ginkgo biloba and CoQ10 are very safe and appropriate for use by nearly all FM patients.*

- <u>Clinical investigation and clinical trial: Oxidative stress, headache symptoms in fibromyalgia and the role of CoQ10 in clinical improvement (*PLoS One* 2012 Apr[515])</u>: The authors introduce this study by noting that FM is a chronic pain syndrome with "unknown etiology" and a wide spectrum of symptoms such as allodynia (perception of pain from stimuli that are not normally painful), debilitating fatigue, joint stiffness, and migraine headaches. The authors note a link between oxidative stress and the clinical symptoms in FM. In this study, the researchers examined oxidative stress and bioenergetic status in blood mononuclear cells (BMCs) and the association with headache symptoms in FM patients. Following this correlative analysis, the authors assessed the effects of oral CoQ10 supplementation on biochemical markers and clinical improvements. In 20 FM patients and 15 healthy controls, a variety of validated clinical and biochemical parameters was assessed; specifically for the biochemical component, measurements were performed for serum CoQ10, catalase, lipid peroxidation (LPO) levels and ATP levels in BMCs. In patients with FM, the authors found lower CoQ10 (CoQ10 deficiency), lower catalase (reduced antioxidant defenses) and lower ATP levels (reduced energy production) in BMCs while FM patients also showed elevated LPO (evidence of free-radical damage) in BMCs. Lower levels of CoQ10 and catalase levels in BMCs correlated with greater severity-frequency of headache. **In this clinical trial using CoQ10 300 mg/d for 3 months, CoQ10 supplementation caused significant reductions in pain and tender points, significant reductions in headache impact, significant elevations in cellular levels of CoQ10, a reduction in malondialdehyde (marker of lipid peroxidation) from 30nmol to 5 nmol (normal 6 nmol), an increase in catalase levels from 35 U/mg to 85 U/mg (normal 96 U/mg), and an increase in BMC production of ATP/energy from 61 nmol/mg to 191 nmol/mg (normal 202 nmol/mg).** Supplementation with CoQ10 300 mg/day divided in three doses for 3 months "restored biochemical parameters and induced a significant improvement in clinical and headache symptoms." *Note by Dr Vasquez: The dose of CoQ10 used clinically is generally approximately 100 mg per day, and occasionally a patient or doctor might decide to use a higher dose, which might be up to 300 mg per day. Higher doses generally provide better results with excellent safety, but CoQ10 tends to be one of the most expensive nutritional supplements and as such the lowest effective dose—again approximately 100 mg/d as the standard—is used. Some patients will not respond to 100 mg/d and will respond well to 300 mg/d; these more challenging patients might also need additional/different treatments, such as supplementation with synergistic nutrients, hormonal correction, xenobiotic depuration, or assertive treatment of dysbiosis/SIBO.*

---

[515] Cordero et al. Oxidative stress correlates with headache symptoms in fibromyalgia: coenzyme Q10 effect on clinical improvement. *PLoS One.* 2012;7(4):e35677

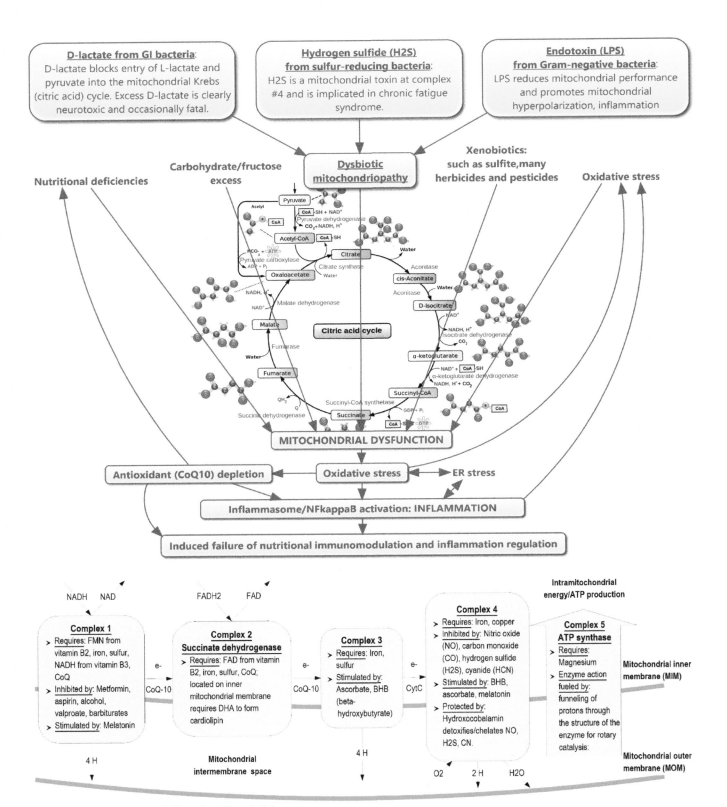

D-lactate from GI bacteria: D-lactate blocks entry of L-lactate and pyruvate into the mitochondrial Krebs (citric acid) cycle. Excess D-lactate is clearly neurotoxic and occasionally fatal.

Hydrogen sulfide (H2S) from sulfur-reducing bacteria: H2S is a mitochondrial toxin at complex #4 and is implicated in chronic fatigue syndrome.

Endotoxin (LPS) from Gram-negative bacteria: LPS reduces mitochondrial performance and promotes mitochondrial hyperpolarization, inflammation

Nutritional deficiencies

Carbohydrate/fructose excess

Dysbiotic mitochondriopathy

Xenobiotics: such as sulfite, many herbicides and pesticides

Oxidative stress

Pyruvate

Acetyl

CoA

CoA -SH + NAD⁺
Pyruvate dehydrogenase
CO₂+NADH, H⁺

Acetyl-CoA   CoA -SH

HCO₃⁻ + ATP
Pyruvate carboxylase
ADP + Pᵢ

Citrate

Citrate synthase

Oxaloacetate   Water

Water

Aconitase

cis-Aconitate

Aconitase   Water

NADH, H⁺
NAD⁺

Malate dehydrogenase

D-Isocitrate

NAD⁺

Malate

Citric acid cycle

NADH, H⁺
Isocitrate dehydrogenase
CO₂

Fumarase

Water

α-ketoglutarate

Fumarate

NAD⁺ + CoA -SH
α-ketoglutarate dehydrogenase
NADH, H⁺+ CO₂

QH₂
Q

Succinyl-CoA

Succinyl-CoA synthetase

Succinate dehydrogenase

Succinate

GDP + Pᵢ

CoA -S   GTP

CoA

MITOCHONDRIAL DYSFUNCTION

Antioxidant (CoQ10) depletion   →   **Oxidative stress**   ↔   **ER stress**

Inflammasome/NFkappaB activation: INFLAMMATION

Induced failure of nutritional immunomodulation and inflammation regulation

Intramitochondrial energy/ATP production

NADH   NAD

Complex 1
➢ Requires: FMN from vitamin B2, iron, sulfur, NADH from vitamin B3, CoQ
➢ Inhibited by: Metformin, aspirin, alcohol, valproate, barbiturates
➢ Stimulated by: Melatonin

e⁻
CoQ-10

FADH2   FAD

Complex 2 Succinate dehydrogenase
➢ Requires: FAD from vitamin B2, iron, sulfur, CoQ; located on inner mitochondrial membrane requires DHA to form cardiolipin

e⁻
CoQ-10

Complex 3
➢ Requires: Iron, sulfur
➢ Stimulated by: Ascorbate, BHB (beta-hydroxybutyrate)

e⁻
CytC

Complex 4
➢ Requires: Iron, copper
➢ Inhibited by: Nitric oxide (NO), carbon monoxide (CO), hydrogen sulfide (H2S), cyanide (HCN)
➢ Stimulated by: BHB, ascorbate, melatonin
➢ Protected by: Hydroxocobalamin detoxifies/chelates NO, H2S, CN.

Complex 5 ATP synthase
➢ Requires: Magnesium
➢ Enzyme action fueled by: funneling of protons through the structure of the enzyme for rotary catalysis:

Mitochondrial inner membrane (MIM)

4 H

Mitochondrial intermembrane space

4 H

O2   2 H   H2O

Mitochondrial outer membrane (MOM)

Reduce mitochondrial protein synthesis: Tetracyclines, chloramphenicol

Cause mtDNA depletion: Adriamycin/doxorubicin, zidovudine, herpes simplex virus

Damage mitochondrial inner membrane: Roundup ® (mixture of glyphosate and solvent/inert chemicals) per *Environ Toxicol Pharmacol* 2012 Sep, *Toxicol In Vitro* 2013 Feb, *Toxicology* 2013 Nov

Microbial debris (LPS) and metabolites (D-lactate and H2S) and the subsequent inflammatory response lead to mitochondrial dysfunction: Nutritional deficiencies, genetic faults, and xenobiotic exposure/accumulation exacerbate mitochondrial impairment and also exacerbate the peripheral and central inflammatory responses. Copyright © 2015 by Dr Alex Vasquez. All rights reserved and enforced; this image may not be used, copied, or distributed without written permission. Citric acid cycle from en.wikipedia.org/wiki/Citric_acid_cycle. "Citric acid cycle with aconitate 2" by Narayanese, WikiUserPedia, YassineMrabet, TotoBaggins licensed under Creative Commons Attribution-Share Alike 3.0. See www.inflammationmastery.com/pain

- **NLRP3 inflammasome is activated in fibromyalgia and reduced by coenzyme Q10** (*Antioxid Redox Signal* 2014 Mar[516]): "Mitochondrial dysfunction was accompanied by increased protein expression of interleukin (IL)-1, NLRP3 (NOD-like receptor family, pyrin domain containing 3) and caspase-1 activation, and an increase of serum levels of proinflammatory cytokines (IL-1 and IL-18). CoQ10 deficiency induced by p-aminobenzoate treatment in blood mononuclear cells and mice showed NLRP3 inflammasome activation with marked algesia. A placebo-controlled trial of CoQ10 in FM patients has shown a reduced NLRP3 inflammasome activation and IL-1 and IL-18 serum levels. ...CONCLUSION: These findings provide new insights into the pathogenesis of FM and suggest that NLRP3 inflammasome inhibition represents a new therapeutic intervention for the disease. ... After CoQ10 supplementation [300 mg/day CoQ10 divided into three doses], NLRP3 and IL-1 gene were downregulated. ... IL-1 and IL-18 serum levels were significantly reduced with respect to placebo." The most complete/consistent model of FMS is that it is caused by SIBO, leading to mitochondrial dysfunction, central sensitization, tryptophan/serotonin/melatonin deficiencies; these interconnections are illustrated later in this chapter and detailed elsewhere.[517]

  - **Mitochondrial dysfunction in CRPS**: Patients with CRPS show evidence of impaired oxygen diffusion and mitochondrial impairment[518], and Tan et al[519] specifically noted that mitochondrial ETC "complex II activity in the CRPS I patients was significantly lower." From a "mitochondrial micromanagement" perspective, one might consider the use of riboflavin 400 mg/d and CoQ10 100-300 mg/d to support ETC complex #2, but obviously the entire mitochondria—indeed the entire body—works together as a unit.

- **Melatonin**: Melatonin is a hormone produced in the pineal gland of the brain; melatonin is synthesized from the neurotransmitter serotonin, and production of both serotonin and melatonin are dependent on the nutritional availability of tryptophan and/or 5-HTP as discussed above. Patients with FM show decreased nocturnal secretion of melatonin.[520] Melatonin benefits FM patients through a wide range of mechanisms, including promotion of restful sleep and reduction in LPS-induced mitochondrial impairment. As a powerful antioxidant, melatonin scavenges oxygen and nitrogen-based reactants generated in mitochondria and thereby limits the loss of intramitochondrial glutathione, the most important component of antioxidant defense; this prevents damage to mitochondrial protein and DNA. **Melatonin increases the activity of Complexes 1 and 4 of the mitochondrial electron transport chain, improving mitochondrial respiration and increasing ATP synthesis** under various physiological and experimental conditions.[521] Successful treatment with melatonin or its precursor tryptophan/5-HTP should not deter the clinician from addressing other contributing or causative problems such as vitamin D deficiency, gastrointestinal dysbiosis including SIBO, magnesium deficiency, and chronic psychoemotional stress. The adult physiologic dose which mimics natural internal (endogenous) production is approximately 200-500 mcg [micrograms] nightly. In adults, supplementation with melatonin has a wide therapeutic index and is used safely and effectively in doses up to 20 to 40 mg [milligrams] nightly.

  - **Case series (n=4): Melatonin therapy in fibromyalgia** (*Journal of Pineal Research* 2006 Jan[522]): Melatonin (3–6 mg per night, administered orally 1 hour before bedtime) has been reported to normalize sleep, alleviate pain and fatigue, and resolve many other clinical manifestations of FM. The authors report, "After 15 days of treatment with melatonin, all patients developed a sleep/wake cycle that was considered normal. They also mentioned a significant reduction of pain. At this time, the patients were taken off hypnotics. Thirty days after the initiation of melatonin, other medications were withdrawn and thereafter they only took melatonin." *Comment by Dr Vasquez: These results are impressive, but—again—the other components of FM such*

[516] Cordero et al. NLRP3 inflammasome is activated in fibromyalgia: the effect of coenzyme Q10. *Antioxid Redox Signal.* 2014 Mar 10;20(8):1169-80

[517] Vasquez A. *Naturopathic Rheumatology and Integrative Inflammology v3.5*, 2014 and *Fibromyalgia in a Nutshell*, 2012

[518] "The mean venous oxygen saturation (S(v)O(2)) value (94.3% ± 4.0%) of the affected limb was significantly higher than S(v)O(2) values found in healthy subjects (77.5% ± 9.8%) pointing to a severely decreased oxygen diffusion or utilization within the affected limb. ... Ultrastructural investigations of soleus skeletal muscle capillaries revealed thickened endothelial cells and thickened basement membranes. Muscle capillary densities were decreased in comparison with literature data. High venous oxygen saturation levels were partially explained by impaired diffusion of oxygen due to thickened basement membrane and decreased capillary density. ...The abnormal skeletal muscle findings points to severe disuse but only partially explain the impaired diffusion of oxygen; mitochondrial dysfunction seems a likely explanation in addition." Tan et al. Impaired oxygen utilization in skeletal muscle of CRPS I patients. *J Surg Res.* 2012 Mar;173(1):145-52

[519] "We observed that mitochondria obtained from CRPS I muscle tissue displayed reduced mitochondrial ATP production and substrate oxidation rates in comparison to control muscle tissue. Moreover, we observed reactive oxygen species evoked damage to mitochondrial proteins and reduced MnSOD levels." Tan et al. Mitochondrial dysfunction in muscle tissue of complex regional pain syndrome type I patients. *Eur J Pain.* 2011 Aug;15(7):708-15

[520] Wikner J, et al. Fibromyalgia—a syndrome associated with decreased nocturnal melatonin secretion. *Clin Endocrinol* (Oxf). 1998 Aug;49(2):179-83

[521] León J, Acuña-Castroviejo D, Escames G, Tan DX, Reiter RJ. Melatonin mitigates mitochondrial malfunction. *J Pineal Res.* 2005 Jan;38(1):1-9

[522] Acuna-Castroviejo D, Escames G, Reiter RJ. Melatonin therapy in fibromyalgia. *J Pineal Res.* 2006 Jan;40(1):98-9

as SIBO and CoQ10 deficiency should also be treated assertively to reduce the risk of relapse and to treat the underlying problems; good healthcare and good self-care should extend beyond mere symptom alleviation.

- ▪ <u>Clinical trial (n=101): Adjuvant use of melatonin for treatment of fibromyalgia</u> (*Journal of Pineal Research.* 2011 Apr[523]): group A (24 patients) treated with 20 mg/day fluoxetine alone; group B (27 patients) treated with melatonin 5 mg alone; group C (27 patients) treated with 20 mg fluoxetine plus 3 mg melatonin; group D (23 patients) treated with 20 mg fluoxetine plus 5 mg melatonin for 8 weeks. "Using melatonin (3 mg or 5 mg/day) in combination with 20 mg/day fluoxetine resulted in significant reduction in both total and different components of Fibromyalgia Impact Questionnaire score compared to the pretreatment values. In conclusion, **administration of melatonin, alone or in a combination with fluoxetine, was effective in the treatment of patients with FMS.**"

- <u>Acetyl-L-carnitine (ALC)</u>: Acetyl-L-carnitine is a form of the amino acid L-carnitine, most notable for its critical role in supporting mitochondrial energy/ATP production by supporting the metabolism (beta oxidation) of fatty acids in the mitochondria. A large study with 102 patients showed that ALC (administered by oral and parenteral routes, 1500 mg/d) was beneficial in patients with fibromyalgia.[524] Given the role of ALC in supporting and improving mitochondrial function, this supplement probably benefits fibromyalgia patients by compensating for LPS-induced skeletal muscle dysfunction.

- <u>D-ribose</u>: D-ribose is a naturally occurring pentose carbohydrate available as a dietary supplement. When administered orally (5 g thrice daily), it safely provides numerous benefits to fibromyalgia patients, according to a recent pilot study with 41 patients.[525] Improvements are seen in energy, sleep, mental clarity, pain intensity, and well-being, as well as global assessment. Among its beneficial mechanisms of action is enhancement of mitochondrial ATP production. Thus, the benefits of D-ribose supplementation may be mediated by restoration or preservation of mitochondrial impairment caused by LPS in fibromyalgia patients.

- <u>Creatine monohydrate</u>: Skeletal muscle levels of phosphocreatine and ATP are reduced in patients with fibromyalgia compared with normal controls; thus, oral supplementation with creatine would appear to be an obvious intervention to restore these depressed levels to normal. Artimal et al[526] reported that a patient with severe refractory fibromyalgia attained sustained alleviation of depression and pain, as well as improvements in sleep and quality of life, following oral administration of creatine monohydrate for 4 weeks (3 grams daily in the first week, then 5 grams daily). Creatine supplementation has been shown to improve ATP production and oxygen utilization in brain and skeletal muscle in humans.[527]

- <u>Oxygen</u>: One-hundred percent oxygen delivered by facial mask at 8 L/min for 10 minutes can help abort an attack of cluster headache. Oxygen is the required electron and proton acceptor of the mitochondrial electron transport chain (ETC) for ATP production; thus, supraphysiologic oxygen, like supraphysiologic doses of mitochondria-specific nutrients, generally improves mitochondrial energy (ATP) production. The model of pain sensitization in so-called "chronic pain syndromes"—specifically migraine, cluster headache, fibromyalgia, myofascial pain syndrome and complex regional pain syndrome (CRPS)—that I have developed includes a tripartite vicious cycle of mitochondrial dysfunction, glial activation, and neuronal hyperexcitation, all of which promote brain inflammation, central sensitization, and perpetuation and amplification of pain. Strong support for this model comes from both its biochemical and physiologic rationale as well as the efficacy of corresponding treatments that address each of the main components: mitochondrial dysfunction, glial activation, neuronal hyperexcitation, brain inflammation.

  Appreciation of the efficacy of oxygen therapy—whether as normobaric (more available and affordable) or hyperbaric (more effective and more expensive; hyperbaric oxygen therapy [HBOT])—in various pain states invites us to revisit the naturopathic profession's hierarchy of therapeutics. Symptomatic therapy clearly has a role in patient care but, in order to avoid repeated use of urgent/emergency care and the creation of unnecessary medical dependency, repeated acute care or even "maintenance therapy" should never replace treatment of the underlying cause(s). Patients need to receive treatment aimed at the underlying pathophysiology so that health is optimized and patients are moved toward better general well-being and disease-specific health. Oxygen

---

[523] Hussain SA, Al-Khalifa II, Jasim NA, Gorial FI. Adjuvant use of melatonin for treatment of fibromyalgia. *J Pineal Res.* 2011 Apr;50(3):267-71
[524] Rossini M, et al. Double-blind, multicenter trial comparing acetyl l-carnitine with placebo in treatment of fibromyalgia patients. *Clin Exp Rheumatol.* 2007 Mar-Apr;25:182-8
[525] Teitelbaum JE, Johnson C, St Cyr J. The use of D-ribose in chronic fatigue syndrome and fibromyalgia: a pilot study. *J Altern Complement Med.* 2006 Nov;12:857-62
[526] Amital D, Vishne T, Rubinow A, Levine J. Observed effects of creatine monohydrate in a patient with depression and fibromyalgia. *Am J Psychiatry.* 2006 Oct;163(10):1840-1
[527] Watanabe A, Kato N, Kato T. Effects of creatine on mental fatigue and cerebral hemoglobin oxygenation. *Neurosci Res.* 2002 Apr;42(4):279-85

therapy is abortive of pain and shows some contribution to breaking the vicious cycles of mitochondrial impairment (immediate treatment of headaches, current-prospective treatment of fibromyalgia and CRPS) but this therapy does not address the other aspects of mitochondrial dysfunction (e.g., CoQ10 deficiency) and does not address the cause (e.g., small intestine bacterial overgrowth [SIBO] in fibromyalgia) and therefore should remain as supplemental, abortive/acute, and adjunctive therapy not as they foundation of therapy. Obviously, hyperbaric therapy makes more money for doctors/clinics and—(except/including) when patients buy their own home hyperbaric units—will therefore receive more press and more endorsement than therapies that are curative and empowering (ie, autonomous, without medical dependence). Given that most patients with persistent inflammation and pain are antioxidant deficient and therefore at increased risk for oxygen toxicity (including subclinical damage), antioxidant repletion should occur prior to oxygen therapy; the idea of administering supraphysiologic doses of oxygen to pull more protons and electrons through an *already damaged* and *pro-inflammatory* and *ROS-generating* electron transport chain is not meritorious, although some will defend it—weakly—on the theoretic basis of hormesis.

- <u>High-flow oxygen therapy for all types of headache</u> (*Am J Emerg Med* 2012 Nov[528]): "We performed a prospective, randomized, double-blinded, placebo-controlled trial of patients presenting to the ED with a chief complaint of headache. The patients were randomized to receive either 100% oxygen via nonrebreather mask at 15 L/min or the placebo treatment of room air via nonrebreather mask for 15 minutes in total. ... A total of 204 patients agreed to participate in the study and were randomized to the oxygen (102 patients) and placebo (102 patients) groups. Patient headache types included tension (47%), migraine (27%), undifferentiated (25%), and cluster (1%). Patients who received oxygen therapy reported significant improvement in visual analog scale scores at all points when compared with placebo: 22 mm vs 11 mm at 15 minutes, 29 mm vs 13 mm at 30 minutes, and 55 mm vs 45 mm at 60 minutes. ... In addition to its role in the treatment of cluster headache, high-flow oxygen therapy may provide an effective treatment of all types of headaches in the ED setting.

- <u>Hyperbaric oxygen therapy for fibromyalgia; randomized n=60, crossover n=24</u> (*PLoS One.* 2015 May[529]): "The HBOT protocol comprised 40 sessions, 5 days/week, 90 minutes, 100% oxygen at 2ATA. ... HBOT in both groups led to significant amelioration of all FMS symptoms, with significant improvement in life quality. Analysis of SPECT imaging revealed rectification of the abnormal brain activity: decrease of the hyperactivity mainly in the posterior region and elevation of the reduced activity mainly in frontal areas. No improvement in any of the parameters was observed following the control period. CONCLUSIONS: The study provides evidence that HBOT can improve the symptoms and life quality of FMS patients. Moreover, it shows that HBOT can induce neuroplasticity and significantly rectify abnormal brain activity in pain related areas of FMS patients." Why would (hyperbaric) oxygen provide more benefit for fibromyalgia than for migraine, given the both are largely due to mitochondrial dysfunction?—Because in migraine, the mitochondrial dysfunction is generally low, and then acute with exacerbations, and it is most notable only in the brain; in contrast, in fibromyalgia, the mitochondrial dysfunction is more moderate-severe and therefore more amenable to treatment during the course of the disease (ie, one does not have to wait for an exacerbation or attack). Also in fibromyalgia, the mitochondrial dysfunction and the pain are both central in the brain as well as peripheral in the muscles; both locations contribute partly to the pain sensations, and oxygen therapy addresses both components, therefore leading to more opportunity for symptomatic improvement.

- <u>Hyperbaric oxygen therapy for fibromyalgia; randomized n=50</u> (*J Int Med Res.* 2004 May[530]): "We conducted a randomized controlled study to evaluate the effect of hyperbaric oxygen (HBO) therapy in FMS (HBO group: n = 26; control group: n = 24). Tender points and pain threshold were assessed before, and after the first and fifteenth sessions of therapy. Pain was also scored on a visual analogue scale (VAS). There was a significant reduction in tender points and VAS scores and a significant increase in pain threshold of the

[528] Ozkurt et al. Efficacy of high-flow oxygen therapy in all types of headache: a prospective, randomized, placebo-controlled trial. *Am J Emerg Med.* 2012 Nov;30(9):1760-4
[529] Efrati et al. Hyperbaric oxygen therapy can diminish fibromyalgia syndrome—prospective clinical trial. *PLoS One.* 2015 May 26;10(5):e0127012
[530] Yildiz et al. A new treatment modality for fibromyalgia syndrome: hyperbaric oxygen therapy. *J Int Med Res.* 2004 May-Jun;32(3):263-7

HBO group after the first and fifteenth therapy sessions. There was also a significant difference between the HBO and control groups for all parameters except the VAS scores after the first session. We conclude that HBO therapy has an important role in managing FMS."

- Hyperbaric oxygen therapy for complex regional pain syndrome (*J Int Med Res.* 2004 May[531]): "In this double-blind, randomized, placebo-controlled study we aimed to assess the effectiveness of hyperbaric oxygen (HBO) therapy for treating patients with complex regional pain syndrome (CRPS). Of the 71 patients, 37 were allocated to the HBO group and 34 to the control (normal air) group. Both groups received 15 therapy sessions in a hyperbaric chamber. Pain, edema and range of motion (ROM) of the wrist were evaluated before treatment, after the 15th treatment session and on day 45. In the HBO group there was a significant decrease in pain and edema and a significant increase in the ROM of the wrist. When we compared the two groups, the HBO group had significantly better results with the exception of wrist extension. In conclusion, HBO is an effective and well-tolerated method for decreasing pain and edema and increasing the ROM in patients with CRPS."

- Hyperbaric oxygen therapy for myofascial pain syndrome (*J Natl Med Assoc* 2009 Jan[532]): "Thirty patients with the diagnosis of MPS were divided into HBO (n=20) and control groups (n=10). Patients in the HBO group received a total of 10 HBO treatments in 2 weeks. Patients in the control group received placebo treatment in a hyperbaric chamber. Pain threshold and visual analogue scale (VAS) measurements were performed immediately before and after HBO therapy and 3 months thereafter. Additionally, Pain Disability Index (PDI) and Short Form 12 Health Survey (SF-12) evaluations were done before HBO and after 3 months. HBO therapy was well tolerated with no complications. In the HBO group, pain threshold significantly increased and VAS scores significantly decreased immediately after and 3 months after HBO therapy. PDI, Mental and Physical Health SF-12 scores improved significantly with HBO therapy after 3 months compared with pretreatment values. In the control group, pain thresholds, VAS score, and Mental Health SF-12 scores did not change with placebo treatment; however, significant improvement was observed in the Physical Health SF-12 test. We concluded that HBO therapy may be a valuable alternative to other methods in the management of MPS."

SOCIOLOGY, SLEEP, STRESS, SOMATIC TREATMENTS, SWEAT/EXERCISE, SPECIAL SUPPLEMENTATION

Common clinical and lifestyle considerations are listed in the following sections.

- Sociology/psychology, and stress management/reduction: Everyone—patients as well as clinicians—can benefit from developing self-awareness, emotional intelligence, and other core life skill and insights; since much of our perception of stress has a psycho-epistemological basis, enhanced self-awareness in this key area can help to deconstruct the phenomenon of stress and its secondary consequences. Because this consideration is self-evident in terms of safety, efficacy, broad applicability, and life-enhancement, specific literature will not be reviewed here.

- Sleep: Sleep deprivation induces immune suppression, enhanced sensitivity to pain, and an objectively documentable proinflammatory state evidenced by increases in serum hsCRP. Patients should be encouraged to optimize sleep by avoiding late-in-the-day exercise, overstimulation, caffeine (which generally has a half-life of six hours), and overuse of bright lights following nightfall; items that are conducive to sleep are having a dark and quiet room, relaxing music or reading, and using melatonin. Enhancement of sleep quality and duration have been shown to alleviate systemic inflammation, tendency toward insulin resistance, and pain perception/sensitivity.

- Sweating and exercise: Obesity/overweight and physical inactivity are consistently associated with elevated risk for and experience of depression, low self-esteem, social isolation, systemic inflammation, cardiometabolic disease and diabetes mellitus type-2, cancers of various types, and inflammatory disorders such as asthma and psoriasis. Weight optimization and physical activity promote enhanced self-confidence, self-efficacy, skill-building, social interaction, and reductions in cause-specific and all-cause mortality. Mechanistically, exercise— defined here as physical activity of sustained duration and intensity to promote diaphoresis/sweating— promotes lipolysis (for mobilization of adipose-stored toxins, weight reduction, and enhanced BHB production

[531] Kiralp et al. Effectiveness of hyperbaric oxygen therapy in the treatment of complex regional pain syndrome. *J Int Med Res.* 2004 May-Jun;32(3):258-62
[532] Kiralp et al A novel treatment modality for myofascial pain syndrome: hyperbaric oxygen therapy. *J Natl Med Assoc.* 2009 Jan;101(1):77-80

for induction of histone acetylation and ECT stimulation), promotes glycolysis (to promote induction of enhanced mitochondrial function and insulin sensitivity), and hyperventilation which results in respiratory alkalosis and secondary urinary alkalinization (which promotes mineral retention, xenobiotic excretion, endorphin elevation, and cortisol reduction). Commonly accepted international guidelines as well as common sense advocate 30-60 minutes of daily exercise that should globally include components such as aerobic training, resistance training, skill-building, balance, and flexibility; intensity, duration, and variety are tailored to patient needs and preferences. Because this consideration is self-evident in terms of safety, efficacy, broad applicability, and life-enhancement, specific literature will not be reviewed here.

- Somatic treatments (chiropractic, acupuncture, osteopathic manipulation, qigong, balneotherapy): In a randomized, controlled clinical trial among 24 female fibromyalgia patients, balneotherapy (warm bath) in daily 20-minute sessions 5 days per week for 3 weeks (total of 15 sessions; water temperature: 96.8°F = 36°C), resulted in statistically significant reductions in measured inflammatory mediators (PGE2, interleukin-1, LTB4) and amelioration of clinical symptoms among treated FM patients.[533] The symptomatic benefits of balneotherapy for FM patients have been corroborated in other trials.[534,535,536] Chiropractic treatment (including spinal manipulation, stretching, soft tissue treatments, and therapeutic ultrasound) has shown modest symptomatic benefit in several fibromyalgia case series and clinical trials.[537,538] A short-term trial showed that osteopathic manipulative therapy with standard medical care was superior to medical care alone for FM patients.[539] Acupuncture (including traditional, nontraditional, and electrical stimulation) also has been found beneficial for fibromyalgia patients.[540,541,542] Acupuncture may relieve fibromyalgia pain by improving regional blood flow, in addition to other mechanisms.[543,544] Because specific needle placement does not appear to be important[545], the conclusion that true acupuncture is ineffective because it may not differ markedly from the results obtained by sham acupuncture[546] may not be logical. A similar conundrum is seen in other clinical trials involving physical interventions such as manual osseous manipulation, wherein authentic treatments and sham treatments may both be effective by virtue of common physiological responses.[547] Qigong was found helpful for 10 fibromyalgia patients, and benefits were still apparent at three months' follow-up.[548]

- Special treatment, somatic treatment—Intramuscular needling and anesthesia: Myofascial pain is commonly received by needing (inserting a sterile needle into the muscle), whether or not the location is specific (e.g., acupuncture) and whether or not anesthetic agents, saline, or nothing (ie, dry needling) accompany the needle; having said that, more accurate localization (e.g., available trigger points or tender points) and the use of anesthetic agents tends to yield better results.

  - Analgesic and anti-hyperalgesic effects of muscle injections with lidocaine or saline in fibromyalgia syndrome. (*Eur J Pain.* 2014 Jul[549]): "We enrolled 62 female patients with FM into a double-blind controlled study of three groups who received 100 or 200 mg of lidocaine or saline injections into both trapezius and gluteal muscles. …[Each subject received 2 muscle injections into the center of each trapezius muscle and 2 injections into the upper medial quadrants of both gluteus maximus muscles. …Each syringe used for muscle injections contained either 5 ml of 1% lidocaine (50 mg) or 5 ml of normal saline.] RESULTS: Primary

[533] Ardiç F, Ozgen M, Aybek H, et al. Effects of balneotherapy on serum IL-1, PGE2 and LTB4 levels in fibromyalgia patients. *Rheumatol Int.* 2007 Mar;27(5):441-6
[534] Evcik D, Kizilay B, Gökçen E. The effects of balneotherapy on fibromyalgia patients. *Rheumatol Int.* 2002 Jun;22(2):56-9
[535] Fioravanti A, Perpignano G, Tirri G, et al. Effects of mud-bath treatment on fibromyalgia patients: a randomized clinical trial. *Rheumatol Int.* 2007 Oct;27(12):1157-61
[536] Dönmez A, Karagülle MZ, Tercan N, et al. SPA therapy in fibromyalgia: a randomised controlled clinic study. *Rheumatol Int.* 2005 Dec;26(2):168-72
[537] Citak-Karakaya I, et al. Short and long-term results of connective tissue manipulation and combined ultrasound therapy in patients with fibromyalgia. *J Manipulative Physiol Ther.* 2006 Sep;29(7):524-8
[538] Blunt KL, et al. The effectiveness of chiropractic management of fibromyalgia patients: a pilot study. *J Manipulative Physiol Ther.* 1997 Jul-Aug;20(6):389-99
[539] Gamber et al. Osteopathic manipulative treatment in conjunction with medication relieves pain associated with fibromyalgia syndrome. *J Am Osteopath Assoc.* 2002 Jun:321-5
[540] Martin DP, et al. Improvement in fibromyalgia symptoms with acupuncture: results of a randomized controlled trial. *Mayo Clin Proc.* 2006 Jun;81(6):749-57
[541] Singh BB, et al. Effectiveness of acupuncture in the treatment of fibromyalgia. *Altern Ther Health Med.* 2006 Mar-Apr;12(2):34-41
[542] Deluze C, Bosia L, Zirbs A, Chantraine A, Vischer TL. Electroacupuncture in fibromyalgia: results of a controlled trial. *BMJ.* 1992 Nov 21;305(6864):1249-52
[543] Sandberg M, Larsson B, Lindberg LG, Gerdle B. Different patterns of blood flow response in the trapezius muscle following needle stimulation (acupuncture) between healthy subjects and patients with fibromyalgia and work-related trapezius myalgia. *Eur J Pain.* 2005 Oct;9(5):497-510
[544] Sandberg M, Lindberg LG, Gerdle B. Peripheral effects of needle stimulation (acupuncture) on skin and muscle blood flow in fibromyalgia. *Eur J Pain.* 2004 Apr;8(2):163-71
[545] Harris RE, Tian X, Williams DA, Tian TX, Cupps TR, Petzke F, Groner KH, Biswas P, Gracely RH, Clauw DJ. Treatment of fibromyalgia with formula acupuncture: investigation of needle placement, needle stimulation, and treatment frequency. *J Altern Complement Med.* 2005 Aug;11(4):663-71
[546] Assefi NP, et al. A randomized clinical trial of acupuncture compared with sham acupuncture in fibromyalgia. *Ann Intern Med.* 2005 Jul 5;143(1):10-9
[547] Mein EA, et al. Manual medicine diversity: research pitfalls and the emerging medical paradigm. *J Am Osteopath Assoc.* 2001 Aug;101(8):441-4
[548] Chen KW, Hassett AL, Hou F, et al. A pilot study of external qigong therapy for patients with fibromyalgia. *J Altern Complement Med.* 2006 Nov;12(9):851-6
[549] Staud et al. Analgesic and anti-hyperalgesic effects of muscle injections with lidocaine or saline in patients with fibromyalgia syndrome. *Eur J Pain.* 2014 Jul;18(6):803-12

mechanical hyperalgesia at the shoulders and buttocks decreased significantly more after lidocaine than saline injections (p = 0.004). Similar results were obtained for secondary heat hyperalgesia at the arms (p = 0.04). After muscle injections, clinical FM pain significantly declined by 38% but was not statistically different between lidocaine and saline conditions. Placebo-related analgesic factors (e.g., patients' expectations of pain relief) accounted for 19.9% of the variance of clinical pain after the injections. ... CONCLUSION: These results suggest that muscle injections can reliably reduce clinical FM pain, and that peripheral impulse input is required for the maintenance of mechanical and heat hyperalgesia of patients with FM. Whereas the effects of muscle injections on hyperalgesia were greater for lidocaine than saline, the effects on clinical pain were similar for both injectates."

- Special supplementation in the treatment of FM—targeting (micro)glia activation and glutaminergic/NMDAr-mediated neuroexcitation: In my previous publications (prior to 2015) and consistent with the bulk of the basic science and clinical research, the emphasis of my fibromyalgia protocol has been on the treatment of SIBO and mitochondrial dysfunction, and the ever-necessary fine-tuning of the treatment protocol per patient. Progressively throughout 2015 as I further developed my understanding of the nuances of glial activation and the increasingly popular "gut-brain" concept (reviewed in printed monograph[550] and CE/CME videos[551]), I have become convinced that we should be—and already have been—addressing the glial activation directly. *How can we have already been doing this if we did not know that we were doing it?*—Simply by using nutrients such as anti-inflammatory fatty acids (e.g., EPA and DHA), nutrient-dense diets with minimal/moderate carbohydrate intake, vitamin and mineral supplementation (especially pyridoxine, magnesium, zinc, and vitamin D), phytonutrients, probiotics, CoQ10 and melatonin). All of these nutrients and substances have safety and efficacy for patients generally and FM patients particularly. What we know now is that these and other nutrients lessen the severity and duration of glial activation—brain inflammation—as well, and they therefore can be used to this effect. As such, I will summarize here that central sensitization is easily understood as a combination of **microglial inflammation**, which results in a) formation of the NMDAr agonist **QUIN**, b) formation of NO- which increases glutamate release while also causing mitochondrial dysfunction, and c) astrocyte activation leading to increased glutaminergic neurotransmission. As such, addressing the microglial activation *directly* while also addressing the dysbiotic and mitochondrial components is expected to enhance efficacy of the overall protocol; further, this discussion enhances our understanding of the mechanisms of action of and the clinical rationale for these interventions.

  - Dousing glial inflammation with vitamin D, fatty acids EPA and DHA, melatonin, phytonutrients: Various specific nutritional supplements and "over the counter remedies" have evidence—per in vitro, experimental, or human studies—to reduce glial inflammation; from these can be selected interventions which safely reduce glial activation in patients. All of these have proven safety for human use; the utility in reducing clinically relevant glial activation is established by the combination of available research plus the response of individual patients. As expected given its numerous anti-inflammatory properties, **DHA** reduces (micro)glia-induced inflammation, and the effect is enhanced with aspirin; the combination of **DHA with (low-dose) aspirin** is increasingly appreciated as synergistically anti-inflammatory and proresolutory, specifically but not exclusively via enhanced production of neuroprotective and anti-inflammatory resolvins.[552] Two paradoxes are worth noting: 1) Although immunostimulatory in the periphery[553], **melatonin reduces glial activation** in experimental models of brain injury.[554] 2) **Vitamin D**

[550] Vasquez A. *Human Microbiome and Dysbiosis in Clinical Disease*. ICHNFM, 2015.
[551] Vasquez A. "Microbiome and Dysbiosis in Clinical Disease" available CE/CME at NutritionAndFunctionalMedicine.org and pay-per-view at vimeo.com/ichnfm/vod_pages
[552] "Docosahexaenoic Acid increased total Glutathione levels in microglia cells and enhanced their anti-oxidative capacity. It reduced production of the pro-inflammatory cytokines TNF-α and IL-6 induced through TLR-3 and TLR-4 activation. Furthermore, it reduced production of Nitric Oxide. Aspirin showed similar anti-inflammatory effects with respect to TNF-α during TLR-3 and TLR-7 stimulation. ... Combination of Aspirin and Docosahexaenoic Acid showed augmentation in total Glutathione production during TLR-7 stimulation as well as a reduction in IL-6, TNF-α and Nitric Oxide. CONCLUSIONS: Collectively, these findings highlight the combination of Docosahexaenoic Acid and Aspirin as a possible measure against inflammation of the nervous system, thus leading to protection against neurodegenerative diseases with an inflammatory etiology." Pettit LK, Varsanyi C, Tadros J, Vassiliou E. Modulating the inflammatory properties of activated microglia with Docosahexaenoic acid and Aspirin. *Lipids Health Dis.* 2013 Feb 11;12:16
[553] This is a clinical trial showing anti-infective efficacy of melatonin, while other articles have specifically documented increases in inflammatory cytokines following melatonin administration. "Administration of melatonin as an adjuvant therapy in the treatment of neonatal sepsis is associated with improvement of clinical and laboratory outcomes." Gitto et al. Effects of melatonin treatment in septic newborns. *Pediatr Res.* 2001 Dec;50(6):756-60
[554] "Melatonin administration was associated with markedly restrained microglial activation, decreased release of proinflammatory cytokines and increased the number of surviving neurons at the site of peri-contusion. Meanwhile, melatonin administration resulted in dephosphorylated mTOR pathway." Ding et al. Melatonin reduced microglial activation and alleviated neuroinflammation induced neuron degeneration in experimental traumatic brain injury. *Neurochem Int.* 2014 Oct;76:23-31

reduces glial activation[555], and this is highly consistent with the clinical benefits seen of vitamin D against depression and other neuropsychiatric conditions, clearly including chronic pain; yet, antimicrobial peptide LL-37, production of which is at least partly dependent on vitamin D adequacy, induces glial-mediated neuroinflammation[556], perhaps thereby explaining the rare and possibly transient/inconsequential exacerbation of "sickness behavior" in some patients upon commencement of vitamin D supplementation. Many **phytonutrients—especially curcumin, quercetin, green tea catechins, baicalein, and luteolin**—show anti-inflammatory and neuroprotective benefits, some of which are mediated via reducing microglial activation/inflammation; we can endlessly debate the bioavailability of agents such as curcuminoids and quercetin, or we can accept them as low-cost high-safety nutrients that merit clinical utilization based on mechanistic studies and successful multicomponent clinical trials.[557,558]

- Alleviating **NO-induced glutaminergic neurotransmission and mitochondrial dysfunction** with **vitamin B12, especially in the form of hydroxocobalamin**: Vitamin B12 in general and hydroxocobalamin in particular bind with nitric oxide (NO-); supplemental (hydroxo)cobalamin has a pharmaconutritional effect of alleviating migraine[559] and low-back pain[560,561], two conditions known to have a component of neuroinflammatory central sensitization. Likely, the clinically observed analgesic effect of (hydroxo)cobalamin is mediated partly if not largely via its "chelation" or "detoxification" of NO-, thereby reducing the mitochondrial dysfunction and NMDAr activation that would have otherwise been triggered by NO-.

- Alleviating **astrocyte-induced and QUIN-triggered glutamate/NMDA receptor activation with pyridoxine, magnesium, zinc**: As previously reviewed, microglial activation promotes NMDAr activation via QUIN and glutamate. Regarding glutamate's activation of the NMDAr, sufficient biochemical, experimental, and clinical data allows us to conclude that we can reduce glutamate's excitatory effect by reducing glutamate itself via supplemental pyridoxine (vitamin B6), either in its active phosphorylated form of P5P (pyridoxal 5'-phosphate) or by supporting its magnesium-dependent requirement for conversion to the active P5P form when pyridoxine itself is used. In addition to promoting conversion of pyridoxine to P5P, magnesium also partly blocks calcium passage through the NMDAr-associated calcium channel (as does zinc) and also offsets the effects of increased intracellular calcium, in addition to supporting mitochondrial function, which is easily compromised by both inflammation and increased intracellular calcium. The clinical benefit of pyridoxine supplementation in migraine headache[562], seizures/epilepsy[563], neuropsychiatric symptoms of premenstrual syndrome (depression, irritability and tiredness)[564] is likely mediated via several different mechanisms, primary among which is the enhanced conversion of glutamate to gamma-amino-butyric acid (GABA), thereby synergistically reducing neuroexcitation and enhancing neuroregulation. A generalized

---

[555] "According to the results of the present study, activated microglia might increase the expression of 1-α-hydroxylase and VDR. 25(OH)D3 is converted into 1,25(OH)2D3 by 1-α-hydroxylase, which then stimulates VDR signaling and inhibits the phosphorylation of p38 in activated microglia. This cascade might inhibit the inflammatory reaction of activated microglia. In conclusion, the present study suggests that vitamin D3 might have an important role in the negative regulation of microglial activation." Hur et al. Regulatory Effect of 25-hydroxyvitamin D3 on Nitric Oxide Production in Activated Microglia. *Korean J Physiol Pharmacol.* 2014 Oct;18(5):397-402

[556] "We blocked the inflammatory stimulant action of LL-37 by removing it with an anti-LL-37 antibody. The inflammatory effect was also prevented by treatment with inhibitors of PKC, PI3K and MEK-1/2 as well as with the intracellular Ca(2+)-chelator, BAPTA-AM. This indicates involvement of these intracellular pathways. Our data suggest that LL-37, in addition to its established roles, may play a role in the chronic neuroinflammation which is observed in neurodegenerative diseases such as Alzheimer's and Parkinson's disease." Lee et al. Human antimicrobial peptide LL-37 induces glial-mediated neuroinflammation. *Biochem Pharmacol.* 2015 Mar 15;94(2):130-41

[557] Blaylock RL, Maroon J. Natural plant products and extracts that reduce immunoexcitotoxicity-associated neurodegeneration and promote repair within the central nervous system. *Surg Neurol Int* 2012;3:19

[558] Bredesen DE. Reversal of cognitive decline: a novel therapeutic program. *Aging* (Albany NY). 2014 Sep;6(9):707-17

[559] "Drugs which directly counteract nitric oxide (NO), such as endothelial receptor blockers, NO-synthase inhibitors, and NO-scavengers, may be effective in the acute treatment of migraine, but are also likely to be effective in migraine prophylaxis. In the underlying pilot study the prophylactic effect of the NO scavenger hydroxocobalamin after intranasal administration in migraine was evaluated. ... 1 mg intranasal hydroxocobalamin daily. ... A reduction in migraine attack frequency of >/ or = 50% was seen in 10 of 19 patients... A reduction of > or = 30% was noted in 63% of the patients. The mean attack frequency in the total study population showed a reduction from 4.7 +/- 1.7 attacks per month to 2.7 +/- 1.6. ." van der Kuy et al. Hydroxocobalamin, a nitric oxide scavenger, in the prophylaxis of migraine: an open, pilot study. *Cephalalgia.* 2002 Sep;22(7):513-9

[560] "The efficacy and safety of parenteral Vitamin B12 in alleviating low back pain and related disability and in decreasing the consumption of paracetamol was confirmed in patients with no signs of nutritional deficiency." Mauro et al. Vitamin B12 in low back pain. *Eur Rev Med Pharmacol Sci.* 2000 May-Jun;4(3):53-8

[561] "Intramuscular methylcobalamin is both an effective and safe method of treatment for patients with nonspecific low back pain, both singly or in combination with other forms of treatment." Chiu et al. The efficacy and safety of intramuscular injections of methylcobalamin in patients with chronic nonspecific low back pain: a randomised controlled trial. *Singapore Med J.* 2011 Dec;52(12):868-73

[562] Sadeghi et al. Effects of pyridoxine supplementation on severity, frequency and duration of migraine attacks in migraine patients with aura. *Iran J Neurol.* 2015 Apr 4:74-80

[563] "An 8-year-old girl treated at our facility for superrefractory status epilepticus was found to have a low pyridoxine level at 5μg/L. After starting pyridoxine supplementation, improvement in the EEG for a 24-hour period was seen. ... A selective pyridoxine deficiency was seen in 94% of patients with status epilepticus (compared to 39.4% in the outpatients) which leads us to believe that there is a relationship between status epilepticus and pyridoxine levels." Dave et al. Pyridoxine deficiency in adult patients with status epilepticus. *Epilepsy Behav.* 2015 Nov;52(Pt A):154-8

[564] Doll H, Brown S, Thurston A, Vessey M. Pyridoxine (vitamin B6) and the premenstrual syndrome: a randomized crossover trial. *J R Coll Gen Pract.* 1989 Sep;39(326):364-8

schematic—mostly direct but very clearly clinically accurate—is provided; the illustration connects NMDAr activation with neuropsychiatric complications while providing insight into clinical remediation.

- In the treatment of pain—including headaches and fibromyalgia—reducing the effects of glutamate-mediated neurotransmission and cellular effects is of very high importance: Excess glutaminergic neurotransmission very clearly promotes anxiety, depression, fibromyalgia pain, myofascial pain and myofascial trigger points[565], migraine and headaches, seizures/epilepsy, and neurodegeneration. Our therapeutic goals are to 1) reduce glutamate levels with vitamin B6 and by avoiding/treating microglial activation, 2) reduce glutamate-triggered influx of calcium with zinc and magnesium, also vitamin D, alkalinization (increased consumption of base-forming foods, such as fruits and vegetables which contain citrate which is converted to bicarbonate to promote alkalinization, one effect of which is to promote magnesium retention, thereby alleviating pain[566]), omega-3 fatty acids such as from fish oil, 3) reduce the effects of glutamate/NMDA receptor activation by counterbalancing with benzodiazepine/GABA receptor activation by promoting conversion of glutamate to GABA and perhaps also by using niacinamide and the botanicals that act as ligands for the GABA receptor.

- Reduce homocysteine levels, and recall that homocysteine may be elevated in the central nervous system (cerebrospinal fluid) of patients with chronic fatigue syndrome and fibromyalgia even when levels in blood/serum/plasma are normal[567]; safety and benefit of folate and vitamin B12 administration have been documented[568]: Homocysteine contributes to NMDA receptor activation resulting in—identically as with glutamate—increased intracellular calcium and neurotoxicity.[569]

  - Folinic acid or methylfolate 2-5 mg/d: Use in combination with other vitamins, especially vitamin B12, in the form of hydroxocobalamin, adenosylcobalamin, or methylcobalamin—cyanocobalamin is obviously to be avoided because of its clinically relevant content of cyanide.

  - Vitamin B12 >2,000 mcg per day orally, or 1-2 mg per week by injection: Use in the form of hydroxocobalamin, adenosylcobalamin, or methylcobalamin—cyanocobalamin is obviously to be avoided because of its clinically relevant content of cyanide.

  - Vitamin B6, pyridoxine 50-250 mg/d: The phosphorylated form (P5P) can also be used; when the HCL form is used, additional attention must be given to magnesium status/supplementation and urinary alkalinization. As a rule, B6 supplementation should always be used with magnesium supplementation.

  - Riboflavin 20-400 mg/d: Small doses of 2 mg/d have been shown to significantly reduce homocysteine levels, and doses of 400 mg/d are common and well-tolerated in the treatment of migraine.

  - Thyroid optimization: Hypothyroidism causes elevated homocysteine and promotes insulin resistance[570] and should be treated appropriately per Chapter 1.

  - NAC 600 mg per day and upward to 500-1,500 mg thrice daily: Doses of NAC 4,800 mg/d have been used with success and safety in the treatment of SLE.

  - Avoidance of homocysteine-elevating factors: High coffee intake (>5 cups per day), ethanol, tobacco smoking, and medications/treatments (such as methotrexate, metformin, niacin and fibrate drugs); fish oil can raise homocysteine levels in some patients. Metformin is well-known to cause malabsorption of vitamin B12 and to thereby exacerbate "diabetic neuropathy" and promote depression and dementia/psychosis.

  - Choline, phosphatidylcholine, lecithin (approximately 2.6 g choline/d): Each TBS (tablespoon, approximately 15 mL) of lecithin contains 275 mg of choline; thus, if the goal is to get to 2.6 g choline, one would need to use 10 TBS (150 mL) per day of granulated lecithin.

  - Betaine, trimethylglycine 6–12 g/day: Effects are weak/modest; likely more relevant for patients taking drugs such as metformin and fibrates that promote loss of betaine in urine.

---

[565] Wang et al. Spatial pain propagation over time following painful glutamate activation of latent myofascial trigger points in humans. *J Pain.* 2012 Jun;13(6):537-45

[566] Vormann et al. Supplementation with alkaline minerals reduces symptoms in patients with chronic low back pain. *J Trace Elem Med Biol.* 2001;15(2-3):179-83

[567] Regland et al. Increased concentrations of homocysteine in the cerebrospinal fluid in patients with fibromyalgia and chronic fatigue syndrome. *Scand J Rheumatol.* 1997;26(4):301-7

[568] Regland et al. Response to vitamin B12 and folic acid in myalgic encephalomyelitis and fibromyalgia. *PLoS One.* 2015 Apr 22;10(4):e0124648

[569] Abushik et al. The role of NMDA and mGluR5 receptors in calcium mobilization and neurotoxicity of homocysteine in trigeminal and cortical neurons and glial cells. *J Neurochem.* 2014 Apr;129(2):264-74

[570] Yang N et al. Novel Clinical Evidence of an Association between Homocysteine and Insulin Resistance in Patients with Hypothyroidism or Subclinical Hypothyroidism. *PLoS One.* 2015 May 4;10(5):e0125922

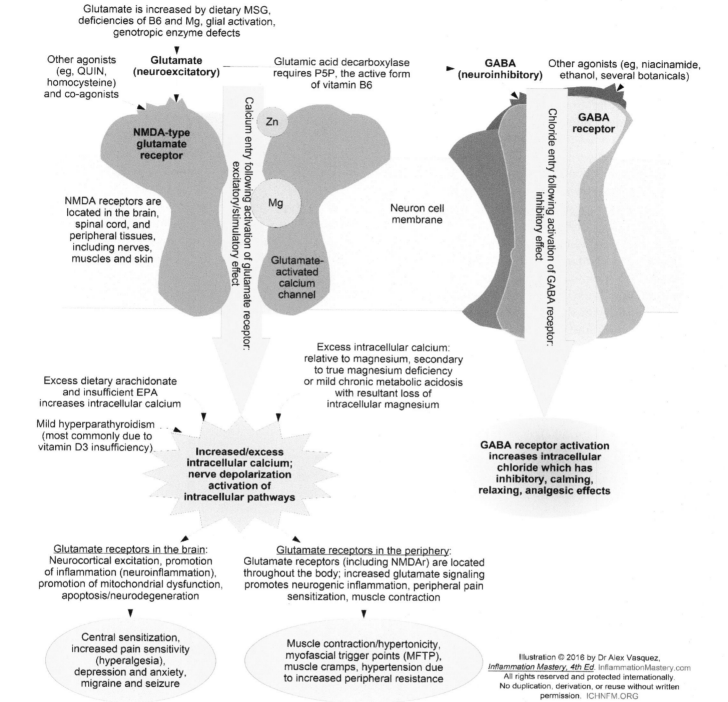

Illustration of the NMDA-type glutamate receptor, its activation, effects, and nutritional modulation: The NMDA receptor is activated by glutamate, QUIN, and other substances which act as agonists (e.g., homocysteine) or co-agonists (e.g., glycine). Different forms of the NMDA receptor exist; thus, the image presented here is a generalized version that is conceptually accurate (rather than all-inclusive; for more details see reviews[571]) and clinically relevant. Neuroexcitatory glutamate is converted to neuroinhibitory GABA by the enzyme glutamic acid decarboxylase, which shows vitamin B6 dose-responsiveness in its reduction of glutamate levels. Magnesium and zinc (and perhaps copper) retard the passage of calcium through this channel, thereby mitigating some of the effects of NMDAr activation. Quenching nitric oxide (for example with hydroxocobalamin), which would otherwise trigger glutamate release, and dousing glial activation are important considerations not included in this illustration. For updates and additional information and explanations, see videos and articles at www.inflammationmastery.com/pain

---

[571] Vyklicky et al. Structure, function, and pharmacology of NMDA receptor channels. *Physiol Res.* 2014;63 Suppl 1:S191-203

| ENDOCRINE IMBALANCE & OPTIMIZATION | Peptide-based and steroid-based hormones have wide-ranging effects beyond those with which they are classically and thus simplistically associated. The "main" hormones that we consider in most chronic inflammatory disorders are the three pro-inflammatory hormones (prolactin, estradiol, and insulin) and the three anti-inflammatory hormones (DHEA, cortisol, and testosterone); each of these hormones can be objectively assessed with serologic testing and modulated with therapeutic intervention. A full thyroid evaluation—including history, physical examination (with particular scrutiny for cold extremities [DDX: hypothyroidism, hypogonadism, vasoconstriction/vaso-obstruction, Raynaud's disorder, peripheral vascular disease, H2S-producing GI dysbiosis], relative bradycardia [DDX, hypothyroidism, heart block, beta-blocker medications], and delayed Achilles reflex return [considered diagnostic of hypothyroidism]), and laboratory evaluation (including TSH, free T4, total or free T3, rT3, and antithyroid antibodies) is warranted in any patient whose concerns include fatigue, depression, systemic inflammation and chronic pain; musculoskeletal manifestations of hypothyroidism include muscle pain, weakness, myopathy, and adhesive capsulitis. The pineal hormone melatonin was discussed in a previous section.

- Testosterone to treat central sensitization of chronic pain in fibromyalgia patients (*Int Immunopharmacol* 2015 Aug[572]): "Considering these mechanisms together, abnormally low testosterone levels are likely to result in amplified ascending/descending facilitation of nociception and reduced descending inhibitory control, resulting in a widening pain field and neuronal plasticity which can turn into the entrenched chronic pain states found in fibromyalgia patients." In this article, the author's review the role of testosterone as an antiinflammatory hormone that reduces glial activation and thereby mitigates the neuro-inflammatory basis (detailed previously) of central sensitization and the resulting pain. Testosterone is well-known to have anti-inflammatory and immunomodulatory properties with clinical utility in rheumatoid arthritis and cluster headache.

- Treatment of pain in fibromyalgia patients with testosterone gel (*Int Immunopharmacol.* 2015 Aug[573]): "Assessment of the typical symptoms of fibromyalgia by patient questionnaire and tender point exam demonstrated significant change in: decreased muscle pain, stiffness, and fatigue, and increased libido during study treatment. These results are consistent with the hypothesized ability of testosterone to relieve the symptoms of fibromyalgia. Symptoms not tightly related to fibromyalgia were not improved."

| XENOBIOTIC ACCUMULATION & DETOXIFICATION | The term "xenobiotics" is generally used to refer to carbon-based foreign chemicals such as persistent organic pollutants (POPs) including herbicides, pesticides, phthalates, parabens, dioxin-related chemicals, and many others; used more casually, the term may also be used to include noncarbon-based foreign substances such as toxic metals like lead, mercury, cadmium, and arsenic. Thus, "xenobiotics" has become somewhat synonymous with "toxins" in both professional-level and vernacular conversations. Laboratory assessments for chemical and metal toxins are commercially available through specialized medical laboratories and are based on analysis of blood and urine. The many biochemical and physiologic components of detoxification/depuration have been reviewed in chapter 4 of this book. Essentially everyone—all humans on the planet worldwide—have biochemical evidence of xenobiotic chemical/metal accumulation, generally with numerous xenobiotics, which have additive and synergistic adverse effects on physiology and health. Thus, scientifically, since xenobiotic accumulation is pandemic, consideration of and treatment for xenobiotic accumulation via therapeutic detoxification programs and lifestyle interventions should be routine. Easy and effective means for promoting detoxification of chemicals and metals include plant-based diet to promote bowel and renal excretion of toxins (via reduced enterohepatic recycling [better microflora, more fiber for adsorption, more frequent fecal excretion] and reduced renal resorption [urinary alkalinization], respectively), NAC for arsenic chelation and GSH production, sweating/exercise (lipolysis promotes mobilization of lipophilic toxins from adipose tissue, diaphoresis promotes direct toxin excretion), sufficient micronutrient and protein intake supports phase 1 and phase 2 of the oxidation and conjugation processes in the liver. Chemical xenobiotics can be bound in the gut during the normal process of enterohepatic recycling/recirculation with periodic or rotational use of activated charcoal, cholestyramine, and chlorella; anecdotal reports from clinical practices support the use of phytochelatin (metal-binding peptides from plants, used by plants for protection from metal toxicity) in the

---

[572] White HD, Robinson TD. A novel use for testosterone to treat central sensitization of chronic pain in fibromyalgia patients. *Int Immunopharmacol.* 2015 Aug;27(2):244-8

[573] White et al. Treatment of pain in fibromyalgia patients with testosterone gel: Pharmacokinetics and clinical response. *Int Immunopharmacol.* 2015 Aug;27(2):249-56

prevention/treatment of metal toxicity in humans but no formal clinical studies have been performed to document the effectiveness of this approach although its safety is clinically appreciated.

- Pilot study: *Chlorella pyrenoidosa* for patients with fibromyalgia syndrome (*Phytother Res* 2000 May[574]): *Chlorella pyrenoidosa* is a unicellular green alga that grows in fresh water. It is a dense source of nutrients, particularly vitamin D (500 IU vitamin D per 1.35 g *Chlorella*). *Chlorella* may have value in treating some fibromyalgia patients, but overall the efficacy is low. Thus, *Chlorella* should not be used as monotherapy for fibromyalgia, although it may be a useful adjunct either as a source of vitamin D, as a means to help modify gut flora, or as an aid in the detoxification of xenobiotics due to its ability to bind ingested and bile-excreted toxins and prevent their absorption and reabsorption in a manner similar to that of cholestyramine, a drug used to bind cholesterol in the gut, promote its excretion, and thereby lower blood cholesterol levels.[575,576,577] This "detoxifying" effect of *Chlorella* in humans is supported by 2 clinical trials showing that nursing mothers who supplement with *Chlorella* during lactation transfer less dioxin in their breast milk compared to nursing mothers who do not consume *Chlorella*.[578,579]

- Clinical investigation: Reduced exposure to xenobiotics (cosmetics) alleviates fibromyalgia (*Journal of Women's Health* 2004 Mar[580]): Women use more cosmetic products than do men, and fibromyalgia is more common in women. Cosmetic products generally contain skin-absorbable xenobiotics with potentially adverse effects; therefore this study was conducted to determine if avoidance of cosmetics would alleviate symptoms of FM. The author of this report describes a prospective, randomized, controlled trial of 48 women with FM (some of whom had a rheumatic condition) who were regular users of cosmetics was carried out to investigate if a reduced use of cosmetics would reduce the symptoms. The patients were told to avoid or completely abstain from using all ointments, creams, skin lotions, pain-relieving liniments, cleaning lotions, oil treatments, hair-coloring chemicals, and tanning lotion; they were also advised to reduce their use of soap and shampoo, both of which—like skin creams—are generally formulated with perfumes and other chemicals and applied to large regions of the body. This research showed that, after 2 years, FM patients who reduced their exposure to chemicals/xenobiotics/cosmetics experienced significant reductions in pain, sleep disturbances, and musculoskeletal stiffness ($p < 0.02$), together with better physical function and improved sense of well-being as measured by the Fibromyalgia Impact Questionnaire (FIQ). Thus, avoiding chemical exposure appears to provide no-cost no-risk therapeutic benefit to FM patients by alleviating pain and improving several indicators of overall health.

Conclusion: In sum, current research indicates that fibromyalgia results from impairment of cellular energy/ATP production (mitochondrial dysfunction) and induction of pain hypersensitivity (peripheral and central sensitization) due to absorbed metabolic toxins from bacterial/microbial overgrowth of the gastrointestinal tract; this is complicated by induction of tryptophan deficiency which is most likely caused by tryptophan degradation by bacterial tryptophanase activity and which leads to serotonin and melatonin insufficiencies, which lead to associated biochemical and clinical consequences, discussed previously. Available studies have shown that SIBO is ubiquitous among fibromyalgia patients and that antimicrobial interventions—whether pharmaceutical or nutritional—are efficacious. Secondary physiological effects such as mitochondrial impairment, pain sensitization, nutritional deficiencies, oxidative stress, and reduced tissue perfusion are treated with combined use of select therapeutics as reviewed previously. Patients presenting with widespread pain should be screened for causative underlying disease; if no other explanation can be found, then the diagnosis of fibromyalgia should be made, and the condition should be treated with the nondrug therapeutics discussed above. The first visit can include history, physical examination, and laboratory tests; initial laboratory assessment should include complete blood count (CBC), metabolic/chemistry panel, serum 25-hydroxyvitamin D, C-reactive protein (CRP), anti-nuclear antibodies

---

[574] Merchant RE, et al. Nutritional supplementation with Chlorella pyrenoidosa for patients with fibromyalgia syndrome: a pilot study. *Phytother Res* 2000 May;14:167-73
[575] Pore RS. Detoxification of chlordecone poisoned rats with chlorella and chlorella derived sporopollenin. *Drug Chem Toxicol.* 1984;7(1):57-71
[576] Morita K, Ogata M, Hasegawa T. Chlorophyll derived from Chlorella inhibits dioxin absorption from the gastrointestinal tract and accelerates dioxin excretion in rats. *Environ Health Perspect.* 2001 Mar;109(3):289-94
[577] Morita K, Matsueda T, Iida T, Hasegawa T. Chlorella accelerates dioxin excretion in rats. *J Nutr.* 1999 Sep;129(9):1731-6
[578] Nakano S, Noguchi T, Takekoshi H, Suzuki G, Nakano M. Maternal-fetal distribution and transfer of dioxins in pregnant women in Japan, and attempts to reduce maternal transfer with Chlorella (Chlorella pyrenoidosa) supplements. *Chemosphere.* 2005 Dec;61(9):1244-55
[579] Nakano et al. Chlorella (pyrenoidosa) supplementation decreases dioxin and increases immunoglobulin a concentrations in breast milk. *J Med Food.* 2007 Mar:134-42
[580] Sverdrup B. Use less cosmetics—suffer less from fibromyalgia? *J Womens Health* (Larchmt). 2004 Mar;13(2):187-94

(ANA), antibodies against cyclic citrullinated proteins (anti-CCP antibodies), ferritin, muscle enzymes aldolase and creatine kinase, and a complete thyroid assessment including TSH, free T4, free T3, total T3, reverse T3 (rT3), and antithyroid peroxidase and antithyroglobulin antibodies. First-day interventions can include dietary optimization, multivitamin-multimineral supplementation (including vitamin D3 and magnesium), tryptophan/5-HTP, CoQ10, mixed tocopherols, and combination fatty acids including gamma-linolenic acid (GLA), eicosapentaenoic acid (EPA) and docosahexaenoic acid (DHA). SIBO should be treated empirically; otherwise, it can be objectively assessed with breath hydrogen and methane testing, stool analysis, culture, microscopy, and parasitology. At follow-up visits, additional assessments and interventions (such as for toxic metals and chronic occult infections) can be used to fine-tune the diagnosis and further discover and define its contributors in order to maximize the patient's response to treatment and promote optimal recovery and health.

MIGRAINE HEADACHES, HYPOTHYROIDISM, AND FIBROMYALGIA:

ASSESSMENTS AND THERAPEUTIC APPROACHES USING INTEGRATIVE CHIROPRACTIC, NATUROPATHIC, OSTEOPATHIC, AND FUNCTIONAL MEDICINE

Objective *real* non-neurologic non-psychiatric abnormalities in fibromyalgia: the case against primary central sensitization.

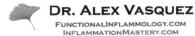

DR. ALEX VASQUEZ
FUNCTIONALINFLAMMOLOGY.COM
INFLAMMATIONMASTERY.COM

Archive: vimeo.com/56334919

MIGRAINE HEADACHES, HYPOTHYROIDISM, AND FIBROMYALGIA:

ASSESSMENTS AND THERAPEUTIC APPROACHES USING INTEGRATIVE CHIROPRACTIC, NATUROPATHIC, OSTEOPATHIC, AND FUNCTIONAL MEDICINE

Is "central sensitization" in fibromyalgia a bunch of c.r.a.p. (Commercial Rationalization Advocating Pharmaceuticals)?

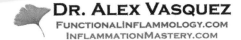

DR. ALEX VASQUEZ
FUNCTIONALINFLAMMOLOGY.COM
INFLAMMATIONMASTERY.COM

Archive: vimeo.com/56437367

Dysbiotic prototypes

Brain—dyscognition: Autointoxication, auto-brewery syndrome, hepatic encephalopathy sin hepatopathy

Brain—pain, fatigue, depression: Fibromyalgia

Inflammation—CIC, various tissues: Dysbiotic arthropathy, dermatitis, vasculitis

Inflammation—joints: Reactive arthritis

Inflammation—skin: Psoriasis

ICHNFM

Fibromyalgia

▸ One of my favorite clinical disorders because it blends 3 of my favorite topics:

1. **Dysbiosis**—these patients have a high prevalence of SIBO, which completely explains every aspect of the condition

2. **Mitochondrial dysfunction**—these patients have mitochondrial dysfunction caused by SIBO

3. **Social (in)justice**—perfectly exemplifies the extent to which the medical profession and medical practice can be easily coopted—hijacked—by the commercial interests of the pharmaceutical industry despite a mountain of research pointing directly to the cause and cure of this condition.

Archive: vimeo.com/139867947

How does small intestinal bacterial/microbial overgrowth (SIBO) cause fibromyalgia?

1. **Bacterial endotoxin/lipopolysaccharide/LPS**: causes inflammation, mitochondrial/muscle impairment, and increased sensitization to pain.

2. **Bacteria-produced D-lactic acid**: neurotoxin and metabolic poison; causes fatigue, muscle pain, dyscognition.

3. **Bacteria-produced hydrogen sulfide (H2S)**: neurotoxin and metabolic poison; causes fatigue, muscle pain, dyscognition.

4. **Bacteria-produced tryptophanase**: leads to tryptophan deficiency (documented in FM patients) and "serotonin deficiency" (pain, fatigue, carbohydrate cravings, depression) and "melatonin deficiency" (sleep disturbance, mitochondrial impairment, oxidative stress, muscle fatigue).

Archive: vimeo.com/56334918

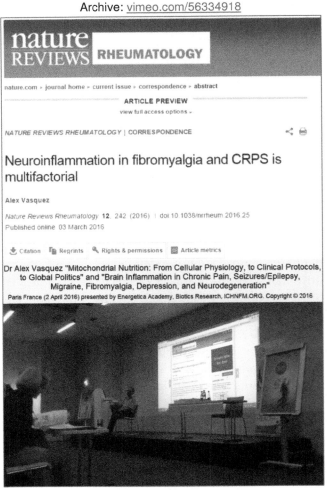

Archive: vimeo.com/161526099

Intracellular Hypercalcinosis: A Functional Nutritional Disorder with Implications Ranging from Myofascial Trigger Points to Affective Disorders, Hypertension, and Cancer

This article was originally published in *Naturopathy Digest* in 2006
naturopathydigest.com/archives/2006/sep/vasquez.php

Introduction: Let us explore the possibility that elevated levels of calcium *within the cell* (intracellular hypercalcinosis) might predispose toward a wide range of clinical problems including migraine, hypertension, myofascial trigger points, inflammation, and cancer. Further, let's review the data showing that several commonly employed nutritional interventions can be used synergistically to counteract and correct this problem. By the time readers complete this article, they will have 1) an understanding of this problem, 2) a protocol for how to correct this problem, and 3) be able to explain the biochemical rationale for using these nutritional protocols in patients who might otherwise be treated with drugs in general and calcium-channel-blocking drugs in particular.

Although prescription drugs are often used by medical doctors in a "willy-nilly manner" (according to Harvard Medical School Professor Dr. Jerry Avorn[581]), let's assume for a moment that legitimate reasons exist for the widespread use of drugs that block calcium channels in cell membranes—the "calcium-channel-blocking drugs." Although it is counterintuitive to promote health by interfering with the body's natural function, calcium-channel-blocking drugs are routinely used in pharmaceutical medicine for a broad range of problems including hypertension, heart rhythm disturbances, bipolar disorder, and anxiety/panic disorders. Widespread medical use of calcium-channel-blocking drugs appears to validate the supposition that excess intracellular calcium is an important contributor to these and perhaps other problems. Therefore, if intracellular hypercalcinosis is the problem, then any safe and cost-effective treatment that can correct this problem should be met with the same widespread acceptance given to calcium-channel-blocking drugs, which are universally accepted and utilized in the allopathic "conventional medicine" society. At the very least, we can generally state that all phenomena that contribute to calcium deficiency result in an increase in intracellular calcium levels (the "calcium paradox") due to the effect of parathyroid hormone, which specifically promotes calcium uptake in cells while mobilizing calcium from bone. Additionally, a few other nutritional influences (such as fatty acid imbalances) modulate cellular calcium balance, and these will be discussed in the section on clinical interventions.

The Problem of Excess Intracellular Calcium: Although the current author is the first to coin the phrase "intracellular hypercalcinosis", several other authors have pointed to the problem of the "calcium paradox" and the means by which *body-wide calcium deficiency* can result in *intracellular calcium overload*, which triggers a cascade of events leading to adverse health effects. Most notably, the work of Takuo Fujita[582,583] stands out in its clarity and specificity in linking intracellular hypercalcinosis with disorders such as hypertension, arteriosclerosis, diabetes mellitus, neurodegenerative diseases, malignancy, and degenerative joint disease.

Mechanisms by which intracellular hypercalcinosis contributes to disease have been defined, at least partially. However, we must remember that nutritional disorders never occur in isolation, and that the effects of intracellular hypercalcinosis observed clinically are overlaid with manifestations of the primary nutritional/metabolic disorder. Stated differently, contrary to what the pharmaceutical paradigm's monotherapeutic use of calcium-channel-blocking drugs would imply, intracellular hypercalcinosis never occurs by itself. For example, if intracellular hypercalcinosis is contributed to by vitamin D3 deficiency, then some of the observed clinical complications of that condition are due to and yet independent from the excess intracellular calcium since the primary problem (vitamin D3 deficiency) causes adverse effects and deficiency symptoms that are independent of its effect on intracellular calcium levels. To better understand the specific effects of excess intracellular calcium, a brief review of a few specific biochemical/physiologic mechanisms by which intracellular hypercalcinosis can contribute to disease is warranted. We must start by realizing that calcium is much more than

---

[581] America the Medicated. cbsnews.com/stories/2005/04/21/health/main689997.shtml
[582] Fujita T. Calcium paradox: consequences of calcium deficiency manifested by a wide variety of diseases. *J Bone Miner Metab.* 2000;18(4):234-6
[583] Fujita et al. Calcium paradox disease: calcium deficiency prompting secondary hyperparathyroidism and cellular calcium overload. *J Bone Miner Metab.* 2000;18(3):109-25

a "bone nutrient" and that it functions as an electrolyte, intracellular messenger, and regulator of cell replication and metabolism. Let's talk about five pathways by which increased intracellular calcium promotes disease:

1. <u>Adverse effects on membrane receptors and intracellular transduction</u>: The concentration of extracellular calcium exceeds the concentration of intracellular calcium by a ratio of 10,000 to one. When intracellular calcium levels rise even slightly, receptors and messaging systems in the cell membrane fail to function optimally. Thereby, increased intracellular calcium can predispose to insulin resistance (via interference with insulin receptors) and can promote neurodegeneration by amplifying the intracellular cascade of effects that follows activation of the brain's NMDA-receptors (excitoneurotoxicity). More specifically, we must note that the recently discovered "calcium-sensing receptor" (CaR, a G protein-coupled plasma membrane receptor) senses minute alterations in serum calcium levels and then ultimately translates these variations into changes in cellular function, notably alterations in cell replication (think cancer) and eicosanoid production (think inflammation).[584,585] Given that CaR are found in a wide range of cell types, including those found in bone, the kidneys, and immune system, we can see a pathway by which alterations in calcium balance could be implicated in a wide range of diseases. CaR-mediated alterations in cell function are likely to be complicated by disorders of vitamin D3 nutrition and metabolism (that commonly complicate disorders of calcium homeostasis), which affect an even wider range of cell types including those of the breast, prostate, ovary, lung, skin, lymph nodes, colon, pancreas, adrenal medulla, brain (pituitary, cerebellum, and cerebral cortex), aortic endothelium, and immune system, including monocytes, transformed B-cells, and activated T-cells. This is an example of the complexity involved in understanding nutrition in general and the effects of nutritional deficiency (always multifaceted) in particular.

2. <u>Mitochondrial failure and cell death</u>: According to the most recent edition of the classic text *Robbins Pathologic Basis of Disease* (pages 15-16), increased intracellular calcium is a major cause of cell death. When calcium levels are increased within the cell, one adverse effect is the inhibition of mitochondrial function. Since calcium is pumped out of the cell in an energy-dependent process, and because dysfunctional mitochondria pour calcium into the intracellular space, calcium-induced mitochondrial failure results in an additional increase in intracellular calcium. Further complicating this problem is the fact that the cell membrane becomes increasingly permeable to calcium as calcium levels increase. Elevated intracellular calcium levels activate enzymes such as ATPase, phospholipase, proteases, and endonucleases that promote cell death.

3. <u>Pro-inflammatory effects of intracellular calcium</u>: The recent finding that intracellular calcium activates NF-kappaB[586] has obvious implications given the pivotal role of NF-kappaB in the promotion of systemic inflammation and diseases such as rheumatoid arthritis.[587] Thus, increased intracellular calcium appears to promote inflammation. This may explain in part how vitamin D3 supplementation (which lowers intracellular calcium levels) exerts its clinically impressive anti-inflammatory and immunomodulatory benefits.[588]

4. <u>Enhanced production of lipid peroxides</u>: Fujita notes that lipid peroxides lead to an increase in cell membrane permeability to calcium, which results in increased intracellular calcium; this activates metabolic pathways that increase oxidative stress, thus leading to a vicious cycle stimulated by the production of additional lipid peroxides. Thus, intracellular hypercalcinosis promotes oxidative stress, which becomes self-perpetuating by this and other mechanisms. Of course, we all know by now that increased production of free radicals contributes to the development of many health problems, such as cancer, cardiovascular disease, arthritis, autoimmunity, diabetes, and other forms of rapid biological aging.

5. <u>Myofascial trigger points, chronic muscle spasm, and increased vascular tone (hypertension)</u>: The release of calcium from the sarcoplasmic reticulum triggers muscle contraction and plays a role in hypertension (hence the use of calcium-channel-blocking drugs in the treatment of hypertension), chronic muscle spasm

[584] Peterlik M, Cross HS. Vitamin D and calcium deficits predispose for multiple chronic diseases. *Eur J Clin Invest.* 2005 May;35(5):290-304

[585] Heaney RP. Long-latency deficiency disease: insights from calcium and vitamin D. *Am J Clin Nutr.* 2003 Nov;78(5):912-9

[586] "Furthermore, a calcium chelator, BAPTA-AM, attenuated the NF-kappaB activation... CONCLUSIONS: Induction of NF-kappaB within 30 min by TNF-alpha- and IL-1beta was mediated through intracellular calcium but not ROS." Chang JW, Kim CS, Kim SB, Park SK, Park JS, Lee SK. Proinflammatory cytokine-induced NF-kappaB activation in human mesangial cells is mediated through intracellular calcium but not ROS: effects of silymarin. *Nephron Exp Nephrol.* 2006;103:e156-65

[587] Tak PP, Firestein GS. NF-kappaB: a key role in inflammatory diseases. *J Clin Invest.* 2001 Jan;107(1):7-11

[588] Timms et al. Circulating MMP9, vitamin D and variation in the TIMP-1 response with VDR genotype: mechanisms for inflammatory damage in chronic disorders? *QJM.* 2002 Dec;95(12):787-96. See also: Vasquez A, Manso G, Cannell J. The clinical importance of vitamin D. *Altern Ther Health Med.* 2004 Sep-Oct;10(5):28-36

(especially when complicated by magnesium deficiency), and the perpetuation of myofascial trigger points.[589] Reducing the levels of cytosolic and sarcoplasmic calcium promotes muscle relaxation.

<u>Nutritional Interventions to Ameliorate Intracellular Hypercalcinosis</u>: Now that we've reviewed the data implicating intracellular hypercalcinosis as a legitimate contributor to a wide range of clinical disorders and diseases, let's explore some nutritional solutions.

1. <u>Correction of vitamin D deficiency</u>: Vitamin D deficiency causes calcium deficiency which increases parathyroid hormone production resulting in increased intracellular calcium levels. Vitamin D deficiency is common (40-80% of most populations) and can be established via history and more objectively by measurement of serum 25-hydroxyl-vitamin D. Replacement doses are in the range of 1,000 IU per day for infants, 2,000 IU per day for children, and 4,000 IU per day for adults.[590] Vitamin D2 (ergocalciferol) should be avoided, and vitamin D3 (cholecalciferol) should be used, preferably in emulsified form to facilitate absorption, especially in older patients and those with impaired digestion and absorption.[591]

2. <u>Reduction in dietary arachidonic acid intake</u>: Arachidonic acid promotes intracellular calcium uptake, as demonstrated in a recent study using human erythrocytes.[592] Rich sources of arachidonic acid include beef, liver, pork, lamb, and cow's milk.

3. <u>Increase intake of eicosapentaenoic acid (EPA)</u>: EPA reduces intracellular calcium levels in experimental models[593] and anticancer, antihypertensive, and anti-inflammatory effects of EPA are seen clinically. One to three grams per day is reasonable for adults.

4. <u>Urinary alkalinization</u>: Diet-induced chronic metabolic acidosis[594] promotes loss of calcium in urine[595] and thus indirectly contributes to calcium deficiency and the resultant rise in parathyroid hormone and intracellular calcium levels. An alkalinizing plant-based Paleo-Mediterranean diet should be the foundational treatment for numerous reasons[596]; however some patients may need to supplement with vegetable culture, potassium citrate, potassium bicarbonate, and/or sodium bicarbonate either regularly or "as needed"/PRN.

5. <u>Ensuring adequate intake of calcium</u>: A healthy diet can supply upwards toward 1,000 mg of calcium per day, and some people may choose to supplement with an additional 500 to 1,500 mg daily. Calcium supplementation should be used with magnesium, vitamin D and other components of the supplemented Paleo-Mediterranean diet.

6. <u>Avoiding other dietary and lifestyle factors that promote calcium loss in urine</u>: Caffeine, sugar, alcohol/ethanol, and psychoemotional stress all increase calcium loss in urine and thus contribute to secondary hyperparathyroidism and intracellular hypercalcinosis.

<u>Conclusions</u>: In this brief article, I have introduced and reviewed important concepts related to diet-induced alterations in cellular calcium balance. Notice that this discussion of calcium has transcended the usual conversation of simple "deficiency" and "excess." What I've done here is review data showing that we can indirectly modulate certain aspects of intracellular nutrition to promote optimal biochemical balance within the cell in order to optimize health and prevent and correct disease and dysfunction. Next time someone tells you that there is no scientific basis for interventional nutrition, sit them down and give them a lecture on causes and treatments for intracellular hypercalcinosis. Tell them it is only the tip of the iceberg, and that they'd be wise to take interventional nutrition seriously. Just because we buy groceries and nutritional supplements without a prescription (for now), this does not mean that these choices are not powerful or lacking in scientific merit. Amazing results can be achieved with diet modification and nutritional/botanical supplementation.

---

[589] Simons DG. Cardiology and myofascial trigger points: Janet G. Travell's contribution. *Tex Heart Inst J*. 2003;30(1):3-7

[590] Vasquez A, Manso G, Cannell J. The clinical importance of vitamin D (cholecalciferol). *Altern Ther Health Med*. 2004 Sep-Oct;10(5):28-36

[591] "The Ca(2+) influx rate varied from 0.5 to 3 nM Ca(2+)/s in the presence of AA and from 0.9 to 1.7 nM Ca(2+)/s with EPA." Soldati L, Lombardi C, Adamo D, Terranegra A, Bianchin C, Bianchi G, Vezzoli G. Arachidonic acid increases intracellular calcium in erythrocytes. *Biochem Biophys Res Commun*. 2002 May 10;293(3):974-8

[592] "The Ca(2+) influx rate varied from 0.5 to 3 nM Ca(2+)/s in the presence of AA and from 0.9 to 1.7 nM Ca(2+)/s with EPA." Soldati L, Lombardi C, Adamo D, Terranegra A, Bianchin C, Bianchi G, Vezzoli G. Arachidonic acid increases intracellular calcium in erythrocytes. *Biochem Biophys Res Commun*. 2002 May 10;293(3):974-8

[593] "This is a consequence of the ability of EPA to release Ca2+ from intracellular stores while inhibiting their refilling via capacitative Ca2+ influx that results in partial emptying of intracellular Ca2+ stores and thereby activation of protein kinase R." Palakurthi SS, Fluckiger R, Aktas H, Changolkar AK, Shahsafaei A, Harneit S, Kilic E, Halperin JA. Inhibition of translation initiation mediates the anticancer effect of the n-3 polyunsaturated fatty acid eicosapentaenoic acid. *Cancer Res*. 2000 Jun 1;60(11):2919-25

[594] Maurer M, Riesen W, Muser J, Hulter HN, Krapf R. Neutralization of Western diet inhibits bone resorption independently of K intake and reduces cortisol secretion in humans. *Am J Physiol Renal Physiol*. 2003 Jan;284(1):F32-40

[595] Sellmeyer et al. Potassium citrate prevents increased urine calcium excretion and bone resorption induced by a high sodium chloride diet. *J Clin Endocrinol Metab*. 2002 May;87(5):2008-12

[596] Vasquez A. A Five-Part Nutritional Protocol that Produces Consistently Positive Results. *Nutritional Wellness* 2005 September inflammationmastery.com/reprints

Allergy—Part 1: Allergic Inflammation

Introduction:

Allergic inflammation is the second of the three major categories of inflammation: ❶ Metabolic, including neuroinflammation, ❷ Allergic, and ❸ Rheumatic/Autoimmune. While exacerbations of allergic disease might necessitate pharmacologic immunosuppression, long-term management of allergic conditions should focus on nutritional immunomodulation (detailed in Chapter 4, Section 3 of *Functional Inflammology* / *Inflammation Mastery*. Failure to normalize the immunophenotype imbalance via nutritional immunomodulation and failure to reduce the total inflammatory load (TIL), especially the mitochondrial and dysbiotic components, are what lead to both pharmacologic dependence and pharmacologic failure in the management of allergic disease. Allergy in general and food allergy in particular are discussed in Chapter 4, Section 1 (op cit), and that information should be used in conjunction with the allergy-specific information in the following sections. Different from the other sections focusing on Clinical Applications, and appropriate for the clinical management of allergic disorders, treatments here are discussed relative to a "hierarchy of therapeutics" which—in the naturopathic medical model—prioritizes treatments which might be sequenced in first, second, third, and fourth groups. Hence the FINDSEX ® acronym and sequence has not been applied to these sections on allergy. Readers and clinicians can mentally mix and intellectually overlay the two approaches—FINSEX ® components and the sequential format here—for a skilled and flexible clinical approach.

Allergy and Food Allergy

"Adverse food reactions" is a broad and general category that includes food allergy, food sensitivity, and food intolerance. The term "food" here means anything that is ingested other than drugs and medications and includes food, drink, additives, preservatives, and dyes. Many studies have underestimated the true prevalence and clinical importance of food allergies because of inconsistent terminology, insensitive/inaccurate laboratory assessments[1], and the assumption that an "apparently healthy" person would only be allergic/sensitive to one or two foods—this is an erroneous assumption considering that many patients with food allergy/sensitivity/intolerance must avoid several (common range 3-10) commonly eaten foods to obtain clinical response and maximal improvement.[2,3] Clinical practice differs from basic research in that we as clinicians must often do what is effective while having neither the need nor the luxury for determining the molecular and physiologic basis for the effectiveness of each treatment in each patient. Clinical research has scientifically proven that *adverse food reactions*—regardless of the underlying mechanism(s) or classification of allergy/intolerance/sensitivity—can exacerbate a wide range of human illnesses, including thyroid disease[4], mental depression[5,6], asthma, rhinitis,[7] recurrent otitis media[8], migraine[9,10,11], attention deficit and hyperactivity disorders[12], epilepsy[13,14,15], gastrointestinal inflammation[16], hypertension[17], joint pain[18,19,20,21,22,23,24] and other health problems.

---

[1] Bindslev-Jensen C, Skov PS, Madsen F, Poulsen LK. Food allergy and food intolerance--what is the difference? *Ann Allergy*. 1994 Apr;72(4):317-20

[2] Grant EC. Food allergies and migraine. *Lancet*. 1979 May 5;1(8123):966-9

[3] Speer F. Multiple food allergy. *Ann Allergy*. 1975 Feb;34(2):71-6

[4] Sategna-Guidetti et al. Prevalence of thyroid disorders in untreated adult celiac disease patients and effect of gluten withdrawal. *Am J Gastroenterol*. 2001 Mar;96(3):751-7

[5] Mills N. Depression and food intolerance: a single case study. *Hum Nutr Appl Nutr*. 1986 Apr;40(2):141-5

[6] Parker G, Watkins T. Treatment-resistant depression: when antidepressant drug intolerance may indicate food intolerance. *Aust N Z J Psychiatry*. 2002;36(2):263-5

[7] Speer F. The allergic child. *Am Fam Physician*. 1975 Feb;11(2):88-94

[8] Juntti H, Tikkanen S, Kokkonen J, Alho OP, Niinimaki A. Cow's milk allergy is associated with recurrent otitis media during childhood. *Acta Otolaryngol*. 1999;119(8):867-73

[9] Monro J, Carini C, Brostoff J. Migraine is a food-allergic disease. *Lancet*. 1984 Sep 29;2(8405):719-21

[10] Egger J, Carter CM, Wilson J, Turner MW, Soothill JF.Is migraine food allergy?A double-blind controlled trial of oligoantigenic diet treatment.*Lancet*1983;2:865-9

[11] Monro J, Brostoff J, Carini C, Zilkha K. Food allergy in migraine. Study of dietary exclusion and RAST. *Lancet*. 1980 Jul 5;2(8184):1-4

[12] Boris M, Mandel FS. Foods and additives are common causes of the attention deficit hyperactive disorder in children. *Ann Allergy*. 1994 May;72(5):462-8

[13] Egger J, Carter CM, Soothill JF, Wilson J. Oligoantigenic diet treatment of children with epilepsy and migraine. *J Pediatr*. 1989;114(1):51-8

[14] Pelliccia et al. Partial cryptogenetic epilepsy and food allergy/intolerance. Reflections on three clinical cases. *Minerva Pediatr*. 1999 May;51(5):153-7

[15] Frediani T, Lucarelli S, Pelliccia A, et al. Allergy and childhood epilepsy: a close relationship? *Acta Neurol Scand*. 2001 Dec;104(6):349-52

[16] Marr HY, Chen WC, Lin LH. Food protein-induced enterocolitis syndrome: report of one case. *Acta Paediatr Taiwan*. 2001;42(1):49-52

[17] Grant EC. Food allergies and migraine. *Lancet*. 1979 May 5;1(8123):966-9

[18] Golding DN. Is there an allergic synovitis? *J R Soc Med*. 1990 May;83(5):312-4

[19] Panush RS. Food induced ("allergic") arthritis: clinical and serologic studies. *J Rheumatol*. 1990 Mar;17(3):291-4

[20] Pacor ML, Lunardi C, Di Lorenzo G, Biasi D, Corrocher R. Food allergy and seronegative arthritis: report of two cases. *Clin Rheumatol*. 2001;20(4):279-81

[21] Schrander JJ, Marcelis C, de Vries MP, van Santen-Hoeufft HM. Does food intolerance play a role in juvenile chronic arthritis? *Br J Rheumatol*. 1997;36(8):905-8

[22] van de Laar MA, van der Korst JK. Food intolerance in rheumatoid arthritis. I. A double blind, controlled trial of the clinical effects of elimination of milk allergens and azo dyes. *Ann Rheum Dis*. 1992 Mar;51(3):298-302

[23] Haugen MA,Kjeldsen-Kragh J, Forre O.A pilot study of the effect of an elemental diet in the management of rheumatoid arthritis.*Clin Exp Rheumatol* 1994;12:275-9

[24] van de Laar MA, Aalbers M, Bruins FG, et al. Food intolerance in rheumatoid arthritis. II. Clinical and histological aspects. *Ann Rheum Dis*. 1992 Mar;51(3):303-6

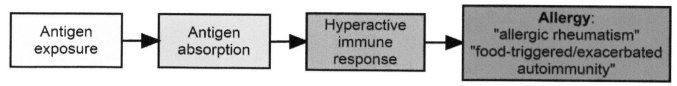

Overly simplistic ideas about allergy lead to overly simplistic drug treatments for allergic disease: This is the popular but inaccurate image that many patients and doctors have about allergy: "Allergy" and "allergic disease" do not result simply/solely from antigen exposure/absorption. The common view of allergic phenomena is incomplete and therefore inaccurate because it fails to include the prerequisite immune dysfunction and complex physiologic interconnections. Allergy should be seen as a reflection of immune dysfunction rather than a simple consequence of allergen exposure and absorption.

"**Food allergy**" generally refers to adverse food reactions that are specifically immunoglobulin-mediated. Classically, food allergy is seen with immediate-onset allergy mediated via IgE antibodies which initiate mast cell degranulation and histamine release. The classic symptoms of immediate-onset allergies are skin rash, abdominal pain, angioedema, and bronchoconstriction. However, many doctors recognize the possibility of IgG-mediated allergies and suggest that these might be responsible for the delayed-onset or "hidden" food allergies which are clinically significant but more subtle and difficult to diagnose than the classic IgE-mediated allergies.

> **Allergy is a manifestation of immune dysfunction; except for urgent or exceptionally recalcitrant cases, simply suppressing the symptoms of this manifestation is neither rational nor adequate treatment if our goal is to provide optimal healthcare by addressing the cause of the problem**
>
> "Allergic disease is a manifestation of a fundamental distortion of the mechanism through which the individual adapts itself on a cellular level to a hostile environment."
>
> Rapaport HG. What to do about the growing problem of pediatric allergy. *J Asthma Res.* 1967 Sep

The binding of antigens with immunoglobulins forms immune complexes that can deposit in parenchymal and synovial tissues where a localized immune response causes inflammation and organ dysfunction. "**Food sensitivity**" refers to immune-mediated adverse food reactions that are not antibody-mediated but are mediated by some other aspect of the immune/inflammatory system. An example of this is the increased production of specific prostaglandins in food-induced irritable bowel syndrome.[25] "**Food intolerance**" refers to adverse food reactions which are associated with poor nutritional status and/or impaired hepatic detoxification and which are *not* immune-mediated. Classic and well-known examples of this category of adverse food reaction include MSG sensitivity (associated with deficiency of vitamin B-6 and subsequent defects in hepatic transamination), tyramine intolerance that can result in hypertension and headaches, and histamine intolerance that can result in bronchoconstriction.[26] Surely, there is some overlap between allergy, sensitivity, and intolerance in some patients, and regardless of the specific mechanism(s) involved, from a practical clinical standpoint, the following facts are self-evident for any doctor working in the field of nutrition:

1. Some people have adverse food reactions from/to the foods that they eat. (This fact is obvious to anyone who has studied nutrition, but in most medical schools where nutrition is not taught, the only adverse food reaction discussed in class is the prototypic anaphylactic reaction [e.g., to peanuts] with possible mention of celiac disease while other forms of long-term and nonclassic food allergies/adversities are not discussed.)
2. Food-induced reactions may be either immediate-onset (i.e., within minutes) or delayed-onset (within days) of eating the triggering food.
3. The same patient might have immediate-onset reactions to food X with symptoms A and B and simultaneously have a delayed-onset reaction to food Y with symptom C.
4. Food X might cause symptoms D and E in one patient and symptoms F and G in another patient.
5. By avoiding allergens and/or improving or "modulating" immune function, many "diseases" resolve *without direct treatment* and the patient experiences an improved state of health.

---

[25] "Food intolerance associated with prostaglandin production is an important factor in the pathogenesis of IBS." Jones VA, McLaughlan P, Shorthouse M, Workman E, Hunter JO. Food intolerance: a major factor in the pathogenesis of irritable bowel syndrome. *Lancet.* 1982 Nov 20;2(8308):1115-7

[26] Wantke et al. Histamine in wine. Bronchoconstriction after a double-blind placebo-controlled red wine provocation test. *Int Arch Allergy Immunol.* 1996 Aug;110(4):397-400

6. Failure to identify and avoid problematic foods combined with failure to correct the underlying immune dysfunction often makes the "disease" recalcitrant to remediation even with "generally effective" treatment. This has been demonstrated in migraine, hypertension[27], and drug-resistant mental depression.[28]

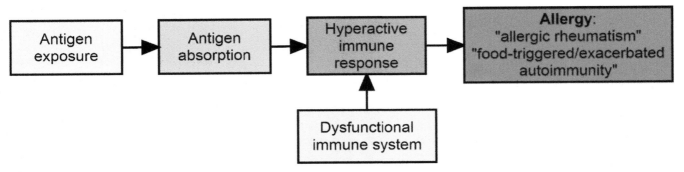

Allergy and allergic disease can only occur in the presence of preexisting immune dysfunction: Therefore, addressing the underlying immune dysfunction is the optimal treatment.

Potential roles of "food allergy" in the induction and perpetuation of autoimmunity and chronic inflammation

Food allergy both *results from* and *contributes to* immune dysfunction and a systemic proinflammatory state. Food allergy contributes to "autoimmunity" and musculoskeletal inflammation via several mechanisms, including but not limited to the following:

1. Stimulation of cytokine release: As will be discussed later, the term "superantigen" classically refers to microbial—viral, bacterial, or fungal—antigens which have the ability to induce production of excessive levels of cytokines and other inflammatory effectors[29], and superantigens appear to be involved in the pathogenesis of inflammatory musculoskeletal disorders such as rheumatoid arthritis.[30,31] In this section I propose that since food allergens appear capable of inducing cytokine production, they should in certain circumstances be considered "dietary superantigens" since they invoke cytokine release similarly as do microbial superantigens. An important distinction here, however, is that microbial superantigens generally stimulate cytokine release as an inherent property in *all* patients, whereas the production of cytokines by dietary (super)antigens is dependent on previous sensitization; thus cytokine production by allergens is patient-dependent and not an inherent property of the allergen itself. Mononuclear cells from egg-allergic patients produce much more proinflammatory cytokine (interferon) than do those from nonallergic patients.[32] Similarly, in children with autism, who commonly demonstrate immune dysfunction and neuroautoimmunity[33], exposure to food allergens greatly increases cytokine release compared to controls.[34] Food allergy, NFkB activation, cytokine release, and increased intestinal permeability form a self-perpetuating vicious cycle because consumption of dietary allergens causes damage to the intestinal mucosa and stimulates NFkB activation and cytokine release which then increases intestinal permeability, thus allowing for increased absorption of dietary and microbial immunogens for the perpetuation and

---

[27] "When an average of ten common foods were avoided there was a dramatic fall in the number of headaches per month, 85% of patients becoming headache-free. The 25% of patients with hypertension became normotensive." Grant EC. Food allergies and migraine. *Lancet.* 1979 May 5;1(8123):966-9

[28] "The prevalence of food intolerance as a contributing factor to depressive disorders requires clarification. Clinicians should be aware of the possible syndrome and that it may be worsened by psychotropic medication." Parker G, Watkins T. Treatment-resistant depression: when antidepressant drug intolerance may indicate food intolerance. *Aust N Z J Psychiatry.* 2002 Apr;36(2):263-5

[29] "The basis of autoimmune disorders due to superantigen is due to greater stimulation of T-lymphocytes and elaborate cytokine production." Hemalatha V, Srikanth P, Mallika M. Superantigens - Concepts, clinical disease and therapy. *Indian J Med Microbiol* 2004;22:204-211

[30] "They also suggest that the etiology of RA may involve initial activation of V beta 14+ T cells by a V beta 14-specific superantigen with subsequent recruitment of a few activated autoreactive v beta 14+ T cell clones to the joints while the majority of other V beta 14+ T cells disappear." Paliard X, West SG, Lafferty JA, Clements JR, Kappler JW, Marrack P, Kotzin BL. Evidence for the effects of a superantigen in rheumatoid arthritis. *Science.* 1991 Jul 19;253(5017):325-9

[31] "Given that binding sites for superantigens have been mapped to the CDR4s of TCR beta chains, the synovial localization of T cells bearing V beta s with significant CDR4 homology indicates that V beta-specific T-cell activation by superantigen may play a role in RA." Howell MD, Diveley JP, Lundeen KA, Esty A, Winters ST, Carlo DJ, Brostoff SW. Limited T-cell receptor beta-chain heterogeneity among interleukin 2 receptor-positive synovial T cells suggests a role for superantigen in rheumatoid arthritis. *Proc Natl Acad Sci U S A.* 1991 Dec 1;88(23):10921-5

[32] "The levels of IFN-gamma production of only IL-2-stimulated or both ovalbumin-stimulated and IL-2-stimulated peripheral blood mononuclear cells from egg-sensitive patients with atopic dermatitis was significantly higher than that of healthy children and that of egg-sensitive patients with immediate allergic symptoms." Shinbara M, Kondo N, Agata H, et al. Interferon-gamma and interleukin-4 production of ovalbumin-stimulated lymphocytes in egg-sensitive children. *Ann Allergy Asthma Immunol.* 1996;77(1):60-6

[33] "Autistic children, but not normal children, had antibodies to caudate nucleus (49% positive sera), cerebral cortex (18% positive sera) and cerebellum (9% positive sera)." Singh VK, Rivas WH. Prevalence of serum antibodies to caudate nucleus in autistic children. *Neurosci Lett.* 2004 Jan 23;355(1-2):53-6

[34] Jyonouchi H, Sun S, Itokazu N. Innate immunity associated with inflammatory responses and cytokine production against common dietary proteins in patients with autism spectrum disorder. *Neuropsychobiology.* 2002;46(2):76-84

exacerbation of allergy and immune dysfunction.[35] Generally speaking, cytokines are proinflammatory and would be expected to contribute to autoimmune disease induction via mechanisms such as bystander activation and increased autoantigen processing regardless of their original stimuli.

2. <u>Immune complex formation and deposition</u>: Dietary antigen-antibody immune complexes are formed following the consumption of allergenic foods by patients with allergy to those foods[36,37] and these anti-food and anti-IgE immune complexes contribute to allergic symptomatology by a mechanism that has been described as "chronic serum sickness."[38] These immune complexes are then deposited in the joints to localize the resultant proinflammatory response. In the study by Carini et al[39], the authors found that patients with food-induced joint pain and inflammation had anti-IgE IgG antibodies which formed large immune complexes that were detectable in synovial fluid and which probably contributed to the arthritis. Anti-IgE IgG antibodies are commonly elevated in patients with allergic/inflammatory diseases such as eczema[40], asthma[41], and Crohn's disease[42] and thus tissue damage in these conditions appears mediated at least in part by anti-immunoglobulin immune complexes (i.e., anti-IgE IgG complexed with IgE) rather than the classic antigen-antibody immune complexes. In this way, food allergies cause joint pain and inflammation by the deposition of immune complexes into the synovium and joint cartilage.[43] Conversely, the consumption of a relatively hypoallergenic diet reduces intake of food antigens and helps reduce IgE levels. This explains, in part, the success of hypoallergenic diets in the treatment of immune-complex-mediated diseases such as mixed cryoglobulinemia[44,45], hypersensitivity vasculitis[46], and leukocytoclastic vasculitis with arthritis.[47] In patients with rheumatoid arthritis, the symptomatic and clinical improvement induced by hypoallergenic diets correlates with reductions in antibodies to food antigens.[48]

3. <u>Damage to the intestinal mucosa with resultant increased absorption of dietary and microbial antigens</u>: Consumption of food allergens increases intestinal permeability[49] and thus amplifies the absorption of intestinal contents—dietary and microbial antigens. Patients with food allergy have "leaky gut" that is

> **Perspective & Context**
>
> This section on the protean clinical manifestations of allergy originally emphasized the relevance of allergy to systemic inflammation, including rheumatic diseases. Clinicians should keep food allergy and intolerance in mind when dealing with a wide range of conditions, including:
> - Thyroid disease
> - Mental depression
> - Fatigue
> - Asthma
> - Rhinitis
> - Recurrent otitis media
> - Migraine
> - Attention deficit and hyperactivity disorders
> - Epilepsy
> - Gastrointestinal inflammation and chronic abdominal pain
> - Hypertension
> - Joint pain and inflammation

---

[35] Ma et al. TNF-alpha-induced increase in intestinal epithelial tight junction permeability requires NF-kappa B activation. Am *J Physiol Gastrointest Liver Physiol*. 2004 Mar;286(3):G367-76 ajpgi.physiology.org/cgi/content/full/286/3/G367

[36] "Antigen entry and the formation of immune complexes occur in atopic subjects after food ingestion. ...Food allergic subjects showed, after food challenge, the presence of IgE and IgG immune complexes, which correlates with the subsequent occurrence of symptoms." Carini C, Brostoff J. Evidence for circulating IgE complexes in food allergy. *Ric Clin Lab*. 1987 Oct-Dec;17(4):309-22

[37] "Following challenge, immune complexes containing IgE, IgG, and antigen are detectable in the circulation. Their appearance correlates with the production of symptoms." Carini C, Brostoff J, Wraith DG. IgE complexes in food allergy. *Ann Allergy*. 1987 Aug;59(2):110-7

[38] Marinkovich V. "Immunology and Food Allergy" in "Applying Functional Medicine in Clinical Practice" hosted by the Institute for Functional Medicine. Seattle,Wa: Mar2005

[39] "In three food-allergic patients IgG anti-IgE was detectable in a complexed form in the serum samples examined before and after food challenge. The finding of IgG anti-IgE autoantibody in a group of patients with allergic arthralgia is quite exciting." Carini et al. Immune complexes in food-induced arthralgia. *Ann Allergy*. 1987 Dec;59(6):422-8

[40] "An IgG type of antibody directed against IgE has been studied in serum from healthy and allergic individuals. ... Significantly raised levels of anti-IgE autoantibody were found in patients suffering from atopic disorders in comparison to the controls." Carini et al. IgG autoantibody to IgE in atopic patients. *Ann Allergy*. 1988 Jan;60(1):48-52

[41] "Significantly enhanced levels of IgE/anti-IgE IC were detected in children with asthma." Ritter C, Battig M, Kraemer R, Stadler BM. IgE hidden in immune complexes with anti-IgE autoantibodies in children with asthma. *J Allergy Clin Immunol*. 1991 Nov;88(5):793-801

[42] "In CD sera no food-specific IgE could be detected, but levels of immune complexes of IgE and IgG anti-IgE autoantibodies were statistically significantly increased compared to healthy controls." Huber et al. IgE/anti-IgE immune complexes in sera from patients with Crohn's disease do not contain food-specific IgE. *Int Arch Allergy Immunol*. 1998 Jan;115(1):67-72

[43] Inman RD. Antigens, the gastrointestinal tract, and arthritis. *Rheum Dis Clin North Am*. 1991 May;17(2):309-21

[44] "CONCLUSION: These data show that an LAC diet decreases the amount of circulating immune complexes in MC and can modify certain signs and symptoms of the disease." Ferri C, Pietrogrande M, Cecchetti R, et al. Low-antigen-content diet in the treatment of patients with mixed cryoglobulinemia. *Am J Med*. 1989 Nov;87(5):519-24

[45] Pietrogrande M, Cefalo A, Nicora F, Marchesini D. Dietetic treatment of essential mixed cryoglobulinemia. *Ric Clin Lab*. 1986 Apr-Jun;16(2):413-6

[46] "In three cases the vasculitis relapsed following the introduction of food additives; in one case with the addition of potatoes and green vegetables (i.e., beans and green peas) and in the last case with the addition of eggs to the diet." Lunardi et al. Elimination diet in the treatment of selected patients with hypersensitivity vasculitis. *Clin Exp Rheumatol*. 1992 Mar-Apr;10(2):131-5

[47] "Described in this report are two children with severe vasculitis caused by specific foods." Businco L, Falconieri P, Bellioni-Businco B, Bahna SL. Severe food-induced vasculitis in two children. *Pediatr Allergy Immunol*. 2002 Feb;13(1):68-71

[48] Hafstrom I, Ringertz B, Spangberg A, et al. A vegan diet free of gluten improves the signs and symptoms of rheumatoid arthritis: the effects on arthritis correlate with a reduction in antibodies to food antigens. *Rheumatology*. 2001 Oct;40(10):1175-9 rheumatology.oxfordjournals.org/cgi/content/full/40/10/1175

[49] "When compared to the control group, the 11 patients of the allergic group presented a normal mannitol urinary excretion (16.5 +/- 13.4%, p = NS, Student's t-test) and an increase in the lactulose excretion (1.36 +/- 0.92%, p < 0.001). Moreover, the allergic group showed a lactulose/mannitol ratio that was significantly different (0.105 +/- 0.071, p < 0.001)." Laudat A, Arnaud P, Napoly A, Brion F. The intestinal permeability test applied to the diagnosis of food allergy in paediatrics. *West Indian Med J*. 1994 Sep;43(3):87-8

exacerbated by consumption of allergenic foods; thus lactulose-mannitol assays can be used to assist the diagnosis of food allergy.[50,51] By increasing intestinal permeability, consumption of dietary antigens serves to exacerbate the adverse effects of gastrointestinal dysbiosis by increasing antigen and (anti)metabolite absorption. Since both dietary allergens and bacterial endotoxin stimulate production of cytokines[52], concomitant exposure to both allergens and intra-intestinal endotoxin leads to an additive increase in proinflammatory cytokine production.[53] Thus, consumption of allergenic foods in the presence of gastrointestinal dysbiosis would be expected to lead to more severe and more diverse adverse physiologic and clinical consequences than would be experienced following exposure to either allergens or dysbiosis alone.

4. <u>Dietary haptenization</u>: Dietary antigens can complex with human tissues to form *neoantigens* that are immunostimulatory. The best example of this appears to be the induction of autoimmunity by wheat-derived gliadin which haptenizes with intestinal tissue transglutaminase and other extracellular matrix proteins and results in the allergic-autoimmune disease celiac disease.[54,55] The finding that gliadin proteins haptenize with collagen and can induce the formation of anti-collagen antibodies in humans[56] makes clear the pathomechanism by which "wheat allergy" can directly precipitate systemic musculoskeletal autoimmunity. Once initiated and perpetuated by dietary gliadin from wheat, additional autoimmunity ensues (perhaps mediated directly by epitope spreading and/or indirectly by deposition of immune complexes) which is directed against various tissues, most notably the thyroid gland[57], brain[58], and musculoskeletal system.[59] Given the association between lupus and celiac disease[60,61,62], we may speculate that "allergy" becomes/triggers "autoimmunity" in certain circumstances and in susceptible patients.

5. <u>Dietary molecular mimicry</u>: Just as microbes produce structures similar to human molecules which then incite a cross-reacting immune response—molecular mimicry (discussed elsewhere in this chapter in the section on dysbiosis)—certain dietary antigens appear capable of inducing cross reactions. For example, Vojdani et al[63] recently demonstrated cross-reactivity between anti-gliadin antibodies and anti-cerebellar antibodies in an experimental model that may partly explain the anti-brain autoimmunity seen in autism. Further expanding this concept of dietary molecular mimicry is the finding that "the virulence factor of C albicans-hyphal wall protein 1 (HWP1)-contains amino acid sequences that are identical or highly homologous to known celiac disease-related alpha-gliadin and gamma-gliadin T-cell epitopes."[64] This raises three interrelated possibilities: 1) that gastrointestinal overgrowth of *Candida albicans* and the

[50] "After ingestion of food allergens by the patients, mean mannitol recovery fell to 11.57% and mean recovery of lactulose rose to 1.04%, both values being significantly different from those obtained in the fasting patients." Andre C, Andre F, Colin L, Cavagna S. Measurement of intestinal permeability to mannitol and lactulose as a means of diagnosing food allergy and evaluating therapeutic effectiveness of disodium cromoglycate. *Ann Allergy.* 1987 Nov;59(5 Pt 2):127-30

[51] "A provocation IPT with food induced significant L/M ratio changes only in the group in which the food was proved to be responsible for the exacerbation of skin lesions." Dupont C, Barau E, Molkhou P, Raynaud F, Barbet JP, Dehennin L. Food-induced alterations of intestinal permeability in children with cow's milk-sensitive enteropathy and atopic dermatitis. *J Pediatr Gastroenterol Nutr.* 1989 May;8(4):459-65

[52] Jyonouchi H, Sun S, Itokazu N. Innate immunity associated with inflammatory responses and cytokine production against common dietary proteins in patients with autism spectrum disorder. *Neuropsychobiology.* 2002;46(2):76-84

[53] "Thus, endotoxin and allergen acting together could play a role in up-regulating the response of the human asthmatic airway to adenosine. However, our data suggest that the interaction would be additive rather than synergistic." Karmouty Quintana H, Mazzoni L, Fozard JR. Effects of endotoxin and allergen alone and in combination on the sensitivity of the rat airways to adenosine. *Auton Autacoid Pharmacol.* 2005 Oct;25(4):167-70

[54] "Our findings firstly demonstrated that gliadin was directly bound to tTG in duodenal mucosa of coeliacs and controls, and the ability of circulating tTG-autoantibodies to recognize and immunoprecipitate the tTG-gliadin complexes." Ciccocioppo R, Di Sabatino A, Ara C, Biagi F, Perilli M, Amicosante G, Cifone MG, Corazza GR. Gliadin and tissue transglutaminase complexes in normal and coeliac duodenal mucosa. *Clin Exp Immunol.* 2003 Dec;134(3):516-24

[55] "Thus, modification of gluten peptides by tTG, especially deamidation of certain glutamine residues, can enhance their binding to HLA-DQ2 or -DQ8 and potentiate T cell stimulation. Furthermore, tTG-catalyzed cross-linking and consequent haptenization of gluten with extracellular matrix proteins allows for storage and extended availability of gluten in the mucosa." Dieterich W, Esslinger B, Schuppan D. Pathomechanisms in celiac disease. *Int Arch Allergy Immunol.* 2003 Oct;132(2):98-108

[56] "Gliadins alpha1-alpha11, gamma1- gamma6, omega1-omega3, and omega5 were substrates for tTG. tTG catalyzed the crosslinking of gliadin peptides with interstitial collagens type I, III and VI. Coeliac patients showed increased antibody titers against the collagens I, III, V and VI." Dieterich et al. Crosslinking to tissue transglutaminase and collagen favours gliadin toxicity in coeliac disease. *Gut.* 2006 Apr; 55(4): 478–484

[57] "Elevated titres of antithyroid antibodies observed in children with coeliac disease (41.1%) in comparison to control group (3.56%) indicate the need for performing the screening tests for antithyroid antibodies in children with CD." Kowalska E, Wasowska-Krolikowska K, Toporowska-Kowalska E. Estimation of antithyroid antibodies occurrence in children with coeliac disease. *Med Sci Monit.* 2000 Jul-Aug;6(4):719-2 medscimonit.com/pub/vol_6/no_4/1240.pdf

[58] Kieslich M, Errazuriz G, Posselt HG, Moeller-Hartmann W, Zanella F, Boehles H. Brain white-matter lesions in celiac disease: a prospective study of 75 diet-treated patients. *Pediatrics.* 2001 Aug/108(2):E21 pediatrics.aappublications.org/cgi/content/full/108/2/e21

[59] "JIA children have an increased prevalence of autoimmune thyroiditis, subclinical hypothyroidism and coeliac disease." Stagi S, Giani T, Simonini G, Falcini F. Thyroid function, autoimmune thyroiditis and coeliac disease in juvenile idiopathic arthritis. *Rheumatology* (Oxford). 2005 Apr;44(4):517-2

[60] Zitouni M, Daoud W, Kallel M, Makni S. Systemic lupus erythematosus with celiac disease: a report of five cases. *Joint Bone Spine.* 2004 Jul;71(4):344-6

[61] Komatireddy GR, Marshall JB, Aqel R, Spollen LE, Sharp GC. Association of systemic lupus erythematosus and gluten enteropathy. *South Med J.* 1995 Jun;88(6):673-6

[62] Rustgi AK, Peppercorn MA. Gluten-sensitive enteropathy and systemic lupus erythematosus. *Arch Intern Med.* 1988 Jul;148(7):1583-4

[63] "This cross-reaction was further confirmed by DOT-immunoblot and inhibition studies. We conclude that a subgroup of patients with autism produce antibodies against Purkinje cells and gliadin peptides, which may be responsible for some of the neurological symptoms in autism." Vojdani A, O'Bryan T, Green JA, Mccandless J, Woeller KN, Vojdani E, Nourian AA, Cooper EL. Immune response to dietary proteins, gliadin and cerebellar peptides in children with autism. *Nutr Neurosci.* 2004 Jun;7(3):151-61

[64] "Subsequently, C albicans might function as an adjuvant that stimulates antibody formation against HWP1 and gluten, and formation of autoreactive antibodies against tissue transglutaminase and endomysium." Nieuwenhuizen et al. Is Candida albicans a trigger in the onset of coeliac disease? *Lancet.* 2003;361(9375):2152-4

resultant elaboration of HWP1 and immunostimulation may result in sensitivity to gluten, particularly as HWP1 and gliadin are both substrates for transglutaminase, 2) that consumption of wheat gluten may trigger sensitivity to *Candida albicans,* and 3) that wheat gluten and *Candida albicans* must both be present for the development of celiac disease and the ensuant autoimmunity. Additional details on the ability of C. *albicans* to contribute to autoimmunity are discussed in the section on dysbiosis.

6. Enhanced processing of autoantigens: Food-allergic patients may produce autoimmunity-stimulating autoantigens following exposure to foods to which they are sensitized. This has been demonstrated in autistic children, exposure of lymphocytes from autistic patients to dietary antigens (gliadin and casein peptides) stimulates production of autoantigens that presumably incite and perpetuate autoimmunity.[65] Thus, at least in autistic patients, we have evidence that food allergy can segue into autoimmunity. This phenomenon is probably not restricted only to autistic patients, as suggested by the association between celiac disease and the systemic autoimmune disease lupus.[66,67,68]

7. Diet-derived xenobiotic immunotoxicity: Foods commonly contain trace amounts of xenobiotics such as pesticides, fungicides, fumigants, fertilizers, preservatives, military propellants such as perchlorate[69], and toxic metals such as mercury. Some of these xenobiotics have been insufficiently studied in humans, while others such as mercury are well-known immunotoxins capable of inducing immune dysfunction which may contribute to autoimmunity. Mercury poisoning/accumulation can occur in humans as a result of consumption of contaminated foods—especially seafood such as shark, swordfish, king mackerel, tilefish, and albacore ("white") tuna[70], and the immunologic effects of organic and/or inorganic mercury include immunosuppression, immunostimulation, formation of antinucleolar antibodies targeting fibrillarin, and formation and deposition of immune-complexes, resulting in a syndrome called "mercury-induced autoimmunity" which can be induced by exposure of susceptible animals to mercury.[71] Mercury/"silver" amalgam dental fillings rank highly among the most significant source of mercury exposure in humans, and implantation of mercury-silver dental amalgams in susceptible animals causes chronic stimulation of the immune system with induction of systemic autoimmunity.[72] Besides being a neurotoxin with no safe exposure limit[73], mercury is known to modify/antigenize endogenous proteins to promote autoimmunity[74], and mercury may also promote autoimmunity by contributing to a pro-inflammatory environment that awakens quiescent autoreactive immunocytes via bystander activation[75] (detailed later). For example, administration of mercury to "susceptible" mice induces autoimmunity via modification of the nucleolar protein *fibrillarin*[76]; noteworthy in this regard is the fact that antifibrillarin antibodies are characteristic of the autoimmune disease scleroderma.[77] Mercury toxicity is commonly encountered in clinical practice (diagnosis and treatment are discussed later), and a recent study published in *JAMA* showed that 8% of American women of childbearing age have sufficient levels of mercury in their bodies to produce neurologic damage in their children.[78] The mercury-based preservative thimerosol is a type-IV (delayed

[65] Vojdani A, Pangborn JB, Vojdani E, Cooper EL. Infections, toxic chemicals and dietary peptides binding to lymphocyte receptors and tissue enzymes are major instigators of autoimmunity in autism. *Int J Immunopathol Pharmacol.* 2003 Sep-Dec;16(3):189-99

[66] Zitouni M, Daoud W, Kallel M, Makni S. Systemic lupus erythematosus with celiac disease: a report of five cases. *Joint Bone Spine.* 2004 Jul;71(4):344-6

[67] Komatireddy GR, Marshall JB, Aqel R, Spollen LE, Sharp GC. Association of systemic lupus erythematosus and gluten enteropathy. *South Med J.* 1995 Jun;88(6):673-6

[68] Rustgi AK, Peppercorn MA. Gluten-sensitive enteropathy and systemic lupus erythematosus. *Arch Intern Med.* 1988 Jul;148(7):1583-4

[69] "The Bush administration has imposed a gag order on the U.S. Environmental Protection Agency from publicly discussing perchlorate pollution, even as two new studies reveal high levels of the rocket-fuel component may be contaminating the nation's lettuce supply." Peter Waldman. Rocket Fuel Residues Found in Lettuce: Bush administration issues gag order on EPA discussions of possible rocket fuel tainted lettuce. *Wall Street Journal.* See organicconsumers.org/toxic/lettuce042903.cfm rhinoed.com/epa's_gag_order.htm peer.org/press/508.html yubanet.com/artman/publish/article_13637.shtml

[70] See cfsan.fda.gov/~dms/admehg3.html for the white-washed version; see ewg.org/issues/mercury/20040319/index.php for a more complete perspective.

[71] Havarinasab S, Hultman P. Organic mercury compounds and autoimmunity. *Autoimmun Rev.* 2005;4(5):270-5 generationrescue.org/pdf/havarinasab.pdf

[72] "We hypothesize that under appropriate conditions of genetic susceptibility and adequate body burden, heavy metal exposure from dental amalgam may contribute to immunological aberrations, which could lead to overt autoimmunity." Hultman P, Johansson U, Turley SJ, Lindh U, Enestrom S, Pollard KM. Adverse immunological effects and autoimmunity induced by dental amalgam and alloy in mice. *FASEB J.* 1994 Nov;8(14):1183-90 fasebj.org/cgi/reprint/8/14/1183

[73] University of Calgary Faculty of Medicine. How Mercury Causes Brain Neuron Degeneration commons.ucalgary.ca/mercury/

[74] Havarinasab S, Hultman P. Organic mercury compounds and autoimmunity. *Autoimmun Rev.* 2005 Jun;4(5):270-5

[75] "It is therefore theoretically possible that compounds present in vaccines such as thiomersal or aluminium hydroxyde can trigger autoimmune reactions through bystander effects." Fournie et al. Induction of autoimmunity through bystander effects. Lessons from immunological disorders induced by heavy metals. *J Autoimmun.* 2001 May;16:319-26

[76] Nielsen JB, Hultman P. Mercury-induced autoimmunity in mice. *Environ Health Perspect.* 2002 Oct;110 Suppl 5:877-81

[77] "Since anti-fibrillarin antibodies are specific markers of scleroderma, the present animal model may be valuable for studies of the immunological aberrations which are likely to induce this autoimmune response." Hultman P, Enestrom S, Pollard KM, Tan EM. Anti-fibrillarin autoantibodies in mercury-treated mice. *Clin Exp Immunol.* 1989 Dec;78:470-7

[78] "However, approximately 8% of women had concentrations higher than the US Environmental Protection Agency's recommended reference dose (5.8 microg/L), below which exposures are considered to be without adverse effects. Women who are pregnant or who intend to become pregnant should follow federal and state advisories on consumption of fish." Schober et al. Blood mercury levels in US children and women of childbearing age, 1999-2000. *JAMA.* 2003 Apr 2;289(13):1667-74

hypersensitivity) sensitizing agent[79], and recent research implicates mercury as an important contributor to the clinical manifestations of autism[80,81] and eczema.[82] Preliminary clinical evidence shows that removal of mercury amalgams, particularly along with implementation of antioxidant therapy and/or mercury chelation, benefits the biochemical status and/or clinical course of autoimmune disease.[83,84] More recently, what has become very clear is that many foods are contaminated with pesticides; glyphosate for example promotes DNA damage, endocrine disruption, mitochondrial dysfunction, and—via its antibiotic effect—gastrointestinal dysbiosis.[85,86,87,88] Pesticide-contaminated foods and drinks should be avoided.

8. Diet-derived dysbiosis: Induction and exacerbation of dysbiosis following chronic consumption of allergenic foods has been reported to occur in humans; this paragraph reviews the three main types of diet induced dysbiosis: ❶ food contamination with problematic microbes, ❷ promotion of gastrointestinal bacterial overgrowth by over-consumption of carbohydrate substrate, and ❸ chronic diet-induced immunosuppression due to nutrient insufficiency or carbohydrate overconsumption. Raw vegetables and salad greens are thoroughly contaminated with bacteria and occasionally other microbes. Food can be contaminated with pathogenic microbes via improper preparation, storage, or handling by chefs with contagious diseases and poor hygiene. An inflammatory "reactive" arthritis can result from consumption of food that is contaminated by microorganisms, most commonly *Salmonella*[89,90,91] and *Campylobacter* species.[92] Long-term autoimmune/inflammatory complications of gastrointestinal infections/colonization sourced from food include Reiter's syndrome, Guillain-Barre syndrome (autoimmunity peripheral demyelinating neuropathy), uveitis, sacroiliitis, and ankylosing spondylitis. Independent and probably more common than the food contamination issues mentioned at the first half of this paragraph is the chronic gastrointestinal dysbiosis—in particular a generalized bacterial overgrowth of the small bowel—that is maintained and perpetuated by overconsumption of carbohydrates in general (starches, rice, sucrose, fructose) and difficult-to-digest carbohydrates in particular (such as those found in milk/lactose, wheat, and potatoes). High-fructose beverages are very popular, and they can promote excess colonic fermentation[93] which would be expected to result in bacterial overgrowth over time. By "feeding" intestinal bacteria with excess carbohydrate and promoting bacterial overgrowth in the intestines, the standard Western/American diet promotes dysbiosis-induced systemic inflammation and chronic musculoskeletal pain; this is particularly relevant for patients with rheumatoid arthritis or fibromyalgia.[94] Thus dietary modification taken in the interest of avoiding common allergens such as milk and wheat quite likely results

[79] "Thimerosal is an important preservative in vaccines and ophthalmologic preparations. The substance is known to be a type IV sensitizing agent. High sensitization rates were observed in contact-allergic patients and in health care workers who had been exposed to thimerosal-preserved vaccines." Westphal et al. Homozygous gene deletions of the glutathione S-transferases M1 and T1 are associated with thimerosal sensitization. *Int Arch Occup Environ Health*. 2000 Aug;73(6):384-8

[80] Vojdani A, Pangborn JB, Vojdani E, Cooper EL. Infections, toxic chemicals and dietary peptides binding to lymphocyte receptors and tissue enzymes are major instigators of autoimmunity in autism. *Int J Immunopathol Pharmacol*. 2003 Sep-Dec;16(3):189-99

[81] Geier DA, Geier MR. A comparative evaluation of the effects of MMR immunization and mercury doses from thimerosal-containing childhood vaccines on the population prevalence of autism. *Med Sci Monit*. 2004 Mar;10(3):PI33-9. Epub 2004 Mar 1. medscimonit.com/pub/vol_10/no_3/3986.pdf

[82] Weidinger et al. Body burden of mercury is associated with acute atopic eczema and total IgE in children from southern Germany. *J Allergy Clin Immunol*. 2004 Aug;114(2):457-9

[83] Prochazkova J, Sterzl I, Kucerova H, Bartova J, Stejskal VD. The beneficial effect of amalgam replacement on health in patients with autoimmunity. *Neuro Endocrinol Lett*. 2004 Jun;25(3):211-8. See also: "The MELISA Test is reproducible, sensitive, specific, and reliable for detecting metal sensitivity in metal-sensitive patients." Valentine-Thon E, Schiwara HW. Validity of MELISA for metal sensitivity testing. *Neuro Endocrinol Lett*. 2003 Feb-Apr;24(1-2):57-64. See also: "The hypothesis that metal exposure from dental amalgam can cause ill health in a susceptible part of the exposed population was supported." Lindh U, Hudecek R, Danersund A, Eriksson S, Lindvall A. Removal of dental amalgam and other metal alloys supported by antioxidant therapy alleviates symptoms and improves quality of life in patients with amalgam-associated ill health. *Neuro Endocrinol Lett*. 2002 Oct-Dec;23(5-6):459-82 nel.edu/23_56/NEL235602A12_Lindh.htm and nel.edu/pdf_w/23_56/NEL235602A12_Lindh_wr.pdf

[84] "This study documents objective biochemical changes following the removal of these fillings along with other dental materials, utilizing a new health care model of multidisciplinary planning and treatment." Huggins HA, Levy TE. Cerebrospinal fluid protein changes in multiple sclerosis after dental amalgam removal. *Altern Med Rev*. 1998 Aug;3(4):295-300

[85] Seneff S, Swanson N Li C. Aluminum and Glyphosate Can Synergistically Induce Pineal Gland Pathology: Connection to Gut Dysbiosis and Neurological Disease. *Agricultural Sciences* 2015; 6, 42-70. dx.doi.org/10.4236/as.2015.61005

[86] Krüger M, Schledorn P, Schrödl W, Hoppe HW, Lutz W, et al. Detection of Glyphosate Residues in Animals and Humans. *J Environ Anal Toxicol* 2014;4: 210

[87] Shehata AA, Schrödl W, Schledorn P, Krüger M. Distribution of glyphosate in chicken organs and its reduction by humic acid supplementation. *J Poult Sci*. 2014;51:333-7

[88] Krüger et al. Glyphosate suppresses the antagonistic effect of Enterococcus spp. on Clostridium botulinum. *Anaerobe*. 2013 Apr;20:74-8

[89] "We describe the case of a patient who became ill with Salmonella Blockley food poisoning while working in Cyprus in August 1994. As his diarrhoea resolved he began to suffer from lower limb joint pains which were diagnosed as acute salmonella reactive arthritis." Wilson IG, Whitehead E. Long-term post-Salmonella reactive arthritis due to Salmonella Blockley. *Jpn J Infect Dis*. 2004 Oct;57(5):210-1

[90] "Reactive joint symptoms after food-borne Salmonella infection may be more frequent than previously thought. The duration of diarrhea is strongly correlated with the occurrence of joint symptoms." Locht et al. High frequency of reactive joint symptoms after an outbreak of Salmonella enteritidis. *J Rheumatol*. 2002 Apr;29(4):767-71

[91] Leirisalo-Repo et al. Long-term prognosis of reactive salmonella arthritis. *Ann Rheum Dis*. 1997 Sep;56(9):516-20 ard.bmjjournals.com/cgi/content/full/56/9/516

[92] "Campylobacter jejuni is the most commonly reported bacterial cause of foodborne infection in the United States. Adding to the human and economic costs are chronic sequelae associated with C. jejuni infection--Guillian-Barre syndrome and reactive arthritis." Altekruse SF, Stern NJ, Fields PI, Swerdlow DL. Campylobacter jejuni--an emerging foodborne pathogen. *Emerg Infect Dis*. 1999 Jan-Feb;5(1):28-35

[93] "RESULTS: The incidence of colonic fermentation after ingesting sports drink, milk, and green tea was five (62.5%), six (75%), and none (0%), respectively in eight subjects." Mitsui T, Shimaoka K, Kanao Y, Kondo T. Colonic fermentation after ingestion of fructose-containing sports drink. *J Sports Med Phys Fitness*. 2001 Mar;41(1):121-3

[94] Vasquez A. *Musculoskeletal Pain: Expanded Clinical Strategies*. Gig Harbor, WA: The Institute for Functional Medicine; 2008

in benefit not only due to antigen avoidance but also due to the reduction in carbohydrate substrate that had been maintaining occult small intestine bacterial overgrowth, with its attendant systemic complications, including mitochondrial impairment and immune activation. [95] Micronutrient deficiencies, particularly of zinc and vitamins D and A, reduce immune system effectiveness and thereby promote mucosal colonization with dysbiotic bacteria; I believe this explains—at least in part—the oft experienced clinical phenomenon of significant improvement in dysbiosis-related diseases when only dietary improvement and

> **Clinical Pearl**
>
> Clinically, the most powerful "antibiotic"—antibacterial and antiviral and antifungal agent—ever discovered is the human immune system. For patients with chronic infections (including but not limited to dysbiosis), one of the first questions to ask is *"Why isn't this patient's immune system doing a better job of eliminating or controlling this infection?"* **Often, patients with chronic infections derive tremendous benefit from dietary improvement and nutritional supplementation, which allows their immune system to function more effectively and thus to clear or better control the infection/dysbiosis.**

nutritional supplementation are used: nutritional repletion empowers the immune system in general to function more effectively, thereby quantitatively and qualitatively reducing the severity of mucosal colonization. High-carbohydrate loads cause a reduction in immune surveillance that lasts for 2-3 hours after consumption.

9. <u>Diet-derived immunodysregulation</u>: Certain foods contain constituents that cause immune dysfunction and the induction or exacerbation of autoimmunity. L-canavanine sulfate is a non-protein amino acid found in alfalfa sprouts which triggers a condition similar to systemic lupus erythematosus in monkeys[96,97] and which may exacerbate SLE in humans.

10. <u>Dietary xenobiotics</u>: Artificial sweeteners, thickeners, flavor enhancers, emulsifiers, and plasticizers can be found in foods, particularly those which are manufactured and processed. Some of these chemicals have the potential to alter immune mechanisms in favor of autoimmunity. These dietary xenobiotics may be particularly relevant for initiating and promoting Crohn's disease.[98]

11. <u>Immunogenicity induced by cooking—the Maillard reaction (non-enzymatic glycosylation)</u>: Heated exposure of lysine, arginine, and tryptophan to reducing sugars such as fructose and lactose results in the non-enzymatic binding (glycosylation) of the sugar with the amino acid. If the amino acid is a component of a protein, then the structure and antigenicity of the protein is altered as it is now a glycoprotein, which may either serve as a neoantigen or may increase the allergenicity of a protein that was previously hypoallergenic, as seen with the roasting of peanuts.[99,100] Glycoproteins formed from the baking and browning of foods are also called *glycotoxins* and are capable of exacerbating inflammation in patients with diabetes.[101] Similar to the formation of glycotoxins is the formation of acrylamide, a possible carcinogen, in fried and baked foods.

Common allergy treatments advocated by the pharmaceutical industry create an overly simplistic and inaccurate view of the allergic process which obfuscates the identification and correction of the underlying processes, only two of which are antigen exposure and histamine release. Nutritionally oriented doctors, too, often emphasize the identification and elimination of allergen exposure as the sole means of addressing allergic diathesis with the presumption that allergen avoidance cures the allergy. These simplistic models and the incomplete treatments based upon them fail to address the underlying cause of the allergic phenomenon: immune dysfunction. Allergic

[95] "RESULTS: The incidence of colonic fermentation after ingesting sports drink, milk, and green tea was five (62.5%), six (75%), and none (0%), respectively in eight subjects." Mitsui T, Shimaoka K, Kanao Y, Kondo T. Colonic fermentation after ingestion of fructose-containing sports drink. *J Sports Med Phys Fitness.* 2001 Mar;41(1):121-3
[96] "L-Canavanine sulfate, a constituent of alfalfa sprouts, was incorporated into the diet and reactivated the syndrome in monkeys in which an SLE-like syndrome had previously been induced by the ingestion of alfalfa seeds or sprouts." Malinow MR, Bardana EJ Jr, Pirofsky B, Craig S, McLaughlin P. Systemic lupus erythematosus-like syndrome in monkeys fed alfalfa sprouts: role of a nonprotein amino acid. *Science.* 1982 Apr 23;216(4544):415-7
[97] "Occurrence of autoimmune hemolytic anemia and exacerbation of SLE have been linked to ingestion of alfalfa tablets containing L-canavanine." Alcocer-Varela J, Iglesias A, Llorente L, Alarcon-Segovia D. Effects of L-canavanine on T cells may explain the induction of systemic lupus erythematosus by alfalfa. *Arthritis Rheum.* 1985 Jan;28(1):52-7
[98] "Various food additives, especially emulsifiants, thickeners, surface-finishing agents and contaminants like plasticizers share structural domains with mycobacterial lipids. It is therefore hypothesized, that these compounds are able to stimulate by molecular mimicry the CD1 system in the gastrointestinal mucosa and to trigger the pro-inflammatory cytokine cascade." Traunmuller F. Etiology of Crohn's disease: Do certain food additives cause intestinal inflammation by molecular mimicry of mycobacterial lipids? *Med Hypotheses.* 2005;65(5):859-64
[99] "Roasted peanuts exhibited a higher level of IgE binding, which was correlated with a higher level of AGE adducts. We concluded that there is an association between AGE adducts and increased IgE binding (i.e., allergenicity) of roasted peanuts." Chung SY, Champagne ET. Association of end-product adducts with increased IgE binding of roasted peanuts. *J Agric Food Chem.* 2001 Aug;49(8):3911-6
[100] "The data presented here indicate that thermal processing may play an important role in enhancing the allergenic properties of peanuts and that the protein modifications made by the Maillard reaction contribute to this effect." Maleki et al.The effects of roasting on the allergenic properties of peanut proteins. *J Allergy Clin Immunol.* 2000 Oct;106:763-8
[101] "A study now reveals that the consumption of foods rich in browned and oxidized products (so-called glycotoxins) induces a chronic inflammatory state in diabetic individuals." Monnier VM, Obrenovich ME. Wake up and smell the maillard reaction. *Sci Aging Knowledge Environ.* 2002 Dec 18;2002(50):pe21

manifestations always require at least two factors: 1) exposure of the antigen to the immune system (antigen absorption) and 2) a dysfunctional immune system that "overreacts" to the otherwise benign antigen. Allergy treatment that fails to address the underlying immune dysfunction is incomplete. Allergy treatment that addresses the underlying immune dysfunction has the opportunity to correct the *total problem*, rather than merely reducing the manifestations of the problem. Therefore, treatment of the allergic diathesis must always address issues of antigen exposure, antigen absorption, *and the dysfunctional immune system* that results in the hyperactive immune response that we call "allergy." Elimination of either antigen exposure or antigen absorption eliminates allergic manifestations, but does not necessarily correct the underlying immune defect(s). Complete correction of the underlying immune defect obviates the need for the identification and avoidance of the allergen. In clinical practice, a combination of both approaches—allergen avoidance and immune modulation—is the most effective approach, affording relatively high effectiveness in symptom reduction even with only modest compliance.

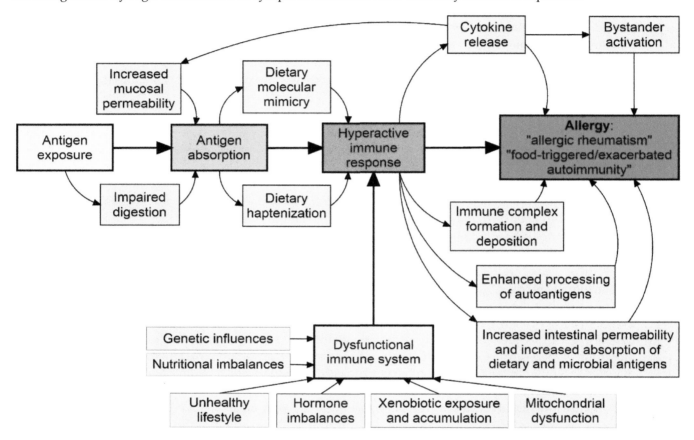

Approaching a More Comprehensive Understanding of "Allergy" and Its Contribution to Immune Dysfunction, Musculoskeletal Inflammation, Autoimmunity, and "Allergic Diseases" such as Asthma: Immune dysfunction contributes to and is perpetuated by inflammation and allergic reactions, thus forming a vicious cycle; of particular noteworthiness is the vicious cycle formed by inflammation in response to immunogen exposure that leads to increased intestinal permeability and thus to additional immunogen (e.g., dietary and microbial) exposure.

Anti-Allergy Orthomolecular Immunomodulation: The Author's Approach to Alleviating Allergy—Introduction and Perspectives Spanning more than 10 years of Protocol Development
My clinical approach to improving immune function in patients with allergy typically started/starts with supplementation of vitamin E, CoQ-10, vitamin B-12, vitamin C, bioflavonoids, honey, and fish oil; readers will appreciate that these are all anti-inflammatory nutrients/foods, all of which—like vitamin B12—have anti-allergy effects that are extensions of and/or different from their traditionally considered nutritional roles. Thereafter, I look at hormones, particularly dehydroepiandrosterone (DHEA), estrogen (quantitative and qualitative), testosterone, and cortisol. I also look at diet and bowel health with respect to putrefaction and intestinal permeability. Although rarely powerful when used in isolation, these treatments when used in combinations tailored to the individual

patient often result in an impressive reduction in allergic manifestations even when allergen avoidance is either not pursued or not feasible. The process of alleviating allergic disorders is, however, arduous and time-consuming unless the doctor uses a group of protocols such as those described herein which address the most common contributing factors to allergic problems. Here I extend my previous three-step process (first published in 2005[102]) into a four-tiered approach (first published in 2009[103]), with the fourth step including selected pharmaceutical drugs. These days—starting in 2012[104] and beyond—the integration of the nutritional immunomodulation protocol (Chapter 4.3) should be used within the initial and foundational management of allergic and other inflammatory disorders; nonetheless, this previous version of the protocol serves useful purposes by providing perspectives and clinical interventions not included in the "nutritional immunomodulation protocol" described as such.

Step 1: From initial patient assessment to the first phase of treatment

In a patient with presumed "allergy" who is in otherwise good health, following a basic health assessment and exclusion of significant disease, I begin by correcting problems that are common to patients with allergy. Minor improvements in allergy symptoms as a result of a low-cost low-risk interventions can be multiplied with a specified group of interventions; we aim for a modest improvement with several treatments rather than a "silver bullet" miracle cure with a single intervention. For example, 10% improvement in symptoms may be insignificant in itself; however a 10% improvement from six interventions results in a 60% improvement and enhances patient confidence long enough for other interventions and assessments to be implemented, if necessary. The goal with the first step of treatment is to correct the most common and most likely problems, namely fatty acid imbalances, micronutrient deficiencies, phytonutrient insufficiencies, and dysbiosis.

- Avoidance of suspected food allergens: The most common allergens are wheat, cow's milk, and eggs; however any patient can be allergic to any food. It is not uncommon for patients to have to avoid up to 10 foods before attaining maximal improvement, and up to 85% of migraine patients can be cured of their headaches by the use of allergy avoidance alone.[105] Food allergy avoidance for 1 month helps achieve symptomatic relief and allows the gut to heal and the immune system to recalibrate. The diet should emphasize consumption of lean meats, fruits, vegetables, nuts, seeds, and berries to ensure a systemic anti-inflammatory effect and increased consumption of anti-inflammatory phytonutrients, especially flavonoids. High-glycemic foods are avoided as are "food additives" such as tartrazine, which is known to exacerbate allergic asthma. Some foods like tuna, certain cheeses and wines are high in histamine; frequent consumption of these foods by an allergic individual is analogous to adding fuel to a fire that the patient is simultaneously trying to extinguish. Recall that in breast-feeding infants, the mother will have to consume a hypoallergenic diet to prevent passage of allergens[106] and allergen-antibody immune complexes[107] in breast milk.

- Rotation diet: While select "offending foods" and exposures should be completely avoided, the remaining foods that are consumed should be rotated in and out of the diet with a periodicity of 3-5 days. Patients should avoid "dietary monotony"[108] by consuming a variety of foods. By rotating different foods in and out of the diet, patients are more likely to consume a nutritious diet and are less likely to develop or perpetuate food allergies.

- CoQ-10: CoQ-10 levels are low in approximately 40% of patients with allergies, according to a small study conducted by Folkers and Pfeiffer.[109] Asthmatics also have lower levels of CoQ-10 compared to healthy people.[110] In an open cross-over randomized clinical trial of patients with persistent mild-moderate asthma

[102] Vasquez A. Improving neuromusculoskeletal health by optimizing immune function and reducing allergic reactions: a review of 16 treatments and a 3-step clinical approach. *Nutritional Perspectives* 2005; October: 27-35, 40 https://ichnfm.academia.edu/AlexVasquez

[103] Vasquez A. *Chiropractic and Naturopathic Mastery of Common Clinical Disorders.* IBMRC, 2009

[104] Vasquez A. *Functional Immunology and Nutritional Immunomodulation: Introduction to...the new FIND SEX Acronym.* 2012

[105] Grant EC. Food allergies and migraine. *Lancet.* 1979 May 5;1(8123):966-9

[106] "In all, clinical disappearance of symptoms was observed after removal of milk from the mother's diet and/or elimination from the child's diet of any cow's-milk-based hypoallergenic formula." Barau E, Dupont C. Allergy to cow's milk proteins in mother's milk or in hydrolyzed cow's milk infant formulas as assessed by intestinal permeability measurements. *Allergy.* 1994 Apr;49(4):295-8

[107] The finding of egg-allergen immune complex in breast milk implies 1) egg protein escapes complete digestion/degradation in the gastrointestinal tract, 2) egg protein is absorbed intact through the mucosa, 3) egg protein escapes filtration by the liver, 4) egg protein stimulates formation IgA immune complexes, and 5) egg-IgA immune complexes are secreted in milk which would then expose the infant to both allergen and immune complex, possibly resulting in clinical disease. Hirose et al. Occurrence of the major food allergen, ovomucoid, in human breast milk as an immune complex. *Biosci Biotechnol Biochem.* 2001 Jun;65(6):1438-40 jstage.jst.go.jp/article/bbb/65/6/1438/_pdf

[108] Pelchat ML, Schaefer S. Dietary monotony and food cravings in young and elderly adults. *Physiol Behav.* 2000 Jan;68(3):353-9

[109] Ye CQ, Folkers K, et al. A modified determination of coenzyme Q10 in human blood and CoQ10 blood levels in diverse patients with allergies. *Biofactors.* 1988 Dec;1:303-6

[110] Gazdik et al. Decreased levels of coenzyme Q(10) in patients with bronchial asthma. *Allergy.* 2002 Sep;57(9):811-4

(n=41; ages 25-50y), daily administration of hydrosoluble CoQ10 120 mg, alpha-tocopherol 400 mg, and vitamin C 250 mg was shown to allow statistically and clinically significant reduction in the required dosage of corticosteroids; however, "Spirometric parameters did not change significantly during the study."[111] In my experience, clinical improvement is commonly seen in allergic patients after supplementation with CoQ-10, within the context of overall diet and lifestyle improvement including vitamin, mineral, and combination fatty acid supplementation. I generally prescribe at least 100 mg and preferably 200 mg per day of CoQ-10 for adults.

- Vitamin C: A clinical trial showed that 2 grams per day of ascorbic acid reduced blood histamine levels by 38%.[112] Cathcart hypothesized that high doses of vitamin C (i.e., bowel tolerance) may impair the adsorption of IgE with allergens and thus retard the allergic cascade from being initiated.[113] Either of these two mechanisms, perhaps in addition to other mechanisms such as stabilization of mast cell membranes (especially when used with bioflavonoids), may explain the anti-allergy effects of ascorbic acid.[114]

- Probiotics: Supplementation with probiotics (beneficial strains of bacteria and yeast) appears to improve intestinal barrier function, promote microecological balance in the gastrointestinal tract, modulate immune function, and thus *via several mechanisms* reduce manifestations/severity of allergic disease.[115,116,117]

- Vitamin E: Vitamin E has been shown to reduce IgE levels in humans and to reduce the manifestations of allergy-related disease.[118] I commonly prescribe 800-2,000 IU per day of mixed tocopherols with approximately 40% gamma tocopherol for patients with allergy.

- Bioflavonoids: Bioflavonoids stabilize mast cell membranes and thus reduce the liberation of histamine. Additionally, quercetin and catechin inhibit the action of histidine decarboxylase, which converts histidine into histamine. Many fruits, vegetables, herbal teas, and honey are excellent sources of flavonoids, which can also be consumed in the form of tablets, capsules, beverages, or whole foods. The efficacy of honey for reducing serum IgE is particularly noteworthy; honey consumption has been shown to significantly reduce (-34%) serum IgE levels in humans.[119] The required dose is 1.2 g of honey per kg body weight. For an individual who weighs about 220 lbs, the correct amount of honey to remain consistent with this study would be approximately 120 grams. Since one tablespoon of honey weighs 21 grams, the dose would be 5-6 tablespoons (one-third cup) of honey per day (again, this dose is for a person weighing 220 lbs). Since each tablespoon of honey contains 64 calories, six tablespoons of this powerful natural anti-inflammatory nutraceutical would add 384 calories to the daily diet; if the remainder of the patient's diet is generally low-carbohydrate (as it generally should be for most patients), then the addition of less than 400 calories is relatively insignificant, especially if the patient also exercises on a daily or near-daily basis (as most patients should). In the context of a low-carb diet and regular exercise, honey can be the before/after carbohydrate source used to fuel the workout or to provide post-exertional glycogen supercompensation. To avoid/minimize consumption of mitochondria-damaging and endocrine-disrupting pesticides, honey and other foods should be organically cultivated; commercial "mass-market" [American] honey has recently

[111] Gvozdjáková et al. Coenzyme Q10 supplementation reduces corticosteroids dosage in patients with bronchial asthma. *Biofactors*. 2005;25(1-4):235-40

[112] "Chemotaxis was inversely correlated to blood histamine (r = -0.32, p = 0.045), and, compared to baseline and withdrawal values, histamine levels were depressed 38% following VC supplementation. ... These data indicate that VC may indirectly enhance chemotaxis by detoxifying histamine in vivo." Johnston CS, Martin LJ, Cai X. Antihistamine effect of supplemental ascorbic acid and neutrophil chemotaxis. *J Am Coll Nutr*. 1992 Apr;11(2):172-6

[113] "Allergic and sensitivity reactions are frequently ameliorated and sometimes completely blocked by massive doses of ascorbate. I now hypothesize that one mechanism in blocking of allergic symptoms is the reducing of the disulfide bonds between the chains in antibody molecules making their bonding antigen impossible." Cathcart RF 3rd. The vitamin C treatment of allergy and the normally unprimed state of antibodies. *Med Hypotheses*. 1986 Nov;21(3):307-21

[114] Bucca C, Rolla G, Oliva A, Farina JC. Effect of vitamin C on histamine bronchial responsiveness of patients with allergic rhinitis. *Ann Allergy*. 1990 Oct;65(4):311-4

[115] Majamaa H, Isolauri E. Probiotics: a novel approach in the management of food allergy. *J Allergy Clin Immunol* 1997 Feb;99(2):179-85

[116] von der Weid T, Ibnou-Zekri N, Pfeifer A. Novel probiotics for the management of allergic inflammation. *Dig Liver Dis*. 2002 Sep;34 Suppl 2:S25-8

[117] "The administration of probiotics, strains of bacteria from the healthy human gut microbiota, have been shown to stimulate antiinflammatory, tolerogenic immune responses, the lack of which has been implied in the development of atopic disorders. Thus probiotics may prove beneficial in the prevention and alleviation of allergic disease." Rautava et al. The development of gut immune responses and gut microbiota: effects of probiotics in prevention and treatment of allergic disease. *Curr Issues Intest Microbiol* 2002 Mar;3:15-22

[118] Tsoureli-Nikita et al. Evaluation of dietary intake of vitamin E in atopic dermatitis: clinical course and evaluation of immunoglobulin E. *Int J Dermatol*. 2002 Mar;41(3):146-50

[119] "Seven men and three women received a strictly controlled regular diet during a 2-week control period, followed by the regular diet supplemented with daily consumption of 1.2 g/kg body weight honey dissolved in 250 ml of water during a 2-week test period. ... Honey reduced serum immunoglobulin E by 34%..." Al-Waili NS. Effects of daily consumption of honey solution on hematological indices and blood levels of minerals and enzymes in normal individuals. *J Med Food*. 2003 Summer;6(2):135-40

been reported as low in antioxidants and commonly contaminated with pesticides, including glyphosate.[120,121]

- <u>Vitamin B-12</u>: Vitamin B-12 has been shown to reduce physiologic manifestations of allergy in ovalbumin-sensitized mice.[122] Since vitamin B-12 is safe, non-toxic, and bioavailable when administered orally in large doses to humans, I commonly prescribe 2,500-5,000 mcg per day for allergic patients for a one-month trial. Although the benefit of vitamin B-12 in patients with sulfite-sensitive asthma is biochemically mediated rather than immunologically mediated[123], this research adds tangential support to the use of high-dose vitamin B-12 in selected patients with allergy (particularly asthma), at least for a short-term clinical trial. Hydroxocobalamin and methylcobalamin are preferred over cyanocobalamin due to the significant content of cyanide in the latter.[124]

Step 2: Additional interventions for moderate or unresponsive allergies.

For patients who do not respond sufficiently to the first phase of treatment, the following interventions can be considered.

- <u>Pancreatic and proteolytic enzymes</u>: Pancreatic enzymes have been shown to alleviate symptoms of food allergy in a controlled clinical trial.[125] Administration of enzyme preparations can alleviate intestinal and extra-intestinal manifestations of food allergy.[126] Proteolytic enzymes are safe and effective for the relief of musculoskeletal pain, as reviewed later in this text and elsewhere.[127] When taken with food, pancreatic/proteolytic enzymes facilitate hydrolysis of proteins, fats, and carbohydrates and are then absorbed into the systemic circulation for an anti-inflammatory effect. Although individual enzymes may be used in isolation, enzyme therapy is generally delivered in the form of polyenzyme preparations containing pancreatin, bromelain, papain, amylase, lipase, trypsin and alpha-chymotrypsin.

- <u>Nuclear transcription factor kappa-B (NFkB) inhibitors</u>: NFkB plays a critical role in the induction of pro-inflammatory genes and is upregulated in allergic disease; its phytonutritional modulation is detailed later in this book and elsewhere.[128] Nutrients that can be used to downregulate inflammatory responses are 1,25-dihydroxyvitamin D3[129,130], curcumin[131] (requires piperine for absorption[132]), lipoic acid[133], green tea[134],

Nutrients and foods that inhibit NFkB
• 1,25-dihydroxyvitamin D3
• Curcumin (requires piperine for absorption)
• Lipoic acid
• Green tea
• Rosemary
• Grape seed extract
• Bee propolis
• Zinc
• Selenium
• Indole-3-carbinol
• N-acetyl-L-cysteine
• Resveratrol
• Isohumulones
• CoQ-10
• Boswellia serrata
• GLA via PPAR-gamma
• Oxidized EPA via PPAR-alpha

---

[120] "More than 70 percent of pollen and honey samples collected from foraging bees in Massachusetts contain at least one neonicotinoid, a class of pesticide..." Feldscher K. Pesticide found in 70 percent of Massachusetts' honey samples. news.harvard.edu/gazette/story/2015/07/pesticide-found-in-70-percent-of-massachusetts-honey-samples/

[121] "Eleven of the tested honey samples were organic; five of the organic honey samples, or forty-five percent (45%), contained glyphosate concentrations above the method LOQ, with a range of 26 to 93 ppb and a mean of 50 ppb. Of the fifty-eight non-organic honey samples, thirty-six samples, or sixty-two percent (62%), contained glyphosate concentrations above the method LOQ, with a range of 17 to 163 ppb and a mean of 66 ppb." Rubio F. Survey of Glyphosate Residues in Honey, Corn and Soy Products. *Journal of Environmental & Analytical Toxicology.* 2014 Nov omicsonline.org/open-access/survey-of-glyphosate-residues-in-honey-corn-and-soy-products-2161-0525.1000249.php?aid=36354

[122] "We infer that Cbl administration significantly reduced the IL-2 concentration, and secondarily the IL-4, IgE and histamine concentrations." Funada U, Wada M, Kawata T, Tanaka N, Tadokoro T, Maekawa A. Effect of cobalamin on the allergic response in mice. *Biosci Biotechnol Biochem* 2000 Oct;64(10):2053-8

[123] Anibarro B, Caballero T, Garcia-Ara C, et al. Asthma with sulfite intolerance in children: a blocking study with cyanocobalamin. *J Allergy Clin Immunol.* 1992 Jul;90(1):103-9

[124] Freeman AG. Cyanocobalamin—a case for withdrawal: discussion paper. *J R Soc Med.* 1992 Nov;85(11):686-7

[125] Raithel M, Weidenhiller M, Schwab D, Winterkamp S, Hahn EG. Pancreatic enzymes: a new group of antiallergic drugs? *Inflamm Res.* 2002 Apr;51 Suppl 1:S13-4

[126] Gaby AR. Pancreatic enzymes block food allergy reactions. *Townsend Letter for Doctors and Patients* 2002; Nov. townsendletter.com/Nov_2002/gabyliteraturereview1102.htm

[127] Vasquez A. Improving overall health while safely and effectively treating musculoskeletal pain. *Nutr Perspect* 2005;28:34-38,40-42 ichnfm.academia.edu/AlexVasquez

[128] Vasquez A. Reducing pain and inflammation naturally - part 4: nutritional and botanical inhibition of NF-kappaB, the major intracellular amplifier of the inflammatory cascade. A practical clinical strategy exemplifying anti-inflammatory nutrigenomics. *Nutritional Perspectives,* July 2005:5-12 ichnfm.academia.edu/AlexVasquez

[129] "1Alpha,25-dihydroxyvitamin D3 (1,25-(OH)2-D3), the active metabolite of vitamin D, can inhibit NF-kappaB activity in human MRC-5 fibroblasts, targeting DNA binding of NF-kappaB but not translocation of its subunits p50 and p65." Harant H, Wolff B, Lindley IJ. 1Alpha,25-dihydroxyvitamin D3 decreases DNA binding of nuclear factor-kappaB in human fibroblasts. *FEBS Lett.* 1998 Oct 9;436(3):329-34

[130] "Thus, 1,25(OH)₂D₃ may negatively regulate IL-12 production by downregulation of NF-kB activation and binding to the p40-kB sequence." D'Ambrosio D, Cippitelli M, Cocciolo MG, Mazzeo D, Di Lucia P, Lang R, Sinigaglia F, Panina-Bordignon P. Inhibition of IL-12 production by 1,25-dihydroxyvitamin D3. Involvement of NF-kappaB downregulation in transcriptional repression of the p40 gene. *J Clin Invest.* 1998 Jan 1;101(1):252-62

[131] "Curcumin, EGCG and resveratrol have been shown to suppress activation of NF-kappa B." Surh et al. Molecular mechanisms underlying chemopreventive activities of anti-inflammatory phytochemicals: down-regulation of COX-2 and iNOS through suppression of NF-kappa B activation. *Mutat Res.* 2001 Sep 1;480-481:243-68

[132] Shoba et al. Influence of piperine on the pharmacokinetics of curcumin in animals and human volunteers. *Planta Med.* 1998 May;64(4):353-6

[133] "ALA reduced the TNF-alpha-stimulated ICAM-1 expression in a dose-dependent manner, to levels observed in unstimulated cells. Alpha-lipoic acid also reduced NF-kappaB activity in these cells in a dose-dependent manner." Lee HA, Hughes DA. Alpha-lipoic acid modulates NF-kappaB activity in human monocytic cells by direct interaction with DNA. *Exp Gerontol.* 2002 Jan-Mar;37(2-3):401-10

[134] "In conclusion, EGCG is an effective inhibitor of IKK activity. This may explain, at least in part, some of the reported anti-inflammatory and anticancer effects of green tea." Yang F, Oz HS, Barve S, de Villiers WJ, McClain CJ, Varilek GW. The green tea polyphenol (-)-epigallocatechin-3-gallate blocks nuclear factor-kappa B activation by inhibiting I kappa B kinase activity in the intestinal epithelial cell line IEC-6. *Mol Pharmacol.* 2001 Sep;60(3):528-33

rosemary[135], grape seed extract[136], bee propolis[137], zinc[138], high-dose selenium[139], indole-3-carbinol[140,141], N-acetyl-L-cysteine[142], resveratrol[143,144], isohumulones from *Humulus lupulus*[145], CoQ-10[146], and acetyl-11-keto-beta-boswellic acid from *Boswellia serrata*.[147] Fatty acids inhibit NF-kappaB *indirectly*; GLA activates PPAR-gamma and thereby inhibits NFkB[148], while (oxidized) EPA activates PPAR-alpha and thus inhibits NFkB.[149]

- **Stress reduction, psychotherapy, deconditioning**: Emotional and social aspects may be particularly important for some patients with allergies. "Allergic" responses to stimuli can be classically conditioned, according to replicable studies in animals[150] and humans.[151] The neurohormonal response to physical-psychological stress predisposes the immune system toward the Th-2 response with subsequent IgE antibody formation and the development of allergy.[152] Höglund et al[153] summarized by stating, "The dominance of Th2 cytokines leads to enhanced Ig class switching to IgE, recruitment of eosinophils to the airways and to down-regulation of cell-mediated immunity, features characteristic of asthmatic and allergic disease." In support of the stress-allergy link, we note published research showing, for example, increased prevalence of allergy in children exposed to the stress of international relocation.[154] Mechanisms by which physical-psychological stress can promote allergy are likely to be very complex, interactive, synergistic, self-perpetuating, and variable among individuals. Documented factors and mechanisms involved include increased mucosal permeability, alterations in flora/microbial quality (species), quantity (numerical counts) and activity (elaboration of virulence factors and changes in phenotypic expression), hypercortisolemia followed by hypocortisolemia, increased secretion of pro-inflammatory corticotrophin releasing factor, reductions in immunomodulating hormones DHEA and testosterone with an increase in pro-inflammatory estrogens and prolactin, alterations in lifestyle such as sugar and pastry binging along with dietary monotony, and the perpetuation and amplification of stress from one aspect of life to another, for example: work stress can cause financial worries which spills over into marital discord and perhaps binge eating and

[135] "These results suggest that carnosol suppresses the NO production and iNOS gene expression by inhibiting NF-kappaB activation, and provide possible mechanisms for its anti-inflammatory and chemopreventive action." Lo AH, Liang YC, Lin-Shiau SY, Ho CT, Lin JK. Carnosol, an antioxidant in rosemary, suppresses inducible nitric oxide synthase through down-regulating nuclear factor-kappaB in mouse macrophages. *Carcinogenesis*. 2002 Jun;23(6):983-91

[136] "Constitutive and TNFalpha-induced NF-kappaB DNA binding activity was inhibited by GSE at doses > or =50 microg/ml and treatments for > or =12 h." Dhanalakshmi et al. Inhibition of NF-kappaB pathway in grape seed extract-induced apoptotic death of human prostate carcinoma DU145 cells. *Int J Oncol*. 2003 Sep;23(3):721-7

[137] "Caffeic acid phenethyl ester (CAPE) is an anti-inflammatory component of propolis (honeybee resin). CAPE is reportedly a specific inhibitor of nuclear factor-kappaB (NF-kappaB)." Fitzpatrick LR, Wang J, Le T. Caffeic acid phenethyl ester, an inhibitor of nuclear factor-kappaB, attenuates bacterial peptidoglycan polysaccharide-induced colitis in rats. *J Pharmacol Exp Ther*. 2001 Dec;299(3):915-20

[138] "Our results suggest that zinc supplementation may lead to downregulation of the inflammatory cytokines through upregulation of the negative feedback loop A20 to inhibit induced NF-kappaB activation." Prasad AS, Bao B, Beck FW, Kucuk O, Sarkar FH. Antioxidant effect of zinc in humans. *Free Radic Biol Med*. 2004 Oct 15;37(8):1182-90

[139] Note that the patients in this study received a very high dose of selenium: 960 micrograms per day. This is at the top—and some would say over the top—of the safe and reasonable dose for long-term supplementation. In this case, th study lasted for three months. "In patients receiving selenium supplementation, selenium NF-kappaB activity was significantly reduced, reaching the same level as the nondiabetic control group. CONCLUSION: In type 2 diabetic patients, activation of NF-kappaB measured in peripheral blood monocytes can be reduced by selenium supplementation, confirming its importance in the prevention of cardiovascular diseases." Faure P, Ramon O, Favier A, Halimi S. Selenium supplementation decreases nuclear factor-kappa B activity in peripheral blood mononuclear cells from type 2 diabetic patients. *Eur J Clin Invest*. 2004 Jul;34(7):475-81

[140] Takada Y, Andreeff M, Aggarwal BB. Indole-3-carbinol suppresses NF-{kappa}B and I{kappa}B{alpha} kinase activation causing inhibition of expression of NF-{kappa}B-regulated antiapoptotic and metastatic gene products and enhancement of apoptosis in myeloid and leukemia cells. *Blood* 2005 July 15; 106(2): 641–649

[141] "Overall, our results indicated that indole-3-carbinol inhibits NF-kappaB and NF-kappaB-regulated gene expression and that this mechanism may provide the molecular basis for its ability to suppress tumorigenesis." Takada Y, Andreeff M, Aggarwal BB. Indole-3-carbinol suppresses NF-kappaB and IkappaBalpha kinase activation, causing inhibition of expression of NF-kappaB-regulated antiapoptotic and metastatic gene products and enhancement of apoptosis in myeloid and leukemia cells. *Blood*. 2005 Jul 15;106(2):641-9

[142] "CONCLUSIONS: Administration of N-acetylcysteine results in decreased nuclear factor-kappa B activation in patients with sepsis, associated with decreases in interleukin-8 but not interleukin-6 or soluble intercellular adhesion molecule-1. These pilot data suggest that antioxidant therapy with N-acetylcysteine may be useful in blunting the inflammatory response to sepsis." Paterson RL, Galley HF, Webster NR. The effect of N-acetylcysteine on nuclear factor-kappa B activation, interleukin-6, interleukin-8, and intercellular adhesion molecule-1 expression in patients with sepsis. *Crit Care Med*. 2003 Nov;31(11):2574-8

[143] "Resveratrol's anticarcinogenic, anti-inflammatory, and growth-modulatory effects may thus be partially ascribed to the inhibition of activation of NF-kappaB and AP-1 and the associated kinases." Manna SK, Mukhopadhyay A, Aggarwal BB. Resveratrol suppresses TNF-induced activation of nuclear transcription factors NF-kappa B, activator protein-1, and apoptosis: potential role of reactive oxygen intermediates and lipid peroxidation. *J Immunol*. 2000 Jun 15;164(12):6509-19

[144] "Both resveratrol and quercetin inhibited NF-kappaB-, AP-1- and CREB-dependent transcription to a greater extent than the glucocorticosteroid, dexamethasone." Donnelly et al. Anti-inflammatory Effects of Resveratrol in Lung Epithelial Cells: Molecular Mechanisms. *Am J Physiol Lung Cell Mol Physiol*. 2004 Jun 4 [Epub ahead of print]

[145] Yajima et al. Isohumulones, bitter acids derived from hops, activate both peroxisome proliferator-activated receptor alpha and gamma and reduce insulin resistance. *J Biol Chem*. 2004 Aug 6;279:33456-62 jbc.org/cgi/content/full/279/32/33456

[146] Ebadi M, Sharma SK, et al. Coenzyme Q10 inhibits mitochondrial complex-1 down-regulation and nuclear factor-kappa B activation. *J Cell Mol Med*. 2004 Apr-Jun;8:213-22

[147] "Overall, our results indicated that AKBA enhances apoptosis induced by cytokines and chemotherapeutic agents, inhibits invasion, and suppresses osteoclastogenesis through inhibition of NF-kappaB-regulated gene expression." Takada Y, Ichikawa H, Badmaev V, Aggarwal BB. Acetyl-11-keto-beta-boswellic acid potentiates apoptosis, inhibits invasion, and abolishes osteoclastogenesis by suppressing NF-kappa B and NF-kappa B-regulated gene expression. *J Immunol*. 2006 Mar 1;176(5):3127-40

[148] "Thus, PPAR gamma serves as the receptor for GLA in the regulation of gene expression in breast cancer cells. " Jiang WG, Redfern A, et al. Peroxisome proliferator activated receptor-gamma (PPAR-gamma) mediates the action of gamma linolenic acid in breast cancer cells. *Prostaglandins Leukot Essent Fatty Acids*. 2000 Feb;62(2):119-27

[149] "...EPA requires PPARalpha for its inhibitory effects on NF-kappaB." Mishra A, Chaudhary A, Sethi S. Oxidized omega-3 fatty acids inhibit NF-kappaB activation via a PPARalpha-dependent pathway. *Arterioscler Thromb Vasc Biol*. 2004 Sep;24(9):1621-7. atvb.ahajournals.org/cgi/content/full/24/9/1621

[150] "In a classical conditioning procedure in which an immunologic challenge was paired with the presentation of an odor, guinea pigs showed a plasma histamine increase when presented with the odor alone. This suggests that the immune response can be enhanced through activity of the central nervous system." Russell et al. Learned histamine release. *Science*. 1984 Aug 17;225(4663):733-4

[151] "A classical Pavlovian paradigm pairing an olfactory cue with allergen challenge for a single training trial was used to produce conditioned histamine release and conditioned nasal airflow decrease in seasonal allergic rhinitis sufferers." Barrett JE, King MG, Pang G. Conditioning rhinitis in allergic humans. *Ann N Y Acad Sci*. 2000;917:853-9

[152] Montoro J, Mullol J, Jáuregui I, et al. Stress and allergy. *J Investig Allergol Clin Immunol*. 2009;19 Suppl 1:40-7 jiaci.org/issues/vol19s1/7.pdf

[153] Höglund et al. Changes in immune regulation in response to examination stress in atopic and healthy individuals. *Clin Exp Allergy*. 2006 Aug;36(8):982-92

[154] "This study suggests that unidentified factors associated with foreign relocation increase the risk of sensitization in predisposed children. Stress might be one factor." Anderzén et al. Stress and sensitization in children: a controlled prospective psychophysiological study of children. *J Psychosom Res*. 1997 Sep;43(3):259-69

drinking all of which synergize with internal neuronal and immunologic imbalances to promote the exacerbation of allergy.

- <u>Eradication of intestinal dysbiosis</u>: I have seen several patients become cured of their "allergies" once we eradicated the dysbiotic bacteria, yeast, amoebas, or other microorganisms from their gastrointestinal tract. Intestinal colonization with harmful bacteria/yeast/protozoa/amebas can cause mucosal injury and result in macromolecular absorption and thus promotes immune sensitization to dietary antigens; in these situations, correction of dysbiosis via eradication of harmful microorganisms can lead to an impressive reduction in food-associated allergic phenomena. Although many indirect mechanisms will be discussed later, the most direct means by which dysbiosis may contribute to "allergy" is via endogenous formation of histamine via bacterial histidine decarboxylase. Galland and Lee[155] reported that eradication of *Giardia lamblia* in patients with chronic digestive complaints lessened the severity of food intolerance/allergy in 54% of patients. The supremely important topic of gastrointestinal dysbiosis is detailed in Chapter 4.

Bacteriology

Beneficial Bacteria

Lactobacillus species	N	4+
Escherichia coli	I	*NG
Bifidobacterium	N	4+

Additional Bacteria

alpha haemolytic Streptococcus	N	3+
gamma haemolytic Streptococcus	N	4+
Citrobacter freundii	P	4+
Klebsiella pneumoniae	P	4+
beta Strep (Not Group A or B)	I	2+

Mycology

Candida krusei	P	4+
Geotrichum capitatum	P	4+

Intestinal dysbiosis as the causative factor in new-onset immediate hypersensitivity reactions to multiple foods, as well as physical and mental fatigue and environmental sensitivity: This 25yoM patient developed numerous complaints clustering around fatigue, neurocognitive dysfunction, and multiple chemical sensitivity following a period of severe psychoemotional stress; new immediate-onset "food allergies" developed against several spices and soy/lecithin. Allergic food reactions/responses included immediate-onset (within seconds) hypersensitivity reactions in the mouth (including a blistering mucosal/labial rash) upon consumption of (previously tolerated) soy. All of the "food allergies", neurocognitive fatigue, and chemical sensitivities vanished upon successful eradication of the intestinal dysbiosis, clearly depicted per the above results on comprehensive microbiologic assessment of the stool. *Citrobacter* and *Klebsiella* are both Gram-negative bacteria implicated in pathogenic inflammatory responses, increased intestinal permeability, and impaired cytochrome p450 activity (general to endotoxin, with some additional specificity for *Klebsiella*). The *Geotrichum* is an unusual yeast associated with immunosuppression, while the *Candida* is known for producing an IgA protease that increases propensity toward dysbiosis and allergy by proteolytic degradation of the first-line IgA defense. Patient was treated with numerous antimicrobial botanicals including berberine and oregano as well as daily first-morning gastrointestinal lavage with ~30 grams ascorbic acid in one liter of water (potent osmotic laxative) with two cups of coffee (peristaltic/gastroprokinetic agent). Other testing at this time showed increased intestinal permeability via elevated lactulose-mannitol ratio, increased fecal beta-glucuronidase (leading to increased enterohepatic recycling, thereby reducing/neutralizing xenobiotic clearance), and a "pathologic" detoxification profile, characterized by (among other markers) markedly elevated caffeine clearance and brutally slow benzoate conjugation; the impaired detoxification is of course consistent with and explanatory for the patient's multiple chemical sensitivities. Among various interventions used over the seven-year course of this patient's illness, the ascorbate-coffee combination (additionally discussed in Chapter 4.2) was clearly the most effective and ultimately—and durably—curative.

---

[155] Galland L, Lee M. Abstract #170 High frequency of giardiasis in patients with chronic digestive complaints. *Am J Gastroenterol* 1989;84:1181

Step 3: Treatment for severe allergies

For some patients with severe allergies, we start with selected treatments from Step 2 or Step 3 on the first visit *in addition to* the treatments included in Step 1. Implementation is customized based on history, examination, laboratory findings, and the doctor's experience and good judgment.

- Calcium and magnesium butyrate: Butyrate is a short-chain fatty acid which can be obtained from 1) a limited number of foods, namely butter, 2) intestinal fermentation of carbohydrates by probiotic bacteria, and 3) use of nutritional supplements. It is increasingly well-established that probiotic bacteria have immune-normalizing and "anti-allergy" effects, and this benefit is probably mediated at least in part by probiotic production of butyrate. The mechanisms of the anti-allergy effect of butyrate are manifold, and as a fatty acid butyrate activates peroxisome-proliferator activated receptor-alpha (PPAR-alpha) and thereby results in an immunomodulatory action and a suppressive effect on NFkB.[156,157] Butyrate is also a primary fuel for enterocytes and may improve enterocyte metabolism for the normalization of intestinal permeability. In the treatment of patients with inflammatory bowel disease, 4 grams per day of orally administered butyrate salts safely improves the action of mesalamine[158] as does topical application of butyrate (via enema) in ulcerative colitis.[159] As a normal dietary component and product of the gastrointestinal tract, supplemental calcium/magnesium salts of butyrate are safe and effective for human consumption at doses of 1,000 – 4,500 mg butyrate per day for the alleviation of allergic diseases.[160,161]

- Purified chondroitin sulfate and glucosamine sulfate: Doctors and patients everywhere should already know that chondroitin sulfate and glucosamine sulfate are safe and effective for the treatment of osteoarthritis. Furthermore, purified chondroitin sulfate is cardioprotective and that it helps to reduce the vessel occlusion characteristic of atherosclerosis.[162] Additionally, new experimental evidence shows that chondroitin sulfate and glucosamine sulfate can inhibit allergic reactions.[163] With this in mind, it is reasonable to speculate that many arthritic patients who respond to glucosamine and chondroitin may actually be responding to the anti-allergy benefits of chondroitin and glucosamine *rather than* or *in addition to* the "cartilage building" properties of these supplements. Furthermore, there is evidence that purified chondroitin sulfate can act as a "decoy" and reduce adhesion of harmful bacteria; the role of harmful gastrointestinal bacteria in the genesis and perpetuation of joint pain and inflammation will be discussed in the next article in this series. For now, suffice to say that occult gastrointestinal infections (i.e., gastrointestinal dysbiosis) are a major contributor to the systemic pain and inflammation seen in conditions such as rheumatoid arthritis and ankylosing spondylitis.

- Hormones: DHEA, progesterone, testosterone, and cortisol tend to be lower in allergic/autoimmune individuals than in healthy controls. I use either serum testing and/or 24-hour urine samples before prescribing hormones, though I will empirically use progesterone in a woman or a 3-month trial of DHEA in a man with allergies if I find sufficient indications and no contraindications. Treatment is customized per patient. I discuss the hormonal contributions to autoimmunity and chronic inflammation in Chapter 4.6 under the heading of "orthoendocrinology." Much of what applies to "allergy" also applies to "autoimmunity" and vise-versa; they are both manifestations of immune dysfunction.[164]

Step 4: Drug treatments

We must acknowledge a place for drug therapy in patients with recalcitrant or severe allergies.

- Prednisone: For patients with allergies that are inconsolable, prednisone becomes a reasonable consideration. The lowest effective dose should be used for the shortest possible period of time.

[156] Zapolska-Downar et al. Butyrate inhibits cytokine-induced VCAM-1 and ICAM-1 expression in cultured endothelial cells: the role of NF-kappaB and PPARalpha. *J Nutr Biochem*. 2004 Apr;15(4):220-8

[157] Luhrs et al. Butyrate inhibits NF-kappaB activation in lamina propria macrophages of patients with ulcerative colitis. *Scand J Gastroenterol*. 2002 Apr;37(4):458-66

[158] Vernia P, Monteleone G, Grandinetti G, Villotti G, Di Giulio E, Frieri G, Marcheggiano A, Pallone F, Caprilli R, Torsoli A. Combined oral sodium butyrate and mesalazine treatment compared to oral mesalazine alone in ulcerative colitis: randomized, double-blind, placebo-controlled pilot study. *Dig Dis Sci*. 2000 May;45(5):976-81

[159] Vernia et al. Topical butyrate improves efficacy of 5-ASA in refractory distal ulcerative colitis: results of a multicentre trial. *Eur J Clin Invest*. 2003;33(3):244-8

[160] Neesby TE. Method for desensitizing the gastrointestinal tract from food allergies. United States Patent 4,721,716. January 26, 1988

[161] Neesby TE. Method for desensitizing the gastrointestinal tract from food allergies. United States Patent 4,735,967. April 5, 1988

[162] Morrison LM, Enrick N. Coronary heart disease: reduction of death rate by chondroitin sulfate A. *Angiology*. 1973 May;24(5):269-87

[163] Theoharides TC, Bielory L. Mast cells and mast cell mediators as targets of dietary supplements. *Ann Allergy Asthma Immunol*. 2004 Aug;93(2 Suppl 1):S24-34

[164] My ideas on immunology and inflammation were first published in *Textbook of Functional Medicine* (2005, 2010) and later matured greatly in *Integrative Rheumatology* (2006), *Rheumatology v3.5* (2014) and later (2016) in the 4th Edition; the information will continue to be developed in future editions.

Discontinuation of treatment that has lasted longer than 4-7 days must be gradual in order to avoid adrenal insufficiency. Topical rather than systemic therapy should be used when appropriate.

- Sodium cromoglycate: Cromoglycate is a mast cell stabilizer which can be applied nasally for allergic rhinitis (Nasalcrom) or taken orally (Gastrocrom) by patients with food allergy to inhibit the local response to type-1 allergies.[165] The drug is poorly absorbed; therefore its anti-allergy effect is mediated at the gastrointestinal mucosa even though the benefits are systemic. Although not officially "approved" in the US for the treatment of food allergy, numerous studies support its use for this purpose.[166] Cromoglycate has been shown to reduce allergy-induced migraine[167] and eczema[168] and prevent the formation of immune complexes following the consumption of allergenic foods. In addition to preventing the allergic phenomena related directly to the consumption of allergenic foods, an additional mechanism of action of sodium cromoglycate is probably that it reduces the allergy-induced increase in intestinal permeability[169] and thereby prohibits absorption of bacterial and other microbial antigens and metabolites; stated differently, some of the manifestations attributed to "food allergy" are probably not mediated by the response to food allergens directly but result from the adverse immunologic and metabolic responses toward gut-derived microbial antigens and metabolites which are absorbed in increased amounts following the consumption of allergenic foods which increase intestinal permeability and absorption of "foreign" and "toxic" intraluminal contents which would have otherwise been excluded. Common doses for children are 100 mg 30 minutes before food (up to 400 mg per day) and 100-200 mg qid for adults 30 minutes before meals. Capsules or ampules should be mixed in plain water before consumption.

- Leukotriene antagonists: Montelukast (Singulair®, Merck) is an orally active leukotriene receptor antagonist that blocks leukotriene D4 from the cysteinyl leukotriene CysLT-1 receptor and thereby reduces vasodilation, eosinophilic inflammation, and vascular hyperpermeability. Montelukast is used in the medical treatment of asthma, rhinitis, and eczema.

Objective means for the identification of allergens: skin-prick testing, serum IgE and IgG assays, double-blind placebo-controlled food challenges, and the elimination and challenge technique

- Skin prick testing: IgE-dependent immediate-onset allergies as assessed with a **skin-prick test** are indicative of immediate-onset allergy to the particular allergen, and provide the identity of the allergen, quantification of the severity of the allergic response, *and evidence of underlying immune dysfunction*. Skin-prick testing does not assess for delayed-onset allergies thus leaving at least one class of adverse food reactions unassessed.

- Allergen-specific serum levels of IgE and IgG: Elevated serum levels of IgE and IgG, which are identified as specific for certain foods, also provide the identity of the allergen *and evidence of underlying immune dysfunction*. These "objective" tools are part of the clinician's repertoire for identifying food allergens, while keeping in mind that both skin-prick testing and serum testing are prone to both false positives and false negatives. Serum IgE testing does not assess IgG-mediated allergies, nor does it assess for sensitivity (immune but not immunoglobulin-mediated responses) or intolerance, which tends to be biochemical rather than immunologic. IgG assays and the subclasses of IgG-4 assays have not gained acceptance for their sensitivity or specificity, even though clinicians order them and patients pay for them.

- Double-blind placebo-controlled food challenge: Another commonly mentioned objective means for identifying food allergens is the "double-blind placebo-controlled food challenge" (DBPCFC) wherein food is administered a double-blind fashion with placebo control generally via either capsules or nasogastric tube. Unfortunately, DBPCFC is commonly considered the gold standard for the identification of particular allergens and the establishment of an allergic diathesis. This is unfortunate because the hospital admission

[165] drugs.com/MMX/Cromolyn_Sodium.html   Accessed November 24, 2005

[166] "Both the clinician's and patient's preferences and the clinician's evaluation of the specific response to challenge showed a significant benefit from SCG." Dannaeus A, Foucard T, Johansson SG. The effect of orally administered sodium cromoglycate on symptoms of food allergy. *Clin Allergy*. 1977 Mar;7(2):109-15

[167] "Immune complexes were not produced in those patients who were protected by sodium cromoglycate. These observations confirm that a food-allergic reaction is the cause of migraine in this group of patients." Monro J, Carini C, Brostoff J. Migraine is a food-allergic disease. *Lancet*. 1984 Sep 29;2(8405):719-21

[168] "The same atopic patients pretreated with oral sodium cromoglycate had less antigen entry, diminished immune-complex formation, and no atopic symptoms." Paganelli et al. Immune complexes containing food proteins in normal and atopic subjects after oral challenge and effect of sodium cromoglycate on antigen absorption. *Lancet*. 1979 Jun 16;1(8129):1270-2

[169] "It is suggested that a local IgE-mediated mechanism acts as a "trigger" for the entry of antigen and the formation of immune complexes by altering the permeability of the gut mucosa. The resulting delayed onset symptoms could be viewed as a form of serum sickness with few or many target organs affected." Carini C, Brostoff J, Wraith DG. IgE complexes in food allergy. *Ann Allergy*. 1987 Aug;59(2):110-7

and associated costs are expensive, cumbersome and therefore inaccessible for most patients. Some patients will have a false-negative response when challenged with isolated foods because of the lack of "accessory antigens", "accomplice antigens", or "bystander antigens."[170] Some patients will have adverse food reactions only when foods are eaten either with *high frequency* or in *specific combinations* or when *gastrointestinal problems* (e.g., dysbiosis or increased intestinal permeability) are present at the same time as the food challenge. For example, while the patient may tolerate eggs alone and wheat alone without the manifestation of allergic symptoms, the additive insult of the combination of both eggs and wheat may cause sufficient intestinal damage and/or immune activation that clinical manifestations become apparent. With single food challenges given with DBPCFC, "real life" situations are not reproduced, and false negative results may erroneously suggest that either the patient has no allergies or that a particular food is not offensive. Furthermore, the scientific sterility of the DBPCFC generally takes the patient out of his/her real life experience and context; the implications for this are obvious when we consider the emotional-social-psychological aspects of immune system hyper-reactivity and/or neurogenic inflammation that underlies the neuropsychological aspect of allergy, mentioned previously in the context of classical/Pavlovian conditioning of allergic responses.[171,172]

- Elimination and challenge: The "elimination and challenge" technique (more accurately described as "avoidance and challenge") requires that the patient first clear the diet of all possible offending foods, either by fasting or by consuming a simple diet of unlikely-to-be-allergenic foods, such as the classic triad of rice, lamb, and pears or a relatively hypoallergenic hydrolyzed formula such as Vivonex. After 7-14 days of elimination (i.e., avoidance) *and the clearing of symptoms thought to be allergy-mediated*, an offending food is reintroduced by intense consumption (i.e., eaten with every meal) for a period of up to two days. Every two to four days, a new food is added back into the diet, and a correlation is searched for between consumption of a given food and the exacerbation of symptoms. If the symptoms do not abate or disappear with the fasting/elimination phase, then confirming the nature of the disorder as allergic is more difficult and determining the identity of the allergen is additionally unlikely. However, in some cases, clinical signs and symptoms that are indeed allergy-mediated will fail to regress significantly during the brief washout period. This is because the underlying tissue damage is too great to be healed in such a short time. A good example is the thyroid disease induced by gluten-containing grains in people with the severe gluten allergy called celiac disease; simply avoiding gluten for 1-2 weeks does not restore endocrine function because the body needs more time to reacquire homeostasis and to heal injured tissues. A common scenario is one in which symptoms remit during fasting/elimination and then return *gradually* rather than *immediately* when the offending food is eaten. In these situations, the most likely explanations are either ❶ a threshold of time was necessary for physiologic abnormalities (e.g., immune complex deposition, increased intestinal permeability, dysbiosis, accumulative immune stimulation) to culminate in the reproduction of symptoms, or ❷ synergistic factors may have to be combined in order to produce the symptoms of allergy, such as the induction of IgE-mediated increased intestinal permeability by food R which then leads to the increased absorption of food S, to which the peripheral immune system then responds with an IgG-mediated reaction with resultant clinical manifestations. In the latter case, food R or food S *when eaten alone or on a rotation basis* may be insufficient to produce allergic manifestations, but the combination of R+S, which would not be identified with skin-prick testing, serum tests, or one-at-a-time DBPCFC, may produce allergic manifestations. Since, in real life, foods are eaten in combination when they cause allergic disease (e.g. a headache or joint pain after eating a hamburger with wheat/gluten, cheese/milk, mayonnaise/egg, and pickle/tartrazine/yeast), a reasonable conclusion is that foods will have to be avoided in specific combinations to attain maximal improvement in allergic symptoms since complex foods probably work synergistically to produce allergic manifestations in affected people. Creating chronological distance between the consumption of allergenic foods explains the success of the **rotation diets** in alleviating allergic manifestations, but it does little to address the underlying immune dysfunction other than to reduce the total allergenic load to which the immune system is exposed. **Intestinal dysbiosis** can also increase intestinal permeability and result in increased absorption of food antigens and depletion of detoxification co-factors, which can mimic or perpetuate immune-mediated food allergies. Correction of this problem can begin to normalize immune function and eliminate symptoms attributed to the consumption of specific foods.

---

[170] "The mechanisms of enhanced permeability to specific and bystander antigens have been delineated as well as the molecular events involved in the sequential phases of allergic reactions." Heyman M. Gut barrier dysfunction in food allergy. *Eur J Gastroenterol Hepatol*. 2005 Dec;17(12):1279-1285

[171] "In a classical conditioning procedure in which an immunologic challenge was paired with the presentation of an odor, guinea pigs showed a plasma histamine increase when presented with the odor alone. This suggests that the immune response can be enhanced through activity of the central nervous system." Russell M, Dark KA, Cummins RW, Ellman G, Callaway E, Peeke HV. Learned histamine release. *Science*. 1984 Aug 17;225(4663):733-4

[172] "A classical Pavlovian paradigm pairing an olfactory cue with allergen challenge for a single training trial was used to produce conditioned histamine release and conditioned nasal airflow decrease in seasonal allergic rhinitis sufferers." Barrett JE, King MG, Pang G. Conditioning rhinitis in allergic humans. *Ann N Y Acad Sci*. 2000;917:853-9

Allergy—Part 2: Asthma & Reactive Airway Disease

Introduction:
While all allergic diseases are important (particularly for the patients who suffer from them), I have chosen to detail asthma because of its increasing frequency, its debilitating nature, the many adverse effects from its medical treatment, and its life-threatening potential. Clinician readers should appreciate that many of the interventions used generally for allergy can apply to asthma, and vice-versa.   Criteria for the evaluation and classification of asthma change frequently; indeed some authorities have called for the abolition of the term "asthma" in favor of the more inclusive and "reactive airway disease" (RAD). Readers wishing to specialize in the treatment of asthma/RAD should consult more than one authoritative source (e.g., a recent clinical specialty textbook and a comprehensive peer-reviewed position paper or clinical practice guideline).

Description & Pathophysiology:

- "Asthma" (Greek: "difficult breathing") refers to a heterogeneous group of airway-pulmonary disorders characterized by the following:
    - Inflammation and histologic changes: Airway epithelium shows increased numbers of activated inflammatory cells including eosinophils, mast cells, macrophages, neutrophils, and T-lymphocytes which produce soluble inflammatory mediators such as cytokines, leukotrienes, and bradykinins. Airway inflammation leads to airway edema, increased vascularity, and disruption of ciliated columnar epithelium—each of these leads to perpetuation of chronic inflammation and airway obstruction. Smooth muscle hyperplasia and hypertrophy, along with increased deposition of collagen contributes to airway constriction and stiffness, both of which contribute to obstruction. Increased mucus production and goblet cell hyperplasia predispose to formation of mucus plugs, which can completely block bronchioles, thus eliminating gas exchange and promoting atelectasis in the corresponding pulmonary segment.
    - Airway hyper-reactivity: Airways are normally reactive to various stimuli; the distinction that characterizes asthma is the severity of the reactivity (overzealous response) and the exquisite sensitivity to triggers—asthmatic airways respond to stimuli at levels which are subthreshold for nonasthmatics. Thus, hyper-reactivity reflects overactivity of the inflammatory response and hypersensitivity to generally innocuous levels bronchoconstrictor stimuli. The speed of the inflammatory response following irritant exposure can be immediate ("immediate asthmatic response") or delayed by 4-6 hours ("late asthmatic response").
    - Reversibility: One of the diagnostic characteristics of asthma is its reversibility with bronchodilator challenge. However, with long-standing severe disease, airway remodeling—which includes smooth muscle hypertrophy/hyperplasia and fibrosis—becomes progressively irreversible. Irreversible airway obstruction is characteristic of COPD—chronic obstructive pulmonary disease—which includes asthma and chronic bronchitis.
    - Airway obstruction: Asthma primarily affects the bronchi rather than the lung parenchyma and alveoli. Thus, the clinical problem is one of *air movement* rather than *gas exchange* per se; although severely impaired air movement does necessarily impair gas exchange even when the alveoli are fully functional. Due to the dynamics of air movement during lung deflation, asthma primarily results in impaired exhalation, resulting in "air trapping" within the lungs and the resultant hyperinflation and secondarily impaired inhalation and efficient gas exchange.
    - Increased prevalence during adolescence: African Americans and children are most affected; the highest death rates due to asthma are seen in young African-Americans aged 15-24 years. "Asthma is the most common chronic pediatric disease."[173] Compared with adults, children show an increased prevalence of allergic/atopic disorders, which many of them will "grow out of" as they get older. Maturation of the immune system in general and the progressively increased elaboration of immunomodulating hormones cortisol, DHEA, testosterone with adrenarche (average age 6-10 years) in particular contribute to the regression of allergy/atopy as young children get older.

---

[173] Witcoff LJ. Pulmonology. In: Brown LJ, Miller LT. (Eds.) *Pediatrics Board Review Series*. Philadelphia: Lippincott Williams and Wilkins; 2005, 268-71

- Increased prevalence in industrialized societies: Asthma affects 7% of the US population (nearly 15 million people, causing more than 5,550 deaths per year), reflecting an increase of 75% from 1960 to 1994.

- Contributors to and triggers for asthma include the following:
  - Chronic sinusitis
  - Diminished β2-adrenergic receptor function: this predisposes to bronchospasm
  - Drug allergens/sensitizers, including prescription drugs with artificial colors that are known to trigger asthma
  - Dust mites and their feces
  - Food allergens
  - Fungi and mold exposure
  - Gastroesophageal reflux
  - Insects such as roaches, pet dander and saliva
  - Obesity—see Chapters 2 and 4.4 for discussion of link between obesity and inflammation
  - Pollen
  - Viral infections
  - Xenobiotic/chemical fumes including urban pollution

Clinical Presentation:

- **The classic triad of asthma includes ❶ persistent wheeze, ❷ persistent dyspnea** (shortness of breath, subjective "chest tightness"), **and ❸ persistent cough.** In the acute care setting, these same manifestations could be caused by inhalation of a foreign object, acute airway inflammation due to chemical-toxic-smoke inhalation injury, or anaphylaxis. Laboratory confirmation of asthma includes a fourth component: induction and reversibility with chemical provocation.
- **Indicators of urgency—implement immediate and aggressive treatment: difficulty talking due to dyspnea, use of accessory muscles if inspiration, pulsus paradoxus (no palpable radial pulse during inhalation), diaphoresis, mental status changes (e.g., agitation or somnolence).**
  - *Pulsus paradoxus*—the paradoxically missing peripheral pulse during inspiration—is may be seen with cardiac tamponade, pericarditis, chronic sleep apnea, croup, asthma and COPD.

Major Differential Diagnoses:

- Acute airway inflammation and angioedema due to chemical-toxic-smoke-aspiration inhalation: This can include gastroesophageal reflux, which may be otherwise asymptomatic, and which may occur unknown to the patient during sleep; relatedly, tracheoesophageal fistula should be considered in infants and post-trauma patients.
- Airway compression due to anatomic anomaly, tumor, or mediastinal lymphadenopathy:
- Allergic bronchopulmonary aspergillosis (ABPA), allergic bronchopulmonary mycosis: Skin allergy test is commonly positive to *Aspergillus fumigatus*.
- Anaphylaxis
- Antitrypsin deficiency: alpha-1-antitrypsin deficiency classically leads to emphysema and hepatic fibrosis.
- Bronchiectasis
- Bronchopulmonary dysplasia
- Cardiac disease and heart failure: "Cardiac asthma"
- Churg-Strauss vasculitis
- Cystic fibrosis
- Eosinophilic pneumonia
- Idiopathic pulmonary fibrosis: Extremely rare in children; more common (but still rare) in older adults in general and particularly those with inflammatory/autoimmune diseases
- Inhalation of a foreign object
- Pneumothorax
- Pulmonary edema: Consider congestive heart failure as a primary cause.

Clinical Assessments:

- **History/subjective**:

  > **Clinical Pearl**
  >
  > During acute exacerbations of asthma, air movement can be so severely reduced that wheezing is not present; in these situations, the more subtle physical examination findings of prolonged exhalation and a global reduction in breath sounds should be pursued.

  - <u>HPI</u>: Episodic wheezing (reversible spontaneously or with treatment), dyspnea, subjective "chest tightness", cough, excess sputum; symptoms may be intermittent or persistent.
  - <u>Associated findings</u>: Nasal congestion, rhinorrhea, polyps; increased prevalence of eczema and otitis media.
  - <u>Common triggers</u>: URI, aspiration, gastroesophageal reflux disorder (GERD), psychoemotional and physical stress, exercise, tobacco smoke, pollution including ozone and sulfur dioxide, menses ("catamenial asthma"); assessment for the head/facial pain and post-nasal drip of chronic sinusitis is particularly important as treatment for chronic sinusitis is very effective in alleviating asthma manifestations.

- **Physical Examination/Objective**: Physical examination and pulmonary function may be essentially normal between exacerbations, especially in younger patients with intermittent disease.
  - <u>Lung auscultation and percussion</u>: Prolonged exhalation, tachypnea, diffuse wheezes, hyperresonance.
  - <u>Spirometry</u>: Clinical assessment of FEV1 and FVC provides the FEV1/FVC ratio, which when reduced indicates the airway obstruction typical of *but not specific for* asthma. Peak expiratory flow measurement can also be used to assess current status and response to treatment.
  - <u>BMI</u>: Overweight patients should follow a diet-exercise-lifestyle program that facilitates weight loss, with its attendant reduction in *total inflammatory load* and improved respiratory function. Weight loss in general and low-carbohydrate diets in particular help alleviate GERD, which is a well-known cause of asthma, particularly adult-onset asthma.

- **Laboratory Assessments**: Always perform a basic laboratory evaluation in essentially all patients, particularly when evaluating them for the first time or if their therapeutic progress is unsatisfactory. This basic laboratory evaluation should include CBC, chemistry/metabolic panel, urinalysis and preferably TSH, vitamin D level, CRP, and ferritin. Just because a patient has a diagnosis of "asthma" (or any other disease) and the same patient has shortness of breath (SOB) or dyspnea on exertion (DOE), this does not mean that the SOB/DOE is due to the asthma; the patient may also have iron deficiency and/or anemia as a cause of or contributor to their symptomatology.
  - <u>CBC</u>: May reveal eosinophilia. Elevated WBC, neutrophils or lymphocytes can indicate infection, whether bacterial or viral, respectively. Elevated RBC consistent with polycythemia can indicate chronic hypoxia, which may be due to chronic severe asthma or another pulmonary, renal, or myeloproliferative disorder.
  - <u>Serum total IgE levels</u>: Increased in some (not all) patients with atopy, parasitosis, ABPA
  - <u>Serum IgE levels for specific allergens</u>
  - <u>Skin testing for IgE/immediate allergy</u>
  - <u>Serum IgG4 levels for specific delayed-onset allergens</u>
  - <u>Urine sulfite</u>: A subset of asthma patients—prototypically those presenting concomitant multiple chemical sensitivity (MCS)—is sensitive to or unable to detoxify various endogenous and exogenous precursors that are ultimately reduced to sulfite. As a result, sulfite levels are increase in the urine and can be measured at abnormally high levels in affected patients. Subsequently, steps can be taken to reduce sulfite intake and/or facilitate in vivo detoxification of sulfite, such as with supraphysiologic doses of vitamin B-12, and perhaps with molybdenum supplementation.
  - <u>Sputum eosinophils</u>: Quantification of eosinophils in induced sputum can guide corticosteroid administration more effectively than clinical assessment for the prevention of exacerbations.
  - <u>Exhaled nitric oxide (eNO)</u>: Measurement of exhaled nitric oxide provides noninvasive assessment of airway inflammation, but conflicting data does not currently clarify the role of eNO in asthma management.
  - <u>Fecal antigen testing for current *Helicobacter pylori* infection</u>: A small percentage of patients with asthma—as with migraine and inflammation/autoimmunity—may have occult *H pylori* infection; eradication of this dysbiosis—especially if combined with regular implementation of the 5-part supplemented Paleo-

Mediterranean diet protocol and other anti-inflammatory health-restorative treatments may reduce their *total inflammatory load* sufficiently to provide objective and subjective improvement in their clinical status.

- **Imaging**:
  - **Chest radiograph** may show hyperinflation and can be used to assess for differential diagnoses such as foreign object, pneumonia, interstitial lung disease, pneumothorax, or lung tumor in appropriate clinical scenarios.
- **Biopsy/Procedure**: Lung biopsy is not used in the diagnosis and management of asthma *per se*; its role in this context would only be in the exclusion/confirmation of another lung disease
  - Arterial blood gases and pulse oximetry may show hypoxemia during exacerbations.
  - Spirometry can be performed in office and at home to assess response to treatment and challenge (e.g., consumption of suspected food allergen) and to monitor for exacerbations.
- **Establishing the Diagnosis**: The diagnosis of asthma is established with demonstration (clinical or historical) of reversible airway obstruction and airway hyper-reactivity. These can be provoked artificially by administration of a bronchoconstrictor (e.g., methacholine, histamine, cold air, exercise; these are considered "nonspecific" and are able to induce bronchoconstriction at levels much lower than those required to induce bronchoconstriction in nonasthmatics) and/or bronchodilator, such as albuterol or epinephrine. Iatrogenic bronchoconstriction should be undertaken only by pulmonary specialists with on-site emergency management capabilities, and such diagnostic challenge should obviously never be undertaken during an already in-process exacerbation or when FEV1 is less than 65% of predicted. **A compatible history of repeated and reversible airway obstruction based on the patient's experience is generally sufficient for diagnosis; this can be further supported with a favorable response to bronchodilator therapy.** In-office spirometry can be used to document and quantify airway obstruction. Lung volume measurements can be assessed by various methods and characteristically show hyperinflation. Arterial blood gases and pulse oximetry may show hypoxemia during exacerbations. Chest radiograph may show hyperinflation and can be used to assess for differential diagnoses such as foreign object, pneumonia, interstitial lung disease, or lung tumor in appropriate clinical scenarios.
  - ***Status asthmaticus*** is any severe acute exacerbation of asthma that is relatively unresponsive to expedient treatment. ***Hyperacute asthma*** **can be rapidly fatal.**
  - **Arterial blood gas analysis showing *progressive/absolute* hypoxemia or hypercarbia portends/indicates a medical emergency. "The combination of an increased PaCO2 and respiratory acidosis may indicate impending respiratory failure and the need for mechanical ventilation."[174]**

Disease Complications:
- Quality of life complications: Inability to participate fully in activities of daily living (ADL), impaired quality of life, social compromise, low self-esteem, lost opportunities, depression.
- Medical complications: Exhaustion, syncope, pneumothorax, respiratory failure, death

Clinical Management: Clinical management of the asthmatic patient is based on assessment of impairment and risk. In this context, impairment includes asthma severity (frequency and intensity) and the resultant functional limitations, while risk includes likelihood of acute exacerbations and chronic decline in lung function due to chronic inflammation, airway remodeling, and decompensation. Experts Chestnut, Murray, and Prendergast[175] state, "A key insight is that these two domains of control may respond differently to treatment: some patients may have minimal impairment yet remain at risk for severe exacerbations, for example, in the setting of an upper respiratory tract infection."
- Home-use peak expiratory flow (PEF) meters: Measurements can be used by patients for self-monitoring, for assessing response to challenges such as stressful events, food allergen consumption, and environmental exposure. The patient can record a daily log or "lung diary" that is given to and used by the clinician to monitor response to treatment. PEF shows diurnal variation (worst in the morning, best in the afternoon), and PEF values can be contrasted to the patient's previous values thereby serving as a true guide to patient status, whether that of improvement or exacerbation. "PEF values less than 200 L/min indicate severe airflow

[174] Chestnut et al. "Pulmonary Disorders." In: McPhee et al. (Eds.) *Current Medical Diagnosis and Treatment 2009, 48th Edition*. McGraw Hill Medical; 2009, 210-228
[175] Chestnut et al. "Pulmonary Disorders." In: McPhee et al. (Eds.) *Current Medical Diagnosis and Treatment 2009, 48th Edition*. McGraw Hill Medical; 2009, 210-228

obstruction."[176] Physicians should give patients a plan of action should pulmonary function decline significantly so that early-stage declinations can be treated before potentially developing into serious exacerbations.

- <u>Written instructions</u>: Patients must receive clearly written instructions for ❶ daily management including schedule of administration for their medication(s) and nutritional supplements and ❷ emergent management including additional doses of treatments and clear instructions—preferably with address, phone number, and map—to the nearest emergency care facility.
- <u>Reserve ("back-up") medication</u>: Patients and clinicians should ensure that treatment is available to the patient at all times and locations: at home, at school, at work, and when traveling. When traveling, patients should have reserve treatment with them, namely medications in their personal carry-on luggage as well as their checked baggage in case one of these is lost or confiscated by airport security; necessary prescriptions should be preauthorized at national pharmacies. The patient has the responsibility to inform the clinician of travel plans and to schedule any necessary office visits before traveling and with enough time for clinical evaluation and the obtainment of laboratory results.

<u>**Treatments**</u>: The two minimal goals of treatment are ❶ **expedient and efficacious control of any acute exacerbations**, and ❷ **convenient and nontoxic control of daily symptoms**. The highest goal of ❸ **optimizing endogenous inflammatory and immune balance so that the asthma resolves** is generally not a consideration in standardized allopathic medicine although is a foremost goal in naturopathic and functional medicine. Clinicians specializing in the treatment of pulmonary disorders should stay abreast with updated treatment guidelines, such as those published by the National Heart, Lung, and Blood Institute (NHLBI) nhlbi.nih.gov/guidelines/asthma and the National Asthma Education and Prevention Program (NAEPP) nhlbi.nih.gov/about/naepp. Further, treatment of status asthmaticus should be managed by emergency medicine personnel trained in and equipped for intubation, artificial ventilation, and parenteral drug administration.

- **Prescription drug treatments per asthma classification/severity**: Inhaled corticosteroids are the "default" treatment for asthma unless it is sufficiently mild and intermittent to be managed with PRN use of bronchodilators, typically inhaled beta-2 agonists (hereafter: beta2-inhaler) such as albuterol; additional drugs include leukotriene synthesis inhibitors, leukotriene receptor blockers, mast cell stabilizers, anti-IgE antibodies, and methylxanthines/theophylline. Drugs are added in a stepwise fashion depending on asthma classification, which is defined by disease frequency and severity, as shown in the following table:

Classification	Frequency & Severity	Drug Management
<u>Intermittent</u>	▪ Daytime symptoms: ≤ 2/wk ▪ Nighttime symptoms: ≤ 2/mo	▪ PRN short-acting beta2-inhaler
<u>Mild persistent</u>	▪ Daytime symptoms: 2-6/wk ▪ Nighttime symptoms: > 2/mo ▪ FEV1 ≥ 80% (normal)	▪ PRN short-acting beta2-inhaler ▪ Scheduled daily use of low-dose inhaled steroid; second-line alternatives include cromolyn, or leukotriene modulator
<u>Moderate persistent</u>	▪ Daytime symptoms: daily ▪ Nighttime symptoms: > 1/wk ▪ FEV1 60-80%	▪ PRN short-acting beta2-inhaler ▪ Medium-dose inhaled steroid <u>or</u> low-dose inhaled steroid and long-acting beta2-inhaler
<u>Severe persistent</u>	▪ Daytime symptoms: continuous ▪ Nighttime symptoms: frequent ▪ FEV1 ≤ 60%	▪ PRN short-acting beta2-inhaler -inhaler ▪ High-dose inhaled steroid ▪ Long-acting beta2-inhaler-inhaler ▪ Systemic steroids

- <u>Cromolyn sodium</u>: Cromolyn acts as a mast cell stabilizer, reducing the elaboration of inflammatory mediators; it is used for long-term management and is not used in the treatment of acute exacerbations.

---

[176] Chestnut et al. "Pulmonary Disorders." In: McPhee et al. (Eds.) Current Medical Diagnosis and Treatment 2009, 48th Edition. New York: McGraw Hill Medical; 2009, 210-228

- Corticosteroids: These "steroids" are either short-acting or long-acting and are delivered by oral, inhalational, and parenteral routes; although they are essential for the management of severe asthma, their chronic use can cause growth retardation in children, as well as immunosuppression, osteoporosis, and a Cushing-like syndrome and metabolic syndrome (i.e., insulin resistance, hypertension, dyslipidemia, and obesity). Importantly, corticosteroid administration increases body losses (mostly through increased urinary excretion) of calcium, magnesium, potassium, and zinc; the iatrogenic magnesium insufficiency exacerbates anxiety and bronchospasm while the zinc insufficiency impairs immune responsiveness and adversely affects hormonal immunomodulation by enhancing the effects of estrogen(s) and impairing the effects of androgens, particularly testosterone. Gvozdjáková et al[177] noted that "Long-term administration of corticosteroids has been shown to result in mitochondrial dysfunction and oxidative damage of mitochondrial and nuclear DNAs" and suggested that this iatrogenic cellular damage might be prevented or ameliorated via supplementation with coenzyme Q10, as discussed below.
- Anticholinergic drugs: Anticholinergic drugs such as atropine and ipratropium bromide block vagal/parasympathetic-mediated bronchoconstriction and thus function as bronchodilators; anticholinergic drugs can be used as second-line bronchodilators in the treatment of severe asthma.
- Anti-IgE antibody (omalizumab): Omalizumab binds to IgE and thus reduces allergic responses; the clinical safety and efficacy profiles are notably good.

- **Dietary interventions**:
    - Food allergens: Some experts would argue that the link between food allergies and asthma is so strong that failure to address the food allergy component of asthma is clinical malpractice. Among the most commonly consumed allergens that exacerbate asthma are cereal grains, "nuts" and peanuts, cow milk, eggs, chocolate (also a source of cow's milk in the case of milk chocolate), fish, tomatoes and other *Solanaceae* nightshade plants (perhaps due in part to the anti-acetylcholinesterase constituent(s)

> **Fast food (e.g., wheat, high-glycemic loads and indexes, GMO foods, AGE components, and high-dose sodium to activate Th17 inflammatory cells) increases the incidence of allergic inflammatory disease: dose-dependent response with asthma**
>
> "CONCLUSIONS: Frequent consumption of hamburgers showed a dose-dependent association with asthma symptoms, and frequent takeaway [fast food] consumption showed a similar association with bronchial hyperresponsiveness."
>
> Wickens et al. Fast foods - are they a risk factor for asthma? *Allergy.* 2005 Dec

promoting parasympathetic bronchoconstriction), food colorings (especially tartrazine [yellow dye #5] which is also found in some asthma medications, as well as some formulations of thyroxine). Early introduction of cereal grains/grasses into the childhood diet promotes development of IgE antibodies against other grasses and airborne pollens[178]; not surprisingly, the risk of atopic/allergic disease correlates directly with the number of solid foods prematurely introduced into an infant's diet.[179] Furthermore, grains are commonly contaminated with additional allergens and immunogens such as mold/fungi/yeast and insects and their feces.

    - Avoidance of proinflammatory foods: Specific food components associated with development and/or exacerbation of asthma include saturated fatty acids and high-carbohydrate calorie-dense foods. Saturated fatty acids promote systemic inflammation *in vivo* by several mechanisms not the least of which is activation of Toll-like receptor 4 which in turn activates NF-kappaB. Similarly, high glucose loads induce oxidative stress, which is well known to deplete antioxidants (some of which have immunomodulating and anti-allergy effects) and to promote systemic inflammation. Childhood food consumption patterns characterized by low intake of magnesium, vitamin E, breast milk, fruits and vegetables, and increased consumption of "fast foods", pasta, and hamburgers increase the risk of asthma.[180,181,182]

---

[177] Gvozdjáková et al. Coenzyme Q10 supplementation reduces corticosteroids dosage in patients with bronchial asthma. *Biofactors.* 2005;25(1-4):235-40
[178] Armentia et al. Early introduction of cereals into children's diets as a risk-factor for grass pollen asthma. *Clin Exp Allergy.* 2001 Aug;31(8):1250-5
[179] Fergusson DM, Horwood LJ, Shannon FT. Early solid feeding and recurrent childhood eczema: a 10-year longitudinal study. *Pediatrics.* 1990 Oct;86(4):541-6
[180] Hijazi N, Abalkhail B, Seaton A. Diet and childhood asthma in a society in transition: a study in urban and rural Saudi Arabia. *Thorax.* 2000 Sep;55(9):775-9
[181] Wickens K, Barry D, Friezema A, Rhodius R, Bone N, Purdie G, Crane J. Fast foods - are they a risk factor for asthma? *Allergy.* 2005 Dec;60(12):1537-41
[182] Awasthi et al. Prevalence and risk factors of asthma and wheeze in school-going children in Lucknow, North India. *Indian Pediatr.* 2004 Dec;41(12):1205-10

- <u>Health-promoting Paleo-Mediterranean Diet (previously described in this text—see Chapter 2):</u> In 2008 Castro-Rodriguez et al[183] concluded, "The Mediterranean diet is an independent protective factor for current wheezing in preschoolers, irrespective of obesity and physical activity."

- <u>Diet modification for weight loss and BMI optimization:</u> Obesity and its associated lifestyle and dietary risk factors correlates with an increased risk factor for asthma by several mechanisms, including: ❶ overconsumption of saturated fatty acids and simple carbohydrates, both of which promote systemic inflammation and oxidant stress, ❷ sedentary lifestyle, as lack of exercise causes a relative increase in systemic inflammation compared to an active lifestyle because exercising muscle releases anti-inflammatory cytokines (myokines), ❸ caloric overload is most easily accomplished by consumption of processed foods such as grain products which are inherently allergenic, ❹ physical enlargement of abdominal contents (i.e., visceral adipose) which retards diaphragmatic descent and thereby reduces respiratory efficiency, ❺ increased elaboration of inflammatory cytokines (adipokines) from adipose tissue, and ❻ enhancement of an inflammatory state via alterations in hormone levels, particularly an increase in *pro-inflammatory* estrogens and reduction in *anti-inflammatory* androgens. Delgado et al[184] wrote, "Most prospective studies show that obesity is a risk factor for asthma and have found a positive correlation between baseline body mass index and the subsequent development of asthma. Furthermore, several studies suggest that whereas weight gain increases the risk of asthma, weight loss improves the course of the illness. ... The treatment of obese asthmatics must include a weight control program."

- <u>Avoidance of sulfite-containing foods for patients with sulfite-sensitive asthma:</u> A subset of asthmatic patients are intolerant to sulfite(s) and suffer exacerbations of asthma following sulfite consumption or, possibly, increased endogenous production. Among the more commonly sulfited foods are lettuce, shrimp, dried fruits (e.g., apricots), white grape juice, dehydrated potatoes (as mashed potatoes), wine, beer, mushrooms, and candy bars (e.g., Mounds). Sodium metabisulfite is used in foods and some medications (e.g., acetaminophen) as a disinfectant, antioxidant, and preservative. Adverse food reactions following consumption of sulfited foods are not always consistent, even when the patient has confirmed sulfite sensitivity based on double-blind capsule/beverage challenge testing. Taylor et al[185] summarized, "The likelihood of a reaction is dependent on the nature of the food, the level of residual sulfite, the sensitivity of the patient, and perhaps on the form of residual sulfite and the mechanism of the sulfite-induced reaction." The clinical application of this information is to consider sulfite sensitivity in asthmatic patients, particularly those with recalcitrant disease and those with other manifestations of impaired sulfur metabolism such as multiple chemical sensitivity (MCS); in these patients, a broader therapeutic

> **Paleo-Mediterranean diet (compared to standard processed food diet) protects against the development of allergy and asthma**
>
> "CONCLUSIONS: The Mediterranean diet is an independent protective factor for current wheezing in preschoolers, irrespective of obesity and physical activity."
>
> Castro-Rodriguez et al. Mediterranean diet as a protective factor for wheezing in preschool children. *J Pediatr.* 2008 Jun

> **Clinical Pearl: Sulfite leads to mast cell degranulation and thus "allergic inflammation" while it also impairs mitochondrial function, thereby promoting chronic/sustained inflammation and metabolic impairment**
>
> "Sulfur dioxide is 1 of 6 environmental pollutants monitored by the Environmental Protection Agency. Its ability to induce bronchoconstriction is well documented. ... Peripheral blood basophils also showed histamine release after exposure to sodium sulfite. ...
> <u>Conclusions</u>: **Sulfite**, the aqueous ion of sulfur dioxide, induces cellular activation, **leading to degranulation in mast cells through a non-IgE-dependent pathway.** The response also differs from IgE-mediated degranulation..."
>
> Collaco et al. Effect of sodium sulfite on mast cell degranulation and oxidant stress. *Ann Allergy Asthma Immunol.* 2006 Apr

---

[183] Castro-Rodriguez et al. Mediterranean diet as a protective factor for wheezing in preschool children. *J Pediatr.* 2008 Jun;152(6):823-8, 828.e1-2

[184] Delgado J, Barranco P, Quirce S. Obesity and asthma. *J Investig Allergol Clin Immunol.* 2008;18(6):420-5

[185] Taylor et al. Sensitivity to sulfited foods among sulfite-sensitive subjects with asthma. *J Allergy Clin Immunol.* 1988 Jun;81(6):1159-67. <u>This is a small clinical trial of eight patients, and most of the findings were inconclusive; this study was funded in large part by the processed food industry</u>: Supported by contributions from the Corn Refiners Association, National Fisheries Institute, National Cherry Growers and Industries Foundation, American Mushroom Institute, National Coalition of Fresh Potato Processors, Dried Fruit Association of California, Northwest Cherry Briners Association, International Food Additives Council, Villa Banfi Foundation, Inc., Frito-Lay, Inc., Del Monte Corp., Larsen Co., Pillsbury, Inc., Basic American Foods, Inc., Campbells, Inc., General Mills, Inc., Prepared Potato Co., Calreco, Inc., T. J. Lipton, Inc., Northern Star Co., Hershey Foods, Inc., R. T. French Co., Stauffer Chemical Co., Universal Foods Corp., and Mead Johnson Co.

approach might include vitamin B-12 supplementation as discussed in a following section, avoidance of sulfited foods, and perhaps more comprehensive detoxification programs.[186]

- **Avoidance of excess sodium chloride**: American/Westernized diets are overladen with sodium chloride. Excess sodium promotes water retention and tissue edema, especially when combined with a high-carbohydrate diet and/or insulin resistance. Sodium promotes induction of the pro-inflammatory Th17 phenotype, known to contribute to asthma.[187] The chloride ion is acidogenic and thus perturbs metabolism, disrupts homeostatic mechanisms, and promotes renal loss of calcium and magnesium—this latter effect promotes inflammation via nutrigenomic mechanisms, including but probably not limited to the development of intracellular hypercalcinosis (discussed elsewhere in this text). Avoidance of sodium chloride appears particularly relevant in the treatment of exercise-induced asthma (EIA).

  - Clinical trial: Both sodium and chloride contribute to the worsening of EIA symptoms: "The NaHCO3 diet lessened the deterioration of post-exercise pulmonary function, but not to the extent of LSD [low-salt diet]. These data suggest that both sodium and chloride contribute to the worsening of EIA symptoms seen after consuming a normal or high NaCl diet."[188] The fact that sodium bicarbonate had less impact on lung function than did sodium chloride shows that the chloride ion promotes bronchoconstriction.

  - Review: A nutritional approach to managing exercise-induced asthma: "Exercise-induced asthma (EIA) is traditionally treated with the use of pharmacotherapy. However, there is now convincing evidence that a variety of dietary factors such as elevated omega-3 polyunsaturated fatty acids and antioxidant intake, and a sodium-restricted diet can reduce this condition."[189]

  - Population-based study: Wheeze and asthma in children are associated with body mass index, sports, television viewing, and diet: "CONCLUSIONS: Our data support the hypothesis that high body weight, spending a lot of time watching television, and a salty diet each independently increase the risk of asthma symptoms in children."[190]

  - Randomized, double-blind crossover study: Dietary salt, airway inflammation, and diffusion capacity in exercise-induced asthma: "CONCLUSION: Our findings indicate that dietary salt loading enhances airway inflammation following exercise in asthmatic subjects, and that small salt-dependent changes in vascular volume and microvascular pressure might have substantial effects on airway function following exercise in the face of mediator-induced increased vascular permeability."[191]

- **Nutritional supplementation** :
  - Magnesium (oral, intravenous, inhaled/nebulized): In addition to serving as a cofactor for hundreds of biochemical enzymatic reactions including ATP production and utilization, magnesium is also necessary for muscle relaxation (implications for muscle cramps, myofascial trigger points, constipation, bronchoconstriction, hypertension, and cardiac contractility) and proper neuronal function (implications for depression, seizures, migraine, neurogenic inflammation, and NMDA receptor modulation). Given that dietary intake of magnesium is low in industrialized societies due to insufficient intake of vegetables and that urinary excretion of magnesium is increased with consumption of corticosteroids, caffeine, sugar, and alcohol, the consistent finding of laboratory-validated magnesium deficiency among a high percentage of outpatients and inpatients is to be expected. **For outpatient management and improved control of asthma and the associated anxiety and respiratory fatigue, magnesium should be a routine supplement to care given its low cost, safety, and collateral benefits.** In the acute setting, oral absorption and secondary tissue distribution would obviously be too slow to be of benefit; in the emergency setting, parenteral administration is required.
    - Clinical trial: Oral magnesium (-glycine) 300 mg/d: A double-blind randomized parallel placebo-controlled trial of children and adolescents with moderate persistent asthma (n=37; ages 7-19y) taking PRN fluticasone and salbutamol investigated the use of magnesium 300 mg/d administered

---

[186] Detoxification processes are reviewed in Chapter 4.7 of *Inflammation Mastery, 4th Edition* (2016) and later versions.
[187] Bedoya et al. Th17 Cells in Immunity and Autoimmunity. Clinical and Developmental Immunology 2013, Article 986789
[188] Mickleborough et al. Dietary chloride as a possible determinant of the severity of exercise-induced asthma. *Eur J Appl Physiol*. 2001 Sep;85(5):450-6
[189] Mickleborough TD. A nutritional approach to managing exercise-induced asthma. *Exerc Sport Sci Rev*. 2008 Jul;36(3):135-44
[190] Corbo et al. Wheeze and asthma in children: associations with body mass index, sports, television viewing, and diet. *Epidemiology*. 2008 Sep;19(5):747-55
[191] Mickleborough TD, Lindley MR, Ray S. Dietary salt, airway inflammation, and diffusion capacity in exercise-induced asthma. *Med Sci Sports Exerc*. 2005 Jun;37(6):904-14

orally in the form of Mg-glycine while the placebo group received only glycine. After 2 months of oral treatment, the Mg-group showed reduced bronchial reactivity as assessed by methacholine challenge, and skin responses to recognized antigens were also decreased. No changes were seen in forced vital capacity (FVC) or forced expiratory volume at first second (FEV1); however, the magnesium group experienced fewer asthma exacerbations and used less salbutamol compared to the placebo group.[192] Improvements in respiratory parameters seen following glycine supplementation in the "placebo" group attenuated more robust statistical differences between groups; glycine may exert therapeutic benefit in asthma ❶ by acting as an inhibitory neurotransmitter in the spinal cord and thereby modulating neurogenic inflammation, ❷ by acting as a precursor to glutathione, or ❸ or by downregulating NF-kappaB and inducible nitric oxide synthetase. In a separate study, Fogarty et al[193] researched the potential roles of amino acids in asthma and found that asthma severity was inversely related to serum glycine levels; thus glycine appears to attenuate asthma.

- Clinical trial: Oral magnesium (citrate) 200-270 mg/d: This randomized double-blind placebo-controlled prospective trial examined the use of magnesium (citrate) 200-290 mg/d for 12 weeks to find a statistically significant reduction in bronchodilator use, leading the authors to conclude, "Long-lasting Mg supplementation is clearly of benefit in mildly to moderately asthmatic children and is recommended as a concomitant drug in stable asthma."[194]

- Clinical trial: Intravenous MgSO4: In a randomized double-blind placebo-controlled study, patients with emergency acute asthma (n=135; ages 18-65y; FEV1 less than 75% predicted both before and after a single albuterol treatment) were treated with inhaled beta-agonists and intravenous (IV) steroids. Thirty minutes after entry, patients received either 2 g IV magnesium sulfate (MgSO4) or IV placebo. Overall, "Hospital admission rates were 35.3% for placebo-treated group and 25.4% for the magnesium-treated group." In patients with moderate asthma (FEV1 25-75%), hospital admission rates were 22.4% (11/49) for the placebo-treated group and 22.2% (10/25) for the magnesium-treated group; thus, no significant improvement in FEV1 was obtained in the moderate group for magnesium-treated patients. In patients with severe asthma (FEV1 < 25%), hospital admission rates were 78.6% (11/14) for the placebo-treated group and 33.3% (7/21) for the magnesium-treated group; also noted was a significant improvement in FEV1 at 120 min and 240 min among the severe asthma patients treated with magnesium. The authors concluded, "Intravenous MgSO4 decreased admission rate and improved FEV1 in patients with acute severe asthma but did not cause significant improvement in patients with moderate asthma."[195]

- Systematic review: Intravenous MgSO4: Review of the 7 of 27 clinical trials that met inclusion criteria lead the authors to conclude, "The use of intravenous magnesium sulfate reduces the rate of hospital admissions and improves pulmonary function in patients with severe acute asthma treated in the emergency department" while no consistent benefit was shown for patients with mild to moderate asthma.[196]

- Systematic review: Intravenous MgSO4: This systematic review of randomized controlled trials was limited to seven trials of acute asthma treated with intravenous magnesium sulfate versus placebo. Overall results showed that benefits of IV MgSO4 included fewer hospital admissions (especially among patients with severe asthma rather than moderate asthma) and nonsignificant improvements in peak expiratory flow rates (PEFR); FEV(1) generally improved by 10% predicted in patients with severe acute asthma. The authors concluded, "Current evidence does not clearly support routine use of intravenous magnesium sulfate in all patients with acute asthma presenting to the ED. However, **magnesium sulfate appears to be safe and beneficial for patients who present with severe acute asthma. Practice guidelines need to be changed to reflect these results.**"[197]

[192] Gontijo-Amaral C, et al. Oral magnesium supplementation in asthmatic children: a double-blind randomized placebo-controlled trial. *Eur J Clin Nutr* 2007;61:54–60
[193] Fogarty A, Broadfield E, Lewis S, Lawson N, Britton J. Amino acids and asthma: a case-control study. *Eur Respir J*. 2004 Apr;23(4):565-8
[194] Bede et al. Urinary magnesium excretion in asthmatic children receiving magnesium supplementation. *Magnes Res*. 2003 Dec;16(4):262-70
[195] Bloch H, Silverman R, Mancherje N, et al. Intravenous magnesium sulfate as an adjunct in the treatment of acute asthma. *Chest*. 1995 Jun;107(6):1576-81
[196] Rowe et al. Magnesium sulfate is effective for severe acute asthma treated in the emergency department. *West J Med*. 2000 Feb;172(2):96
[197] Rowe et al. Intravenous magnesium sulfate treatment for acute asthma in emergency department: a systematic review of the literature. *Ann Emerg Med*. 2000 Sep;36:181-90

- Systematic review: Inhaled/nebulized MgSO4: Six trials involving 296 patients were included in this review; four studies compared nebulized "MgSO4 + beta2-agonist" to "beta2-agonist alone", and two studies compared "MgSO4 alone" to "beta2-agonist alone." The authors concluded, "Nebulised inhaled magnesium sulfate in addition to beta2-agonist in the treatment of an acute asthma exacerbation, appears to have benefits with respect to improved pulmonary function in patients with severe asthma and there is a trend towards benefit in hospital admission."[198]

o Selenium: Selenium's (Se) prominent biological functions include ❶ antioxidant activity via its role as a cofactor for glutathione peroxidase, which regenerates reduced glutathione from glutathione disulfide, ❷ anti-inflammatory activity based on the elimination of hydroperoxide (arachidonic acid 5-hydroperoxide [5-hydroperoxyeicosatetraenoic acid, 5-HPETE] is the leukotriene-A4 precursor formed from arachidonate by 5-lipoxygenase) and downregulation of NF-kappaB, ❸ facilitating the conversion of T4 to T3, ❹ downregulation of estrogenic activity, and ❺ clinically significant antiviral effects. Routine supplemental dose is 200 mcg/d (most commonly either as selenomethionine or sodium selenite), while higher doses of approximately 800 mcg/d are also safe for long-term use but are generally reserved for acute treatment of viral infections or for the treatment of debilitating conditions such as chronic lymphedema. Given that asthmatic patients consistently show lower serum levels of selenium, reduced activity of glutathione peroxidase, and increased oxidative stress, routine supplementation with selenium is justified to reverse these negative biochemical parameters.

  - Clinical trial: Selenium 200 mcg/d for two years: A pilot study of 17 steroid-dependent asthmatics (n=17; ages 30-74y) used selenium 200 mcg/d for 24 months to effect reduced consumption of inhaled and systemic corticosteroids; clinical improvement correlated with the elevation of Se levels both in plasma and erythrocytes, and no adverse effects were noted.[199]

  - Clinical trial: Sodium selenite 100 mcg/d for 14 weeks: This double-blind clinical trial among asthmatic patients (n=24) effected significant increases in serum Se and platelet GSH-Px activity, significant reduction in the irreversible platelet aggregation induced by 5 mumol/l ADP, and significant clinical improvement in the Se-supplemented group as assessed by "assembled clinical evaluation" rather than reliance upon individual isolated parameters.[200] Sodium selenite tends to have a faster onset of action than other forms of selenium, and this—along with the use of the composite clinical evaluation rather than reliance on a single parameter—may explain the success of this clinical trial despite its low dose and short duration.

  - Clinical trial: Yeast-sourced selenium 100 mcg for 24 weeks: In a clinical trial with 197 patients, treatment with selenium 100 mcg/d for 6 months increased plasma selenium levels by 48% but provided no clinical benefit in adult asthmatic patients, the majority of whom were concomitantly treated with steroids[201]; faults with this trial include the subtherapeutic dosage (i.e., a daily dose of 800 mcg would have been more reasonable) and the fact that the selenium was sourced from yeast, to which some of the patients may have been allergic.

- Coenzyme Q10 (CoQ10): CoQ10 is an endogenous antioxidant, immunomodulator, and essential component of the mitochondrial electron transport chain; deficiency of CoQ10 may be a primary cause of or secondary effect of various disease states. Supplementation with CoQ10 has been shown in human clinical trials to ameliorate hypertension, congestive heart failure, migraine headaches, Parkinson's disease, and some cases of allergy, HIV disease, and cancer. The safety of chronic oral administration of CoQ10 in doses of 100-300 mg/d is exceedingly well established. Patients with corticosteroid-dependent asthma (n=56) were shown to have significantly lower concentrations of CoQ10 in plasma (0.34 micromol/l) and whole blood (0.33 micromol/l) compared with levels seen in healthy volunteers (0.52 and 0.50 micromol/l, respectively).[202]

  - Clinical trial: CoQ10, alpha-tocopherol, and ascorbic acid: In an open cross-over randomized clinical trial of patients with persistent mild-moderate asthma (n=41; ages 25-50y), daily administration of

[198] Blitz et al. Inhaled magnesium sulfate in the treatment of acute asthma. *Cochrane Database Syst Rev*. 2005 Oct 19;(4):CD003898

[199] Gazdik et al. Decreased consumption of corticosteroids after selenium supplementation in corticoid-dependent asthmatics. *Bratisl Lek Listy*. 2002;103(1):22-5 [Data from Medline abstract]

[200] Hasselmark L, Malmgren R, Zetterström O, Unge G. Selenium supplementation in intrinsic asthma. *Allergy*. 1993 Jan;48(1):30-6

[201] Shaheen et al. Randomised, double blind, placebo-controlled trial of selenium supplementation in adult asthma. *Thorax*. 2007 Jun;62(6):483-90

[202] Gazdík F, Gvozdjáková A, Nádvorníková R, et al. Decreased levels of coenzyme Q(10) in patients with bronchial asthma. *Allergy*. 2002 Sep;57(9):811-4

hydrosoluble CoQ10 120 mg, alpha-tocopherol 400 mg, and vitamin C 250 mg was shown to allow statistically and clinically significant reduction in the required dosage of corticosteroids; however, "Spirometric parameters did not change significantly during the study."[203]

- <u>Vitamin B6 (pyridoxine)</u>: A clear majority of young patients with asthma show endogenous defects in tryptophan metabolism, as evidenced by abnormal elevations in urinary kynurenic acid (KA) and xanthurenic acid (XA) acid following oral tryptophan administration.[204] This defect can be partially corrected by administration of high-dose pyridoxine, leading to clinical benefit.

  - <u>Clinical trial: Pyridoxine 100-200 mg/d in children</u>: The authors of this two-part study first showed that asthmatic patients had elevated urinary xanthurenic and kynurenic acid levels, which were reduced following supplementation 50-100 mg of pyridoxine; clinical benefit was seen in patients receiving pyridoxine 100 mg/d (not 50 mg/d). The second part of the study was a double-blind trial with 76 asthmatic children treated with pyridoxine 200 mg/d for five months; clinical benefits included significant improvement in asthma following pyridoxine therapy and reduction in dosage of bronchodilators and corticosteroids, leading the authors to conclude, "The data suggest that these children with severe bronchial asthma had a metabolic block in tryptophan metabolism, which was benefited by long-term treatment with large doses of pyridoxine."[205]

  - <u>Clinical trial: Pyridoxine 50 mg/d in adults</u>: Fifteen adult asthmatic patients showed lower levels of erythrocyte pyridoxal phosphate (PLP) compared to 16 control patients. Oral supplementation of seven asthmatics with pyridoxine 100 mg/d produced dramatic decreases in frequency and severity of wheezing and asthmatic attacks.[206]

- <u>Vitamin B-12 (hydroxocobalamin)</u>: Vitamin B-12 serves numerous physiologic and pharmacologic roles, and the complexities of absorption, transport, and metabolism subject this nutrient to manifold errors of metabolism as well as pervasive misunderstandings by clinicians. Relevant to the treatment of asthma, vitamin B-12 particularly its hydroxocobalamin form is a nitric oxide scavenger and sulfite chelator. A subset of asthmatic patients are intolerant to sulfite(s) and suffer exacerbations of asthma following sulfite consumption or increased endogenous production; vitamin B-12 can be used to chelate or "detoxify" sulfite and thus ameliorate asthma exacerbations. This clinical benefit to vitamin B-12 supplementation is not reliant upon the patient being vitamin B-12 deficient; thus documentation of low serum vitamin B-12 or elevated methylmalonic acid is unnecessary prior to treatment. Oral vitamin B-12 is exceptionally safe when given orally in doses of 2,000-6,000 mcg/d; fruit-tasting chewable tablets increase compliance among children and adults.

  - <u>Clinical trial: Cyanocobalamin 1,500 mcg prior to metabisulfite challenge</u>: In this small proof-of-principle study, five asthmatic children with metabisulfite intolerance confirmed by oral challenge testing were pretreated with 1.5 mg of oral cyanocobalamin prior to sulfite rechallenge. Following vitamin B-12 administration, four of the five patients were protected from metabisulfite-induced bronchospasm.[207]

- <u>Bioflavonoids</u>: As previously mentioned in the section on diet, increased intake of fruits and vegetables reduces risk and severity of asthma; certainly this occurs by many mechanisms, including ❶ increased intake of vitamin C, ❷ increased intake of magnesium, ❸ systemic alkalinization which promotes renal retention of magnesium and urinary excretion of xenobiotics, ❹ increased intake of phytonutrients and bioflavonoids, most of which have biologically relevant antioxidant and anti-inflammatory action. Given that most botanicals have an alkalinizing effect due to the virtual lack of sodium chloride and the high amounts of potassium, magnesium, and citrate (which is converted to bicarbonate in the body), and given that plants are rich sources of bioflavonoids which as a group have antioxidant and anti-inflammatory properties and respective clinical benefits, clinicians and patients can choose from a wide range of plant-based dietary patterns and plant-derived nutritional supplements. Many standardized concentrated

[203] Gvozdjáková et al. Coenzyme Q10 supplementation reduces corticosteroids dosage in patients with bronchial asthma. *Biofactors*. 2005;25(1-4):235-40
[204] Collipp PJ, Chen SY, Sharma RK, Balachandar V, Maddaiah VT. Tryptophane metabolism in bronchial asthma. *Ann Allergy*. 1975 Sep;35(3):153-8
[205] Collipp PJ, Goldzier S III, Weiss N, et al. Pyridoxine treatment of childhood bronchial asthma. *Ann Allergy* 1975;35:93–7
[206] Reynolds RD, Natta CL. Depressed plasma pyridoxal phosphate concentrations in adult asthmatics. *Am J Clin Nutr* 1985;41:684–8
[207] Añíbarro B, Caballero T, García-Ara C, et al. Asthma with sulfite intolerance in children: a blocking study with cyanocobalamin. *J Allergy Clin Immunol*. 1992 Jul;90:103-9

bioflavonoid products are commercially available as nutritional supplements, and many of the available and popular botanical medicines (e.g., *Ginkgo biloba*) and medical foods (e.g., green tea, honey) owe at least part of their clinical benefit to their flavonoid content. Among the many clinically utilized bioflavonoid products, Pycnogenol is a proprietary mixture of water-soluble bioflavonoids extracted from French maritime pine; the main constituents of

Pycnogenol are phenolic compounds including the monomers catechin, epicatechin, and taxifolin and condensed flavonoids such as procyanidins and proanthocyanidins.

- Clinical trial: Pycnogenol 1 mg/lb/d in two divided doses: A randomized placebo-controlled double-blind trial among patients with mild-to-moderate asthma (n=60; age 6-18y) was conducted for 3 months found that patients receiving Pycnogenol 1 mg/lb/d in two divided doses had significant improvement in pulmonary functions, reductions in asthma symptoms, reduction or discontinuation of rescue inhalers, and reduction of urinary leukotrienes.[208]
- Clinical experience with *Crataegus* tincture or solid extract in the treatment of asthma: "Administration of a tincture of solid extract preparation of *Crataegus spp* to patients with asthma has proven remarkably effective in the clinical setting. ... While Crataegus is a powerful tool in the treatment of asthma, it should not be used alone if complete healing is expected to take place. Basic naturopathic therapies that address nutritional needs, allergies, adrenal function, and immune and liver function should always be considered."[209]

- "Vitamin E": "Vitamin E" intake has shown a protective inverse association with asthma in several epidemiologic studies. Food-sourced "vitamin E" would be expected to provide benefits superior to those obtained from the use of supplemental "vitamin E" when the later contains synthetic or isolated tocopherol isomers, namely DL-tocopherol or D-alpha-tocopherol, respectively, both of which may serve to promote inflammation and/or block intestinal absorption of the more potent anti-inflammatory gamma-tocopherol. Thus, the finding that "Dietary supplementation with vitamin E adds no benefit to current standard treatment in adults with mild to moderate asthma" by Pearson et al[210] in 2007 was not surprising given their use of D-alpha-tocopherol 500 mg (746 IU) per day; had the researchers used mixed tocopherols with a high concentration of gamma-tocopherol, their patients may have benefited.
- Vitamin C: Asthma patients may show a relative insufficiency of vitamin C as measured by serum vitamin C levels. Higher intakes of vitamin C protect against the development and progression of asthma.
  - Randomized, placebo controlled double-blind crossover trial: Ascorbic acid supplementation attenuates exercise-induced bronchoconstriction in patients with asthma: Eight subjects with exercise-induced bronchoconstriction (EIB) entered the study on their usual diet and were placed on either 2 weeks of ascorbic acid supplementation (1500 mg/day) or placebo, followed by a 1-week washout period, before crossing over to the non-supplemented group. "Results: The ascorbic acid diet significantly reduced (p < 0.05) the maximum fall in post-exercise FEV1 (-6.4 +/- 2.4%) compared to usual (-14.3 +/- 1.6%) and placebo diet (-12.9 +/- 2.4%). Asthma symptoms scores significantly improved (p<0.05) on the ascorbic acid diet compared to the placebo and usual diet. Post-exercise FENO, LTC4-E4 and 9alpha, 11beta-PGF2 concentration was significantly lower (p<0.05) on the ascorbic acid diet compared to the placebo and usual diet. CONCLUSION: Ascorbic acid supplementation provides a protective effect against exercise-induced airway narrowing in asthmatic subjects."[211]
  - Placebo-controlled clinical trial: Ascorbic acid lowers histamine and improves neutrophil chemotaxis: Histamine is immunosuppressive, pro-inflammatory, and capable of inducing

[208] Lau BH, Riesen SK, Truong KP, et al. Pycnogenol as an adjunct in the management of childhood asthma. *J Asthma* 2004;41:825–32
[209] Frances D. Crataegus for asthma: case studies. *Journal of Naturopathic Medicine* 1998: 8; 20-24
[210] Pearson PJ, Lewis SA, Britton J, Fogarty A. Vitamin E supplements in asthma: a parallel group randomised placebo controlled trial. *Thorax.* 2004 Aug;59(8):652-6
[211] Tecklenburg et al. Ascorbic acid supplementation attenuates exercise-induced bronchoconstriction in patients with asthma. *Respir Med.* 2007 Aug;101(8):1770-8

bronchoconstriction. Ten subjects ingested a placebo during weeks 1, 2, 5 and 6, and 2 g/day of vitamin C [VC] during weeks 3 and 4. "Plasma ascorbate rose significantly following VC administration compared to baseline and withdrawal values. Neutrophil chemotaxis rose 19% (NS) during VC administration, and fell 30% after VC withdrawal, but these changes were not correlated to plasma ascorbate levels. Chemotaxis was inversely correlated to blood histamine ($r = -0.32$, $p = 0.045$), and, compared to baseline and withdrawal values, histamine levels were depressed 38% following VC supplementation. … These data indicate that VC may indirectly enhance chemotaxis by detoxifying histamine in vivo."[212]

- <u>Iodine, iodide</u>: Iodine is a nonmetal trace element (I_2) which is called iodide (I^{-1}) in the ionic form; clinicians can recall this difference in nomenclature by remembering that the elemental form of ends with "N" as in *iodine* and *natural*, whereas the ionic form in which the iodine atoms have been separated has a "D" as in *iodide* and *divided*. Both iodine and iodide can be consumed by humans, and some experts state that optimal intake of this nutrient should include both the diatomic iodine and the ionic iodide; because of this, and because of the interconversion between the diatomic and ionic forms the conjugate "iodine-iodide" will be used here while "iodide" will be used when this form is specifically cited, as it tends to be the more commonly discussed and biologically active form of this nutrient and element. Iodide has a wide range of biologic effects beyond functioning as a requisite component of thyroxine and triiodothyronine; iodide affects gene expression, hormone receptor activity, hormone metabolism, mucus viscosity, microbial survival (directly through microbicidal action and indirectly through enhanced antimicrobial effectiveness of the phagocytic respiratory burst), and oxidant-antioxidant balance. Iodide can function as an antioxidant because it is a reducing agent that can neutralize reactive oxygen species such as hydrogen peroxide via the formation of iodo-compounds. The antioxidant biochemical mechanism of iodides[213] is probably one of the most ancient mechanisms of defense from poisonous reactive oxygen species, used by blue-green algae for more than three billion years: (Iodo-Compounds* include iodo-tyrosine/histidine/lipids/carbons.)

$$2\ I^- + Peroxidase + H_2O_2 + Tyro/Hist/Lipid/Carbons \rightarrow Iodo\text{-}Compounds^* + H_2O + 2\ e^- \text{(antioxidants)}$$

An increasing number of clinicians are using combination iodine-iodide products either in liquid or tablet form to provide approximately 12 mg/d—this is consistent with the average daily intake of iodine-iodide countries such as Japan with a high intake of seafood. Adverse effects for which to monitor include biochemical thyroid dysfunction, goiter, and acneiform skin lesions. Clinical data on the use of iodine/iodide against asthma is limited, even though it was a popular treatment among clinicians prior to onslaught of new drugs and the powerful marketing campaigns that accompanied them. Formulations of iodine/iodide are natural, nonpatentable, and of comparatively low profit for manufacturers compared to patented drugs and delivery systems.

- <u>Letter and report of clinical experience: Iodides in bronchial asthma (*J Allergy Clin Immunol* 1981 Jun[214])</u>: Whether administered orally or intravenously, "the iodides appeared in the saliva in about 5 to 10 minutes and in the bronchial secretions within 15 to 30 minutes. The increased salivation by these patients seemed to us to increase the probability that the iodide in adequate amounts can be effective expectorants because they are eliminated by the bronchial mucosa. Their usefulness for this purpose can be attested to by many physicians including myself who have used this drug in the treatment of asthma for many years."
- <u>Controlled study of iodotherapy for childhood asthma (*J Allergy* 1966 Sep[215])</u>: Patients received KI—potassium iodide—in doses of "900 and 300 mg daily." "…in the population as a whole, asthmatic symptoms were improved by KI particularly at the high dose level." The authors estimate that 64% of patients benefited from iodide supplementation.

- **Hormonal modulation**: The "Orthoendocrinology" protocol detailed in Chapter 4.6 can be reasonably employed in any patient with chronic inflammatory disease—this includes allergy and autoimmunity. In

---

[212] Johnston CS, Martin LJ, Cai X. Antihistamine effect of supplemental ascorbic acid and neutrophil chemotaxis. *J Am Coll Nutr* 1992 Apr;11(2):172-6

[213] wikipedia.org/wiki/Iodide Accessed June 29, 2009

[214] Tuft L. Iodides in bronchial asthma. *J Allergy Clin Immunol*. 1981 Jun;67(6):497

[215] Falliers CJ, McCann WP, Chai H, Ellis EF, Yazdi N. Controlled study of iodotherapy for childhood asthma. *J Allergy*. 1966 Sep;38(3):183-92

summary, serum measurement of prolactin, DHEA, cortisol, testosterone (free and total), and estradiol is performed and any abnormalities are corrected. With specific regard to allergy and asthma, DHEA has clearly received the most attention and literature support as a safe and effective intervention. Women with menstrual exacerbations of asthma may benefit from administration of progesterone either orally, by injection, or over-the-counter in transdermal preparations; progesterone has immune-modulating effects, is a precursor to cortisol, and has anti-estrogen benefits.

- Low serum dehydroepiandrosterone sulfate concentration is an indicator of adrenocortical suppression in asthmatic children treated with inhaled steroids: "In conclusion, inhaled steroid treatment suppresses dehydroepiandrosterone sulfate production in a dose-dependent manner. Monitoring of serum dehydroepiandrosterone sulfate concentrations can be used as a practical method to follow adrenocortical function and to detect its suppression during inhaled steroid treatment in children."[216] One of the important practical implications of this study is that it supports the use of serum DHEA-sulfate testing as a means for monitoring adrenal function. The ideal test for measuring adrenal reserve is the assay of serum cortisol before and after an injection of ACTH; however this test requires ACTH prescription (not available to all clinicians), ACTH injection (ACTH is often difficult to procure, and injections are poorly tolerated by many patients, especially children), and two phlebotomies for serum cortisol measurement. The simple measurement of serum DHEA-sulfate may suffice for an expedient quantification of adrenal function.

- Effects of dehydroepiandrosterone on Th2 cytokine production in peripheral blood mononuclear cells from asthmatics: "CONCLUSIONS: DHEA suppressed both Th1 and Th2 responses, with a Th1 bias, and the degree of suppression was associated with the severity of AHR [airway hyperresponsiveness] or atopy. Therefore, DHEA may be a useful therapy for asthma."[217]

- Clinical experience with low-dose DHEA in asthmatics: "I have seen two female patients with long-standing asthma who had clinical improvement after receiving 10 mg/day of DHEA. In one of these patients, chronic nasal polyps also disappeared, much to the surprise of her otolaryngologist."[218]

- Case reports: Severe premenstrual asthma alleviated with intramuscular progesterone: "Three patients with severe premenstrual exacerbations of asthma are reported. None had responded to conventional treatment, including high-dose corticosteroids. In all cases there was a striking fall premenstrually in peak flow rate. The addition of intramuscular progesterone (100 mg daily in two cases and 600 mg twice a week in one) to the regimen eliminated the premenstrual dips in peak flow, and daily doses of prednisolone were reduced in the three patients."[219]

- **Physical medicine and manipulation**: Essentially all clinical trials of manipulative therapy have shown benefit in subjective and/or objective markers of respiration. The two main problems seen in this research are ❶ the near-impossibility of having an adequate control group, and ❷ the political manipulation of the conclusions by medical journals that have a strong history of bias against natural and non-drug and non-surgical treatments. With regard to the former of these two problems, for obvious reasons clinicians should appreciate the difficulty in conducting a placebo-controlled study with manipulation, particularly if that "placebo" involves physical contact or any soft-tissue manipulation.

  - Review: Research pitfalls and manual medicine diversity versus the emerging medical paradigm (J Am Osteopath Assoc. 2001 Aug[220]): "Recent studies published in leading medical journals have concluded that chiropractic treatment is not particularly helpful for relieving asthma and migraine symptoms because even though study participants showed notable improvement in symptoms, those subjects who received sham manual medicine treatments also showed improvement. Yet the sham treatment received by control groups in these studies is reminiscent in many ways of traditional osteopathic manipulation. This seems to represent not only a failure to recognize the value of many manual medicine techniques but also an ignorance of the broad spectrum of manual medicine techniques used by various practitioners, from osteopathic physicians to chiropractors to physical therapists. Such blind spots compromise research

[216] Kannisto S, Korppi M, Remes K, Voutilainen R. Serum dehydroepiandrosterone sulfate concentration as an indicator of adrenocortical suppression in asthmatic children treated with inhaled steroids. *J Clin Endocrinol Metab.* 2001 Oct;86(10):4908-12

[217] Choi et al. Effects of dehydroepiandrosterone on Th2 cytokine production in peripheral blood mononuclear cells from asthmatics. *Korean J Intern Med.* 2008 Dec;23(4):176-81

[218] Gaby AR. Dehydroepiandrosterone: Biological Effects and Clinical Significance. *Alt Med Rev* 1996;1(2):60-69

[219] Beynon HL, Garbett ND, Barnes PJ. Severe premenstrual exacerbations of asthma: effect of intramuscular progesterone. *Lancet.* 1988 Aug 13;2(8607):370-2

[220] Mein EA, et al. Manual medicine diversity: research pitfalls and the emerging medical paradigm. *J Am Osteopath Assoc.* 2001 Aug;101(8):441-4

methodology with regard to manual medicine studies, which could, in turn, diminish the role of manual medicine in clinical practice."

- Cochrane review: Manual therapy for asthma (*Cochrane Database Syst Rev* 2005 Apr[221]): "AUTHORS' CONCLUSIONS: There is insufficient evidence to support the use of manual therapies for patients with asthma. There is a need to conduct adequately-sized RCTs that examine the effects of manual therapies on clinically relevant outcomes. Future trials should maintain observer blinding for outcome assessments, and report on the costs of care and adverse events. Currently, there is insufficient evidence to support or refute the use of manual therapy for patients with asthma."

- Randomized controlled trial: Effects of osteopathic manipulative treatment (OMT) on pediatric patients with asthma (*J Am Osteopath Assoc* 2005 Jan[222]): "The authors conducted a randomized controlled trial attempting to demonstrate the therapeutic relevance of OMT in the pediatric asthma population. With a confidence level of 95%, results for the OMT group showed a statistically significant improvement of 7 L per minute to 9 L per minute for peak expiratory flow rates. These results suggest that OMT has a therapeutic effect among this patient population."

- Clinical trial: Quantifiable effects of osteopathic manipulative techniques on patients with chronic asthma (*J Am Osteopath Assoc* 2002 Jul[223]): "Measurements of both upper thoracic and lower thoracic forced respiratory excursion statistically increased after osteopathic manipulative procedures compared with sham procedures. Changes in peak expiratory flow rates and asthma symptoms were not statistically significant."

- Spinal manipulative therapy (SMT) is not simply a physical intervention (*J Manipulative Physiol Ther* 2001 Jul[224]): "CONCLUSION: After 3 months of combining chiropractic SMT with optimal medical management for pediatric asthma, the children rated their quality of life substantially higher and their asthma severity substantially lower. These improvements were maintained at the 1-year follow-up assessment. There were no important changes in lung function or hyperresponsiveness at any time. The observed improvements are unlikely as a result of the specific effects of chiropractic SMT alone, but other aspects of the clinical encounter that should not be dismissed readily."

- *New England Journal of Medicine* contradicts positive results with negative conclusions in study of chiropractic manipulation in the treatment of asthma (*N Engl J Med* 1998 Oct[225]): "RESULTS: Eighty children (38 in the active-treatment group and 42 in the simulated-treatment group) had outcome data that could be evaluated. There were small increases (7 to 12 liters per minute) in peak expiratory flow in the morning and the evening in both treatment groups, with no significant differences between the groups in the degree of change from base line (morning peak expiratory flow, P=0.49 at two months and P=0.82 at four months). Symptoms of asthma and use of 3-agonists decreased and the quality of life increased in both groups, with no significant differences between the groups. There were no significant changes in spirometric measurements or airway responsiveness. CONCLUSIONS: In children with mild or moderate asthma, the addition of chiropractic spinal manipulation to usual medical care provided no benefit."

- An osteopathic approach to asthma (*J Am Osteopath Assoc* 1999 May[226]): "Five areas involving asthma management are reviewed and involve a failure to do the following: (1) identify disease instability and progression; (2) adopt an optimal pharmacologic treatment plan; (3) identify and help the patient avoid

---

An osteopathic approach to asthma

"Five areas involving asthma management are reviewed and involve a failure to do the following:
1. Identify disease instability and progression;
2. Adopt an optimal pharmacologic treatment plan;
3. Identify and help the patient avoid environmental triggers;
4. Evaluate and treat certain disruptive psychodynamic issues; and
5. Use essential non-pharmacologic modes of therapy such as osteopathic manipulation, nutritional considerations, physical training, and controlled breathing techniques that may help to favorably modify the asthma disease process."

Rowane et al. An osteopathic approach to asthma. *J Am Osteopath Assoc.* 1999 May

---

[221] Hondras MA, Linde K, Jones AP. Manual therapy for asthma. *Cochrane Database Syst Rev.* 2005 Apr 18;(2):CD001002
[222] Guiney PA, et al. Effects of osteopathic manipulative treatment on pediatric patients with asthma: a randomized controlled trial. *J Am Osteopath Assoc.* 2005 Jan;105(1):7-12
[223] Bockenhauer et al. Quantifiable effects of osteopathic manipulative techniques on patients with chronic asthma. *J Am Osteopath Assoc.* 2002 Jul;102(7):371-5
[224] Bronfort G, et al. Chronic pediatric asthma and chiropractic spinal manipulation. *J Manipulative Physiol Ther.* 2001 Jul-Aug;24(6):369-77
[225] Balon J, et al. A comparison of active and simulated chiropractic manipulation as adjunctive treatment for childhood asthma. *N Engl J Med.* 1998 Oct 8;339(15):1013-20
[226] Rowane WA, Rowane MP. An osteopathic approach to asthma. *J Am Osteopath Assoc.* 1999 May;99(5):259-64

environmental triggers; (4) evaluate and treat certain disruptive psychodynamic issues; and (5) use essential non-pharmacologic modes of therapy such as osteopathic manipulation, nutritional considerations, physical training, and controlled breathing techniques that may help to favorably modify the asthma disease process."

- Randomized clinical trial: Chronic asthma and chiropractic spinal manipulation (*Clin Exp Allergy* 1995 Jan[227]): "Using the cross-over analysis, no clinically important or statistically significant differences were found between the active and sham chiropractic interventions on any of the main or secondary outcome measures. Objective lung function did not change during the study, but over the course of the study, non-specific bronchial hyperreactivity (n-BR) improved by 36% (P = 0.01) and patient-rated asthma severity decreased by 34% (P = 0.0002) compared with the baseline values."

- **Environmental interventions**: Beyond dietary allergen avoidance, the patient's residential, occupational, and recreational environments can be remediated to effect a reduction in immunogen exposure; effective reduction in immunogen exposure leads to pathologic and clinical improvements in asthma patients. Attention to the patient's sleeping area is particularly important and commonly overlooked; this is an area where patients spend 8-10 hours each night, and allergen exposure here can have effects throughout the day.
  - Use allergen/pollen-reducing air filters; change them on a regular basis each 1-2 months.
  - Replace old pillows and mattress with nonallergenic varieties, or have the older pillows/mattress covered with an allergen barrier, such as a vinyl enclosure.
  - Remediate or ventilate any mold-prone areas in the bathroom, kitchen, basement, attic, walls, or utility area. Use portable HEPA filtration machines in rooms where the patient spends prolonged periods of time.
  - Strongly consider removing/replacing the old carpet and pad, which might be permeated with allergens, antigens, dust mites, animal dander, etc. Hardwood, cement, laminate, or bamboo floors are much easier to keep clean of allergens/antigens than is carpet.
  - Clothes and linens can be machine washed with a detergent solution containing eucalyptus oil to eliminate dust mites. The combination of 1) hot water, 2) detergent, and 3) eucalyptus oil is an effective and method to kill dust mites and remove additional allergens. As validated by research published in *Journal of Allergy and Clinical Immunology*[228], this is an effective technique for killing and eliminating dust mites from clothing and bed sheets. Suitable detergents include "Bi-O-Klean Hand Dishwashing Liquid" or "Kit liquid dishwashing detergent concentrate" since they meet the criteria for the selection of a detergent for this purpose. 1) When mixed, the oil-detergent mixture should dissolve to form a clear homogenous solution, and 2) five mL (1 teaspoon) of the mixture stirred with 200 mL (6 oz.) of water should form a "milky, opaque solution that is stable (does not "break oil") for at least 10 minutes." Eucalyptus oil should not be applied to the skin or taken internally.
  - Use of a dehumidifier and adequate moisture ventilation can be important for homes/rooms that accumulate moisture. The steam from bathing and cooking areas should be vented outdoors so that moisture does not accumulate inside the living area. Moisture is necessary for dust mites to live and to create allergens; if the air is very moist then the allergy-producing activities of the dust mites are stimulated. Conversely, by reducing the humidity in the air, we are able to impair the dust mites and thus reduce the amount of dust mite feces—this is an important allergen for many asthmatics. In some instances, reducing the amount of moisture in the air by use of an electric dehumidifier may be necessary to help reduce the amount of both dust allergen and mold in a home.

- **Avoidance of aspirin and inhibitors of cyclooxygenase**: Inhibition of cyclooxygenase shunts free arachidonate into leukotriene formation via 5-lipoxygenase, thereby exacerbating the leukotriene-mediated inflammation of asthma.

- **Treatment of chronic sinusitis—See Chapter 4.2 subsection on sinorespiratory dysbiosis**: Chronic sinusitis exacerbates asthma by direct and indirect mechanism; the direct mechanism is the irritation of the respiratory pathway via post-nasal drip of inflammatory and antigenic secretions, while the indirect mechanism is the contribution to systemic inflammation. Treatment of chronic sinusitis effectively alleviates asthma for many patients; not surprisingly, most research studies have used pharmaceutical antibacterial drugs for this purpose.

---

[227] Nielsen et al. Chronic asthma and chiropractic spinal manipulation: a randomized clinical trial. *Clin Exp Allergy*. 1995 Jan;25(1):80-8
[228] Tovey ER, McDonald LG. A simple washing procedure with eucalyptus oil for controlling house dust mites and their allergens in clothing and bedding. *J Allergy Clin Immunol*. 1997 Oct;100(4):464-6

Clinically, the use of once-twice daily nasal lavage is very effective for the treatment of chronic sinusitis; the solution is 1 cup warm *sterile* water salinated with 0.5-1 teaspoon sodium chloride with 0.5 teaspoon baking soda administered via the nostrils by way of a bulb syringe or neti pot. Patient selection is relevant to prevent choking or aspiration; the procedure is awkward at first but becomes much more acceptable with practice. Nasal-sinus lavage is reviewed in Chapter 4 in Section 2, in the subsection on sinorespiratory dysbiosis.

- Clinical trial: Concomitant chronic sinusitis treatment in children with mild asthma: the effect on bronchial hyperresponsiveness (*Chest* 2003 Mar[229]): Among 61 children with mild asthma and allergic rhinitis, 41 were found to have chronic bacterial sinusitis, too—this finding stresses the importance of doctors' continual searching for and refining the details of their patient assessment. The treatment group received amoxicillin-clavulanate for 6 weeks and then with nasal saline solution irrigation for 6 weeks. Clinical improvement included the following: "After aggressive treatment for sinusitis, it was found that the provocative concentration of methacholine causing a 20% fall in FEV(1) of children with mild asthma and sinusitis was significantly higher after treatment. CONCLUSION: The results suggest that every asthmatic patient needs to [be] carefully evaluate[d] to determine whether the patient has concomitant sinusitis. Respiratory infections that meet criteria for sinusitis, even if they do not exacerbate asthma, should be treated. It is suggested that sinusitis should always be kept in mind as a possible inducible factor for BHR [bronchial hyperresponsiveness], and that aggressive treatment of chronic sinusitis is indicated when dealing with an asthmatic patient who shows an unpredictable response to appropriate treatment. Moreover, the findings of this study provide more evidence for an association between sinusitis and asthma with respect to BHR."

- Clinical trial: Improvement of clinical and immunopathologic parameters in asthmatic children treated for concomitant chronic rhinosinusitis (*Ann Allergy Asthma Immunol* 1997 Jul[230]): Eighteen children with moderate asthma (ages 5-12y) who were poorly controlled by high doses of inhaled corticosteroids and who also had chronic rhinosinusitis were treated with a combination of amoxicillin and clavulanate (20 mg/kg twice daily) and fluticasone propionate aqueous nasal spray (100 microg/d) for 14 days. A short course of oral corticosteroids was also prescribed (deflazacort, 1 mg/kg daily for 2 days, 0.5 mg/kg daily for 4 days, and 0.25 mg/kg daily for 4 days). "RESULTS: A negative endoscopy result was demonstrated in 15 children after treatment. Symptoms and respiratory function significantly improved after treatment and 1 month later; 8 children had intermittent asthma and 10 had mild asthma. A significant reduction of inflammatory cell numbers was detected in all asthmatic children. Interleukin 4 levels significantly decreased (P < 0.001), whereas interferon-y levels increased (P < 0.001)—[This latter finding indicates a shift from Th-2 to a Th-1 pattern of inflammation.]. CONCLUSION: Treatment of chronic rhinosinusitis is able to improve symptoms and respiratory function in asthmatic children, reducing inflammatory cells and reversing the cytokine pattern from a Th2 toward a Th1 profile."

- Clinical trial: Improvement of bronchial hyperresponsiveness in asthmatic children treated for concomitant sinusitis (*Ann Allergy Asthma Immunol* 1997 Jul[231]): This open label, randomized trial in forty-six atopic and 20 normal children used 30 days of treatment with nasal saline, sulfamethoxazole-trimethoprim, antihistamine/decongestant, and five days of prednisone. "RESULTS: The only patients with increase in methacholine PC20 were patients with rhinitis and asthma with opacified maxillary sinuses at entry and who at 30 days had normal sinus radiographs (P < .05). CONCLUSION: In this study, children with allergic rhinitis and sinusitis with asthma improved their bronchial hyperresponsiveness to methacholine and decreased their symptoms with appropriate response of their sinuses to clinical therapy." In sum, this study showed that asthmatic patients with occult sinusitis achieved clinical benefit—improved lung function—following resolution of the sinusitis with the 30-day use of nasal saline, oral antibiotics, antihistamine/decongestant, and five days of prednisone.

- **Psychosocial interventions**: Stress reduction, relationship optimization, resolution of past hurts and dysfunctional relationships should be included in any *truly* holistic healthcare plan for any condition, and of course this includes asthma.

---

[229] Tsao et al. Concomitant chronic sinusitis treatment in children with mild asthma: the effect on bronchial hyperresponsiveness. *Chest.* 2003 Mar;123(3):757-64
[230] Tosca et al. Improvement of clinical and immunopathologic parameters in asthmatic children treated for concomitant chronic rhinosinusitis. *Ann Allergy Asthma Immunol.* 2003 Jul;91(1):71-8
[231] Oliveira et al. Improvement of bronchial hyperresponsiveness in asthmatic children treated for concomitant sinusitis. *Ann Allergy Asthma Immunol.* 1997 Jul;79(1):70-4

- Clinical trial—Humorous movie (*Physiol Behav* 2004 Jun[232]): In this cross-over placebo-controlled trial of asthmatic patients (asthma n=35; control n=35) who were sensitive to either house dust mite (n=20) or epigallocatechin gallate (EGCg) (n=15), reduced bronchial responsiveness was noted among the asthmatic patients but not the control patients following watching a humorous movie. The author concluded, "Viewing a humorous film significantly reduced bronchial responsiveness to methacholine or EGCg, while viewing a nonhumorous film failed to do so in [asthma] patients…. These findings indicate that viewing a humorous film may be useful in the treatment and study of BA [bronchial asthma]." This study was published in 2004; the humorous film used was "Modern Times" featuring Charlie Chaplin released in 1936.
- Systematic review of psychological interventions for children with asthma (*Pediatr Pulmonol* 2007 Feb[233]): "Twelve studies, involving 588 children, were included in the review; however, study quality was poor and sample sizes were frequently small. A meta-analysis was performed on two studies, examining the effects of relaxation therapy on PEFR which favored the treatment group (SD 0.82, CI 0.41-1.24). ... This review was unable to draw firm conclusions for the role of psychological interventions for children with asthma. ... The absence of an adequate evidence base is demonstrated, highlighting the need for well-conducted RCTs in this area."

---

[232] Kimata H. Effect of viewing a humorous vs. nonhumorous film on bronchial responsiveness in patients with bronchial asthma. *Physiol Behav*. 2004;81(4):681-4
[233] Yorke et al. A systematic review of psychological interventions for children with asthma. *Pediatr Pulmonol*. 2007 Feb;42(2):114-24

Rheumatoid Arthritis, RA

Introduction:

Rheumatoid arthritis (RA) is one of the most common and "most classic" systemic autoimmune diseases. Despite its name, RA affects much more than the musculoskeletal system: rheumatoid lung, rheumatoid kidney disease, and other systemic, vasculitic, and (sub)cutaneous complications are not uncommon. Readers should begin to recognize the "patterns of inflammation" that result in distinct diagnostic labels are simply "variations on a theme" based on a finite number of identifiable and modifiable factors, which are largely amenable to nonpharmacologic interventions.

   Rheumatoid arthritis and psoriasis are very similar conditions—different patterns of inflammation—and these conditions and their respective assessments and treatments should be viewed as prototypical for other conditions; as such, and especially considering that these conditions are very common in clinical practice, a reasonable assumption will be made that readers will have studied these sections so that some facts and concepts will not have to be unnecessarily repeated throughout the book for each condition that follows a similar pattern of pathogenesis and resolution.

Description/pathophysiology:

- Description in a nutshell: RA is a relatively common, persistent, symmetric, destructive, systemic inflammatory "autoimmune" disease chiefly characterized by peripheral arthritis but which may also affect the proximal joints (e.g., hips and shoulders), the axial skeleton (e.g., spine—notably the atlantoaxial joint—as well as the sacroiliac joints), and internal organs (e.g., "rheumatoid lung") and vascular system (e.g., rheumatoid vasculitis).

- Basic pathology: A pathogenic hallmark of the disease is immune complex formation and intra-articular deposition with resultant release of cytokines and other pro-inflammatory mediators. Immune complexes are important instigators of rheumatoid arthritis and vasculitis, and rheumatoid factor (RF) antibodies are important contributors to these immune complexes.[1,2] The chronic/sustained inflammation leads to synovial thickening, villous hypertrophy (pannus formation), and intraarticular colonization with activated lymphocytes and plasma cells. The localized immunocytes cause inflammation and tissue destruction via elaboration of matrix metalloproteinases (including collagenases), prostaglandins, and cytokines such as IL-1.

- Prevalence: Affects 0.8-1% of all populations: considered the second most common rheumatic diagnosis[3] after "osteoarthritis", many cases of which are actually genetic hemochromatosis, one of the most common hereditary conditions in humans (heterozygote frequency: 1:7; homozygote frequency 1:200-250).
  - Musculoskeletal disorders and iron overload disease (*Arthritis Rheum* 1996 Oct[4]—full text provided within this textbook): "Arthropathy affects up to 80% of iron-overloaded patients and is often the only manifestation of the disease. ... Thus, since iron overload affects such a large portion of the population and arthropathy is a common manifestation of this disorder, patients with musculoskeletal symptoms should be screened for iron overload."

- Introduction to standard allopathic medical perspective and treatment: From the allopathic perspective, RA is seen as a chronic "idiopathic" inflammatory disorder primarily affecting the peripheral joints but also affecting the axial skeleton and internal organs; it is generally treated with NSAIDs and other "anti-inflammatory" and immunosuppressive drugs, which are palliative and have no chance of providing cure. The standard sequential protocol is as follows: NAIDs and acetaminophen, prednisone, methotrexate, (perhaps sulfasalazine and hydroxychloroquine), then—ever more commonly prescribed—the "biologics", which may be followed by newer experimental and immunoparalytic drugs; this routine protocol has value in the acute suppression of inflammation, but it is notoriously expensive, wrought with adverse effects, and ineffective for the authentic treatment of rheumatoid arthritis, as noted in the landmark 2012 article cited here:
  - Sustained rheumatoid arthritis remission is uncommon in *medical* practice (*Arthritis Res Ther* 2012 Mar[5]): "This study shows that in clinical practice, a minority of RA patients are in sustained remission. ... Other studies have described sustained remission in daily practice as uncommon, being reached by only

[1] Beers MH, Berkow R (eds). *Merck Manual. 17th Edition*. Whitehouse Station; Merck Research Laboratories: 1999, page 416
[2] Jonsson T, Valdimarsson H. What about IgA rheumatoid factor in rheumatoid arthritis? *Ann Rheum Dis*. 1998 Jan;57(1):63-4 ard.bmjjournals.com/cgi/content/full/57/1/63
[3] Hardin JG, Waterman J, Labson LH. Rheumatic disease: Which diagnostic tests are useful? *Patient Care* 1999; March 15: 83-102
[4] Vasquez A. Musculoskeletal disorders and iron overload disease: comment on the American College of Rheumatology guidelines for the initial evaluation of the adult patient with acute musculoskeletal symptoms. *Arthritis Rheum*. 1996 Oct;39(10):1767-8. See full-text at ichnfm.academia.edu/AlexVasquez
[5] Prince et al. Sustained rheumatoid arthritis remission is uncommon in clinical practice. *Arthritis Res Ther*. 2012 Mar 19;14(2):R68 arthritis-research.com/content/14/2/R68

17% to 36% of RA patients for up to 6 months. These studies did not evaluate time in remission beyond 6 months. A recent study investigated the probability of remaining in remission up to 24 months, according to the ACR/EULAR, SDAI, and CDAI remission criteria in two different cohorts. They also concluded that long-term remission is rare, considering that probability of a remission lasting 2 years was 6-14%." Despite the constant barrage of new drugs, shiny brochures, polished advertisments, and self-agrandizing announcements of "progress", medical drug-based treatment of autoimmunity is impressively ineffective for long-term management and generally makes zero attempt to accomplish cure of these medically-proclaimed "incurable" conditions. Medical practice has largely been co-opted by the pharmaceutical sales model; most doctors these days do not look for authentic solutions to complex problems, and they have been convinced that "medical management" (i.e., diagnosis and testing followed by long-term medicalization and polypharmacy) is the epitome and axiom of medical practice.[6]

- <u>Introduction to naturopathic medicine and functional medicine perspective and treatment</u>: From the perspective of naturopathic medicine and functional medicine, the condition is considered highly amenable to treatment provided that such treatment is multifaceted and addresses the allergic, dysbiotic, nutritional, mitochondrial, endocrinologic, and immunophenotypic components of this multifaceted phenomenon.
- <u>Etiological considerations include</u>:
  - <u>Genetic predisposition and HLA-DR</u>: HLA-DR4 is positive in 70% of RA patients, compared to 28% of control patients. "Genetic risk factors do not fully account for the incidence of RA, suggesting that environmental factors also play a role in the etiology of the disease. ...[C]limate and urbanization have a major impact on the incidence and severity of RA in groups of similar genetic background."[7]
  - <u>Urbanization / Western lifestyle</u>: Urbanization is a risk factor for the development of rheumatic disease.[8,9] Urbanization is associated with increased risk of vitamin D deficiency and increased exposure to nutritionally-depleted multiallergenic genetically-modified AGE-laden phytonutrient-deficient prohyperglycemic "convenience foods", sleep disturbances, and exposure to particulate debris (i.e., pollution from diesel and other petrochemical combustion); each of these factors has been shown in animal models or human trials to promote systemic inflammation.
  - <u>Female gender / estrogen</u>: Women are affected 2-3x more often than men. Male RA patients tend to have relative reductions in DHEA and testosterone and relative excess of estrogen and prolactin. Predisposing factors for women include vitamin D deficiency, higher prolactin and estrogen/dysestrogenism (pro-inflammatory) with "relative insufficiency" of testosterone (anti-inflammatory), and the anatomically shorter urethra which predisposes the female urinary tract to recurrent microbial colonization.
  - <u>Tobacco/cigarette smoke</u>: Habitual tobacco/cigarette smoking increases exposure to reactive oxygen species, vasoactive/vasoconstrictive substances, carcinogens, and bacterial endotoxin. Tobacco leaves are noted for their high surface area which—unfortunately for smokers—serves as a deposition reservoir for both ambient radioactive particles[10,11] as well as Gram-negative bacteria, Gram-positive bacteria, and fungi[12]; thereby, tobacco smoking increases exposure to radioactive particles as well as microbial debris (e.g., endotoxin, exotoxin, and bacterial DNA). Thus, the finding that tobacco smoking—particularly from cigarette smoke which is inhaled deeply into the lungs in contrast with cigar smoke which is generally inhaled only into the mouth and pharynx—is a major risk factor for the development of

---

[6] Ely et al. Analysis of questions asked by family doctors regarding patient care. *BMJ*. 1999 Aug 7;319(7206):358-61

[7] Fauci AS, Braunwald E, Isselbacher KJ, et al., eds. *Harrison's Principles of Internal Medicine. 14th Ed*. New York, NY: McGraw-Hill; 1998, page 1881

[8] "In particular, a significantly lower prevalence of RA in rural areas compared with urban cohorts has led to the hypothesis that environmental factors associated with urbanization may be involved in disease pathogenesis." Adebajo A, Davis P. Rheumatic diseases in African blacks. *Semin Arthritis Rheum*. 1994 Oct;24(2):139-53

[9] "The general impression is that rheumatoid arthritis (RA) has a lower prevalence and a milder course in developing countries. Epidemiological studies from different regions show that varying prevalence is possibly related to urbanization." Kalla et al. Rheumatoid arthritis in the developing world. *Best Pract Res Clin Rheumatol*. 2003 Oct;17(5):863-75

[10] "Tobacco leaves are large and have sticky exudates that retain the radon decay products once they deposit on the leaves." Savidou A, Kehagia K, Eleftheriadis K. Concentration levels of 210Pb and 210Po in dry tobacco leaves in Greece. *J Environ Radioact*. 2006;85(1):94-102

[11] "Leaf tobacco contains minute amounts of lead 210 (210Pb) and polonium 210 (210Po), both of which are radioactive carcinogens and both of which can be found in smoke from burning tobacco. Tobacco smoke also contains carcinogens that are nonradioactive. People who inhale tobacco smoke are exposed to higher concentrations of radioactivity than nonsmokers. Deposits of 210Pb and alpha particle-emitting 210Po form in the lungs of smokers, generating localized radiation doses far greater than the radiation exposures humans experience from natural sources. This radiation exposure, delivered to sensitive tissues for long periods of time, may induce cancer both alone and synergistically with nonradioactive carcinogens." Kilthau GF. Cancer risk in relation to radioactivity in tobacco. *Radiol Technol*. 1996 Jan-Feb;67(3):217-22

[12] "Cured tobacco in diverse types of cigarettes is known to harbor a plethora of bacteria (Gram-positive and Gram-negative), fungi (mold, yeast), spores, and is rich in endotoxin (lipopolysaccharide). Reviewed herein are recent observations of the authors' team and other investigators that support the hypothesis that lung inflammation of long-term smokers may be attributed in part to tobacco-associated bacterial and fungal components that have been identified in tobacco and tobacco smoke." Pauly et al. Review: Is lung inflammation associated with microbes and microbial toxins in cigarette tobacco smoke? *Immunol Res*. 2010 Mar;46(1-3):127-36

rheumatoid arthritis and other systemic inflammatory/autoimmune/autoinflammatory disorders is consistent with the microbial/dysbiotic model discussed later in this section.

- Cigarette smoking and inflammation (*J Dent Res* 2012 Feb[13]): "**CS [cigarette smoking] impairs innate defenses against pathogens, modulates antigen presentation, and promotes autoimmunity.** ... Potential mechanisms by which CS promotes rheumatoid arthritis include the release of intracellular proteins from ROS-activated or injured cells, augmentation of auto-reactive B-cell function, altered presentation of antigens by CS-impaired antigen-presenting cells, altered regulatory T-cell functions, and T-cell activation by antigens found in CS." Additionally, tobacco use can alter the oral microbiome and/or promote gingivitis which promotes microbial translocation; the oxidative stress of smoked tobacco promotes nutrient deficiency via oxidative destruction/utilization of immunomodulating nutrients such as ascorbate and tocopherols.

o Occult viral, bacterial or parasitic infections/colonizations are common in autoimmune diseases:

- Viral: **Cytomegalovirus and rubella viruses have been cultured from the synovium in patients with rheumatoid arthritis.** "...some viral diseases, such as parvovirus, chronic hepatitis B virus and hepatitis C virus infections, can produce long-lasting rheumatic symptoms. ... Some evidence suggests hepatitis C virus as a possible trigger to rheumatoid arthritis."[14] The implications of this data are not perfectly clear; however, possibilities (which may coexist) include: 1) virus *directly* provoking joint destruction, 2) virus *indirectly* provoking joint destruction, such as via immune complexes, 3) noncausal, coincidental finding, 4) inability of RA patients to clear this infection due to immunologic deficits which accompany immune dysfunction. Remember, "Unhealthy people are unhealthy" which is to say that they generally demonstrate multiple abnormalities in addition to their index disease, and an *associated* abnormality does not imply a *causal* relationship. Sick people—those who are metabolically/immunologically impaired—tend to enter vicious cycles that can amplify the original illness and lead to the genesis of new, additive health problems. Additionally, given that nutritional deficiencies—pandemic in the general population and even more common in patients with chronic illness (due to malabsorption, hypermetabolism of immune activation, and nutrient losses and malabsorption due to pharmaceutical drugs, etc)—promote viral mutagenesis and replication, the possibility exists that enhanced viral replication in patients with RA/autoimmunity is a surrogate marker for nutritional deficiency; relatedly, enhanced viral replication might be a surrogate marker for enhanced activity of the NFkB pathway, which is upregulated in inflammatory responses and which promotes viral replication. More likely from this author's perspective is the probability that increased viral replication/presence is—regardless of primary etiology—a likely contributor to the total microbial load (TML) and total inflammatory/antigenic load (TIL, TAL) that perpetuates chronic/sustained immune activation and which thus drives systemic inflammation and the clinical manifestation of autoimmunity.

- Bacterial (specific species and generalized SIBO—small intestine bacterial overgrowth): RA is associated with gastrointestinal and genitourinary colonization with *Proteus mirabilis.*[15,16] Approximately 40% of patients with rheumatoid arthritis have bacterial overgrowth of the small bowel, and the severity of bacterial overgrowth correlates positively with the severity of the musculoskeletal inflammation, suggesting the probability of a causal relationship.[17] Relatedly, clinicians should recall that peptidoglycans, bacterial cell wall debris, endotoxins, indole, skatole and numerous other gut-derived "toxins" can promote joint inflammation.[18,19] **Animal models have demonstrated that gut-derived metabolites can cause inflammatory degenerative**

Prototypic multifocal dysbiosis in RA
• <u>Nasopharynx</u>: *Streptococcus pyogenes*
• <u>Gastrointestinal</u>: *Eubacterium aerofaciens* and (likely) segmented filamentous bacteria, in addition to generalized SIBO; some patients will have a specific "parasitic rheumatism" to a particular microbe, such as *Citrobacter* or *Endolimax*
• <u>Genitourinary</u>: *Proteus mirabilis*

---

[13] Lee et al. Cigarette smoking and inflammation: cellular and molecular mechanisms. *J Dent Res.* 2012 Feb;91(2):142-9 ncbi.nlm.nih.gov/pmc/articles/PMC3261116/
[14] Siegel LB, Gall EP. Viral infection as a cause of arthritis. *Am Fam Physician* 1996 Nov 1;54(6):2009-15
[15] Ebringer A, Rashid T, Wilson C. Rheumatoid arthritis: proposal for the use of anti-microbial therapy in early cases. *Scand J Rheumatol* 2003;32(1):2-11
[16] Rashid et al. Proteus IgG antibodies and C-reactive protein in English, Norwegian and Spanish patients with rheumatoid arthritis. *Clin Rheumatol* 1999;18(3):190-5
[17] "Eight (32%) of the patients with RA had hypochlorhydria or achlorhydria... A high frequency of small intestinal bacterial overgrowth was found in patients with RA; it was associated with a high disease activity and observed in patients with hypochlorhydria or achlorhydria and in those with normal acid secretion." Henriksson AE, Blomquist L, Nord CE, Midtvedt T, Uribe A. Small intestinal bacterial overgrowth in patients with rheumatoid arthritis. *Ann Rheum Dis.* 1993 Jul;52(7):503-10
[18] Simelyte et al. Bacterial cell wall-induced arthritis: chemical composition and tissue distribution of four Lactobacillus strains. *Infect Immun.* 2000 Jun;68(6):3535-40
[19] Toivanen P. Normal intestinal microbiota in the aetiopathogenesis of rheumatoid arthritis. *Ann Rheum Dis.* 2003 Sep;62(9):807-11 ard.bmjjournals.com/cgi/reprint/62/9/807

arthritis that resembles rheumatoid arthritis.[20,21] **The dysbiotic contribution to rheumatoid arthritis is likely to be both *qualitative* (related to specific inciting microbes) and *quantitative* (related to total, nonspecific bacterial overgrowth of the gut and multifocal mucosal colonization).** Accordingly, research published in 2007 showed that dietary modification was comparable in benefit to prednisolone, supporting the model that gastrointestinal dysfunction—namely, food allergic reactions (and probably intestinal dysbiosis)—is a major etiologic component of rheumatoid arthritis, at least in its initial stages; the authors concluded, "**This study supports the concept that rheumatoid arthritis may be a reaction to a food antigen(s) and that** the disease process starts within the intestine."[22]

- Parasitic: Gastrointestinal parasite infections, such as with *Endolimax nana*[23] and other microbes such a *Giardia lamblia*, can induce a systemic inflammatory response that mimics rheumatoid arthritis and is cured with parasite eradication.

Clinical presentations:

- Course: Variable course with exacerbations and remissions; the general trend is one of progressive joint destruction and systemic inflammation-induced damage.
- Presentation: The disease begins slowly in 2/3 of patients and can be slow to reach a diagnostic threshold—generally takes 9 months between initial onset and diagnosis; may affect only one joint initially. 10% have acute-onset polyarthritis. RA can affect any age, either gender, and clinical presentations will vary.
  - o 2-3x more common in women than men.
  - o Age of onset is typically 25-50 years of age.
  - o "Peripheral symmetric polyarthropathy" is a classic description for RA; but this same description can be applied to many cases of hemochromatosis and SLE as well.
  - o Palpable joint swelling with synovitis and effusion.
  - o Morning stiffness > 1 hour.
  - o Typical autoimmune systemic manifestations: fatigue, malaise, low-grade fever, anorexia, and weight loss—note that all of these clinical presentations are manifestations of immune activation in general and increased cytokine production in particular.
- Musculoskeletal:
  - o The joints most commonly affected are the wrists, MCP, PIP, MTP (metatarsophalangeal) joints, and knees (Baker's cyst is common). In severe or advanced disease, essentially any joint in the body—including the TMJ and upper cervical spine—can be involved.
  - o Most common at PIP, MCP joints, wrists (i.e., "knuckles and wrists").
  - o Upper cervical spine involvement can lead to atlantoaxial instability—upper cervical spine manipulation is contraindicated until atlantoaxial instability has been excluded clinically or radiographically.
  - o Periarticular muscle atrophy and osteoporosis—due to inflammation and disuse.
  - o Generalized osteoporosis is common due to inflammation, disuse/deconditioning, hypogonadism, and drug effects.
  - o Advanced complications include radial deviation of the wrists and ulnar deviation of the fingers, swan neck deformity (PIP hyperextension with DIP hyperflexion), and boutonniere deformity (PIP hyperflexion with DIP hyperextension).
- Skin: Rheumatoid nodules (subcutaneous inflammatory granulomas) are seen in up to 30% of patients. These are also rarely seen in patients with hemochromatoic arthropathy mimicking RA.[24]
- Arteries and vessels: Rheumatoid vasculitis leads to impaired circulation, causing necrosis of affected tissues/organs: fingers, skin, internal organs, and nerves (peripheral neuropathy).
- Pulmonary manifestations: Dyspnea, pulmonary nodules, fibrosis; more common in men.
- Eye: Complications are seen in 1% of patients but can lead to rapid blindness.
- Other autoimmune diseases: Up to 20% of patients with RA develop Sjogren's syndrome. SLE, MS, Hashimoto's thyroiditis, and mixed connective tissue disease can easily co-exist with RA.

---

[20] Nakoneczna I, Forbes JC, Rogers KS. The arthritogenic effect of indole, skatole and other tryptophan metabolites in rabbits. *Am J Pathol*. 1969 Dec;57(3):523-38
[21] Rogers KS, Forbes JC, Nakoneczna I. Arthritogenic properties of lipophilic, aryl molecules. *Proc Soc Exp Biol Med*. 1969 Jun;131(2):670-2
[22] Podas et al. Is rheumatoid arthritis a disease that starts in intestine? Pilot study comparing an elemental diet with oral prednisolone. *Postgrad Med J*. 2007 Feb;83(976):128-31
[23] "Endolimax nana grew on stool culture. Both the patient's diarrhea and arthritis responded effectively to therapy with metronidazole. The diagnosis of parasitic rheumatism was made in retrospect." Burnstein SL, Liakos S. Parasitic rheumatism presenting as rheumatoid arthritis. *J Rheumatol*. 1983 Jun;10(3):514-5
[24] "These manifestations which are common to rheumatoid arthritis may be seen in hemochromatotic arthropathy." Bensen WG, Laskin CA, Little HA, Fam AG. Hemochromatotic arthropathy mimicking rheumatoid arthritis. A case with subcutaneous nodules, tenosynovitis, and bursitis. *Arthritis Rheum*. 1978 Sep-Oct;21(7):844-8

Major differential diagnoses:

- Osteoarthritis (OA): OA tends to be monoarticular or oligoarticular rather than polyarticular; OA is generally only minimally inflammatory (except after the progression of joint destruction) whereas RA is clearly more inflammatory as assessed clinically and serologically (with ESR or CRP). OA is more likely to be asymmetric whereas RA is nearly always symmetric (except in cases of stroke, paralysis, or peripheral nerve lesion due to interference with neurogenic inflammation). Lab tests such as ANA, RF, and CCP antibodies are expected to be normal in OA; CRP and ESR may be moderately elevated in severe OA but inflammatory markers are generally much lower than the levels seen in RA.

- SLE: Differentiated by nonerosive arthritis, anti-DS-DNA antibodies, anti-Smith antibodies, low serum complement, the classic "butterfly rash", and an earlier and more frequent development of mucosal, serosal, vasculitic and renal complications.

- Septic arthritis: Differentiated by monoarthritis, fever, and purulent joint aspiration.
  - Septic arthritis may complicate pre-existing rheumatoid arthritis, and patients with RA appear to be predisposed to septic arthritis: Reasons for this septic predisposition include immune dysfunction, use of prednisone or other immunosuppressant medications, and concomitant obesity and/or diabetes. **Patients may lack the classic systemic manifestations of septic arthritis (fever, chills, leukocytosis) due to age, disease, or pharmaceutical immunosuppression.**[25,26] Patients may have concomitant respiratory or urinary tract infections, which makes the clinical presentation even more unclear. Treatment may require systemic antibiotics (oral or intravenous) and joint lavage with antibiotics.[27] **Failure to diagnose and treat septic arthritis promptly may result in deformity, disability, or death.**

- Hemochromatosis and iron overload: Given its high frequency and multifarious clinical presentations, iron overload is an essential diagnostic consideration in patients with rheumatic disease.[28,29] Doctors must test serum ferritin and transferrin saturation (along with CRP) as discussed in Chapter 1.

- Reactive arthritis: Differentiated by the recent history of infection, greatly increased prevalence of HLA-B27, and the presence of uveitis/iritis, sacroiliac and lumbar involvement, predominant acute/subacute-onset inflammation of the heels, knees, hips. *Perspective from DrV*: I think rheumatoid arthritis should be considered a variant of reactive arthritis, with RA being triggered by multifocal dysbiosis (several subclinical infections) whereas the latter is triggered by a single true infection.

- Gout and other crystal-induced arthropathy: Asymmetric arthritis, negatively birefringent crystals demonstrated with joint aspiration.

- Arthritis related to viral infection: Such as parvovirus and hepatitis C[30]; clinical correlation with appropriate serologies are warranted.

- Psoriatic arthritis: Skin lesions, nail pitting, asymmetric arthritis, negative RF and CCP. Rarely, the joint inflammation of psoriatic arthritis precedes the expected dermatologic lesions: well-demarcated erythematous patches covered with silvery scales.

- Adult Still's disease: Diagnosis relies on *all of the following*: high fevers (>102.2°F), arthralgia/arthritis, RF<80, ANA<1:100, *plus two of the following*: skin rash (generalized and confluent red papules and plaques), pleuritis/pericarditis, WBC count >15,000 cells/mm³, and hepatomegally/spenomegally/lymphadenopathy.

- Ewing's sarcoma: An aggressive bone malignancy that typically presents in children and young adults with periarticular bone pain and fever which can mimic inflammatory monoarthritis.

---

[25] "Many patients lacked distinctive features of joint sepsis (fever, chills) and only one half had leukocytosis." Blackburn WD Jr, Dunn TL, Alarcon GS. Infection versus disease activity in rheumatoid arthritis: eight years' experience. *South Med J.* 1986 Oct;79(10):1238-41

[26] "Pain and loss of motion in the affected joint were prominent, but toxic features of pyogenic infections—hectic fever, chills, sweats, local warmth, or erythema--were conspicuously absent. Two patients had moderate fever and three patients had mild leukocytosis." Kraft SM, Panush RS, Longley S. Unrecognized staphylococcal pyarthrosis with rheumatoid arthritis. *Semin Arthritis Rheum.* 1985 Feb;14(3):196-201

[27] Septic arthritis complicating rheumatoid arthritis was due to Staphylococcus aureus (12 cases) and Escherichia coli (1 case). Recommended treatment: "The authors recommend as the treatment of choice: systemic antibiotic therapy and immediate arthrotomy followed by through-and-through irrigation with fluid containing the appropriate antibiotics." Gristina AG, Rovere GD, Shoji H. Spontaneous septic arthritis complicating rheumatoid arthritis. *J Bone Joint Surg Am.* 1974 Sep;56(6):1180-4

[28] Vasquez A. Musculoskeletal disorders and iron overload disease: comment on the American College of Rheumatology guidelines for the initial evaluation of the adult patient with acute musculoskeletal symptoms. *Arthritis Rheum.* 1996 Oct;39(10):1767-8

[29] "These manifestations which are common to rheumatoid arthritis may be seen in hemochromatotic arthropathy." Bensen WG, Laskin CA, Little HA, Fam AG. Hemochromatotic arthropathy mimicking rheumatoid arthritis. A case with subcutaneous nodules, tenosynovitis, and bursitis. *Arthritis Rheum.* 1978 Sep-Oct;21(7):844-8

[30] Siegel LB, Gall EP. Viral infection as a cause of arthritis. *Am Fam Physician* 1996 Nov 1;54(6):2009-15

Clinical assessment:
- **History/subjective**:
    - Systemic manifestations (eg, fatigue, lassitude) with symmetric peripheral polyarthropathy.
    - Morning stiffness lasting more than 30-60 minutes is common.
- **Physical examination/objective**:
    - Assess joints, especially the distal/peripheral joints of the wrists/hands and ankles/feet. Remember that the initial manifestation of RA, like all inflammatory arthropathies, can affect any joint in the body, including the atlantoaxial joint. Flexion contractures and ulnar deviation of the fingers are common, classic findings of developed disease.
    - Clinically assess patient for exclusion of other diseases. Some patients with RA will develop other autoimmune diseases, especially hypothyroidism and Sjogren's syndrome.
- **Laboratory assessments**: Goals of laboratory testing are 1) exclude serious life-threatening conditions (e.g., septic arthritis), 2) quantitatively and qualitatively assess patient's health status, 3) determine nature and severity of underlying diseases and disorders for which correction can contribute to an overall improvement in immune function and reduction in total inflammatory load.
    - **CCP: Cyclic citrullinated protein antibody; Citrullinated protein antibodies (CPA); anti-CCP antibodies: anti-cyclic citrullinated peptide antibody**: Anti-CCP antibodies have 95-98% specificity for RA[31] and has become the laboratory standard for evaluating the diagnosis and prognosis of RA.[32] The best current data indicates that anti-CCP antibodies are sensitive and specific for RA[33], and clinicians should use this test in the diagnosis of RA.[34] Anti-CCP antibodies with a positive rheumatoid factor (RF) is termed "composite/conjugate seropositivity" and appears to be more specific than isolated anti-CCP or RF positivity.[35]
    - C-reactive protein: CRP can be used to support the diagnosis (as it indicates inflammation) and can be used to monitor the disease and the response to treatment.[36]
    - Erythrocyte sedimentation rate: ESR is elevated in 90% of patients and can be used to support the diagnosis (as it indicates inflammation) and can be used to monitor the disease and the response to treatment.[37]
    - Complete blood count: CBC may reveal anemia of chronic disease, anemia due to NSAID-related gastrointestinal bleeding, or suggest nutritional deficiencies (namely B12 and folic acid as discussed in Chapter 1); elevated WBC suggests infection and requires clinical correlation.
    - Ferritin: As an acute phase reactant, serum ferritin is elevated by inflammation; as a marker for iron status, serum ferritin is elevated by iron overload and lowered by iron deficiency. Transferrin saturation and serum iron should be low in RA due to inflammation, whereas they are commonly elevated in patients with iron overload. In order to determine the acute phase contribution to an elevated ferritin level, an independent marker of inflammation such as CRP or ESR should be tested simultaneously. When in doubt, iron overload can be excluded with diagnostic phlebotomy, liver MRI, liver

> **CCP antibodies: the single best laboratory test for the early detection, diagnosis, and monitoring of RA**
>
> "The anti-CCP test is more specific than the commonly used RF test (95% versus less than 90%) and has a comparable sensitivity (more than 70%). ... In conclusion, testing for anti-CCP autoantibodies is widely accepted as an indispensable tool for diagnosis and early treatment in the management of rheumatoid arthritis patients."
>
> van Venrooij et al. *Ann N Y Acad Sci* 2008 Nov

[31] Hill J, Cairns E, Bell DA. The joy of citrulline: new insights into the diagnosis, pathogenesis, and treatment of rheumatoid arthritis. *J Rheumatol*. 2004 Aug;31(8):1471-3

[32] "We conclude that, at present, the antibody response directed to citrullinated antigens has the most valuable diagnostic and prognostic potential for RA." van Boekel MA, et al. Autoantibody systems in rheumatoid arthritis: specificity, sensitivity and diagnostic value. *Arthritis Res*. 2002;4(2):87-93 arthritis-research.com/content/4/2/87

[33] "Serum antibodies reactive with citrullinated proteins/peptides are a very sensitive and specific marker for rheumatoid arthritis." Migliorini P, Pratesi F, Tommasi C, Anzilotti C. The immune response to citrullinated antigens in autoimmune diseases. *Autoimmun Rev*. 2005 Nov;4(8):561-4

[34] "The anti-CCP test is more specific than the commonly used RF test (95% versus less than 90%) and has a comparable sensitivity (more than 70%). ... In conclusion, testing for anti-CCP autoantibodies is widely accepted as an indispensable tool for diagnosis and early treatment in the management of rheumatoid arthritis patients." van Venrooij WJ, van Beers JJ, Pruijn GJ. Anti-CCP Antibody, a Marker for the Early Detection of Rheumatoid Arthritis. *Ann N Y Acad Sci*. 2008 Nov;1143:268-85

[35] "...our findings suggest that a positive anti-CCP antibody result does not necessarily exclude SLE in African American patients presenting with inflammatory arthritis. In such patients, the additional assessment of IgA-RF or IgM-RF isotypes may be of added value since composite seropositivity appears to be nearly exclusive to patients with RA." Mikuls et al. Anti-cyclic citrullinated peptide antibody and rheumatoid factor isotypes in African Americans with early rheumatoid arthritis. *Arthritis Rheum*. 2006 Sep;54:3057-9

[36] Gabay C, Kushner I. Acute-phase proteins and other systemic responses to inflammation. *N Engl J Med*. 1999 Feb 11;340(6):448-54

[37] Klippel JH (ed). *Primer on the Rheumatic Diseases. 11th Edition*. Atlanta: Arthritis Foundation. 1997 page 94

biopsy (especially if liver enzymes are elevated), or the response to therapeutic phlebotomy.[38]

- o Rheumatoid factor: RF is positive in 70-80% of patients with RA but is not specific and is not necessary for the diagnosis of RA. RF provides "supportive evidence" for the diagnosis of RA only in the presence of corresponding clinical manifestations. High RF levels indicate more severe disease and worse prognosis. IgA-RF appears to have clinical superiority over other forms of RF.[39] RF is seen in 5% of apparently healthy people, and it is present in some patients with iron overload, thus making the distinction between RA and hemochromatoic arthropathy all the more difficult.[40] Diseases (other than RA) associated with RF positivity include iron overload, chronic infections, hepatitis, sarcoidosis, and bacterial endocarditis.

- o Thyroid assessment: Hypothyroidism can mimic systemic rheumatic disease by causing an inflammatory oligoarthropathy and myopathy, complete with elevations of CRP and ESR.[41] Overt or imminent hypothyroidism is suggested by TSH greater than 2 mU/L[42] or 3 mU/L[43], low T4 or T3, and/or the presence of anti-thyroid peroxidase antibodies (anti-TPO).[44] This author's current practice is—for the laboratory evaluation of hypothyroidism—to assess the full spectrum of thyroid indexes: THS, free T4, free or total T3, reverse T3 (rT3), and the antithyroid antibodies: anti-thyroglobulin and anti-thyroid peroxidase (anti-TPO).

- o Complete hormone assessment: Patients with RA commonly show elevations of prolactin and estradiol along with insufficiencies of testosterone, cortisol, and DHEA. These can be tested in serum, and early-morning serum cortisol is more accurate than late-day cortisol. Other options and details are provided in the following section under *Treatments* and in the section in Chapter 4 on *Orthoendocrinology*.

- o Lactulose-mannitol assay for "leaky gut": Increased intestinal permeability (IP) is a common contributor to and complication of many inflammatory/rheumatic/chronic diseases including psoriasis[45], Behcet's disease[46], ankylosing spondylitis[47] and seronegative spondyloarthritis[48], enteropathic spondyloarthropathy and oligoarticular juvenile idiopathic arthritis[49], lupus[50], and chronic congestive heart failure.[51] This test may be used for the evaluation of gastrointestinal mucosal integrity, which simultaneously serves as a barometer of overall health and when elevated can indicate the presence of a variety of intestinal disorders, including celiac disease, food allergies, and GI dysbiosis. Thus, an elevated lactulose:mannitol ratio is *sensitive* but not *specific* for the presence of intestinal disorders. See discussion in Chapter 1. Use of this test in RA is at the discretion of the clinician and patient, as most patients can be reasonably assumed to have increased intestinal permeability and thereafter treated empirically; the value—if any—of this test in RA is in monitoring response to treatment.

- o Comprehensive stool analysis and comprehensive parasitology with bacterial and fungal culture and sensitivity: **All patients with rheumatoid arthritis should be considered to have gastrointestinal dysbiosis until proven otherwise** by ❶ dysbiosis laboratory assessment (including comprehensive stool testing with parasitology *performed by a specialty laboratory*), and ❷ response to anti-dysbiosis treatment

---

[38] "Therapeutic phlebotomy is used to remove excess iron and maintain low normal body iron stores, and it should be initiated in men with serum ferritin levels of 300 microg/L or more and in women with serum ferritin levels of 200 microg/L or more, regardless of the presence or absence of symptoms." Barton et al. Management of hemochromatosis. Hemochromatosis Management Working Group. *Ann Intern Med*. 1998 Dec 1;129(11):932-9

[39] Jonsson T, Valdimarsson H. What about IgA rheumatoid factor in rheumatoid arthritis? *Ann Rheum Dis*. 1998 Jan;57(1):63-4 ard.bmjjournals.com/cgi/content/full/57/1/63

[40] "These manifestations which are common to rheumatoid arthritis may be seen in hemochromatotic arthropathy." Bensen WG, Laskin CA, Little HA, Fam AG. Hemochromatotic arthropathy mimicking rheumatoid arthritis. A case with subcutaneous nodules, tenosynovitis, and bursitis. *Arthritis Rheum*. 1978;21(7):844-8

[41] Bowman et al. Bilateral adhesive capsulitis, oligoarthritis and proximal myopathy as presentation of hypothyroidism. *Br J Rheumatol*. 1988;27(1):62-4

[42] Weetman AP. Hypothyroidism: screening and subclinical disease. *BMJ*. 1997 Apr 19;314(7088):1175-8 bmj.bmjjournals.com/cgi/content/full/314/7088/1175

[43] "Now AACE encourages doctors to consider treatment for patients who test outside the boundaries of a narrower margin based on a target TSH level of 0.3 to 3.0. AACE believes the new range will result in proper diagnosis for millions of Americans who suffer from a mild thyroid disorder, but have gone untreated until now." American Association of Clinical Endocrinologists (AACE). 2003 Campaign Encourages Awareness of Mild Thyroid Failure, Importance of Routine Testing aace.com/pub/tam2003/press.php November 26, 2005

[44] Beers MH, Berkow R (eds). *Merck Manual. 17th Edition*. Whitehouse Station; Merck Research Laboratories 1999 Page 96

[45] Humbert P, Bidet A, Treffel P, Drobacheff C, Agache P. Intestinal permeability in patients with psoriasis. *J Dermatol Sci*. 1991 Jul;2(4):324-6

[46] Fresko I, et al. Intestinal permeability in Behcet's syndrome. *Ann Rheum Dis*. 2001 Jan;60(1):65-6

[47] Vaile et al. Bowel permeability and CD45RO expression on circulating CD20+ B cells in patients with ankylosing spondylitis and their relatives. *J Rheumatol* 1999 Jan:128-35

[48] Di Leo et al. Effect of Helicobacter pylori and eradication therapy on gastrointestinal permeability. Implications for patients with seronegative spondyloarthritis. *J Rheumatol*. 2005 Feb;32(2):295-300

[49] Picco P, et al. Increased gut permeability in juvenile chronic arthritides. A multivariate analysis of the diagnostic parameters. *Clin Exp Rheumatol*. 2000 Nov-Dec;18(6):773-8

[50] "Fourteen cases of primary lupus-associated protein-losing enteropathy have now been reported in the English-language literature." Perednia DA, Curosh NA. Lupus-associated protein-losing enteropathy. *Arch Intern Med*. 1990 Sep;150(9):1806-10

[51] "Chronic heart failure patients had a 35% increase of small intestinal permeability (lactulose/mannitol ratio: 0.023 vs. 0.017 …, p = 0.006), a 210% increase of large intestinal permeability (sucralose excretion: 0.62 … vs. 0.20), and a 29% decrease of D-xylose absorption, indicating bowel ischemia (26.7% vs. 37.4%, p = 0.003)." Sandek A, Bauditz J, Swidsinski A, et al. Altered intestinal function in patients with chronic heart failure. *J Am Coll Cardiol*. 2007 Oct 16;50(16):1561-9

which minimally includes the combination of <u>anti-dysbiosis dietary modification</u> (nutritional supplementation, plant-based diet, low-fermentation, high-fiber, superadequate protein and phytonutrients) <u>with antimicrobial drugs or botanicals</u>, commonly including berberine (500mg BID-TID for 3 months), emulsified time-released oil of oregano (200mg TID for 6 weeks[52]), Augmentin (2,000mg BID for variable durations of days to months to years—supportively, note successful use of long-term penicillin in the treatment of psoriasis[53]), azithromycin (500mg every other day for variable durations of days to months to years[54]), ciprofloxacin (short course only to avoid exacerbation/induction of tendonopathy), and metronidazole. Since 2013, I have become impressed by the efficacy of low-dose oral vancomycin 125-250mg PO QD; as a nonabsorbed antibiotic, the drug remains in the gut and is effective against segmented filamentous bacteria (SFB) which have been shown in several animal experiments to induce Th-17 effector cells which promote chronic arthritis/autoimmunity. A **three-sample comprehensive stool analysis and parasitology examination** performed by a **specialty laboratory** is strongly recommended as a minimal component of basic care. In lieu of *or preferably in addition to* a comprehensive parasitology test, patients can be treated for 4-8 weeks with broad-spectrum antimicrobial treatment (including an anti-dysbiosis diet) that is effective against gram-positive and gram-negative bacteria, aerobes and anaerobes, yeast, protozoa and amebas. For additional details, see Chapter 4.2 for details on dysbiosis.

- **Imaging**:
  - Radiographic changes are not seen in early disease and only have utility for clarifying diagnostic uncertainty later in the disease, screening for complications such as atlantoaxial instability, or for pre-operative assessment in patients who are candidates for joint repair or replacement.
  - Radiographic findings when clustered are relatively specific in developed disease: soft tissue swelling, periarticular osteoporosis, joint space narrowing due to loss of cartilage, **marginal erosions**, ulnar/lateral deviation of the fingers, and subluxation and dislocation may occur.

- **Establishing the diagnosis**:
  - The diagnosis is established by pattern recognition of the typical clinical manifestations and laboratory abnormalities and reasonable exclusion of protean diseases such as hepatitis C, SLE, and iron overload.

Complications:

- Disease complications are common and range from the inconveniences of pain and inflammation for patients with milder disease to the major complications of joint deformity, occupational and social disability, serious cardiovascular/renal/pulmonary/cerebral complications (due mostly to inflammation, fibrosis, and vasculitis), infections (especially septic arthritis), depression, and suicide. Adding drug side-effects atop these manifold

---

2010 American College of Rheumatology/European League against Rheumatism classification criteria

<u>Screening</u>: Patients with at least 1 joint and definite clinical synovitis which is not explained by another disease.

<u>A score of ≥6 is needed for classification of definite RA</u>:
- Score 1 large joint: 0
- 2–10 large joints: 1
- 1–3 small joints (with or without large joints): 2
- 4–10 small joints (with or without large joints): 3
- >10 joints (at least 1 small joint): 5

<u>Serology</u>: At least 1 test is needed:
- Negative RF (rheumatoid factor) and negative ACPA (anticitrullinated protein antibody): 0
- Low positive RF or low positive ACPA: 2
- High positive RF or high positive ACPA: 3

<u>Acute phase reactants</u>: At least 1 result is needed.
- Normal CRP (C-reactive protein) and normal ESR: 0
- Abnormal CRP or ESR: 1

<u>Duration of symptoms</u>: (self-reported)
- <6 weeks: 0
- ≥6 weeks: 1

Although patients with a score <6/10 are not classifiable as having RA, their status can be reassessed and the criteria might be fulfilled cumulatively over time.

onlinelibrary.wiley.com/doi/10.1002/art.27580/pdf
ncbi.nlm.nih.gov/pmc/articles/PMC3077961/pdf/nihms266537.pdf
unboundmedicine.com/5minute/view/5-Minute-Clinical-Consult/116053/all/Arthritis_Rheumatoid__RA

---

[52] "Oil of Mediterranean oregano *Oreganum vulgare* was orally administered to 14 adult patients whose stools tested positive for enteric parasites, *Blastocystis hominis*, *Entamoeba hartmanni* and *Endolimax nana*. After 6 weeks of supplementation with 600 mg emulsified oil of oregano daily, there was complete disappearance of *Entamoeba hartmanni* (four cases), *Endolimax nana* (one case), and *Blastocystis hominis* in eight cases. Also, *Blastocystis hominis* scores declined in three additional cases. Gastrointestinal symptoms improved in seven of the 11 patients who had tested positive for *Blastocystis hominis*." Force M, Sparks WS, Ronzio RA. Inhibition of enteric parasites by emulsified oil of oregano in vivo. *Phytother Res.* 2000 May;14(3):213-4
[53] Saxena VN, Dogra J. Long-term use of penicillin for the treatment of chronic plaque psoriasis. *Eur J Dermatol.* 2005 Sep-Oct;15(5):359-6
[54] Saxena VN, Dogra J. Long-term oral azithromycin in chronic plaque psoriasis: a controlled trial. *Eur J Dermatol.* 2010 May-Jun;20(3):329-33

disease complications makes managing the disease more difficult for doctors, and enduring the disease more difficult for patients.

- Mild disease results in mild symptoms and manageable impact on ADL (activities of daily living) and QOL (quality of life). Severe disease is painful, less responsive to treatment, disfiguring and generally devastating. Treatments that are inefficacious, unavailable, prohibitively expensive, or complicated by significant side effects contribute to despair. **RA patients are at increased risk for social isolation, depression, and suicide**[55]; these sociopsychiatric complications can be attributed to chronic pain, neuropsychiatric effects of inflammatory cytokines, therapeutic nihilism, adverse drug effects (e.g., NSAID- and steroid-induced psychosis), cerebral vasculitis, and nutritional deficiencies (e.g., EPA, DHA, vitamin D, zinc) in patients not cared for by competent integrative clinicians.

- Decreased life expectancy by 3-7 years, mostly due to infection, gastrointestinal bleeding, and cardiorenal complications.

- Patients with systemic inflammatory diseases are at increased risk for cardiovascular disorders (including hypertension, accelerated atherosclerosis, vasculitis) and renal complications (secondary to hypertension, vasculitis, immune complex deposition, NSAIDs and other drugs).

Clinical management:

- <u>Routine assessment, surveillance for complications, compliance, consultation, laboratory follow-up, access to treatments</u>: Clinical visits should include surveillance for subjective and objective indicators of disease progression/remission, treatment compliance (including overzealous compliance with its risk of adverse toxic effects or unnecessary expense, or undercompliance with attendant hazards of inefficacy and disease exacerbation), and overall health status. Questions are answered, and problems addressed. Necessary consultations are scheduled as needed; the referring provider sends a narrative letter and ensures that the patient has a scheduled appointment. Review and anticipatory scheduling of laboratory tests should be performed. Access to treatments should be verified. Appropriate documentation is mandatory.

- <u>Standard medical treatments</u>:
  - <u>Discouraging the discouragement of "nutritional quackery"</u>: According to the *Merck Manual* (1999), "Food and diet quackery is common and should be discouraged."[56] In contrast to this allopathic rhetoric, the biomedical literature strongly supports the use of nutritional interventions for **direct benefits** (e.g., anti-inflammatory, analgesic, immunomodulatory, and drug-sparing effects) and **indirect benefits** (e.g., cardiorenal protection, alleviation of depression).
  - <u>NSAIDs as first-line treatment</u>: NSAIDS provide temporary pain relief while contributing to increased intestinal permeability, gastrointestinal hemorrhage, liver toxicity (dose-response relationship), renal toxicity (dose-response relationship) possible exacerbation of food allergies[57], and accelerated destruction of articular structures (especially indomethacin).[58,59,60]
  - <u>Immunosuppression with prednisone, methotrexate, or other DMARD (disease-modifying antirheumatic drugs)</u>: **Despite the clinical drawbacks, philosophical inadequacies, and steep financial consequences, pharmacologic immunosuppression has a role in the management of patients with autoimmunity when their disease flares and threatens vital structures, particularly the heart, kidneys, and nervous system.** A common sequence of medicalization used by rheumatologists is:

---

[55] "Rheumatoid arthritis (RA) is a somatic disorder, which is known to be associated with major depression, and prevalences exceeding even 40% have been reported [5, 6]. Recently, Treharne et al. [7] showed that 11% of hospital out-patients with RA had experienced suicidal ideation." Timonen M, Viilo K, Hakko H, Särkioja T, Ylikulju M, Meyer-Rochow VB, Väisänen E, Räsänen P. Suicides in persons suffering from rheumatoid arthritis. *Rheumatology.* 2003 Feb;42(2):287-91

[56] Beers MH, Berkow R (eds). *The Merck Manual. 17th Edition.* Whitehouse Station; Merck Research Laboratories: 1999, page 419

[57] Abbreviations: cow's milk beta-lactoglobulin absorption (BLG), acetylsalicylic acid (ASA), disodium chromoglycate (DSCG). "ASA administration strongly increased BLG absorption, not prevented by DSCG pretreatment. ... Our results suggest that prolonged treatment with nonsteroidal anti-inflammatory drugs induces an increase of food antigen absorption, apparently not related to anaphylaxis mediator release, with possible clinical effects." Fagiolo U, Paganelli R, Ossi E, Quinti I, Cancian M, D'Offizi GP, Fiocco U. Intestinal permeability and antigen absorption in rheumatoid arthritis. Effects of acetylsalicylic acid and sodium chromoglycate. *Int Arch Allergy Appl Immunol.* 1989;89(1):98-102

[58] "At…concentrations comparable to those… in the synovial fluid of patients treated with the drug, several NSAIDs suppress proteoglycan synthesis… These NSAID-related effects on chondrocyte metabolism … are much more profound in osteoarthritic cartilage than in normal cartilage, due to enhanced uptake of NSAIDs by the osteoarthritic cartilage." Brandt KD. Effects of nonsteroidal anti-inflammatory drugs on chondrocyte metabolism in vitro and in vivo. *Am J Med.* 1987 Nov 20; 83: 29-34

[59] "The case of a young healthy man, who developed avascular necrosis of head of femur after prolonged administration of indomethacin, is reported here." Prathapkumar KR, Smith I, Attara GA. Indomethacin induced avascular necrosis of head of femur. *Postgrad Med J.* 2000 Sep; 76(899): 574-5

[60] "This highly significant association between NSAID use and acetabular destruction gives cause for concern, not least because of the difficulty in achieving satisfactory hip replacements in patients with severely damaged acetabula." Newman et al. Acetabular bone destruction related to non-steroidal anti-inflammatory drugs. *Lancet.* 1985; 2: 11-4

- Begin first-visit treatment with daily/PRN low-dose prednisone (5-7.5 mg/day) and weekly methotrexate (7.5-15 mg/week, with daily folic acid to improve efficacy and reduce toxicity),
- Eventually add hydroxychloroquine and/or sulfasalazine as disease progresses,
- When the patient becomes "resistant to treatment" add either an oral immunosuppressant or one of the "biologics" such as the parenterally-administered TNF/cytokine blockers: etanercept, infliximab, adalimumab, etc.

Such a drug protocol might easily cost $50,000 per year and carry complications such as increased risk and severity of opportunistic infections (especially tuberculosis), exacerbation of heart failure, and increased risk for lymphoma and—less commonly—SLE and CNS demyelination similar to multiple sclerosis. Immunosuppression with corticosteroids/prednisone promotes bacterial overgrowth of the small bowel in humans[61], and animal studies have demonstrated increased bacterial translocation following prednisone administration[62]; recall that intestinal bacterial overgrowth/translocation are both pro-inflammatory and arthritogenic. Prednisone also causes mitochondrial dysfunction, which exacerbates fatigue and inflammation.

- o <u>Surgery</u>: Surgery is used for deformities and other orthopedic complications, including atlantoaxial instability and protrusio acetabuli.

- | <u>**FOOD & NUTRITION**</u>: 5-part "supplemented Paleo-Mediterranean diet" (SPMD, 5pSPMD) | The 5-part "supplemented Paleo-Mediterranean diet" (SPMD—reviewed in Chapter 4) consists of ❶ foundational plant-based low-carbohydrate diet of fruits, vegetables, nuts, seeds, berries and lean sources of protein, ❷ multivitamin and multimineral supplementation, ❸ physiologic doses of vitamin D3 (range 2,000-10,000 IU/d), ❹ combination fatty acid therapy (CFAT) with n3-ALA, n6-GLA, n3-EPA, n3-DHA, and phytochemical-rich olive oil which contains n9-oleate, and ❺ probiotics.

  - o <u>Avoidance of pro-inflammatory foods</u>: Pro-inflammatory foods act *directly* and *indirectly* to promote and exacerbate systemic inflammation. *Direct* mechanisms include the activation of Toll-like receptors and NFkB, while *indirect* mechanisms include depleting the body of anti-inflammatory nutrients and dietary displacement of more nutrient-dense anti-inflammatory foods. Arachidonic acid (found in cow's milk, beef, liver, pork, and lamb) is the direct precursor to pro-inflammatory prostaglandins and leukotrienes[63] and pain-promoting isoprostanes.[64] Saturated fats promote inflammation by activating/enabling pro-inflammatory Toll-like receptors, which are otherwise "specific" for inducing pro-inflammatory responses to microorganisms.[65] Consumption of saturated fat in the form of cream creates marked oxidative stress and lipid peroxidation that lasts for at least 3 hours postprandially.[66] Corn oil rapidly activates NFkB (in hepatic Kupffer cells) for a pro-inflammatory effect[67]; similarly, consumption of PUFA and linoleic acid promotes antioxidant depletion and may thus promote oxidation-mediated inflammation via activation of NFkB. Linoleic acid causes intracellular oxidative stress and calcium influx and results in increased NFkB-stimulated transcription of pro-inflammatory genes.[68] High glycemic foods cause oxidative stress[69,70] and inflammation via activation of NFkB and other mechanisms—e.g.,

---

[61] "A 63-year-old man with systemic lupus erythematosus and selective IgA deficiency developed intractable diarrhoea the day after treatment with prednisone, 50 mg daily, was started. The diarrhoea was considered to be caused by bacterial overgrowth and was later successfully treated with doxycycline." Denison H, Wallerstedt S. Bacterial overgrowth after high-dose corticosteroid treatment. *Scand J Gastroenterol*. 1989 Jun;24(5):561-4

[62] "These bacteria also translocated to the mesenteric lymph nodes in mice injected with cyclophosphamide or prednisone." Berg RD, Wommack E, Deitch EA. Immunosuppression and intestinal bacterial overgrowth synergistically promote bacterial translocation. *Arch Surg*. 1988 Nov;123(11):1359-64

[63] Vasquez A. New Insights into Fatty Acid Supplementation and Eicosanoid Production and Gene Expression. *Nutr Perspect* 2005; Jan:5-16 ichnfm.academia.edu/AlexVasquez

[64] Evans et al. Isoprostanes, novel eicosanoids that produce nociception and sensitize rat sensory neurons. *J Pharmacol Exp Ther*. 2000 Jun;293(3):912-20

[65] Lee et al. Saturated fatty acids not unsaturated fatty acids induce expression of cyclooxygenase-2 mediated through Toll-like receptor 4. *J Biol Chem* 2001 May;276:16683-9

[66] "The increase in ROS generation lasted 3 h after cream intake and 1 h after protein intake." Mohanty et al. Both lipid and protein intakes stimulate increased generation of reactive oxygen species by polymorphonuclear leukocytes and mononuclear cells. *Am J Clin Nutr*. 2002 Apr;75(4):767-72

[67] Rusyn et al. Corn oil rapidly activates nuclear factor-kappaB in hepatic Kupffer cells by oxidant-dependent mechanisms. *Carcinogenesis*. 1999 Nov;20(11):2095-100

[68] "Exposing endothelial cells to 90 micromol linoleic acid/L for 6 h resulted in a significant increase in lipid hydroperoxides that coincided wih an increase in intracellular calcium concentrations." Hennig B, et al. Linoleic acid activates nuclear transcription factor-kappa B (NF-kappa B) and induces NF-kappa B-dependent transcription in cultured endothelial cells. *Am J Clin Nutr*. 1996 Mar;63(3):322-8 ajcn.org/cgi/reprint/63/3/322

[69] Mohanty et al. Glucose challenge stimulates reactive oxygen species (ROS) generation by leucocytes. *J Clin Endocrinol Metab*. 2000 Aug;85(8):2970-3 Glucose/carbohydrate and saturated fat consumption appear to be the two biggest offenders in the food-stimulated production of oxidative stress. The effect by protein is much less. "CONCLUSIONS: Both fat and protein intakes stimulate ROS generation. The increase in ROS generation lasted 3 h after cream intake and 1 h after protein intake. Cream intake also caused a significant and prolonged increase in lipid peroxidation." Mohanty et al. Both lipid and protein intakes stimulate increased generation of reactive oxygen species by polymorphonuclear leukocytes and mononuclear cells. *Am J Clin Nutr*. 2002 Apr;75(4):767-72

[70] Koska et al. Insulin, catecholamines, glucose and antioxidant enzymes in oxidative damage during different loads in healthy humans. *Physiol Res*. 2000;49 Suppl 1:S95-100

white bread causes inflammation[71] as does *a high-fat high-carbohydrate fast-food-style breakfast.*[72] High glycemic foods suppress immune function[73,74] and thus promote the perpetuation of microbial colonization and dysbiosis. Delivery of a high carbohydrate load to the gastrointestinal lumen promotes bacterial overgrowth[75,76], which is inherently pro-inflammatory[77,78] and which appears to be myalgenic in humans[79] at least in part due to the ability of endotoxin to impair muscle function.[80] Overconsumption of high-carbohydrate low-phytonutrient grains, potatoes, and manufactured foods displaces phytonutrient-dense foods such as fruits, vegetables, nuts, seeds, and berries which contain more than 8,000 phytonutrients, many of which have antioxidant and thus anti-inflammatory actions.[81,82]

- o Avoidance of allergenic foods: **Gluten-free vegetarian diets benefit patients with rheumatoid arthritis.**[83] Any patient may be allergic to any food, even if the food is generally considered a health-promoting food. Generally speaking, the most notorious allergens are wheat, citrus (especially citrus *juice* due to the industrial use of fungal hemicellulases), cow's milk, eggs, peanuts, chocolate, and yeast-containing foods. According to a study in patients with migraine, some patients will have to avoid as many as 10 specific foods in order to become symptom-free.[84] **Celiac disease can present with inflammatory oligoarthritis that resembles rheumatoid arthritis and which remits with avoidance of wheat/gluten.** The inflammatory arthropathy of celiac disease has preceded bowel symptoms and/or an accurate diagnosis by as many as 3-15 years.[85,86] Clinicians must explain to their patients that celiac disease and wheat allergy are two different clinical entities and that exclusion of one does not exclude the other, and in neither case does mutual exclusion obviate the promotion of intestinal bacterial overgrowth (i.e., pro-inflammatory dysbiosis) by indigestible wheat oligosaccharides.

- o Gluten-free vegetarian/vegan diet: **Gluten-free vegetarian diets benefit patients with rheumatoid arthritis.**[87] Vegetarian/vegan diets show high safety and variable efficacy in the treatment of various inflammatory disorders.[88,89,90,91] The benefits of gluten-free vegetarian diets are well documented, and the mechanisms of action are well elucidated, including reduced intake of pro-inflammatory linoleic[92] and

[71] "The present study shows that high GI carbohydrate, but not low GI carbohydrate, mediates an acute proinflammatory process as measured by NF-kappaB activity." Dickinson et al. High glycemic index carbohydrate mediates an acute proinflammatory process as measured by NF-kappaB activation. *Asia Pac J Clin Nutr.* 2005;14 Suppl:S120

[72] Aljada et al. Increase in intranuclear nuclear factor kappaB and decrease in inhibitor kappaB in mononuclear cells after a mixed meal. *Am J Clin Nutr.* 2004 Apr;79(4):682-90

[73] Sanchez A, Reeser JL, Lau HS, et al. Role of sugars in human neutrophilic phagocytosis. *Am J Clin Nutr.* 1973 Nov;26(11):1180-4

[74] "Postoperative infusion of carbohydrate solution leads to moderate fall in the serum concentration of inorganic phosphate. ... The hypophosphatemia was associated with significant reduction of neutrophil phagocytosis, intracellular killing, consumption of oxygen and generation of superoxide during phagocytosis." Rasmussen A, Segel E, Hessov I, Borregaard N. Reduced function of neutrophils during routine postoperative glucose infusion. *Acta Chir Scand.* 1988 Jul-Aug;154(7-8):429-33

[75] Ramakrishnan T, Stokes P. Beneficial effects of fasting and low carbohydrate diet in D-lactic acidosis associated with short-bowel syndrome. *JPEN J Parenter Enteral Nutr.* 1985 May-Jun;9(3):361-3

[76] Gottschall E. *Breaking the Vicious Cycle: Intestinal Health through Diet.* Kirkton Press; Rev edition (August 1, 1994)

[77] Lin HC. Small intestinal bacterial overgrowth: a framework for understanding irritable bowel syndrome. *JAMA.* 2004 Aug 18;292(7):852-8

[78] Lichtman et al. Reactivation of arthritis induced by small bowel bacterial overgrowth in rats. *Infect Immun.* 1995 Jun;63(6):2295-301

[79] Pimentel et al. A link between irritable bowel syndrome and fibromyalgia may be related to findings on lactulose breath testing. *Ann Rheum Dis.* 2004 Apr;63:450-2

[80] Bundgaard et al. Endotoxemia stimulates skeletal muscle Na+-K+-ATPase and raises blood lactate under aerobic conditions in humans. *Am J Physiol Heart Circ Physiol.* 2003 Mar;284(3):H1028-34 ajpheart.physiology.org/cgi/reprint/284/3/H1028

[81] "We propose that the additive and synergistic effects of phytochemicals in fruit and vegetables are responsible for their potent antioxidant and anticancer activities, and that the benefit of a diet rich in fruit and vegetables is attributed to the complex mixture of phytochemicals present in whole foods." Liu RH. Health benefits of fruit and vegetables are from additive and synergistic combinations of phytochemicals. *Am J Clin Nutr.* 2003 Sep;78(3 Suppl):517S-520S

[82] Seaman DR. The diet-induced proinflammatory state: a cause of chronic pain and other degenerative diseases? *J Manipulative Physiol Ther.* 2002;25(3):168-79

[83] "The immunoglobulin G (IgG) antibody levels against gliadin and beta-lactoglobulin decreased in the responder subgroup in the vegan diet-treated patients, but not in the other analysed groups." Hafstrom et al. A vegan diet free of gluten improves the signs and symptoms of rheumatoid arthritis: the effects on arthritis correlate with a reduction in antibodies to food antigens. *Rheumatology* (Oxford). 2001 Oct;40(10):1175-9 rheumatology.oxfordjournals.org/cgi/content/abstract/40/10/1175

[84] Grant EC. Food allergies and migraine. *Lancet.* 1979 May 5;1(8123):966-9

[85] "We report six patients with coeliac disease in whom arthritis was prominent at diagnosis and who improved with dietary therapy. Joint pain preceded diagnosis by up to three years in five patients and 15 years in one patient." Bourne et al. Arthritis and coeliac disease. *Ann Rheum Dis.* 1985 Sep;44(9):592-8

[86] "A 15-year-old girl, with synovitis of the knees and ankles for 3 years before a diagnosis of gluten-sensitive enteropathy, is described." Pinals RS. Arthritis associated with gluten-sensitive enteropathy. *J Rheumatol.* 1986 Feb;13(1):201-4

[87] "The immunoglobulin G (IgG) antibody levels against gliadin and beta-lactoglobulin decreased in the responder subgroup in the vegan diet-treated patients, but not in the other analysed groups." Hafstrom et al. A vegan diet free of gluten improves the signs and symptoms of rheumatoid arthritis: the effects on arthritis correlate with a reduction in antibodies to food antigens. *Rheumatology* (Oxford). 2001 Oct;40(10):1175-9 rheumatology.oxfordjournals.org/cgi/content/abstract/40/10/1175

[88] "After four weeks at the health farm the diet group showed a significant improvement in number of tender joints, Ritchie's articular index, number of swollen joints, pain score, duration of morning stiffness, grip strength, erythrocyte sedimentation rate, C-reactive protein, white blood cell count, and a health assessment questionnaire score." Kjeldsen-Kragh et al. Controlled trial of fasting and one-year vegetarian diet in rheumatoid arthritis. *Lancet.* 1991 Oct 12;338(8772):899-902

[89] "During fasting, arthralgia was less intense in many subjects. In some types of skin diseases (pustulosis palmaris et plantaris and atopic eczema) an improvement could be demonstrated during the fast. During the vegan diet, both signs and symptoms returned in most patients, with the exception of some patients with psoriasis who experienced an improvement." Lithell et al. A fasting and vegetarian diet treatment trial on chronic inflammatory disorders. *Acta Derm Venereol.* 1983;63(5):397-403

[90] Tanaka et al. Vegetarian diet ameliorates symptoms of atopic dermatitis through reduction of the number of peripheral eosinophils and of PGE2 synthesis by monocytes. *J Physiol Anthropol Appl Human Sci.* 2001 Nov;20(6):353-61 jstage.jst.go.jp/article/jpa/20/6/20_353/_article/-char/en

[91] "For the patients who were randomised to the vegetarian diet there was a significant decrease in platelet count, leukocyte count, calprotectin, total IgG, IgM rheumatoid factor (RF), C3-activation products, and the complement components C3 and C4 after one month of treatment." Kjeldsen-Kragh J, Mellbye OJ, Haugen M, Mollnes TE, Hammer HB, Sioud M, Forre O. Changes in laboratory variables in rheumatoid arthritis patients during a trial of fasting and one-year vegetarian diet. *Scand J Rheumatol.* 1995;24(2):85-93

[92] Rusyn et al. Corn oil rapidly activates nuclear factor-kappaB in hepatic Kupffer cells by oxidant-dependent mechanisms. *Carcinogenesis.* 1999 Nov;20(11):2095-100

arachidonic acids[93], iron[94], common food antigens[95], gluten[96] and gliadin[97,98], pro-inflammatory sugars[99] and increased intake of omega-3 fatty acids, micronutrients[100], and anti-inflammatory and antioxidant phytonutrients.[101] Vegetarian diets also effect subtle yet biologically and clinically important changes—both *qualitative* and *quantitative*—in intestinal flora[102,103] that correlate with clinical improvement.[104] Patients who rely on the Paleo-Mediterranean diet (which is inherently omnivorous) can use vegetarian *meals* on a daily basis or for days at a time—for example, by having a daily vegetarian meal, or one week per month of vegetarianism. Some (not all) patients can use a purely vegetarian diet long-term provided that nutritional needs (especially protein and cobalamin) are consistently met.

o Routine carbohydrate restriction, periodic short-term fasting: Whether the foundational diet is Paleo-Mediterranean, vegetarian, vegan, or a combination of all of these, autoimmune/inflammatory patients will still benefit from periodic fasting, whether on a weekly (e.g., every Saturday), monthly (every first week or weekend of the month, or every other month), or yearly (1-2 weeks of the year) basis. The diet should generally be low in carbohydrates in order to promote ketogenesis and to retard SIBO. Since consumption of food—particularly "unhealthy" (i.e., high-fat, high-sugar, allergenic, nutritionally depleted, AGE-laden) foods—induces an inflammatory effect[105], abstinence from food provides a relative anti-inflammatory effect. Fasting indeed provides a distinct anti-inflammatory benefit and may help "re-calibrate" metabolic and homeostatic mechanisms by breaking self-perpetuating "vicious cycles"[106] that autonomously promote inflammation independent of pro-inflammatory stimuli. Water-only fasting is completely hypoallergenic (assuming that the patient is not sensitive to chlorine, fluoride, or other contaminants), and subsequent re-introduction of foods provides the ideal opportunity to identify offending foods. Fasting deprives intestinal microbes of substrate[107], stimulates intestinal B-cell immunity[108], improves the bactericidal action of neutrophils[109], reduces lysozyme release and leukotriene formation[110], and ameliorates intestinal hyperpermeability.[111] Fasting and carbohydrate avoidance also promote endogenous production of beta-hydroxybutyrate (bHB) which promotes histone acetylation for induction of a rejuvenative phenotype while bHB also stimulates complexes 3 and 4 of the mitochondrial

[93] Vasquez A. New Insights into Fatty Acid Supplementation and Its Effect on Eicosanoid Production and Genetic Expression. *Nutritional Perspectives* 2005; January: 5-16

[94] Dabbagh AJ, Trenam CW, Morris CJ, Blake DR. Iron in joint inflammation. *Ann Rheum Dis.* 1993 Jan;52(1):67-73

[95] Hafstrom et al. A vegan diet free of gluten improves the signs and symptoms of rheumatoid arthritis: the effects on arthritis correlate with a reduction in antibodies to food antigens. *Rheumatology* (Oxford). 2001 Oct;40(10):1175-9 rheumatology.oxfordjournals.org/cgi/reprint/40/10/1175

[96] "The data provide evidence that dietary modification may be of clinical benefit for certain RA patients, and that this benefit may be related to a reduction in immunoreactivity to food antigens eliminated by the change in diet." Hafstrom I, Ringertz B, et al. A vegan diet free of gluten improves the signs and symptoms of rheumatoid arthritis: the effects on arthritis correlate with a reduction in antibodies to food antigens. *Rheumatology* (Oxford). 2001 Oct;40(10):1175-9

[97] "Despite the increased AGA [antigliadin antibodies] positivity found distinctively in patients with recent-onset RA, none of the RA patients showed clear evidence of coeliac disease." Paimela L, Kurki P, Leirisalo-Repo M, Piirainen H. Gliadin immune reactivity in patients with rheumatoid arthritis. Clin Exp Rheumatol. 1995 Sep-Oct;13(5):603-7

[98] "The median IgA antigliadin ELISA index was 7.1 (range 2.1-22.4) for the RA group and 3.1 (range 0.3-34.9) for the controls (p = 0.0001)." Koot et al. Elevated level of IgA gliadin antibodies in patients with rheumatoid arthritis. *Clin Exp Rheumatol.* 1989 Nov-Dec;7(6):623-6

[99] Seaman DR. The diet-induced proinflammatory state: a cause of chronic pain and other degenerative diseases? *J Manipulative Physiol Ther.* 2002 Mar-Apr;25(3):168-79

[100] Hagfors L, Nilsson I, Skoldstam L, Johansson G. Fat intake and composition of fatty acids in serum phospholipids in a randomized, controlled, Mediterranean dietary intervention study on patients with rheumatoid arthritis. *Nutr Metab* (Lond). 2005 Oct 10;2:26 nutritionandmetabolism.com/content/2/1/26

[101] Liu. Health benefits of fruit and vegetables from additive and synergistic combinations of phytochemicals. *Am J Clin Nutr* 2003:517S-520S ajcn.org/cgi/content/full/78/3/517S

[102] "Significant alteration in the intestinal flora was observed when the patients changed from omnivorous to vegan diet. ... This finding of an association between intestinal flora and disease activity may have implications for our understanding of how diet can affect RA." Peltonen et al. Changes of faecal flora in rheumatoid arthritis during fasting and one-year vegetarian diet. *Br J Rheumatol.* 1994 Jul;33(7):638-43

[103] Toivanen P, Eerola E. A vegan diet changes the intestinal flora. *Rheumatology* (Oxford). 2002 Aug;41(8):950-1 rheumatology.oxfordjournals.org/cgi/reprint/41/8/950

[104] "We conclude that a vegan diet changes the faecal microbial flora in RA patients, and changes in the faecal flora are associated with improvement in RA activity." Peltonen et al. Faecal microbial flora and disease activity in rheumatoid arthritis during a vegan diet. *Br J Rheumatol.* 1997 Jan;36(1):64-8 rheumatology.oxfordjournals.org/cgi/reprint/36/1/64

[105] Aljada et al. Increase in intranuclear nuclear factor kappaB and decrease in inhibitor kappaB in mononuclear cells after a mixed meal. *Am J Clin Nutr.* 2004 Apr;79(4):682-90

[106] "The ability of therapeutic fasts to break metabolic vicious cycles may also contribute to the efficacy of fasting in the treatment of type 2 diabetes and autoimmune disorders." McCarty MF. A preliminary fast may potentiate response to a subsequent low-salt, low-fat vegan diet in the management of hypertension - fasting as a strategy for breaking metabolic vicious cycles. *Med Hypotheses.* 2003 May;60(5):624-33

[107] Ramakrishnan et al. Beneficial effects of fasting and low carbohydrate diet in D-lactic acidosis associated with short-bowel syndrome. *JPEN J Parenter Enteral Nutr.* 1985 May-Jun;9(3):361-3

[108] Trollmo C, Verdrengh M, Tarkowski A. Fasting enhances mucosal antigen specific B cell responses in rheumatoid arthritis. *Ann Rheum Dis.* 1997 Feb;56(2):130-4

[109] "An association was found between improvement in inflammatory activity of the joints and enhancement of neutrophil bactericidal capacity. Fasting appears to improve the clinical status of patients with RA." Uden AM, Trang L, Venizelos N, Palmblad J. Neutrophil functions and clinical performance after total fasting in patients with rheumatoid arthritis. *Ann Rheum Dis.* 1983 Feb;42(1):45-51

[110] "We thus conclude that a reduced ability to generate cytotaxins, reduced release of enzyme, and reduced leukotriene formation from RA neutrophils, together with an altered fatty acid composition of membrane phospholipids, may be mechanisms for the decrease of inflammatory symptoms that results from fasting." Hafstrom et al. Effects of fasting on disease activity, neutrophil function, fatty acid composition, and leukotriene biosynthesis in patients with rheumatoid arthritis. *Arthritis Rheum.* 1988 May;31(5):585-92

[111] "The results indicate that, unlike lactovegetarian diet, fasting may ameliorate the disease activity and reduce both the intestinal and the non-intestinal permeability in rheumatoid arthritis." Sundqvist T, et al. Influence of fasting on intestinal permeability and disease activity in patients with rheumatoid arthritis. *Scand J Rheumatol.* 1982;11(1):33-8

electron transport chain (mETC) for enhanced mitochondrial function and efficiency. **In case reports and clinical trials, short-term fasting (or protein-sparing fasting) has been documented as safe and effective treatment for SLE[112], RA[113], and non-rheumatic diseases such as chronic severe hypertension[114], moderate hypertension[115], obesity[116,117], type-2 diabetes[118], and epilepsy.[119]**

- o <u>Broad-spectrum fatty acid therapy with ALA, EPA, DHA, GLA and oleic acid</u>: Fatty acid supplementation should be delivered in the form of combination therapy with ALA, GLA, DHA, and EPA. Given at doses of 3,000 – 9,000 mg per day, ALA from flaxseed oil has impressive anti-inflammatory benefits demonstrated by its ability to halve prostaglandin production in humans.[120] **Numerous studies have demonstrated the benefit of GLA in the treatment of rheumatoid arthritis when used at doses between 500 mg – 4,000 mg per day.[121,122] Fish oil provides EPA and DHA which have well-proven anti-inflammatory benefits in rheumatoid arthritis[123,124,125] and lupus.[126,127]** ALA, EPA, DHA, and GLA need to be provided in the form of supplements; when using high doses of therapeutic oils, *liquid* supplements that can be mixed in juice or a smoothie are generally more convenient and palatable than are *capsules*. For example, at the upper end of oral fatty acid administration, the patient may be consuming as much as one-quarter cup per day of fatty acid supplementation; this same dose administered in the form of pills would require at least 72 capsules to attain the equivalent doses of ALA, EPA, DHA, and GLA. Therapeutic amounts of oleic acid can be obtained from generous use of olive oil, preferably on fresh vegetables. Supplementation with polyunsaturated fatty acids warrants increased intake of antioxidants from diet, from fruit and vegetable juices, and from properly formulated supplements. Since patients with systemic inflammation are generally in a pro-oxidative state, consideration must be given to the timing and starting dose of fatty acid supplementation and the need for antioxidant protection; some patients should start with a low dose of fatty acid supplementation until inflammation and the hyperoxidative state have been reduced. Clinicians must realize that fatty acids are not clinically or biochemically interchangeable and that one fatty acid does not substitute for another; each of the health-promoting fatty acids—ALA, GLA, EPA, DHA, and oleic acid—must be supplied in order for its benefits to be obtained; imbalanced supplementation causes or exacerbates biochemical imbalances and produces suboptimal results.[128]
- o <u>Vitamin D3 supplementation with physiologic doses and/or tailored to serum 25(OH)D levels</u>: Vitamin D deficiency is common in the general population and is even more common in patients with chronic illness and chronic musculoskeletal pain.[129] Correction of vitamin D deficiency supports normal immune function against infection and provides a clinically significant anti-inflammatory[130] and analgesic benefit

[112] Fuhrman et al. Brief case reports of medically supervised water-only fasting associated with remission of autoimmune disease. *Altern Ther Health Med* 2002 Jul-Aug:112,110-1
[113] "Association was found between improvement in inflammatory activity of joints and enhancement of neutrophil bactericidal capacity. Fasting appears to improve the clinical status of patients with RA." Uden et al. Neutrophil functions and clinical performance after total fasting in patients with rheumatoid arthritis. *Ann Rheum Dis* 1983 Feb:45-51
[114] "The average reduction in blood pressure was 37/13 mm Hg, with the greatest decrease being observed for subjects with the most severe hypertension. Patients with stage 3 hypertension (those with systolic blood pressure greater than 180 mg Hg, diastolic blood pressure greater than 110 mm Hg, or both) had an average reduction of 60/17 mm Hg at the conclusion of treatment." Goldhamer A, Lisle D, Parpia B, Anderson SV, Campbell TC. Medically supervised water-only fasting in the treatment of hypertension. *J Manipulative Physiol Ther*. 2001 Jun;24(5):335-9 healthpromoting.com/335-339Goldhamer115263.QXD.pdf
[115] "RESULTS: Approximately 82% of the subjects achieved BP at or below 120/80 mm Hg by the end of the treatment program. The mean BP reduction was 20/7 mm Hg, with the greatest decrease being observed for subjects with the highest baseline BP." Goldhamer et al. Medically supervised water-only fasting in the treatment of borderline hypertension. *J Altern Complement Med*. 2002 Oct;8(5):643-50
[116] Vertes V, Genuth SM, Hazelton IM. Supplemented fasting as a large-scale outpatient program. *JAMA*. 1977 Nov 14;238(20):2151-3
[117] Bauman WA, et al. Early and long-term effects of acute caloric deprivation in obese diabetic patients. *Am J Med*. 1988 Jul;85(1):38-46
[118] Goldhamer AC. Initial cost of care results in medically supervised water-only fasting for treating high blood pressure and diabetes. *J Altern Complement Med*. 2002 Dec;8(6):696-7 healthpromoting.com/Articles/pdf/Study%2032.pdf
[119] "The ketogenic diet should be considered as alternative therapy for children with difficult-to-control seizures. It is more effective than many of the new anticonvulsant medications and is well tolerated by children and families when it is effective." Freeman JM, Vining EP, Pillas DJ, Pyzik PL, Casey JC, Kelly LM. The efficacy of the ketogenic diet-1998: a prospective evaluation of intervention in 150 children. *Pediatrics*. 1998 Dec;102(6):1358-63 pediatrics.aappublications.org/cgi/reprint/102/6/1358
[120] Adam et al. Effect of alpha-linolenic acid in human diet on linoleic acid metabolism and prostaglandin biosynthesis. *J Lipid Res*. 1986 Apr;27:421-6 jlr.org/cgi/reprint/27/4/421
[121] "Other results showed a significant reduction in morning stiffness with gamma-linolenic acid at 3 months and reduction in pain and articular index at 6 months with olive oil." Brzeski et al. Evening primrose oil in patients with rheumatoid arthritis and side-effects of non-steroidal anti-inflammatory drugs. *Br J Rheumatol*. 1991 Oct;30(5):370-2
[122] Rothman D, DeLuca P, Zurier RB. Botanical lipids: effects on inflammation, immune responses, and rheumatoid arthritis. *Semin Arthritis Rheum*. 1995 Oct;25(2):87-96
[123] Adam O, et al. Anti-inflammatory effects of a low arachidonic acid diet and fish oil in patients with rheumatoid arthritis. *Rheumatol Int*. 2003 Jan;23(1):27-36
[124] Lau CS, Morley KD, Belch JJ. Effects of fish oil supplementation on non-steroidal anti-inflammatory drug requirement in patients with mild rheumatoid arthritis--a double-blind placebo controlled study. *Br J Rheumatol*. 1993 Nov;32(11):982-9
[125] Kremer et al. Fish-oil fatty acid supplementation in active rheumatoid arthritis. A double-blinded, controlled, crossover study. *Ann Intern Med*. 1987 Apr;106(4):497-503
[126] Walton AJ, et al. Dietary fish oil and the severity of symptoms in patients with systemic lupus erythematosus. *Ann Rheum Dis*. 1991 Jul;50(7):463-6
[127] Duffy et al. The clinical effect of dietary supplementation with omega-3 fish oils and/or copper in systemic lupus erythematosus. *J Rheumatol*. 2004 Aug;31(8):1551-6
[128] Vasquez A. New Insights into Fatty Acid Supplementation and Its Effect on Eicosanoid Production and Genetic Expression. *Nutritional Perspectives* 2005; January: 5-16
[129] Plotnikoff GA, Quigley JM. Prevalence of severe hypovitaminosis D in patients with persistent, nonspecific musculoskeletal pain. *Mayo Clin Proc*. 2003 Dec;78(12):1463-70
[130] Timms PM, Mannan N, Hitman GA, Noonan K, Mills PG, Syndercombe-Court D, Aganna E, Price CP, Boucher BJ. Circulating MMP9, vitamin D and variation in the TIMP-1 response with VDR genotype: mechanisms for inflammatory damage in chronic disorders? *QJM*. 2002 Dec;95(12):787-96 qjmed.oxfordjournals.org/cgi/content/full/95/12/787

in patients with back pain[131] and limb pain.[132] Reasonable daily doses for children and adults are 1,000-2,000 and 4,000 IU, respectively.[133] Deficiency and response to treatment are monitored with serum 25(OH)vitamin D while safety is monitored with serum calcium; inflammatory granulomatous diseases and certain drugs such as hydrochlorothiazide greatly increase the propensity for hypercalcemia and warrant increment dosing and frequent monitoring of serum calcium. Vitamin D2 (ergocalciferol) is not a human nutrient and should not be used in clinical practice.

- **INFECTIONS & DYSBIOSIS: ❶ antimicrobial treatments, ❷ immunorestoration, ❸ immunotolerance via Treg induction** Essentially all autoimmune/rheumatic disorders are associated with microbial colonization and intolerance to same; the presence of persistent microbial colonization is *prima facie* evidence of immunosuppression. The eight areas of multifocal dysbiosis are: ❶ sinorespiratory, ❷ orodental, ❸ gastrointestinal, ❹ genitourinary, ❺ tissue/blood, ❻ dermal, ❼ environmental, and ❽ endomicrobial.

  - Gastrointestinal dysbiosis: **All patients with rheumatoid arthritis have gastrointestinal dysbiosis until proven otherwise by the combination of 1) three-sample comprehensive parasitology examinations performed by a specialty laboratory and 2) clinical response to at least two 2-4 week courses of broad-spectrum antimicrobial treatment.** Yeast, bacteria, and parasites are treated as indicated based on identification and sensitivity results from comprehensive parasitology assessments. Patients taking immunosuppressant drugs such as corticosteroids/prednisone have increased risk of intestinal bacterial overgrowth and translocation.[134,135] Dysbiotic loci should be investigated as discussed in Chapter 4.2.

    - Cell wall fragments from major residents of the human intestinal flora induce chronic arthritis in rats (*J Rheumatol* 1989 Aug[136]): "A single intraperitoneal injection of cell wall fragments from *Eubacterium aerofaciens* or *Bifidobacterium* species induced persistent chronic arthritis, in contrast to those from *Eubacterium rectale*, *Clostridium* species and *Lactobacillus leichmanii*. The results show that cell wall fragments of major residents from the human fecal flora can induce chronic arthritis in the rat and support the hypothesis that normal human intestinal flora plays a role in the induction of arthritis in man."

    - Normal intestinal microbiota in the etiopathogenesis of rheumatoid arthritis (*Ann Rheum Dis* 2003 Sep[137]): The ability of bacterial cell walls to induce chronic, erosive arthritis was first described in the rat by using *Streptococcus pyogenes*. Self-perpetuating arthritis, closely resembling human rheumatoid arthritis by histological criteria, develops in susceptible rat strains after a single intraperitoneal injection of the bacterial cell wall. In addition to *Streptococcus pyogenes*, several bacterial species representing *Lactobacillus*, *Bifidobacterium*, *Eubacterium*, *Collinsella*, and *Clostridium* have been observed to have a similar ability.

  - Orodental dysbiosis: The systemic inflammatory response triggered by subclinical oral/dental "infections" is now believed to exacerbate conditions associated with inflammation, such as cardiovascular disease and diabetes mellitus.[138] Patients with RA have heightened antibody levels against common oral bacteria. IgG levels against *Porphyromonas gingivalis*, *Prevotella melaninogenica*, *Bacteroides forsythus*, and *Prevotella intermedia* were found to be significantly higher in RA patients when compared with those of controls.[139] In the first human clinical trial to test the hypothesis that treatment of orodental dysbiosis would provide subjective and objective clinical benefits for patients with RA, AlKatma et al[140] showed that **periodontal treatment consisting of scaling/root planing and oral hygiene instruction reduced symptom scores and ESR levels in patients with RA.**

[131] Al Faraj S, Al Mutairi K. Vitamin D deficiency and chronic low back pain in Saudi Arabia. *Spine*. 2003 Jan 15;28(2):177-9
[132] Masood et al. Persistent limb pain and raised serum alkaline phosphatase earliest markers of subclinical hypovitaminosis D. *Indian J Physiol Pharmacol*. 1989 Oct-Dec; 259-61
[133] Vasquez et al. Clinical importance of vitamin D: paradigm shift for all healthcare providers. *Altern Ther Health Med*. 2004 Sep;10(5):28-36 ichnfm.academia.edu/AlexVasquez
[134] "A 63-year-old man with systemic lupus erythematosus and selective IgA deficiency developed intractable diarrhoea the day after treatment with prednisone, 50 mg daily, was started. The diarrhoea was considered to be caused by bacterial overgrowth and was later successfully treated with doxycycline." Denison H, Wallerstedt S. Bacterial overgrowth after high-dose corticosteroid treatment. *Scand J Gastroenterol*. 1989 Jun;24(5):561-4
[135] "These bacteria also translocated to the mesenteric lymph nodes in mice injected with cyclophosphamide or prednisone." Berg RD, Wommack E, Deitch EA. Immunosuppression and intestinal bacterial overgrowth synergistically promote bacterial translocation. *Arch Surg*. 1988 Nov;123(11):1359-64
[136] Severijnen AJ, et al. Cell wall fragments from major residents of the human intestinal flora induce chronic arthritis in rats. *J Rheumatol*. 1989 Aug;16(8):1061-8
[137] Toivanen P. Normal intestinal microbiota in the aetiopathogenesis of rheumatoid arthritis. *Ann Rheum Dis*. 2003 Sep;62(9):807-11
[138] Amar S, Han X. The impact of periodontal infection on systemic diseases. *Med Sci Monit*. 2003 Dec;9(12):RA291-9 medscimonit.com/pub/vol_9/no_12/3776.pdf
[139] Ogrendik M, Kokino S, Ozdemir F, Bird PS, Hamlet S. Serum antibodies to oral anaerobic bacteria in patients with rheumatoid arthritis. *MedGenMed*. 2005 Jun 16;7(2):2
[140] "There was a statistically significant difference in DAS28 (4.3 +/- 1.6 vs. 5.1 +/- 1.2) and erythrocyte sedimentation rate (31.4 +/- 24.3 vs. 42.7 +/- 22) between the treatment and the control groups." Al-Katma MK, et al. Control of periodontal infection reduces the severity of active rheumatoid arthritis. *J Clin Rheumatol*. 2007 Jun;13(3):134-7

- Genitourinary dysbiosis: Microbial contamination of the genitourinary tract can cause a systemic pro-inflammatory arthritogenic response in susceptible individuals; **in a study of 234 patients with inflammatory arthritis, 44% of patients had subclinical genitourinary colonization, mostly due to *Chlamydia, Mycoplasma*, or *Ureaplasma*.**[141]

- **NUTRITIONAL IMMUNOMODULATION: Treg induction for modulation of Th-1/2/17 inflammation** Nutrients and therapeutic approaches that promote Treg or IL-10 induction and/or Th-17, IL-17 suppression include 1) mitochondrial optimization and mTOR suppression, 2) biotin, 3) vitamin E, 4) sodium avoidance, 5) transgenic/GMO food avoidance, 6) probiotics, 7) lipoic acid, 8) vitamin A, 9) inflammation reduction, 10) vitamin D, 11) fatty acid supplementation with GLA and n3, 12) infection and dysbiosis remediation, 13) green tea EGCG. Acronym: MiBESTPLAIDFIG, as detailed and substantiated in Chapter 4.

- **DYSMETABOLISM & DYSFUNCTIONAL MITOCHONDRIA: MitoDys, ERS-UPR, AGE/RAGE, hyperglycemia and ceramide** The major clinical considerations in this section are mitochondrial dysfunction, endoplasmic reticulum stress, unfolded protein response, TLR activation, and the dysmetabolic effects of sustained hyperglycemia and hyperinsulinemia and resultant oxidative stress, inflammation, RAGE activation, and accumulation of AGE, palmitate and ceramide. The review of this information in Chapter 4 covered approximately 30 interventions relevant to dysmetabolism, mitochondrial dysfunction, ERS-UPR, etc; these will not be reviewed here except to mention those most commonly, easily, empirically, synergistically, and effectively used: 1) low-carbohydrate diet with 2) moderate exercise, 3) CoQ-10, 4) acetyl-carnitine with 5) lipoic acid, 6) NAC, 7) resveratrol, and 8) melatonin.

- **STYLE OF LIVING (LIFESTYLE) & SPECIAL CONSIDERATIONS: S**leep optimization, **S**ocioPsychology, **S**tress management/avoidance, **S**omatic treatments, **S**pecial **S**upplementation, **S**weat/exercise, **S**auna/detoxification, **S**urgery, **S**tamp your passport and vacate current reality, **S**ensory deprivation therapy This is a buffet of mostly lifestyle-based interventions yet also including considerations such as somatic treatments, additional supplementation, and surgery.

  - Self-expression and therapeutic writing: Limited evidence indicates that self-expressive writing can significantly reduce symptomatology in patients with RA.[142]

- **ENDOCRINE IMBALANCE & OPTIMIZATION: Prolactin, Insulin, Estrogen, DHEA, Cortisol, Testosterone, Thyroid** Common hormonal imbalances seen among autoimmune/inflammatory patients are: ❶ *elevated* prolactin, ❷ *elevated* estrogen, ❸ *elevated* insulin, and ❹ *reduced* DHEA, ❺ *reduced* cortisol, and ❻ *reduced* testosterone; see Chapter 4 for discussion of these hormones and respective interventions. Thyroid evaluation (patient + labs) should be comprehensive, as discussed in Chapter 1, with a low threshold for empiric treatment.

  - Estradiol: Men with rheumatoid arthritis show an excess of estradiol and a decrease in DHEA, and the excess estrogen is proportional to the degree of inflammation.[143]

  - Testosterone (insufficiency): Androgen deficiencies predispose to, are exacerbated by, and contribute to autoimmune/inflammatory disorders. **A large proportion of men with SLE or RA have low testosterone**[144,145] and suffer the effects of hypogonadism: fatigue, weakness, depression, slow healing, low libido, and difficulties with sexual performance. Testosterone levels may rise following DHEA

---

[141] "Urogenital swab cultures showed a microbial infection in 44% of the patients with oligoarthritis (15% Chlamydia, 14% Mycoplasma, 28% Ureaplasma), whereas in the control group only 26% had a positive result (4% Chlamydia, 7% Mycoplasma, 21% Ureaplasma)." Erlacher et al. Reactive arthritis: urogenital swab culture is the only useful diagnostic method for the detection of the arthritogenic infection in extra-articularly asymptomatic patients with undifferentiated oligoarthritis. *Br J Rheumatol*. 1995 Sep;34(9):838-42

[142] "Rheumatoid arthritis patients in the experimental group showed improvements in overall disease activity (a mean reduction in disease severity from 1.65 to 1.19 [28%] on a scale of 0 [asymptomatic] to 4 [very severe] at the 4-month follow-up; P=.001), whereas control group patients did not change." Smyth JM, Stone AA, Hurewitz A, Kaell A. Effects of writing about stressful experiences on symptom reduction in patients with asthma or rheumatoid arthritis: a randomized trial. *JAMA*. 1999 Apr 14;281(14):1304-9

[143] "RESULTS: DHEAS and estrone concentrations were lower and estradiol was higher in patients compared with healthy controls. DHEAS differed between RF positive and RF negative patients. Estrone did not correlate with any disease variable, whereas estradiol correlated strongly and positively with all measured indices of inflammation." Tengstrand B, Carlstrom K, Fellander-Tsai L, Hafstrom I. Abnormal levels of serum dehydroepiandrosterone, estrone, and estradiol in men with rheumatoid arthritis: high correlation between serum estradiol and current degree of inflammation. *J Rheumatol*. 2003 Nov;30(11):2338-43

[144] Karagiannis A, Harsoulis F. Gonadal dysfunction in systemic diseases. *Eur J Endocrinol*. 2005 Apr;152(4):501-13 eje-online.org/cgi/content/full/152/4/501

[145] "...patients with rheumatoid arthritis showed significantly lower serum testosterone and derived free testosterone concentrations and significantly higher serum LH and FSH concentrations compared with controls." Gordon et al. Androgenic status and sexual function in men with rheumatoid arthritis and ankylosing spondylitis. *Q J Med* 1986 Jul;671-9

supplementation (especially in women) and can be elevated in men by the use of anastrozole/Arimidex. Transdermal testosterone such as Androgel, Testim, or compounded formula can be applied as indicated.

- o DHEA (insufficiency / supraphysiologic supplementation): DHEA is an anti-inflammatory and immunoregulatory hormone that is commonly deficient in patients with autoimmunity and inflammatory arthritis.[146] DHEA levels are suppressed by prednisone[147], and DHEA supplementation has been shown to reverse the osteoporosis and loss of bone mass induced by corticosteroid treatment.[148] DHEA shows no acute or subacute toxicity even when used in supraphysiologic doses, even when used in sick patients. For example, in a study of 32 patients with HIV, DHEA doses of 750 mg – 2,250 mg per day were well-tolerated and produced no dose-limiting adverse effects.[149] This lack of toxicity compares favorably with any and all so-called "antirheumatic" drugs, nearly all of which show impressive comparable toxicity. **When used at doses of 200 mg per day, DHEA safely provides clinical benefit for patients with various autoimmune diseases, including ulcerative colitis, Crohn's disease[150], and SLE.[151]** In patients with SLE, DHEA supplementation allows for reduced dosing of prednisone (thus avoiding its adverse effects) while providing symptomatic improvement.[152] Optimal clinical response appears to correlate with serum levels that are supraphysiologic[153], and therefore treatment may be implemented with little regard for initial/baseline DHEA levels provided that the patient is free of contraindications, particularly high risk for sex-hormone-dependent malignancy. Other than mild adverse effects predictable with any androgen (namely voice deepening, transient acne, and increased facial hair), DHEA supplementation does not cause serious adverse effects[154], and it is appropriate for routine clinical use particularly when 1) the dose of DHEA is kept as low as possible, 2) duration is kept as short as possible, 3) other interventions are used to address the underlying cause of the disease, 4) the patient is deriving benefit, and 5) the risk-to-benefit ratio is favorable. Astute clinicians should anticipate that DHEA supplementation can increase testosterone and estradiol levels—the former with benefit and the latter with detriment in patients with autoimmunity; thus, serum levels of DHEA, testosterone, and estradiol (and potentially other estrogen metabolites) need to be reevaluated if DHEA is added to the daily regimen. Commonly, rheumatic patients will show an increase in estradiol following use of DHEA, and these over-producers of estrogen ("rapid converters") should be co-treated with an aromatase inhibitor if DHEA supplementation elevates estrogen levels, especially if testosterone levels are low.

- o Prolactin and antiprolactin treatments: Patients with RA and SLE have higher basal and stress-induced levels of prolactin compared with normal controls.[155,156] Men with RA have higher serum levels of prolactin, and these levels correlate with the severity and duration of the disorder.[157,158] Serum prolactin

---

[146] "DHEAS concentrations were significantly decreased in both women and men with inflammatory arthritis (IA) (P < 0.001)." Dessein et al. Hyposecretion of the adrenal androgen dehydroepiandrosterone sulfate and its relation to clinical variables in inflammatory arthritis. *Arthritis Res.* 2001;3(3):183-8 arthritis-research.com/content/3/3/183

[147] "Basal serum DHEA and DHEAS concentrations were suppressed to a greater degree than was cortisol during both daily and alternate day prednisone treatments. ...Thus, adrenal androgen secretion was more easily suppressed than was cortisol secretion by this low dose of glucocorticoid, but there was no advantage to alternate day therapy." Rittmaster et al. Effect of daily and alternate day low dose prednisone on serum cortisol and adrenal androgens in hirsute women. *J Clin Endocrinol Metab.* 1988 Aug;67(2):400-3

[148] "CONCLUSION: Prasterone treatment prevented BMD loss and significantly increased BMD at both the lumbar spine and total hip in female patients with SLE receiving exogenous glucocorticoids." Mease PJ, Ginzler EM, Gluck OS, Schiff M, Goldman A, Greenwald M, Cohen S, Egan R, Quarles BJ, Schwartz KE. Effects of prasterone on bone mineral density in women with systemic lupus erythematosus receiving chronic glucocorticoid therapy. *J Rheumatol.* 2005 Apr;32(4):616-21

[149] "Thirty-one subjects were evaluated and monitored for safety and tolerance. The oral drug was administered three times daily in doses ranging from 750 mg/day to 2,250 mg/day for 16 weeks. ... The drug was well tolerated and no dose-limiting side effects were noted." Dyner TS, Lang W, Geaga J, et al. An open-label dose-escalation trial of oral dehydroepiandrosterone tolerance and pharmacokinetics in patients with HIV disease. *J Acquir Immune Defic Syndr.* 1993 May;6(5):459-65

[150] "CONCLUSIONS: In a pilot study, dehydroepiandrosterone was effective and safe in patients with refractory Crohn's disease or ulcerative colitis." Andus T, et al. Patients with refractory Crohn's disease or ulcerative colitis respond to dehydroepiandrosterone: a pilot study. *Aliment Pharmacol Ther.* 2003 Feb;17(3):409-14

[151] "CONCLUSION: The overall results confirm that DHEA treatment was well-tolerated, significantly reduced the number of SLE flares, and improved patient's global assessment of disease activity." Chang DM, Lan JL, Lin HY, Luo SF. Dehydroepiandrosterone treatment of women with mild-to-moderate systemic lupus erythematosus: a multicenter randomized, double-blind, placebo-controlled trial. *Arthritis Rheum.* 2002 Nov;46(11):2924-7

[152] "CONCLUSION: Among women with lupus disease activity, reducing the dosage of prednisone to < or = 7.5 mg/day for a sustained period of time while maintaining stabilization or a reduction of disease activity was possible in a significantly greater proportion of patients treated with oral prasterone, 200 mg once daily, compared with patients treated with placebo." Petri et al. Effects of prasterone on corticosteroid requirements of women with systemic lupus erythematosus. *Arthritis Rheum.* 2002 Jul;46(7):1820-9

[153] "CONCLUSION: The clinical response to DHEA was not clearly dose dependent. Serum levels of DHEA and DHEAS correlated only weakly with lupus outcomes, but suggested an optimum serum DHEAS of 1000 microg/dl." Barry NN, McGuire JL, van Vollenhoven RF. Dehydroepiandrosterone in systemic lupus erythematosus: relationship between dosage, serum levels, and clinical response. *J Rheumatol.* 1998 Dec;25(12):2352-6

[154] Tierney ML. McPhee SJ, Papadakis MA. *Current Medical Diagnosis and Treatment 2006. 45th edition.* New York: Lange Medical Books: 2006, page 1721

[155] Dostal et al. Serum prolactin stress values in patients with systemic lupus erythematosus. *Ann Rheum Dis.* 2003 May;62(5):487-8 ard.bmjjournals.com/cgi/content/full/62/5/487

[156] "RESULTS: A significantly higher rate of elevated PRL levels was found in SLE patients (40.0%) compared with the healthy controls (14.8%). No proof was found of association with the presence of anti-ds-DNA or with specific organ involvement. Similarly, elevated PRL levels were found in RA patients (39.3%)." Moszkorzova L, Lacinova Z, Marek J, Musilova L, Dohnalova A, Dostal C. Hyperprolactinaemia in patients with systemic lupus erythematosus. *Clin Exp Rheumatol.* 2002 Nov-Dec;20(6):807-12

[157] "CONCLUSION: Men with RA have high serum PRL levels and concentrations increase with longer disease evolution and worse functional stage." Mateo L, Nolla JM, Bonnin MR, Navarro MA, Roig-Escofet D. High serum prolactin levels in men with rheumatoid arthritis. *J Rheumatol.* 1998 Nov;25(11):2077-82

[158] "Male patients affected by RA showed high serum PRL levels. The serum PRL concentration was found to be increased in relation to the duration and the activity of the disease. Serum PRL levels do not seem to have any relationship with the BMD, at least in RA." Seriolo B, Ferretti V, Sulli A, Fasciolo D, Cutolo M. Serum prolactin concentrations in male patients with rheumatoid arthritis. *Ann N Y Acad Sci.* 2002 Jun;966:258-62

is the standard assessment of prolactin status. Since elevated prolactin may be a sign of pituitary tumor, assessment for headaches, visual deficits, and other abnormalities of pituitary hormones (e.g., GH and TSH) should be performed; CT or MRI must be considered. Patients with prolactin levels less than 100 ng/mL and normal CT/MRI findings can be managed conservatively with effective prolactin-lowering treatment and annual radiologic assessment (less necessary with favorable serum response).[159, see review 160] Specific treatment options include the following:

- Thyroid hormone: Hypothyroidism frequently causes hyperprolactinemia which is reversible upon effective treatment of hypothyroidism. Obviously therefore, thyroid status should be evaluated in all patients with hyperprolactinemia. Thyroid assessment and treatment is reviewed in Chapter 4 and later in this section.

- *Vitex astus-cagnus* and other supporting botanicals and nutrients: **Vitex lowers serum prolactin in humans**[161,162] **via a dopaminergic effect.**[163] Vitex is considered safe for clinical use; mild and reversible adverse effects possibly associated with Vitex include nausea, headache, gastrointestinal disturbances, menstrual disorders, acne, pruritus and erythematous rash. No drug interactions are known, but given the herb's dopaminergic effect it should probably be used with some caution in patients treated with dopamine antagonists such as the so-called antipsychotic drugs.[164,165] Bone[166] stated that daily doses can range from 500 mg to 2,000 mg DHE (dry herb equivalent) and can be tailored to the suppression of prolactin. Due at least in part to its content of L-dopa, *Mucuna pruriens* **shows clinical dopaminergic activity** as evidenced by its effectiveness in Parkinson's disease[167]; up to 15-30 gm/d of mucuna has been used clinically but doses will be dependent on preparation and phytoconcentration. **Triptolide and other extracts from *Tripterygium wilfordii* Hook F exert clinically significant anti-inflammatory action in patients with rheumatoid arthritis**[168,169] **and also offer protection to dopaminergic neurons.**[170,171] Ironically, even though tyrosine is the nutritional precursor to dopamine with evidence of clinical effectiveness (e.g., narcolepsy[172], enhancement of memory[173] and cognition[174]), **supplementation with tyrosine appears to actually increase rather**

[159] Beers MH, Berkow R (eds). *Merck Manual. 17ᵗʰ Edition*. Whitehouse Station; Merck Research Laboratories 1999 Page 77-78

[160] Serri O, Chik CL, Ur E, Ezzat S. Diagnosis and management of hyperprolactinemia. *CMAJ*. 2003 Sep 16;169(6):575-81 cmaj.ca/cgi/content/full/169/6/575

[161] "Since AC extracts were shown to have beneficial effects on premenstrual mastodynia serum prolactin levels in such patients were also studied in one double-blind, placebo-controlled clinical study. Serum prolactin levels were indeed reduced in the patients treated with the extract." Wuttke W, Jarry H, Christoffel V, Spengler B, Seidlova-Wuttke D. Chaste tree (Vitex agnus-castus)--pharmacology and clinical indications. *Phytomedicine*. 2003 May;10(4):348-57

[162] German abstract from Medline: "The prolactin release was reduced after 3 months, shortened luteal phases were normalised and deficits in the luteal progesterone synthesis were eliminated." Milewicz A, Gejdel E, Sworen H, Sienkiewicz K, Jedrzejak J, Teucher T, Schmitz H. [Vitex agnus castus extract in the treatment of luteal phase defects due to latent hyperprolactinemia. Results of a randomized placebo-controlled double-blind study] *Arzneimittelforschung*. 1993 Jul;43(7):752-6

[163] "Our results indicate a dopaminergic effect of Vitex agnus-castus extracts and suggest additional pharmacological actions via opioid receptors." Meier B, Berger D, Hoberg E, Sticher O, Schaffner W. Pharmacological activities of Vitex agnus-castus extracts in vitro. *Phytomedicine*. 2000 Oct;7(5):373-81

[164] "The majority of patients in each group discontinued their assigned treatment owing to inefficacy or intolerable side effects or for other reasons." Lieberman JA, Stroup TS, McEvoy JP, Swartz MS, Rosenheck RA, Perkins DO, Keefe RS, Davis SM, Davis CE, Lebowitz BD, Severe J, Hsiao JK; Clinical Antipsychotic Trials of Intervention Effectiveness (CATIE) Investigators. Effectiveness of antipsychotic drugs in patients with chronic schizophrenia. *N Engl J Med*. 2005 Sep 22;353(12):1209-23

[165] Whitaker R. The case against antipsychotic drugs: a 50-year record of doing more harm than good. *Med Hypotheses*. 2004;62(1):5-13

[166] "In conditions such as endometriosis and fibroids, for which a significant estrogen antagonist effect is needed, doses of at least 2 g/day DHE may be required and typically are used by professional herbalists." Bone K. New Insights into Chaste Tree. *Nutritional Wellness* 2005 November nutritionalwellness.com/archives/2005/nov/11_bone.php

[167] "CONCLUSIONS: The rapid onset of action and longer on time without concomitant increase in dyskinesias on mucuna seed powder formulation suggest that this natural source of L-dopa might possess advantages over conventional L-dopa preparations in the long term management of PD." Katzenschlager R, et al. Mucuna pruriens in Parkinson's disease: a double blind clinical and pharmacological study. *J Neurol Neurosurg Psychiatry*. 2004 Dec;75(12):1672-7

[168] "The ethanol/ethyl acetate extract of TWHF shows therapeutic benefit in patients with treatment-refractory RA. At therapeutic dosages, the TWHF extract was well tolerated by most patients in this study." Tao X, Younger J, Fan FZ, Wang B, Lipsky PE. Benefit of an extract of Tripterygium Wilfordii Hook F in patients with rheumatoid arthritis: a double-blind, placebo-controlled study. *Arthritis Rheum*. 2002 Jul;46(7):1735-43

[169] "The EA extract of TWHF at dosages up to 570 mg/day appeared to be safe, and doses > 360 mg/day were associated with clinical benefit in patients with RA." Tao et al. A phase I study of ethyl acetate extract of the Chinese antirheumatic herb Tripterygium wilfordii hook F in rheumatoid arthritis. *J Rheumatol*. 2001 Oct;28(10):2160-7

[170] "Our data suggests that triptolide may protect dopaminergic neurons from LPS-induced injury and its efficiency in inhibiting microglia activation may underlie the mechanism." Li et al. Triptolide, a Chinese herbal extract, protects dopaminergic neurons from inflammation-mediated damage through inhibition of microglial activation. *J Neuroimmunol*. 2004 Mar;148(1-2):24-31

[171] "Moreover, tripchlorolide markedly prevented the decrease in amount of dopamine in the striatum of model rats. Taken together, our data provide the first evidence that tripchlorolide acts as a neuroprotective molecule that rescues MPP+ or axotomy-induced degeneration of dopaminergic neurons, which may imply its therapeutic potential for Parkinson's disease." Li FQ, Cheng et al. Neurotrophic and neuroprotective effects of tripchlorolide, an extract of Chinese herb Tripterygium wilfordii Hook F, on dopaminergic neurons. *Exp Neurol*. 2003 Jan;179(1):28-37

[172] "Of twenty-eight visual analogue scales rating mood and arousal, the subjects' ratings in the tyrosine treatment (9 g daily) and placebo periods differed significantly for only three (less tired, less drowsy, more alert)." Elwes et al. Treatment of narcolepsy with L-tyrosine: double-blind placebo-controlled trial. *Lancet*. 1989 Nov 4;2(8671):1067-9

[173] "Ten men and 10 women subjects underwent these batteries 1 h after ingesting 150 mg/kg of l-tyrosine or placebo. Administration of tyrosine significantly enhanced accuracy and decreased frequency of list retrieval on the working memory task during the multiple task battery compared with placebo." Thomas JR, Lockwood PA, Singh A, Deuster PA. Tyrosine improves working memory in a multitasking environment. *Pharmacol Biochem Behav*. 1999 Nov;64(3):495-500

[174] "Ten subjects received five daily doses of a protein-rich drink containing 2 g tyrosine, and 11 subjects received a carbohydrate rich drink with the same amount of calories (255 kcal)." Deijen et al. Tyrosine improves cognitive performance and reduces blood pressure in cadets after one week of a combat training course. *Brain Res Bull*. 1999 Jan 15;48(2):203-9

than decrease prolactin levels[175]; therefore tyrosine should be used cautiously (if at all) in patients with systemic inflammation and elevated prolactin. Furthermore, the finding that **high-protein meals stimulate prolactin release**[176] may partly explain the benefits of vegetarian diets in the treatment of systemic inflammation; since vegetarian diets are comparatively low in protein compared to omnivorous diets, they may lead to a relative reduction in prolactin production due to lack of protein-induced prolactin stimulation.

- Bromocriptine: Bromocriptine has long been considered the pharmacologic treatment of choice for elevated prolactin.[177] Typical dose is 2.5 mg per day (effective against lupus[178]); gastrointestinal upset and sedation are common.[179] Clinical intervention with bromocriptine appears warranted in patients with RA, SLE, reactive arthritis, psoriatic arthritis, and probably multiple sclerosis and uveitis.[180] Data supporting bromocriptine vicariously supports cabergoline, the preferred agent.

- Cabergoline/Dostinex: Cabergoline/Dostinex is a newer dopamine agonist with few adverse effects; typical dose starts at 0.5 mg per week (0.25 mg twice per week).[181] Several studies have indicated that cabergoline is safer and more effective than bromocriptine for reducing prolactin levels[182] and the dose can often be reduced after successful prolactin reduction, allowing for reductions in cost and adverse effects.[183] Although fewer studies have been published supporting the antirheumatic benefits of cabergoline than bromocriptine, its antirheumatic benefits have been documented in a case report of a patient with unremitting RA[184] and more recently in a controlled trial.[185]

- | **XENOBIOTIC ACCUMULATION & DETOXIFICATION: Chemical avoidance, nutritional support for detoxification pathways, urine alkalinization** | The clinical relevance and pathogenic mechanisms of xenobiotic accumulation are irrefutably well documented and described. Clinical assessments include history, physical examination, and laboratory assessment (using serum, whole blood, urine or—rarely yet accurately—fat biopsy), and response to treatment. Treatments include nutritional support for Phases 1 and 2 of detoxification (e.g., oxidation and conjugation) and excretion via bile and urine; for the latter, urinary alkalinization is generally recommended. Chemical toxins can be bound in the gut using activated charcoal, cholestyramine, or *Chlorella*—all of these three treatments have documented safety and effectiveness for promoting removal/clearance of chemical xenobiotics. Clinically and empirically, phytochelatin (plant-derived peptides that bind toxic metals) concentrates appear safe and effective despite lack of conclusive published data supporting clinical use.

---

[175] "Tyrosine (when compared to placebo) had no effect on any sleep related measure, but it did stimulate prolactin release." Waters et al. A comparison of tyrosine against placebo, phentermine, caffeine, and D-amphetamine during sleep deprivation. *Nutr Neurosci.* 2003;6(4):221-35

[176] "Whereas carbohydrate meals had no discernible effects, high protein meals induced a large increase in both PRL and cortisol; high fat meals caused selective release of PRL." Ishizuka et al. Pituitary hormone release in response to food ingestion: evidence for neuroendocrine signals from gut to brain. *J Clin Endocrinol Metab.* 1983 Dec;57(6):1111-6

[177] Beers MH, Berkow R (eds). *Merck Manual. 17th Edition.* Whitehouse Station; Merck Research Laboratories 1999 Page 77-78

[178] "A prospective, double-blind, randomized, placebo-controlled study compared BRC at a fixed daily dosage of 2.5 mg with placebo... Long term treatment with a low dose of BRC appears to be a safe and effective means of decreasing SLE flares in SLE patients." Alvarez-Nemegyei et al. Bromocriptine in systemic lupus erythematosus: a double-blind, randomized, placebo-controlled study. *Lupus.* 1998;7(6):414-9

[179] Serri O, Chik CL, Ur E, Ezzat S. Diagnosis and management of hyperprolactinemia. *CMAJ.* 2003 Sep 16;169(6):575-81 cmaj.ca/cgi/content/full/169/6/575

[180] "...clinical observations and trials support the use of bromocriptine as a nonstandard primary or adjunctive therapy in the treatment of recalcitrant RA, SLE, Reiter's syndrome, and psoriatic arthritis and associated conditions unresponsive to traditional approaches." McMurray RW. Bromocriptine in rheumatic and autoimmune diseases. *Semin Arthritis Rheum.* 2001 Aug;31(1):21-32

[181] Serri O, Chik CL, Ur E, Ezzat S. Diagnosis and management of hyperprolactinemia. *CMAJ.* 2003 Sep 16;169(6):575-81 cmaj.ca/cgi/content/full/169/6/575

[182] "CONCLUSION: These data indicate that cabergoline is a very effective agent for lowering the prolactin levels in hyperprolactinemic patients and that it appears to offer considerable advantage over bromocriptine in terms of efficacy and tolerability." Sabuncu T, Arikan E, Tasan E, Hatemi H. Comparison of the effects of cabergoline and bromocriptine on prolactin levels in hyperprolactinemic patients. *Intern Med.* 2001 Sep;40(9):857-61

[183] "Cabergoline also normalized PRL in the majority of patients with known bromocriptine intolerance or -resistance. Once PRL secretion was adequately controlled, the dose of cabergoline could often be significantly decreased, which further reduced costs of therapy." Verhelst et al. Cabergoline in the treatment of hyperprolactinemia: a study in 455 patients. *J Clin Endocrinol Metab.* 1999 Jul;84(7):2518-22 jcem.endojournals.org/cgi/content/full/84/7/2518

[184] Erb N, Pace AV, Delamere JP, Kitas GD. Control of unremitting rheumatoid arthritis by the prolactin antagonist cabergoline. *Rheumatology* (Oxford). 2001 Feb;40(2):237-9 rheumatology.oxfordjournals.org/cgi/content/full/40/2/237

[185] Mobini et al. The effect of cabergoline on clinical and laboratory findings in active rheumatoid arthritis. *Iran Red Crescent Med J.* 2011 Oct;13(10):749-50

| Clinical Case | **Exemplary case of clinical and laboratory evidence of reversal of "severe, aggressive, drug-resistant" rheumatoid arthritis in a 51yoWF following implementation of the Functional Inflammology Protocol**: This summarizes the 13-month clinical outcome of the first patient treated with the updated functional inflammology protocol after its revision and expansion in March 2012.[186] After being diagnosed accurately by a rheumatologist—for this patient very clearly met diagnostic criteria—this patient presented for care following notably inefficacious treatment with the full medicopharmaceutical antirheumatic protocol comprised of NSAIDs, prednisone (she had only minimal response to prednisone >60mg/d), methotrexate, hydroxychloroquine, and "biologics" including etanercept/Enbrel; she was now being recommended to start newer "experimental" drugs. Following the failure of medical treatment, the patient was treated at the teaching clinic of a naturopathic college where her treatments included a clinician-supervised 26-day water-only fast, which resulted in the loss of 30 pounds (13.6 kilograms) but provided no clinical benefit for the rheumatoid arthritis. [Note: I/Dr Vasquez treat this patient at no charge. Dr William J Beakey of Professional Co-Op Services (Professionalco-op.com) generously donated these laboratory tests for collaborative/research purposes. Biotics Research Corporation (BioticsResearch.com) generously donated nutritional supplements for this patient.]

<u>March 2012—severe symptoms and CCP >250</u>: Patient reports suffering significantly with joint pain and lower extremity edema; foundational nutritional protocol[187] is implemented with antidysbiotic/antimicrobial intervention limited to emulsified oregano oil 600mg/d, mitochondrial support and the nutritional immunomodulation protocol. CCP level at this time is beyond laboratory testing limits, measured simply as "greater than" 250 units.

CCP Antibodies IgG/IgA	>250	High	units	0 – 19
			Negative	<20
			Weak positive	20 – 39
			Moderate positive	40 – 59
			Strong positive	>59

<u>January 2013—mild symptoms and CCP 195</u>: Few modifications are made for the first 9 months and patient feels progressively better, but wants to "move to the next level of improvement" because—despite feeling and functioning significantly better solely with dietary and nutritional interventions—patient still notes exacerbations of pain, particularly following extended manual farm labor. At this time, labs are drawn showing an impressive reduction in CCP levels from "greater than" 250 units to 195 units, correlating with a reduction of at least 22%. At this time, patient was commenced on additional treatments including cabergoline, oral vancomycin, and azithromycin.

CCP Antibodies IgG/IgA	195	High	units	0 – 19
			Negative	<20
			Weak positive	20 – 39
			Moderate positive	40 – 59
			Strong positive	>59

<u>April 2013—virtually normal, CCP 54</u>: Patient continues to improve clinically; her subjective and objective clinical improvements (including additional loss of 30 pounds [13.6 kilograms] and reduction in hand swelling necessitating resizing of wedding ring) correlate nicely with the reduction in CCP levels, which have reduced from >250 units to 54 units, for a reduction of more than 78%. Thus, by objective physical and laboratory criteria, this patient appears to be experiencing authentic reversal—cure—of her disease due to the functional inflammology protocol.

CCP Antibodies IgG/IgA	54	High	units	0 – 19
			Negative	<20
			Weak positive	20 – 39
			Moderate positive	40 – 59
			Strong positive	>59

---

[186] Vasquez A. *Functional Immunology and Nutritional Immunomodulation*. 2012 createspace.com/3899760 and updated as *F.I.N.D. S.E.X® The Easily Remembered Acronym for the Functional Inflammology Protocol*. 2013 createspace.com/4234627

[187] Vasquez A. Revisiting the Five-Part Nutritional Wellness Protocol: Supplemented Paleo-Mediterranean Diet. *Nutr Perspect* 2011 Jan ichnfm.academia.edu/AlexVasquez

Psoriasis & Psoriatic Arthritis

Introduction:

Psoriasis is my favorite condition to treat; successful implementation of the Functional Inflammology protocol can lead to such rapid resolution of long-term skin lesions that objective improvement is clearly and objectively demonstrable—providing irrefutable proof of efficacy while immediately improving the patient's quality of life, sense of efficacy, and self-esteem.

    From this chapter onward, readers should use the information in Chapter 4—detailing the concepts and implementation of the Functional Inflammology protocol—and apply those concepts and interventions to the clinical conditions in the book and encountered in clinical practice.

Description/pathophysiology:

- Psoriatic arthritis is an inflammatory arthropathy seen in patients with psoriasis that can have both peripheral (e.g., hands and feet) and axial (i.e., spine and sacroiliac joints) manifestations. This condition has frequently been referred to as *psoriatic rheumatism* or *rheumatic psoriasis*.

- Similar to reactive arthritis and rheumatoid arthritis; strongly associated with streptococcal infections as well as staphylococcal infections.[188] Although many researchers have contributed to the literature which establishes psoriasis as a disease of multifocal dysbiosis, to the best of my knowledge the work of Patricia W. Noah PhD is exceptionally noteworthy; her 1990 review published in *Seminars in Dermatology*[189] is required reading for doctors wishing to gain independent *peer-reviewed* confirmation that **multifocal dysbiosis is the major initiator and perpetuator of this systemic autoimmune inflammatory disorder.** In this particular article, Dr Noah documents the experience of her group at the College of Medicine at the University of Tennessee, their anti-dysbiosis protocol, and its success in the treatment of psoriasis.

- **Psoriasis and psoriatic arthritis must be considered an autoimmune diseases** based on the findings of autoantibodies directed against dermal structures—stratum corneum[190] and keratinocytes[191]—and antibody-dependent and antibody-independent immune-mediated tissue destruction. Although stratum corneum antibodies are found in healthy patients without consequence, what makes them uniquely pathogenic in psoriasis is their tissue penetration in lesioned skin, their ability to bind with autoantigens, and their activation of complement.[192,193]

Clinical presentations:

- Dermal lesions are generally described as well demarcated erythematous patches with silvery scales. Lesions may be widespread or comparatively minor. Patients may have *hidden* dermal lesions on scalp or in gluteal cleft; clinical examination in patients with oligoarthritis can search for dermal psoriatic lesions while assessing for cutaneous dysbiosis. Rarely, nail pitting is the only cutaneous lesion.

- Chronologic association of *dermal psoriasis* with *psoriatic arthritis*:
  - 7-30% of patients with (dermal) psoriasis develop psoriatic arthritis
  - In 70% of patients, *dermal psoriasis* precedes *psoriatic arthritis* by several years
  - In 15% of patients, *dermal psoriasis* and *psoriatic arthritis* occur at the same time

---

[188] Klippel JH (ed). *Primer on the Rheumatic Diseases. 11th Edition.* Atlanta: Arthritis Foundation. 1997 page 176

[189] Noah PW. The role of microorganisms in psoriasis. *Semin Dermatol.* 1990 Dec;9(4):269-76

[190] "... titers of IgG anti-SC autoantibodies in psoriatic patients were not specifically higher than in normal controls but were more variable, indicating that their circulating levels are dependent on a delicate balance between consumption at inflammatory sites and a secondary increase due to SC-antigen release following inflammation." Tagami H, Iwatsuki K, Yamada M. Profile of anti-stratum corneum autoantibodies in psoriatic patients. *Arch Dermatol Res.* 1983;275(2):71-5

[191] "It seems that autoantibodies, although they do not appear to participate in the pathogenesis of psoriasis, are an important feature, and that skin antigens, which appear in lesional immature keratinocytes, cross-react with S. pyogenes and contribute to the autoimmune process in psoriasis." Perez-Lorenzo et al. Autoantibodies to autologous skin in guttate and plaque forms of psoriasis and cross-reaction of skin antigens with streptococcal antigens. *Int J Dermatol.* 1998 Jul;37(7):524-31. The authors found that all psoriasis patients had dermal autoantibodies and that these antibodies reacted specifically with endogenous dermal antigens; thus their finding that "Deposits of immunoglobulin G (IgG) were not detected in the lesions" is unexpected and inexplicable. This statement from their research is inconsistent with the findings of other research groups, and—specifically—must be placed in a context of other articles, most notably "... titers of IgG anti-SC autoantibodies in psoriatic patients were not specifically higher than in normal controls but were more variable, indicating that their circulating levels are dependent on a delicate balance between consumption at inflammatory sites and a secondary increase due to SC-antigen release following inflammation." Tagami et al. Profile of anti-stratum corneum autoantibodies in psoriatic patients. *Arch Dermatol Res.* 1983;275(2):71-5.

[192] "The stratum corneum (SC) antibodies are present in all human sera as seen by indirect immunofluorescence (IF) staining... IF tests with proper controls showed that the SC antigen in psoriatic scales is coated not only with IgG but in a majority of the lesions also with complement." Beutner EH, Jarzabek-Chorzelska M, Jablonska S, Chorzelski TP, Rzesa G. Autoimmunity in psoriasis. A complement immunofluorescence study. *Arch Dermatol Res.* 1978 Apr 7;261(2):123-34

[193] "Indirect immunofluorescent (IF) tests on sections of normal human skin reveal presence of antibodies to stratum corneum in most normal human sera. ...Direct IF tests of psoriatic lesions revealed presence of in vivo bound IgG as well as other immunoglobulins and complement in stratum corneum." Beutner et al. Studies in immunodermatology. VI. IF studies of autoantibodies to stratum corneum and of in vivo fixed IgG in stratum corneum of psoriatic lesions. *Int Arch Allergy Appl Immunol.* 1975;48(3):301-23

- o In 15% of patients, *psoriatic arthritis* precedes *dermal psoriasis*—this 'reverse presentation' is particularly common in children
- Onset may be gradual (70%) or acute (30%)
- In some patients the onset and disease can be of such severity that hospitalization is required.
- Peripheral joint involvement is more common in women; spinal involvement is more common in men, particularly in association with HLA-B27
- Peak onset age 30-55 years
- Musculoskeletal manifestations: prevalence: hands > feet > sacroiliac > spine
  - o Oligoarticular peripheral arthropathy—distal interphalangeal (DIP) joints are notably affected
  - o Peripheral polyarthritis: distribution may be symmetric or asymmetric
  - o Arthritis mutilans: total destruction of the phalanges and meta-tarsals/carpals
  - o Spinal and sacroiliac involvement: may affect any portion of the spine in a random fashion—lumbar spondylitis and sacroiliitis are more common than atlantoaxial instability; spinal involvement is more common in patients positive for HLA-B27
  - o Enthesitis: inflammation at the junction of tendons to bones, classically noted at the Achilles tendon
- Systemic manifestations and complications
  - o Conjunctivitis, uveitis: seen in 30%
  - o Nail pitting may or may not be present; other findings may include transverse ridging, thickening, flaking and brittleness
  - o Aortic insufficiency
  - o Pulmonary fibrosis
  - o Swelling of the fingers and hands

Major differential diagnoses:
- <u>Ankylosing spondylitis</u>: does not occur with dermal psoriatic lesions
- <u>Rheumatoid arthritis</u>: differentiated from rheumatoid arthritis by 1) skin lesions, 2) absence of rheumatoid nodules, 3) negative rheumatoid factor
- <u>Hemochromatosis</u>: non-inflammatory peripheral arthropathy
- <u>Reactive arthritis</u>: does not classically occur with dermal psoriatic lesions
- <u>Septic arthritis</u>: e.g., infected psoriatic skin lesion predisposing to septicemia with resultant joint infection
- <u>HIV infection</u>: increased prevalence of psoriasis[194] especially associated with "an explosive onset of psoriasis and psoriatic arthritis"[195]

Clinical assessments:
- **History/subjective**:
  - o Inquire about the clinical presentations listed above
  - o Family and personal history of psoriasis is often positive
  - o Historical risk factors for psoriasis include bacterial pharyngitis and stressful life events[196]
- **Physical examination/objective**:
  - o Psoriasis—sharply demarcated erythematous plaque with silver scales
  - o Neuromusculoskeletal examination as indicated—see *Integrative Orthopedics*[197]
  - o Assess blood pressure and perform screening physical examination

---

[194] Beers MH, Berkow R (eds). *Merck Manual. 17th Edition*. Whitehouse Station; Merck Research Laboratories 1999 page 448
[195] Klippel JH (ed). *Primer on the Rheumatic Diseases. 11th Edition*. Atlanta: Arthritis Foundation. 1997 page 176
[196] "The study confirmed that recent pharyngeal infection is a risk factor for guttate psoriasis... Finally, the study added evidence to the belief that stressful life events may represent risk factors for the onset of psoriasis." Naldi et al; Psoriasis Study Group of Italian Group for Epidemiological Research in Dermatology. Family history of psoriasis, stressful life events, and recent infectious disease are risk factors for first episode of acute guttate psoriasis: results of a case-control study. *J Am Acad Dermatol*. 2001 Mar:433-8
[197] Vasquez A. *Integrative Orthopedics, 3rd Edition*, 2012

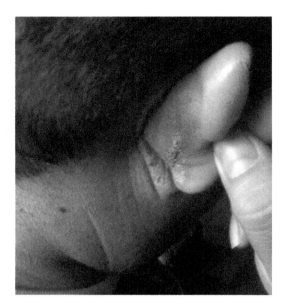 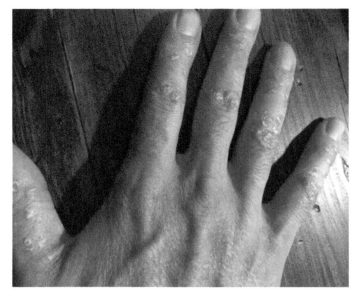

Images of Psoriasis with Two Different Types of Arthritis—Both Cases Present the Classic Dermal Manifestations of Erythematous Patches with While/Silvery Scales, Indicating Dermal Hyperproliferation: _Image left_: 34yoM with a solitary psoriasis patch virtually hidden behind his right ear, previous diagnosis was confirmed by dermatologist as a "classic psoriasis flare" after the patient was given a single dose of "penicillin" (possibly amoxicillin) for dental procedure prophylaxis; of very important note is that this patient also had confirmed rheumatoid arthritis with seropositivity for both RF and CCP, portending more aggressive disease; this patient also has thyroid autoimmunity, for a total of three different autoimmune diseases: 1) psoriasis, 2) rheumatoid arthritis, and 3) thyroiditis. _Image left_: 39yoM with psoriasis and psoriatic arthritis; nail pitting was evident in the toenails, but not the fingernails.

- **Laboratory assessments**:
    - <u>ANA</u>: Antinuclear antibodies are present in 47% of patients with psoriatic arthritis, further supporting the "autoimmune" description of this disease.[198]
    - <u>Rheumatoid factor</u>: RF is negative: positive RF suggests concomitant RA along with psoriasis.
    - <u>Chemistry/metabolic panel with uric acid</u>: Assess for overall status and elevated uric acid, the latter may be increased due to rapid skin turnover.
    - <u>Cardiovascular risk factors, especially homocysteine</u>: Patients with psoriasis have increased incidence of cardiovascular disease and as such should receive additional screening and care with regard to cardiovascular risk—including lifestyle risks such as obesity, sedentariness, smoking—and especially homocysteine.
    - <u>Ferritin</u>: Assess ferritin preferably with transferrin saturation and CRP to exclude iron overload, especially with any arthropathy.
    - <u>CRP</u>: Generally elevated; can be used to track progression/remission of the disease
    - <u>HLA-B27</u>: Present in 40% of patients with psoriatic arthritis; correlates with increased severity of disease, including increased CRP, increased propensity for sacroiliitis, and more extensive joint destruction.[199]
    - <u>HIV serologic testing</u>: Especially for patients with severe disease and/or sudden onset.
    - <u>Lactulose/mannitol assay for "leaky gut"</u>: Patients with psoriasis have increased intestinal permeability.[200]
    - <u>Dysbiosis assessments</u>
        - <u>Gastrointestinal dysbiosis</u>: Comprehensive stool and parasitology testing must include bacterial/yeast culture; antigen or antibody testing for _H. pylori_ is recommended; patients with psoriasis have shown a greatly increased prevalence of _H. pylori_ compared with controls[201], and the

---

[198] "RESULTS: 44/94 (47%) patients with PsA were ANA positive (>/=1/40); 13/94 (14%) had a clinically significant titre of >/=1/80. Three per cent had dsDNA antibodies, 2% had RF and anti-Ro antibodies, 1% had anti-RNP antibodies, and none had anti-La or anti-Smith antibodies." Johnson et al. Autoantibodies in biological agent naive patients with psoriatic arthritis. _Ann Rheum Dis_. 2005 May;64(5):770-2

[199] Tsai et al. Relationship between human lymphocyte antigen-B27 and clinical features of psoriatic arthritis. _J Microbiol Immunol Infect_. 2003 Jun;36(2):101-4

[200] "The 24-h urine excretion of 51Cr-EDTA from psoriatic patients was 2.46 +/- 0.81%. These results differed significantly from controls (1.95 +/- 0.36%; P less than 0.05)." Humbert et al. Intestinal permeability in patients with psoriasis. _J Dermatol Sci_. 1991 Jul;2:324-6

[201] "In the current study, 20 (40%), psoriatic patients and 5 (10%) patients of control group demonstrated H. pylori antibodies... Although our study supports a causal role of H. pylori in the pathogenesis of psoriasis..." Qayoom S, Ahmad QM. Psoriasis and helicobacter pylori. _Indian J Dermatol Venereol Leprol_ 2003;69:133-134 ijdvl.com/

authors of this study suggested a causal association; likewise intestinal colonization with yeasts including *Candida albicans* and *Geotrichum candidum* are found much more commonly in psoriatics than controls.[202] Stressing the importance of this association, Waldman et al[203] wrote, "Our results reinforce the hypothesis that *C. albicans* is one of the triggers to both exacerbation and persistence of psoriasis. We propose that in psoriatics with a significant quantity of *Candida* in feces, an antifungal treatment should be considered as an adjuvant treatment of psoriasis."

> **Microbial colonization contributes to psoriasis**
>
> "We have repeatedly observed psoriatic flares associated with microbial infection, sequestered antigen, and colonization. **Removal of these microbial foci results in clearing of the disease.**"
>
> Noah P. The role of microorganisms in psoriasis. *Semin Dermatol.* 1990 Dec

- Dermal dysbiosis: Skin/nail culture, Giemsa staining, culture lesioned skin on blood agar, MacConkey agar, Sabouraud plates.[204]
- Sinorespiratory dysbiosis: Nasal swab and culture, throat culture for bacteria and yeasts.[205]
- Genitourinary dysbiosis: Culture and sensitivity testing for all organisms from clean catch specimens; assessment of sexual partners is advised.[206]
- Orodental dysbiosis: Culture of dentures and oral cavity for yeast and bacteria.
- Environmental dysbiosis: Examination, culture, and/or thorough cleaning of wigs, shoes, furniture, whirlpool/pool water.[207]

- **Imaging**:
  - Imaging is generally unnecessary. Radiographic findings of advanced joint disease are characteristic and can aid in differential diagnosis; findings such as the osteolytic "pencil-in-cup" and "marginal erosions" are characteristic and differentiate psoriatic arthropathy from other conditions. Radiographic changes in the spine may be severe even when the patient has mild or no symptoms—assess the spine radiographically before initiating spinal manipulative therapy. Note that inflammatory changes such as facet ankylosis and atlantoaxial instability may occur and could potentially complicate manipulative therapy.[208] Myelocompressive atlantoaxial subluxation has been reported as the presenting manifestation of psoriatic arthropathy.[209] Remarkably, Lee and Lui[210] published that, "...atlantoaxial subluxation without high cervical myelopathy has been reported in 45% of cases of psoriatic spondylitis."
- **Establishing the diagnosis**:
  - Psoriasis: Clinical exam reveals erythematous patches with silvery scales—this classic finding is common and may present as a singular lesion in an obscure location, such as behind the ear, at the hairline at the back of the neck, or in the gluteal cleft.
  - Psoriatic arthritis: Psoriasis with arthritis after the exclusion of RA, iron overload, AS, and HIV; psoriatic arthritis classicall associates with pitting of the nails.

---

[202] Candida albicans (and other yeasts) was detected in 68% of psoriatics,70% of eczematics, 54% of the controls. Qualitative analysis revealed a predominance of Candida albicans. Geotrichum candidum occurred in 22% of psoriatics, 10% of eczematics, and 3% of controls. Buslau et al. Fungal flora of human faeces in psoriasis and atopic dermatitis. *Mycoses.* 1990 Feb;33(2):90-4

[203] "Our results reinforce the hypothesis that C. albicans is one of the triggers to both exacerbation and persistence of psoriasis. We propose that in psoriatics with a significant quantity of Candida in faeces, an antifungal treatment should be considered as an adjuvant treatment of psoriasis." Waldman et al. Incidence of Candida in psoriasis--a study on the fungal flora of psoriatic patients. *Mycoses.* 2001 May;44(3-4):77-8

[204] Noah PW. The role of microorganisms in psoriasis. *Semin Dermatol.* 1990 Dec;9(4):269-76

[205] Noah PW. The role of microorganisms in psoriasis. *Semin Dermatol.* 1990 Dec;9(4):269-76

[206] Noah PW. The role of microorganisms in psoriasis. *Semin Dermatol.* 1990 Dec;9(4):269-76

[207] Noah PW. The role of microorganisms in psoriasis. *Semin Dermatol.* 1990 Dec;9(4):269-76

[208] Laiho K, Kauppi M. The cervical spine in patients with psoriatic arthritis. *Ann Rheum Dis.* 2002 Jul;6:650-2 ard.bmjjournals.com/cgi/content/full/61/7/650

[209] "We report severe upward axial dislocation and acquired basilar impression as a presenting manifestation of psoriatic arthropathy." Kaplan et al. Atlantoaxial subluxation in psoriatic arthropathy. *Ann Neurol.* 1988 May;23(5):522-4

[210] "...atlantoaxial subluxation without high cervical myelopathy has been reported in 45% of cases of psoriatic spondylitis." Lee ST, Lui TN. Psoriatic arthritis with C-1-C-2 subluxation as a neurosurgical complication. *Surg Neurol.* 1986 Nov;26(5):428-30

Vitamin D, 1,25 + 25-Hydroxy

Test	Low	Normal	High	Reference Range	Units
Calcitriol(1,25 Di-Oh Vit D)			115.8	10.0-75.0	pg/mL
Vitamin D, 25-Hydroxy		53.1		30.0-100.0	ng/mL

Cmp14+Egfr

Test	Low	Normal	High	Reference Range	Units
Glucose, Serum		90		65-99	mg/dL
Bun		20		6-20	mg/dL
Creatinine, Serum		0.93		0.76-1.27	mg/dL
Egfr If Nonafricn Am		104		>59	mL/min/1.73
Egfr If Africn Am		120		>59	mL/min/1.73
Bun/Creatinine Ratio			22	8-19	1
Sodium, Serum		142		134-144	mmol/L
Potassium, Serum		4.8		3.5-5.2	mmol/L
Chloride, Serum		99		97-108	mmol/L
Carbon Dioxide, Total		26		18-29	mmol/L
Calcium, Serum		9.7		8.7-10.2	mg/dL

Cbc/Diff Ambiguous Default

Test	Low	Normal	High	Reference Range	Units
Wbc		5.8		3.4-10.8	x10E3/uL
Rbc		5.26		4.14-5.80	x10E6/uL

Ldh

Test	Low	Normal	High	Reference Range	Units
Ldh		123		121-224	IU/L

Homocyst(E)Ine, Plasma

Test	Low	Normal	High	Reference Range	Units
Homocyst(E)Ine, Plasma		10.7		0.0-15.0	umol/L

Laboratory results for an adult patient with psoriasis and psoriatic arthritis: Abnormally increased conversion of 25-OH-cholecalciferol to 1,25-diOH-cholecalciferol is due expression of 25-hydroxyvitamin D3-1alpha-hydroxylase (1-OHase) in inflammatory tissue/cells. Note that serum calcium is normal, so no immediate threat is present (i.e., hypercalcemia) but of course the clinician has the responsibility to ❶ monitor periodically, ❷ inform the patient of symptoms of hypercalcemia such as headache and abdominal pain, and ❸ search for any predictive risk factors such as renal insufficiency or occult leukemia/lymphoma that could precipitate hypercalcemia. Assessment for hyperparathyroidism (eg, iPTH) is reasonable but not completely necessary; likewise, cancer screening is not absolutely indicated, as it would be in the case of idiopathic hypercalcemia. Also noted is the elevated homocysteine, common in patients with psoriasis; increased cell turnover—dermal hyperproliferation—likely contributes to draining/catabolizing nutrients such as folate. Since this patient's 25-OH-D is plenty sufficient, I had the patient temporarily reduce/discontinue vitamin D supplementation to reduce risk of hypercalcemia given that he is clearly vitamin D sufficient.

<u>Complications</u>:
- Infection of skin lesions, may progress to septicemia or septic arthritis
- Atlantoaxial instability
- Cosmetic and functional deformity
- Pain
- Destructive and crippling arthritis
- Depression, social isolation, pain, reduced quality of life: **"Patients with psoriasis reported reduction in physical functioning and mental functioning comparable to that seen in cancer, arthritis, hypertension, heart disease, diabetes, and depression."**[211]

<u>Clinical management</u>:
- Referral if clinical outcome is unsatisfactory or if serious complications are evident.

<u>Treatments</u>:
- <u>Medical treatments</u>: The goal of medical treatment is to suppress inflammation and dermal proliferation; no consideration is given to searching for and addressing the underlying cause(s) of the disorder because the disease is considered idiopathic.[212] Medical textbooks describe the treatment as merely targeted toward the symptoms, e.g., "Treatment [of psoriatic arthritis] is symptomatic."[213]
  - <u>For dermal psoriasis</u>:
    - Prescription topical steroids
    - Topical coal tars and hydrocarbons: carcinogenic
    - UV-B radiation: kills active lymphocytes in skin and results in short-term superficial disappearance of psoriatic skin lesions
    - PUVA: psoralen with UV-A radiation; may result in cataracts and skin cancer
    - Methotrexate
    - Etretinate: a severely teratogenic retinoid
  - <u>For psoriatic arthritis</u>: Medical treatments for psoriatic arthritis are essentially the same as for rheumatoid arthritis[214] and are generally noncurative and "symptomatic."[215]
    - <u>Etretinate</u>: a severely teratogenic retinoid
    - <u>PUVA</u>: psoralen with UV-A radiation; may result in cataracts and skin cancer
    - <u>Corticosteroids</u> are not highly effective
    - <u>Antimalarial drugs</u> (commonly used against systemic lupus erythematosus) frequently exacerbate psoriasis
    - <u>Methotrexate</u>: Used for recalcitrant psoriatic arthritis.[216]
    - <u>TNF inhibitors</u>: Etanercept 25 mg subcutaneously twice weekly, or infliximab 5 mg/kg every other month. These drugs are clinically effective from the perspective of anti-inflammation, but they are associated with increased risks for lymphoma, infections, congestive heart failure, demyelinating diseases, and systemic lupus erythematosus.

- **FOOD & NUTRITION: 5-part "supplemented Paleo-Mediterranean diet" (5pSPMD)** The 5-part "supplemented Paleo-Mediterranean diet" (SPMD—reviewed in Chapter 4) consists of ❶ foundational plant-based low-carbohydrate diet of fruits, vegetables, nuts, seeds, berries and lean sources of protein, ❷ multivitamin and multimineral supplementation, ❸ physiologic doses of vitamin D3 (range 2,000-10,000 IU/d), ❹ combination fatty acid therapy (CFAT) with n3-ALA, n6-GLA, n3-EPA, n3-DHA, and phytochemical-rich olive oil which contains n9-oleate, and ❺ probiotics.

[211] "Patients with psoriasis reported reduction in physical functioning and mental functioning comparable to that seen in cancer, arthritis, hypertension, heart disease, and depression." Rapp et al. Psoriasis causes as much disability as other major medical diseases. *J Am Acad Dermatol* 1999 Sep;41(3 Pt 1):401-7
[212] Lookingbill DP, Marks JG, eds. *Principles of Dermatology*. Philadelphia: W.B. Saunders, 1986: 138
[213] Tierney ML. McPhee SJ, Papadakis MA. *Current Medical Diagnosis and Treatment 2006. 45th edition*. New York; Lange Medical: 2006, pages 851-855
[214] Beers MH, Berkow R (eds). *Merck Manual. 17th Edition*. Whitehouse Station; Merck Research Laboratories 1999 page 448
[215] Tierney ML. McPhee SJ, Papadakis MA. *Current Medical Diagnosis and Treatment 2006. 45th edition*. New York; Lange Medical: 2006, pages 851-855
[216] Tierney ML. McPhee SJ, Papadakis MA. *Current Medical Diagnosis and Treatment 2006. 45th edition*. New York; Lange Medical: 2006, pages 851-855

o <u>Vitamin D3 supplementation with physiologic doses and/or tailored to serum 25(OH)D levels</u>: Vitamin D deficiency is common in the general population and is even more common in patients with chronic illness and chronic musculoskeletal pain.[217] Vitamin D3 can be applied topically and is about as effective as topical steroids in the treatment of psoriatic skin lesions.[218] Correction of vitamin D deficiency supports normal immune function against infection and provides a clinically significant anti-inflammatory[219] and analgesic benefit in patients with back pain[220] and limb pain.[221] Reasonable daily doses for children and adults are 2,000 and 4,000 IU, respectively, as defined by Vasquez, et al.[222] Deficiency and response to treatment are monitored with serum 25(OH)vitamin D while safety is monitored with serum calcium; inflammatory granulomatous diseases and certain drugs such as hydrochlorothiazide increase the propensity for hypercalcemia and warrant increment dosing and frequent monitoring of serum calcium.

o <u>Alcohol/ethanol avoidance</u>: Consumption of alcoholic beverages—even in low doses—increases intestinal permeability and exacerbates psoriasis. Psoriatics should avoid ethanol consumption[223]; wheat/grain antigens are immunogenic, ethanol exacerbates intestinal hyperpermeability, and some patients are sensitive to brewer's yeast.

o <u>Gluten-free vegetarian diet</u>: Vegetarian/vegan diets have a place in the treatment plan of all patients with autoimmune/inflammatory disorders[224], including psoriasis and psoriatic arthritis[225]; this is also true for patients for whom long-term exclusive reliance on a meat-free vegetarian diet is either not appropriate or not appealing. No legitimate scientist or literate clinician doubts the antirheumatic power and anti-inflammatory advantages of vegetarian diets, whether used short-term or long term.[226] The benefits of gluten-free vegetarian diets are well documented, and the mechanisms of action are well elucidated, including reduced intake of proinflammatory linoleic[227] and arachidonic acids[228], iron[229], common food antigens[230], gluten[231] and gliadin[232,233], proinflammatory sugars[234] and increased intake of omega-3 fatty acids and micronutrients[235], and anti-inflammatory and anti-oxidant phytonutrients[236]; vegetarian diets also effect profound changes—both *qualitative* and *quantitative*—in intestinal flora[237,238] that correlate with clinical improvement.[239] Patients who rely on the Paleo-Mediterranean Diet can use vegetarian meals, on a daily basis or for days at a time, for example, by having a daily vegetarian meal, or one week per month of vegetarianism. Of course, some (not all) patients can use a purely vegetarian diet long-term provided

[217] Plotnikoff GA, Quigley JM. Prevalence of severe hypovitaminosis D in patients with persistent, nonspecific musculoskeletal pain. *Mayo Clin Proc.* 2003 Dec;78(12):1463-70

[218] Lookingbill DP, Marks JG, eds. *Principles of dermatology.* Philadelphia: W.B. Saunders, 1986: 141

[219] Timms et al. Circulating MMP9, vitamin D and variation in TIMP-1 response with VDR genotype. *QJM.* 2002 Dec;95(12):787-96

[220] Al Faraj S, Al Mutairi K. Vitamin D deficiency and chronic low back pain in Saudi Arabia. *Spine.* 2003 Jan 15;28(2):177-9

[221] Masood et al. Persistent limb pain and raised serum alkaline phosphatase earliest markers of subclinical hypovitaminosis D. *Indian J Physiol Pharmacol* 1989 Oct:259-61

[222] Vasquez et al. The clinical importance of vitamin D (cholecalciferol): a paradigm shift for all healthcare providers. *Altern Ther Health Med.* 2004 Sep-Oct;10(5):28-36

[223] "We recommend that clinicians discourage patients with psoriasis from consuming alcohol, especially during periods of disease exacerbation." Behnam SM, Behnam SE, Koo JY. Alcohol as a risk factor for plaque-type psoriasis. *Cutis.* 2005 Sep;76(3):181-5

[224] "After four weeks at the health farm the diet group showed a significant improvement in number of tender joints, Ritchie's articular index, number of swollen joints, pain score, duration of morning stiffness, grip strength, erythrocyte sedimentation rate, C-reactive protein, white blood cell count, and a health assessment questionnaire score." Kjeldsen-Kragh et al. Controlled trial of fasting and one-year vegetarian diet in rheumatoid arthritis. *Lancet.* 1991 Oct 12;338(8772):899-902

[225] "During the vegan diet, both signs and symptoms returned in most patients, with the exception of some patients with psoriasis who experienced an improvement." Lithell et al. A fasting and vegetarian diet treatment trial on chronic inflammatory disorders. *Acta Derm Venereol.* 1983;63(5):397-403

[226] "For the patients who were randomised to the vegetarian diet there was a significant decrease in platelet count, leukocyte count, calprotectin, total IgG, IgM rheumatoid factor (RF), C3-activation products, and the complement components C3 and C4 after one month of treatment." Kjeldsen-Kragh et al. Changes in laboratory variables in rheumatoid arthritis patients during a trial of fasting and one-year vegetarian diet. *Scand J Rheumatol.* 1995;24(2):85-93

[227] Rusyn I, Bradham CA, Cohn L, Schoonhoven R, Swenberg JA, Brenner DA, Thurman RG. Corn oil rapidly activates nuclear factor-kappaB in hepatic Kupffer cells by oxidant-dependent mechanisms. *Carcinogenesis.* 1999 Nov;20(11):2095-100 carcin.oxfordjournals.org/cgi/content/full/20/11/2095

[228] Vasquez A. New Insights into Fatty Acid Supplementation and Its Effect on Eicosanoid Production and Genetic Expression. *Nutritional Perspectives* 2005; January: 5-16

[229] Dabbagh AJ, Trenam CW, Morris CJ, Blake DR. Iron in joint inflammation. *Ann Rheum Dis.* 1993 Jan;52(1):67-73

[230] Hafstrom I, et al. A vegan diet free of gluten improves the signs and symptoms of rheumatoid arthritis: the effects on arthritis correlate with a reduction in antibodies to food antigens. *Rheumatology* (Oxford). 2001 Oct;40(10):1175-9 rheumatology.oxfordjournals.org/cgi/reprint/40/10/1175

[231] "The data provide evidence that dietary modification may be of clinical benefit for certain RA patients, and that this benefit may be related to a reduction in immunoreactivity to food antigens eliminated by the change in diet." Hafstrom et al. A vegan diet free of gluten improves the signs and symptoms of rheumatoid arthritis: the effects on arthritis correlate with a reduction in antibodies to food antigens. *Rheumatology* (Oxford). 2001 Oct;40(10):1175-9

[232] "Despite the increased AGA [antigliadin antibodies] positivity found distinctively in patients with recent-onset RA, none of the RA patients showed clear evidence of coeliac disease." Paimela L, Kurki P, Leirisalo-Repo M, Piirainen H. Gliadin immune reactivity in patients with rheumatoid arthritis. Clin Exp Rheumatol. 1995 Sep-Oct;13(5):603-7

[233] "The median IgA antigliadin ELISA index was 7.1 (range 2.1-22.4) for the RA group and 3.1 (range 0.3-34.9) for the controls (p = 0.0001)." Koot et al. Elevated level of IgA gliadin antibodies in patients with rheumatoid arthritis. *Clin Exp Rheumatol.* 1989 Nov-Dec;7(6):623-6

[234] Seaman DR. The diet-induced proinflammatory state: a cause of chronic pain and other degenerative diseases? *J Manipulative Physiol Ther.* 2002 Mar-Apr;25(3):168-79

[235] Hagfors et al. Fat intake and composition of fatty acids in serum phospholipids in a randomized, controlled, Mediterranean dietary intervention study on patients with rheumatoid arthritis. *Nutr Metab* (Lond). 2005 Oct 10;2:26 nutritionandmetabolism.com/content/2/1/26

[236] Liu RH. Health benefits of fruit and vegetables are from additive and synergistic combinations of phytochemicals. *Am J Clin Nutr* 2003;78(3 Suppl):517S-520S

[237] "Significant alteration in the intestinal flora was observed when the patients changed from omnivorous to vegan diet. ... This finding of an association between intestinal flora and disease activity may have implications for our understanding of how diet can affect RA." Peltonen et al. Changes of faecal flora in rheumatoid arthritis during fasting and one-year vegetarian diet. *Br J Rheumatol.* 1994 Jul;33(7):638-43

[238] Toivanen P, Eerola E. A vegan diet changes the intestinal flora. *Rheumatology* (Oxford). 2002 Aug;41(8):950-1 rheumatology.oxfordjournals.org/cgi/reprint/41/8/950

[239] "We conclude that a vegan diet changes the faecal microbial flora in RA patients, and changes in the faecal flora are associated with improvement in RA activity." Peltonen et al. Faecal microbial flora and disease activity in rheumatoid arthritis during a vegan diet. *Br J Rheumatol.* 1997 Jan;36(1):64-8 rheumatology.oxfordjournals.org/cgi/reprint/36/1/64

that nutritional needs (especially protein and cobalamin) are consistently met. One particular advantage to low-protein diets in psoriasis is that the relative reduction in amino acid availability should serve to reduce polyamine formation. Formed from amino acids via ornithine decarboxylase and other enzymes, polyamines stimulate dermal hyperproliferation and are elevated in patients with psoriasis.[240] Effective psoriasis treatments are associated with a reduction in dermal/urinary polyamine levels, and, conversely, reducing polyamine formation—via either dietary manipulation or antibiologic/pharmaceutical drugs—is associated with clinical improvements in patients with psoriasis.

- **INFECTIONS & DYSBIOSIS: ❶ antimicrobial treatments, ❷ immunorestoration, ❸ immunotolerance via Treg induction** Essentially all autoimmune/rheumatic disorders are associated with microbial colonization and intolerance to same; the presence of persistent microbial colonization is *prima facie* evidence of immunosuppression. The eight areas of multifocal polydysbiosis are: ❶ sinorespiratory, ❷ orodental, ❸ gastrointestinal, ❹ genitourinary, ❺ tissue/blood, ❻ dermal, ❼ environmental, and ❽ endomicrobial.

  o <u>Psoriatogenic multifocal dysbiosis—overview of and homage to the work of Patricia Noah PhD</u>: In a very intensive investigation into the role of bacteria, yeast/fungi, and viruses in the pathogenesis of psoriasis, Noah[241] assessed microflora of 297 psoriasis patients by culture and serologic tests. Culture samples for aerobic bacteria, yeast, and dermatophytes were taken from the throat, urine, and skin surfaces from scalp, ears, chest, face, axillary, submammary, umbilical, upper back, inguinal crease, gluteal-fold, perirectal, vaginal, pubis, penis, scrotal, leg, hands, feet, finger, and toenail areas. More than 15 different microbes were causatively associated with exacerbation of psoriasis; this finding is entirely logical and is consistent with the 'idiopathic' nature of the illness and why Koch-indoctrinated researchers and clinicians have failed to understand the microbial contribution to autoimmune/inflammatory diseases. Given that each of the microbes listed (see shaded box on upcoming page) is a *common*—but not necessarily *optimal*—inhabitant of human surfaces and orifices, it is possible to see how their synergism *particularly in a genetically susceptible patient with hormonal imbalances and a proinflammatory lifestyle/diet* could tip the scales in favor of systemic inflammation and the picture/illusion of autoimmunity. Of the more than 15 categories/subspecies listed as causative microbes, what if only seven of these common "commensals" were present in a systemically-genetically-nutritionally-hormonally-emotionally predisposed patient, and each contributed only 5% to the pathophysiology of a patient's psoriasis? We would have already arrived at 35% of the psoriatic

Microorganisms causally associated with psoriasis
1. Streptococcal groups A (including Streptococcus pyogenes), B, C, D, F, G, S viridans, S pneumoniae
2. Klebsiella pneumoniae, oxytoca
3. Escherichia coli
4. Enterobacter cloacae, E aerogenes, E agglomerans
5. Proteus mirabilis, P vulgaris
6. Citrobacter freundii, C diversus
7. Morganella morganii
8. Pseudomonas aeruginosa, P maltiphilia, P putida
9. Serratia marcescens
10. Acinetobacter calbio aceticus, A luoffi
11. Flavobacterium species
12. CDC groups Ve-1, Ve-2, E-o2
13. Bacillus subtilis, B cereus
14. Staphylococcus aureus
15. Candida albicans, C parapsilosis
16. Torulopsis/Candida glabrata
17. Rhodotorula spp.
18. H. pylori*

See Noah P. The role of microorganisms in psoriasis. *Semin Dermatol.* 1990;9:269
* Qayoom S, Ahmad QM. Psoriasis and helicobacter pylori. *Indian J Dermatol Venereol Leprol* 2003;69:133-134

pathogenesis, leaving 10% each for hormones, diet, allergy, nutrition, xenobiotic accumulation (present in everyone[242,243]). While these numbers and percentages are purely speculative, I left 15% for "idiopathic" to keep researchers and clinicians alert to new possibilities and to placate the therapeutic and epidemiologic nihilists that have so far dominated the field of rheumatology with their "unknown cause" rhetoric. Each cause—each contributor to disease—may in itself be "clinically insignificant" but when additive and synergistic influences coalesce, we find ourselves confronted with an "idiopathic disease"

---

[240] "Psoriasis lesions showed increased ornithine decarboxylase activity compared with uninvolved skin." Lowe et al. Cutaneous polyamines in psoriasis. *Br J Dermatol.* 1982 Jul;107(1):21-5

[241] Noah PW. The role of microorganisms in psoriasis. *Semin Dermatol.* 1990 Dec;9(4):269-76

[242] "Although the use of HCB as a fungicide has virtually been eliminated, detectable levels of HCB are still found in nearly all people in the USA." Robinson et al. An evaluation of hexachlorobenzene body-burden levels in the general population of the USA. *IARC Sci Publ* 1986;77:183-92

[243] "Many U.S. residents carry toxic pesticides in their bodies above government assessed "acceptable" levels." Pesticide Action Network North America (PANNA). Chemical Trespass: Pesticides in Our Bodies and Corporate Accountability. panna.org/campaigns/docsTrespass/chemicalTrespass2004.dv.html

and the decision to choose between the only two available options: 1) despair in the failure of our "one cause, one disease, one drug" paradigm, or 2) appreciate that numerous influences work together to disrupt physiologic function and produce the biologic dysfunction that we experience as disease.

Microbial antigens evoke psoriasis and autoimmunity

"RESULTS: The predicted microbial product appeared heavily in lesional epidermis, but unexpectedly also as a thin deposit along the skin basement membrane zone (SBMZ) of apparently unaffected skin. Staining was negative for nonpsoriatic subjects. CONCLUSIONS: The findings support a direct effect of microbial antigen in psoriasis."

Noah et al. Skin basement membrane zone: a depository for circulating microbial antigen evoking psoriasis and autoimmunity. *Skinmed.* 2006 Mar-Apr

o Gastrointestinal dysbiosis: Patients with psoriasis have shown a greatly increased prevalence of *H. pylori*[244] and *Candida albicans*[245] and *Geotrichum candidum*.[246]

o Sinorespiratory and dermal dysbiosis: Sinorespiratory and dermal dysbiosis in patients with is *qualitatively* (increased prevalence in psoriatics compared with healthy controls) and *quantitatively* (increased prevalence of toxin-producing strains compared to those found in controls) associated with the severity of the disease.[247] Patients with psoriasis show an increased rate of nasal/dermal colonization with *Staphylococcus aureus*[248,249], a microbe known to produce several powerfully inflammatory antigens, toxins, and superantigens, and nasal colonization with which appears causally associated with the inflammatory/autoimmune disorder ANCA-associated vasculitis.[250,251] A study by Bartenjev et al[252] showed that subclinical streptococcal/staphylococcal infections were detected in 68% of psoriasis patients and in only 11 % of the control group; these authors encouraged searching for and eliminating microbial infections as an important aspect of the management of psoriasis. Supportively, other researchers[253] have found that infection with *S pyogenes* can initiate and/or exacerbate guttate psoriasis; therefore streptococcal throat infections should be treated assertively and early to avoid triggering an exacerbation of psoriasis.[254] *Streptococcus pyogenes* is a very likely trigger of psoriasis[255]; chronic penicillin treatment leads to clinical improvement of recalcitrant psoriasis.[256] Patients with guttate psoriasis have increased oropharyngeal colonization with *Streptococcus hemolyticus* compared with controls.[257] Similar to Behcet's disease[258], the dermal lesions of psoriasis are commonly colonized by

---

[244] "In the current study, 20 (40%), psoriatic patients and 5 (10%) patients of control group demonstrated H. pylori antibodies... Although our study supports a causal role of H. pylori in the pathogenesis of psoriasis, a large scale study is needed to confirm the findings." Qayoom S, Ahmad QM. Psoriasis and helicobacter pylori. *Indian J Dermatol Venereol Leprol* 2003;69:133-134 ijdvl.com/

[245] "Our results reinforce the hypothesis that C. albicans is one of the triggers to both exacerbation and persistence of psoriasis. We propose that in psoriatics with a significant quantity of Candida in faeces, an antifungal treatment should be considered as an adjuvant treatment of psoriasis." Waldman et al. Incidence of Candida in psoriasis--a study on the fungal flora of psoriatic patients. *Mycoses.* 2001 May;44(3-4):77-8

[246] Candida albicans (and other yeasts) was detected in 68% of psoriatics, 70% of eczematics, 54% of the controls. Qualitative analysis revealed a predominance of Candida albicans. Geotrichum candidum occurred in 22% of psoriatics, 10% of eczematics, and 3% of controls. Buslau et al. Fungal flora of human faeces in psoriasis and atopic dermatitis. *Mycoses.* 1990 Feb;33(2):90-4

[247] "In this study, S aureus was present in more than 50% of patients with AD and PS. We found that the severity of AD and PS significantly correlated to enterotoxin production of the isolated S aureus strains." Tomi et al. Staphylococcal toxins in patients with psoriasis, atopic dermatitis, and erythroderma, and in healthy control subjects. *J Am Acad Dermatol.* 2005 Jul;53(1):67-72

[248] "In this study, S aureus was present in more than 50% of patients with AD and PS. We found that the severity of AD and PS significantly correlated to enterotoxin production of the isolated S aureus strains." Tomi et al. Staphylococcal toxins in patients with psoriasis, atopic dermatitis, and erythroderma, and in healthy control subjects. *J Am Acad Dermatol.* 2005 Jul;53(1):67-72

[249] "The nasal carriage rate of Staphylococcus aureus in psoriatics was higher than the control groups." Singh et al. Bacteriology of psoriatic plaques. *Dermatologica.* 1978:21-7

[250] Brons RH, Bakker HI, Van Wijk RT, et al. Staphylococcal acid phosphatase binds to endothelial cells via charge interaction; a pathogenic role in Wegener's granulomatosis? *Clin Exp Immunol.* 2000 Mar;119(3):566-73 blackwell-synergy.com/doi/abs/10.1046/j.1365-2249.2000.01172.x

[251] Popa et al. Staphylococcus aureus and Wegener's granulomatosis. *Arthritis Res.* 2002;4(2):77-9 arthritis-research.com/content/4/2/77

[252] "Subclinical streptococcal and/or staphylococcal infections were detected in 68 % of tested patients and in only 11 % of the control group. The results of this study indicate that subclinical bacterial infections of the upper respiratory tract may be an important factor in provoking a new relapse of chronic plaque psoriasis. Searching for, and eliminating, microbial infections could be of importance in the treatment of psoriasis." Bartenjev et al. Subclinical microbial infection in patients with chronic plaque psoriasis. *Acta Derm Venereol Suppl* (Stockh). 2000;(211):17-8

[253] "This study confirms the strong association between prior infection with S pyogenes and guttate psoriasis but suggests that the ability to trigger guttate psoriasis is not serotype specific." Telfer et al. The role of streptococcal infection in the initiation of guttate psoriasis. *Arch Dermatol.* 1992 Jan;128(1):39-42

[254] "CONCLUSIONS: This study confirms anecdotal and retrospective reports that streptococcal throat infections can cause exacerbation of chronic plaque psoriasis." Gudjonsson et al. Streptococcal throat infections and exacerbation of chronic plaque psoriasis: a prospective study. *Br J Dermatol.* 2003 Sep;149(3):530-4

[255] "These findings justify the hypothesis that S pyogenes infections are more important in the pathogenesis of chronic plaque psoriasis than has previously been recognized, and indicate the need for further controlled therapeutic trials of antibacterial measures in this common skin disease." El-Rachkidy et al. Increased Blood Levels of IgG Reactive with Secreted Streptococcus pyogenes Proteins in Chronic Plaque Psoriasis. *J Invest Dermatol.* 2007 Mar 8

[256] "Total duration of the study was two years. Initially benzathine penicillin 1.2 million units, was given I.M. AST fortnightly. After 24 weeks benzathine penicillin was reduced to 1.2 million units once a month... Significant improvement in the PASI score was noted from 12 weeks onwards. All patients showed excellent improvement at 2 years." Saxena VN, Dogra J. Long-term use of penicillin for the treatment of chronic plaque psoriasis. *Eur J Dermatol.* 2005 Sep-Oct;15(5):359-62

[257] "A high incidence of Streptococcus hemolyticus culture was observed in the guttate psoriatic group compared with the plaque psoriasis and control groups." Zhao et al. Acute guttate psoriasis patients have positive streptococcus hemolyticus throat cultures and elevated antistreptococcal M6 protein titers. *J Dermatol.* 2005;32(2):91-6

[258] "At least one type of microorganism was grown from each pustule. Staphylococcus aureus (41/70, 58.6%, p = 0.008) and Prevotella spp (17/70, 24.3%, p = 0.002) were significantly more common in pustules from BS patients, and coagulase negative staphylococci (17/37, 45.9%, p = 0.007) in pustules from acne patients. CONCLUSIONS: The pustular lesions of BS are not usually sterile." Hatemi et al. The pustular skin lesions in Behcet's syndrome are not sterile. *Ann Rheum Dis.* 2004 Nov;63(11):1450-2

proinflammatory microbes including *Staphylococcus aureus*.[259] More conclusively, Villeda-Gabriel et al[260] and Perez-Lorenzo et al[261] showed that antibodies against *Streptococcus pyogenes* cross-react (perhaps via molecular mimicry or epitope spreading) with dermal antigens; additionally, Muto et al[262] showed that antibodies against streptococcal cell wall proteins could bind with nuclei and cytoplasm of cells from skin and synovium. Thus, psoriasis is indeed a microbe-induced autoimmune disease by virtue of these cross-reacting endogenous antibodies that bind with nuclear, dermal, and articular antigens. Patients with psoriasis have elevated serum levels of antibodies against streptococcal M12 protein[263], and patients with psoriatic arthritis have a heightened inflammatory response to staphylococcal superantigens.[264]

- o Antimicrobial treatments for (gastrointestinal) dysbiosis commonly include but are not limited to the following: Doses listed are for adults. Combination therapy generally allows for lower doses of each intervention to be used. Severe dysbiosis often requires weeks or months of treatment. Drugs are not necessarily more effective than natural treatments; in fact, often the botanicals work when the pharmaceuticals do not. See introductory review at the start of this chapter as well as details provided in Chapter 4 for details on anti-dysbiotic treatments.

  - St. John's Wort (*Hypericum perforatum*): *Hypericum* may prove to be a useful botanical for the treatment of psoriasis due to the combination of its antidepressant and antimicrobial benefits. Hyperforin from *Hypericum perforatum* also shows impressive antibacterial action, particularly against gram-positive bacteria such as *Staphylococcus aureus*, *Streptococcus pyogenes*, *Streptococcus agalactiae*[265] and perhaps *Helicobacter pylori*.[266] Up to 600 mg three times per day of a 3% hyperforin standardized extract is customary in the treatment of depression.

  - Topical antimicrobials: Treating the dermal lesions of psoriatic arthritis may help break the vicious cycles of (super)antigen absorption which perpetuates immune dysfunction. A variety of botanical and pharmaceutical creams are available. *In vitro* evidence supports the use of equal parts honey, olive oil, and beeswax against *Staph aureus* and *Candida albicans*.[267] Topical *Mahonia/Berberis* is effective for dermal psoriasis.[268] A topical gel containing artemesinin is also available for clinical use, and animal studies have demonstrated systemic absorption from topical application[269]; its use in humans with psoriasis has not been studied. Relatedly if not tangentially, topical honey is better than acyclovir against oral and genital herpes; apply *qid* for 15 minutes.[270]

[259] "S aureus was present in more than 50% of patients with AD and PS. We found that the severity of AD and PS significantly correlated to enterotoxin production of the isolated S aureus strains." Tomi et al. Staphylococcal toxins in patients with psoriasis, atopic dermatitis, and erythroderma. *J Am Acad Dermatol*. 2005 Jul;53(1):67-72

[260] "The recognition by immunoblot of streptococcal antigens by serum of guttate psoriasis patients, the presence of autoantibodies against their own skin, and recognition of the same skin antigens by anti-streptococcal rabbit antibodies confirm the participation of the immune system and of streptococcal infections in guttate psoriasis." Villeda-Gabriel G, et al. Recognition of Streptococcus pyogenes and skin autoantigens in guttate psoriasis. *Arch Med Res*. 1998 Summer;29(2):143-8

[261] "It seems that autoantibodies, although they do not appear to participate in the pathogenesis of psoriasis, are an important feature, and that skin antigens, which appear in lesional immature keratinocytes, cross-react with S. pyogenes and contribute to the autoimmune process in psoriasis." Perez-Lorenzo R, Zambrano-Zaragoza JF, Saul A, Jimenez-Zamudio L, Reyes-Maldonado E, Garcia-Latorre E. Autoantibodies to autologous skin in guttate and plaque forms of psoriasis and cross-reaction with skin antigens with streptococcal antigens. *Int J Dermatol*. 1998 Jul;37(7):524-31. The authors found that all psorais paitents had dermal autoantiboes and that these antibodies reacted specifically with endogenous dermal antigens; thus their finding that "Deposits of immunoglobulin G (IgG) were not detected in the lesions" is unexpected and inexplicable. This statement from their research is inconsistent with the findings of other research groups, and—specifically—must be placed in a context of other articles, most notably "… titers of IgG anti-SC autoantibodies in psoriatic patients were not specifically higher than in normal controls but were more variable, indicating that their circulating levels are dependent on a delicate balance between consumption at inflammatory sites and a secondary increase due to SC-antigen release following inflammation." Tagami H, Iwatsuki K, Yamada M. Profile of anti-stratum corneum autoantibodies in psoriatic patients. *Arch Dermatol Res*. 1983;275(2):71-5

[262] "Monoclonal antibodies directed against type 12 Group A streptococcal cell wall antigens cross-react with nuclei and cytoplasm of cells from skin and synovium from controls, uninvolved skin of psoriatics and psoriatic plaques." Muto et al. Immune response to Streptococcus pyogenes and the susceptibility to psoriasis. *Australas J Dermatol*. 1996 May;37 Suppl 1:S54-5

[263] "Patients with psoriasis had high serum titres of antibody against the M12 (C-region) streptococcal antigen compared to controls." Muto et al. Immune response to Streptococcus pyogenes and the susceptibility to psoriasis. *Australas J Dermatol*. 1996 May;37 Suppl 1:S54-5

[264] "Our data raised the possibility that staphylococcal superantigens may also play an exacerbating role in PA." Yamamoto T, Katayama I, Nishioka K. Peripheral blood mononuclear cell proliferative response against staphylococcal superantigens in patients with psoriasis arthropathy. *Eur J Dermatol*. 1999 Jan-Feb;9(1):17-21

[265] Schempp et al. Antibacterial activity of hyperforin from St John's wort against multiresistant Staphylococcus aureus and gram-positive bacteria. *Lancet*. 1999 Jun;353:2129

[266] "A butanol fraction of St. John's Wort revealed anti-Helicobacter pylori activity with MIC values ranging between 15.6 and 31.2 microg/ml." Reichling J, Weseler A, Saller R. A current review of the antimicrobial activity of Hypericum perforatum L. *Pharmacopsychiatry*. 2001 Jul;34 Suppl 1:S116-8

[267] "Honey, beeswax and olive oil mixture (1:1:1, v/v) is useful in the treatment of diaper dermatitis, psoriasis and eczema... CONCLUSIONS: Honey and honey mixture apparently could inhibit growth of S. aureus or C. albicans." Al-Waili NS. Mixture of honey, beeswax and olive oil inhibits growth of Staphylococcus aureus and Candida albicans. *Arch Med Res*. 2005 Jan-Feb;36(1):10-3

[268] "Taken together, these clinical studies conducted by several investigators in several countries indicate that Mahonia aquifolium is a safe and effective treatment of patients with mild to moderate psoriasis." Gulliver WP, Donsky HJ. A report on three recent clinical trials using Mahonia aquifolium 10% topical cream and a review of the worldwide clinical experience with Mahonia aquifolium for the treatment of plaque psoriasis. *Am J Ther*. 2005 Sep-Oct;12:398-406

[269] "This paper reports results of pharmacokinetic studies of this preparation when applied onto a fixed area of the shaved skin of mice and rabbits. ..The drug was found to be easily absorbed from the skin." Zhao et al. [The pharmacokinetics of a transdermal preparation of artesunate in mice and rabbits] [Article in Chinese] *Yao Xue Xue Bao*. 1989;24(11):813-6

[270] Al-Waili NS. Topical honey application vs. acyclovir for the treatment of recurrent herpes simplex lesions. *Med Sci Monit*. 2004 Aug;10(8):MT94-8

- Sarsaparilla (*Smilax* spp): A clinical trial published in the *New England Journal of Medicine* in 1942 documented benefit of a sarsaparilla compound in psoriasis.[271] The proposed mechanism of action includes the binding of bacterial endotoxins, preventing their local action and systemic absorption.

- Commonly used antibiotic/antifungal drugs: The most commonly employed drugs for intestinal bacterial overgrowth are described here.[272] Treatment duration is generally at least 2 weeks and up to 8 weeks, depending on clinical response and the severity and diversity of the intestinal overgrowth. With all anti*bacterial* treatments, use empiric anti*fungal* treatment to prevent yeast overgrowth; some patients benefit from antifungal treatment that is continued for *months* and occasionally *years*. Drugs can generally be coadministered with natural antibiotics/antifungals for improved efficacy. Treatment can be guided by identification of the dysbiotic microbes and the results of culture and sensitivity tests.

  - Penicillin: Chronic penicillin treatment leads to clinical improvement of recalcitrant psoriasis; benefits are seen when treatment is continued for at least 12 weeks, according to a clinical trial of treatment lasting for two years.[273]

  - Metronidazole: 250-500 mg BID-QID (generally limit to 1.5 g/d); metronidazole has systemic bioavailability and effectiveness against a wide range of dysbiotic microbes, including protozoans, amebas/Giardia, *H. pylori*, *Clostridium difficile* and most anaerobic gram-negative bacilli.[274] Adverse effects are generally limited to stomatitis, nausea, diarrhea, and—rarely and/or with long-term use—peripheral neuropathy, dizziness, and metallic taste; the drug must not be consumed with alcohol. Metronidazole resistance by *Blastocystis hominis* and other parasites has been noted.

  - Erythromycin: 250-500 mg TID-QID; this drug is a widely used antibiotic that also has intestinal promotility benefits (thus making it an ideal treatment for intestinal bacterial overgrowth associated with or caused by intestinal dysmotility/hypomotility such as seen in scleroderma[275,276]). Do not combine erythromycin with the promotility drug cisapride due to risk for serious cardiac arrhythmia.

Antimicrobial treatment for psoriasis

"Patients are questioned, examined, and subjected to microbiologic laboratory investigations in an attempt to identify possibly relevant microorganisms, and then are treated with antibiotics. ... Results obtained with this approach compare favorably with those achieved with more usual anti-psoriasis treatments. We recommend that a microbiologic investigation and a trial of antimicrobial treatment should precede any plan to treat psoriasis patients with anything more than the simplest topical agents."

Rosenberg EW, Noah PW, Skinner RB Jr. Microorganisms and psoriasis. *J Natl Med Assoc.* 1994 Apr

Long-term penicillin for psoriasis

"Significant improvement in the PASI score was noted from 12 weeks onwards. All patients showed excellent improvement at 2 years. Patients tolerated the therapy well. Controlled studies are needed to further confirm the benefits of long-term use of benzathine penicillin in the treatment of psoriasis."

Saxena VN, Dogra J. Long-term use of penicillin for treatment of chronic plaque psoriasis. *Eur J Dermatol.* 2005 Sep

Long-term azithromycin for psoriasis

"30 randomly selected patients with moderate to severe chronic plaque psoriasis received azithromycin for 48 weeks as a single oral 500 mg daily dose for 4 days with a gap of 10 days (total 24 such courses). ... Though the trial concluded at 48 weeks, patients in the azithromycin-arm were followed for another year to observe any relapse. A significant improvement in PASI score was noted from 12 weeks in the majority of patients in the azithromycin group. At the end of 48 weeks, 18 patients (60%) showed excellent improvement, while 6 patients (20%) showed good improvement and 4 patients (13.33%) showed mild improvement. ... An exacerbation in lesions was reported in 5 cases (16.66%) in the group receiving azithromycin. These exacerbations also responded by continuing the same treatment. ...Patients tolerated the therapy well."

Saxena VN, Dogra J. Long-term oral azithromycin in chronic plaque psoriasis. *Eur J Dermatol.* 2010 May

---

[271] Thurmon FM. The treatment of psoriasis with a sarsaparilla compound. *N Engl J Med* 1942; 227 (4): 128-33

[272] Saltzman JR, Russell RM. Nutritional consequences of intestinal bacterial overgrowth. *Compr Ther.* 1994;20(9):523-30

[273] "Total duration of the study was two years. Initially benzathine penicillin 1.2 million units, was given I.M. AST fortnightly. After 24 weeks benzathine penicillin was reduced to 1.2 million units once a month... Significant improvement in the PASI score was noted from 12 weeks onwards. All patients showed excellent improvement at 2 years." Saxena VN, Dogra J. Long-term use of penicillin for the treatment of chronic plaque psoriasis. *Eur J Dermatol.* 2005 Sep-Oct;15(5):359-62

[274] Tierney ML. McPhee SJ, Papadakis MA. *Current Medical Diagnosis and Treatment 2006. 45th edition.* New York; Lange Medical: 2006, pages 1578-1577

[275] "Prokinetic agents effective in pseudoobstruction include metoclopramide, domperidone, cisapride, octreotide, and erythromycin. ... The combination of octreotide and erythromycin may be particularly effective in systemic sclerosis." Sjogren RW. Gastrointestinal features of scleroderma. *Curr Opin Rheumatol.* 1996 Nov;8(6):569-75

[276] "Erythromycin accelerates gastric and gallbladder emptying in scleroderma patients and might be helpful in the treatment of gastrointestinal motor abnormalities in these patients." Fiorucci et al. Effect of erythromycin administration on upper gastrointestinal motility in scleroderma patients. *Scand J Gastroenterol.* 1994 Sep;29(9):807-13

- **NUTRITIONAL IMMUNOMODULATION: Treg induction for modulation of Th-1/2/17 inflammation** Nutrients and therapeutic approaches that promote Treg or IL-10 induction and/or Th-17, IL-17 suppression include 1) mitochondrial optimization and mTOR suppression, 2) biotin, 3) vitamin E, 4) sodium avoidance, 5) transgenic/GMO food avoidance, 6) probiotics, 7) lipoic acid, 8) vitamin A, 9) inflammation reduction, 10) vitamin D, 11) fatty acid supplementation with GLA and n3, 12) infection and dysbiosis remediation, 13) green tea EGCG. Acronym: MiBESTPLAIDFIG.

- **DYSMETABOLISM & DYSFUNCTIONAL MITOCHONDRIA: MitoDys, ERS-UPR, AGE/RAGE, hyperglycemia and ceramide** The major clinical considerations in this section are mitochondrial dysfunction, endoplasmic reticulum stress, unfolded protein response, TLR activation, and the dysmetabolic effects of sustained hyperglycemia and hyperinsulinemia and resultant oxidative stress, inflammation, RAGE activation, and accumulation of AGE, palmitate and ceramide. The review of this information in Chapter 4 covered approximately 30 interventions relevant to dysmetabolism, mitochondrial dysfunction, ERS-UPR, etc; these will not be reviewed here except to mention those most commonly, easily, empirically, synergistically, and effectively used: 1) low-carbohydrate diet with 2) moderate exercise, 3) CoQ-10, 4) acetyl-carnitine with 5) lipoic acid, 6) NAC, 7) resveratrol, and 8) melatonin.
  - Carnitine / fumarate: Fumaric acid 250-500 mg 3 times a day was advocated by Wright and Gaby[277], who advised beginning with a low dose and slowly increasing the dose over a period of weeks. Flushing and hypoglycemia may occur; serial measurements of liver and kidney function tests are mandatory since fumarate has been reported to cause liver and/or renal damage. **Carnitine appears to have anti-inflammatory action via its corticosteroid receptor agonist properties[278,279] and has been reported as beneficial in a case of psoriatic arthritis.**[280]

- **STYLE OF LIVING (LIFESTYLE) & SPECIAL CONSIDERATIONS: Sleep optimization, SocioPsychology, Stress management/avoidance, Somatic treatments, Special Supplementation, Sweat/exercise, Sauna/detoxification, Surgery, Stamp your passport and vacate current reality, Sensory deprivation therapy** This is a buffet of mostly lifestyle-based interventions yet also including considerations such as somatic treatments, additional supplementation, and surgery.
  - Folinic acid or methylfolate 5-20 mg per day: Patients with psoriasis have reduced folate status and elevated homocysteine levels.[281] Wright and Gaby recommended 50-150 mg per day of folic acid for psoriatics.[282] Folic acid has antiproliferative and anti-inflammatory effects mediated by nutrigenomic mechanisms. Folic acid, along with other vitamins and nutrients, may also help alleviate the biochemical aspect of the depression that is common in patients with psoriasis. Always supplement with vitamin B-12 in form of hydroxocobalamin or methylcobalamin (e.g., 2,000 mcg per day) when using high-dose folic acid. Most clinicians no longer use folic acid due to is causation of intracellular oxidative stress and association with malignancy; instead, folinic acid and methylated folate are preferred.
  - Topical *Berberis/Mahonia*: Topical *Berberis/Mahonia* is effective for dermal psoriasis.[283] Very obviously, topical treatments do not address the underlying problems in psoriasis and should therefore only be used for symptomatic/cosmetic improvement within the context of an overall treatment plan designed to correct the underlying/internal imbalances.
  - Topical *Capsicum annuum, Capsicum frutescens* (Cayenne pepper, hot chili pepper): Topical capsaicin has proven beneficial for alleviating the pruritus of psoriasis, presumably by depleting cutaneous neurons of

---

[277] Gaby A, Wright JV. *Nutritional Protocols*. 1998 by Nutrition Seminars

[278] "Accumulating evidence from both animal and human studies indicates that pharmacologic doses of L-carnitine (LCAR) have immunomodulatory effects resembling those of glucocorticoids (GC)." Manoli I, et al. Modulatory effects of L-carnitine on glucocorticoid receptor activity. *Ann N Y Acad Sci.* 2004 Nov;1033:147-57

[279] "Taken together, our results suggest that pharmacological doses of L-carnitine can activate GRalpha and, through this mechanism, regulate glucocorticoid-responsive genes, potentially sharing some of the biological and therapeutic properties of glucocorticoids."Alesci et al. L-carnitine: A nutritional modulator of glucocorticoid receptor functions. *FASEB J.* 2003 Aug;17(11):1553-5. Epub 2003 Jun 17 fasebj.org/cgi/reprint/02-1024fjev1

[280] Afeltra et al. Clinical improvement in psoriatic arthritis symptoms during treatment for infertility with carnitine. *Clin Exp Rheumatol.* 2004 Jan-Feb;22(1):138

[281] "The mean levels of serum tHcy, fibrinogen, fibronectin, sICAM, PAI-1 and AuAb-oxLDL were increased in patients whereas tPA, vitamin B(12) and folate levels were decreased significantly." Vanizor Kural et al. Plasma homocysteine and its relationships with atherothrombotic markers in psoriatic patients. *Clin Chim Acta.* 2003 Jun;332:23-30

[282] Gaby A, Wright JV. *Nutritional Protocols*. 1998 Nutrition Seminars

[283] "Taken together, these clinical studies conducted by several investigators in several countries indicate that Mahonia aquifolium is a safe and effective treatment of patients with mild to moderate psoriasis." Gulliver WP, Donsky HJ. A report on three recent clinical trials using Mahonia aquifolium 10% topical cream and a review of the worldwide clinical experience with Mahonia aquifolium for the treatment of plaque psoriasis. *Am J Ther.* 2005 Sep-Oct;12:398-406

substance P.[284] Very obviously, topical treatments do not address the underlying problems in psoriasis and should therefore only be used for symptomatic/cosmetic improvement within the context of an overall treatment plan designed to correct the underlying/internal imbalances.

- o Spinal manipulation: Many years ago I read a published case report of a female patient who experienced acute onset of psoriasis following trauma received during a skiing accident. Her psoriasis resolved promptly following a series of treatments of chiropractic spinal manipulative therapy.
- o Hydrotherapy, local hyperthermia: Hot bath hyperthermia (or heating pads[285]) improves skin lesions and lessens pruritus in the majority of patients with psoriasis.[286] The dermatologic improvements following hyperthermia can be objectively documented clinically and histologically/microscopically.[287]

- • **ENDOCRINE IMBALANCE & OPTIMIZATION: Prolactin, Insulin, Estrogen, DHEA, Cortisol, Testosterone, Thyroid** | Common hormonal imbalances seen among autoimmune/inflammatory patients are: ❶ *elevated* prolactin, ❷ *elevated* estrogen, ❸ *elevated* insulin, and ❹ *reduced* DHEA, ❺ *reduced* cortisol, and ❻ *reduced* testosterone; see Chapter 4 for discussion of these hormones and respective interventions. Thyroid evaluation (patient + labs) should be comprehensive, as discussed in Chapter 1, with a low threshold for empiric treatment.
  - o Melatonin: Melatonin is a pineal hormone with well-known sleep-inducing and immunomodulatory properties, and it is commonly administered in doses of 1-40 mg in the evening, before bedtime. Its exceptional safety is well documented. Although psoriatic patients appear to have lost the physiologic nocturnal peak of melatonin[288], the role of supplemental melatonin in the treatment of patients with psoriasis has not been researched; however clinicians may reasonably decide to add this to their patients' treatment plan as appropriate. In contrast to implementing treatment with high doses of 20-40 mg, starting with a relatively low dose (e.g., 1-5 mg) and increasing as tolerated is recommended. Melatonin (20 mg hs) appears to have cured two patients with drug-resistant sarcoidosis[289] and 3 mg provided immediate short-term benefit to a patient with multiple sclerosis.[290] Immunostimulatory anti-infective action of melatonin was demonstrated in a clinical trial wherein septic newborns administered 20 mg melatonin showed significantly increased survival over nontreated controls[291]; given that psoriasis is associated with many subclinical infections, melatonin may provide therapeutic benefit by virtue of its anti-infective properties.
  - o Prolactin (excess): According to clinical trials with small numbers of patients, whether prolactin levels are high or not, treatment with prolactin-lowering treatment (such as bromocriptine[292]) appears beneficial in patients with psoriatic arthritis. Serum prolactin is the standard assessment of prolactin status. Since elevated prolactin may be a sign of pituitary tumor, assessment for headaches, visual deficits, other abnormalities of pituitary hormones (e.g., GH and TSH) should be performed and CT or MRI must be considered. Patients with prolactin levels less than 100 ng/mL and normal CT/MRI findings can be managed conservatively with effective prolactin-lowering treatment and annual radiologic assessment (less necessary with favorable serum response).[293, see review 294] Patients with RA and SLE have higher basal

[284] "CONCLUSION: Topically applied capsaicin effectively treats pruritic psoriasis, a finding that supports a role for substance P in this disorder." Ellis CN, et al. A double-blind evaluation of topical capsaicin in pruritic psoriasis. *J Am Acad Dermatol* 1993 Sep;29(3):438-42

[285] Urabe H, Nishitani K, Kohda H. Hyperthermia in the treatment of psoriasis. *Arch Dermatol.* 1981 Dec;117(12):770-4

[286] "These results indicate that simple repetitive water bath hyperthermia alone is effective in the treatment of psoriatic lesions in heatable locations." Boreham DR, Gasmann HC, Mitchel RE. Water bath hyperthermia is a simple therapy for psoriasis and also stimulates skin tanning in response to sunlight. *Int J Hyperthermia.* 1995 Nov-Dec;11(6):745-54

[287] "Electron microscopy of psoriatic skin prior to and after local hyperthermia revealed both temporary and gradual changes following treatment." Imayama S, Urabe H. Human psoriatic skin lesions improve with local hyperthermia: an ultrastructural study. *J Cutan Pathol.* 1984 Feb;11(1):45-52

[288] "Our results show that psoriatic patients had lost the nocturnal peak and usual circadian rhythm of melatonin secretion. Levels of melatonin were significantly lower than in controls at 2 a.m., and higher at 6 and 8 a.m. and at 12 noon." Mozzanica et al. Plasma melatonin levels in psoriasis. *Acta Derm Venereol.* 1988;68(4):312-6

[289] Cagnoni ML, Lombardi A, Cerinic MC, Dedola GL, Pignone A. Melatonin for treatment of chronic refractory sarcoidosis. *Lancet.* 1995 Nov 4;346(8984):1229-30

[290] "…administration of melatonin (3 mg, orally) at 2:00 p.m., when the patient experienced severe blurring of vision, resulted within 15 minutes in a dramatic improvement in visual acuity and in normalization of the visual evoked potential latency after stimulation of the left eye." Sandyk R. Diurnal variations in vision and relations to circadian melatonin secretion in multiple sclerosis. *Int J Neurosci.* 1995 Nov;83(1-2):1-6

[291] Gittoet al. Effects of melatonin treatment in septic newborns. *Pediatr Res.* 2001 Dec;50(6):756-60 pedresearch.org/cgi/content/full/50/6/756

[292] "In 2 cases of psoriatic arthritis, adding bromocriptine to gold salts and nonsteroidal anti-inflammatory drug was followed by a drastic efficacy with spectacular improvement in clinical, biological and occupational status. Because none of the cases had hyperprolactinaemia, bromocriptine acted probably had an intrinic anti-inflammatory effect independent of its antiprolactinic effect." Eulry et al. [Blood prolactin under the effect of protirelin in spondylarthropathies. Treatment trial of 4 cases of reactive arthritis and 2 cases of psoriatic arthritis with bromocriptine. French] *Ann Med Interne* (Paris). 1996;147(1):15-9

[293] Beers MH, Berkow R (eds). *Merck Manual. 17th Edition.* Whitehouse Station; Merck Research Laboratories 1999 Page 77-78

[294] Serri O, Chik CL, Ur E, Ezzat S. Diagnosis and management of hyperprolactinemia. *CMAJ.* 2003 Sep 16;169(6):575-81 cmaj.ca/cgi/content/full/169/6/575

and stress-induced levels of prolactin compared with normal controls.[295,296] A normal serum prolactin level does not necessarily exclude the use of prolactin-lowering intervention, especially since many autoimmune patients have latent hyperprolactinemia which may not be detected with random serum measurement of prolactin. Bromocriptine has long been considered the pharmacologic treatment of choice for elevated prolactin.[297] Bromocriptine appears to benefit most patients with psoriasis/psoriatic arthritis, according to a small Italian study[298] and three case reports in the French literature.[299] Typical dose is 2.5 mg per day (effective against lupus[300]); gastrointestinal upset and sedation are common.[301] Clinical intervention with bromocriptine appears warranted in patients with RA, SLE, reactive arthritis, psoriatic arthritis, and probably multiple sclerosis and uveitis.[302] A normal serum prolactin level does not necessarily exclude the use of prolactin-lowering intervention, especially since many autoimmune patients have latent hyperprolactinemia which may not be detected with random serum measurement of prolactin. Cabergoline/Dostinex is a newer dopamine agonist with few adverse effects; typical dose starts at 0.5 mg per week (0.25 mg twice per week).[303] Several

> **Estrogen promotes inflammation**
>
> "We report a patient with severe psoriatic arthritis in whom the severity of both the arthritis and psoriasis fluctuated with the menstrual cycle. These features failed to improve with standard therapy, but there was a prompt response to treatment which suppressed estrogen secretion."
>
> Stevens et al. Cyclical psoriatic arthritis responding to anti-oestrogen therapy. *Br J Dermatol.* 1993 Oct

studies have indicated that cabergoline is safer and more effective than bromocriptine for reducing prolactin levels[304] and the dose can often be reduced after successful prolactin reduction, allowing for reductions in cost and adverse effects.[305] Although fewer studies have been published supporting the antirheumatic benefits of cabergoline than those supporting bromocriptine; its antirheumatic benefits have indeed been documented.[306]

o Estrogen (excess): Although the classic pattern in patients with autoimmunity is elevated estrogen (generally considered immunodysregulatory) and reduced testosterone (generally considered anti-inflammatory and immunoregulatory), data in patients with psoriatic arthritis is inadequate to extend this otherwise consistent and successful generalization to this group. On the contrary, Stevens et al[307] published a case report of a woman with recalcitrant psoriasis and psoriatic arthritis who responded very well to anti-estrogen treatment. The small amount of data available actually suggests that estrogen may be beneficial (reduction in skin lesions with pregnancy) and that testosterone (in one woman who developed psoriasis following a testosterone-containing hormonal implant following oophorectomy) could exacerbate the disease.

o Testosterone (insufficiency): Androgen deficiencies predispose to, are exacerbated by, and contribute to autoimmune/inflammatory disorders. Female patients with psoriasis have lower levels of testosterone

[295] Dostal C, et al. Serum prolactin stress values in patients with systemic lupus erythematosus. *Ann Rheum Dis.* 2003 May;62(5):487-8

[296] "RESULTS: A significantly higher rate of elevated PRL levels was found in SLE patients (40.0%) compared with the healthy controls (14.8%). No proof was found of association with the presence of anti-ds-DNA or with specific organ involvement. Similarly, elevated PRL levels were found in RA patients (39.3%)." Moszkorzova L, Lacinova Z, Marek J, Musilova L, Dohnalova A, Dostal C. Hyperprolactinaemia in patients with systemic lupus erythematosus. *Clin Exp Rheumatol.* 2002 Nov-Dec;20(6):807-12

[297] Beers MH, Berkow R (eds). *Merck Manual. 17th Edition.* Whitehouse Station; Merck Research Laboratories 1999 Page 77-78

[298] "Bromocriptin was shown to be effective in 13 of our 18 psoriatic patients." Valentino A, Fimiani M, Bilenchi R, Castelli A, Francini G, Gonnelli S, Gennari C, Andreassi L. [Therapy with bromocriptine and behavior of various hormones in psoriasis patients] *Boll Soc Ital Biol Sper.* 1984 Oct 30;60(10):1841-4. Italian.

[299] "All three were treated with bromocriptine (5 mg/d in 2 doses) after verification of normal baseline and protirelin-stimulation prolactin levels. There was a beneficial effect in nocturnal pain relief, morning stiffness, the Lee and Ritchie scores and biological markers of inflammation." Eulry F, Mayaudon H, Lechevalier D, Bauduceau B, Ariche L, Ouakil H, Crozes P, Magnin J. [Treatment of rheumatoid psoriasis with bromocriptine] *Presse Med.* 1995 Nov 18;24(35):1642-4. French.

[300] "A prospective, double-blind, randomized, placebo-controlled study compared BRC at a fixed daily dosage of 2.5 mg with placebo... Long term treatment with a low dose of BRC appears to be a safe and effective means of decreasing SLE flares in SLE patients." Alvarez-Nemegyei J, Cobarrubias-Cobos A, Escalante-Triay F, Sosa-Munoz J, Miranda JM, Jara LJ. Bromocriptine in systemic lupus erythematosus: a double-blind, randomized, placebo-controlled study. *Lupus.* 1998;7(6):414-9

[301] Serri O, Chik CL, Ur E, Ezzat S. Diagnosis and management of hyperprolactinemia. *CMAJ.* 2003 Sep 16;169(6):575-81 cmaj.ca/cgi/content/full/169/6/575

[302] "...clinical observations and trials support the use of bromocriptine as a nonstandard primary or adjunctive therapy in the treatment of recalcitrant RA, SLE, Reiter's syndrome, and psoriatic arthritis and associated conditions unresponsive to traditional approaches." McMurray RW. Bromocriptine in rheumatic and autoimmune diseases. *Semin Arthritis Rheum.* 2001 Aug;31(1):21-32

[303] Serri O, Chik CL, Ur E, Ezzat S. Diagnosis and management of hyperprolactinemia. *CMAJ.* 2003 Sep 16;169(6):575-81

[304] "CONCLUSION: These data indicate that cabergoline is a very effective agent for lowering the prolactin levels in hyperprolactinemic patients and that it appears to offer considerable advantage over bromocriptine in terms of efficacy and tolerability." Sabuncu T, Arikan E, Tasan E, Hatemi H. Comparison of the effects of cabergoline and bromocriptine on prolactin levels in hyperprolactinemic patients. *Intern Med.* 2001 Sep;40(9):857-61

[305] "Cabergoline also normalized PRL in the majority of patients with known bromocriptine intolerance or -resistance. Once PRL secretion was adequately controlled, the dose of cabergoline could often be significantly decreased, which further reduced costs of therapy." Verhelst et al. Cabergoline in the treatment of hyperprolactinemia: a study in 455 patients. *J Clin Endocrinol Metab.* 1999 Jul;84(7):2518-22 jcem.endojournals.org/cgi/content/full/84/7/2518

[306] Erb et al. Control of unremitting rheumatoid arthritis by the prolactin antagonist cabergoline. *Rheumatology.* 2001 Feb;40(2):237-9

[307] "We report a patient with severe psoriatic arthritis in whom the severity of both the arthritis and psoriasis fluctuated with the menstrual cycle. These features failed to improve with standard therapy, but there was a prompt response to treatment which suppressed oestrogen secretion." Stevens HP, Ostlere LS, Black CM, Jacobs HS, Rustin MH. Cyclical psoriatic arthritis responding to anti-oestrogen therapy. *Br J Dermatol.* 1993 Oct;129(4):458-60

compared to those seen in healthy controls.[308] A large proportion of men with lupus or RA have low testosterone[309] and suffer the effects of hypogonadism: fatigue, weakness, depression, slow healing, low libido, and difficulties with sexual performance. Testosterone levels may rise following DHEA supplementation (especially in women) and can be elevated in men by the use of anastrozole/Arimidex. Otherwise, transdermal testosterone such as Androgel or Testim can be applied as indicated.

- o DHEA: DHEA is an anti-inflammatory and immunoregulatory hormone that is commonly deficient in patients with autoimmunity and inflammatory arthritis.[310] However, the role of DHEA in psoriatic arthritis *en masse* is unclear due to conflicting data. One study showed that patients with psoriasis did not show evidence of DHEA insufficiency[311], while other studies—especially in the German literature—have consistently documented low serum and intracellular levels of DHEA.[312] DHEA levels should be measured in these patients—especially those with severe disease, deficiencies should be treated unless contraindicated, and therapeutic trials are not unreasonable.

- • XENOBIOTIC ACCUMULATION & DETOXIFICATION: Chemical avoidance, nutritional support for detoxification pathways, urine alkalinization The clinical relevance and pathogenic mechanisms of xenobiotic accumulation are irrefutably well documented and described. Clinical assessments include history, physical examination, and laboratory assessment (using serum, whole blood, urine or—rarely yet accurately—fat biopsy), and response to treatment. Treatments include nutritional support for Phases 1 and 2 of detoxification (e.g., oxidation and conjugation) and excretion via bile and urine; for the latter, urinary alkalinization is generally recommended. Chemical toxins can be bound in the gut using activated charcoal, cholestyramine, or *Chlorella*—all of these three treatments have documented safety and effectiveness; clinically and empirically, phytochelatin (plant-derived peptides that bind toxic metals) concentrates appear safe and effective despite lack of conclusive published data supporting clinical use.

  - o Detoxification support: Cytochrome P450 (Cyp450) defects (phenotypic—not genotropic—in this research) have been noted in patients with psoriasis and correlate with the severity of the disease.[313] Assuming a causal relationship, one can speculate as to the nature and direction of that relationship:

    - ▪ Cause of disease: Perhaps the detoxification defects lead to xenobiotic accumulation which alters immune function in favor of xenobiotic immunotoxicity: resulting in immune impairment and exaggerated inflammatory response.
    - ▪ Effect of disease: Perhaps the inflammation or oxidative stress or nutritional deficiencies of psoriasis is/are the cause of the detoxification defects.
    - ▪ Shared causality: Perhaps the increased total bacterial load impairs Cyp450 via LPS and also causes the inflammatory dysfunction that precipitates psoriasis.
    - ▪ Nonexclusivity, additive/synergistic effects: All of the above.

---

[308] "The testosterone levels and LH/FSH ratio were significantly lower in the psoriatic group." Pietrzak A, Lecewicz-Torun B, Jakimiuk A. Lipid and hormone profile in psoriatic females. *Ann Univ Mariae Curie Sklodowska* [Med]. 2002;57(2):478-83

[309] Karagiannis A, Harsoulis F. Gonadal dysfunction in systemic diseases. *Eur J Endocrinol*. 2005 Apr;152(4):501-13 eje-online.org/cgi/content/full/152/4/501

[310] "DHEAS concentrations were significantly decreased in both women and men with inflammatory arthritis (IA) (P < 0.001)." Dessein PH, et al. Hyposecretion of the adrenal androgen dehydroepiandrosterone sulfate and its relation to clinical variables in inflammatory arthritis. *Arthritis Res*. 2001;3(3):183-8 arthritis-research.com/content/3/3/183

[311] "Assessing the patients by group, the mean DHEAS level was markedly lower in the pemphigoid/pemphigus than in the psoriasis and OA patients (geometric mean 600 vs. 2130 and 2100 nmol/l, respectively; p < 0.001)." de la Torre B, Fransson J, Scheynius A. Blood dehydroepiandrosterone sulphate (DHEAS) levels in pemphigoid/pemphigus and psoriasis. *Clin Exp Rheumatol*. 1995 May-Jun;13(3):345-8

[312] "The effects of this dehydroepiandrosterone deficiency are changes in the humoral regulation of events in growth and proliferation in patients with psoriasis." Holzmann H, Benes P, Morsches B. [Dehydroepiandrosterone deficiency in psoriasis. Hypothesis on the etiopathogenesis of this disease. German] *Hautarzt*. 1980 Feb;31(2):71-5

[313] "Low CYP2C activity was associated with severe psoriasis, poor metaboliser status occurring in 50% of the severe group, but in none of the mild cases, p < 0.01." Helsby NA, et al. Hepatic cytochrome P450 CYP2C activity in psoriasis: studies using proguanil as a probe compound. *Acta Derm Venereol* 1998 Mar;78(2):81-3

Systemic Lupus Erythematosus: "SLE" or "Lupus"

Introduction:
As was said to me once by a Vice President of one of the largest hospital systems in Texas, SLE is a "big league" disease with numerous and potentially fatal complications; it is not to be taken lightly. Best interests of both doctor and patient are served by having a rheumatologist and/or internist as part of the care team. SLE is the prototype of multiorgan autoimmunity, mediated by a combination of cellular and humoral factors especially including immune-complex deposition and localized inflammation in the vascular system (vasculitis), skin (dermatitis), joints (arthritis) and kidneys (nephritis).

Description/pathophysiology:

- SLE as the prototype of multisystem autoimmune disease: SLE is the prototype of multisystem autoimmune disease, characterized by a chronic progressive course with remissions and relapses; as the prototype of multiorgan "idiopathic" autoimmunity, SLE will serve to model facts and concepts that are applicable to other conditions. The skin, joints, kidneys, serosal membranes (pleura, pericardium, peritoneum), and vascular system are the most prominent targets of inflammatory attack; however, any cell and tissue may be damaged, either directly or indirectly. Autoantibodies (and resultant immune complexes) against a wide range of

Immune complex pathophysiology
Consecutive linking of antigen and antibody results in formation of immune complexes which are predisposed for deposition in joints, skin, kidneys, and vasculature. Immune complex deposition results in focal and atopic (distant from site of antigen exposure) inflammatory damage of surrounding tissue via local activation of complement pathway and local inflammation, including recruitment of neutrophils and monocytes which release free radicals and autolytic lysosomal enzymes.

endogenous/self targets are pathogenic in SLE; however, **the current pathologic paradigm places ultimate responsibility on CD4+ helper T-cells—i.e., e.g., the Th1, Th2, Th17, and Treg cells discussed in Chapter 4—** rather than the antibody-producing B-cells/plasma cells. Tissue damage in SLE is largely mediated by **autoantibodies—particularly anti-nuclear antibodies (ANA)—** and the resulting **immune complexes**, cryoglobulins, and the subsequent inflammatory cascade.[314,315,316,317] **Patients with SLE have impaired ability to clear immune complexes via hepatic and splenic routes**[318,319]; therapeutic implications are discussed below. **SLE is considered a type-3 hypersensitivity disease because it is largely mediated by immune complex deposition** and secondary activation of the complement cascade and other inflammatory pathways.

- Allopathic perspective = "idiopathic": This condition is generally considered "idiopathic" in most cases, though in some patients the disease is induced by pharmaceutical drugs (especially hydralazine, procainamide, D-penicillamine) and is then generally reversible upon discontinuation of the drug. Most people with complement deficiencies (a group of congenital immune defects) develop SLE. Other precipitating/contributing factors include ultraviolet light exposure, chemical exposure, and possibly consumption of alfalfa sprouts (based on animal data[320] and very little human data). Abnormal hormone metabolism has also been noted and may play a role in the pathogenesis as described in the section on *orthoendocrinology*—Chapter 4.6.

- Integrative/functional/naturopathic perspective = multifactorial: Numerous—not innumerable—factors contribute to SLE pathogenesis; these are well represented within the FINDSEX™ of the functional inflammology protocol.

- The role of microbes, especially viral infections: The cytokine pattern and many of the pathogenic features of SLE have pointed toward "a viral etiology" for many years; one is simultaneously challenged with the paradox

[314] Tierney ML. McPhee SJ, Papadakis MA (eds). *Current Medical Diagnosis and Treatment 2006. 45th edition*. New York; Lange Medical Books: 2006, pages 833-837
[315] Suzuki et al. Development of pathogenic anti-DNA antibodies in patients with systemic lupus erythematosus. *FASEB J*. 1997 Oct;11:1033-8 fasebj.org/cgi/reprint/11/12/1033
[316] "Pisetsky DS. Antibody responses to DNA in normal immunity and aberrant immunity. *Clin Diagn Lab Immunol*. 1998 Jan;5(1):1-6 cvi.asm.org/cgi/reprint/5/1/1
[317] Sikander FF, Salgaonkar DS, Joshi VR. Cryoglobulin studies in systemic lupus erythematosus. *J Postgrad Med* [serial online] 1989 [cited 2005 Nov 2];35:139-43
[318] "These observations support the hypothesis that IC handling is abnormal in SLE." Davies KA, Peters AM, Beynon HL, Walport MJ. Immune complex processing in patients with systemic lupus erythematosus. In vivo imaging and clearance studies. *J Clin Invest*. 1992 Nov;90(5):2075-83
[319] "These results indicate that Fc-mediated clearance of ICs is defective in patients with SLE and suggest that ligation of ICs by Fc receptors is critical for their efficient binding and retention by the fixed MPS in the liver." Davies et al. Defective Fc-dependent processing of immune complexes in patients with systemic lupus erythematosus. *Arthritis Rheum*. 2002 Apr;46(4):1028-38
[320] "L-Canavanine sulfate, a constituent of alfalfa sprouts, was incorporated into the diet and reactivated the syndrome in monkeys in which an SLE-like syndrome had previously been induced by the ingestion of alfalfa seeds or sprouts." Malinow et al. Systemic lupus erythematosus-like syndrome in monkeys fed alfalfa sprouts: role of a nonprotein amino acid. *Science*. 1982 Apr 23;216(4544):415-7

of wanting to accept this as plausible and wanting to reject it as yet another *undefined* and therefore *useless* and therefore *idiopathic* allopathic description of disease pathogenesis. With more currently available research however, I think the viral hypothesis—or more accurately the *poly*viral and polymicrobial model—is gaining credible and clinically usable merit. I will outline this territory as I see it:

- o Increased and/or altered total microbial load (TML): Some evidence has shown that SLE patients have evidence of increased microbial loads—both bacterial and viral. For example, patients with SLE, psoriasis, Wegener's, and eczema have all shown increased nasal carriage of *Staphylococcus aureus*. Even if no immune abnormalities were present, increased antigenic exposure would be expected to result in increased humor antibody response and the formation of more—perhaps a pathogenic "excess" of—immune complexes; if the immune system were hyperresponsive, say due to vitamin D deficiency and the resulting lack of Treg induction, then the situation would only get worse as the causes of immune hyperresponsiveness become additive or synergistic. Obviously, the TML contributes directly and powerfully to the TIL—total inflammatory load.

- o Impaired immune complex clearance: Impaired clearance of immune complexes would—of course—complicate the aforementioned problems associated with increased TML and TIL; in fact, the result would be a positive/upward dissociation of the TIL from the TML as the inflammatory consequences become greater than normal/proportionate.

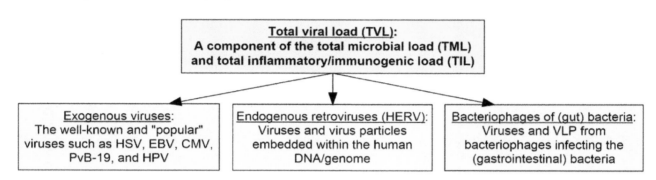

The total viral load (TVL): TVL contributes to TML (total microbial load) and thus to the TIL (total inflammatory load), to which are added the TCL (total carbohydrate load) and TXL (total xenobiotic load).

- o Viruses, part 1—Known/popular "epigenomic" viruses: I categorize as "known" and/or "popular" those viruses that we commonly consider, such as Epstein-Bar virus (EBV), parvovirus B-19 (PvB19), cytomegalovirus (CMV), human papilloma virus (HPV) and other such viruses as we generally consider clinically and/or studied in whatever medical school we as clinicians attended. These have been described as epigenomic and/or exogenous viruses because they are close to but not part of the human genome—"epi" is a Greek-derived prefix denoting "above, on, over, nearby, upon"; these *epigenomic* viruses are contrasted with the *endogenous* viruses that are integrally "built in" to the human DNA. All four viruses mentioned in the previous sentence have been associated with autoimmunity; more recently has arrived the data supporting our new appreciation that "autoimmune patients" *may well be* and *generally are* "actively infected" with many of these viruses simultaneously—this is well-documented now in scleroderma, patients with which show active and "ectopic" (unusual locations) infections simultaneously with EBV, PvB19, and CMV. *Helicobacter pylori* may play a powerful role as a synergistic bioagent via its ability to *simultaneously* and *paradoxically* cause immunosuppression (thereby allowing other microbes to flourish) and systemic inflammation[321]; in this manner, the bacterial infection is permissive to and perhaps necessary for the autoimmune-inducing vasculopathic and fibrogenic viral infections (see section on Scleroderma for pathology details). An important concept to remember is that viral infections promote other viral infections—transactivation—via direct genomic enhancement of viral replication, by promoting a favorable cytokine environment for viral replication, and/or by stimulating

---

[321] "Infectious agents such as Helicobacter pylori (Hp) may cause chronic inflammation and autoimmune reactivity in susceptible subjects. The results of in vitro experiments performed with lymphocytes from Hp infected patients indicate that Hp can cause immunosuppression which might be eliminated by successful eradication therapy." Hybenova et al. The role of environmental factors in autoimmune thyroiditis. *Neuro Endocrinol Lett.* 2010;31(3):283-9

NFkB which is commonly "hijacked" by viruses to promote viral replication; therefore activation or suppression of any virus can be said to contribute *indirectly* to the activation or suppression, respectively, of other viral populations.[322] Relatedly and as will be discussed in the following section on endogenous viruses, replication of exogenous/epigenomic viruses—such as influenza virus and herpes simplex type-1—increases expression of endogenous viruses.

> **Rationale for anti-viral therapy for treating autoimmunity**
>
> "Cited epidemiologic and experimental evidence suggests that increased replication of epigenomic viral pathogens such as Epstein-Barr Virus (EBV) in chronic human autoimmune diseases such as rheumatoid arthritis (RA), systemic lupus erythematosus (SLE), and multiple sclerosis (MS) may activate endogenous human retroviruses (HERV) as a pathologic mechanism."
>
> Dreyfus DH. Autoimmune disease: A role for new anti-viral therapies? *Autoimmun Rev*. 2011 Dec

- **Epstein-Barr virus in the pathogenesis of some autoimmune disorders (*Eur J Microbiol Immunol* 2011 Dec[323])**: "Moreover, many observations indicate that EBV contributes also to the pathomechanism of SLE. However, this contribution differs from the relationship between EBV and MS, as shown by the lack of any increase in the risk of SLE after IM [infectious mononucleosis]. In SLE, EBV serology is quantitatively and qualitatively different from the normal response - that is, EBV viral load is higher and a strong cross-reaction can be detected between certain EBV antigens and autoantigens of pathological importance."

- **Lupus and Epstein-Barr (*Curr Opin Rheumatol* 2012 Jul[324])**: "SLE patients have a dysregulated immune response against EBV. EBV antigens exhibit structural molecular mimicry with common SLE antigens and functional molecular mimicry with critical immune-regulatory components. SLE patients, from a number of unique geographic regions, are shown to have higher rates of EBV seroconversion, especially against early EBV antigens, suggesting frequent viral reactivation. SLE patients also have increased EBV viral loads and impaired EBV-specific CD8 cytotoxic T cells, with impaired cytokine responses to EBV in lupus patients. ... Recent advances demonstrate SLE-specific serologic responses, gene expression, viral load, T-cell responses, humoral fine specificity, and molecular mimicry with EBV, further supporting potential roles for EBV in lupus etiology and pathogenesis."

- **HTLV (human T-lymphotropic virus) in SLE (*Clin Immunol.* 2002 Feb[325])**: "SLE patients produce high titer antibodies to various retroviral proteins, including Gag, Env, and Nef of HIV and HTLV (human T-lymphotropic virus), in the absence of overt retroviral infection. ... In particular, we consider the role of HTLV-1-related endogenous sequence (HRES-1) in SLE. We propose that molecular mimicry between HRES-1 and the small ribonucleoprotein complex initiates the production of autoantibodies, leading to immune complex formation, complement fixation, and pathological tissue deposition."

o **Viruses, part 2—Human endogenous retroviruses (endoretroviruses, HERVs or ERVs)**: Human DNA is "pre-loaded" with remnants of viral infections that have coursed through and been transmitted from parents to offspring for millions of years; these endogenous viral genomes implanted into human DNA are now known to undergo reactivation with the production of immunogenic viral remnants and the anticipated inflammatory immune response. As mentioned previously related to exogenous viral transactivation, replication of exogenous/epigenomic viruses—such as influenza virus and herpes simplex type-1—increases expression of endogenous viruses[326]; as such, one method to reduce/control activation of HERVs is to suppress replication of exogenous viruses. HERV activation is inhibited by

---

[322] White et al. Reciprocal transactivation between HIV-1 and other human viruses. *Virology.* 2006 Aug 15;352(1):1-13
[323] Füst G. The role of the Epstein-Barr virus in the pathogenesis of some autoimmune disorders - Similarities and differences. *Eur J Microbiol Immunol* (Bp). 2011 Dec;1:267-78
[324] James JA, Robertson JM. Lupus and Epstein-Barr. *Curr Opin Rheumatol.* 2012 Jul;24(4):383-8
[325] Adelman MK, Marchalonis JJ. Endogenous retroviruses in systemic lupus erythematosus: candidate lupus viruses. *Clin Immunol.* 2002 Feb;102(2):107-16
[326] "Since viral infections have previously been reported to transactivate retroviral long terminal repeat regions we examined the basal expression of HERV-W elements and following infections by influenza A/WSN/33 and Herpes simplex 1 viruses in human cell-lines. ... Subsets of HERV-W elements were transactivated by viral infection in the different cell-lines. Transcriptional activation of these elements, including that encoding syncytin, was dependent on viral replication and was not induced by antiviral responses." Nellaker et al. Transactivation of elements in the human endogenous retrovirus W family by viral infection. *Retrovirology.* 2006 Jul 6;3:44

DNA methylation; conversely, DNA hypomethylation is consistently associated with SLE in humans and animals.[327,328]

- Human endogenous retroviruses in the development of autoimmune diseases (*Int Rev Immunol* 2010 Aug[329]): In 2010, Balada et al provided a succinct and authoritative summary of HERVs and their relationship to the pathogenesis of autoimmunity: "Retroviruses can exist in an endogenous form, in which viral sequences are integrated into the human germ line and are vertically transmitted in a Mendelian fashion. Human endogenous retroviruses (HERVs), probably representing footprints of ancient germ-cell retroviral infections, occupy about 1% of the human genome. … Although some of these elements show mutations and deletions, some HERVs are transcriptionally active and produce functional proteins. Some medical conditions, such as cancer and autoimmune diseases, are linked to the transcription of some of the HERVs genes, to the expression of HERVs proteins (that may act as superantigens, for example), and/or to the development of antibodies against them that might cross-react with our own proteins. Their genetic sequences may also be, totally or partially, integrated into genes that regulate the immune response. These mechanisms could give rise to autoimmune diseases, such as lupus erythematosus, insulin-dependent diabetes mellitus, multiple sclerosis, Sjögren's syndrome, and rheumatoid arthritis, among others."

> **HERV-autoimmunity associations**
> - Rheumatoid arthritis: expression of multiple ERVs detected in RA patients; HERV-K10 shows molecular mimicry
> - Juvenile RA: HERV-K10
> - Multiple sclerosis: MS-associated retroviral element (MRSV)-type HERV-W; increased expression of the env RNA and protein expression in the blood and brain cells of MS patients; also clear increase in HERV-H/F family HERV-Fc1 activity and RNA production; HERV-K18 on chromosome 1 is a risk factor for MS
> - Psoriasis: Increased expression of HERV-W, K, E, and variant ERV-9/HERV-W
> - Lupus: Hypomethylation of HERV-E and HERV-K
>
> Mechanisms for HERV-induced autoimmune diseases:
> - Molecular mimicry (HERV-K10)
> - Superantigen production (HERV-K)
> - LTR (long terminal repeat)-mediated alterations of gene expression
> - Antigenicity and immune complex formation
>
> Activation of HERVs:
> - DNA hypomethylation
> - Transactivation

Clear and complete as that is, readers might reasonably want additional sources of support, and I have provided samples of such here:

- Human endogenous retroviruses in the pathogenesis of autoimmune diseases (*Med Sci Monit* 2012 Jun[330]): "This theory takes into account the existence in the human genome, since approximately 40 million years, of so-called human endogenous retroviruses (HERVs), which are transmitted to descendants vertically by the germ cells. It was recently established that these generally silent sequences perform some physiological roles, but occasionally become active and influence the development of some chronic diseases like diabetes, some neoplasms, chronic diseases of the nervous system (e.g., sclerosis multiplex), schizophrenia and autoimmune diseases."
- Endogenous retroviral pathogenesis in lupus (*Curr Opin Rheumatol* 2010 Sep[331]): "ERV proteins may trigger lupus through structural and functional molecular mimicry, whereas the accumulation of ERV-derived nucleic acids stimulates interferon and anti-DNA antibody production in SLE."
- Autoimmune disease treatment with anti-viral therapies (*Autoimmun Rev* 2011 Dec[332]): "Cited epidemiologic and experimental evidence suggests that increased replication of epigenomic viral pathogens such as Epstein-Barr Virus (EBV) in chronic human autoimmune diseases such as rheumatoid arthritis (RA), systemic lupus Erythematosus (SLE), and multiple sclerosis (MS) may activate endogenous human retroviruses (HERV) as a pathologic mechanism. … Other [drug] anti-viral therapies of chronic autoimmune diseases, such as retroviral integrase inhibitors, could be effective, although not without risk." This article provides support and rationale for using antiviral

---

[327] "This raises the possibility that HERV demethylation participates in the pathogenesis of SLE." Renaudineau et al. Epigenetics and autoimmunity, with special emphasis on methylation. *Keio J Med.* 2011;60(1):10-6
[328] "Hypomethylation of HERV-E and HERV-K was also observed in SLE patients." Katoh et al. Association of endogenous retroviruses and long terminal repeats with human disorders. *Front Oncol.* 2013 Sep 11;3:234
[329] Balada E et al. Implication of human endogenous retroviruses in the development of autoimmune diseases. *Int Rev Immunol.* 2010 Aug;29(4):351-70
[330] Brodziak et al. The role of human endogenous retroviruses in the pathogenesis of autoimmune diseases. *Med Sci Monit.* 2012 Jun;18(6):RA80-8
[331] Perl et al. Endogenous retroviral pathogenesis in lupus. *Curr Opin Rheumatol.* 2010 Sep;22(5):483-92
[332] Dreyfus DH. Autoimmune disease: A role for new anti-viral therapies? *Autoimmun Rev.* 2011 Dec;11(2):88-97

therapies in the treatment of autoimmunity; since anti-viral drugs nearly always have limited effectiveness and an excess of adverse effects and high cost while natural antiviral agents are safer and more broadly effective, the therapeutic choice is very clear.

- Role of endogenous retroviruses in murine SLE—an established animal model of human SLE[333] (*Autoimmun Rev* 2010 Nov[334]): "Among the principal targets of the autoantibodies produced in murine SLE are nucleic acid-protein complexes and the envelope glycoprotein gp-70 of endogenous retroviruses. Recent studies have revealed that the innate receptor TLR-7 plays a pivotal role in the development of a wide variety of autoimmune responses against DNA- and RNA-containing nuclear antigens… Moreover, the demonstration that TLR-7 is involved in the acute phase expression of serum gp70 uncovers an additional pathogenic role of TLR7 in murine lupus nephritis by promoting the expression of nephritogenic gp-70 autoantigen." Thus this animal model proves with molecular detail the cause-and-effect relationship between ERVs and SLE and further points to TLR-7 as a necessary byway for nephritogenic autoantigen expression; parallels to human SLE and according therapeutic interventions are likely. While most readers should already appreciate that TLRs recognize pathogen-associated molecular patterns (PAMPs) expressed on infectious agents (and saturated fatty acids for TLR-4, as discussed in Chapter 4) and mediate the specific PAMP-TLR expression of inflammatory cytokines for immune defense responses, what is important to note here is that TLR-7 recognizes single-stranded RNA in endosomes, a common feature of viral genomes internalized within macrophages and dendritic cells; in this manner, TLR-7 is poised to be the mediator of virus-induced HERV transactivation with resultant production of pathogenic autoantigens.

- Selective antibody reactivity with peptides from human endogenous retroviruses—HERVs—and nonviral poly(amino acids) in patients with systemic lupus erythematosus (*Arthritis Rheum* 1996 Oct[335]): "Measurement by immunoassay revealed increased frequencies of antiretroviral antibodies against 2 peptides derived from the env gene of the type C-like class, which includes ERV-9 and HERV-H, and against 2 peptides from the gag region of human T-lymphotropic virus type I-related endogenous sequence 1, in patients with SLE. Antibodies to 2 nonviral peptides, polyhistidine and polyproline, were also overrepresented in patient sera. In 1 patient, longitudinal data obtained over a period of 12 years indicated that the concentrations of certain antiretroviral antibodies varied according to disease activity. CONCLUSION: Reactivity to certain type C HERV-derived antigens was found among patients with SLE. This reactivity could be explained by increased exposure to cross-reactive epitopes from essentially complete type C HERVs."

- Endogenous retroviruses in systemic lupus erythematosus: candidate lupus viruses (*Clin Immunol.* 2002 Feb[336]): "SLE patients produce high titer antibodies to various retroviral proteins, including Gag, Env, and Nef of HIV and HTLV (human T-lymphotropic virus), in the absence of overt retroviral infection. … In particular, we consider the role of HTLV-1-related endogenous sequence (HRES-1) in SLE. We propose that molecular mimicry between HRES-1 and the small ribonucleoprotein complex initiates the production of autoantibodies, leading to immune complex formation, complement fixation, and pathological tissue deposition."

Thus given that HERVs are 100% pervasive among humans and give rise to active transcription to HERV proteins, superantigens and the resulting antibodies—noting that microbial proteins + superantigens + antibodies = the perfect recipe for immune complex disease, made even worse among persons (e.g., lupus patients) with an inability to clear immune complexes—the most important question then becomes *what steps can be taken to suppress/repress/hamper HERV replication? Can we use the same effective antiviral treatments which already have available (in the previously listed antiviral protocol)?* Obviously, since we are not dealing with free viral particles, some of the previously mentioned antiviral treatments will

---

[333] "Murine models are useful tools for the study of the etiology of lupus. A multitude of models exist, each sharing a subset of attributes with SLE observed in humans. In addition, each model affords the study of different aspects of lupus pathogenesis." Perry et al. Murine Models of Systemic Lupus Erythematosus. *J Biomed Biotech* 2011; 271694
[334] Baudino et al. Role of endogenous retroviruses in murine SLE. *Autoimmun Rev.* 2010 Nov;10(1):27-34
[335] Bengtsson et al. Selective antibody reactivity with peptides from human endogenous retroviruses and nonviral poly(amino acids) in patients with systemic lupus erythematosus. *Arthritis Rheum.* 1996 Oct;39(10):1654-63
[336] Adelman MK, Marchalonis JJ. Endogenous retroviruses in systemic lupus erythematosus: candidate lupus viruses. *Clin Immunol.* 2002 Feb;102(2):107-16

have no effect because the mechanisms are irrelevant (such as selenium's prevention of immune-escape by reducing viral mutagenesis) or cannot reach within the nucleus to have effect (such as the virucidal activity of zinc ions, or the binding-inactivating effect of glycyrrhetinic acid to HSV particles). Given that "the virus" is already and permanently embedded/encoded within the human genome, the most immediate and obvious solutions would be those of promoting DNA methylation to silence HERV long terminal repeats (LTR, not to be confused with TLR for Toll-like receptors) and to prevent/reduce active transcription of those HERV LTR via transcription factors like NFkB and/or a pro-inflammatory cytokine milieu. This is to say, the

means would most likely have to be ❶ *contra* DNA transcription, most notably via the promotion of DNA methylation, ❷ reducing any contribution of viral transactivation, ❸ reducing any contribution of inflammatory (e.g., TLR-7 pathway) and stress-induced (trans)activation.

- Blocking HERV transcription by promoting DNA methylation: "There has been a reasonable prediction that aberrant LTR activation could trigger malignant disorders and autoimmune responses if epigenetic changes including DNA hypomethylation occur in somatic cells. ... Hypomethylation of HERV-E and HERV-K was also observed in SLE patients."[337]

  - Clinical implementation of optimal DNA methylation: For optimization of DNA methylation, methyl-donating/transferring nutrients such as folate (used clinically as folinic acid and/or methylfolate), betaine, and (methyl)cobalamin are necessary but not sufficient. Other nutrients—particularly vitamin D3—play critical and complex roles, promoting methylation of some DNA regions and demethylation of others[338]; in the case of vitamin D, we note consistent epidemiologic and clinical experimental research showing that vitamin D3 protects against and treats inflammatory/autoimmune diseases. The complexity of nutrients, in this case vitamin D3, is demonstrated by the observation that vitamin D causes complex changes in gene expression at different locations and likely under different circumstances; vitamin D and activation of its receptor correlate with DNA methylation and the *conceptual opposite* DNA demethylation (occurring at different DNA sites), while also promoting histone acetylation of some regions and histone deacetylation of others.[339] Lastly and very importantly, clinicians have to think beyond nutrients and methylating nutrients to fully appreciate and optimize DNA methylation, given that this process is potently impacted by numerous environmental factors, including xenobiotic/toxin exposure, ultraviolet (UV) light exposure, and drug exposure (e.g., procainamide, hydralazine); again noted is the fact that SLE patients show global hypomethylation of DNA[340] therefore suggesting that the patients need a combination of nutritional optimization (adding methyl-active nutrients such as folinic acid, cobalamin, and cholecalciferol) and environmental optimization (subtracting injurious agents such as UV light, xenobiotics and drugs) in order to optimize DNA methylation patterns and balance.

- Blocking HERV transcription by blocking exogenous virus replication—Rationale for autoimmune disease treatment with anti-viral therapies: "Cited epidemiologic and experimental evidence suggests that increased replication of epigenomic viral pathogens such as Epstein-Barr Virus (EBV) in chronic human autoimmune diseases such as rheumatoid arthritis (RA), systemic lupus

---

[337] Katoh et al. Association of endogenous retroviruses and long terminal repeats with human disorders. *Front Oncol.* 2013 Sep 11;3:234

[338] "Alterations in DNA methylation lead to aberrant gene expression and disruptions of genomic integrity, which contribute to development and progression of diseases. Vitamin D can regulate these processes; the mechanisms behind need further investigations." Fetahu et al. Vitamin D and the epigenome. *Front Physiol.* 2014 Apr 29;5:164

[339] "These changes involve the methylation of genomic DNA and/or reversible post-translational modifications of histone proteins, such as acetylation or deacetylation at exposed lysine residues." Carlberg C. Genome-wide (over)view on the actions of vitamin D. *Front Physiol.* 2014 Apr 29;5:167

[340] "The mechanisms causing altered DNA methylation in autoimmunity, aging and carcinogenesis are incompletely characterized but include exposure to environmental agents and drugs, diet, altered signaling in pathways regulating DNA methyltransferase expression and changes in endogenous regulatory mechanisms. ... Initial studies demonstrated that T cells from patients with active lupus had globally hypomethylated DNA. ... Treating normal T cells with DNA methylation inhibitors is sufficient to cause a lupus-like disease in animal models, so exposure to exogenous DNA methylation inhibitors might similarly contribute to the development of autoimmunity. In support of this, the two drugs most frequently implicated in causing a lupus-like disease, procainamide and hydralazine, have been reported to inhibit DNA methylation...and induce autoreactivity in human and murine T lymphocytes." Richardson BC. Role of DNA methylation in the regulation of cell function: autoimmunity, aging and cancer. *J Nutr.* 2002 Aug;132(8 Sup):2401S-2405S

Erythematosus (SLE), and multiple sclerosis (MS) may activate endogenous human retroviruses (HERV) as a pathologic mechanism."[341]

- Blocking HERV transcription by blocking exogenous virus replication: "Herpes simplex viruses are known to transactivate retroviral regulatory LTR regions of both exogenous and endogenous human retroviruses..."[342]

- Blocking HERV transcription by blocking nonspecific cellular stress and inflammation: "Induction of cellular stress responses through serum deprivation did however, to some extent, mimic the effects of virus infection in terms of transcription of HERV-W elements. ... Environmental stressors can modulate the transcriptional activities of certain HERV-W elements which could thereby be markers for such insults."[343]

o Viruses, part 3— Bacteriophages, especially of the gastrointestinal bacteria: The fact that the lumen of the gastrointestinal tract is loaded with bacteria is well known; progressively, all healthcare providers and researchers are appreciating that bacterial imbalances (quantitative) and metabolic/behavioral disturbances (qualitative) contribute to various disease via multiple mechanisms, as reviewed in the section on dysbiosis in Chapter 4. The next step in our understanding of dysbiosis is what I have referred to previously as microbial dysbiosis—infections within microbes. Bacteriophages are viruses that infect bacteria, and the gastrointestinal bacteria, which are themselves susceptible to innumerable quantitative and qualitative imbalances, are susceptible to viral infections. Thus, any complete understanding of

> **Bacteriophages (also called "phages" or "virus-like particles" or VLP): mechanisms of contribution to dysbiosis, inflammation, and autoimmunity**
>
> - Bacteriophages ("viruses that infect bacteria") are the most abundant biological entities on earth; they outnumber bacteria by 10x; more than 1,200 genotypes found within the human gastrointestinal tract
> - The gut virome is dominated by these prokaryotic viruses that prey on gut bacteria; since the reproductive capability of all phage particles is unknown, describing them as "viruses" is discouraged in preference for "virus-like particles" (VLP)
> - Bacteriophages influence bacterial diversity and "population structure" via "destabilization of bacterial communities"; the infectious and lytic nature of bacteriophages will obviously influence survival and death of specific populations of bacteria while the effects of lysogeny result directly in more viral particles and death of bacteria with release of bacterial and viral immunogens. Conversely, human gut bacteriophage populations do not change impressively with the corresponding bacterial colonizations (exception seen with *Faecalibacterium prausnitzii* which has a proportionate phage population) within physiologic norms (longitudinal stability); the majority of phages seem to correspond (34-41%) to the *Firmicutes* phylum of bacteria.
> - Bacteriophages participate in gene transfer and genome reorganization; they also carry numerous antibiotic resistance genes: multidrug efflux transporters (n = 355), vancomycin resistance genes (n = 129), tetracycline resistance genes (n = 18), and beta-lactamases (n = 16).
> - VLP sequences represent 4% to 17% of the total DNA from human stool; this quantitative minority of DNA material could have profound pathological implications for conditions characterized by anti-nuclear antibodies and the resulting immune complexes. Viral particles from intestinal bacteriophages are certainly absorbed and would thereafter contribute to 1) primary inflammation, and almost certainly to 2) transactivation of HERVs, 3) cross-reactivity to DNA (e.g., ANA), and 4) immune complex deposition.
> - Patients with the "autoimmune disease" Crohn's disease harbor many more bacteriophages per biopsy sample (2.1-4.1 billion) than do healthy controls (1.2 billion).
> - Phage populations are modified via dietary change (*Genome Res* 2012 Oct); but the implications are not clear.

dysbiosis must also consider the role of bacteriophages; these will be reviewed via the following survey of the literature.

- Dysbiosis in inflammatory bowel disease via bacteriophages (*Gut.* 2008 Mar[344]): In this excellent and brief report by Lepage et al, the authors propose that bacteriophage-mediated or bacteriophage-induced inflammatory dysbiosis may play a role in inflammatory bowel disease; and they note that bacteriophages outnumber bacteria 10-fold "in many natural ecosystems." Bacteriophages are diverse, with more than 1,200 genotypes found within the human gastrointestinal tract; per biopsy

---

[341] Dreyfus DH. Autoimmune disease: A role for new anti-viral therapies? *Autoimmun Rev.* 2011 Dec;11(2):88-97

[342] Nellaker et al. Transactivation of elements in the human endogenous retrovirus W family by viral infection. *Retrovirology.* 2006 Jul 6;3:44

[343] Nellaker et al. Transactivation of elements in the human endogenous retrovirus W family by viral infection. *Retrovirology.* 2006 Jul 6;3:44

[344] Lepage et al. Dysbiosis in inflammatory bowel disease: a role for bacteriophages? *Gut.* 2008 Mar;57(3):424-5

sample from the human gastrointestinal tract, an average of 1.2 billion (1.2×10^9) virus-like particles (VLP) are quantifiable and dominated by the families *Siphoviridae*, *Myoviridae* and *Podoviridae*. Patients with the "autoimmune disease" Crohn's disease (CD) harbor many more VLP per biopsy sample (2.1-4.1 billion) than do healthy controls (1.2 billion).

- Human gut virome: inter-individual variation and response to diet (*Genome Res.* 2011 Oct[345]): "VLP sequences represent a minority of the total DNA from stool, in the range of from 4% to 17%"; while this may be a *numerical* minority the physiologic and immunogenic significance could be massive. This article provides technical information and demonstrates phage response to diet, but the clinical implications and the authors' presentation of data are not clear.

o Viruses, part 4—Bacterial synergism via NFkB activation and immunosuppression:
  - Bacterial promotion of viral replication via inflammatory pathways: Bacterial debris such as DNA and LPS are known to trigger inflammatory responses via TLR and NFkB; activation of NFkB—the proinflammatory transcription factor often "hijacked" by viruses to promote their own replication— promotes viral replication. Thus, increased total bacterial load (TBL, such as SIBO) would be expected to promote viral replication.
  - Bacterial promotion of viral replication via immunosuppression: As a specific example, *Helicobacter pylori* may play a powerful role as a synergistic bioagent for the microbial promotion of autoimmunity via its ability to *simultaneously* and *paradoxically* cause immunosuppression (thereby allowing other microbes to flourish) and systemic inflammation[346]; in this manner, the bacterial infection is permissive to and perhaps necessary for the autoimmune-inducing vasculopathic and fibrogenic viral infections (see section on Scleroderma for pathology details).

Clinical presentations:

- Subtypes and overlapping presentations: As shown in the diagram below, SLE has several subtypes which can present exclusively or in combination, ie, a patient may have classic SLE with no skin lesions, skin lesions without fulminant SLE, or classic SLE with one or more types of skin lesions.

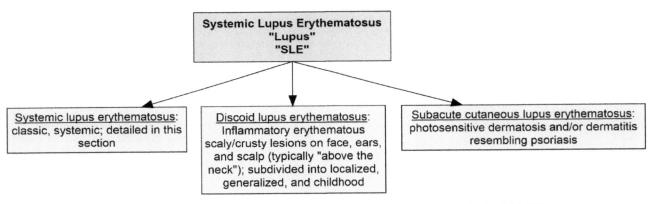

Graphic above illustrating different disease subtypes that fall under the label of SLE/lupus

- Gender: 85-90% of new patients are women in their childbearing years (frequency: 1 per 700 women); the ratio of women to men is 9:1 except among prepubertal children and older/postmenopausal men and women in which the ratio is 2:1.[347] The much higher prevalence of the disorder among women of childbearing age compared to men of the same age (11:1) implicates sex hormones and hormonal fluctuations as causative factors that predispose young women to this disorder.
- 4x more common in women of African descent (1 per 250) than Caucasian women (1 per 1000).[348] The increased prevalence of SLE in dark-skinned women may be due at least in part to their higher prevalence of vitamin D

[345] Minot et al. The human gut virome: inter-individual variation and dynamic response to diet. *Genome Res.* 2011 Oct;21(10):1616-25

[346] "Infectious agents such as Helicobacter pylori (Hp) may cause chronic inflammation and autoimmune reactivity in susceptible subjects. The results of in vitro experiments performed with lymphocytes from Hp infected patients indicate that Hp can cause immunosuppression which might be eliminated by successful eradication therapy." Hybenova et al. The role of environmental factors in autoimmune thyroiditis. *Neuro Endocrinol Lett.* 2010;31(3):283-9

[347] Manzi S. Epidemiology of systemic lupus erythematosus. *Am J Manag Care.* 2001 Oct;7(16 Suppl):S474-9 ajmc.com/files/articlefiles/A01_131_2001octManziS474_9.pdf

[348] Tierney ML. McPhee SJ, Papadakis MA. *Current Medical Diagnosis and Treatment 2006. 45th edition.* New York; Lange Medical Books: 2006, pages 833-837

deficiency, which unquestionably predisposes to inflammation, immune dysfunction, and the clinical manifestation of autoimmunity.[349] Although administration of vitamin D3 to cholecalciferol-deficient adults clearly has anti-inflammatory action[350,351], important windows of opportunity appear to occur *in utero* and within the first few postnatal months and years; for example, administration of vitamin D to **infants** reduces the subsequent incidence of type-1 *autoimmune-mediated* diabetes by 78%.[352] Vitamin D sufficiency appears to support immune function and thereby reduce the acquisition of infectious diseases[353]; thus, vitamin D may exert an anti-*rheumatic* benefit by exerting an anti-*infectious* benefit; i.e., by preventing the dysbiotic infections that may serve to trigger autoimmunity. Given the strength of evidence supporting the routine use of vitamin D3 supplementation in infants, children, and adults, healthcare providers should ensure adequate vitamin D status in their patients[354,355,356] for the treatment and prevention of long-latency deficiency diseases[357] and alleviation of systemic inflammation.[358]

- Positive family history of the disease is common: daughters of a mother with SLE have a 1 in 40 prevalence of SLE, whereas sons have a 1 in 250 prevalence
- Clinical course may be slow or acute, involving many organ systems or only one, and is characterized by exacerbations and remissions
- **Classic autoimmune systemic manifestations: fatigue, malaise, low-grade fever, anorexia, weight loss, peripheral polyarthritis**. Septicemia and septic arthritis should always be considered in patients with SLE, especially those taking immunosuppressive drugs and those experiencing what appears to be an exacerbation of the disease.
  - o Skin:
    - Malar "butterfly" rash over the cheeks and bridge of the nose: this is a classic manifestation of the disease but is seen in less than half of SLE patients
    - Photosensitivity: erythematous skin rash develops readily on sun-exposed areas
    - Hair loss
    - Nail infarcts, periungual erythema, splinter hemorrhages
    - Purpura
  - o Musculoskeletal:
    - 90% of patients have polyarthralgia—most commonly affecting the peripheral joints of the hands, wrists, knees, feet
    - Polymyalgia, myositis, and myopathy; avascular necrosis due to corticosteroids
  - o Renal/kidney:
    - Immune complex-mediated glomerulonephritis: 50% of patients have clinical nephritis, hematuria, and proteinuria; renal function commonly declines during exacerbation of disease and then improves with disease remission
    - **Renal failure is a leading cause of death in patients with SLE**[359]
  - o CNS:
    - 70% have EEG abnormalities
    - **Neuropsychiatric lupus (secondary to vasculitis, neuroinflammation, and immune-mediated alterations in [dopaminergic] neurotransmission) requires specialist care and has been described as a medical emergency**[360]: Characteristics include psychosis, seizures, transient ischemic attacks, severe depression, delirium, confusion. Exclude adverse drug effect (especially corticosteroid psychosis), infection, hypertension, and hyponatremia.

[349] Cantorna MT. Vitamin D and autoimmunity: is vitamin D status an environmental factor affecting autoimmune disease prevalence? *Proc Soc Exp Biol Med.* 2000;223:230-3
[350] Timms et al. Circulating MMP9, vitamin D and variation in TIMP-1 response with VDR genotype: mechanisms for inflammatory damage chronic disorders? *QJM* 2002:787-96
[351] Van den Berghe G, et al. Bone turnover in prolonged critical illness: effect of vitamin D. *J Clin Endocrinol Metab.* 2003;88(10):4623-32
[352] "Children who regularly took recommended dose of vitamin D (2000 IU daily) had a RR of 0.22 (0.05-0.89) compared with those who regularly received less than recommended amount." Hypponen et al. Intake of vitamin D and risk of type 1 diabetes: birth-cohort study. *Lancet* 2001;358:1500-3: very important article
[353] Wayse V, et al. Association of subclinical vitamin D deficiency with severe acute lower respiratory infection in Indian children under 5 y. *Eur J Clin Nutr.* 2004;58(4):563-7
[354] Vasquez A, Manso G, Cannell J. The clinical importance of vitamin D (cholecalciferol). *Altern Ther Health Med.* 2004 Sep;10(5):28-36 ichnfm.academia.edu/AlexVasquez
[355] Heaney RP. Vitamin D, nutritional deficiency, and the medical paradigm. *J Clin Endocrinol Metab.* 2003 Nov;88(11):5107-8
[356] Hollis BW, Wagner CL. Assessment of dietary vitamin D requirements during pregnancy and lactation. *Am J Clin Nutr.* 2004 May;79:717-26
[357] Heaney RP. Long-latency deficiency disease: insights from calcium and vitamin D. *Am J Clin Nutr.* 2003;78(5):912-9 jcem.endojournals.org/cgi/content/full/88/11/5107
[358] Timms et al. Circulating MMP9, vitamin D and variation in TIMP-1 response with VDR genotype. *QJM.* 2002;95:787-96
[359] Suzuki et al. Development of pathogenic anti-DNA antibodies in patients with systemic lupus erythematosus. *FASEB J* 1997 Oct;11:1033-8
[360] McInnes I, Sturrock R. Rheumatological emergencies. *Practitioner.* 1994 Mar;238(1536):220-4

- Headaches, migraine, stroke
- Peripheral and cranial neuropathies, transverse myelitis
- Increased risk for meningitis when immunosuppressive therapy is used.
  - o Cardiovascular and circulation:
    - Vasculitis
    - Thrombosis and **increased risk for myocardial infarction**
    - Pericarditis, myocarditis: may result in sudden death, heart failure, arrhythmias
    - Hypertension due to renal injury
    - Raynaud's phenomenon—periodic vasospasm affecting the hands and fingers
    - Antiphospholipid antibody syndrome—a major cause of complications
  - o Lungs/pulmonary:
    - Pneumonitis: presents with fever, cough, dyspnea—important to **assess with radiographs and exclude infection**
    - Pleurisy, pleural effusion; **alveolar hemorrhage can be life-threatening**
  - o Hematologic/CBC abnormalities:
    - Leukopenia, lymphopenia, thrombocytopenia, anemia
    - Immune complexes: Immune complexes are elevated in patients with active SLE[361]
  - o Gastrointestinal:
    - Nausea
    - Diarrhea
    - **Intestinal/mesenteric vasculitis and infarct—surgical emergency**—postprandial abdominal pain, cramps, vomiting, diarrhea
    - Pancreatitis
    - Increased intestinal permeability, occasionally protein-losing enteropathy results[362]
  - o Eyes:
    - **Retinal vasculitis (look for exudates with fundoscopic examination) can cause blindness in days— treat as an emergency**
    - Other manifestations include conjunctivitis, photophobia, blurred vision
  - o Other:
    - Edema—may be seen with cardiac or renal damage
    - Lymphadenopathy
    - Mucocutaneous ulcerations
    - Increased risk of miscarriage and congenital heart block

Major differential diagnoses:
- Infection
- Cancer, lymphoma
- RA or other autoimmune disease such as scleroderma, vasculitis, sarcoidosis
- Iron overload
- Fibromyalgia
- Porphyria cutanea tarda
- Drug hypersensitivity and drug-induced lupus: SLE is differentiated from drug-induced lupus by the following characteristics of drug-induced lupus: 1) temporal association with drug/medication use; remission of disease following drug discontinuation, and 2) lack of fully characteristic pattern of clinical and laboratory manifestations: lack of renal and CNS involvement, lack of hypocomplementemia and anti-native DNA antibodies. Clinicians must exclude drug-induced lupus before making diagnosis of SLE.

---

[361] Suzuki N, Mihara S, Sakane T. Development of pathogenic anti-DNA antibodies in patients with systemic lupus erythematosus. *FASEB J*. 1997 Oct;11(12):1033-8
[362] "Fourteen cases of primary lupus-associated protein-losing enteropathy have now been reported in the English-language literature." Perednia DA, Curosh NA. Lupus-associated protein-losing enteropathy. *Arch Intern Med*. 1990 Sep;150(9):1806-10

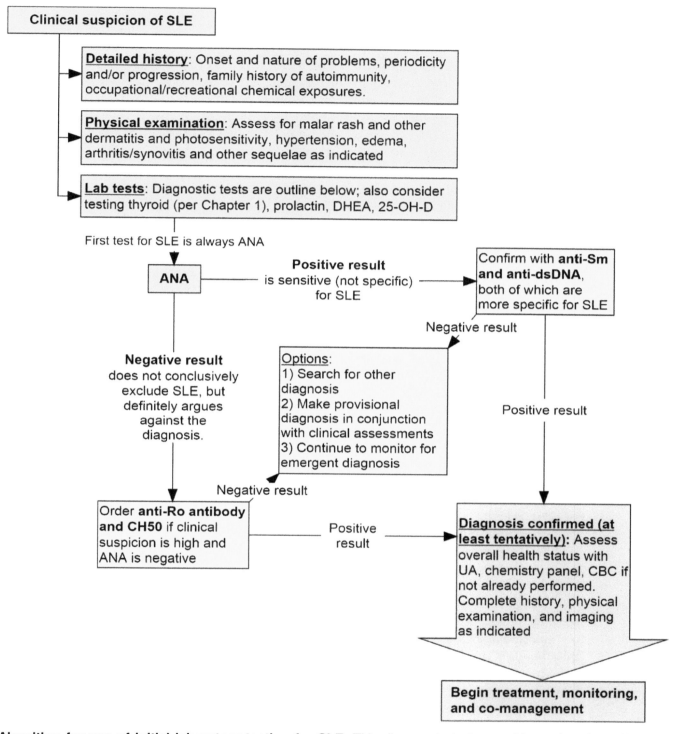

Algorithm for use of initial laboratory testing for SLE: This diagram is to be used in conjunction with other information presented in this book and any new published guidelines; however, this information will likely always remain clinically relevant and reasonably useful.

Clinical assessments:
- **History and physical examination**: consistent with the clinical presentations listed previously
- **Laboratory assessments**:
  - Comprehensive laboratory evaluation: Use other tests (e.g. and especially, metabolic/chemistry panel, UA, CBC, etc.) to assess for complications and concomitant disease.

- ANA—anti-nuclear antibodies: ANA is the best screening test and has been described as positive in 100% of SLE patients[363] despite the acknowledged existence of ANA-negative SLE. ANA levels correlate with disease activity. Previous editions of standard medical textbooks reported that this test was less than 100% sensitive for SLE; it may be that improvements in laboratory analysis now account for the 100% sensitivity. A positive ANA test result—even with a high titer—does not necessarily indicate that the patient has SLE, especially if no other signs or symptoms are present. ANA are directed against the following four targets: ❶ DNA, ❷ histones, ❸ non-histone proteins bound to RNA, ❹ nucleolar antigens.
    - Anti-double stranded (DS, native) DNA antibodies (anti-dsDNA): Positive in ~60% of patients; specific (not sensitive) for SLE; when positive, anti-dsDNA levels correlate with disease activity.
    - Anti-Sm (anti-Smith) antibodies: Positive in ~30% of patients; specific (not sensitive) for SLE.[364]
    - Anti-histone antibodies: Seen in drug-induced lupus.
    - Anti-Ro antibodies (SSA: Sjogren's syndrome antibodies): Seen with cutaneous SLE, Sjogren's syndrome, and neonatal lupus.[365]
- CRP: Sensitive indicator of inflammation *except in SLE* where CRP levels can be normal even with severe active disease.[366,367]
- ESR: Not useful in all patients with SLE.[368]
- Complement levels (CH50): Complement levels are lowered in accord with complement pathway activation by immune complexes; levels tend to normalize when disease is in remission.
- Inherited complement deficiencies: 6% of SLE patients has an inherited/genetic deficiency in one or more complement proteins. Deficiency of C1q, C2, or **C4** appears to result in inability to clear immune complexes and thus results in exacerbation of disease manifestations due to immune complex deposition. C1q deficiency may impair clearance of apoptotic cells and thus promote antigenicity toward nuclear debris via—for example—activation of DAMP (damage-associated molecular pattern) receptors.
- HLA-DR2 and HLA-DR3: These are more common in patients with SLE than in the general population.
- Serologic testing for syphilis (VDRL): A false-positive test for syphilis is characteristic of SLE and is a reflection of antiphospholipid antibodies.
- Antiphospholipid and Anticardiolipin antibodies: Antiphospholipid antibodies (directed against plasma proteins complexed to phospholipids) are seen in 40-50% of SLE patients. Antiphospholipid antibodies are associated with significantly increased risk for venous and arterial thrombosis. In SLE patients with antiphospholipid antibodies, treatment with anticoagulants such as warfarin/coumadin are commonly used (see INR below):
    - Anticardiolipin antibodies: This is one of several types of antiphospholipid antibodies; also used in syphilis serologic testing, and therefore SLE patients with anticardiolipin antibodies may have false positive result for syphilis. Anticardiolipin antibodies interfere with the PT (partial thromboplastin) test and are thus occasionally called "lupus anticoagulant"—this factitious anticoagulation is purely an *in vitro* phenomenon and is misleading since these same patients actually have a hypercoagulable state that predisposes them to arterial and venous thromboses. Readers attentive to the information on mitochondrial will have also noted that the phospholipid cardiolipin is located on the mitochondrial inner membrane, where it serves as an anchor for the enzyme succinate dehydrogenase; this data suggests an important role for mitochondrial dysfunction in SLE: a fact which is now very well proven, although not widely known by many practicing clinicians.
    - INR: International Normalized Ratio is a standardized quantification of Prothrombin Time (PT), which is a measure of clotting/bleeding tendency. INR is used to monitor dosing of warfarin/coumadin; generally the INR should be kept between 2.0-3.0.[369]
- Comprehensive testing for celiac disease and wheat allergy: Some patients diagnosed with "systemic lupus erythematosus" actually have autoimmunity and systemic inflammation due to occult celiac

[363] Tierney ML. McPhee SJ, Papadakis MA. *Current Medical Diagnosis and Treatment 2006, 45th edition*. New York; Lange Medical Books: 2006, pages 833-837
[364] Shojania K. Rheumatology: 2. What laboratory tests are needed? *CMAJ*. 2000 Apr 18;162(8):1157-63 cmaj.ca/cgi/content/full/162/8/1157
[365] Shojania K. Rheumatology: 2. What laboratory tests are needed? *CMAJ*. 2000 Apr 18;162(8):1157-63
[366] Deodhar SD. C-reactive protein: the best laboratory indicator available for monitoring disease activity. *Cleve Clin J Med* 1989 Mar-Apr;56(2):126-30
[367] Gabay C, Kushner I. Acute-phase proteins and other systemic responses to inflammation. *N Engl J Med*. 1999 Feb 11;340(6):448-54
[368] Klippel JH (ed). *Primer on the Rheumatic Diseases. 11th Edition*. Atlanta: Arthritis Foundation. 1997 page 94
[369] Tierney ML. McPhee SJ, Papadakis MA. *Current Medical Diagnosis and Treatment 2006, 45th edition*. New York; Lange Medical Books: 2006, pages 833-837

disease. These patients achieve clinical remission after avoiding gluten/gliadin-containing grains such as wheat.[370,371] More than 23% of patients with SLE have anti-gliadin antibodies.[372] In addition to IgA and IgG anti-gliadin antibodies, serologic testing for celiac disease includes IgA and IgG antiendomysial and anti-transglutaminase antibodies which should be interpreted along with a test for total serum IgA to identify those patients with selective IgA deficiency.

- **Imaging**:
  - Imaging is used to in the assessment of complications and exclusion of concomitant diseases.
  - The arthritis of SLE is typically mild (compared to rheumatoid arthritis) and is nondeforming.

Establishing the diagnosis:

- Clinical presentation and lab tests; more positives = more confident diagnosis.

Qualification for a diagnosis of SLE requires quantification of at least four of these eleven criteria:
1. Malar/cheek rash
2. Discoid rash
3. Photosensitivity
4. Ulcerations of oral mucosa
5. Joint pain and inflammation not attributable to other disease or trauma
6. Serositis: Inflammation of the serous tissues, which line the lungs (pleura), heart (pericardium), and the inner lining of the abdomen (peritoneum) and associated organs
7. Renal disease (any of the following): >3+ proteinuria measured by dipstick; cellular casts; proteinuria >0.5 grams per day
8. CNS involvement: seizures or psychosis without other cause
9. Hematologic abnormalities (any of the following): hemolytic anemia, leucopenia (45%), lymphopenia, thrombocytopenia (30%), anemia of chronic disease
10. Positive ANA

11. Additional serologic tests (any of the following):
    ○ Positive LE cell prep
    ○ Anti-native DNA antibody (50%)
    ○ Anti-Sm antibody (20%)
    ○ False-positive test for syphilis (25%)

Life-threatening complications and medical urgencies/emergencies:

- **Infection**—Infections are now the leading cause of death in patients with SLE[373]
- **SLE complications: renal failure and CNS involvement**
- **Stroke, myocardial infarction**—Increased risk with male gender and antiphospholipid antibodies
- Septic arthritis
- Thromboembolism
- 10-year survival is >85%[374]

Overview of clinical management:

- **The clinical course of the disease is variable, marked by exacerbations and remissions. Life-threatening complications can develop rapidly and must be managed effectively to prevent patient morbidity and practitioner liability.**
- Treat patient safely and effectively. If you cannot get good results, refer them to someone who can. Refer if clinical outcome is unsatisfactory or if serious complications are possible. Stable patients are seen every 3-6

---

[370] "The immunological profile of IgA deficiency and/or raised double stranded DNA in the absence of antinuclear factor together with raised inflammatory markers and symptoms suggestive of an immune diathesis should alert the physician to the possibility of gluten sensitivity." Hadjivassiliou et al. Gluten sensitivity masquerading as systemic lupus erythematosus. *Ann Rheum Dis.* 2004 Nov;63(11):1501-3 ard.bmjjournals.com/cgi/content/full/63/11/1501

[371] "Villous atrophy on duodenal biopsy specimens with a favorable response to a gluten-free diet was noted in all five patients." Zitouni et al. Systemic lupus erythematosus with celiac disease: a report of five cases. *Joint Bone Spine.* 2004 Jul;71(4):344-6

[372] "Twenty-four of 103 (23.3%) systemic lupus erythematosus patients tested positive for either antigliadin antibody, whereas none of the 103 patients tested positive for antiendomysial antibody." Rensch et al. The prevalence of celiac disease autoantibodies in patients with systemic lupus erythematosus. *Am J Gastroenterol.* 2001 Apr;96(4):1113-5 For the authors to state that these patients did not have celiac disease simply because their intestinal biopsies were normal is inconsistent with the modern paradigm of celiac disease which acknowledges that the disease can be present in the absence of gastrointestinal lesions.

[373] Tierney ML. McPhee SJ, Papadakis MA. *Current Medical Diagnosis and Treatment 2006. 45th edition.* New York; Lange Medical Books: 2006, pages 833-837

[374] Tierney ML. McPhee SJ, Papadakis MA. *Current Medical Diagnosis and Treatment 2006. 45th edition.* New York; Lange Medical Books: 2006, pages 833-837

months for monitoring of disease activity, re-examination, and treatment recalibration.[375] Patients must understand that acute exacerbations and/or new symptoms—especially fever—must be evaluated promptly.

- Treatment must be customized to the patient and must be flexible to accommodate the natural exacerbations and remissions of the disease.
- To the extent possible, discourage use of NSAIDs since these drugs exacerbate joint destruction, renal impairment, and increased intestinal permeability which increases exposure to dietary and microbial antigens.

<u>**Treatments**</u>: The standard medical protocol centers on and starts with (new drugs are always being developed and added): prednisone, Plaquenil and immunoparalytic and immunosuppressive drugs.

- <u>Drug treatments</u>:
  - **NSAIDs**: For joint pain[376] despite adverse effects on the gut[377], joints[378,379,380] and kidneys.
  - **Antimalarial drug: hydroxychloroquine/Plaquenil**): Adverse effects include retinal damage, neuropathy, myopathy. As with anticonvulsant drugs, hydroxychloroquine/Plaquenil interferes with conversion of 25-hydroxycholecalciferol to the more active 1-25-dihydroxycholecalciferol[381]; this would be expected to exacerbate immune dysfunction, inflammation, hypertension, and depression.
  - **Danazol is an androgenic corticosteroid**: particularly used against thrombocytopenia
  - **Immunosuppression** with <u>prednisone</u> (promotes bacterial overgrowth and osteoporosis), <u>cyclophosphamide</u> (especially for renal involvement), <u>mycophenolate mofetil</u>, <u>azathioprine</u>, or other DMARD (disease-modifying antirheumatic drugs) is commonly used, particularly for the more serious complications of the disease such as those affecting the brain, heart, lungs, and kidneys. **Despite the clinical drawbacks and philosophical inadequacies, pharmacologic immunosuppression has a role in the management of patients with autoimmunity when their disease flares and threatens vital structures, particularly the heart, brain, and kidneys.**
  - **Anticoagulant drugs such as warfarin** are used for patients with antiphospholipid antibodies and resultant thrombotic complications.

- **FOOD & NUTRITION**: 5-part "supplemented Paleo-Mediterranean diet" (SPMD) The 5-part "supplemented Paleo-Mediterranean diet" (SPMD—reviewed in Chapter 4) consists of ❶ foundational plant-based low-carbohydrate diet of fruits, vegetables, nuts, seeds, berries and lean sources of protein, ❷ multivitamin and multimineral supplementation, ❸ physiologic doses of vitamin D3 (range 2,000-10,000 IU/d), ❹ combination fatty acid therapy (CFAT) with n3-ALA, n6-GLA, n3-EPA, n3-DHA, and phytochemical-rich olive oil which contains n9-oleate, and ❺ probiotics.
  - <u>Gluten avoidance</u>: Celiac disease can present with inflammatory oligoarthritis that resembles rheumatoid arthritis and which remits with avoidance of wheat/gluten; the inflammatory arthropathy of celiac disease has preceded bowel symptoms and/or an accurate diagnosis by as many as 3-15 years.[382,383] Some patients diagnosed with "systemic lupus erythematosus" actually have autoimmunity and systemic inflammation due to occult celiac disease, and they achieve remarkable improvement—complete remission of systemic inflammation and the ability to discontinue all anti-inflammatory drugs—after

---

[375] Manzi S. Epidemiology of systemic lupus erythematosus. *Am J Manag Care* 2001 Oct;7(16Sup):S474-9 ajmc.com/files/articlefiles/A01_131_2001octManziS474_9.pdf
[376] Tierney ML. McPhee SJ, Papadakis MA. *Current Medical Diagnosis and Treatment 2006. 45th edition*. New York; Lange Medical Books: 2006, pages 833-837
[377] Abbreviations: cow's milk beta-lactoglobulin absorption (BLG), acetylsalicylic acid (ASA), disodium chromoglycate (DSCG). "ASA administration strongly increased BLG absorption, not prevented by DSCG pretreatment. In normal controls treated with a single dose of ASA we obtained similar results. Our results suggest that prolonged treatment with nonsteroidal anti-inflammatory drugs induces an increase of food antigen absorption, apparently not related to anaphylaxis mediator release, with possible clinical effects." Fagiolo et al. Intestinal permeability and antigen absorption in rheumatoid arthritis. Effects of acetylsalicylic acid and sodium chromoglycate. *Int Arch Allergy Appl Immunol.* 1989;89(1):98-102
[378] "At...concentrations comparable to those... in the synovial fluid of patients treated with the drug, several NSAIDs suppress proteoglycan synthesis...." Brandt KD. Effects of nonsteroidal anti-inflammatory drugs on chondrocyte metabolism in vitro and in vivo. *Am J Med.* 1987 Nov 20; 83(5A): 29-34
[379] "This highly significant association between NSAID use and acetabular destruction gives cause for concern, not least because of the difficulty in achieving satisfactory hip replacements in patients with severely damaged acetabula." Newman NM, Ling RS. Acetabular bone destruction related to non-steroidal anti-inflammatory drugs. *Lancet.* 1985 Jul 6; 2(8445): 11-4
[380] Vidal y Plana et al. Articular cartilage pharmacology: In vitro studies on glucosamine and non steroidal anti-inflammatory drugs. *Pharmacol Res Commun.* 1978 Jun;10:557-69
[381] "Half the SLE and FM patients had 25(OH)-vitamin D levels < 50 nmol/l, a level at which PTH stimulation occurs. Our data suggest that in SLE patients HCQ might inhibit conversion of 25(OH)-vitamin D to 1,25(OH)2-vitamin D." Huisman et al. Vitamin D levels in women with systemic lupus erythematosus and fibromyalgia. *J Rheumatol.* 2001 Nov;28(11):2535-9
[382] "We report six patients with coeliac disease in whom arthritis was prominent at diagnosis and who improved with dietary therapy. Joint pain preceded diagnosis by up to three years in five patients and 15 years in one patient." Bourne JT, et al. Arthritis and coeliac disease. *Ann Rheum Dis.* 1985 Sep;44(9):592-8
[383] "A 15-year-old girl, with synovitis of the knees and ankles for 3 years before a diagnosis of gluten-sensitive enteropathy, is described." Pinals RS. Arthritis associated with gluten-sensitive enteropathy. *J Rheumatol.* 1986 Feb;13(1):201-4

avoiding gluten/gliadin-containing grains, most notoriously, wheat.[384] In a study of 103 SLE patients, more than 23% of SLE patients had anti-gliadin antibodies.[385]

o <u>Short-term fasting</u>: In case reports and clinical trials, short-term fasting (or protein-sparing fasting) has been documented as safe and effective treatment for SLE[386], RA[387], and non-rheumatic diseases such as chronic severe hypertension[388], moderate hypertension[389], obesity[390,391], type-2 diabetes[392], and epilepsy.[393] The combination of energy restriction and fish oil supplementation was shown highly beneficial in an animal model of SLE.[394]

o <u>Broad-spectrum fatty acid therapy with ALA, EPA, DHA, GLA and oleic acid</u>: Fish oil provides EPA and DHA which have well-proven anti-inflammatory benefits when used in the treatment of SLE.[395,396,397] Fatty acid supplementation should be delivered in the form of combination therapy with ALA, GLA, DHA, and EPA. Given at doses of 3,000 – 9,000 mg per day, ALA from flax oil has impressive anti-inflammatory benefits demonstrated by its ability to halve prostaglandin production in humans.[398] Numerous studies have demonstrated the benefit of GLA in the treatment of rheumatoid arthritis when used at doses between 500 mg – 4,000 mg per day.[399,400] Fish oil provides EPA and DHA which have well-proven anti-inflammatory benefits in RA[401,402,403] and SLE.[404,405]

o <u>Vitamin D3 supplementation with physiologic doses and/or tailored to serum 25(OH)D levels</u>: Vitamin D deficiency is common in the general population and is even more common in patients with chronic illness and chronic musculoskeletal pain.[406] **At least 50% of patients with SLE are deficient in vitamin D[407]**, and even more would be found deficient if stricter and more appropriate criteria are used.

---

[384] "The immunological profile of IgA deficiency and/or raised double stranded DNA in the absence of antinuclear factor together with raised inflammatory markers and symptoms suggestive of an immune diathesis should alert the physician to the possibility of gluten sensitivity." Hadjivassiliou M, Sanders DS, Grunewald RA, Akil M. Gluten sensitivity masquerading as systemic lupus erythematosus. *Ann Rheum Dis.* 2004 Nov;63(11):1501-3 ard.bmjjournals.com/cgi/content/full/63/11/1501

[385] "Twenty-four of 103 (23.3%) systemic lupus erythematosus patients tested positive for either antigliadin antibody, whereas none of the 103 patients tested positive for antiendomysial antibody." Rensch et al. The prevalence of celiac disease autoantibodies in patients with systemic lupus erythematosus. *Am J Gastroenterol.* 2001 Apr;96(4):1113-5. For the authors to state that these patients did not have celiac disease simply because their intestinal biopsies were normal seems to indicate that the authors were ignorant of the modern paradigm of celiac disease which acknowledges that the disease can be present in the absence of gastrointestinal lesions.

[386] Fuhrman et al. Brief case reports of medically supervised, water-only fasting associated with remission of autoimmune disease. *Altern Ther Health Med.* 2002 Jul;8:112, 110-1

[387] "An association was found between improvement in inflammatory activity of the joints and enhancement of neutrophil bactericidal capacity. Fasting appears to improve the clinical status of patients with RA." Uden AM, Trang L, Venizelos N, Palmblad J. Neutrophil functions and clinical performance after total fasting in patients with rheumatoid arthritis. *Ann Rheum Dis.* 1983 Feb;42(1):45-51

[388] "The average reduction in blood pressure was 37/13 mm Hg, with the greatest decrease being observed for subjects with the most severe hypertension. Patients with stage 3 hypertension (those with systolic blood pressure greater than 180 mm Hg, diastolic blood pressure greater than 110 mg Hg, or both) had an average reduction of 60/17 mm Hg at the conclusion of treatment." Goldhamer et al. Medically supervised water-only fasting in the treatment of hypertension. *J Manipulative Physiol Ther.* 2001 Jun;24(5):335-9

[389] "RESULTS: Approximately 82% of the subjects achieved BP at or below 120/80 mm Hg by the end of the treatment program. The mean BP reduction was 20/7 mm Hg, with the greatest decrease being observed for subjects with the highest baseline BP." Goldhamer AC, Lisle DJ, Sultana P, Anderson SV, Parpia B, Hughes B, Campbell TC. Medically supervised water-only fasting in the treatment of borderline hypertension. *J Altern Complement Med.* 2002 Oct;8(5):643-50

[390] Vertes V, Genuth SM, Hazelton IM. Supplemented fasting as a large-scale outpatient program. *JAMA.* 1977 Nov 14;238(20):2151-3

[391] Bauman WA, Schwartz E, Rose HG, et al. Early and long-term effects of acute caloric deprivation in obese diabetic patients. *Am J Med.* 1988 Jul;85(1):38-46

[392] Goldhamer AC. Initial cost of care results in medically supervised water-only fasting for treating high blood pressure and diabetes. *J Altern Complement Med.* 2002 Dec;8(6):696-7

[393] "The ketogenic diet should be considered as alternative therapy for children with difficult-to-control seizures. It is more effective than many of the new anticonvulsant medications and is well tolerated by children and families when it is effective." Freeman et al. The efficacy of the ketogenic diet-1998: a prospective evaluation of intervention in 150 children. *Pediatrics.* 1998 Dec;102(6):1358-63 pediatrics.aappublications.org/cgi/reprint/102/6/1358

[394] "In conclusion, our data strongly indicate that ER and FO maintain antioxidant status and GSH:GSSG ratio, thereby protecting against renal deterioration from oxidative insults during ageing." Kelley et al. A fish oil diet rich in eicosapentaenoic acid reduces cyclooxygenase metabolites, and suppresses lupus in MRL-lpr mice. *J Immunol.* 1985 Mar;134(3):1914-9

[395] "No major side effects were noted, and it is suggested that dietary modification with additional marine oil may be a useful way of modifying disease activity in systemic lupus erythematosus." Walton et al. Dietary fish oil and the severity of symptoms in patients with systemic lupus erythematosus. *Ann Rheum Dis.* 1991 Jul;50(7):463-6

[396] "CONCLUSION: In the management of SLE, dietary supplementation with fish oil may be beneficial in modifying symptomatic disease activity." Duffy et al. The clinical effect of dietary supplementation with omega-3 fish oils and/or copper in systemic lupus erythematosus. *J Rheumatol.* 2004 Aug;31(8):1551-6

[397] "Oral supplementation of EPA and DHA induced prolonged remission of SLE in 10 consecutive patients without any side-effects. These results suggest that n-3 fatty acids, EPA and DHA, are useful in the management of SLE and possibly, other similar collagen vascular diseases." Das UN. Beneficial effect of eicosapentaenoic and docosahexaenoic acids in the management of systemic lupus erythematosus and its relationship to the cytokine network. *Prostaglandins Leukot Essent Fatty Acids.* 1994 Sep;51(3):207-13

[398] Adam O, Wolfram G, Zollner N. Effect of alpha-linolenic acid in the human diet on linoleic acid metabolism and prostaglandin biosynthesis. *J Lipid Res.* 1986 Apr;27(4):421-6

[399] "Other results showed a significant reduction in morning stiffness with gamma-linolenic acid at 3 months and reduction in pain and articular index at 6 months with olive oil." Brzeski et al. Evening primrose oil in patients with rheumatoid arthritis and side-effects of non-steroidal anti-inflammatory drugs. *Br J Rheumatol.* 1991 Oct;30(5):370-2

[400] Rothman D, DeLuca P, Zurier RB. Botanical lipids: effects on inflammation, immune responses, and rheumatoid arthritis. *Semin Arthritis Rheum.* 1995 Oct;25(2):87-96

[401] Adam et al. Anti-inflammatory effects of a low arachidonic acid diet and fish oil in patients with rheumatoid arthritis. *Rheumatol Int.* 2003 Jan;23(1):27-36

[402] Lau et al. Effects of fish oil supplementation on non-steroidal anti-inflammatory drug requirement in patients with mild rheumatoid arthritis. *Br J Rheumatol* 1993 Nov:982-9

[403] Kremer et al. Fish-oil fatty acid supplementation in active rheumatoid arthritis. A double-blinded, controlled, crossover study. *Ann Intern Med.* 1987 Apr;106(4):497-503

[404] Walton et al. Dietary fish oil and the severity of symptoms in patients with systemic lupus erythematosus. *Ann Rheum Dis.* 1991 Jul;50(7):463-6

[405] Duffy et al. The clinical effect of dietary supplementation with omega-3 fish oils and/or copper in systemic lupus erythematosus. *J Rheumatol.* 2004 Aug;31(8):1551-6

[406] Plotnikoff GA, Quigley JM. Prevalence of severe hypovitaminosis D in patients with persistent, nonspecific musculoskeletal pain. *Mayo Clin Proc.* 2003 Dec;78(12):1463-70

[407] "Half the SLE and FM patients had 25(OH)-vitamin D levels < 50 nmol/l, a level at which PTH stimulation occurs. Our data suggest that in SLE patients HCQ might inhibit conversion of 25(OH)-vitamin D to 1,25(OH)2-vitamin D." Huisman et al. Vitamin D levels in women with systemic lupus erythematosus and fibromyalgia. *J Rheumatol.* 2001 Nov;28(11):2535-9

- **INFECTIONS & DYSBIOSIS: ❶ antimicrobial treatments, ❷ immunorestoration, ❸ immunotolerance via Treg induction** Essentially all autoimmune/rheumatic disorders are associated with microbial colonization and intolerance to same; the presence of persistent microbial colonization is *prima facie* evidence of immunosuppression. The eight areas of dysbiosis (multifocal) are: ❶ sinorespiratory, ❷ orodental, ❸ gastrointestinal, ❹ urogenital/genitourinary, ❺ parenchymal/tissue, ❻ microbial, ❼ dermal/cutaneous, and ❽ environmental. Dysbiotic loci should be investigated as discussed previously in Chapter 4. Recall that patients with lupus have abnormal gastrointestinal bacteria (decreased colonization resistance[408]), and some evidence suggests that gastrointestinal bacteria in these patients may translocate into the systemic circulation to induce formation of antibodies that cross-react with double-stranded DNA to produce the clinical manifestations of the disease.[409,410] Each cause—each contributor to disease—may in itself be "clinically insignificant" but when numerous "insignificant" additive and synergistic influences coalesce, we find ourselves confronted with an "idiopathic disease." We must then decide between the only two available options: 1) despair in the failure of our "one cause, one disease, one drug" paradigm, or 2) appreciate that numerous influences work together to disrupt physiologic function and produce the biologic dysfunction that we experience as disease. Experimental evidence shows that exposure to single-stranded bacterial DNA can provoke formation of antibodies to single-stranded mammalian DNA. Human patients with SLE have a reduced ability to bind bacterial DNA with antibodies, thus allowing normal/ambient levels of bacterial DNA to provoke an ongoing inflammatory response.[411] Recall from Chapter 4 that stimulation of inflammation by bacterial DNA is one of the 17 pathomechanisms of autoimmune/inflammation induction by multifocal dysbiosis
  - Sinorespiratory/nasopharyngeal and dermal dysbiosis: **Increased nasal colonization with *Staphylococcus aureus* has been noted in patients with SLE.**[412]
  - Gastrointestinal dysbiosis: Yeast, bacteria, and parasites are treated as indicated based on identification and sensitivity results from comprehensive parasitology assessments.

- **NUTRITIONAL IMMUNOMODULATION: Treg induction for modulation of Th-1/2/17 inflammation** Nutrients and therapeutic approaches that promote Treg or IL-10 induction and/or Th-17, IL-17 suppression include 1) mitochondrial optimization and mTOR suppression, 2) biotin, 3) vitamin E, 4) sodium avoidance, 5) transgenic/GMO food avoidance, 6) probiotics, 7) lipoic acid, 8) vitamin A, 9) inflammation reduction, 10) vitamin D, 11) fatty acid supplementation with GLA and n3, 12) infection and dysbiosis remediation, 13) green tea EGCG. Acronym: MiBESTPLAIDFIG as reviewed in Chapter 4.

- **DYSMETABOLISM & DYSFUNCTIONAL MITOCHONDRIA: MitoDys, ERS-UPR, AGE/RAGE, hyperglycemia and ceramide** The major clinical considerations in this section are mitochondrial dysfunction, endoplasmic reticulum stress, unfolded protein response, TLR activation, and the dysmetabolic effects of sustained hyperglycemia and hyperinsulinemia and resultant oxidative stress, inflammation, RAGE activation, and accumulation of AGE, palmitate and ceramide. The review of this information in Chapter 4 covered approximately 30 interventions relevant to dysmetabolism, mitochondrial dysfunction, ERS-UPR, etc; these will not be reviewed here except to mention those most commonly, easily, empirically, synergistically, and effectively used: 1) low-carbohydrate diet with 2) moderate exercise, 3) CoQ-10, 4) acetyl-carnitine with 5) lipoic acid, 6) NAC, 7) resveratrol, and 8) melatonin.
  - Mitochondrial hyperpolarization and ATP depletion in patients with systemic lupus erythematosus (*Arthritis Rheum* 2002 Jan[413]): "Mitochondrial hyperpolarization and the resultant ATP depletion sensitize T cells for necrosis, which may significantly contribute to inflammation in patients with SLE."

[408] "Colonization Resistance (CR)...tended to be lower in active SLE patients than in healthy individuals. This could indicate that in SLE more and different bacteria translocate across the gut wall due to a lower CR. Some of these may serve as polyclonal B cell activators or as antigens cross-reacting with DNA." Apperloo-Renkema et al. Host-microflora interaction in systemic lupus erythematosus (SLE): colonization resistance of the indigenous bacteria of the intestinal tract. *Epidemiol Infect.* 1994;112(2):367-73

[409] "The lower IgG antibacterial antibody titres in active SLE might possibly result from sequestration of these IgG antibodies in immune complexes, indicating a possible role for antibacterial antibodies in exacerbations of SLE." Apperloo-Renkema et al. Host-microflora interaction in systemic lupus erythematosus (SLE): circulating antibodies to the indigenous bacteria of the intestinal tract. *Epidemiol Infect.* 1995 Feb;114(1):133-41

[410] Pisetsky DS. Antibody responses to DNA in normal immunity and aberrant immunity. *Clin Diagn Lab Immunol.* 1998 Jan;5(1):1-6 cdli.asm.org/cgi/content/full/5/1/1

[411] Pisetsky DS. Antibody responses to DNA in normal immunity and aberrant immunity. *Clin Diagn Lab Immunol.* 1998 Jan;5(1):1-6 cdli.asm.org/cgi/content/full/5/1/1

[412] Medline abstract from Polish research: "In 9 from 14 patients with (64.3%) a.b. very massive growth of Staphylococcus aureus in culture from vestibulae of the nose swab was, in other cultures very massive growth of physiological flora was seen. ...clinical significance of asymptomatic bacteriuria and pathogenic bacteria colonisation of nostrils as a precedence to symptomatic infections needs further investigations." Koseda-Dragan et al. [Asymptomatic bacteriuria in women diagnosed with systemic lupus erythematosus (SLE)] *Pol Arch Med Wewn.* 1998 Oct;100(4):321-30.

[413] Gergely et al. Mitochondrial hyperpolarization and ATP depletion in patients with systemic lupus erythematosus. *Arthritis Rheum.* 2002 Jan;46(1):175-90

- **STYLE OF LIVING (LIFESTYLE) & SPECIAL CONSIDERATIONS:** <u>S</u>leep optimization, <u>S</u>ocioPsychology, <u>S</u>tress management/avoidance, <u>S</u>omatic treatments, <u>S</u>pecial <u>S</u>upplementation, <u>S</u>weat/exercise, <u>S</u>auna/detoxification, <u>S</u>urgery, <u>S</u>tamp your passport and vacate current reality, <u>S</u>ensory deprivation therapy

This is a buffet of mostly lifestyle-based interventions yet also including considerations such as somatic treatments, additional supplementation, and surgery.

- o <u>Cardiovascular disease (CVD) risk reduction</u>: Patients with SLE have an increased risk of cardiovascular disease due to the synergistic effects of inflammation, oxidative stress, antiphospholipid antibodies, and elevated homocysteine. Obviously, the risk for CVD will be exacerbated if the SLE patient has other risk factors such as tobacco use, diabetes, obesity, hypertension, or physical inactivity. Therapeutic and interventional considerations specific to the prevention of cardiovascular disease include but are not limited to the following:
  - <u>Cardioprotective diet</u>: Paleo-Mediterranean diet
  - <u>Fatty acid supplementation</u>: Combination fatty acid supplementation with ALA, GLA, EPA, DHA[414,415]
  - <u>Magnesium supplementation</u>: > 200 mg up to bowel tolerance
- o <u>Treatments to lower homocysteine</u>: Doses given here for various treatments are for adults:
  - <u>Folic acid</u>: 5-10 mg, should be used with high-dose vitamin B-12
  - <u>Hydroxocobalamin</u>: 2,000-6,000 mcg/d orally, or 1,000-4,000 mcg/wk by injection
  - <u>Pyridoxine</u>: 250 mg/day with meals, co-administered with magnesium (e.g., >200 mg/d)
  - <u>NAC</u>: 600 mg tid
  - <u>Betaine/ trimethylglycine</u>: 1-2 grams tid (>6 grams daily when used alone)
  - <u>Lecithin</u>: 2.6 g choline/d (as phosphatidylcholine) decreased mean fasting plasma homocysteine by 18%.[416] Attaining this high dose might require as many as 45 capsules of commercially available supplements; an equivalent dose in the form of powdered lecithin granules delivered in a smoothie may be better tolerated than the capsules.
- o <u>**N-Acetyl-Cysteine (NAC) for antioxidant, antiviral, and mitochondrial-protective benefits**</u>: NAC provides cysteine for GSH production. NAC also inhibits NFkB. NAC inhibits viral replication (e.g., HIV) more effectively than and independently from its conversion to GSH. Recently, NAC at relatively high doses of 4,800mg/d in divided doses was shown to modulate mitochondrial hyperpolarization (by dissociating the generally resultant mTOR activation) and lead to very important clinical and immunological improvements in patients with SLE; NAC was shown to be safe and well-tolerated by all SLE patients up to 2.4g/d with reversible nausea in 33% of patients receiving 4.8g/d. This study by Lai, Hanczko, Bonilla, et al[417] is truly a landmark contribution and advance in the field

> **Mechanistic and clinical proof of anti-rheumatic benefit of NAC**
>
> "Similar to the effect of rapamycin, **suppression of mTOR by NAC was accompanied by increased FoxP3 expression in CD4+/CD25+ T cells**. These results suggest that the effect of NAC on the immune system is 1) cell type-specific and 2) it occurs through disconnecting the activation of mTOR from the elevation of Δψm in lupus T cells, similar to the effect of rapamycin."
>
> Lai et al. N-acetylcysteine reduces disease activity by blocking mammalian target of rapamycin in T cells from systemic lupus erythematosus patients. *Arthritis Rheum.* 2012 Sep

of rheumatology and immunology because it proves 1) that mitochondrial dysfunction directly leads to an autoimmune phenotype, and 2) that inhibition of mTOR by NAC is safe and effective in patients with SLE; important insights from this remarkable work are as follows:
  - NAC 4,800mg/d proved safe and clinically beneficial in patients with SLE, leading to reductions in disease activity and ANA levels.

[414] Vasquez A. New Insights into Fatty Acid Supplementation and Its Effect on Eicosanoid Production and Genetic Expression. *Nutritional Perspectives* 2005; January: 5-16
[415] Laidlaw M, Holub BJ. Effects of supplementation with fish oil-derived n-3 fatty acids and gamma-linolenic acid on circulating plasma lipids and fatty acid profiles in women. *Am J Clin Nutr.* 2003 Jan;77(1):37-42 ajcn.org/cgi/content/full/77/1/37
[416] Olthof MR, Brink EJ, Katan MB, Verhoef P. Choline supplemented as phosphatidylcholine decreases fasting and postmethionine-loading plasma homocysteine concentrations in healthy men. *Am J Clin Nutr.* 2005 Jul;82(1):111-7
[417] Lai et al. NAC reduces disease activity by blocking mammalian target of rapamycin in T cells from systemic lupus erythematosus patients. *Arthritis Rheum* 2012 Sep:2937-46

- Mitochondrial hyperpolarization (MHP) causes mTOR activation which in turn suppresses the expression of the FoxP3 transcription factor necessary for induction of T-regulatory cells. Note that the mTOR activation is the cause of the FoxP3 suppression; ironically, NAC actually increases MHP but dissociates it from mTOR by having a greater effect on and via mTOR suppression. The nutritional supplement NAC works in a similar manner as does the immunosuppressive drug rapamycin, with a mechanism of suppression of mTOR and the effect of enhancing endogenous anti-inflammatory immunomodulation via CD4+ CD25+ FoxP3+ T-regulatory cells. Stated again and differently, NAC paradoxically worsens mitochondrial hyperpolarization in patients with SLE but does so at the same time that it has a more significant impact on mTOR; NAC's rapamycin-like targeting of mTOR dissociates mitochondrial hyperpolarization from mTOR activation. The reduction in mTOR activity (which is of greater consequence than the increase in MIM polarization) allows enhanced expression of FoxP3 for increased elaboration of T-regulatory cells, thereby providing endogenous immunoregulation.
- "MHP of lupus T cells, which most prominently affects DN [double-negative, autoimmunity-promoting] T cells, was associated with resistance to activation-induced apoptosis. In 27 SLE patients receiving daily NAC doses of 1.2 g, 2.4 g, and 4.8 g considered together, both **spontaneous and CD3/CD28-induced apoptosis of DN T cells were markedly increased** and the **expansion of these cells was effectively reversed**. The **elimination of DN T cells, which are known promote anti-DNA autoantibody production by B cells**, is likely to contribute to reduced anti-DNA titers and to the efficacy of NAC.
- "The therapeutic importance of NAC for SLE is reflected by: 1) achieving clinical improvement in two validated disease activity scores within 3 months; 2) diminishing fatigue (21), which is considered the most disabling symptom in a majority of SLE patients (22); 3) absence of significant side-effects; and 4) affordability of this medication. A monthly supply of 600-mg NAC capsules (120–240 capsules) costs $15–$30 on the retail market. This sharply contrasts with average annual direct medical costs estimated to be ~$22,580 per patient in 2009.Thus, the cost of NAC at $180–$360/year would be negligible in comparison to the overall expenditures to society and the expected benefit in reducing the need for vastly more expensive medications burdened with potentially serious side-effects."

o Oral enzyme therapy with proteolytic/pancreatic enzymes: Polyenzyme supplementation is used to ameliorate the pathophysiology induced by immune complexes, such as the related condition rheumatoid arthritis.[418]

o CoQ10 (antihypertensive, renoprotective, and probably immunomodulatory): CoQ10 is a powerful antioxidant with a wide margin of safety and excellent clinical tolerability. At least four studies have documented its powerful blood-pressure-lowering ability, which often surpasses the clinical effectiveness of antihypertensive drugs.[419,420,421,422] Furthermore, at least two published papers[423,424] and one case report[425] advocate that CoQ10 has powerful renoprotective benefits. CoQ10 levels are low in patients with allergies[426], and the symptomatic relief that many allergic patients experience following supplementation with CoQ10 suggests that CoQ10 has an immunomodulatory effect. Common doses start at > 100 mg per day with food; doses of 200 mg per day are not uncommon, and doses up to 1,000 mg per day are clinically well tolerated though the high financial toll resembles that of many pharmaceutical drugs.

[418] Galebskaya et al. Human complement system state after wobenzyme intake. *Vestnik Moskovskogo Universiteta (Seriya 2: Khimiya)*. 2000:41(6 Suppl): 148-149 chem.msu.ru/eng/journals/vmgu/00add/148.pdf
[419] Burke et al. Randomized, double-blind, placebo-controlled trial of coenzyme Q10 in isolated systolic hypertension. *South Med J*. 2001 Nov;94(11):1112-7
[420] Singh et al. Effect of hydrosoluble coenzyme Q10 on blood pressures and insulin resistance in hypertensive patients coronary artery disease. *J Hum Hypertens* 1999 Mar:203-8
[421] Digiesi et al. Coenzyme Q10 in essential hypertension. *Mol Aspects Med*. 1994;15 Suppl:s257-63
[422] Langsjoen P, Langsjoen P, Willis R, Folkers K. Treatment of essential hypertension with coenzyme Q10. *Mol Aspects Med*. 1994;15 Suppl:S265-72
[423] Singh et al. Randomized, double-blind placebo-controlled trial of coenzyme Q10 in chronic renal failure: discovery of a new role. *J Nutr Environ Med* 2000;10:281-8
[424] Singh et al. Randomized, Double-blind, Placebo-controlled Trial of Coenzyme Q10 in Patients with End-stage Renal Failure. *J Nutr Environ Med* 2003;13: 13–22
[425] Singh RB, Singh MM. Effects of CoQ10 in new indications with antioxidant vitamin deficiency. *J Nutr Environ Med* 1999; 9:223-228
[426] Ye CQ, Folkers K, et al. A modified determination of coenzyme Q10 in human blood and CoQ10 blood levels in diverse patients with allergies. *Biofactors*. 1988 Dec;1:303-6

○ Anti-autoantibody interventions: Patients with SLE have impaired ability to clear immune complexes via hepatic and splenic routes.[427,428] Given that anti-DNA and related immune complexes and cryoglobulins are considered the most fundamental abnormalities in the pathogenesis of this disorder, we can explore at least three routes of clinical intervention based on this limited focus. First, therapeutic interventions might be used that inhibit the *de novo* formation of autoantibodies, particularly those that are directed against double-stranded DNA. This could be accomplished via bio-logical immunomodulation, pharmacologic/anti-biological immunosuppression, or by removing the underlying stimuli and predisposing factors ("etiologic approach"). Second, treatments might be implemented to nullify or diminish the adverse effects of these antibodies. Third, we might use interventions that remove the autoantibodies that are formed so that they are not significantly available to contribute to disease pathogenesis. As discussed previously in the section on treatments for multifocal dysbiosis, at least two primary mechanisms exist for the removal of autoantibody-containing immune complexes, namely 1) phagocytosis and proteolytic degradation by macrophages embedded in the liver and spleen, and 2) transport via hepatocytes directly into the bile for excretion. IgG double-stranded DNA antibodies are consumed and proteolytically/oxidatively/enzymatically degraded by monocytes/phagocytes[429] while IgA-containing immune complexes are preferentially consumed by hepatocytes and exported intact into the bile for excretion.

- **ENDOCRINE IMBALANCE & OPTIMIZATION: Prolactin, Insulin, Estrogen, DHEA, Cortisol, Testosterone, Thyroid** Hormonal imbalances seen among autoimmune/inflammatory patients are: ❶ *elevated* prolactin, ❷ *elevated* estrogen, ❸ *elevated* insulin, and ❹ *reduced* DHEA, ❺ *reduced* cortisol, and ❻ *reduced* testosterone; see Chapter 4 for discussion of these hormones and respective interventions. Thyroid evaluation (patient + labs) should be comprehensive, as discussed in Chapter 1, with a low threshold for empiric treatment.

  ○ Melatonin: Melatonin is a pineal hormone with well-known sleep-inducing and immunomodulatory properties, and it is commonly administered in doses of 1-40 mg in the evening, before bedtime. Starting with a relatively low dose (e.g., 1-5 mg) and increasing as tolerated is recommended. Melatonin (20 mg hs) appears to have cured two patients with drug-resistant sarcoidosis[430] and 3 mg provided immediate short-term benefit to a patient with multiple sclerosis.[431]

  ○ Prolactin (excess): **Prolactin has proinflammatory and immunodysregulatory actions and is commonly elevated—either overtly or latently—in patients with inflammatory/autoimmune disease.** Accordingly prolactin-lowering treatment shows safety and effectiveness in the treatment of numerous inflammatory/autoimmune diseases; often these results are noted even when the patient's prolactin level was not initially elevated, suggesting the alleviation of latent hyperprolactinemia and/or an inherent anti-inflammatory action of the prolactin-lowering treatment. According to clinical trials with small numbers of patients, whether prolactin levels are high or not, prolactin-lowering treatment (such as bromocriptine) appears highly beneficial when used with other anti-rheumatic treatments ("...**drastic efficacy with spectacular improvement** in clinical, biological and occupational status..."[432]) in patients with psoriatic arthritis. Serum prolactin is the standard assessment of prolactin status. Since elevated prolactin may be a sign of pituitary tumor, assessment for headaches, visual deficits, other abnormalities of pituitary hormones (e.g., GH and TSH) should be performed and CT or MRI must be considered. Patients with

---

[427] "These observations support the hypothesis that IC handling is abnormal in SLE." Davies et al. Immune complex processing in patients with systemic lupus erythematosus. *J Clin Invest*. 1992 Nov;90(5):2075-83

[428] "These results indicate that Fc-mediated clearance of ICs is defective in patients with SLE and suggest that ligation of ICs by Fc receptors is critical for their efficient binding and retention by the fixed MPS in the liver." Davies et al. Defective Fc-dependent processing of immune complexes in patients with systemic lupus erythematosus. *Arthritis Rheum*. 2002 Apr;46(4):1028-38

[429] "In the presence of U937 [monocytic] cells, both the AHP-anti-dsDNA and C3b-opsonized ICs were rapidly removed from the erythrocytes; at 37 degrees C, more than half of the complexes were removed in 2 minutes." Craig et al. Clearance of anti-double-stranded DNA antibodies: the natural immune complex clearance mechanism. *Arthritis Rheum*. 2000 Oct;43(10):2265-75

[430] Cagnoni ML, Lombardi A, Cerinic MC, Dedola GL, Pignone A. Melatonin for treatment of chronic refractory sarcoidosis. *Lancet*. 1995 Nov 4;346(8984):1229-30

[431] "...administration of melatonin (3 mg, orally) at 2:00 p.m., when the patient experienced severe blurring of vision, resulted within 15 minutes in a dramatic improvement in visual acuity and in normalization of the visual evoked potential latency after stimulation of the left eye." Sandyk R. Diurnal variations in vision and relations to circadian melatonin secretion in multiple sclerosis. *Int J Neurosci*. 1995 Nov;83(1-2):1-6

[432] Abstract from article in French: "In 2 cases of psoriatic arthritis, adding bromocriptine to gold salts and nonsteroidal anti-inflammatory drug was followed by a drastic efficacy with spectacular improvement in clinical, biological and occupational status. Because none of the cases had hyperprolactinaemia, bromocriptine acted probably had an intrinic anti-inflammatory effect independent of its antiprolactinic effect." Eulry et al. [Blood prolactin under the effect of protirelin in spondylarthropathies. Treatment trial of 4 cases of reactive arthritis and 2 cases of psoriatic arthritis with bromocriptine] *Ann Med Interne* (Paris). 1996;147(1):15-9. French

prolactin levels less than 100 ng/mL and normal CT/MRI findings can be managed conservatively with effective prolactin-lowering treatment and annual radiologic assessment (less necessary with favorable serum response).[433, see review 434] **Patients with RA and SLE have higher basal and stress-induced levels of prolactin compared with normal controls.**[435,436] A normal serum prolactin level does not necessarily exclude the use of prolactin-lowering intervention, especially since many autoimmune patients have **latent hyperprolactinemia** which may not be detected with random serum measurement of prolactin. Vitex lowers serum prolactin in humans[437,438] via a dopaminergic effect.[439] Due at least in part to its content of L-dopa, *Mucuna pruriens* shows clinical dopaminergic activity as evidenced by its effectiveness in Parkinson's disease[440]; up to 15-30 gm/d of mucuna has been used clinically but doses will be dependent on preparation and phytoconcentration. Clinical intervention with bromocriptine appears warranted in patients with RA, SLE, reactive arthritis, psoriatic arthritis, and probably multiple sclerosis and uveitis.[441] A normal serum prolactin level does not necessarily exclude the use of prolactin-lowering intervention, especially since many autoimmune patients have latent hyperprolactinemia which may not be detected with random serum measurement of prolactin. Cabergoline/Dostinex is a newer dopamine agonist with few adverse effects; typical dose starts at 0.5 mg per week (0.25 mg twice per week).[442] Several studies have indicated that cabergoline is safer and more effective than bromocriptine for reducing prolactin levels[443] and the dose can often be reduced after successful prolactin reduction, allowing for reductions in cost and adverse effects.[444] Although fewer studies have been published supporting the antirheumatic benefits of cabergoline than those supporting bromocriptine; its antirheumatic benefits have indeed been documented.[445]

- o Cruciferous vegetables, DIM, I3C: In a short-term study using I3C in patients with SLE, I3C supplementation at 375 mg per day was well tolerated and resulted in modest treatment-dependent clinical improvement as well as favorable modification of estrogen metabolism away from 16-alpha-hydroxyestrone and toward 2-hydroxyestrone.[446]

- o DHEA: DHEA is an anti-inflammatory and immunoregulatory hormone that is commonly deficient in patients with autoimmunity, including polymyalgia rheumatica, SLE, RA, and inflammatory arthritis.[447,448] DHEA levels are suppressed by prednisone[449], and DHEA has been shown to reverse the

[433] Beers MH, Berkow R (eds). *Merck Manual. 17th Edition*. Whitehouse Station; Merck Research Laboratories 1999 Page 77-78

[434] Serri O, Chik CL, Ur E, Ezzat S. Diagnosis and management of hyperprolactinemia. *CMAJ*. 2003 Sep 16;169(6):575-81 cmaj.ca/cgi/content/full/169/6/575

[435] Dostal et al. Serum prolactin stress values in patients with systemic lupus erythematosus. *Ann Rheum Dis*. 2003 May;62(5):487-8 ard.bmjjournals.com/cgi/content/full/62/5/487

[436] "RESULTS: A significantly higher rate of elevated PRL levels was found in SLE patients (40.0%) compared with the healthy controls (14.8%). No proof was found of association with the presence of anti-ds-DNA or with specific organ involvement. Similarly, elevated PRL levels were found in RA patients (39.3%)." Moszkorzova L, Lacinova Z, Marek J, et al. Hyperprolactinaemia in patients with systemic lupus erythematosus. *Clin Exp Rheumatol*. 2002 Nov-Dec;20(6):807-12

[437] "Since AC extracts were shown to have beneficial effects on premenstrual mastodynia serum prolactin levels in such patients were also studied in one double-blind, placebo-controlled clinical study. Serum prolactin levels were indeed reduced in the patients treated with the extract." Wuttke W, Jarry H, Christoffel V, Spengler B, Seidlova-Wuttke D. Chaste tree, Vitex agnus-castus—pharmacology and clinical indications. *Phytomedicine*. 2003 May;10(4):348-57

[438] German abstract from Medline: "The prolactin release was reduced after 3 months, shortened luteal phases were normalised and deficits in the luteal progesterone synthesis were eliminated." Milewicz et al. [Vitex agnus castus extract in the treatment of luteal phase defects due to latent hyperprolactinemia. Results of a randomized placebo-controlled double-blind study] *Arzneimittelforschung*. 1993 Jul;43(7):752-6

[439] "Our results indicate a dopaminergic effect of Vitex agnus-castus extracts and suggest additional pharmacological actions via opioid receptors." Meier B, Berger D, Hoberg E, Sticher O, Schaffner W. Pharmacological activities of Vitex agnus-castus extracts in vitro. *Phytomedicine*. 2000 Oct;7(5):373-81

[440] "CONCLUSIONS: The rapid onset of action and longer on time without concomitant increase in dyskinesias on mucuna seed powder formulation suggest that this natural source of L-dopa might possess advantages over conventional L-dopa preparations in the long term management of PD." Katzenschlager et al. Mucuna pruriens in Parkinson's disease: a double blind clinical and pharmacological study. *J Neurol Neurosurg Psychiatry*. 2004 Dec;75(12):1672-7

[441] "...clinical observations and trials support the use of bromocriptine as a nonstandard primary or adjunctive therapy in the treatment of recalcitrant RA, SLE, Reiter's syndrome, and psoriatic arthritis and associated conditions unresponsive to traditional approaches." McMurray RW. Bromocriptine in rheumatic and autoimmune diseases. *Semin Arthritis Rheum*. 2001 Aug;31(1):21-32

[442] Serri O, Chik CL, Ur E, Ezzat S. Diagnosis and management of hyperprolactinemia. *CMAJ*. 2003 Sep 16;169(6):575-81 cmaj.ca/cgi/content/full/169/6/575

[443] "CONCLUSION: These data indicate that cabergoline is a very effective agent for lowering the prolactin levels in hyperprolactinemic patients and that it appears to offer considerable advantage over bromocriptine in terms of efficacy and tolerability." Sabuncu et al. Comparison of the effects of cabergoline and bromocriptine on prolactin levels in hyperprolactinemic patients. *Intern Med*. 2001 Sep;40(9):857-61

[444] "Cabergoline also normalized PRL in the majority of patients with known bromocriptine intolerance or -resistance. Once PRL secretion was adequately controlled, the dose of cabergoline could often be significantly decreased, which further reduced costs of therapy." Verhelst et al. Cabergoline in the treatment of hyperprolactinemia: a study in 455 patients. *J Clin Endocrinol Metab*. 1999 Jul;84(7):2518-22 jcem.endojournals.org/cgi/content/full/84/7/2518

[445] Erb N, Pace AV, Delamere JP, Kitas GD. Control of unremitting rheumatoid arthritis by the prolactin antagonist cabergoline. *Rheumatology* (Oxford). 2001 Feb;40(2):237-9

[446] "Women with SLE can manifest a metabolic response to I3C and might benefit from its antiestrogenic effects." McAlindon TE, Gulin J, Chen T, Klug T, Lahita R, Nuite M. Indole-3-carbinol in women with SLE: effect on estrogen metabolism and disease activity. *Lupus*. 2001;10(11):779-83

[447] "The low levels found in patients with PM:TA are in accordance with those previously reported in immune-mediated diseases such as systemic lupus erythematosus (SLE) and rheumatoid arthritis, suggesting that diminution of DHEAS is a constant endocrinologic feature in these categories of patients." Nilsson et al. Blood dehydroepiandrosterone sulphate (DHEAS) levels in polymyalgia rheumatica/giant cell arteritis and primary fibromyalgia. *Clin Exp Rheumatol*. 1994 Jul-Aug;12(4):415-7

[448] "DHEAS concentrations were significantly decreased in both women and men with inflammatory arthritis (IA) (P < 0.001)." Dessein et al. Hyposecretion of the adrenal androgen dehydroepiandrosterone sulfate and its relation to clinical variables in inflammatory arthritis. *Arthritis Res*. 2001;3(3):183-8 arthritis-research.com/content/3/3/183

[449] "Basal serum DHEA and DHEAS concentrations were suppressed to a greater degree than was cortisol during both daily and alternate day prednisone treatments. ...Thus, adrenal androgen secretion was more easily suppressed than was cortisol secretion by this low dose of glucocorticoid, but there was no advantage to alternate day therapy." Rittmaster et al. Effect of daily and alternate day low dose prednisone on serum cortisol and adrenal androgens in hirsute women. *J Clin Endocrinol Metab*. 1988 Aug;67(2):400-3

osteoporosis and loss of bone mass induced by corticosteroid treatment.[450] DHEA shows no acute or subacute toxicity even when used in supraphysiologic doses, even when used in sick patients. For example, in a study of 32 patients with HIV, DHEA doses of 750 mg – 2,250 mg per day were well-tolerated and produced no dose-limiting adverse effects.[451] This lack of toxicity compares favorably with any and all so-called "antirheumatic" drugs, nearly all of which show impressive comparable toxicity. High-dose supplemental DHEA has benefits in the treatment of SLE that are comparable to those obtained with antimalarial drugs.[452] When used at doses of 200 mg per day, DHEA safely provides clinical benefit for patients with various autoimmune diseases, including ulcerative colitis, Crohn's disease[453], and SLE.[454] In patients with SLE, DHEA supplementation allows for reduced dosing of prednisone (thus avoiding its adverse effects) while providing symptomatic improvement.[455] Optimal clinical response appears to correlate with serum levels that are supraphysiologic[456], and therefore treatment may be implemented with little regard for initial/baseline DHEA levels provided that the patient is free of contraindications, particularly high risk for sex-hormone-dependent malignancy. Other than mild adverse effects predictable with any androgen (namely voice deepening, transient acne, and increased facial hair), DHEA supplementation does not cause serious adverse effects[457], and it is appropriate for routine clinical use particularly when 1) the dose of DHEA is kept as low as possible, 2) duration is kept as short as possible, 3) other interventions are used to address the underlying cause of the disease, 4) the patient is deriving benefit, and 5) the risk-to-benefit ratio is favorable.

- **XENOBIOTIC ACCUMULATION & DETOXIFICATION: Chemical avoidance, nutritional support for detoxification pathways, urine alkalinization** The clinical relevance and pathogenic mechanisms of xenobiotic accumulation are irrefutably well documented and described. Clinical assessments include history, physical examination, and laboratory assessment (using serum, whole blood, urine or—rarely yet accurately—fat biopsy), and response to treatment. Treatments include nutritional support for Phases 1 and 2 of detoxification (e.g., oxidation and conjugation) and excretion via bile and urine; for the latter, urinary alkalinization is generally recommended. Chemical toxins can be bound in the gut using activated charcoal, cholestyramine, or *Chlorella*—all of these three treatments have documented safety and effectiveness; clinically and empirically, phytochelatin (plant-derived peptides that bind toxic metals) concentrates appear safe and effective despite lack of conclusive published data supporting clinical use. Mercury exposure via working in a dental office is one of the greatest occupational risks ever identified for the development of SLE in humans.

---

[450] "CONCLUSION: Prasterone treatment prevented BMD loss and significantly increased BMD at both the lumbar spine and total hip in female patients with SLE receiving exogenous glucocorticoids." Mease et al. Effects of prasterone on bone mineral density in women with systemic lupus erythematosus receiving chronic glucocorticoid therapy. *J Rheumatol*. 2005 Apr;32(4):616-21

[451] "Thirty-one subjects were evaluated and monitored for safety and tolerance. The oral drug was administered three times daily in doses ranging from 750 mg/day to 2,250 mg/day for 16 weeks. ... The drug was well tolerated and no dose-limiting side effects were noted." Dyner et al. An open-label dose-escalation trial of oral dehydroepiandrosterone tolerance and pharmacokinetics in patients with HIV disease. *J Acquir Immune Defic Syndr*. 1993 May;6(5):459-65

[452] Tierney ML. McPhee SJ, Papadakis MA. Current Medical Diagnosis and Treatment 2006. 45th edition. New York; Lange Medical Books: 2006, pages 833-837

[453] "CONCLUSIONS: In a pilot study, dehydroepiandrosterone was effective and safe in patients with refractory Crohn's disease or ulcerative colitis." Andus et al. Patients with refractory Crohn's disease or ulcerative colitis respond to dehydroepiandrosterone: a pilot study. *Aliment Pharmacol Ther*. 2003 Feb;17(3):409-14

[454] "CONCLUSION: The overall results confirm that DHEA treatment was well-tolerated, significantly reduced the number of SLE flares, and improved patient's global assessment of disease activity." Chang DM, Lan JL, Lin HY, Luo SF. Dehydroepiandrosterone treatment of women with mild-to-moderate systemic lupus erythematosus: a multicenter randomized, double-blind, placebo-controlled trial. *Arthritis Rheum*. 2002 Nov;46(11):2924-7

[455] "CONCLUSION: Among women with lupus disease activity, reducing the dosage of prednisone to < or = 7.5 mg/day for a sustained period of time while maintaining stabilization or a reduction of disease activity was possible in a significantly greater proportion of patients treated with oral prasterone, 200 mg once daily, compared with patients treated with placebo." Petri et al; GL601 Study Group. Effects of prasterone on corticosteroid requirements of women with systemic lupus erythematosus: a double-blind, randomized, placebo-controlled trial. *Arthritis Rheum*. 2002 Jul;46(7):1820-9

[456] "CONCLUSION: The clinical response to DHEA was not clearly dose dependent. Serum levels of DHEA and DHEAS correlated only weakly with lupus outcomes, but suggested an optimum serum DHEAS of 1000 microg/dl." Barry et al. Dehydroepiandrosterone in systemic lupus erythematosus: relationship between dosage, serum levels, and clinical response. *J Rheumatol*. 1998 Dec;25(12):2352-6

[457] Tierney ML. McPhee SJ, Papadakis MA. *Current Medical Diagnosis and Treatment 2006. 45th edition*. New York; Lange Medical Books: 2006, page 1721

Scleroderma & Systemic Sclerosis

Introduction:

Scleroderma and systemic sclerosis are related conditions of either dermal or dermal+systemic fibrosis, respectively. A reasonable conceptualization is that of an inflammation/ROS-driven fibrotic response; the solution then—of course—is to address the disease-specific and patient-specific causes of excess inflammation and immune imbalance. The vicious cycles of nutritional deficiency, gastrointestinal dysbiosis, and persistent active viral infections must be addressed.

Description/pathophysiology:

- Overview: Generally considered "idiopathic" from the allopathic medical perspective; for example, a 2008 article published by the American Academy of Family Physicians introduces the topic in this manner, providing a brief description along with undermining any possible desire to treat the cause of the illness via the promulgation that the cause is officially declared to be unknown: "Systemic sclerosis (systemic scleroderma) is a chronic connective tissue disease of unknown etiology that causes widespread microvascular damage and excessive deposition of collagen in the skin and internal organs."[458] The terms *scleroderma* and *systemic sclerosis* are used somewhat interchangeably; yet, as these terms suggest, *scleroderma* is properly assigned to disease that is limited to the skin, while *systemic sclerosis* denotes visceral involvement in addition to skin changes. *Scleroderma* will be the default term in this section for linguistic expediency; because the initials "SS" can equally suggest Sjogren's syndrome as well as systemic sclerosis, the initials *SSc* will be used to denote systemic sclerosis—again interchangeably with *scleroderma*.

- **Characterized by fibrosis of the skin and internal organs, including the esophagus, intestines, lung, heart, and kidneys.** The condition can be mild and limited to the skin only, or it can be systemic and rapidly fatal due to internal organ involvement.

- Main subtypes:
  1. Limited, cutaneous scleroderma—60% of cases: Primarily affecting the skin, especially of the fingers and face; distribution often described as distal to the neck, elbows and knees; major complications are GERD, Raynaud's, and pulmonary hypertension, notably "Patients with limited cutaneous systemic sclerosis have the greatest risk of pulmonary arterial hypertension."[459]
     - CREST syndrome—variant of limited/cutaneous scleroderma: Calcinosis, Raynaud's phenomenon, esophageal dysmotility/dysfunction, sclerodactyly, telangiectasia
  2. Diffuse, systemic sclerosis—35% of cases: Characterized by systemic fibrosis of skin and internal organs, especially interstitial lung disease; may rapidly progress to death via scleroderma renal crisis.
  3. Systemic sclerosis sine scleroderma—approximately 5% of patients with systemic sclerosis: Characteristic internal organ manifestations of the disease without skin thickening.
  4. Localized/linear scleroderma and morphea: Primarily affects children, not associated with Raynaud phenomenon or significant internal organ involvement.
  5. Mixed connective tissue disease and "overlap syndromes"—less common: Combination of scleroderma with another autoimmune disease, such as dermatomyositis (sclerodermatomyositis) or RA, SLE, etc.
  6. Scleroderma secondary to xenobiotic immunotoxicity—rare: Scleroderma can result from exposure to vinyl chloride, silicone, petroleum products, toxic oil syndrome, solvents, cocaine, and pesticides.

- Patients with scleroderma have evidence of **increased oxidative stress** demonstrated by a doubling of urinary isoprostane excretion.[460] Oxidative stress *results from* and *contributes to* systemic inflammation because 1) increased immune activity results in elaboration of oxidants, and 2) oxidative stress upregulates NFkB (and other pathways) for additive immune activation; oxidative stress and inflammation both contribute to tissue fibrosis.

---

[458] Hinchcliff M, Varga J. Systemic sclerosis/scleroderma: a treatable multisystem disease. *Am Fam Physician*. 2008 Oct 15;78(8):961-8
[459] Hinchcliff M, Varga J. Systemic sclerosis/scleroderma: a treatable multisystem disease. *Am Fam Physician*. 2008 Oct 15;78(8):961-8
[460] "CONCLUSION: This study provides evidence of enhanced lipid peroxidation in both SSc and UCTD, and suggests a rationale for antioxidant treatment of SSc." Cracowski et al. Enhanced in vivo lipid peroxidation in scleroderma spectrum disorders. *Arthritis Rheum* 2001 May;44(5):1143-8

Clinical presentations:

- <u>Classic presentation</u>: "The typical patient is a young or middle-age woman with a history of Raynaud phenomenon who presents with skin induration and internal organ dysfunction."[461] 4x more common in women, general age of onset is 20-40 years. More than 95% of scleroderma/SSc patients have Raynaud's phenomenon, thereby giving this clinical manifestation a considerable degree of importance in the initial/historical assessment.
- <u>Skin changes</u>: Hyperpigmentation, tightness, tightness and thickening of the face results in "mask-like face", telangiectasia, may also have depigmentation; dermal pitting (mild) and ulceration (more severe) of fingertips; swelling and thickening of the fingers is termed sclerodactyly.
- <u>Soft tissue calcification</u>: Especially in the hands; systemic calcification is also seen.
- <u>Polyarthralgia</u>: Affects 90% of patients; flexion contractures of the joints due to fibrosis is also common.
- <u>Autonomic dysfunction: Raynaud's phenomenon</u>: Seen in 90% of patients and often precedes sclerodermatous manifestations by a period of up to 5 years; the high level of overlap among these two conditions suggests a common etiology—the factor most strongly associated with both conditions and especially Raynaud's is *H pylori* infection, discussed later in this section on SSc and also in the section on Raynaud's.
- <u>Pulmonary</u>: Dyspnea, pulmonary hypertension.
- <u>Cardiac</u>: Arrhythmias, CHF, hypertension, ECG abnormalities—may be fatal.
- <u>Renal</u>: Renal failure is a leading cause of death—see renal assessments in Chapter 1. "Scleroderma renal crisis develops in 3 to 10 percent of all patients with systemic sclerosis and in 10 to 20 percent of those with rapidly progressive diffuse cutaneous systemic sclerosis; the greatest risk occurs within the first three years of the disease. … Patients with scleroderma renal crisis characteristically present with sudden-onset accelerated hypertension that is often associated with progressive oliguric renal failure with proteinuria, microangiopathic anemia, and microscopic hematuria. Ten to 15 percent of patients with scleroderma renal crisis are normotensive, but hypertensive when compared with their baseline blood pressure measurements."[462]
- <u>GI disturbances</u>:
  - Esophageal dysfunction and dysphagia eventually occur in most patients; histologic/biopsy examination reveals degeneration of intestinal nerves, vessels, and smooth muscle.[463]
  - Greatly increased risk for Barrett's esophagus (33% of all scleroderma patients) with a notably low risk of esophageal adenocarcinoma.
  - Slow intestinal transit—intestinal hypomotility in scleroderma promotes bacterial overgrowth of the small bowel, which probably contributes to the pathogenesis of the disease via the pro-inflammatory and immune activating effects discussed in Chapter 4. Treatment of bacterial overgrowth with antibiotics (ciprofloxacin 500 mg bid[464]) or promotility drugs (octreotide[465]) is effective treatment for scleroderma according to published case reports; **such research supports the hypothesis that intestinal dysbiosis— namely bacterial overgrowth—is an important contributor to the perpetuation of scleroderma.**

Major differential diagnoses:

- <u>Parkinson's disease</u>: Mask-like face
- <u>Other autoimmune disorders</u>: Overlap syndromes, mixed connective tissue diseases
- <u>Amyloidosis</u>: Primary or secondary forms; often leads to skin thickening due to amyloid deposition however skin generally remains soft and more edematous-like than induration-like
- <u>Nephrogenic systemic fibrosis</u>: "Nephrogenic systemic fibrosis (NSF) is a fibrosing disorder, recently described in patients with advanced chronic kidney disease, usually after exposure to gadolinium (Gd)-based contrast agents, characterized by progressive fibrotic involvement mainly of the skin. At clinical examination, the

---

[461] Hinchcliff M, Varga J. Systemic sclerosis/scleroderma: a treatable multisystem disease. *Am Fam Physician.* 2008 Oct 15;78(8):961-8
[462] Hinchcliff M, Varga J. Systemic sclerosis/scleroderma: a treatable multisystem disease. *Am Fam Physician.* 2008 Oct 15;78(8):961-8
[463] "We found ultrastructural signs of axonal degeneration and cytoskeletal abnormalities in the bundles of unmyelinated fibers. There was also focal degeneration of smooth muscle cells, often in association with the presence of partially degranulated mast cells." Malandrini et al. Autonomic nervous system and smooth muscle cell involvement in systemic sclerosis: ultrastructural study of 3 cases. *J Rheumatol.* 2000 May;27(5):1203-6
[464] Over KE, Bucknall RC. Regression of skin changes in a patient with systemic sclerosis following treatment for bacterial overgrowth with ciprofloxacin. *Br J Rheumatol.* 1998 Jun;37(6):696 rheumatology.oxfordjournals.org/cgi/reprint/37/6/696a
[465] "After 8 months of treatment, normal weight was obtained and skin induration was spectacularly reduced and pigmentation returned to a normal state." Descamps et al. Global improvement of systemic scleroderma under long-term administration of octreotide. *Eur J Dermatol* 1999 Sep;9(6):446-8

cutaneous findings of NSF may partly resemble those of systemic sclerosis. However, the different topographic distribution of the skin thickening and hardening, usually involving the limbs and trunk, whilst sparing the face, the lack of serologic abnormalities and the distinctive histopathological findings allow this new disease entity to be distinguished from systemic sclerosis and other scleroderma-like fibrosing disorders (scleromyxedema, scleredema, eosinophilic fasciitis, etc.)."[466]

- Vinyl chloride disease: exposure to vinyl chloride (VC) monomer, a volatile substance mostly used for polyvinyl chloride (PVC) synthesis produces a scleroderma-like disorder that may be complicated by vasculitic and neurologic sequelae.[467,468,469]
- Dermal infections and other diseases: Zygomycosis, sporotrichosis, cutaneous lymphoma
- Toxic oil syndrome: A syndrome of incapacitating myalgias, marked peripheral eosinophilia, pulmonary infiltrates, and increased prevalence of scleroderma and neurologic disorders following consumption of contaminated oil.[470]

Clinical assessments:
- **History/subjective**:
  - o Symptoms and complications from dermal induration/hardening and fibrosis
  - o Intestinal and digestive complaints
  - o Areas affected, ROM, ADL, QOL
  - o Xenobiotic exposure: Occupational exposure to silica is associated with scleroderma; some cases appear to be linked to silicone breast implants[471] (controversial[472]) and anti-silicate antibodies may be valuable for documenting humoral response to silicone.[473] Clinicians should ask about any history of iatrogenic, occupational, recreational or domestic xenobiotic exposure, such as to organic solvents[474], pesticides, epoxy resins[475], and other immunotoxins.[476] Use of cocaine may cause or exacerbate scleroderma.[477]
- **Physical examination/objective**: routine, including the following:
  - o Dermal exam, including nailfold capillaroscopy: Symptoms and complications from dermal induration/hardening, swelling, fibrosis, and calcium deposition: swollen fingers, tight skin on face and hands, dermal ulcerations and hypopigmentation. The "colors of Raynaud's phenomenon" are white (vasospasm), blue-purple (ischemia), and red (hyperemia).
    - ▪ Nailfold capillaroscopy—viewed clinically with magnifying lens: Reveals microvascular changes consistent with autoimmunity and autoimmune-expedited cardiovascular disease. Per Cutolo et al[478], "Raynaud's phenomenon (RP) represents the most frequent clinical aspect of cardio/microvascular involvement and is a key feature of several autoimmune rheumatic diseases. Moreover, RP is associated in a statistically significant manner with many coronary diseases. In normal conditions or in primary RP (excluding during the cold-exposure test), the normal nailfold

[466] Rota et al. Nephrogenic systemic fibrosis: an unusual scleroderma-like fibrosing disorder. *Rheumatol Int*. 2010 Aug;30(10):1389-91
[467] "Occupational exposure to vinyl chloride monomers is known to induce Raynaud's phenomenon, periportal fibrosis, liver angiosarcoma and scleroderma-like syndrome." Serratrice et al. A case of polymyositis with anti-histidyl-t-RNA synthetase (Jo-1) antibody syndrome following extensive vinyl chloride exposure. *Clin Rheumatol* 2001;20:379-82
[468] "An unusual case of systemic sclerosis occurring in a patient exposed to the vinyl chloride monomer (VCM) is presented." Ostlere et al. Atypical systemic sclerosis following exposure to vinyl chloride monomer. A case report and review of the cutaneous aspects of vinyl chloride disease. *Clin Exp Dermatol*. 1992 May;17(3):208-10
[469] "Angiosarcoma of the liver, Raynaud's phenomenon, scleroderma-like lesions, acroosteolysis and neuritis are known to be typical vinyl chloride-associated manifestations (VC disease)." Magnavita N, Bergamaschi A, Garcovich A, Giuliano G. Vasculitic purpura in vinyl chloride disease: a case report. *Angiology*. 1986 May;37(5):382-8
[470] "In 1981, in Spain, the ingestion of an oil fraudulently sold as olive oil caused an outbreak of a previously unrecorded condition, later known as toxic oil syndrome (TOS), clinically characterized by intense incapacitating myalgias, marked peripheral eosinophilia, and pulmonary infiltrates." Gelpi et al; WHO/CISAT Scientific Committee for the Toxic Oil Syndrome. The Spanish toxic oil syndrome 20 years after its onset: multidisciplinary review of scientific knowledge. *Environ Health Perspect*. 2002 May;110(5):457-64
[471] "...idiopathic form of scleroderma and related conditions. CONCLUSION. These findings suggest that ANA positivity is relatively common in individuals with silicone breast implants, and may support the existence of autoimmune mechanisms in the pathogenesis of the clinical manifestations seen in this population." Cuellar ML, Scopelitis E, Tenenbaum SA, et al. Serum antinuclear antibodies in women with silicone breast implants. *J Rheumatol*. 1995 Feb;22(2):236-40
[472] "Neither the case-control studies nor the other epidemiologic data support the hypothesis that scleroderma is associated with or causally related to breast implants." Whorton D, Wong O. Scleroderma and silicone breast implants. *West J Med* 1997 Sep;167(3):159-65
[473] Shen GQ, Ojo-Amaize EA, Agopian MS, Peter JB.Silicate antibodies in women with silicone breast implants: development of an assay for detection of humoral immunity. *Clin Diagn Lab Immunol*. 1996 Mar;3(2):162-6 cdli.asm.org/cgi/reprint/3/2/162?view=reprint&pmid=8991630
[474] "We describe a sclerodermatous syndrome in a middle-aged man who had worked with a wide variety of organic solvents over a prolonged period." Bottomley WW, et al. A sclerodermatous syndrome with unusual features following prolonged occupational exposure to organic solvents. *Br J Dermatol* 1993 Feb;128(2):203-6
[475] "A new occupational disorder characterized by skin sclerosis is described. This disease developed acutely in workmen exposed to the vapor of epoxy resins." Yamakage A, et al. Occupational scleroderma-like disorder occurring in men engaged in the polymerization of epoxy resins. *Dermatologica*. 1980;161(1):33-44
[476] "There is growing concern about the association between systemic sclerosis and certain environmental and occupational risk factors, including exposures to vinyl chloride, adulterated cooking oils, L-tryptophan, silica, silicone breast implants, organic solvents, and other agents such as epoxy resins, pesticides, and hand/arm vibration." Nietert PJ, Silver RM. Systemic sclerosis: environmental and occupational risk factors. *Curr Opin Rheumatol* 2000 Nov;12(6):520-6
[477] "It has been reported that cocaine may initiate scleroderma in an already susceptible individual or unmask it at an earlier age in subclinical disease." Attoussi S, Faulkner ML, Oso A, Umoru B. Cocaine-induced scleroderma and scleroderma renal crisis. *South Med J* 1998 Oct;91(10):961-3
[478] Cutolo M, Sulli A, Secchi ME, Paolino S, Pizzorni C. Nailfold capillaroscopy is useful for the diagnosis and follow-up of autoimmune rheumatic diseases. A future tool for the analysis of microvascular heart involvement? *Rheumatology* (Oxford). 2006 Oct;45 Suppl 4:iv43-6 rheumatology.oxfordjournals.org/content/45/suppl_4/iv43.full.pdf

capillaroscopic pattern shows a regular disposition of the capillary loops along with the nailbed. On the contrary, in subjects suffering from secondary RP, one or more alterations of the capillaroscopic findings should alert the physician of the possibility of a connective tissue disease not yet detected. Nailfold capillaroscopy (NV) represents the best method to analyze microvascular abnormalities in autoimmune rheumatic diseases. Architectural disorganization, giant capillaries, hemorrhages, loss of capillaries, angiogenesis and avascular areas characterize >95% of patients with overt scleroderma (SSc)."

- o Range of motion (ROM): Limited range of motion is characteristic secondary to a "straight jacket" effect secondary to tightened and fibrotic skin; reduced neck extension is termed "platysma sign"
- o Abdominal exam: Abdominal exam, gastrointestinal motility
- o Pulmonary exam: Pulmonary examination and auscultation; needs to be complemented by additional diagnostic testing. "Dyspnea is a late manifestation of systemic sclerosis–related lung disease; however, lung involvement is common and is the leading cause of death in patients with systemic sclerosis. ... Thus, routine screening with pulmonary function tests and Doppler echocardiography in all patients is essential for the early detection of interstitial lung disease and pulmonary arterial hypertension, respectively."[479]
- o Cardiovascular exam: Assessment for hypertension is mandatory
- **Laboratory assessments**: *lab assessments are only minimally supportive for the diagnosis, but are helpful to monitor for complications*
    - o Urinalysis: Screen for renal compromise as previously detailed
    - o Chemistry panel: Assess for renal and liver status, electrolytes, etc.
    - o CBC: May reveal anemia due to malabsorption-induced deficiencies of B12, folate, iron, hypoproliferation due to inflammation (i.e., the anemia of chronic disease).
    - o Rheumatoid factor: positive in 33%
    - o Breath hydrogen/methane for SIBO: This test is used to assess for bacterial overgrowth; it is not a perfect test and it delays treatment (dietary, antimicrobial) that should generally be implemented regardless of the results of this test.
    - o Lactulose and mannitol assay for "leaky gut" and malabsorption: Abnormal results are likely due to bacterial overgrowth and/or celiac disease with resultant malabsorption and increased intestinal permeability.[480]
    - o Fecal calprotectin—assessment for gastrointestinal involvement: "Fecal calprotectin (F-calprotectin) is increased in a majority of patients with SSc. It correlates with objective and clinically important features of GI disease, and fecal concentrations do not vary with plasma concentrations. We suggest that F-calprotectin is a promising objective non-invasive biomarker of GI involvement in SSc."[481]
    - o Leukocyte antigens: Increased prevalence of HLA-DR5 and HLA-DR1
    - o *Helicobacter pylori* detection: Given the increased prevalence of *Helicobacter pylori* infection[482,483], the addition of antigen testing onto a comprehensive stool analysis and comprehensive parasitology examination is recommended.
    - o Comprehensive stool analysis and comprehensive parasitology: essential
    - o **ANA (nucleolar): Positive in up to 96% of patients with scleroderma;** nucleolar pattern is most specific
    - o **Anticentromere antibody**: Positive in 50% with CREST; generally—relatively speaking—portends disease course more limited to dermal involvement[484]; correlates with and requires monitoring for pulmonary arterial hypertension

---

[479] Hinchcliff M, Varga J. Systemic sclerosis/scleroderma: a treatable multisystem disease. *Am Fam Physician*. 2008 Oct 15;78(8):961-8
[480] "Coeliac disease may account for malabsorption in scleroderma patients even when test suggest bacterial overgrowth." Marguerie C, Kaye S, Vyse T, Mackworth-Young C, Walport MJ, Black C. Malabsorption caused by coeliac disease in patients who have scleroderma. *Br J Rheumatol*. 1995 Sep;34(9):858-61
[481] Andréasson et al. Faecal calprotectin: a biomarker of gastrointestinal disease in systemic sclerosis. *J Intern Med*. 2011 Jul;270(1):50-7
[482] "Thus, risk for gastric diseases caused by HP infection is enhanced in patients with systemic sclerosis compared with white healthy, asymptomatic persons examined in other studies." Reinauer et al. Helicobacter pylori in patients with systemic sclerosis: detection with the 13C-urea breath test and eradication. *Acta Derm Venereol*. 1994 Sep;74(5):361-3
[483] "Patients with SSc have H. pylori infection at a higher prevalence than the general population." Yazawa et al. High seroprevalence of Helicobacter pylori infection in patients with systemic sclerosis: association with esophageal involvement. *J Rheumatol*. 1998 Apr;25(4):650-3
[484] Ho KT, Reveille JD. The clinical relevance of autoantibodies in scleroderma. *Arthritis Res Ther*. 2003;5(2):80-93 arthritis-research.com/content/5/2/80

- o **Anti-SCL-70 antibodies = anti-topoisomerase-1 antibodies**: Positive in 20-30% of patients; specific for scleroderma; portends disease course with internal organ involvement, particularly of the lungs; correlates with rapidly progressive skin thickening, scleroderma renal crisis, pulmonary fibrosis
  - o Antifibrillarin antibodies: seen in a small portion (~4%) of patients with scleroderma and correlates with internal organ involvement[485]
  - o Antimitochondrial antibodies, assessment for primary biliary cirrhosis: 225 Japanese SSc patients were retrospectively examined for PBC-associated autoantibodies, anti-mitochondrial M2 antibodies (AMA), anti-sp100 antibodies (anti-sp100), and anti-gp210 antibodies (anti-gp210); findings included that "37 (16.4%) had AMA, 13 (5.8%) had anti-sp100, and 3 (1.3%) had anti-gp210. Three patients were positive for both AMA and anti-sp100, and 2 were positive for both AMA and anti-gp210. PBC was found in 22 (9.8%) patients positive for AMA with or without anti-sp100 or anti-gp210, but not in those with anti-sp100 or anti-gp210 without AMA. Furthermore, 13 patients lacking these three antibodies were diagnosed with or suspected of PBC by liver biopsy and/or their clinical manifestation. Multivariable analysis revealed that AMA and anti-centromere antibodies were independently associated with PBC in SSc patients, while anti-sp100 and anti-gp210 were not. CONCLUSIONS: This study has demonstrated even higher prevalence of both PBC-associated autoantibodies and PBC in the Japanese SSc population than in the Caucasian SSc population. AMA and anti-centromere antibodies are likely to indicate increasing risk of PBC in SSc patients."[486]
- **Imaging**:
  - o ECG abnormalities are common and can include ventricular ectopy, which is correlated with sudden cardiac death
  - o Radiography, pulmonary function tests, and CT imaging may be used to detect fibrosing alveolitis and scleroderma-associated pulmonary decline
- **Establishing the diagnosis**:
  - o Clinical assessment is sufficient in patients with classic full-blown disease
  - o Combination of serologic evidence of autoimmunity and dermal induration

Complications:

- **General: Generalized fibrosis leads to thickening of skin (most obvious), obliteration of the lumen of small arteries (most pathologic), and reduced intestinal motility.**
- Cardiopulmonary and renal: Sudden cardiac death, pulmonary fibrosis/hypertension/failure, hypertension secondary to scleroderma-induced renal damage, renal insufficiency/failure.
- Gastrointestinal: 33% of patients will develop Barrett's esophagus and are at increased risk for cancer; periodic endoscopic surveillance is warranted; referral to gastroenterologist is recommended. To the extent possible, acid-blocking (proton pump-inhibiting) drugs should be avoided because the iatrogenic hypochlorhydria will exacerbate the small bowel bacterial overgrowth and thereby perpetuate the systemic inflammatory state. Malabsorption and resultant malnutrition are due to intestinal hypomotility and SIBO/dysbiosis; from the medical perspective—which in this case is largely correct except for failure to include dietary modification, "Antibiotics, including rifaximin (Xifaxan), and correction of nutritional deficiencies are the mainstays of therapy for intestinal overgrowth."[487] Nonpharmacologic treatments for SIBO include dietary modification especially exclusion of high-fermentation foods (such as sucrose, lactose, wheat, potatoes), berberine 1,000-1,500 mg/d, oregano oil (time-released emulsified) 300-600 mg/d, and ascorbate and magnesium to promote bowel clearance.
- Cancer: Increased incidence of breast and lung cancer

[485] "AFA identifies young SSc patients with frequent internal organ involvement, especially pulmonary hypertension, myositis and renal disease." Tormey VJ, Bunn CC, Denton CP, Black CM. Anti-fibrillarin antibodies in systemic sclerosis. *Rheumatology*. 2001 Oct;40(10):1157-62 rheumatology.oxfordjournals.org/cgi/content/full/40/10/1157
[486] Imura-Kumada K et al. High prevalence of primary biliary cirrhosis and disease-associated autoantibodies in Japanese patients with systemic sclerosis. *Mod Rheumatol*. 2012 Nov;22(6):892-8
[487] Hinchcliff M, Varga J. Systemic sclerosis/scleroderma: a treatable multisystem disease. *Am Fam Physician*. 2008 Oct 15;78(8):961-8

Clinical management:

- Address underlying causative contributors; apply Functional Inflammology protocol.
- Monitor for complications such as systemic hypertension, pulmonary hypertension, renal failure.
  - All patients with systemic sclerosis are advised to check their blood pressure at home on a regular basis. Any persistent elevations should prompt medical evaluation and treatment with ACEi.
- Referral if clinical outcome is unsatisfactory or if serious complications are possible/evident.
- Treat complications such as HTN and GERD.

> **Diagnostic evaluation for SSc: Additional rationale for specialist comanagement**
>
> "Clinical evaluation and laboratory testing, along with pulmonary function testing, Doppler echocardiography, and high-resolution computed tomography of the chest [single-photon emission CT for detection of cardiocirculatory abnormalities], establish the diagnosis and detect visceral involvement."
>
> Hinchcliff, Varga. *Am Fam Physician*. 2008 Oct

Treatments:

- **Drug treatments**: "Treatment of progressive systemic sclerosis is symptomatic and supportive. ... Prednisone has little or no role in the treatment of scleroderma."[488] Per 2008 review, "No disease-modifying agent has been proven to prevent or reverse fibrosis, although retrospective studies and case series show that d-penicillamine (Cuprimine), mycophenolate mofetil (Cellcept), and cyclophosphamide (Cytoxan) may be effective in some patients"[489]; other allopathic treatments have been reviewed in articles freely available on-line.[490]
  - Prednisone or other corticosteroid is used for myositis, MCTD, and arthritis; known to exacerbate renal disease when administered in high doses, i.e., greater than 15 mg/d.
  - Penicillamine started at 250 mg/d and gradually increased to 0.5-1.0 g/d can reduce dermal and systemic involvement
  - Tetracycline: one gram per day for bacterial overgrowth[491]
  - ACE inhibitors are the drugs of choice for scleroderma renal disease and hypertension
  - Calcium channel blockers and angiotensin-II receptor blockers for Raynaud phenomenon
  - Endothelin-1 receptor blockers and phosphodiesterase-5 inhibitors for pulmonary arterial hypertension
- **FOOD & NUTRITION: 5-part "supplemented Paleo-Mediterranean diet" (SPMD)** The 5-part "supplemented Paleo-Mediterranean diet" (SPMD—reviewed in Chapter 4) consists of ❶ foundational plant-based low-carbohydrate diet of fruits, vegetables, nuts, seeds, berries and lean sources of protein, ❷ multivitamin and multimineral supplementation, ❸ physiologic doses of vitamin D3 (range 2,000-10,000 IU/d), ❹ combination fatty acid therapy (CFAT) with n3-ALA, n6-GLA, n3-EPA, n3-DHA, and phytochemical-rich olive oil which contains n9-oleate, and ❺ probiotics.
  - Supplemented Paleo-Mediterranean diet: The health-promoting diet of choice for the majority of people is a diet based on abundant consumption of fruits, vegetables, seeds, nuts, omega-3 and monounsaturated fatty acids, and lean sources of protein such as lean meats, fatty cold-water fish, soy and whey proteins. Although this diet is the most-nutrient dense diet available, rational supplementation with vitamins, minerals, and health promoting fatty acids (i.e., ALA, GLA, EPA, DHA) makes this the best practical diet that can possibly be conceived and implemented. **For scleroderma patients whose diets have habitually been low in fiber, dietary improvement which increases fiber consumption should be implemented slowly to avoid phytobezoar formation and intestinal obstruction[492]; consumption of water/fluids with meals is reasonable, as is periodic or regular use of osmotic laxative and stool-softening agents such as magnesium and ascorbate.** The specifications of the specific carbohydrate diet detailed by Gottschall[493] are met with adherence to the Paleo diet by Cordain.[494] The combination of both approaches will give patients an excellent combination of informational

[488] Tierney ML. McPhee SJ, Papadakis MA (eds). *Current Medical Diagnosis and Treatment. 35th edition*. Stamford: Appleton and Lange, 1996 page 747
[489] Hinchcliff M, Varga J. Systemic sclerosis/scleroderma: a treatable multisystem disease. Am Fam Physician. 2008 Oct 15;78(8):961-8
[490] Sapadin AN, Fleischmajer R. Treatment of scleroderma. *Arch Dermatol*. 2002 Jan;138(1):99-105. archderm.ama-assn.org/cgi/content/full/138/1/99
[491] Beers MH, Berkow R (eds). *Merck Manual. 17th Edition*. Whitehouse Station; Merck Research Laboratories 1999 Page 433
[492] Gough et al. Dietary advice in systemic sclerosis: the dangers of a high fibre diet. *Ann Rheum Dis*. 1998;57(11):641-2 ard.bmjjournals.com/cgi/content/full/57/11/641
[493] Gotschall E. *Breaking the Vicious Cycle: Intestinal health though diet*. Kirkton Press; Rev edition (August, 1994) scdiet.com
[494] Cordain L: *The Paleo Diet*. John Wiley & Sons Inc., New York 2002 thepaleodiet.com/

understanding and culinary versatility. In accord with both of these dietary programs, the diet must remain free of gluten-containing grains such as wheat, since **some patients with scleroderma have celiac disease**[495,496], and since **wheat, like most grains (except rice), promotes bacterial overgrowth of the intestine due to its high quantity of indigestible oligosaccharides.**[497] Patients with facial involvement and resulting restricted oral aperture will need to use smaller bites of food; consider using a food processor, smoothies—same applies for patients with esophageal dysmotility or restriction.

- o <u>Overt malnutrition, micronutrient deficiencies, increased oxidative stress are common in SSc</u>: SSc patients often show overt malnutrition, deficiencies of folate, cobalamin, lipoate, iron, copper, selenium, ascorbic acid, tocopherols, carnitine, and beta-carotene, and enhanced oxidative stress.[498] Very importantly, deficiency of antioxidants in general and selenium in particular is expected to result in enhanced viral replication and mutagenicity, an important realization considering the important role that viral infections appear to play in disease pathogenesis. From a practical clinical standpoint, iron status should be tested with ferritin while other nutritional deficiencies are—generally—treated empirically as discussed in chapters 1 and 4; individual testing of each nutrient is impractical, unnecessarily expensive, and an inappropriate use of time/effort/focus/money. Testing for vitamin B-12 status is notoriously inaccurate, and empiric treatment with 2,000 mcg/d PO is generally warranted for patients with suspected deficiency; however, given the high prevalence of malabsorption in patients with scleroderma/SSc, consideration should be given to laboratory assessments and parenteral administration.

- o <u>Daily use of a broad-spectrum high-potency multivitamin and multimineral supplement</u>: **Vitamin and mineral supplementation is important for patients with scleroderma.** Vitamin supplementation (particularly with pyridoxine and riboflavin) appears warranted in patients with **systemic sclerosis** based on a small (n=5) study that documented the normalization of aberrant tryptophan metabolism in most patients following the administration of pyridoxine with riboflavin; the authors concluded that this was evidence of combined vitamin deficiency in patients with scleroderma.[499] This combined deficiency is not surprising given the high incidence of bacterial overgrowth and malabsorption in scleroderma patients. Deficiencies of ascorbate and selenium have also been documented in patients with scleroderma.[500] Reduced folate and cobalamin and elevated homocysteine have also been noted in patients with scleroderma.[501]

- o <u>Avoidance of allergenic foods</u>: Any patient may be allergic to any food, even if the food is generally considered a health-promoting food. Generally speaking, the most notorious allergens are wheat, citrus (especially juice due to the industrial use of fungal hemicellulases), cow's milk, eggs, peanuts, chocolate, and yeast-containing foods; according to a study in patients with migraine, some patients will have to avoid as many as 10 specific foods in order to become symptom-free.[502] **Celiac disease is not uncommon in patients with scleroderma, and their scleroderma diagnosis may precede the recognition of celiac disease by many years.**[503,504] Clinicians must explain to their patients that celiac disease and wheat allergy

[495] "Coeliac disease may account for malabsorption in scleroderma patients even when test suggest bacterial overgrowth." Marguerie et al. Malabsorption caused by coeliac disease in patients who have scleroderma. *Br J Rheumatol.* 1995 Sep;34(9):858-61

[496] Gomez-Puerta et al. Coeliac disease associated with systemic sclerosis. *Ann Rheum Dis.* 2004 Jan;63(1):104-5 ard.bmjjournals.com/cgi/content/full/63/1/104

[497] "Short-chain fructooligosaccharides occur in a number of edible plants, such as chicory, onions, asparagus, wheat... Short-chain fructooligosaccharides, to a large extent, escape digestion in the human upper intestine and reach the colon where they are totally fermented mostly to lactate, short chain fatty acids (acetate, propionate and butyrate), and gas, like dietary fibres." Bornet et al. Nutritional aspects of short-chain fructooligosaccharides: natural occurrence, chemistry, physiology and health implications. *Dig Liver Dis.* 2002 Sep;34 Suppl 2:S111-20

[498] "Half of the patients had a subnormal arm muscle circumference, and two patients also had a subnormal triceps skinfold thickness, indicating severe malnutrition. The concentration of ascorbic acid, alpha-tocopherol, carotene, selenium, and also the proportion of linoleic acid (18:2) in serum phosphatidylcholine was lower in patients than in control subjects." Lundberg et al. Dietary intake and nutritional status in patients with systemic sclerosis. *Ann Rheum Dis.* 1992 Oct;51(10):1143-8 "Selenium levels were lower in patients than in controls (p=0.012). Within the patient cohort, copper correlated inversely with the total skin score (r=-0.52, p=0.03). Our findings provide further evidence that lipid peroxidation is increased and antioxidant capacity is reduced in SSc." Tikly et al. Lipid peroxidation and trace elements in systemic sclerosis. *Clin Rheumatol.* 2006 May;25(3):320-4. "In Raynaud's phenomenon (RP) and Systemic Sclerosis (SSc), a reduced concentration of ascorbic acid, alpha-tocopherol and beta-carotene as well as low values of Selenium have been reported." Simonini et al. Emerging potentials for an antioxidant therapy as a new approach to the treatment of systemic sclerosis. *Toxicology.* 2000 Nov 30;155(1-3):1-15. Famularo et al. Carnitine deficiency in scleroderma—letter. *Immunology Today* 1999 May; 246

[499] "But the simultaneous administration of pyridoxine and nicotinamide to three of these patients normalized the excretory picture after tryptophan loading." De Antoni et al. Tryptophan metabolism "via" nicotinic acid in patients with scleroderma. *Acta Vitaminol Enzymol.* 1976;30(4-6):134-9

[500] "Plasma ascorbic acid was reduced in all 3 groups of patients: median level 10.6 mg/l in controls, 4.8 mg/l in PRP (p < 0.01), 2.5 mg/l in lSSc (p < 0.01) and 6.8 mg/l in dSSc (p < 0.05). A reduction in serum selenium was especially found in dSSc (median 75 micrograms/l compared to 100 micrograms/l in controls, p < 0.05)." Herrick et al. Micronutrient antioxidant status in patients with primary Raynaud's phenomenon and systemic sclerosis. *J Rheumatol.* 1994 Aug;21(8):1477-83

[501] "Patients with SSc had higher Hcy and vWF concentrations than those with RP or controls. Folic acid and vitamin B12 were lower in SSc than in RP or controls." Marasini et al. Homocysteine concentration in primary and systemic sclerosis associated Raynaud's phenomenon. *J Rheumatol.* 2000 Nov;27(11):2621-3

[502] Grant EC. Food allergies and migraine. *Lancet.* 1979 May 5;1(8123):966-9

[503] Gomez-Puerta et al. Coeliac disease associated with systemic sclerosis. *Ann Rheum Dis.* 2004 Jan;63(1):104-5 ard.bmjjournals.com/cgi/content/full/63/1/104

[504] "Coeliac disease may account for malabsorption in scleroderma patients even when test suggest bacterial overgrowth." Marguerie et al. Malabsorption caused by coeliac disease in patients who have scleroderma. *Br J Rheumatol.* 1995 Sep;34(9):858-61

are two different clinical entities and that exclusion of one does not exclude the other, and in neither case does mutual exclusion obviate the **promotion of intestinal bacterial overgrowth (i.e., proinflammatory dysbiosis) by indigestible wheat oligosaccharides**. Rapid implementation of high fiber diets may precipitate bowel obstruction.[505]

o Vitamin D3 supplementation with physiologic doses and/or tailored to serum 25(OH)D and serum calcium levels : Vitamin D deficiency is common in the general population and is even more common in patients with chronic illness and chronic musculoskeletal pain.[506] Correction of vitamin D deficiency provides a clinically significant anti-inflammatory and immunomodulatory benefit.[507] **Oral administration of active vitamin D3 (1,25-dihydroxyvitamin D) has led to clinical improvement in patients with scleroderma**.[508] Reasonable daily doses for children and adults are 2,000 and 4,000 IU, respectively, as defined by Vasquez, et al.[509] Deficiency and response to treatment are monitored with serum 25(OH)vitamin D while safety is monitored with serum calcium; inflammatory granulomatous diseases and certain drugs such as hydrochlorothiazide greatly increase the propensity for hypercalcemia and warrant increment dosing and frequent monitoring of serum calcium.

o Broad-spectrum fatty acid therapy with ALA, EPA, DHA, GLA and oleic acid: "Sophisticated manipulation of EFA metabolism" may prove clinically beneficial for **scleroderma** patients according to a review by the late David Horrobin[510]; however, a six-month clinical trial of fatty acid supplementation showed no benefit[511], thus proving the ineffectiveness of one-dimensional intervention and of fatty acid supplementation in a condition known to have a high prevalence of untreated malabsorption. Nonetheless, as part of a *comprehensive program*, fatty acid supplementation should be delivered in the form of combination therapy with ALA, GLA, DHA, and EPA. Fish oil provides EPA and DHA which have well-proven anti-inflammatory benefits in rheumatoid arthritis[512,513,514] and lupus.[515,516] ALA, EPA, DHA, and GLA need to be provided in the form of supplements; when using high doses of therapeutic oils, liquid supplements that can be mixed in juice or a smoothie are generally more convenient and palatable than capsules. Therapeutic amounts of oleic acid can be obtained from generous use of olive oil, preferably on fresh vegetables. Supplementation with polyunsaturated fatty acids warrants increased intake of antioxidants from diet, fruit and vegetable juices, and properly formulated supplements; since patients with systemic inflammation are generally in a pro-oxidative state, consideration must be given to the timing and starting dose of fatty acid supplementation and the need for antioxidant protection.

o Probiotics for the treatment of systemic sclerosis-associated gastrointestinal bloating/ distention (*Clin Exp Rheumatol.* 2011 Mar[517]): "We compared the GIT 2.0 scores at baseline and after 2 months of use of Align (Bifidobacterium infantis; 10^9 CFU per capsule) or Culturelle (Lactobacillus GG; 10^9 CFU per capsule) using paired t-test and calculated effect size (ES). Significant improvement in total GIT 2.0 score (ES = 0.82), reflux (ES = 0.33), bloating/distention (ES = 1.76), and emotional scales (ES = 0.18) were reported after two months of daily probiotic use. This pilot study suggests probiotics significantly improve the reflux, distention/ bloating, and total GIT scales in SSc patients. As hypothesized, the largest effect was seen in distention/bloating scale. Probiotics may be useful for treatment of SSc-associated distention/ bloating."

[505] Gough et al. Dietary advice in systemic sclerosis: the dangers of a high fibre diet. *Ann Rheum Dis.* 1998 Nov;57(11):641-2 ard.bmjjournals.com/cgi/content/full/57/11/641

[506] Plotnikoff GA, Quigley JM. Prevalence of severe hypovitaminosis D in patients with persistent, nonspecific musculoskeletal pain. *Mayo Clin Proc.* 2003 Dec;78(12):1463-70

[507] Timms et al. Circulating MMP9, vitamin D and variation in the TIMP-1 response with VDR genotype: mechanisms for inflammatory damage in chronic disorders? *QJM.* 2002 Dec;95(12):787-96 qjmed.oxfordjournals.org/cgi/content/full/95/12/787

[508] "After the treatment period (6 months to 3 years), a significant improvement, as compared with baseline values, was observed. No serious side-effects were observed." Humbert et al. Treatment of scleroderma with oral 1,25-dihydroxyvitamin D3: evaluation of skin involvement using non-invasive techniques. *Acta Derm Venereol.* 1993 Dec;73(6):449-51

[509] Vasquez et al. Clinical importance of vitamin D: a paradigm shift with implications for all healthcare providers. *Altern Ther Health Med.* 2004 Sep-Oct;10(5):28-36

[510] "Controlled clinical trials of supplementation with gamma-linolenic acid (GLA) as evening primrose oil (Efamol) in both primary Sjogren's syndrome and systemic sclerosis have given positive results." Horrobin DF. Essential fatty acid and prostaglandin metabolism in Sjogren's syndrome, systemic sclerosis and rheumatoid arthritis. *Scand J Rheumatol Suppl* 1986;61:242-5

[511] "Dietary essential fatty acids have no role in the treatment of vascular symptoms in established systemic sclerosis." Stainforth et al. Clinical aspects of the use of gamma linolenic acid in systemic sclerosis. *Acta Derm Venereol* 1996 Mar;76(2):144-6

[512] Adam et al. Anti-inflammatory effects of a low arachidonic acid diet and fish oil in patients with rheumatoid arthritis. *Rheumatol Int.* 2003 Jan;23(1):27-36

[513] Lau et al. Effects of fish oil supplementation on non-steroidal anti-inflammatory drug requirement in patients with mild rheumatoid arthritis. *Br J Rheumatol.* 1993 Nov:982-9

[514] Kremer et al. Fish-oil fatty acid supplementation in active rheumatoid arthritis. A double-blinded, controlled, crossover study. *Ann Intern Med.* 1987 Apr;106(4):497-503

[515] Walton et al. Dietary fish oil and the severity of symptoms in patients with systemic lupus erythematosus. *Ann Rheum Dis.* 1991 Jul;50(7):463-6

[516] Duffy et al. The clinical effect of dietary supplementation with omega-3 fish oils and/or copper in systemic lupus erythematosus. *J Rheumatol.* 2004 Aug;31(8):1551-6

[517] Frech et al. Probiotics for the treatment of systemic sclerosis-associated gastrointestinal bloating/ distention. *Clin Exp Rheumatol.* 2011 Mar-Apr;29(2 Suppl 65):S22-5

- **INFECTIONS & DYSBIOSIS: ❶ antimicrobial treatments, ❷ immunorestoration, ❸ immunotolerance via Treg induction** Essentially all autoimmune/rheumatic disorders are associated with microbial colonization and intolerance to same; the presence of persistent microbial colonization is *prima facie* evidence of immunosuppression. The eight areas of dysbiosis (multifocal) are: ❶ sinorespiratory, ❷ orodental, ❸ gastrointestinal, ❹ urogenital/genitourinary, ❺ parenchymal/tissue, ❻ microbial, ❼ dermal/cutaneous, and ❽ environmental. What emerges from the research on SSc and microbes is a complex model of microbial interplay where in some microbes infect vascular cells (e.g., parvovirus B19, EBV, CMV) where as other microbes promote the necessary cytokine response to promote fibrosis (e.g., EBV, *H pylori*, parvovirus B19); readers will find in the following table sufficient evidence to justify testing for viral and bacterial infections and treating, either specifically or empirically. See antiviral protocol in Chapter 4.2, second section, which is reprinted from my book *Antiviral Strategies and Immune Nutrition* (2014). Microbial contributions to scleroderma/SSC include:
  - **Gastrointestinal dysbiosis and SIBO** (small intestinal bacterial overgrowth): "The prevalence of SIBO was 43.1% in our SSc patients. ... Our study underscores that SIBO often occurs in SSc patients."[518] A growing body of literature implicates infectious agents in the etiology of **scleroderma**.[519] Regarding dermal dysbiosis, several articles by Cantwell et al[520,521] suggest epidermal and/or intradermal dysbiosis with pleomorphic bacteria, specifically acid-fast cell-wall-deficient mycobacteria. Regarding gastrointestinal dysbiosis, at the very least, we must acknowledge that 1) **bacterial overgrowth of the small bowel is common (33%) in patients with scleroderma**[522] due to impaired gastrointestinal motility, 2) **scleroderma patients show increased levels of deconjugating bacteria**[523], which inactivate bile acids and promote enterohepatic recirculation of endogenous and exogenous toxins, 3) **these patients have a high incidence of *Helicobacter pylori* infection (66% of patients with scleroderma, 78% of patients with scleroderma and Sicca syndrome**[524]), and 4) approximately **44% of scleroderma patients have esophageal overgrowth of *Candida albicans*.**[525] For these and other reasons (detailed in Chapter 4), **patients with scleroderma are presumed to have gastrointestinal dysbiosis until proven otherwise by the combination of 1) three-sample comprehensive parasitology examinations performed by a specialty laboratory and 2) clinical response to at least two 2-4 week courses of broad-spectrum antimicrobial treatment.** Yeast, bacteria, and parasites are treated as indicated based on identification and sensitivity results from comprehensive parasitology assessments. Breath hydrogen/methane testing is inferior to stool testing because it does not allow for identification and sensitivity testing of microbes. Other dysbiotic loci should be investigated as discussed in Chapter 4 in the section on multifocal dysbiosis. Attentive readers may have already surmised that treatment of gastrointestinal dysbiosis in patients with long-standing scleroderma is likely to be particularly difficult due to the neuropathic and myopathic **intestinal dysmotility**[526] **that will serve to perpetuate bacterial overgrowth and dysbiosis, thus necessitating vigilant and long-term treatment**; understanding and due persistence on the part of physician and patient are necessary to see this treatment through to completion—a combination of

---

[518] Marie et al. Small intestinal bacterial overgrowth in systemic sclerosis. *Rheumatology* (Oxford). 2009 Oct;48(10):1314-9

[519] "...increasing evidence has accumulated to implicate infectious agents in the etiology of systemic sclerosis (SSc)... ...increased antibody titers, a preponderance of specific strains in patients with SSc, and evidence of molecular mimicry inducing autoimmune responses suggest mechanisms by which infectious agents may contribute to the development and progression of SSc." Hamamdzic et al. The role of infectious agents in the pathogenesis of systemic sclerosis. *Curr Opin Rheumatol*. 2002 Nov;14(6):694-8

[520] Disabling pansclerotic morphea (DPM): "The organism could be identified as Staphylococcus epidermidis, but it also had stages of growth with morphologic forms more characteristic of a Corynebacterium-like or actinomycetelike microbe." Cantwell et al. Pleomorphic, variably acid-fast bacteria in an adult patient with disabling pansclerotic morphea. *Arch Dermatol*. 1984 May;120(5):656-61

[521] "Variably acid-fast coccoid forms, suggestive of cell wall deficient forms of mycobacteria, were observed in the dermis in microscopic sections of skin from six patients with generalized scleroderma, 10 patients with localized scleroderma (morphea), and four patients with lichen sclerosus et atrophicus (LSA)." Cantwell AR Jr. Histologic observations of pleomorphic, variably acid-fast bacteria in scleroderma, morphea, and lichen sclerosus et atrophicus. *Int J Dermatol*. 1984 Jan-Feb;23(1):45-52

[522] "Eight patients (33%) had significant bacterial counts: > 10(5) colony forming units per ml (cfu/ml) of jejunal fluid." Kaye et al. Small bowel bacterial overgrowth in systemic sclerosis: detection using direct and indirect methods and treatment outcome. *Br J Rheumatol*. 1995 Mar;34(3):265-9

[523] "Our results demonstrated that some of the bacterial species that overgrow in the upper small intestine of patients with progressive systemic sclerosis can deconjugate bile acids, and that a shift to neutral pH in gastric juice, may promote the bacterial overgrowth related to their impaired peristaltic activity." Shindo et al. Deconjugation ability of bacteria isolated from the jejunal fluid of patients with progressive systemic sclerosis and its gastric pH. *Hepatogastroenterology*. 1998 Sep-Oct;45(23):1643-50

[524] "Urease test demonstrated the presence of HP in 23 patients out of 35 (66%); 12 of them were negative to colonization. A Sicca syndrome, with abnormal Schirmers test and dry mouth was detected in 66% of the patients. 78% of the patients with Sicca syndrome had a concomitant HP infection..." Farina et al. High incidence of Helicobacter pylori infection in patients with systemic sclerosis: association with Sicca Syndrome. *Int J Immunopathol Pharmacol*. 2001 May;14(2):81-85

[525] "Esophageal mucosal brushings from 51 consecutive patients with progressive systemic sclerosis (PSS) (group I), 18 PSS patients continuously treated with high-dose ranitidine or omeprazole (group II), 34 controls referred to the outpatient clinic for endoscopy (group III), and 10 patients receiving long-term potent antireflux therapy for idiopathic gastroesophageal reflux (group IV) were cultured for Candida albicans. There were 44%, 89%, 9%, and 0% Candida albicans culture-positive patients in groups I through IV, respectively." Hendel et al. Esophageal candidosis in progressive systemic sclerosis: occurrence, significance, and treatment with fluconazole. *Scand J Gastroenterol*. 1988 Dec;23(10):1182-6

[526] "We found ultrastructural signs of axonal degeneration and cytoskeletal abnormalities in the bundles of unmyelinated fibers. There was also focal degeneration of smooth muscle cells, often in association with the presence of partially degranulated mast cells." Malandrini et al. Autonomic nervous system and smooth muscle cell involvement in systemic sclerosis: ultrastructural study of 3 cases. *J Rheumatol*. 2000 May;27(5):1203-6

pharmaceutical/botanical antimicrobials and promotility agents, including the universally safe and effective osmotic laxative magnesium, is reasonable. By this time, readers should appreciate the clinical implications of SIBO (as discussed in Chapter 4), including but not limited to malabsorption due to damage to the intestinal mucosa and mucosal enzymes, increased intestinal permeability, increased bacterial translocation, microbial mitochondriopathy, systemic inflammation, activation of DAMP, PAMP, and TLR receptors—all of these pro-inflammatory effects should be expected to promote the oxidative stress, autoimmunity, and fibrosis that characterize SSc.

- Octreotide (prescription drug): Descamps et al[527] describe the case of a 53-year-old black woman with progressive and severe systemic scleroderma, with diffuse skin sclerosis, myositis with intestinal pseudo-obstruction and bacterial overgrowth who experienced a "spectacular" normalization of clinical status and skin induration following several months of octreotide (75 mug/d). This drug is a somatostatin analog used in the treatment of acromegaly[528] and it also promotes intestinal motility and thus reduces dysbiotic intestinal bacterial overgrowth in patients with scleroderma.[529] Efficacy of octreotide in improving clinical manifestations of scleroderma is probably mediated *at least in part* by reducing the pro-inflammatory effects of dysbiotic intestinal bacterial overgrowth, which can be addressed by other means as well.

- Ciprofloxacin: Over and Bucknall[530] published a case report of a progressive scleroderma patient who experienced marked clinical improvement and biopsy-proven regression of skin changes following administration of ciprofloxacin 500 mg bid which was eventually reduced to 250 mg/d. This case report strongly supports the theory that intestinal dysbiosis is a major contributor to scleroderma. As with all antibacterial treatments, use empiric antifungal treatment with Nystatin 500,000 units bid and/or emulsified oregano 150 mg tid-qid.[531,532]

- *Artemisia annua*: Artemisinin has been safely used for centuries in Asia for the treatment of malaria, and it also has effectiveness against anaerobic bacteria due to the pro-oxidative sesquiterpene endoperoxide.[533,534] I commonly use artemisinin at 200 mg per day in divided doses for adults with dysbiosis. Evidence of past/current *H. pylori* infection is common (~40-60%) in patients with scleroderma[535], and some doctors—such as Jonathan V Wright MD—have reported anecdotally that *Artemisia annua* helps eradicate *H. pylori*. Conversely, we might reasonably look for a non-pro-oxidative treatment alternative to Artemisia, such as mastic.

- Erythromycin: 250-500 mg TID-QID; this drug is a widely used antibiotic that also has intestinal promotility benefits (thus making it an ideal treatment for intestinal bacterial overgrowth associated with or caused by intestinal dysmotility/hypomotility such as seen in scleroderma[536,537]). Do not combine erythromycin with the promotility drug cisapride due to risk for serious cardiac arrhythmia.

- Nystatin: Nystatin 500,000 units bid with food; duration of treatment begins with a minimum duration of 2-4 weeks and may continue as long as the patient is deriving benefit.

  o **Cytomegalovirus—Induction of vasculopathy via direction infection and induction of pro-inflammatory cytokines, molecular mimicry**: CMV causes experimental vasculopathy resembling SSc; interestingly and consistent with my (DrV) model of dysbiosis which appreciates immunosuppression as (pre)requisite, experimental CMV-induced vasculopathy requires immunosuppression: "A viral agent known for its

---

[527] "After 8 months of treatment, normal weight was obtained and skin induration was spectacularly reduced and pigmentation returned to a normal state." Descamps et al. Global improvement of systemic scleroderma under long-term administration of octreotide. *Eur J Dermatol* 1999 Sep;9(6):446-8

[528] us.sandostatin.com/info/about/home.jsp Accessed December 16, 2005

[529] "Octreotide stimulates intestinal motility in normal subjects and in patients with scleroderma. In such patients, the short-term administration of octreotide reduces bacterial overgrowth and improves abdominal symptoms." Soudah et al. Effect of octreotide on intestinal motility and bacterial overgrowth in scleroderma. *N Engl J Med* 1991 Nov:1461-7

[530] Over et al. Regression of skin changes in a patient with systemic sclerosis following treatment for bacterial overgrowth with ciprofloxacin. *Br J Rheumatol.* 1998 Jun;37(6):696

[531] Stiles JC, Sparks W, Ronzio RA. The inhibition of Candida albicans by oregano. *J Applied Nutr* 1995;47:96–102

[532] Force M, Sparks WS, Ronzio RA. Inhibition of enteric parasites by emulsified oil of oregano in vivo. *Phytother Res.* 2000 May;14(3):213-4

[533] Dien et al. Effect of food intake on pharmacokinetics of oral artemisinin in healthy Vietnamese subjects. *Antimicrob Agents Chemother.* 1997 May;41(5):1069-72

[534] Giao et al. Artemisinin for treatment of uncomplicated falciparum malaria: is there a place for monotherapy? *Am J Trop Med Hyg.* 2001 Dec;65(6):690-5

[535] "Patients with SSc have H. pylori infection at a higher prevalence than the general population." Yazawa et al. High seroprevalence of Helicobacter pylori infection in patients with systemic sclerosis: association with esophageal involvement. *J Rheumatol.* 1998 Apr;25(4):650-3

[536] "Prokinetic agents effective in pseudoobstruction include metoclopramide, domperidone, cisapride, octreotide, and erythromycin. ... The combination of octreotide and erythromycin may be particularly effective in systemic sclerosis." Sjogren RW. Gastrointestinal features of scleroderma. *Curr Opin Rheumatol.* 1996 Nov;8(6):569-75

[537] "Erythromycin accelerates gastric and gallbladder emptying in scleroderma patients and might be helpful in the treatment of gastrointestinal motor abnormalities in these patients." Fiorucci et al. Effect of erythromycin administration on upper gastrointestinal motility in scleroderma patients. *Scand J Gastroenterol.* 1994 Sep;29(9):807-13

ability to damage vessel walls is cytomegalovirus (CMV). … Infected immunocompetent animals exhibited only perivascular inflammation, suggesting that infection and immunosuppression were co-requisites of [vasculopathy] neointima formation. … Induction of TGF-β1, the canonical pro-fibrotic cytokine, by human CMV (HCMV) was reported by other authors (16), implicating that a primary endothelial cell infection by HCMV may induce myofibroblast activation in the vessel wall under the effect of this cytokine."[538] "…higher prevalence of IgA antihuman cytomegalovirus antibodies in patients with SSc. … CMV infection may play a part in SSc pathogenesis due to its ability to infect both endothelial and monocyte/macrophage cells and through the upregulation of fibrogenic cytokines and induction of immune dysregulation. … association between increased serum levels of CMV-specific antibodies and the prevalence of SSc-related autoantibodies in patients with SSc. … Molecular mimicry is a mechanism that may explain the pathogenicity of antibodies against viral proteins in SSc. Infection with HCMV may generate a host-antiviral response that is self-reactive toward autoantigens and endothelial cells."[539] Vulnerably to CMV-induced SSc may include genetic factors and fetomaternal/transfusional microchimerism, noted to be more common in women with SSc.

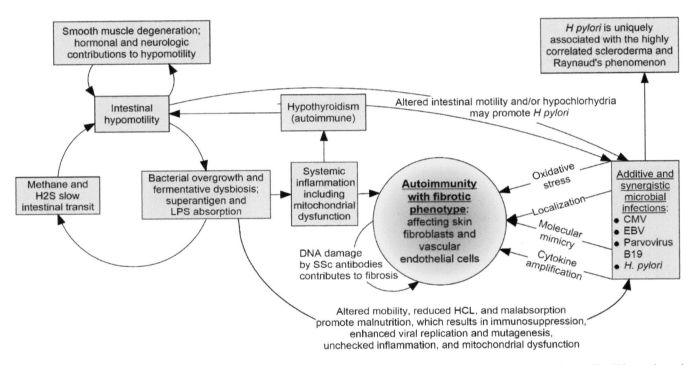

Polymicrobial and inflammatory aspects of scleroderma: diagram by Vasquez; quotes from Radić et al and Svegliati et al: "Systemic sclerosis is an autoimmune disease characterized by vascular obliteration, excessive extracellular matrix deposition and fibrosis of the connective tissues of the skin, lungs, gastrointestinal tract, heart, and kidneys. The pathogenesis of systemic sclerosis is extremely complex; at present, no single unifying hypothesis explains all aspects. Over the last 20 years increasing evidence has accumulated to implicate infectious agents in the etiology of systemic sclerosis. Increased antibody titers, a preponderance of specific strains in patients with systemic sclerosis, and evidence of molecular mimicry inducing autoimmune responses suggest mechanisms by which infectious agents may contribute to the development and progression of systemic sclerosis."[540] "Trichostatin A, an HDAC inhibitor, prevented WIF-1 loss, β-catenin induction, and collagen accumulation in an experimental fibrosis model. Our findings suggest that oxidative DNA damage induced by SSc autoreactive antibodies enables Wnt activation that contributes to fibrosis."[541]

[538] Moroncini et al. Role of viral infections in the etiopathogenesis of systemic sclerosis. *Clin Exp Rheumatol.* 2013 Mar-Apr;31(2 Suppl 76):3-7
[539] Radić et al. Infectious disease as aetiological factor in the pathogenesis of systemic sclerosis. *Neth J Med.* 2010 Nov;68(11):348-53
[540] Radić M, Martinović Kaliterna D, Radić J. Infectious disease as aetiological factor in the pathogenesis of systemic sclerosis. *Neth J Med.* 2010 Nov;68(11):348-53
[541] Svegliati et al. Oxidative DNA damage induces ATM-mediated transcriptional suppression of Wnt inhibitor WIF-1 in systemic sclerosis and fibrosis. *Sci Signal* 2014 Sept;ra84

o **Epstein-Barr virus**—Localized infection in skin fibroblasts and endothelial cells, upregulation of cytokine production: "Here we show that EBV establishes infection in the majority of fibroblasts and endothelial cells in the skin of SSc patients, characterized by the expression of the EBV noncoding small RNAs (EBERs) and the increased expression of immediate-early lytic and latency mRNAs and proteins. We report that EBV is able to persistently infect human SSc fibroblasts in vitro, inducing an aberrant innate immune response in infected cells. EBV-Toll-like receptor (TLR) aberrant activation induces the expression of selected IFN-regulatory factors (IRFs), IFN-stimulated genes (ISGs), transforming growth factor-β1 (TGFβ1), and several markers of fibroblast activation, such as smooth muscle actin and Endothelin-1, and all of these genes play a key role in determining the profibrotic phenotype in SSc fibroblasts. These findings imply that EBV infection occurring in mesenchymal, endothelial, and immune cells of SSc patients may underlie the main pathological features of SSc including autoimmunity, vasculopathy, and fibrosis, and provide a unified disease mechanism represented by EBV reactivation."[542]

o **Parvovirus B19**—Induction of fibrosis: "The presence of parvovirus B19 DNA was demonstrated in a significant percentage of bone marrow biopsies from SSc patients and was never detected in the control group. ... These patients showed the most severe active endothelial injury and perivascular inflammation. ...incubation with parvovirus B19-containing serum induced an invasive phenotype in normal human synovial fibroblasts."[543] Note that bone marrow-derived fibrocytes are involved in the pathogenesis of SSC; therefore, the strong positive correlation between B19 positivity and SSc and the negative correlation seen with B19 negativity and health suggests a likelihood of direct cause and effect.

o *Helicobacter pylori,* **especially the virulent CagA strain**—Induction of systemic inflammation and cytokine response:

"...despite the absence of a difference in *H. pylori* infection rates between SSc patients and control subjects, 90% of patients with SSc were infected with the virulent CagA strain compared with only 37% of the infected control subjects..." "Our data suggest that *H. pylori* infection correlates with severity of skin, gastrointestinal, and joint/tendon involvement in SSc patients. *H. pylori*-positive SSc patients showed higher severity score compared to *H. pylori*-negative. Therefore, *H. pylori* infection may play a role in the pathogenesis of SSc and also can provide some prognostic information."[544] "There are two general lines of evidence implicating bacterial infections in the pathogenesis of SSc. One is anecdotal evidence that treatment with antibiotics relieves SSc symptoms in some patients. The other is that graft-versus-host disease, which is recognized as having many similarities to SSc, cannot be induced in germ-free animals

---

CMV meets pathogenic criteria for SSc
- Direct infection of endothelial cells and immune cells
- Induction of pro-fibrotic cytokines
- Higher levels of CMV antibodies in SSc patients
- Exact molecular mimicry between HCMV late protein UL94 and human endothelial cell surface integrin–NAG-2 protein complex
- Cross-reacting CMV-endothelial antibodies kill endothelial cells and cause fibrosis
- Anti-UL94 antibodies bind to dermal fibroblasts and convert them to a scleroderma phenotype

Moroncini et al. *Clin Exp Rheumatol.* 2013 Mar

EBV meets pathogenic criteria for SSc
- Majority of SSc patients show active infection in vascular and dermal cells
- Virus-induced gene induction promotes the profibrotic scleroderma phenotype

Farina et al. *J Invest Dermatol.* 2014 Apr

PvB19 meets pathogenic criteria for SSc
- Direct infection of endothelial cells, immune cells, and dermal epithelial cells
- Induction of pro-fibrotic cytokines
- Bone marrow infection is seen in many SSc patients, correlates directly with disease severity, and is never noted in health patients; bone marrow fibrocytes contribute to SSc.
- PvB19 infection triggers formation of multiple autoantibodies: nuclear antigens (ANA), rheumatoid factor (RF), neutrophils cytoplasmic antigens, mitochondrial antigens (AMA), smooth muscle, gastric parietal antigens and phospholipids.

Moroncini et al. *Clin Exp Rheumatol.* 2013 Mar

---

[542] Farina et al. Epstein-Barr virus infection induces aberrant TLR activation pathway and fibroblast-myofibroblast conversion in scleroderma. *J Invest Dermatol.* 2014 Apr:954-64
[543] Radić et al. Infectious disease as aetiological factor in the pathogenesis of systemic sclerosis. *Neth J Med.* 2010 Nov;68(11):348-53
[544] Radić et al. Is Helicobacter pylori infection a risk factor for disease severity in systemic sclerosis? *Rheumatol Int.* 2013 Nov;33(11):2943-8

and is significantly reduced in children pre-treated with antibiotics to eradicate their normal bacterial flora."[545]

- o *Toxoplasma gondii* **and hepatitis B virus**: "Patients with SSc had elevated IgM and IgG against *Toxoplasma gondii* and against CMV. Higher titers were also detected against the hepatitis B virus core protein (recombinant HBc antigen) using MONOLISA anti-HBc Plus commercial kit (Bio-Rad). A significantly higher rate of IgM antibodies against the capsid antigen of the EBV was detected in SSc patients compared with healthy controls, as well."[546]

- o <u>**Clinical implications of polymicrobial dysbiosis in scleroderma**</u>: At the risk of redundancy and stating what should be obvious by now to readers who have studied the material in this book—especially chapter 4—here I will outline the implications of the information presented up to this point in this section on scleroderma/SSc. Quite obviously, the typical patient with scleroderma has multiple active microbial infections/colonizations and is therefore—by definition—demonstrating immunosuppression. Thus, two of the three components of my three-part dysbiosis model are established in SSC, and the third component—nutritional immunomodulation—is discussed in the following section. Given the solid data demonstrating polyviral activity for what I will describe as "popular viruses"—EBV, CMV, PvB19—we should reasonably assume that increased transcription of other viruses such as HSV (type-1 in 50% of the adult population; type-2 in 20% of the adult population) and the HERVs—human indigenous retroviruses—is also occurring. Serologic, newer generation PCR testing, and specialty tests—such as western blot for HSV infections—should ideally be performed to assess for the presence and severity/level of viral replication. Per previous discussions, clinicians must appreciate the **total microbial load (TML)** and not simply the presence/absence of these infections; bacterial quantifications—especially *H pylori*—must also be made if the initial laboratory evaluation is to be considered partly complete. Thereafter, the antimicrobial mission becomes on of search and destroy, using a combination of direct antiviral/antimicrobial agents as well as immunorestoration. My opinion and perspective is that antiviral pharmaceutic drugs—which by definition target single pathways in single viruses and are therefore easily bypassed by viral mutations and which have limited efficacy on the **total viral load (TVL)**, respectively—are of limited clinical value but may still be used if found efficacious in individual patients; any failure of pharmacologic antiviral intervention in autoimmunity does not refute the viral etiology of autoimmunity but is rather to be expected from the failure to effectively address the larger viral load and to restore various aspects of disturbed homeodynamics. Attention should be directed toward a global or generalized antiviral approach to reduce TVL for various categories of viruses *concretely* and TVL *conceptually*, reasonably described here as ❶ <u>common/popular viruses</u>—these are the common viruses most commonly considered by clinicians and patients and for which we have readily available diagnostic tests, namely HIV, HBV, HCV, HSV 1 and 2, CMV, EBV, PvB19; readers should note from the above that SSC patients show viral infections that are not simply *more active* but are *active in different locations* compared to nonSSC persons, ❷ <u>human endogenous retroviruses</u>—viruses permanently embedded in the human genome, for which laboratory assessments are generally not clinically available; clinicians should consider this category to be an occult contributor to the TVL and thus TML and thus **TIL**—total inflammatory/immunogenic load, ❸ <u>bacteriophage load</u>—the **total bacterial load (TBL)** of the body and in particular the biomass in the intestines houses the bacteria-specific viruses known as bacteriophages, and these viruses-specific-for-bacteria contribute significantly to the TML of the gut in particular; thus, consideration to reducing/improving TBL in the gut would be expected to reduce the TVL as well, benignly promoting a reduction in the TIL, ❹ <u>other means of reducing TVL—reducing inflammation and bacterial load</u>: Bacterial debris such as LPS/endotoxin, other viral infections (via "transactivation"), and any other inflammatory stimuli that activate NFkB would be expected to promote viral replication via the NFkB pathway and other pathways that are "hijacked" or reappropriated[547] by viruses to promote their replication. In this manner, reducing the TBL lowers the TVL and thus the TIL. Extending the

[545] Radić et al. Infectious disease as aetiological factor in the pathogenesis of systemic sclerosis. *Neth J Med.* 2010 Nov;68(11):348-53

[546] Arnson et al. The role of infections in the immunopathogensis of systemic sclerosis--evidence from serological studies. *Ann N Y Acad Sci.* 2009 Sep;1173:627-32

[547] "As viruses evolve under the highly selective pressures of the immune system, they acquire the capacity to target critical steps in the host cell life, hijacking vital cellular functions to promote viral pathogenesis. Many viruses have evolved mechanisms to target the NF-kB pathway to facilitate their replication, cell survival, and evasion of immune responses." Hiscott et al. Hostile takeovers: viral appropriation of the NF-kappaB pathway. *J Clin Invest.* 2001 Jan;107(2):143-51

understanding and implications: Understanding this helps clinicians and researchers make sense of the confusion seen particularly in the research on CFS [caused by SIBO and GI dysbiosis] which is commonly complicated by evidence of increased viral replication; what I think is occurring here is that bacterial debris/LPS from SIBO is promoting viral replication via pathways including NFkB. Problematically, the LPS from SIBO also contributes to other problems such as impairment of cytochrome p450 which leads to xenobiotic accumulation and the resulting multiple chemical sensitivity [MCS], the persistent low-grade inflammatory and oxidative state which impairs the HPA axis and mitochondrial function; SIBO can cause deficiency of tryptophan and thus serotonin and perhaps melatonin via bacterial tryptophanase and deficiency of vitamin B-12 due to increased binding/chelation of B-12 with H2S.

- **NUTRITIONAL IMMUNOMODULATION: Treg induction for modulation of Th-1/2/17 inflammation**
Nutrients and therapeutic approaches that promote Treg or IL-10 induction and/or Th-17, IL-17 suppression include 1) mitochondrial optimization and mTOR suppression, 2) biotin, 3) vitamin E, 4) sodium avoidance, 5) transgenic/GMO food avoidance, 6) probiotics, 7) lipoic acid, 8) vitamin A, 9) inflammation reduction, 10) vitamin D, 11) fatty acid supplementation with GLA and n3, 12) infection and dysbiosis remediation, 13) green tea EGCG. Acronym: MiBESTPLAIDFIG.
  - <u>Vitamin E</u>: Morelli et al[548] describe a 60-year-old woman with **systemic sclerosis** complicated by hypertension, renal failure, and heart failure; although allopathic drug treatments were of no benefit, **the addition of "vitamin E (600 mg daily)" lead to rapid and significant clinical improvement.** Ayres and Mihan[549] wrote that vitamin E was effective in the clinical management of scleroderma, discoid lupus erythematosus[550], porphyria cutanea tarda, several types of vasculitis, and polymyositis.[551] Given that vitamin E is not a single compound but rather a family of closely related tocopherols, most clinicians prefer to use a source of "mixed tocopherols" inclusive of alpha, beta, delta, and—perhaps most importantly—gamma tocopherol.[552] Vitamin E has a wide margin of safety and although daily doses are kept in the range of 400-1200 IU, doses up to 3,200 IU are generally considered non-toxic. Tocopherols are now known to provide an anti-inflammatory immunomodulatory effect by elevating cAMP and thereby reducing TNF-alpha and increasing IL-10 as reviewed in Chapter 4 in the section on Nutritional Immunomodulation.

- **DYSMETABOLISM & DYSFUNCTIONAL MITOCHONDRIA: MitoDys, ERS-UPR, AGE/RAGE, hyperglycemia and ceramide** The major clinical considerations in this section are mitochondrial dysfunction, endoplasmic reticulum stress, unfolded protein response, TLR activation, and the dysmetabolic effects of sustained hyperglycemia and hyperinsulinemia and resultant oxidative stress, inflammation, RAGE activation, and accumulation of AGE, palmitate and ceramide. The review of this information in Chapter 4 covered approximately 30 interventions relevant to dysmetabolism, mitochondrial dysfunction, ERS-UPR, etc; these will not be reviewed here except to mention those most commonly, easily, empirically, synergistically, and effectively used: 1) low-carbohydrate diet with 2) moderate exercise, 3) CoQ-10, 4) acetyl-carnitine with 5) lipoic acid, 6) NAC, 7) resveratrol, and 8) melatonin.
  - <u>Mitochondrial dysfunction in scleroderma—a cause of a fibrotic phenotype</u>: My (DrV) intuitive sense is that mitochondrial dysfunction—likely induced by bacteria, viruses and/or xenobiotic exposure—induces a fibrotic phenotype in scleroderma patients; research data supporting this concept is indirect.

---

[548] "Casually, vitamin E (600 mg daily) was added. After 6 months, clinical manifestations of heart failure were disappeared and the echocardiogram showed a normally-sized left ventricle with normal wall motion." Morelli et al. Systemic sclerosis (scleroderma). A case of recovery of cardiomyopathy after vitamin E treatment. *Minerva Cardioangiol.* 2001 Apr;49(2):127-30
[549] "Among the diseases that were successfully controlled were a number in the autoimmune category, including scleroderma, discoid lupus erythematosus, porphyria cutanea tarda, several types of vasculitis, and polymyositis." Ayres S Jr, Mihan R. Is vitamin E involved in the autoimmune mechanism? *Cutis.* 1978 Mar;21(3):321-5
[550] "Despite conflicting opinions, our personal experience and a number of reviewed clinical reports indicate that vitamin E, properly administered in adequate doses, is a safe and effective treatment for chronic discoid lupus erythematosus, and may be of value in treating other types of the disease." Ayres S Jr, Mihan R. Lupus erythematosus and vitamin E: an effective and nontoxic therapy. *Cutis.* 1979;23(1):49-52, 54
[551] "She then made a dramatic improvement when large doses of vitamin E (d, alpha-tocopheryl acetate) were administered." Killeen RN, Ayres S Jr, Mihan R. Polymyositis: response to vitamin E. *South Med J.* 1976 Oct;69(10):1372-4
[552] Jiang et al. gamma-tocopherol, the major form of vitamin E in the US diet, deserves more attention. *Am J Clin Nutr.* 2001 Dec;74(6):714-22 ajcn.org/cgi/content/full/74/6/714

However, noted is the observation that worsening systemic inflammation (measured by hsCRP) correlates with antimitochondrial antibodies in patients with scleroderma.[553]

- o Liver giant mitochondria: an almost constant lesion in systemic scleroderma (*Virchows Arch A Pathol Anat Histol* 1977 Jun[554]): "Liver electron microscopic studies were performed in 14 patients with systemic scleroderma. In 13 of these patients, giant mitochondria were demonstrated in the hepatocytes. This ultrastructural abnormality was present whatever the type and duration of the disease and was also present even when the liver was histologically normal. The mechanism of formation of giant mitochondria in systemic scleroderma is unknown."

- o Carnitine: According to the final sentence in a short report by Famularo et al[555], "Interestingly, early uncontrolled studies reported that the administration of L-carnitine had a favorable impact on the course of the disease in and this improvement was paralleled by a reduction in serum immunoglobulin levels." The use of carnitine is reviewed in Chapter 4 in the section on mitochondrial dysfunction.

- • STYLE OF LIVING (LIFESTYLE) & SPECIAL CONSIDERATIONS: This is a buffet of mostly lifestyle-based interventions including considerations such as somatic treatments, additional supplementation, and surgery.

  - o Special supplementation—PABA (para-amino benzoic acid): **Ninety percent of patients treated with PABA experience clinical benefit, especially skin softening.[556] PABA therapy prolongs survival in patients with scleroderma.[557]** "Potaba" is a well-tolerated prescription form of PABA.[558] Wright and Gaby[559] recommend "PABA, 2-3 g, 4 times a day." A 2006 review by Gaby[560] noted that PABA administered as potassium para-aminobenzoate (KPAB) was able to preserve pulmonary function and improve survival at five years (88.5% versus 69.8%) and 10 years (76.6% versus 56.6%) among patients treated with 12-12.5 g per day for three months to 20.6 years (average, 4.2 years). Adverse effects attributable to PABA are dose-dependent and include low blood sugar, rash, fever, and liver damage; one case of fatal toxic hepatitis has been reported. Adverse effects may be seen with doses approximating or exceeding eight grams per day; thus serial serum chemistries (e.g., monthly at first, then bimonthly, then quarterly) are warranted, especially when using high doses.

  - o Special supplementation—*Centella asiatica* (Gotu cola): This botanical has been reported to favorably influence scleroderma.[561] Available forms include teas, tinctures, standardized capsules/tablets, topical ointments, and injectable preparations. The **proprietary product "Madecassol" containing madecassic acid, asiatic acid and asiaticoside has been used in several studies and has demonstrated clinical benefit in scleroderma**[562]; some preparations of this product apparently contain nitrofural, a topically and orally active antibiotic. Contact dermatitis has been reported.

  - o CoQ10: CoQ10 is a powerful antioxidant with a wide margin of safety and excellent clinical tolerability. **At least four studies have documented its powerful blood-pressure-lowering ability, which often surpasses the clinical effectiveness of antihypertensive drugs.[563,564,565,566] Furthermore, at least two published papers[567,568] and one case report[569] advocate that CoQ10 has powerful renoprotective and**

[553] "Occurrence rate of anti-mitochondria antibody in high-sensitivity CRP elevated SSc patients (8/14, 57.1%) was significantly elevated compared with that of high-sensitivity CRP low SSc patients (3/26, 11.5%) (P < 0.01). These results led us to conclusion that elevated high-sensitivity CRP shows relation to the occurrence of anti-mitochondria antibody." Ohtsuka T. Relation between elevated high-sensitivity C-reactive protein and anti-mitochondria antibody in patients with systemic sclerosis. *J Dermatol.* 2008 Feb:70-5
[554] Feldmann et al. Hepatocyte giant mitochondrion: an almost constant lesion in systemic scleroderma. *Virchows Arch A Pathol Anat Histol.* 1977 Jun 23;374(3):215-27
[555] Famularo et al. Carnitine deficiency in scleroderma—letter. *Immunology Today* 1999 May; 246
[556] "Ninety percent of 224 patients treated with KPAB experienced mild, moderate, or marked skin softening." Zarafonetis CJ, Dabich L, Skovronski JJ, DeVol EB, Negri D, Yuan W, Wolfe R. Retrospective studies in scleroderma: skin response to potassium para-aminobenzoate therapy. *Clin Exp Rheumatol.* 1988 Jul-Sep;6(3):261-8
[557] "For the entire group an estimated 81.4% survived 5 years from diagnosis and 69.4% survived 10 years. …adequate treatment with potassium para-aminobenzoate (Potaba KPAB) was associated with improved survival (p less than 0.01); 88.5% 5 year survival rate and 76.6% 10 year survival rate for adequately treated patients." Zarafonetis et al. Retrospective studies in scleroderma: effect of potassium para-aminobenzoate on survival. *J Clin Epidemiol.* 1988;41(2):193-205
[558] glenwood-llc.com/potaba.html
[559] Gaby A, Wright JV. *Nutritional Protocols.* 1998 by Nutrition Seminars.
[560] Gaby AR. Natural remedies for scleroderma. *Altern Med Rev.* 2006 Sep;11(3):188-95
[561] "Titrated extract of Centella asiatica (TECA) contains three principal ingredients, asiaticoside (AS), asiatic acid (AA), and madecassic acid (MA). These components are known to be clinically effective on systemic scleroderma, abnormal scar formation, and keloids." Hong et al. Advanced formulation and pharmacological activity of hydrogel of the titrated extract of C. asiatica. *Arch Pharm Res.* 2005 Apr;28(4):502-8
[562] "Madecassol is effective and well tolerated and therefore recommended for oral and local use in combined treatment of SS adn FS." Guseva et al. [Madecassol treatment of systemic and localized scleroderma]. *Ter Arkh.* 1998;70(5):58-61. Article in Russian; information from abstract.
[563] Burke et al. Randomized, double-blind, placebo-controlled trial of coenzyme Q10 in isolated systolic hypertension. *South Med J.* 2001 Nov;94(11):1112-7
[564] Singh et al. Effect of hydrosoluble coenzyme Q10 on blood pressures and insulin resistance in hypertensive patients with CAD. *J Hum Hypertens.* 1999 Mar;13(3):203-8
[565] Digiesi et al. Coenzyme Q10 in essential hypertension. *Mol Aspects Med.* 1994;15 Suppl:s257-63
[566] Langsjoen P, Langsjoen P, Willis R, Folkers K. Treatment of essential hypertension with coenzyme Q10. *Mol Aspects Med.* 1994;15 Suppl:S265-72
[567] Singh et al. Randomized, double-blind placebo-controlled trial of coenzyme Q10 in chronic renal failure: discovery of a new role. *J Nutr Environ Med* 2000;10:281-8
[568] Singh et al. Randomized, Double-blind, Placebo-controlled Trial of Coenzyme Q10 in Patients with End-stage Renal Failure. *J Nutr Environ Med* 2003:13;13–22
[569] Singh RB, Singh MM. Effects of CoQ10 in new indications with antioxidant vitamin deficiency. *J Nutr Environ Med* 1999; 9:223-228

renorestorative benefits. CoQ10 levels are low in patients with allergies[570], and the symptomatic relief that many allergic patients experience following supplementation with CoQ10 suggests that CoQ10 has an immunomodulatory effect. Common doses start at > 100 mg per day with food; doses of 200 mg per day are not uncommon, and doses up to 1,000 mg per day are clinically well tolerated though the high financial toll approximates that of many pharmaceutical drugs.

- Coenzyme Q supplementation in pulmonary arterial hypertension (*Redox Biol* 2014 Jul[571]): In this controlled clinical trial, 300 mg daily of the reduced form of CoQ-10 were given to eight PAH patients. "Cardiac parameters improved with CoQ supplementation, although 6-minute walk distances and BNP levels did not significantly change. Consistent with improved mitochondrial synthetic function, hemoglobin increased and red cell distribution width (RDW) decreased in PAH patients with CoQ, while hemoglobin declined slightly and RDW did not change in healthy controls. In contrast, metabolic and redox parameters, including lactate, pyruvate and reduced or oxidized glutathione, did not change in PAH patients with CoQ. In summary, CoQ improved hemoglobin and red cell maturation in PAH, but longer studies and/or higher doses with a randomized placebo-controlled controlled design are necessary to evaluate the clinical benefit of this simple nutritional supplement."

○ N-acetyl-cysteine (NAC): **Oxidative stress promotes a fibrotic phenotype in scleroderma fibroblasts, which was normalized by administration of NAC *in vitro*.**[572] NAC is well-tolerated, inhibits NFkB, functions as an antioxidant, is a powerful and clinically important antiviral agent, and promotes detoxification via hepatoprotection and glutathione conjugation. In patients with scleroderma/SSC, studies using oral and IV NAC have been performed; benefits include improved hepatic (one-day study[573]), renal (one-day study[574]), and brachial/digital (three-year study[575]) perfusion following IV NAC.

- Measurement of clinical change in progressive systemic sclerosis: a 1 year double-blind placebo-controlled trial of N-acetylcysteine (*Ann Rheum Dis.* 1979 Aug[576]): "Identically appearing 500 mg capsules of NAC or placebo were dispensed. ... Therapy was begun with 2-4 capsules daily and increased to a maximum of 20 capsules daily given in equally divided doses over a 2-month period. If the full dose was not tolerated, the highest tolerated dose was used. ... In the NAC-treated group, [pulmonary] residual volume increased significantly. Oral aperture increased significantly in the NAC-treated group and latex titers decreased statistically significantly."

- Long-term N-acetylcysteine therapy in systemic sclerosis interstitial lung disease (*Int J Immunopathol Pharmacol* 2011 Jul[577]): "The primary endpoints of this study were changes between baseline and month 24 in single-breath carbon monoxide diffusing capacity (DLco). The secondary endpoints were: vital capacity (VC), forced expired volume in 1 sec (FEV1), total lung capacity (TLC), scores of high resolution computed tomography (HRCT) of the chest, number of adverse effects. In this study, we retrospectively investigated data from SSc patients who had undergone therapy with high-dose *intravenous* N-acetylcysteine (NAC) at a dosage of 15 mg/Kg/h for 5 consecutive hours every 14 days. After NAC therapy median values of DLco (69.5 vs 77.7%), VC (99 vs 101.3%) and TLC (93 vs 98.3%) significantly increased. We did not observe any significant changes from baseline in FEV1 value and HRTC score. The improvement in lung function was more evident in SSc patients

[570] Ye CQ, Folkers K, et al. A modified determination of coenzyme Q10 in human blood and CoQ10 blood levels in diverse patients with allergies. *Biofactors*. 1988 Dec;1:303-6

[571] Sharp et al. Coenzyme Q supplementation in pulmonary arterial hypertension. *Redox Biol.* 2014 Jul 31;2:884-91

[572] "Treatment of SSc fibroblasts with the membrane-permeant antioxidant N-acetyl-L-cysteine inhibited ROS production, and this was accompanied by decreased proliferation of these cells and down-regulation of alpha1(I) and alpha2(I) collagen messenger RNA." Sambo et al. Oxidative stress in scleroderma: maintenance of scleroderma fibroblast phenotype by the constitutive up-regulation of reactive oxygen species generation through the NADPH oxidase complex pathway. *Arthritis Rheum* 2001 Nov;44(11):2653-64

[573] "In an open-label study 40 patients with systemic sclerosis (SSc) were treated with 15 mg/kg/hour intravenous N-acetylcysteine for 5 consecutive hours in a single day. ... The results of our study demonstrate that NAC is able to increase HFV and total liver perfusion after a single infusion in SSc patients with low disease activity and severity scores." Rosato et al. N-acetylcysteine infusion improves hepatic perfusion in the early stages of systemic sclerosis. *Int J Immunopathol Pharmacol.* 2009 Jul-Sep;22(3):763-72

[574] "In an open-label study 40 patients with systemic sclerosis (SSc) were treated with N-acetylcysteine (NAC) iv infusion over 5 consecutive hours, at a dose of 0.015 g x kg(-1) x h(-1). ... In patients with low disease severity NAC ameliorates vascular renal function." Rosato et al. N-acetylcysteine infusion reduces the resistance index of renal artery in the early stage of systemic sclerosis. *Acta Pharmacol Sin.* 2009 Sep;30(9):1283-8

[575] "The aim of this study was to report long-term outcome (median follow-up 3 years) in a prospective study of a cohort of 50 consecutive patients with SSc who received N-acetylcysteine (NAC) infusional therapy every 2 weeks. ... In conclusion, long-term therapy with NAC, in patients with SSc, has a durable effectiveness on ischemic ulcers and Raynaud's phenomenon." Rosato et al. The treatment with N-acetylcysteine of Raynaud's phenomenon and ischemic ulcers therapy in sclerodermic patients: a prospective observational study of 50 patients. *Clin Rheumatol.* 2009 Dec;28(12):1379-84

[576] Furst et al. Measurement of clinical change in progressive systemic sclerosis. *Ann Rheum Dis.* 1979 Aug;38(4):356-61

[577] Rosato et al. Long-term N-acetylcysteine therapy in systemic sclerosis interstitial lung disease: a retrospective study. *Int J Immunopathol Pharmacol.* 2011 Jul-Sep;24:727-33

without radiological signs of pulmonary fibrosis than in patients with pulmonary fibrosis. In SSc patients with mild-moderate pulmonary fibrosis intravenous NAC administration slows the rate of deterioration of DLco, VC and TLC. In conclusion, this retrospective study demonstrates that long-term therapy with intravenous NAC ameliorates pulmonary function tests in SSc patients."

- Comprehensive antioxidation: **As previously mentioned, patients with scleroderma have evidence of increased oxidative stress demonstrated by a doubling of urinary isoprostane excretion.**[578] Oxidative stress results from and contributes to systemic inflammation because 1) increased immune activity results in elaboration of oxidants, and 2) oxidative stress upregulates NFkB (and other pathways) for additive immune activation. *Antioxidant supplementation* alone is clinically and biochemically inferior to a *comprehensive program* that includes both antioxidant supplementation and dietary modification (i.e., the supplemented Paleo-Mediterranean diet, as described previously) that includes heavy reliance upon fruits, vegetables, low-glycemic juices, nuts, seeds, and berries for their additive and synergistic antioxidant benefits.[579]

  - In vitro modulation of collagen type I, fibronectin and dermal fibroblast function and activity, in systemic sclerosis by the antioxidant epigallocatechin-3-gallate (*Rheumatology* 2010 Nov[580]): Dermal fibroblasts from a cell line (AG), healthy individuals (CON) and SSc patients were treated with EGCG, one of the main constituents of green tea. "The results suggest that the antioxidant, EGCG, can reduce ECM production, the fibrotic marker CTGF and inhibit contraction of dermal fibroblasts from SSc patients. Furthermore, EGCG was able to suppress intracellular ROS, ERK1/2 kinase signaling and NFkB activity. Taken together, EGCG may be a possible candidate for therapeutic treatment aimed at reducing both oxidant stress and the fibrotic effects associated with SSc."

- Oral enzyme therapy with proteolytic/pancreatic enzymes: Polyenzyme supplementation is used to ameliorate the pathophysiology induced by immune complexes.[581] Immune complexes are detected in the majority of patients with scleroderma[582] and correlate with disease severity and visceral involvement.[583] Orally administered polyenzyme preparations have an "immune stimulating" action[584] and promote degradation of microbial biofilms and increased immune and antimicrobial penetration into infectious foci.[585] Given that maldigestion, malabsorption, and pancreatic insufficiency are not uncommon in patients with scleroderma[586], enzymes may be given with food for optimal benefit.

- Esophageal dysfunction and GERD in scleroderma—specific treatments:

  - Low carbohydrate diet, specific carbohydrate diet: The gastroesophageal dysfunction that contributes to the high incidence of Barrett's esophagus is likely the result of a confluence of different factors: neurogenic, myogenic, and dysbiotic. With regard to the latter, clinicians must be diligent in the eradication of small intestine bacterial overgrowth, since microbial products of fermentation lead to relaxation of the so-called lower esophageal sphincter.[587,588] This is why diets low in carbohydrate and fermentable fibers (such as those found in grains)—in other words: **"low fermentation diets"**—are effective in the treatment of esophageal reflux; low-carbohydrate diets deprive gut microbes of substrate for fermentation into metabolites that relax the lower esophageal

[578] "CONCLUSION: This study provides evidence of enhanced lipid peroxidation in both SSc and UCTD, and suggests a rationale for antioxidant treatment of SSc." Cracowski et al. Enhanced in vivo lipid peroxidation in scleroderma spectrum disorders. *Arthritis Rheum* 2001 May;44(5):1143-8

[579] Liu RH. Health benefits of fruit and vegetables are from additive and synergistic combinations of phytochemicals. *Am J Clin Nutr*. 2003 Sep;78(3 Suppl):517S-520S

[580] Dooley et al. Modulation of collagen type I, fibronectin and dermal fibroblast function and activity, in systemic sclerosis by the antioxidant epigallocatechin-3-gallate. *Rheumatology* 2010 Nov;49(11):2024-36

[581] Galebskaya et al. Human complement system state after wobenzyme intake. *Vestnik Moskovskogo Universiteta (Seriya 2: Khimiya)*. 2000:41(6 Suppl): 148-149 chem.msu.ru/eng/journals/vmgu/00add/148.pdf

[582] "Serum immune complexes were measured in 92 patients with progressive systemic sclerosis, and elevated levels were found as follows: Raji cell assay 72% (59% after pronase treatment of Raji cell), agarose gel electrophoresis 52%, and C1q binding 24%." Seibold JR, Medsger TA Jr, Winkelstein A, Kelly RH, Rodnan GP. Immune complexes in progressive systemic sclerosis (scleroderma). *Arthritis Rheum*. 1982 Oct;25(10):1167-73

[583] "Patients with SS showed an incidence of circulating immune complexes comparable to that found in SLE, with 20 patients (58.5%),…associated with both elevation of serum IgG and IgA levels and extensive visceral involvement by the disease." Hughes et al. Immune complexes in systemic sclerosis; detection by C1q binding, K-cell inhibition and Raji cell radioimmunoassays. *J Clin Lab Immunol*. 1983 Mar;10(3):133-8

[584] Zavadova et al. Stimulation of reactive oxygen species production and cytotoxicity in human neutrophils in vitro and after oral administration of a polyenzyme preparation. *Cancer Biother*. 1995 Summer;10(2):147-52

[585] "The enzymes were shown to inhibit the biofilm formation. When applied to the formed associations, the enzymes potentiated the effect of antibiotics on the bacteria located in them." Tets VV, et al. [Impact of exogenic proteolytic enzymes on bacteria][Article in Russian] *Antibiot Khimioter*. 2004;49(12):9-13

[586] Of 20 patients: "Three patients had very low levels of tryptic activity in their intestinal juice and only nine had results which were unequivocally normal." Cobden I, Axon AT, Rowell NR. Pancreatic exocrine function in systemic sclerosis. *Br J Dermatol* 1981 Aug;105(2):189-93

[587] "Colonic fermentation of indigestible carbohydrates increases the rate of TLESRs [transient lower esophageal sphincter relaxations], the number of acid reflux episodes, and the symptoms of GERD." Piche et al. Colonic fermentation influences lower esophageal sphincter function in gastroesophageal reflux disease. *Gastroenterology*. 2003 Apr;124(4):894-902

[588] Piche et al. Modulation by colonic fermentation of LES function in humans. *Am J Physiol Gastrointest Liver Physiol*. 2000 Apr;278(4):G578-84

sphincter and thereby contribute to symptomatic improvement in patients with gastroesophageal reflux.[589] This is part of the reason why the diet for these patients must be as low as possible in the difficult-to-digest and easy-to-ferment carbohydrates that are common in the Standard American Diet (SAD) from corn, potatoes, wheat, and disaccharides such as lactose and sucrose; see *Breaking the Vicious Cycle*[590] by Elaine Gottschall for more details and recipes for the specific carbohydrate diet. Similarly, a low-carbohydrate Atkins-type diet[591] might also be considered, particularly for short-term use and particularly if modified away from proinflammatory saturated fats and arachidonic acid. As emphasized previously, high-fiber diets increase the risk for bowel obstruction in scleroderma patients, especially if implemented rapidly; slow implementation of dietary fiber increase along with an osmotic stool softener such as magnesium and/or ascorbate is advised.

- Alginate: Alginate is a processed extract from seaweed that is the active ingredient in the FDA-approved OTC anti-heartburn drug Gaviscon.[592] When mixed with stomach acid, alginate forms a foam "raft" that creates a barrier of protection for the esophagus, and it significantly reduces the number of acidic reflux events. Clinical studies have proven the effectiveness of alginate for treating GERD; however pure supplements of sodium alginate may be preferred over Gaviscon due to the latter's inclusion of aluminum (hydroxide)[593], a metal correlated with adverse effects and increased risk for neurologic disease. Alginate is also said to bind toxic metals and may therefore reduce enterohepatic recirculation of these proinflammatory immunotoxins.

- Betaine hydrochloric acid (betaine HCL): Many patients with gastroesophageal reflux are cured with the administration of supplemental HCL. Although the addition of acid rather than the suppression of acid goes against the well-funded acid-blocking drug paradigm, the truth remains that—*physiologically*—gastric emptying is promoted by acidification and—*clinically*—the treatment works for a significant number of patients with GERD. Furthermore, correction of hypochlorhydria by supplementation with betaine HCL helps to reduce bacterial/yeast counts in the stomach and upper intestine, thereby alleviating GERD by reducing the bacteria/yeast available for fermentation; recall that microbial fermentation is one of the primary driving influences for GERD/reflux.[594]

- GLA: Numerous studies have documented the anti-cancer effects of GLA, and these have specifically been documented in esophageal cancer cell lines.[595] Thus, GLA consumption may help protect against the development of esophageal cancer, in addition to its important anti-inflammatory and vasodilating actions.

- Vitamin B12: Vitamin B-12 levels are low in patients with malabsorption, and vitamin B-12 administration (4,000 mcg/d orally, or 1,000-2,000 mcg intramuscularly/ 2-3 times weekly) can promote intestinal motility.

- Raynaud's phenomenon—specific treatments: See section/minimonograph toward the end of this chapter.

- **ENDOCRINE IMBALANCE & OPTIMIZATION: Prolactin, Insulin, Estrogen, DHEA, Cortisol, Testosterone, Thyroid** Common hormonal imbalances seen among autoimmune/inflammatory patients are: ❶ *elevated* prolactin, ❷ *elevated* estrogen, ❸ *elevated* insulin, and ❹ *reduced* DHEA, ❺ *reduced* cortisol, and ❻ *reduced* testosterone; see Chapter 4 for discussion of these hormones and respective interventions. Thyroid evaluation (patient + labs) should be comprehensive, as discussed in Chapter 1, with a low threshold for empiric treatment.

---

[589] "The 5 individuals described in these case reports experienced resolution of GERD symptoms after self-initiation of a low-carbohydrate diet." Yancy et al. Improvement of gastroesophageal reflux disease after initiation of a low-carbohydrate diet: five brief case reports. *Altern Ther Health Med.* 2001 Nov-Dec;7(6):120, 116-9

[590] Gotschall E. *Breaking the Vicious Cycle: Intestinal health though diet.* Kirkton Press; Rev edition (August, 1994) scdiet.com/

[591] Atkins RC. *Dr. Atkins' New Diet Revolution (revised and updated).* New York: Avon Books, 1999

[592] "For this population, sodium alginate was assessed as significantly superior by both investigators and patients at week two (p < 0.001 and p = 0.004, respectively) and at week four (p = 0.001 and p < 0.001, respectively)." Chatfield S. A comparison of the efficacy of the alginate preparation, Gaviscon Advance, with placebo in the treatment of gastro-oesophageal reflux disease. *Curr Med Res Opin.* 1999;15(3):152-9

[593] gaviscon.com/info.htm

[594] "Colonic fermentation of indigestible carbohydrates increases the rate of TLESRs [transient lower esophageal sphincter relaxations], the number of acid reflux episodes, and the symptoms of GERD." Piche et al. Colonic fermentation influences lower esophageal sphincter function in gastroesophageal reflux disease. *Gastroenterology.* 2003 Apr;124(4):894-902

[595] "A statistically highly significant growth-suppressive effect of the prostaglandin precursor gamma-linolenic acid (GLA) on MG63 human osteogenic sarcoma and oesophageal carcinoma cells in culture was found." Booyens et al. The effect of gamma-linolenic acid on the growth of human osteogenic sarcoma and oesophageal carcinoma cells in culture. *S Afr Med J.* 1984 Feb 18;65(7):240-2

- High incidence of thyroid disorders in systemic sclerosis (*J Clin Endocrinol Metab* 2013 Jul[596]): "Our study shows a high incidence of new cases of hypothyroidism and thyroid dysfunction in female sclerodermic patients. Female sclerodermic patients, who are at high risk (a borderline high [even if in the normal range] TSH value, anti-thyroperoxidase antibody positivity, and a hypoechoic and small thyroid) should have periodic thyroid function follow-up."
- Low DHEA sulphate serum levels in premenopausal systemic sclerosis (*Clin Exp Rheumatol* 2001 Jan[597]): "Mean serum levels of DHEAS in SSc women of childbearing age were significantly lower than in controls (0.87 +/- 0.85 microgram/ml versus 2.75 +/- 0.42 micrograms/ml; p < 0.001). On the contrary, no difference was found between postmenopausal women and controls. A reduction below the 95% confidence limits was found in 10 out of 11 patients of childbearing age and in 8 out of 29 postmenopausal women, respectively. In 5 out of 11 patients of childbearing age taking steroids for their SSc (< 10 mg/daily) DHEAS levels were significantly lower than in patients not taking steroids (p = 0.01. ... Our data show that, as in other autoimmune diseases, low serum DHEAS is a feature of premenopausal SSc patients. More extensive prospective studies are needed to define the exact role of DHEAS dysregulation in SSc."
- High prolactin and low dehydroepiandrosterone sulphate serum levels correlate with disease activity in patients with severe systemic sclerosis (*Br J Rheumatol.* 1997 Apr[598]): "Compared to SSc with <9 disease manifestations, patients with > or =9 disease manifestations had higher PRL (P = 0.044), higher soluble interleukin 2 receptor (sIL-2R, P = 0.004) and vascular cell adhesion molecule (sVCAM, P = 0.044), and lower DHEAS (P = 0.029). PRL (R(Rank) = 0.490, P = 0.003) and DHEAS (R(Rank) = -0.399, P = 0.013) were significantly correlated with the number of disease manifestations. The inverse correlation between PRL and DHEAS showed a trend (P = 0.059). PRL correlated with sIL-2R (R(Rank) = 0.553, P = 0.001) and sVCAM (R(Rank) = 0.520, P = 0.002). The number of disease manifestations and sIL-2R correlated significantly (R(Rank) = 0.463, P = 0.006)."
- Melatonin: **In an *in vitro* study with fibroblasts from normal and scleroderma patients, melatonin was shown to inhibit fibroblast proliferation**[599]; future trials may demonstrate that melatonin has an antifibrotic/antisclerodermatous benefit. Melatonin is a pineal hormone with well-known sleep-inducing and immunomodulatory properties, and it is commonly administered in doses of 1-40 mg in the evening, before bedtime. Its exceptional safety is well documented. In contrast to implementing treatment with high doses of 20-40 mg, starting with a relatively low dose (e.g., 1-5 mg) and increasing as tolerated is recommended. Melatonin (20 mg hs) appears to have cured two patients with drug-resistant sarcoidosis[600] and 3 mg provided immediate short-term benefit to a patient with multiple sclerosis.[601] Immunostimulatory anti-infective action of melatonin was demonstrated in a clinical trial wherein septic newborns administered 20 mg melatonin showed significantly increased survival over nontreated controls[602]; **given that scleroderma is associated with subclinical "infections", melatonin may provide therapeutic benefit by virtue of its anti-infective properties.**
- Estrogen (excess): **Research suggests that estrogen is immunodysregulatory and an important contributor to autoimmune disease**, perhaps explaining the greatly higher incidence of autoimmune diseases in women compared to men. So-called **"estrogen-replacement therapy" used in postmenopausal women increases the risk for lupus and scleroderma.**[603] Men with rheumatoid arthritis show an excess of estradiol and a decrease in DHEA, and the excess estrogen is proportional to the degree of inflammation.[604] Serum estradiol is commonly used to assess estrogen status; estrogens can also be

[596] Antonelli et al. Incidence of thyroid disorders in systemic sclerosis: results from a longitudinal follow-up. *J Clin Endocrinol Metab.* 2013 Jul;98(7):E1198-202

[597] La Montagna, et al. Dehydroepiandrosterone sulphate serum levels in systemic sclerosis. *Clin Exp Rheumatol.* 2001 Jan-Feb;19(1):21-6

[598] Straub et al. High prolactin and low dehydroepiandrosterone sulphate serum levels in patients with severe systemic sclerosis. *Br J Rheumatol.* 1997 Apr;36(4):426-32

[599] "These results suggest that MLT, at higher dosages, is a potent inhibitor of the proliferation of fibroblasts derived from the skin of healthy and SSc patients." Carossino AM, et al. Effect of melatonin on normal and sclerodermic skin fibroblast proliferation. *Clin Exp Rheumatol.* 1996 Sep-Oct;14(5):493-8.

[600] Cagnoni et al. Melatonin for treatment of chronic refractory sarcoidosis. *Lancet.* 1995 Nov 4;346(8984):1229-30

[601] "...administration of melatonin (3 mg, orally) at 2:00 p.m., when the patient experienced severe blurring of vision, resulted within 15 minutes in a dramatic improvement in visual acuity and in normalization of the visual evoked potential latency after stimulation of the left eye." Sandyk R. Diurnal variations in vision and relations to circadian melatonin secretion in multiple sclerosis. *Int J Neurosci.* 1995 Nov;83(1-2):1-6

[602] Gitto et al. Effects of melatonin treatment in septic newborns. *Pediatr Res.* 2001 Dec;50(6):756-60 pedresearch.org/cgi/content/full/50/6/756

[603] "These studies indicate that estrogen replacement therapy in postmenopausal women increases the risk of developing lupus, scleroderma, and Raynaud disease..." Mayes MD. Epidemiologic studies of environmental agents and systemic autoimmune diseases. *Environ Health Perspect.* 1999 Oct;107 Suppl 5:743-8

[604] "DHEAS and estrone concentrations were lower and estradiol was higher in patients compared with healthy controls. DHEAS differed between RF positive and RF negative patients. Estrone did not correlate with any disease variable, whereas estradiol correlated strongly and positively with all measured indices of inflammation." Tengstrand et al. Abnormal levels of serum dehydroepiandrosterone, estrone, and estradiol in men with rheumatoid arthritis: high correlation between serum estradiol and current degree of inflammation. *J Rheumatol.* 2003 Nov;30(11):2338-43

measured in 24-hour urine samples. Interventions to combat high estrogen levels may include any effective combination of the following:

- **Weight loss and weight optimization**: In overweight patients, weight loss is the means to attaining the goal of weight optimization; the task is not complete until the body mass index is normalized/optimized. Excess adiposity and obesity raise estrogen levels due to high levels of aromatase (the hormone that makes estrogen) in adipose tissue; weight optimization and loss of excess fat helps normalize hormone levels and reduce inflammation.
- **Avoidance of ethanol**: Estrogen production is stimulated by ethanol intake.
- **Consider surgical correction of varicocele in affected men**: Men with varicocele have higher estrogen levels due to temperature-induced alterations in enzyme function in the testes; surgical correction of the varicocele lowers estrogen levels.
- **"Anti-estrogen diet"**: Foods and supplements such as green tea, DIM, I3C, licorice, and a high-fiber "anti-estrogenic diet" can also be used; monitoring clinical status and serum estradiol will prove or disprove efficacy.
- **Anastrozole/Arimidex**: In our office, we commonly measure serum estradiol in men and administer the aromatase inhibitor anastrozole/Arimidex 1 mg (2-3 doses per week) to men whose estradiol level is greater than ~20 picogram/mL; we consider estradiol 10-24 picogram/mL to be optimal for a man.[605] Clinical studies using anastrozole/Arimidex in men have shown that aromatase blockade lowers estradiol and raises testosterone[606]; generally speaking, this is exactly the result that we want in patients with severe systemic autoimmunity. Frequency of dosing is based on serum and clinical response. Letrozole/Femara is another aromatase inhibitor, one that should generally be avoided due to its underreported and underappreciated ability to block androgen receptors.

- **XENOBIOTIC ACCUMULATION & DETOXIFICATION: Chemical avoidance, nutritional support for detoxification pathways, urine alkalinization** The clinical relevance and pathogenic mechanisms of xenobiotic accumulation are irrefutably well documented and described. Clinical assessments include history, physical examination, and laboratory assessment (using serum, whole blood, urine or—rarely yet accurately—fat biopsy), and response to treatment. Treatments include nutritional support for Phases 1 and 2 of detoxification (e.g., oxidation and conjugation) and excretion via bile and urine; for the latter, urinary alkalinization is generally recommended. Chemical toxins can be bound in the gut using activated charcoal, cholestyramine, or *Chlorella*—all of these three treatments have documented safety and effectiveness; clinically and empirically, phytochelatin (plant-derived peptides that bind toxic metals) concentrates appear safe and effective despite lack of conclusive published data supporting clinical use.
  - **Xenobiotic immunotoxicity**: Given that **antifibrillarin antibodies are specifically seen in patients with scleroderma**[607] and that **mercury exposure induces antifibrillarin autoimmunity in susceptible mice**[608], clinicians may be justified in searching for and treating evidence of mercury exposure in patients with autoimmunity in general and scleroderma in particular. Detailed history, dental examination for mercury-containing amalgams, and post-DMSA urine metal analysis are suggested.

---

[605] Male Hormone Modulation Therapy, Page 4 Of 7: lef.org/protocols/prtcl-130c.shtml Accessed October 30, 2005
[606] "These data demonstrate that aromatase inhibition increases serum bioavailable and total testosterone levels to the youthful normal range in older men with mild hypogonadism." Leder et al. Effects of aromatase inhibition in elderly men with low or borderline-low serum testosterone levels. *J Clin Endocrinol Metab.* 2004 Mar;89:1174-80
[607] "Since anti-fibrillarin antibodies are specific markers of scleroderma, the present animal model may be valuable for studies of the immunological aberrations which are likely to induce this autoimmune response." Hultman et al. Anti-fibrillarin autoantibodies in mercury-treated mice. *Clin Exp Immunol.* 1989 Dec;78(3):470-7
[608] Nielsen et al. Mercury-induced autoimmunity in mice. *Environ Health Perspect.* 2002 Oct;110 Sup 5:877-81 ehp.niehs.nih.gov/docs/2002/suppl-5/877-881nielsen/abstract.html

Vasculitic Diseases

Introduction:

Vasculitic diseases are largely considered to be mediated by deposition of circulating immune complexes (CIC) into/on the vascular endothelium, resulting in a localized activation of cell-mediated inflammation and activation of the complement cascade. From an allopathic perspective, these conditions are generally considered idiopathic and thus necessarily requiring long-term immunosuppression, in various forms.

From the perspective of logic and with a desire to deconstruct complex clinical phenomena, one can approach diseases that are mediated by immune complex deposition by deciphering the components into their elemental parts. For example, given that most vasculitic disease are mediated by endothelial deposition of immune complexes, and that immune complexes are chains of antigens and antibodies, one can then ask "*What are the major sources of antigens to which the immune system is exposed*?" and the correct answers are: "*Self, diet, microbes.*" One can then ponder the source of the antibodies, and ask if the presumed overproduction of antibodies is a *qualitative* problem or a *quantitative* problem, i.e., "Is the immune system 'wrong' in making antibodies to an antigen to which it is exposed [qualitative problem, error in action], *or* is the immune system 'correct' in its action but simply over-producing antibodies to perhaps otherwise benign antigens, whether these are self, diet, and/or microbes [quantitative problem, error in regulation]? From these questions, we arrive at answers other than crisis management and perpetual medicalization and pharmacologic immunosuppression; we arrive at the opportunity to reduce exposure to antigens from self (via antioxidant therapy to prevent molecular alteration of "self" structures), food (via food allergy avoidance and healing of intestinal hyperpermeability, and microbes (reducing dysbiosis and total microbial load [TML]) while also reducing the likely overzealous production of corresponding immunoglobulins via nutritional immunomodulation: induction of Treg for the reciprocal inhibition Th1, Th2, and Th17.

Description/pathophysiology, and clinical presentations:

- "Vasculitis" refers to a heterogeneous group of inflammatory disorders primarily affecting blood vessels, particularly the arteries and arterioles. Although the underlying pathomechanisms are similar among different disorders, these diseases differ in the location/size and number of affected vessels, and thus the clinical presentations and complications differ accordingly. Polymyalgia rheumatica / giant cell arteritis, ANCA vasculitis, and Behcet's disease are subtypes of vasculitis that are discussed in their respective chapters. As shown in the table at the right, several subtypes of vasculitis can be categorized based on the size/location of the vessel affected, and whether or not the cause of the vasculitis has been determined.

- Systemic manifestations are comparable to many other autoimmune disorders: insidious onset of fever, malaise, weight loss, generalized aches/pains.

- The autoimmune and immune-mediated pathogenesis of the vasculitides includes the following:
  - Antibody-antigen binding: *Example*: Goodpasture syndrome.
  - Delayed hypersensitivity reactions: Especially in lesions characterized with granulomas formation. *Example*: temporal arteritis.

Overview of common vasculopathic disorders
Primary vasculitides
Large vessel diseases
▪ Takayasu's arteritis
▪ Behcet's disease
Medium vessel diseases
▪ Polyarteritis nodosa
▪ Buerger's disease
▪ Giant cell arteritis
Small vessel diseases
Immune-complex mediated
▪ Cutaneous leukocystoclastic vasculitis
▪ Henoch-Schonlein purpura
▪ Cryoglobulinemia
ANCA-associated disorders
▪ ANCA vasculitis
▪ Microscopic polyangiitis: microscopic polyarteritis, leukocytoclastic vasculitis ; variants include allergic granulomatosis and angiitis also known as Churg-Strauss syndrome
Secondary vasculitides
▪ Infections, dysbiosis
▪ Other autoimmune disease
▪ Crohn's disease or ulcerative colitis
▪ Cancer
▪ Drug reactions
▪ Food allergies

  - Deposition of circulating immune complexes: The majority of the vasculitides are characterized by intra-arterial deposition of circulating immune complexes, which provoke activation of the complement cascade and leukocyte migration and activation for the resultant vascular damage, which often includes necrosis, fibrinous occlusion, and thrombosis. *Example*: acute arteritis in SLE.

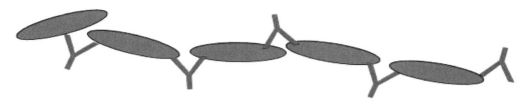

Schematized illustration of an immune complex: Immunoglobulins/antibodies—represented by the Y-shaped molecule—and antigens such as molecular fragments and peptides—represented by the ovoid molecule—form "chains" of alternating antigens-and-antibodies which in the circulation become lodged in the skin (dermatitis), vascular endothelium (vasculitis), kidney (nephritis), serosal surfaces (serositis), and synovial joints (arthritis). Readers must note that the location of the immune complex deposition is "innocent"; in immune complex disease, the location of the inflammation and complement activation (i.e., skin, vascular endothelium, kidney, synovial joints, serosa, and synovial joints) is simply a convenient molecular depot for the circulating immune complexes (CIC). Once deposited and following sufficient accumulation, immune complexes incite activation of the complement cascade and a local cell-mediated immune response, which causes local tissue inflammation and progressive destruction. Thus, for example, the joint or the skin or the kidney will be inflamed, but the actual problem of excess antigen exposure originated elsewhere, and the corresponding excess antibody production may have simply been a normal physiologic response to antigen exposure or may have been facilitated by a pro-inflammatory state and—synergistically yet distinctly—immunophenotypic imbalance.

Major differential diagnoses:

- Infection
- Cancer, especially leukemia, lymphoma, and multiple myeloma
- Autoimmunity: Concomitant or independent
- Trauma or abuse: Numerous unexplainable bruises/purpura may indicate abuse
- Adverse drug reaction
- Atherosclerosis, peripheral vascular disease, aneurysm

Clinical assessments:

- **History/subjective**:
  - See clinical presentations
- **Physical examination/objective**:
  - General physical examination with emphasis placed on symptomatic regions, circulatory examination, and dermal lesions
- **Laboratory assessments**:
  - Chemistry/metabolic panel: Assess for complications, especially renal insufficiency
  - Urinalysis: Assess for renal involvement
  - CRP/ESR: Generally elevated
  - Serum immune complexes: Most vasculopathies are due to immune complex deposition: Immune Complexes Reference Range (Raji cell technique, quantitative analysis):
    - Normal: ≤ 15.0 µg Eq/mL
    - Equivocal: 15.1-19.9 µg Eq/mL
    - Positive: ≥20.0 µg Eq/mL
  - Testing for multifocal dysbiosis: As discussed in Chapter 4
  - ANA
  - CH50: Complement levels may be low during exacerbations of immune complex mediated disease as the complement cascade is activated and complement proteins are consumed in the process, thus leading to a reduction in serum levels.
  - ANCA: Many of the vasculopathies, particularly those affecting the small vessels, are characterized by the presence of anti-neutrophilic cytoplasmic autoantibodies (ANCA), which can be segregated into two distinct subtypes: ❶ **cytoplasmic-ANCA** (C-ANCA, major antigen: proteinase 3) associated with Wegener granulomatosis, and ❷ **perinuclear-ANCA** (P-ANCA, major antigen: myeloperoxidase)

associated with microscopic polyangiitis, or Churg-Strauss syndrome. Clinicians should note that neither P-ANCA nor C-ANCA is specific for a particular diagnosis, and that 10% of patients with biopsy-proved small vessel vasculitis do not show either ANCA subtype. In patients with small vessel vasculitis, levels of ANCA correlate with disease severity, especially C-ANCA in patients with Wegener granulomatosis.

- **Imaging and biopsy**:
  - Angiography is commonly used in the evaluation of vasculitic syndromes affecting larger vessels; Doppler ultrasound imaging can also be used.
  - Biopsy of dermal lesions, superficial arteries, and other tissues can support the diagnosis
- **Establishing the diagnosis**:
  - Based on clinical, laboratory, and biopsy/imaging findings

Major complications:

- Tissue necrosis: Complications depend on location of hypoxia and can include dermal necrosis, myocardial infarction, stroke, and intestinal infarction
- Infection secondary to immunosuppression
- Renal damage

Clinical management:

- Exacerbations are best managed pharmaceutically with appropriate immunosuppression. Patients may require hospital admission.
- An overview/survey of various inflammatory vascular disorders is presented on the following two pages.

Timely referral and comanagement
Generally speaking, patients with these conditions should be co-managed with a specialist (e.g., Internal Medicine, Rheumatology) because complications such as transverse myelitis and vascular occlusion leading to distal tissue ischemia—blindness, digital necrosis, mesenteric ischemia—can present quickly and require immediate immunosuppression in a hospital setting.

Overview of Vasculitic Diseases

Vasculitis subtype	Unique characteristics	Assessment and treatment considerations
Giant Cell (Temporal) Arteritis (outlined here and detailed in following subsection before the therapeutics section): Three subtypes exist along a continuum: • Granulomatous vasculitis (2/3 of cases) • Leukocytic infiltration of vessel wall • Intimal fibrosis with lumenal narrowing	• GCA is the most common form of vasculitis; elevated ESR is classic • Granulomatous inflammation of medium and small arteries, particularly of the head; involvement of the aorta (giant cell aortitis) is a rare variant • Jaw claudication is highly suggestive • Classic presentation includes headache and facial pain; 50% of patients have PMR: polymyalgia rheumatica	• Biopsy is the gold standard for diagnosis, although it may be normal in one-third of patients due to lesion focality/locality. • **Patients can transition from asymptomatic to blind—vision loss due to occlusion of ophthalmic artery—within days; therefore, this condition is generally considered a medical emergency/urgency mandating immediate implementation of prednisone, typically starting at 60 mg/d or 1 mg/kg/d.**
Wegener granulomatosis (outlined here and detailed in following subsection before the therapeutics section): • Affects small arteries all the way through to veins	• Granulomatous vasculitis affecting the upper respiratory tract	• Most patients have C-ANCA (cytoplasmic anti-proteinase 3 antibodies); small percentage of patients have P-ANCA (perinuclear anti-myeloperoxidase antibodies)

Overview of Vasculitic Diseases—*continued*

Vasculitis subtype	Unique characteristics	Assessment and treatment considerations
Takayasu arteritis: "pulseless disease" • Leukocytic infiltration of the vasa vasorum followed by medial fibrosis and granulomatosis	• Granulomatous vasculitis of large and medium arteries • Fibrous thickening of the aortic arch and occlusion of large arteries • Presentation typically includes neuro-ocular disturbances, reduced arm pulses; may include aortic valve insufficiency, and hypertension due to renal artery stenosis	• Clinical assessment with aortogram
Polyarteritis nodosa (PAN): • Immune-complex vasculitis • 10-30% of patients have Hepatitis B—testing for hepatitis B is mandatory[609] • Generally fatal if untreated; estimated 5-year survival 13% • Without treatment, only 20% of patients survive 5 years; with treatment, survival improves to 60-90% at 5 years	• Necrotizing vasculitic ischemia of numerous systems, thrombosis and ischemia at sites distal to lesion • <u>Gut</u>: abdominal pain, nausea, vomiting exacerbated by eating (due to ischemia) • <u>Nerves</u>: mononeuritis multiplex, vasculitic neuropathy; foot drop is most common manifestation • <u>Skin</u>: dermal lesions include sharply-demarcated nodules, erythema, and ulceration; lesions are **non-palpable** and are in **different stages** of development • <u>Kidneys</u>: hypertension due to renal involvement • *Pulmonary involvement is rare* • Can be categorized as *infectious and ANCA-negative* or *noninfectious and P-ANCA-positive*	• Clinical presentation is varied depending on location of arterial lesion(s) and severity of systemic inflammation; typical population is young adults • Anemia, elevated ESR, leukocytosis • Autoantibodies commonly normal or low-positive • Diagnosis is established with biopsy or angiogram • <u>Pharmacotherapy</u>: prednisone: 60 mg/d; pulsed methylprednisolone: 1 gram IV daily for 3 days; cyclophosphamide or other immunosuppressant drug • Plasmapheresis • Treatment of underlying hepatitis: must balance immunosuppression with anti-infective treatments
Mixed cryoglobulinemia: • Many patients have underlying hepatitis C • Many patient respond to avoidance of foods to which they are allergic	• Purpura • Peripheral neuropathy • Glomerulonephritis • Abdominal pain • Hepatitis • May have pulmonary involvement	• Diagnosis is based on clinical picture and serology for cryoglobulins • Testing for and treatment of underlying hepatitis is essential • Immunosuppression may exacerbate viral replication • **Avoidance of food allergens is highly beneficial**[610,611]

[609] Tierney ML. McPhee SJ, Papadakis MA (eds). *Current Medical Diagnosis and Treatment 2006. 45th edition*. New York; Lange Medical Books: 2006, pages 844-850
[610] "CONCLUSION: These data show that an LAC diet decreases the amount of circulating immune complexes in MC and can modify certain signs and symptoms of the disease." Ferri C, Pietrogrande M, Cecchetti R, et al. Low-antigen-content diet in the treatment of patients with mixed cryoglobulinemia. *Am J Med*. 1989 Nov;87:519-24
[611] Pietrogrande M, Cefalo A, Nicora F, Marchesini D. Dietetic treatment of essential mixed cryoglobulinemia. *Ric Clin Lab*. 1986 Apr-Jun;16(2):413-6

Vasculitis subtype	Unique characteristics	Assessment and treatment considerations
<u>Henoch-Schonlein</u> <u>purpura</u>: IgA vasculitis Note: These terms are easy to intermix and confuse: ▪ <u>Buerger's disease</u>: thromboangiitis obliterans ▪ <u>Berger's disease</u>: IgA nephropathy	▪ Dermal purpura ▪ Abdominal pain ▪ Arthritis ▪ Hematuria associated with renal involvement; IgA nephropathy (Berger's disease) is generally considered a glomerular variant of Henoch-Schonlein purpura	▪ The disease is generally self-limiting to 1-6 weeks, subsiding without complications if renal involvement is mild ▪ Monitor renal function ▪ No generally effective allopathic treatment is known
<u>Microscopic polyangiitis,</u> <u>microscopic polyarteritis,</u> <u>leukocytoclastic vasculitis</u>: ▪ Affects small arterioles, capillaries, and venules; affected organs may include skin, lung, brain, heart, and kidneys (necrotizing glomerulonephritis) ▪ Associated with relatively acute events, such as infection (including dysbiosis), drug administration, cancer, or administration of foreign protein	▪ Necrotizing vasculitis ▪ Dermal lesions are differentiated from those of PAN because lesions of leukocytoclastic vasculitis are all at the **same stage of development** (due to acute event) and these lesions are **palpable due to acute inflammation** ▪ P-ANCA is generally positive ▪ Immune complexes are *not* characteristic of the vascular lesions	▪ P-ANCA is generally positive ▪ "In general, the disease responds well to removal of the offending agent."[612]
<u>Churg-Strauss syndrome,</u> <u>allergic granulomatous</u> <u>angiitis</u>: affects small arteries all the way through to veins; variant of leukocytoclastic vasculitis	▪ Eosinophilia with bronchial asthma and sinusitis; mimics allergic sinusitis and allergic asthma ▪ Pulmonary and splenic vessel involvement; granulomas ▪ Associated with Henoch-Schonlein purpura, essential mixed cryoglobulinemia, and vasculitis of malignancy	▪ ANCA, particularly P-ANCA ▪ Eosinophilia
<u>Kawasaki disease;</u> <u>mucocutaneous lymph</u> <u>node syndrome</u>: affects small-large arteries, classically the coronary arteries of children	▪ Arteritis of the coronary arteries in children ▪ Mucocutaneous lymph node syndrome	▪ Coronary angiography ▪ High-dose aspirin therapy

---

[612] Mitchell RN, et al. *Pocket Companion to Robbins and Cotran Pathologic Basis of Disease, 7ᵗʰ Edition*. Philadelphia: Saunders Elsevier: 2006, page 279

Brief Mention / Additional Emphasis

Polymyalgia Rheumatica (PMR), Giant Cell Arteritis (GCA, previously Temporal Arteritis)

Introduction:
Giant cell arteritis (previously called temporal arteritis) and polymyalgia rheumatica are related conditions characterized histopathologically by inflammatory occlusion of small arteries and arterioles in the upper body: head, neck, shoulders. The possibility of arterial occlusion leading to blindness due to occlusion of the ophthalmic artery mandates early implementation of immunosuppressive prednisone (generally at 60mg/d or 1mg/kg/d). These patients must be co-managed with an Internal Medicine or Rheumatology specialist, while components of the Functional Inflammology protocol are appropriately applied.

Description/pathophysiology:

- This group of tightly related and largely synonymous disorders is described as "idiopathic" by medical textbooks.
- **Polymyalgia rheumatica (PMR)**: This disorder typically presents with painful inflammation of the shoulder/neck and hip muscles along with systemic manifestations of fever, malaise, and weight loss. When present in isolation (i.e., not with giant cell arteritis), it does not lead to blindness, and the condition responds to low-dose (10-20 mg) prednisone.
- **Giant Cell Arteritis (GCA):** When treated allopathically, GCA requires higher daily doses (40-60 mg) of prednisone than PMR. GCA can result in rapid-onset blindness and therefore any evidence of ocular involvement in a patient with GCA must be treated as a medical emergency. **Indeed, the diagnosis of GCA itself is considered urgent due to ability of blindness to occur rapidly and without warning.** GCA was previously called temporal arteritis. Approximately 50% of patients with GCA have PMR.

Clinical presentations:

- Pain and stiffness in proximal muscle groups: shoulders, neck, and hips; weakness—if any—is secondary to pain, disuse atrophy, drug side-effect (e.g., "steroid myopathy"), or other concomitant disorder. Presentations are consistent with muscle/tissue ischemia due to the underlying panarteritis which results in vessel occlusion: head pain, jaw claudication, blindness.
- Generally presents after age 50 years. The later age of onset helps distinguish PMR from fibromyalgia, which generally affects young adult patients between the ages of 20-40 years.
- 2x more common in women than in men.
- Typical autoimmune systemic manifestations: fatigue, malaise, fever, anorexia, and weight loss.
- Patients may have high fever and chills with disease initiation and/or exacerbation.

Major differential diagnoses:

- Fibromyalgia: ESR is normal, age of onset is nearly always before 50 years.
- Dermatomyositis, polymyositis: These conditions cause muscle weakness, which is characteristically absent in patients with PMR. Muscle enzymes are elevated in patients with dermatomyositis/polymyositis but are normal in patients with PMR.
- Cancer, particularly multiple myeloma
- Hypothyroidism: Hypothyroidism can easily mimic PMR by producing an inflammatory myopathy that affects the shoulder muscles and which remits following normalization of thyroid status.
- Rheumatoid arthritis, SLE, vasculitis, or other autoimmune disorder
- Infection: WBC count is normal in GCA/PMR and is generally elevated in patients with severe infection.
- Cervical spondylosis: Normal ESR and no anemia

Clinical assessments:

- **History/subjective:**
  - See clinical presentations
- **Physical examination/objective:**
  - Palpate pulses for strength and symmetry:
    - Carotid artery in the anterior neck
    - Axillary/brachial in the axilla and inner arm, respectively
    - Radial pulse at the distal radius
    - Aorta in the abdomen
    - Femoral pulses in the groin
    - Dorsalis pedis and posterior tibial arteries at the ankle/foot
- **Laboratory assessments:**
  - ESR: Most patients will have a very high ESR > 50 mm/h.
  - CBC: Anemia is common.
  - Chemistry/metabolic panel: Hepatic alkaline phosphatase is elevated in 20% of patients.
  - RF: generally negative
  - Muscle enzymes: are almost always normal.
  - Protein in urine, serum protein electrophoresis: No evidence of proteinuria or monoclonal gammopathy, as seen in MM.
- **Imaging:**
  - Not generally indicated except when looking for complications or concomitant disease
- **Establishing the diagnosis:**
  - PMR is a clinical diagnosis based on 1) painful inflammation of the shoulder/neck and hip muscles along with 2) systemic manifestations of fever, malaise, and weight loss and 3) the absence of evidence supporting an alternate diagnosis.[613]
  - GCA is classically diagnosed following biopsy of the temporal artery.
  - Pattern recognition (proximal muscle pain with no other explanation) and evidence of inflammation in an elderly patient when other diseases have been ruled out.

Complications:

- GCA can lead to blindness.
- Dry cough is seen in some patients and may be the presenting complaint.
- Mononeuritis multiplex may cause (shoulder) paralysis.
- Aneurysms of the thoracic aorta are 17x more common in patients with GCA than the general population

Clinical management:

- Assess for temporal arteritis—educate patient about the significance of the onset of eye symptoms, headache, and jaw claudication.
- A few patients treated with prednisone will have permanent remission within 2 years.

Treatments: Use this section in association with previously mentioned assessments and interventions.

    Drug treatments: This condition requires early implementation of prednisone immunosuppression; comanagement with a specialist—Internal Medicine or Rheumatology—is mandatory.

- Prednisone: 10-20 mg per day for PMR should result in "dramatic improvement" within 72 hours.[614] Prednisone dose for GCA is typically 60 mg per day at the start of treatment in order to prevent one of the most feared complications—blindness. Dose is tapered after clinical remission. Low-dose aspirin appears to reduce the risk of blindness and stroke in GCA patients.

---

[613] Tierney ML. McPhee SJ, Papadakis MA. *Current Medical Diagnosis and Treatment. 35th edition*. Stamford: Appleton and Lange, 1996 page 751. Tierney ML. McPhee SJ, Papadakis MA (eds). *Current Medical Diagnosis and Treatment 2006. 45th edition*. New York; Lange Medical Books: 2006, pages 486
[614] Tierney ML. McPhee SJ, Papadakis MA (eds). *Current Medical Diagnosis and Treatment 2006. 45th edition*. New York; Lange Medical Books: 2006, pages 487

Brief Mention / Additional Emphasis

ANCA-associated vasculitis, ANCA vasculitis (formerly known as Wegener's granulomatosis)

Introduction:

ANCA-associated vasculitis, formerly named Wegener's granulomatosis and here abbreviated as "ANCA vasculitis" avoid the unnecessary redundancy of the word "associated", is a granulomatous and vasculitic disease with a high mortality. Insight into the molecular basis of the condition—electrostatic haptenization of the *Staphylococcus aureus* enzyme acid phosphatase with endothelial cells—provides brilliant insight into the disease and its treatment. The possible role of other microbes, along with other factors such as immunophenotype imbalance should be intuitive by this time to readers who have read the other chapters.

Description/pathophysiology:

- This inflammatory condition generally begins with granulomatous involvement of the upper or lower respiratory tract and then progresses to systemic vasculitis and glomerulonephritis.
- Biopsy of nasopharyngeal/pulmonary/renal lesions reveals granulomatous/inflammatory tissue.
- Allopathic textbooks generally describe this condition as *idiopathic*, although the condition is increasingly associated with occult sinorespiratory dysbiosis with *Staphylococcus aureus*.[615,616] Additionally, *Klebsiella aerogenes, Haemophilus influenzae,* and *Bacillus subtilis* have been implicated.[617]
- Immune complexes contribute to pathophysiology

Clinical presentations:

- Twice as common in males as in females
- Sinorespiratory symptoms:
  - Mucosal ulcerations/friability, hemorrhagic rhinorrhea
  - Persistent sinusitis; increased incidence of otitis media
  - Cough, hemoptosis due to intraalveolar hemorrhage, pleuritis
- Renal complications are inevitable without effective/immunosuppressive treatment
- Typical autoimmune systemic manifestations: fatigue, malaise, low-grade fever, anorexia, and weight loss, polyarthritis.

Eponymic retractions: replacing of Reiter's syndrome with "reactive arthritis" and of Wegener's granulomatosus with "ANCA-associated vasculitis" or "granulomatosis with polyangiitis"

Reiter and Wegener were both actively involved in war crimes and support of Nazi atrocities during World War 2, and they have both been stripped of their eponymic recognition.
- Reiter's syndrome is now "reactive arthritis",
- Wegener's granulomatosus is now "ANCA-associated vasculitis" or "granulomatosis with polyangiitis"

Scheinberg MA. Nazi past and changes in disease names: the Wegener's disease case. *Rev Bras Reumatol* 2012 Mar. Panush et al. Retraction of the suggestion to use the term "Reiter's syndrome" sixty-five years later. *Arthritis Rheum* 2007 Feb

---

Major differential diagnoses:

- Extramedullary plasmacytoma of multiple myeloma (typically occurs in the nasopharyngeal region)
- Sinus infection
- Lung cancer
- Tuberculosis
- Septicemia or septic arthritis
- Lymphoma
- Other systemic/inflammatory disorder such as lupus (ANA and low complement)
- Bacterial endocarditis

Clinical assessments:

- **History/subjective**: See clinical presentations.

---

[615] Brons RH, Bakker HI, Van Wijk RT, et al. Staphylococcal acid phosphatase binds to endothelial cells via charge interaction; a pathogenic role in Wegener's granulomatosis? *Clin Exp Immunol*. 2000 Mar;119(3):566-73 blackwell-synergy.com/doi/abs/10.1046/j.1365-2249.2000.01172.x
[616] Popa ER, et al. Staphylococcus aureus and Wegener's granulomatosis. *Arthritis Res*. 2002;4(2):77-9 arthritis-research.com/content/4/2/77
[617] George J, et al. Infections and Wegener's granulomatosis—a cause and effect relationship? *QJM*. 1997 May;90(5):367-73 qjmed.oxfordjournals.org/cgi/reprint/90/5/367

- **Physical examination/objective**:
  - Examination of oral and nasal mucosa
  - Pulmonary auscultation
  - Dermatologic screen for cutaneous vasculitis
- **Laboratory assessments**:
  - Urinalysis for assessment of renal status
  - Chemistry/metabolic panel for BUN and creatinine, etc.
  - Microbial assessments—reviewed in Chapters 1 and 4.
  - Nasal culture for *Staphylococcus aureus*[618] and other bacterial or fungal contaminants
  - Complement levels are normal or elevated
  - ESR/CRP is elevated
  - CBC may reveal leukocytosis and anemia
  - **ANA (antinuclear antibodies) are generally absent**
  - **ANCA are almost always present and strongly support the diagnosis of this condition. The finding of the more specific C-ANCA is 97% specific for the diagnosis of ANCA vasculitis.**[619] Interestingly, ANCA can also be induced by gastrointestinal parasitic infections.
- **Imaging**: Generally not required; only indicated as needed
- **Establishing the diagnosis**: Based on clinical, serologic, and biopsy findings.
  - Respiratory tract symptoms and mucosal lesions; biopsy of granulomas.
  - C-ANCA: Positive C-ANCA result can replace biopsy in a patient with a clinical picture of ANCA vasculitis.[620]

Complications:
- Severe anemia requiring blood transfusion
- Secondary bacterial infections on ulcerated mucosa
- Respiratory and renal failure
- Hypoxic complications due to vasculitis

Clinical management:
- Referral to internist/rheumatologist for additional treatment and defensive management as indicated. Unless you are a specialist, you need to have a specialist as part of the care team who can help you manage acute exacerbations which can occur with any autoimmune/inflammatory disease.

Therapeutic considerations: Medical treatment routinely includes the following:[621]
- Cyclophosphamide: 1-2 mg/kg/d PO or IV: associated with increased risk for cancer, particularly bladder cancer
- Prednisone: 1 mg/kg/d po; use the lowest dose possible
- Methotrexate: pulse treatment < 20-30 mg per week po
- **Antibiotic treatment: Bactrim / trimeth-sulfa 160/800 up to 480/2400 mg/d po**
- Blood transfusions for anemia
- **Assessment for multifocal dysbiosis: emphasis on gastrointestinal and sinorespiratory dysbiosis**
  - *Staphylococcus aureus*: Produces an antigenic acid phosphatase which haptenizes with endothelial cells for the induction of autoimmune vasculitis in ANCA vasculitis.[622]
    - Drugs: Antimicrobial treatment—typically with Bactrim—to eradicate *Staphylococcus aureus* results in clinical remission of the "autoimmune" disease, thus proving the microbe-rheumatic link.[623]
    - Herbs: Hyperforin from *Hypericum perforatum* shows in vitro effectiveness against *Staphylococcus aureus*.[624]

[618] Brons RH, Bakker HI, Van Wijk RT, et al. Staphylococcal acid phosphatase binds to endothelial cells via charge interaction; a pathogenic role in Wegener's granulomatosis? *Clin Exp Immunol*. 2000 Mar;119(3):566-73 blackwell-synergy.com/doi/abs/10.1046/j.1365-2249.2000.01172.x P
[619] Beers MH, Berkow R (eds). *The Merck Manual. Seventeenth Edition*. Whitehouse Station; Merck Research Laboratories 1999 Page 443
[620] Shojania K. Rheumatology: 2. What laboratory tests are needed? *CMAJ*. 2000 Apr 18;162(8):1157-63 cmaj.ca/cgi/content/full/162/8/1157
[621] Beers MH, Berkow R (eds). *Merck Manual. 17th Edition*. Whitehouse Station; Merck Research Laboratories 1999 Page 443
[622] Brons et al. Staphylococcal acid phosphatase binds to endothelial cells via charge interaction in Wegener's granulomatosis? *Clin Exp Immunol*. 2000 Mar;119(3):566-73
[623] Popa ER, et al. Staphylococcus aureus and Wegener's granulomatosis. *Arthritis Res*. 2002;4(2):77-9 arthritis-research.com/content/4/2/077
[624] Schempp et al. Antibacterial activity of hyperforin from St John's wort, against multiresistant Staphylococcus aureus and gram-positive bacteria. *Lancet*. 1999 Jun;353:2129

- ▪ <u>Topical antiseptic</u>: Intranasal 5% povidone iodine is highly effective against *Staphylococcus aureus*; Among 1,697 patients undergoing arthroplasty or spine fusion surgery, 5% povidone iodine proved better tolerated, safer, less expensive and more effective with greater compliance compared with intranasal mupirocin.[625]
   - ○ *Entamoeba histolytica*: *Entamoeba histolytica* induces formation of antineutrophil cytoplasmic antibodies (ANCA).[626] Stool testing with a specialty laboratory is recommended.
   - ○ <u>Other microbes such as *Klebsiella aerogenes, Haemophilus influenzae* and *Bacillus subtilis*</u>: These have also been implicated in ANCA vasculitis.[627]
- • <u>Vitamin D3 supplementation with physiologic doses and/or tailored to serum 25(OH)D levels</u>: Since ANCA vasculitis is a *granulomatous* disease, caution and frequent monitoring must be employed when optimizing vitamin D status to avoid hypercalcemia; ANCA vasculitis can result in hypercalcemia mediated by elevated 1,25-dihydroxyvitamin D [1,25(OH)2D].[628] A reasonable clinical approach would be to start with testing of serum 25(OD)D, serum 1,25(OH)2D, and serum calcium (See Chapter 1 for review of Laboratory Association); thereafter, if necessary, start with a relatively low dose cholecalciferol 1,000-2,000 IU/d following the exclusion of hypercalcemia. Thereafter, serum calcium can be measured at 2 weeks, 4 weeks, 6 weeks, 8 weeks, and monthly/periodically thereafter.
- • <u>Assess for heavy metals, especially mercury</u>: Exposure to mercury and lead is associated with increased risk of developing ANCA vasculitis.[629] Consider urine toxic metal assessment following 10-30 mg/kg DMSA as described in Chapter 4 and as described elsewhere for the assessment of heavy metals in patients with autism.[630]
- • <u>Proteolytic enzymes</u>: ANCA vasculitis is mediated in large part by IgG and IgA immune complexes, which directly contribute to vasculitis and nephritis.[631] Polyenzyme supplementation has been used to ameliorate the pathophysiology induced by immune complexes in other conditions.[632]

- • <u>FOOD & NUTRITION: 5-part "supplemented Paleo-Mediterranean diet" (SPMD)</u> The 5-part "supplemented Paleo-Mediterranean diet" (SPMD—reviewed in Chapter 4) consists of ❶ foundational plant-based low-carbohydrate diet of fruits, vegetables, nuts, seeds, berries and lean sources of protein, ❷ multivitamin and multimineral supplementation, ❸ physiologic doses of vitamin D3 (range 2,000-10,000 IU/d), ❹ combination fatty acid therapy (CFAT) with n3-ALA, n6-GLA, n3-EPA, n3-DHA, and phytochemical-rich olive oil which contains n9-oleate, and ❺ probiotics.
   - ○ <u>Avoidance of allergenic, inflammatory, and SIBO-promoting foods</u>: Hypoallergenic diets can benefit patients with immune-complex-mediated diseases such as mixed cryoglobulinemia[633,634], hypersensitivity vasculitis[635], and leukocystoclastic vasculitis with arthritis.[636] Any patient may be allergic to any food, even if the food is generally considered a health-promoting food. Generally speaking, the most notorious allergens are wheat, citrus (especially juice due to the industrial use of fungal hemicellulases), cow's milk, eggs, peanuts, chocolate, and yeast-containing foods. According to a study

[625] London S. Nasal povidone-iodine cuts postop infections. *Internal Medicine News Digital Network* 2012 Nov. internalmedicinenews.com/news/conference-news/idweek-2012/single-article/nasal-povidone-iodine-cuts-postop-infections/fabb79e1a44f38b7318f060284a6018f.html

[626] George J, Levy Y, Kallenberg CG, Shoenfeld Y. Infections and Wegener's granulomatosis—a cause and effect relationship? *QJM.* 1997 May;90(5):367-73

[627] George J, Levy Y, Kallenberg CG, Shoenfeld Y. Infections and Wegener's granulomatosis—a cause and effect relationship? *QJM.* 1997 May;90(5):367-73

[628] "Furthermore, in view of this case and two other recently reported cases, we believe that Wegener's granulomatosis must be definitively added to the list of granulomatous diseases that are responsible for 1,25(OH)2D-mediated hypercalcemia." Bosch et al. Vitamin D metabolite-mediated hypercalcemia in Wegener's granulomatosis. *Mayo Clin Proc.* 1997 May;72(5):440-4

[629] "Results suggest that mercury and perhaps lead exposure were positively associated with WG as compared with either control group, although the number of patients exposed was small… CONCLUSION: We conclude that heavy metal exposure and a prior history of allergy may play a role in the etiopathogenesis of Wegener's granulomatosis." Albert D, et al. Wegener's granulomatosis: Possible role of environmental agents in its pathogenesis. *Arthritis Rheum.* 2004 Aug 15;51(4):656-64

[630] Bradstreet et al. A case-control study of mercury burden in children with autistic spectrum disorders. *J Am Physicians Surgeons* 2003; 8: 76-79 jpands.org/vol8no3/geier.pdf

[631] "RESULTS: Four of 11 biopsies taken at initial presentation and four of 21 biopsies taken at the onset of a relapse of WG showed IgG and/or IgA containing immune deposits in the subepidermal blood vessels. …CONCLUSION: A substantial number of skin biopsies showed immune deposits during active disease. These results could support the hypothesis that immune complexes may trigger vasculitic lesions in WG." Brons et al. Detection of immune deposits in skin lesions of patients with Wegener's granulomatosis. *Ann Rheum Dis.* 2001 Dec;60(12):1097-102 ard.bmjjournals.com/cgi/content/full/60/12/1097

[632] Galebskaya et al. Human complement system state after wobenzyme intake. *Vestnik Moskovskogo Universiteta (Seriya 2: Khimiya).* 2000:41(6 Suppl): 148-149 chem.msu.ru/eng/journals/vmgu/00add/148.pdf

[633] "CONCLUSION: These data show that an LAC diet decreases the amount of circulating immune complexes in MC and can modify certain signs and symptoms of the disease." Ferri C, Pietrograndc M, Cecchetti R, et al. Low-antigen-content diet in the treatment of patients with mixed cryoglobulinemia. *Am J Med.* 1989 Nov;87:519-24

[634] Pietrograndc M, Cefalo A, Nicora F, Marchesini D. Dietetic treatment of essential mixed cryoglobulinemia. *Ric Clin Lab.* 1986 Apr-Jun;16(2):413-6

[635] "In three cases the vasculitis relapsed following the introduction of food additives; in one case with the addition of potatoes and green vegetables (i.e., beans and green peas) and in the last case with the addition of eggs to the diet." Lunardi et al. Elimination diet in the treatment of selected patients with hypersensitivity vasculitis. *Clin Exp Rheumatol.* 1992 Mar-Apr;10(2):131-5

[636] "Described in this report are two children with severe vasculitis caused by specific foods." Businco et al. Severe food-induced vasculitis in two children. *Pediatr Allergy Immunol.* 2002 Feb;13(1):68-71

in patients with migraine, some patients will have to avoid as many as 10 specific foods in order to become symptom-free.[637] The severe wheat allergy *celiac disease* can present with inflammatory oligoarthritis[638,639], and celiac disease can also present as cryoglobulinemia and vasculitis[640], cutaneous leukocystoclastic vasculitis[641], including cerebral vasculitis[642] and pediatric stroke.[643] High glycemic foods suppress immune function[644,645] and thus promote the perpetuation of infection/dysbiosis. Delivery of a high carbohydrate load to the gastrointestinal lumen promotes bacterial overgrowth[646,647], which is inherently pro-inflammatory[648,649] and which promotes immune complex formation. Wheat consumption induces formation for immune complexes in virtually everyone (i.e., people who are "apparently healthy")[650], including as expected (but certainly not limited to) patients with dermatitis herpetiformis.[651] Vegetarian/vegan diets have a place in the treatment plan of all patients with autoimmune/inflammatory disorders[652,653]; this is also true for patients for whom long-term exclusive reliance on a meat-free vegetarian diet is either not appropriate or not appealing. No legitimate scientist or literate clinician doubts the antirheumatic power and anti-inflammatory advantages of vegetarian diets, whether used short-term or long term.[654] Patients who rely on the Paleo-Mediterranean Diet can use vegetarian meals, on a daily basis or for days at a time, for example, by having a daily vegetarian meal, or one week per month of vegetarianism. Of course, some (not all) patients can use a purely vegetarian diet long-term provided that nutritional needs (especially protein and cobalamin) are consistently met.

Wheat and circulating immune complexes in "healthy" disease-free persons: clinical findings relevant to vasculitis

- Circulating immune complexes (CICs) in blood are associated with autoimmune-diseases such as systemic lupus erythematosus, immune complex glomerulonephritis, rheumatoid arthritis and vasculitis. However, slightly increased serum concentrations of such CICs are sometimes also found in healthy individuals. The objective of the current study was to assess whether food antigens could play a role in the formation of CICs.
- MATERIAL AND METHODS: A total of **352 (265 F, 87 M), so far, healthy individuals** were tested for CICs containing C1q and immunoglobulin G (IgG) as well as for gliadin IgG antibodies using the ELISA technique.
- RESULTS: In our study, 15.3% (54/352) of the patients presented with elevated CIC concentrations (above 50 microg/ml) and 6.5% (23/352) of the study population were positive for gliadin IgG antibodies (above 20 U/ml). **CIC concentration levels were significantly higher in the group with elevated gliadin IgG antibodies** (CIC median: 49.0 microg/ml) **compared with the group with normal levels of gliadin IgG antibodies** (CIC median: 30.0 microg/ml; Mann-Whitney U-test, U=1992; p <0.001). ...
- CONCLUSIONS: **The results of this study indicate that certain food antigens (e.g. gluten) could play a role in the formation of CICs.** ...

Eisenmann et al. *Scand J Gastroenterol.* 2009

---

[637] Grant EC. Food allergies and migraine. *Lancet.* 1979 May 5;1(8123):966-9
[638] "We report six patients with coeliac disease in whom arthritis was prominent at diagnosis and who improved with dietary therapy. Joint pain preceded diagnosis by up to three years in five patients and 15 years in one patient." Bourne et al. Arthritis and coeliac disease. *Ann Rheum Dis.* 1985 Sep;44(9):592-8
[639] "A 15-year-old girl, with synovitis of the knees and ankles for 3 years before a diagnosis of gluten-sensitive enteropathy, is described." Pinals RS. Arthritis associated with gluten-sensitive enteropathy. *J Rheumatol.* 1986 Feb;13(1):201-4
[640] "Immunosuppressive treatment led to a normalization of transaminase levels and resolved the cryoglobulinaemic vasculitis. In addition, the patient exhibited low ferritin and iron levels, which led to the diagnosis of coeliac disease." Biecker E, Stieger M, Zimmermann A, Reichen J. Autoimmune hepatitis, cryoglobulinaemia and untreated coeliac disease: a case report. *Eur J Gastroenterol Hepatol.* 2003 Apr;15(4):423-7
[641] "A 38 year old female, with chronic uncontrolled coeliac disease, presented with the rare complication of cutaneous leucocytoclastic vasculitis." Meyers S, Dikman S, Spiera H, Schultz N, Janowitz HD. Cutaneous vasculitis complicating coeliac disease. *Gut.* 1981 Jan;22(1):61-4
[642] "A 51-year-old white man with celiac disease presented with seizures unresponsive to medical therapy." Rush PJ, Inman R, Bernstein M, Carlen P, Resch L. Isolated vasculitis of the central nervous system in a patient with celiac disease. *Am J Med.* 1986 Dec;81(6):1092-4
[643] "Because celiac disease is a potentially treatable cause of cerebral vasculopathy, serology-specifically antitissue transglutaminase antibodies-should be included in the evaluation for cryptogenic stroke in childhood, even in absence of typical gut symptoms." Goodwin et al. Celiac disease and childhood stroke. *Pediatr Neurol* 2004 Aug;31:139-42
[644] Sanchez A, Reeser JL, Lau HS, et al. Role of sugars in human neutrophilic phagocytosis. *Am J Clin Nutr.* 1973 Nov;26(11):1180-4
[645] "Postoperative infusion of carbohydrate solution leads to moderate fall in the serum concentration of inorganic phosphate. ... The hypophosphatemia was associated with significant reduction of neutrophil phagocytosis, intracellular killing, consumption of oxygen and generation of superoxide during phagocytosis." Rasmussen A, Segel E, Hessov I, Borregaard N. Reduced function of neutrophils during routine postoperative glucose infusion. *Acta Chir Scand.* 1988 Jul-Aug;154(7-8):429-33
[646] Ramakrishnan T, Stokes P. Beneficial effects of fasting and low carbohydrate diet in D-lactic acidosis associated with short-bowel syndrome. *JPEN J Parenter Enteral Nutr.* 1985 May-Jun;9(3):361-3
[647] Gottschall E. *Breaking the Vicious Cycle: Intestinal Health through Diet.* Kirkton Press; Rev edition (August 1, 1994)
[648] Lin HC. Small intestinal bacterial overgrowth: a framework for understanding irritable bowel syndrome. *JAMA.* 2004 Aug 18;292(7):852-8
[649] Lichtman et al. Reactivation of arthritis induced by small bowel bacterial overgrowth in rats: role of cytokines, bacteria, and bacterial polymers. *Infect Immun.* 1995 Jun;63(6):2295-301
[650] Eisenmann A, Murr C, Fuchs D, Ledochowski M. Gliadin IgG antibodies and circulating immune complexes. *Scand J Gastroenterol.* 2009;44(2):168-71
[651] Zone JJ, et al. Induction of IgA circulating immune complexes after wheat feeding in dermatitis herpetiformis patients. *J Invest Dermatol.* 1982 May;78(5):375-80
[652] "After four weeks at the health farm the diet group showed a significant improvement in number of tender joints, Ritchie's articular index, number of swollen joints, pain score, duration of morning stiffness, grip strength, erythrocyte sedimentation rate, white blood cell count, and a health assessment questionnaire score." Kjeldsen-Kragh J, et al. Controlled trial of fasting and one-year vegetarian diet in rheumatoid arthritis. *Lancet.* 1991 Oct 12;338(8772):899-902
[653] "During the vegan diet, both signs and symptoms returned in most patients, with the exception of some patients with psoriasis who experienced an improvement." Lithell H, et al. A fasting and vegetarian diet treatment trial on chronic inflammatory disorders. *Acta Derm Venereol.* 1983;63(5):397-403
[654] "For the patients who were randomised to the vegetarian diet there was a significant decrease in platelet count, leukocyte count, calprotectin, total IgG, IgM rheumatoid factor (RF), C3-activation products, and the complement components C3 and C4 after one month of treatment." Kjeldsen-Kragh et al. Changes in laboratory variables in rheumatoid arthritis patients during a trial of fasting and one-year vegetarian diet. *Scand J Rheumatol.* 1995;24(2):85-93

- **INFECTIONS & DYSBIOSIS: ❶ antimicrobial treatments, ❷ immunorestoration, ❸ immunotolerance via Treg induction** Essentially all autoimmune/rheumatic disorders are associated with microbial colonization and intolerance to same; the presence of persistent microbial colonization is *prima facie* evidence of immunosuppression. The eight areas of dysbiosis (multifocal) are: ❶ sinorespiratory, ❷ orodental, ❸ gastrointestinal, ❹ urogenital/genitourinary, ❺ parenchymal/tissue, ❻ microbial, ❼ dermal/cutaneous, and ❽ environmental. The following survey of the literature serves to remind clinicians of possible underlying infectious contributions to vasculitic diseases:

  o Viral infections associated with Kawasaki disease (*J Formos Med Assoc.* 2014 Mar[655]): "We enrolled 226 children with KD and 226 age- and sex-matched healthy children from February 2004 to March 2010. Throat and nasopharyngeal swabs were taken for both viral isolation and polymerase chain reaction (PCR) for various viruses. ...Cases of KD had a significantly higher positive rate of viral isolation in comparison with the control group (7.5% vs. 2.2%, p = 0.02). Compared with the control group, cases of KD were more likely to have overall positive rates of viral PCR (50.4% vs. 16.4%, p < 0.001) and for various viruses including enterovirus (16.8% vs. 4.4%, p < 0.001), adenovirus (8.0% vs. 1.8%, p = 0.007), human rhinovirus (26.5% vs. 9.7%, p < 0.001), and coronavirus (7.1% vs. 0.9%, p = 0.003)."

  o Ischemic retinal vasculitis in an 18-year-old man with chickenpox infection (*Clin Ophthalmol.* 2014 Feb[656]): "We report a case of a healthy 18-year-old man who presented with unilateral ischemic retinal vasculitis 10 days after the onset of chickenpox. ... Fundus imaging, optical coherence tomography, fundus fluorescence angiography, and electrophysiologic studies confirmed the diagnosis of retinal vasculitis, which led to generalized retinal ischemia."

  o Antineutrophil cytoplasmic antibody-associated vasculitis associated with Epstein-Barr virus infection (*Infection* 2014 Jun[657]): "Although a previous study indicated that there was a high positive rate of ANCA in the sera positive for IgM antibodies to EBV and EBV infection might trigger the relapse of AAV, this is the first case of incipient AAV associated with acute EBV infection. One possible explanation might be that EBV infection stimulated the production of ANCA."

  o Cytomegalovirus-related necrotizing vasculitis mimicking Henoch-Schönlein syndrome (*Clin Exp Rheumatol.* 2014 May[658]): "The causative role of viral infection was revealed by the presence of CMV DNA in patient's blood and positive IgG titer against the virus. ... Our report suggests that CMV vasculitis is probably more frequent than previously thought, even in immunocompetent patients, with a protean clinical presentation, mimicking other types of vasculitides."

  o Hepatitis C virus infection and its rheumatologic implications. *Gastroenterol Hepatol* 2014 May[659]): "Symptoms of HCV infection and rheumatic diseases may be similar and include arthralgia, myalgia, arthritis, and vasculitis. ...It is imperative to distinguish whether symptoms such as arthralgia, myalgia, and arthritis occur in patients with HCV infection due to primary chronic HCV infection or to a newly developed rheumatologic disease process."

  o Vasculitis and anaphylactoid shock induced in mice by cell wall extract of the fungus Candida metapsilosis (*Pol J Microbiol.* 2014[660]): "Our results show that intraperitoneal injection of cell wall extracts induced severe coronary arteritis, and intravenous injection induced acute anaphylactoid shock similar to extracts from Candida albicans (C. albicans)."

  o Varicella zoster virus in the temporal artery of a patient with giant cell arteritis (*J Neurol Sci.* 2013 Dec[661]): "We recently detected varicella zoster virus (VZV) in the temporal arteries (TA) of 5/24 patients with clinically suspect giant cell arteritis (GCA) whose TAs were GCA-negative pathologically; in those GCA-negative, VZV+TAs, virus antigen predominated in the arterial adventitia, but without medial necrosis and multinucleated giant cells. During our continuing search for VZV antigen in GCA-negative TAs, in

[655] Chang et al. Viral infections associated with Kawasaki disease. *J Formos Med Assoc.* 2014 Mar;113(3):148-54
[656] Poonyathalang et al. Ischemic retinal vasculitis in an 18-year-old man with chickenpox infection. *Clin Ophthalmol.* 2014 Feb 24;8:441-3
[657] Xu et al. Antineutrophil cytoplasmic antibody-associated vasculitis associated with Epstein-Barr virus infection: a case report and review of the literature. *Infection.* 2014 Jun;42(3):591-4
[658] D'Alessandro et al. Cytomegalovirus-related necrotising vasculitis mimicking Henoch-Schönlein syndrome. *Clin Exp Rheumatol.* 2014 May-Jun;32(3 Suppl 82):S73-5
[659] Sayiner et al. Hepatitis C virus infection and its rheumatologic implications. *Gastroenterol Hepatol* 2014 May;10(5):287-93
[660] Tada et al. Vasculitis and anaphylactoid shock induced in mice by cell wall extract of the fungus Candida metapsilosis. *Pol J Microbiol.* 2014;63(2):223-30
[661] Nagel et al. Varicella zoster virus in the temporal artery of a patient with giant cell arteritis. *J Neurol Sci.* 2013 Dec 15;335(1-2):228-30

the TA of one subject, we found abundant VZV antigen, as well as VZV DNA, in multiple regions (skip areas) of the TA spanning 350 [micrometers], as well as in skeletal muscle adjacent to the infected TA."

- o Is giant cell arteritis an infectious disease? (*Presse Med.* 2004 Nov[662]): "Simultaneous occurrence of peaks of GCA/PMR and respiratory infections have been observed in Denmark. Several viruses have been suspected as triggers and assessed by serological testing, PCR or immunostaining on temporal artery biopsies, or both techniques: the hepatitis B virus can be ruled out, as well as Herpes simplex 1 and 2, Herpes varicellae, Epstein-Barr virus and cytomegalovirus. Recent studies focused on parainfluenza virus, Parvovirus B19 and Chlamydia pneumoniae. Immunological studies suggest, at the origin of the inflammatory reaction leading to the typical pathological features of giant cell arteritis, the existence of a triggering antigen of unknown nature activating T-cells in the artery wall."

> | **Endocrine imbalance in PMR/GCA** |
> |---|
> | "Patients with PMR/GCA with new-onset active disease before steroid treatment have inappropriately normal cortisol levels regarding the ongoing inflammation, and significantly lower levels of DHEAS compared to the age- and sex-matched healthy control subjects. These data support the existence of a relative adrenal hypofunction in PMR and GCA." |
> | Narvaez et al. *J Rheumatol* 2006;33:1293-8 |

- **NUTRITIONAL IMMUNOMODULATION: Treg induction for modulation of Th-1/2/17 inflammation** Nutrients and therapeutic approaches that promote Treg or IL-10 induction and/or Th-17, IL-17 suppression include 1) mitochondrial optimization and mTOR suppression, 2) biotin, 3) vitamin E, 4) sodium avoidance, 5) transgenic/GMO food avoidance, 6) probiotics, 7) lipoic acid, 8) vitamin A, 9) inflammation reduction, 10) vitamin D, 11) fatty acid supplementation with GLA and n3, 12) infection and dysbiosis remediation, 13) green tea EGCG. Acronym: MiBESTPLAIDFIG.

- **DYSMETABOLISM & DYSFUNCTIONAL MITOCHONDRIA: MitoDys, ERS-UPR, AGE/RAGE, hyperglycemia and ceramide** The major clinical considerations in this section are mitochondrial dysfunction, endoplasmic reticulum stress, unfolded protein response, TLR activation, and the dysmetabolic effects of sustained hyperglycemia and hyperinsulinemia and resultant oxidative stress, inflammation, RAGE activation, and accumulation of AGE, palmitate and ceramide. The review of this information in Chapter 4 covered approximately 30 interventions relevant to dysmetabolism, mitochondrial dysfunction, ERS-UPR, etc; these will not be reviewed here except to mention those most commonly, easily, empirically, synergistically, and effectively used: 1) low-carbohydrate diet with 2) moderate exercise, 3) CoQ-10, 4) acetyl-carnitine with 5) lipoic acid, 6) NAC, 7) resveratrol, and 8) melatonin. See extensive review in Chapter 4.4.

- **STYLE OF LIVING (LIFESTYLE) & SPECIAL CONSIDERATIONS:** This is a buffet of mostly lifestyle-based interventions yet also including considerations such as somatic treatments, additional supplementation, and surgery. See Chapter 4, Section 5 for details.

- **ENDOCRINE IMBALANCE & OPTIMIZATION: Prolactin, Insulin, Estrogen, DHEA, Cortisol, Testosterone, Thyroid** Common hormonal imbalances seen among autoimmune/inflammatory patients are: ❶ *elevated* prolactin, ❷ *elevated* estrogen, ❸ *elevated* insulin, and ❹ *reduced* DHEA, ❺ *reduced* cortisol, and ❻ *reduced* testosterone; see Chapter 4 for discussion of these hormones and respective interventions. Thyroid evaluation (patient + labs) should be comprehensive, as discussed in Chapter 1, with a low threshold for empiric treatment.

  - o Orthoendocrinology and Dysendocrinism: Assess prolactin, cortisol, DHEA, free and total testosterone, serum estradiol, and thyroid status (e.g., TSH, T4, *and* anti-thyroid peroxidase antibodies). Correct as indicated (see Chapter 4). **Prolactin levels are typically elevated in patients with PMR and correlate with clinical symptomatology.**[663] Adrenal hypofunction in patients with PR/GCA is suggested by the relative insufficiencies of cortisol and DHEA.[664] **DHEA (insufficiency and supraphysiologic supplementation):** Patients with autoimmunity should be tested for DHEA insufficiency by

---

[662] Duhaut P, Bosshard S, Ducroix JP. Is giant cell arteritis an infectious disease? *Presse Med.* 2004 Nov 6;33(19 Pt 2):1403-8
[663] Straub RH, Georgi J, Helmke K, Vaith P, Lang B. In polymyalgia rheumatica serum prolactin is positively correlated with the number of typical symptoms but not with typical inflammatory markers. *Rheumatology* (Oxford). 2002 Apr;41(4):423-9 rheumatology.oxfordjournals.org/cgi/content/full/41/4/423
[664] "Patients with PMR/GCA with new-onset active disease before steroid treatment have inappropriately normal cortisol levels regarding the ongoing inflammation, and significantly lower levels of DHEAS compared to the age- and sex-matched healthy control subjects. These data support the existence of a relative adrenal hypofunction in PMR and GCA." Narvaez et al. Low serum levels of DHEAS in untreated polymyalgia rheumatica/giant cell arteritis. *J Rheumatol.* 2006 Jul;33(7):1293-8. Epub 2006 Jun 15

measurement of serum DHEA-sulfate; insufficiencies should generally be corrected except in cases of concomitant hormone-responsive cancer such as breast cancer or prostate cancer. The rationale for using high-dose DHEA in patients with autoimmune diseases is reviewed in Chapter 4.

- **XENOBIOTIC ACCUMULATION & DETOXIFICATION: Chemical avoidance, nutritional support for detoxification pathways, urine alkalinization** The clinical relevance and pathogenic mechanisms of xenobiotic accumulation are irrefutably well documented and described. Clinical assessments include history, physical examination, and laboratory assessment (using serum, whole blood, urine or—rarely yet accurately— fat biopsy), and response to treatment. Treatments include nutritional support for Phases 1 and 2 of detoxification (e.g., oxidation and conjugation) and excretion via bile and urine; for the latter, urinary alkalinization is generally recommended. Chemical toxins can be bound in the gut using activated charcoal, cholestyramine, or *Chlorella*—all of these three treatments have documented safety and effectiveness; clinically and empirically, phytochelatin (plant-derived peptides that bind toxic metals) concentrates appear safe and effective despite lack of conclusive published data supporting clinical use.

Spondyloarthropathies: Axial Inflammatory Conditions
Ankylosing spondylitis
Reactive arthritis (previously Reiter's syndrome)
Enteropathic spondyloarthropathy, enteropathic arthritis

Axial inflammation as yet another *pattern of inflammation*
Spinal/axial inflammatory conditions are patterns of inflammation with etiologic factors consistent with the pattern reviewed throughout this textbook and surveyed in Chapter 4; likewise therefore, similar therapeutic concepts are applicable. As always, pharmacologic immunosuppression may be urgently needed if a patient experiences exacerbation or inflammatory complication; however, routine "chronic" pharmacologic immunosuppression offers no hope of authentically curing the disease and correcting the underlying imbalances: it only suppresses manifestations of underlying physiologic imbalances.

Description/pathophysiology:

- Inflammatory arthropathies affecting the spine and sacroiliac joints are termed "spondyloarthropathies" and like other arthritic conditions are termed *seronegative* if not related to rheumatoid arthritis in general and RF positivity in particular. **The spondyloarthropathies differ in some aspects of their etiologies, affected populations, clinical presentations, and treatment; however—regarding etiology and treatment—the similarities far outnumber the differences.** Regarding clinical management, from both allopathic and integrative/naturopathic perspectives, the treatment and management of these different conditions is virtually identical, save for a few important nuances.

- Spondyloarthropathies and reactive arthritis differ from the classic pattern of other autoimmune conditions in that 1) most patients affected are male, 2) they are highly correlated with HLA-B27, 3) serologic evidence of autoimmunity is generally absent, 4) they are strongly associated with dysbiosis, infections, and/or occult or overt enteropathy.[665,666]

- Some variation exists in the conditions that are included under the heading of *Spondyloarthropathies*. Most medical textbooks include four disorders under the heading of spondyloarthropathies: 1) ankylosing spondylitis, 2) psoriatic arthritis, 3) reactive arthritis, and 4) enteropathic spondyloarthropathy (ES), while a few others go on to include 5) juvenile spondyloarthropathy, and 6) rheumatoid arthritis. Psoriatic arthritis (PsA) and rheumatoid arthritis (RA) are detailed in their own chapters in this book and therefore will not be discussed in great detail here.

- Although ankylosing spondylitis (AS) is the prototype of the spondyloarthropathies, reactive arthritis (ReA) is the best-known and most well accepted model for microbe-induced musculoskeletal autoimmunity. Despite nearly overwhelming research demonstrating that all of these conditions are triggered by exposure to microbes, major medical textbooks[667] still describe these conditions as *idiopathic*. Enteropathic arthritis and enteropathic spondyloarthropathy (EAES) demonstrate how gastrointestinal dysbiosis, hormonal imbalances, increased intestinal permeability ("leaky gut"), and non-musculoskeletal systemic inflammation can spill-over into peripheral and axial arthritis. As detailed in the separate chapter on psoriasis and psoriatic arthritis (PsA), PsA is clearly a microbe-triggered disease, and its similarity to AS suggests a common physiologic etiology. The common themes that weave these disorders together are 1) dysbiosis-induced musculoskeletal inflammation, 2) hormonal imbalances, and 3) increased intestinal/mucosal permeability—the latter is the most voluminous route of absorption of arthritogenic antigens, immunogens, and antimetabolites—see Chapter 4 for overview and details.

- All of these conditions are *systemic* inflammatory disorders that show clear evidence of immune-mediated tissue damage and are therefore worthy of being dubbed *autoimmune*. The systemic nature of these disorders carries important clinical implications because both doctor and patient need to be aware of *non-musculoskeletal*

---

665 Colmegna I, Cuchacovich R, Espinoza LR. HLA-B27-associated reactive arthritis: pathogenetic and clinical considerations. *Clin Microbiol Rev*. 2004 Apr;17(2):348-69
666 Ringrose JH. HLA-B27 associated spondyloarthropathy, an autoimmune disease based on crossreactivity between bacteria and HLA-B27? *Ann Rheum Dis*. 1999 Oct;:598-610
667 Klippel JH (ed). *Primer on the rheumatic diseases. 11th edition*. Atlanta: Arthritis Foundation; 1997, page 181

complications. Non-musculoskeletal complications of these disorders include renal failure secondary to amyloidosis[668,669], cardiovascular and pulmonary complications, and increased risk of trauma, violent death, poisonings, and alcohol misuse.[670,671,672] Not surprisingly, the risk of pulmonary, renal, neurologic, ocular and cardiac complications is increased in patients with long-standing and severe disease.

Differentiating Characteristics of the Spondyloarthropathies

Condition	Etiopathogenesis	Unique presentation	Specific emphasis
Ankylosing spondylitis	• *Allopathic*: idiopathic • *Integrative*: dysbiosis is paramount	• Insidious onset of low-back pain in young patient • Ankylosis begins in lumbopelvis and can progress to thorax, neck, hips and knees. • 90% positive HLA-B27	• *Allopathic*: anti-inflammatory drugs • *Integrative*: Antidysbiosis and orthoendocrinology are treatment cornerstones
Reactive arthritis (previously Reiter's syndrome[673])	• *Allopathic*: infection-triggered arthritis • *Integrative*: infection-triggered arthritis in a patient with dietary and endocrinologic predispositions.	• Classically associated with a recent infection, particularly a genitourinary infection or gastrointestinal infection. • Inflammation is characteristically located at the low-back, iris, and heels. • 75% positive HLA-B27	• Antimicrobial treatment for acute and chronic infections is the mainstay of treatment although in a large percentage of patients the arthropathy continues despite apparent clearance of the primary infection.
Enteropathic spondylo-arthropathy, enteropathic arthritis	• *Allopathic*: idiopathic • *Integrative*: dysbiosis-triggered arthritis in a patient with dietary and endocrinologic predispositions	• Arthropathy of the peripheral joints and/or spine in a patient with inflammatory bowel disease—Crohn's disease or ulcerative colitis • 50% positive HLA-B27	• *Allopathic*: anti-inflammatory drugs • *Integrative*: Antidysbiosis and orthoendocrinology are treatment cornerstones • Treatment is similar to other treatments except with a greater focus on addressing the intestinal lesions

---

[668] "The mechanism of death in these patients was secondary amyloidosis in 19, cardiovascular complications in six, fracture of the spine in one, and it was not known in one patient. Excess deaths due to circulatory, gastrointestinal and renal diseases, and violence were also observed." Lehtinen K. Mortality and causes of death in 398 patients admitted to hospital with ankylosing spondylitis. *Ann Rheum Dis*. 1993 Mar;52(3):174-6

[669] "During an outbreak of Yersinia pseudotuberculosis III, one of two HLA-B27 positive brothers developed reactive arthritis (ReA), mild at first, but later severely destructive and ultimately fatal. The reactivation of ReA was possibly triggered by an oral polio vaccine. The cause of death was severe secondary amyloidosis." Yli-Kerttula T, Mottonen T, Toivanen A. Different course of reactive arthritis in two HLA-B27 positive brothers with fatal outcome in one. *J Rheumatol*. 1997 Oct;24(10):2047-50

[670] "A marked sex-associated effect was noted among deaths caused by injuries/poisoning, since 6 of the deaths occurred in men and only 1 was in a woman. CONCLUSION: Patients with PsA are at an increased risk of death compared with the general population." Gladman DD, Farewell VT, Wong K, Husted J.Mortality studies in psoriatic arthritis: results from a single outpatient center. II. Prognostic indicators for death. *Arthritis Rheum*. 1998 Jun;41(6):1103-10

[671] "The 4 leading causes of death were diseases of the circulatory (36.2%) or respiratory (21.3%) system, malignant neoplasms (17.0%), and injuries/poisoning (14.9%). The SMR for the female cohort was 1.59, and for the men, it was 1.65, indicating a 59% and 65% increase in the death rate, respectively. Deaths due to respiratory causes were particularly increased in these patients." Wong K, Gladman D, Long JA, Farewell VT. Mortality studies in psoriatic arthritis: results from a single outpatient clinic. I. Causes and risk of death. *Arthritis Rheum*. 1997 Oct;40(10):1868-72

[672] "Subjects with ankylosing spondylitis (AS) have an increased incidence of deaths from accidents and violence, which is due in part, but perhaps not entirely, to the vulnerability of the affected spine to fractures… Uncontrolled use of alcohol is an important determinant in the surplus of deaths from accidents and violence in Finnish patients with AS." Myllykangas-Luosujarvi et al. Increased incidence of alcohol-related deaths from accidents and violence in subjects with ankylosing spondylitis. *Br J Rheumatol*. 1998 Jun;37(6):688-90

[673] The term "Reiter's syndrome" has fallen out of favor due to the increasing acknowledgement that Dr Hans Reiter was affiliated with Nazi atrocities during World War II. See the following for additional information: "During World War II, Reiter, a physician leader of the Nazi party, authorized medical experiments on concentration camp prisoners." Lu DW, Katz KA. Declining use of the eponym "Reiter's syndrome" in the medical literature, 1998-2003. *J Am Acad Dermatol*. 2005 Oct;53(4):720-3 and "There is more than ample evidence that Hans Reiter, whose name has been eponymously linked to a rheumatologic syndrome, was a Nazi war criminal. He was responsible for heinous atrocities that violated the precepts of humanity, ethics, and professionalism." Panush et al. The tainted legacy of Hans Reiter. *Semin Arthritis Rheum*. 2003 Feb;32(4):231-6

Differentiating Characteristics of the Spondyloarthropathies—*continued*

Condition	Etiopathogenesis	Unique presentation	Specific emphasis
Juvenile spondylo-arthropathy	• *Allopathic*: idiopathic • *Integrative*: dysbiosis[674]	• Generally occurs in boys aged 8-18 years • Peripheral arthritis (90%) is more common than spondylitis (50%)	• *Allopathic*: anti-inflammatory drugs • *Integrative*: Antidysbiosis
Psoriatic arthritis	• *Allopathic*: idiopathic • *Integrative*: Food allergies and dysbiosis are paramount	• Arthropathy of the peripheral joints and/or spine in a patient with psoriasis • 50% positive HLA-B27	• *Allopathic*: anti-inflammatory drugs • *Integrative*: Antidysbiosis and orthoendocrinology are treatment cornerstones
Rheumatoid arthritis	• *Allopathic*: idiopathic • *Integrative*: dysbiosis-triggered arthritis in a patient with dietary and endocrinologic predisposition	• Inflammatory peripheral arthropathy generally precedes axial joints • Sacroiliac joints are generally spared • RF is frequently positive	• *Allopathic*: anti-inflammatory drugs • *Integrative*: Antidysbiosis and orthoendocrinology are treatment cornerstones

Clinical presentations:

- Musculoskeletal:
  - <u>Pain and limited motion in the low-back sacroiliac joints</u>: This is an aspect of all of the spondyloarthropathies, especially AS and ReA. Back pain is generally worse in the morning and alleviated by motion, including passive motion such as spinal manipulation.
  - <u>Thoracic spine pain and decreased rib expansion/excursion</u>: Although it typically begins in the lumbar spine and sacroiliac joints, AS commonly progresses to involve the thoracic spine and rib cage. Decreased mobility of the ribs limit respiration, and thus respirometry is used in the clinical assessment of patients with AS.
  - <u>Neck pain</u>: particularly common in RA and AS, two conditions associated with spontaneous atlantoaxial instability
  - <u>Atlantoaxial instability</u>: May be the presenting manifestation of AS[675] and is a common long-term complication of RA. Particularly in patients with neck pain and/or long-standing inflammation, cervical radiographs including APOM and measurement of the atlantodental interval should be performed before the clinical use of forceful cervical spine manipulation as well as esophageal/tracheal endoscopy.
  - <u>Enthesopathies</u>: Inflammation at the site of ligament insertion into bone—classically seen at the insertion of the Achilles' tendon at the calcaneus—is a characteristic finding and complaint in patients with ReA.
  - <u>Non-erosive asymmetrical peripheral arthritis</u>: 50% of patients with AS experience a temporary peripheral arthritis, while in 25% of patients the peripheral arthritis is permanent.
- <u>Pulmonary</u>: Pleurisy (painful inflammation of the pleural lining of the internal thoracic cavity) may be a complication of nearly all rheumatic/inflammatory disorders. Patients with AS may develop pulmonary fibrosis.
- <u>Cardiac</u>: "Spondylitic heart disease" is seen in patients with AS and commonly includes atrioventricular conduction defects and aortic regurgitation.[676]

---

[674] "Our findings provide clear evidence of ReA diagnosis following an acute M. pneumoniae infection that in four patients progressed to chronic jSpA. Our results suggest that detecting M. pneumoniae-specific antibodies in serological screening of jSpA patients might be useful." Harjacek et al. Juvenile spondyloarthropathies associated with Mycoplasma pneumoniae infection. *Clin Rheumatol*. 2006 Jan 4;:1-6

[675] Thompson et al. Spontaneous atlantoaxial subluxation as a presenting manifestation of juvenile ankylosing spondylitis. A case report. *Spine* 1982 Jan-Feb;7(1):78-9

[676] Tierney ML. McPhee SJ, Papadakis MA (eds). *Current Medical Diagnosis and Treatment 2006. 45th edition*. New York; Lange Medical Books: 2006, pages 851-855

- <u>GI tract</u>: Oral ulcers, intestinal inflammation, increased intestinal permeability
- <u>Skin/mucosal lesions</u>: Dermal lesions are particularly common in patients with ReA and PsA. Psoriatic lesions are typically well-demarcated erythematous patches with white/silvery scales. Dermal lesions of ReA can include pustular lesions on the feet and hands (palmoplantar pustulosis) in addition to genital lesions in patients with sexually transmitted diseases.
- <u>Renal complications</u>: These can be seen in nearly all rheumatic disorders, either as a result of the systemic inflammation (particularly immune complexes), amyloidosis, or as a result of NSAIDs or other pharmaceutical drugs.
- <u>Neurological complications</u>: Cerebral necrosis, corticosteroid psychosis, and transverse myelitis may occur. Atlantoaxial subluxation can present with myelopathic signs.
- <u>Ocular complications</u>: Anterior uveitis is seen in ~25% of patients with AS and is a characteristic finding in patients with ReA.

Major differential diagnoses:

- Initial evaluation of patients with spondyloarthropathy must include consideration of numerous differential diagnoses which may mimic or co-exist with inflammatory spondyloarthropathy. See table of *Differential Diagnoses* at the end of this chapter, as well as *algorithm for patient assessment and management*. Useful categories during the evaluation of low-back pain include the following:
  - <u>Serious organic diseases requiring immediate attention</u>: Metastatic disease, viscerosomatic referral, osteomyelitis/discitis, aortic aneurysm.
  - <u>Serious musculoskeletal disorders requiring immediate attention</u>: Recent fracture (pathologic fracture, osteoporosis, compression fracture, fall from a height, major motor vehicle accident), cauda equina syndrome, and severe radiculopathy (i.e., severe pain or progressive muscular deficits).
  - <u>Rheumatologic disorders affecting the low back and pelvis</u>: Ankylosing spondylitis, reactive arthritis, enteropathic spondyloarthropathy, psoriatic arthritis, rheumatoid arthritis, and fibromyalgia.
  - <u>Psychogenic</u>: Emotional overlay, symptom amplification, secondary gain, depression.
  - <u>Benign musculoskeletal disorders requiring conservative treatment and monitoring</u>: Muscle spasm, facet irritation, disc injuries causing radiculitis or radiculopathy, self-limiting inflammation due to injury.
  - <u>Functional, metabolic, allergic or nutritional causes of low-back pain</u>: Food allergies, obesity leading to a systemic inflammatory state as well as biomechanical stress on the lumbar spine, vitamin D deficiency[677], acidifying diet[678] (i.e., the Standard American Diet[679,680]).

---

[677] Al Faraj S, Al Mutairi K. Vitamin D deficiency and chronic low back pain in Saudi Arabia. *Spine*. 2003 Jan 15;28(2):177-9
[678] "The results show that a disturbed acid-base balance may contribute to the symptoms of low back pain. The simple and safe addition of an alkaline multimineral preparate was able to reduce the pain symptoms in these patients with chronic low back pain." Vormann et al. Supplementation with alkaline minerals reduces symptoms in patients with chronic low back pain. *J Trace Elem Med Biol*. 2001;15(2-3):179-83
[679] Seaman DR. The diet-induced proinflammatory state: a cause of chronic pain and other degenerative diseases? *J Manipulative Physiol Ther*. 2002 Mar-Apr;25(3):168-79
[680] Cordain L. *The Paleo Diet*. John Wiley & Sons Inc., New York 2002

Low Back Pain: Differential Diagnostic Considerations

	DDX Category	Examples:
V	Vascular	Aortic aneurysm
	Visceral referral	Pancreatic disease/cancer
I	Infectious	Ankylosing spondylitis, reactive arthritis
	Inflammatory	Rheumatoid arthritis
	Immunologic	Psoriatic arthritis
		Enteropathic spondyloarthropathy
		Lymphoma, leukemia
		Bone/ tissue infections
		Gastrointestinal disease
		Kidney infection
		Psoriatic arthritis
		Herpes zoster
N	Neurologic	Metastatic disease, primary bone tumors, multiple myeloma
	Nutritional	Herpes zoster
	New growth: neoplasia, pregnancy	Cauda equina syndrome
D	Deficiency	Degenerative joint/spine disease
	Degenerative	Congenital malformations of bones/ viscera
	Developmental	Scoliosis
		Postural syndromes
		Disc herniation
		Varicose veins in the leg mimicking sciatica
I	Iatrogenic (drug related)	Anticoagulants predispose to epidural or spinal cord bleeding[681]
	Intoxication	Prednisone use promotes osteoporosis and spinal fractures
	Idiosyncratic	Excess alcohol consumption[682]
C	Congenital	Congenital malformations of bones: hemivertebrae, leg length inequality, etc.
A	Allergy	Ankylosing spondylitis
	Autoimmune	Fractures, injuries
	Abuse	
T	Trauma	Fractures: injuries to vertebrae, ribs, muscles
E	Endocrine	Diabetes mellitus
	Exposure	
S	"Subluxation", somatic dysfunction	Segmental dysfunction of lumbar spine and pelvis
	Structural	Muscle tension
	Stress	
	Secondary gain	
M	Mental	Anxiety
	Malpractice	Depression
	Mental disorder	Endometriosis, hematocolpos[683]
	Malignancy	Ovarian tumor
	Metabolic disease	Nephrolithiasis
	Menstrual	Metastasis to spine
	Myofascial	Myofascial trigger points in quadratus lumborum, piriformis, iliacus, psoas

---

[681] Souza TA. *Differential Diagnosis for the Chiropractor: Protocols and Algorithms*. Gaithersburg: Aspen Publications. 1997 page 110
[682] "Alcohol abuse was significantly more frequent among the male low back patients." Sandstrom J, Andersson GB, Wallerstedt S. The role of alcohol abuse in working disability in patients with low back pain. *Scand J Rehabil Med*. 1984;16(4):147-9
[683] London NJ, Sefton GK. Hematocolpos. An unusual cause of sciatica in an adolescent girl. *Spine*. 1996 Jun 1;21(11):1381-2

Specific differential diagnoses
- Mechanical low back pain, traumatic low back pain, spinal strain/sprain
- Cauda equina syndrome
- Vitamin D deficiency: Vitamin D deficiency causes inflammation and low-back pain. Measure 25(OH)vitamin D in serum or supplement with 4,000-10,000 IU daily for at least three months[684] unless contraindicated by drugs (e.g., hydrochlorothiazide) or hypercalcemic condition (e.g., sarcoidosis, cancer, or hyperparathyroidism, etc.).[685]
- Spinal degeneration, degenerative arthritis of the spine
- Spinal fracture: Patients with AS may experience fracture following trivial "injury" such as rolling over in bed: **"Fracture should be suspected whenever a [AS] patient complains of new back pain."[686]**
- Osteitis condensans ilii
- Cancer, malignant disease
- Vertebral osteomyelitis, infectious discitis
- Developmental/congenital sacralization of the lumbar vertebrae
- Other autoimmune disease
- Lung disease: Asthma, COPD, bronchitis, tuberculosis
- Iron overload: Hemochromatosis may resemble ankylosing spondylitis clinically and radiographically.[687]
- Fibromyalgia: ESR, CRP, thyroid tests, ANA and most other 'basic' tests are normal; assess and treat for bacterial overgrowth of the small bowel.[688]
- Diffuse idiopathic skeletal hyperostosis (DISH): DISH generally affects the longitudinal ligaments of the spine rather than the intervertebral discs. Cervical involvement generally precedes that of the lumbar spine, and the condition is strongly associated with diabetes mellitus.

Clinical assessments:
- **History/subjective**: See clinical presentations
  - **Typical presentation is that of dull achy pain in the low-back—worse in the morning and improving as the day progresses and/or with activity.**
  - **Systemic manifestations may or may not be present in the early stages of disease.**
- **Physical examination/objective**:
  - ROM, neurologic assessments; orthopedic assessments
  - Specialty examinations may be indicated:
    - Eye exam: For retinal and anterior chamber abnormalities; external exam for scleritis
    - Genital examination and/or assessment for UTI and STDs: Indicated in patients with ReA due to high association with sexually transmitted diseases. Urethral swab for culture and DNA probes are commonly indicated.
    - Cardiopulmonary assessment: Common considerations include auscultation, measurement of thoracic excursion, and spirometry. Chest radiographs may be indicated.
    - Neurologic examination: A screening neurologic examination should be performed as part of the initial assessment of all patients and more detailed examinations are carried out when indicated.
    - Schober test: Draw a line over the spinous process of L5, then mark a line 10 cm above and 5 cm below; with lumbar flexion, the total distance should increase from 15 cm to 20 cm—less than 5 cm excursion indicates spinal rigidity, consistent with AS.
    - Occiput-to-wall distance: This assessment can be used to quantify progression/regression of cervical flexion in patients with AS.
    - Chest expansion: Use tape measure around lower thorax; measure chest circumference before and after inhalation; use along with spirometry to monitor thoracic stiffness in patients with AS.

[684] Al Faraj S, Al Mutairi K. Vitamin D deficiency and chronic low back pain in Saudi Arabia. *Spine.* 2003 Jan 15;28(2):177-9
[685] Vasquez et al. The clinical importance of vitamin D: a paradigm shift with implications for all healthcare providers. *Altern Ther Health Med.* 2004 Sep-Oct;10(5):28-36
[686] Harley JB, Scofield RH. The spectrum of ankylosing spondylitis. *Hosp Pract (Off Ed)* 1995 Jul 15;30(7):37-43, 46
[687] Bywaters EGL, Hamilton EBD, Williams R. The spine in idiopathic hemochromatosis. *Ann Rheum Dis* 1971; 30: 453-65
[688] Pimentel M, et al. A link between irritable bowel syndrome and fibromyalgia may be related to findings on lactulose breath testing. *Ann Rheum Dis.* 2004 Apr;63:450-2

- **Laboratory assessments:**
  - ESR or CRP: These are generally elevated, and neither test is superior to the other in the assessment of patients with AS. One study[689] used a unique approach to differentiate active disease from inactive disease in patients with AS; they added ESR value (mm/h) and CRP value (mg/L) and classified patients as having active inflammatory disease if the total was greater than thirty (30).
  - Rheumatoid factor (RF): Characteristically **negative** *by definition* in patients with sero**negative** spondyloarthropathies. Positivity suggests rheumatoid spondylitis or concomitant RA with another spondyloarthropathy.
  - CBC: Look for evidence of true *infection* (in contrast to *dysbiosis*); also assess for anemia, which may be secondary to renal failure, NSAID gastropathy, chronic inflammation, or nutritional inadequacy.
  - Comprehensive metabolic panel: Assess as indicated for complications and concomitant disease.
  - Comprehensive stool analysis with comprehensive parasitology: **All patients with AS, RA, and PsA have gastrointestinal dysbiosis until proven otherwise.** Use of comprehensive stool tests should be the standard of care for all patients with AS, RA, PsA, and of course those with enteropathic spondyloarthropathy. Patients with ReA due to gastroenteritis or those whose primary infection has not been identified/eliminated are also obvious candidates for stool testing; the most commonly implicated microbes are *Salmonella*, *Shigella*,

Microorganisms clinically or molecularly associated with induction of seronegative spondyloarthropathy, ankylosing spondylitis, and reactive arthritis
• *Campylobacter* spp
• *Chlamydia trachomatis*
• *Citrobacter freundii*
• *E. coli*
• *Giardia lamblia*
• *Helicobacter pylori*
• *Klebsiella pneumoniae*
• *Mycoplasma* spp
• *Proteus mirabilis*
• *Salmonella typhimurium*
• *Shigella flexneri*
• *Shigella sonnei*
• *Staphylococcus aureus*
• *Streptococcus pyogenes*
• *Ureaplasma* spp
• *Yersinia enterocolitica*

  and *Yersinia*. Regarding the etiopathogenesis of AS, the most commonly implicated microbes are *Klebsiella* and *E. coli*. However, it is more accurate to see that microbes incite autoimmunity/inflammation by numerous mechanisms and that exposure to numerous microbes—each one of which *in isolation* may be innocuous—in combination leads to additive and synergistic proinflammatory effects, as reviewed in Chapter 4 in the section on multifocal dysbiosis and elsewhere in a recent publication by the current author.[690]
  - Serologic and genital tests for sexually transmitted diseases: These tests are particularly indicated in patients with ReA due to the frequent association of this disorder with genitourinary infections, particularly those caused by *Chlamydia*. Numerous articles have shown that patients with long-term idiopathic oligoarthritis harbor "silent infections"—otherwise known as dysbiosis—in the genitourinary and gastrointestinal tracts; the most commonly identified organisms are *Chlamydia trachomatis*, *Yersinia*, *Salmonella*, *Mycoplasma*, and *Ureaplasma*.[691,692]
  - Serum vitamin D: Measure 25(OH)vitamin D in all patients and/or begin empiric treatment with physiologic doses of vitamin D3. Emulsified cholecalciferol is particularly efficacious in older patients and those with malabsorption due to enteropathy.[693] According to research by Falkenbach et al[694], **"Patients with ankylosing spondylitis may have extremely low levels of 25(OH)D."** Vitamin D deficiency appears common in patients with low-back pain[695], limb pain[696], chronic persistent

[689] Maki-Ikola O, Lehtinen K, Nissila M, Granfors K. IgM, IgA and IgG class serum antibodies against Klebsiella pneumoniae and Escherichia coli lipopolysaccharides in patients with ankylosing spondylitis. *Br J Rheumatol* 1994 Nov;33(11):1025-9

[690] Vasquez A. Nutritional Botanical Treatments against "Silent Infections" and Gastrointestinal Dysbiosis. *Nutritional Perspectives* 2006; Jan ichnfm.academia.edu/AlexVasquez

[691] "Urogenital swab cultures showed a microbial infection in 44% of the patients with oligoarthritis (15% Chlamydia, 14% Mycoplasma, 28% Ureaplasma), whereas in the control group only 26% had a positive result (4% Chlamydia, 7% Mycoplasma, 21% Ureaplasma)." Erlacher et al. Reactive arthritis: urogenital swab culture is the only useful diagnostic method for the detection of the arthritogenic infection in extra-articularly asymptomatic patients with undifferentiated oligoarthritis. *Br J Rheumatol*. 1995 Sep;34(9):838-42

[692] Fendler C, et al. Frequency of triggering bacteria in patients with reactive arthritis and undifferentiated oligoarthritis and the relative importance of the tests used for diagnosis. *Ann Rheum Dis*. 2001 Apr;60(4):337-43 ard.bmjjournals.com/cgi/content/full/60/4/337

[693] Vasquez A. Subphysiologic Doses of Vitamin D are Subtherapeutic: Comment on the Study by The Record Trial Group. *The Lancet* Published on-line May 6, 2005

[694] "Patients with ankylosing spondylitis may have extremely low levels of 25(OH)D." Falkenbach et al. Serum 25-hydroxyvitamin D and parathyroid hormone in patients with ankylosing spondylitis before and after a three-week rehabilitation treatment at high altitude during winter and spring. *Wien Klin Wochenschr*. 2001 Apr 30;113(9):328-32

[695] Al Faraj S, Al Mutairi K. Vitamin D deficiency and chronic low back pain in Saudi Arabia. *Spine*. 2003 Jan 15;28(2):177-9

[696] Masood H, Narang AP, Bhat IA, Shah GN. Persistent limb pain and raised serum alkaline phosphatase the earliest markers of subclinical hypovitaminosis D in Kashmir. *Indian J Physiol Pharmacol*. 1989 Oct-Dec;33(4):259-61

musculoskeletal pain[697], and in general medical patients.[698] [699] In our review of the literature[700], we concluded that **optimal serum 25(OH)-vitamin D levels should be defined as 40 – 65 ng/mL (100 - 160 nmol/L)** and that, "Until proven otherwise, the balance of the research clearly indicates that oral supplementation in the range of 1,000 IU per day for infants, 2,000 IU per day for children and **4,000 IU per day for adults** is safe and reasonable to meet physiologic requirements, to promote optimal health, and to reduce the risk of several serious diseases. Safety and effectiveness of supplementation are assured by periodic monitoring of serum 25(OH)D and serum calcium." Vitamin D supplementation 5,000 – 10,000 IU per day for adults was shown to alleviate low-back pain after 3 months in nearly all patients with low initial serum levels of vitamin D.[701]

- o <u>Testing for multifocal dysbiosis</u>: If the intestinal and genitourinary tracts appear clear of infection following direct testing, then empiric antimicrobial treatment should be considered. Following this, searching for other loci of infection—namely the mouth, throat, nose, sinuses, lungs, and skin—should be pursued as discussed in Chapter 4.
- o <u>HLA-B27</u>: This marker is seen with increased prevalence in patients with AS and ReA. The test can be used to support the diagnosis, particularly early in the course of the illness when radiographs are *negative*.
- o <u>Hormone assessments</u>: These should be performed as detailed in Chapter 4.6 and/or as indicated per patient.

- **<u>Imaging</u>**:
  - o <u>Plain radiographs</u>: In contrast to most of the other rheumatic disorders wherein radiographs are generally unnecessary in early stages of the disease, plain radiographs are of tremendous value in the assessment of spondylitis and sacroiliitis and are generally diagnostic once the diagnostic threshold has been crossed; i.e., they may be negative in early disease, but become positive after a given amount of time, which varies per patient and per disease. Characteristic initial findings in AS are lumbar syndesmophytes and sacroiliitis.
  - o <u>MRI and CT imaging</u>: Generally reserved for the evaluation of spinal stenosis and inflammatory myelopathy. **CT imaging is more sensitive than plain radiography for the initial evaluation of sacroiliitis**.[702] Also used for assessment of other complications as indicated.

- **<u>Establishing the diagnosis</u>**:
  - o Inflammatory spondyloarthropathy as a general term can be diagnosed with a combination of serologic, clinical, and radiographic findings. The subtype of spondyloarthropathy—AS, ReA, PsA, RA, ES, etc—is then distinguished based on the details of the clinical history (e.g., inflammatory bowel disease or recent infection), presentation, clinical findings, serologic tests, and radiographic characteristics.

<u>Complications</u>:

- Chronic pain, significant physical limitations and significant morbidity
- Renal failure, secondary to amyloidosis or medications such as sulfasalazine or NSAID's
- Spinal fracture (in patients with spinal ankylosis following minor trauma)
- Respiratory insufficiency
- Permanent disability due to rigid spinal flexion secondary to bony ankylosis resulting in loss of spinal motion
- Neurologic compromise: due to spinal stenosis, transverse myelopathy, atlantoaxial subluxation, cauda equina fibrosis, or cauda equina syndrome

<u>Clinical management</u>:

- Referral if clinical outcome is unsatisfactory or as otherwise indicated.

---

[697] Plotnikoff GA, Quigley JM. Prevalence of severe hypovitaminosis D in patients with persistent, nonspecific musculoskeletal pain. *Mayo Clin Proc.* 2003 Dec;78(12):1463-70
[698] Thomas et al. Hypovitaminosis D in medical inpatients. *N Engl J Med.* 1998 Mar 19;338(12):777-83
[699] Kauppinen-Makelin et al. A high prevalence of hypovitaminosis D in Finnish medical in- and outpatients. *J Intern Med.* 2001 Jun;249(6):559-63
[700] Vasquez A, Manso G, Cannell J. The Clinical Importance of Vitamin D (Cholecalciferol). *Alternative Therapies in Health and Medicine* InflammationMastery.com/reprints
[701] Al Faraj S, Al Mutairi K. Vitamin D deficiency and chronic low back pain in Saudi Arabia. *Spine.* 2003 Jan 15;28(2):177-9
[702] Tierney ML. McPhee SJ, Papadakis MA. <u>*Current Medical Diagnosis and Treatment 2006. 45th edition*</u>. New York; Lange Medical Books: 2006, pages 851-855

Treatments[703]

- NSAIDs, especially indomethacin 25-50 mg thrice daily—"side effects" of indomethacin include headache, giddiness, psychosis, depression, nausea, vomiting, gastric ulcer, and renal impairment. Sulfasalazine: 1,000 mg twice daily.
- Corticosteroids are notably ineffective in the treatment of spondyloarthropathy, though they are commonly used against complications such as uveitis.
- TNF inhibitors: Etanercept 25 mg subcutaneously twice weekly, or infliximab 5 mg/kg every other month. These drugs are clinically effective from the perspective of anti-inflammation, but they are associated with increased risks for lymphoma, serious infections including pulmonary tuberculosis, congestive heart failure, demyelinating diseases, and systemic lupus erythematosus.
- Methotrexate: Used for recalcitrant psoriatic arthritis.[704]

- FOOD & NUTRITION: 5-part "supplemented Paleo-Mediterranean diet" (SPMD) The 5-part "supplemented Paleo-Mediterranean diet" (SPMD—reviewed in Chapter 4) consists of ❶ foundational plant-based low-carbohydrate diet of fruits, vegetables, nuts, seeds, berries and lean sources of protein, ❷ multivitamin and multimineral supplementation, ❸ physiologic doses of vitamin D3 (range 2,000-10,000 IU/d), ❹ combination fatty acid therapy (CFAT) with n3-ALA, n6-GLA, n3-EPA, n3-DHA, and phytochemical-rich olive oil which contains n9-oleate, and ❺ probiotics.
  - o The use of a low starch diet in the treatment of patients suffering from ankylosing spondylitis: alleviation of dysbiosis and immune complex formation via nutritional intervention (*Clin Rheumatol* 1996 Jan[705]): "The majority of ankylosing spondylitis (AS) patients not only possess HLA-B27, but during active phases of the disease have elevated levels of total serum IgA, suggesting that a microbe from the bowel flora is acting across the gut mucosa. .... Furthermore AS patients from 10 different countries have been found to have elevated levels of specific antibodies against Klebsiella bacteria. It has been suggested that these Klebsiella microbes, found in the bowel flora, might be the trigger factors in this disease and therefore reduction in the size of the bowel flora could be of benefit in the treatment of AS patients. Microbes from the bowel flora depend on dietary starch for their growth and therefore a reduction in starch intake might be beneficial in AS patients. A "low starch diet" involving a reduced intake of "bread, potatoes, cakes and pasta" has been devised and tested in healthy control subjects and AS patients. The "low starch diet" leads to a reduction of total serum IgA in both healthy controls as well as patients, and furthermore to a decrease in inflammation and symptoms in the AS patients."

- INFECTIONS & DYSBIOSIS: ❶ antimicrobial treatments, ❷ immunorestoration, ❸ immunotolerance via Treg induction Essentially all autoimmune/rheumatic disorders are associated with microbial colonization and intolerance to same; the presence of persistent microbial colonization is *prima facie* evidence of immunosuppression. The eight areas of dysbiosis (multifocal) are: ❶ sinorespiratory, ❷ orodental, ❸ gastrointestinal, ❹ urogenital/genitourinary, ❺ parenchymal/tissue, ❻ microbial, ❼ dermal/cutaneous, and ❽ environmental.
  - o Rational assumption of polymicrobial dysbiosis: The association of spondyloarthropathies and reactive arthritis with microbial infection/colonization is so strong and consistent throughout decades of research that a review or substantiation here, notwithstanding a few relevant samples, would be superfluous; rather, the 3-part anti-dysbiosis protocols and concepts reviewed in Chapter 4 should be implemented. See also the laboratory (microbial) assessments and concepts in Chapter 1. The examples that follow should be viewed concretely for the data provided, but also as metaphorical and representative of the microbe-autoimmunity connection.
  - o Helicobacter pylori eradication therapy on gastrointestinal permeability in seronegative spondyloarthritis (*J Rheumatol.* 2005 Feb[706]): "Disruption of intestinal barrier function, followed by increased antigen load, may possibly trigger joint inflammation. In seronegative spondyloarthritis (SpA)

[703] Tierney ML. McPhee SJ, Papadakis MA. *Current Medical Diagnosis and Treatment 2006. 45th edition.* New York; Lange Medical Books: 2006, pages 851-855
[704] Tierney ML. McPhee SJ, Papadakis MA. *Current Medical Diagnosis and Treatment 2006. 45th edition.* New York; Lange Medical Books: 2006, pages 851-855
[705] Ebringer A, Wilson C. The use of a low starch diet in the treatment of patients suffering from ankylosing spondylitis. *Clin Rheumatol.* 1996 Jan;15 Suppl 1:62-66
[706] Di Leo et al. Effect of Helicobacter pylori and eradication therapy on gastrointestinal permeability. Implications for patients with seronegative spondyloarthritis. *J Rheumatol.* 2005 Feb;32(2):295-300

both gut inflammation and altered intestinal permeability have been reported. We evaluated ...20 SpA patients, 30 patients with endoscopic gastritis (EndG), and 35 healthy controls... H. pylori affected GI permeability in both SpA and EndG patients. After eradication therapy, sucrose excretion remained increased in SpA and reverted to normal in EndG patients, whereas lactulose/mannitol test became comparable to controls in both groups. SpA patients taking chronic NSAID had increased gastroduodenal permeability only when H. pylori-positive. In SpA patients, GI permeability did not correlate with clinical activity or biochemical inflammation. CONCLUSION: In SpA, H. pylori and NSAID contribute to impaired GI permeability. Eradication therapy may help to maintain epithelial barrier function and possibly influence clinical improvement in patients with SpA."

- o Reactive arthritis responding to antiretroviral therapy in an HIV-1-infected individual (*Int J STD AIDS.* 2012 May[707]): "Reactive arthritis (ReA) is an autoimmune seronegative spondyloarthropathy that occurs in response to a urogenital or enteric infection. Several studies have reported a link between ReA and HIV infection. We report a case of an HIV-1-infected patient diagnosed with a disabling ReA who failed to respond to conventional therapy but whose symptoms resolved rapidly after starting antiretroviral therapy (ART)."

- o Human immunodeficiency virus associated spondyloarthropathy (*Ann Rheum Dis.* 2001 Jul[708]): "In this case report a patient is described with severe HIV associated reactive arthritis, who on magnetic resonance imaging and sonographic imaging of inflamed knees had extensive polyenthesitis and adjacent osteitis. The arthritis deteriorated despite conventional antirheumatic treatment, but improved dramatically after highly active antiretroviral treatment, which was accompanied by a significant rise in CD4 T lymphocyte counts."

- o Reactive arthritis: urogenital swab culture is the only useful diagnostic method for the detection of the arthritogenic infection in extra-articularly asymptomatic patients with undifferentiated oligoarthritis (*Br J Rheumatol.* 1995 Sep[709]): "Reactive arthritis (ReA) is a seronegative oligoarthritis triggered by a preceding extra-articular infection. ... In a retrospective study, we evaluated the usefulness of urogenital swab cultures, serology and stool culture to identify infections in 234 patients with undifferentiated oligoarthritis. One hundred and forty-four patients complaining about joint pain who had no sign or history of inflammatory arthritis served as controls. Urogenital swab cultures showed a microbial infection in 44% of the patients with oligoarthritis (15% Chlamydia, 14% Mycoplasma, 28% Ureaplasma), whereas in the control group only 26% had a positive result (4% Chlamydia, 7% Mycoplasma, 21% Ureaplasma). A Chlamydia IgG-antibody titer > or = 1:256 was found in 22% of the patients in the oligoarthritis group and in 9% of the controls (P < 0.01). However, for only half of Chlamydia IgG-positive patients could a Chlamydia infection be confirmed by urogenital swab culture. Twenty-one per cent of patients with oligoarthritis vs 23% of the controls had positive antibody titers for Salmonella (not significant), 15% vs 5% for Yersinia (P < 0.05) and 17% vs 3% for Borrelia IgG (P < 0.01). In two patients, stool cultures were positive for Campylobacter. Urogenital swab culture is a sensitive diagnostic method to identify the triggering infection in ReA."

- **NUTRITIONAL IMMUNOMODULATION: Treg induction for modulation of Th-1/2/17 inflammation** Nutrients and therapeutic approaches that promote Treg or IL-10 induction and/or Th-17, IL-17 suppression include 1) mitochondrial optimization and mTOR suppression, 2) biotin, 3) vitamin E, 4) sodium avoidance, 5) transgenic/GMO food avoidance, 6) probiotics, 7) lipoic acid, 8) vitamin A, 9) inflammation reduction, 10) vitamin D, 11) fatty acid supplementation with GLA and n3, 12) infection and dysbiosis remediation, 13) green tea EGCG. Acronym: MiBESTPLAIDFIG.

- **DYSMETABOLISM & DYSFUNCTIONAL MITOCHONDRIA: MitoDys, ERS-UPR, AGE/RAGE, hyperglycemia and ceramide** The major clinical considerations in this section are mitochondrial dysfunction, endoplasmic reticulum stress, unfolded protein response, TLR activation, and the dysmetabolic effects of

[707] Scott et al. Reactive arthritis responding to antiretroviral therapy in an HIV-1-infected individual. *Int J STD AIDS.* 2012 May;23(5):373-4
[708] McGonagle et al. Human immunodeficiency virus associated spondyloarthropathy. *Ann Rheum Dis.* 2001 Jul;60(7):696-8
[709] Erlacher et al. Reactive arthritis: urogenital swab culture is the only useful diagnostic method for the detection of the arthritogenic infection in extra-articularly asymptomatic patients with undifferentiated oligoarthritis. *Br J Rheumatol.* 1995 Sep;34(9):838-42

sustained hyperglycemia and hyperinsulinemia and resultant oxidative stress, inflammation, RAGE activation, and accumulation of AGE, palmitate and ceramide. The review of this information in Chapter 4 covered approximately 30 interventions relevant to dysmetabolism, mitochondrial dysfunction, ERS-UPR, etc; these will not be reviewed here except to mention those most commonly, easily, empirically, synergistically, and effectively used: 1) low-carbohydrate diet with 2) moderate exercise, 3) CoQ-10, 4) acetyl-carnitine with 5) lipoic acid, 6) NAC, 7) resveratrol, and 8) melatonin.

- **STYLE OF LIVING (LIFESTYLE) & SPECIAL CONSIDERATIONS:** Sleep optimization, SocioPsychology, Stress management/avoidance, Somatic treatments, Special Supplementation, Sweat/exercise, Sauna/detoxification, Surgery, Stamp your passport and vacate current reality, Sensory deprivation therapy
This is a buffet of mostly lifestyle-based interventions yet also including considerations such as somatic treatments, additional supplementation, and surgery.

- **ENDOCRINE IMBALANCE & OPTIMIZATION:** Prolactin, Insulin, Estrogen, DHEA, Cortisol, Testosterone, Thyroid Common hormonal imbalances seen among autoimmune/inflammatory patients are: ❶ *elevated* prolactin, ❷ *elevated* estrogen, ❸ *elevated* insulin, and ❹ *reduced* DHEA, ❺ *reduced* cortisol, and ❻ *reduced* testosterone; see Chapter 4 for discussion of these hormones and respective interventions. Thyroid evaluation (patient + labs) should be comprehensive, as discussed in Chapter 1, with a low threshold for empiric treatment.

- **XENOBIOTIC ACCUMULATION & DETOXIFICATION:** Chemical avoidance, nutritional support for detoxification pathways, urine alkalinization The clinical relevance and pathogenic mechanisms of xenobiotic accumulation are irrefutably well documented and described. Clinical assessments include history, physical examination, and laboratory assessment (using serum, whole blood, urine or—rarely yet accurately—fat biopsy), and response to treatment. Treatments include nutritional support for Phases 1 and 2 of detoxification (e.g., oxidation and conjugation) and excretion via bile and urine; for the latter, urinary alkalinization is generally recommended. Chemical toxins can be bound in the gut using activated charcoal, cholestyramine, or *Chlorella*—all of these three treatments have documented safety and effectiveness; clinically and empirically, phytochelatin (plant-derived peptides that bind toxic metals) concentrates appear safe and effective despite lack of conclusive published data supporting clinical use.

Sjögren Syndrome/Disease

Introduction:

Sjögren Syndrome/Disease is a sustained inflammatory disorder characterized by inflammatory and destructive lymphocytic infiltrates in exocrine organs, leading to failure of these glands and the resultant complications reviewed in the section that follows. Common to other inflammatory and autoimmune disorders, the condition is multifactorial in accord with most of the categories addressed by the Functional Inflammology protocol and recalled by the FINDSEX acronym detailed in Chapter 4 and the accompanying videos. Readers are expected to have read Chapters 1 and 4 so that this chapter can focus on the more salient points specific for Sjögren Syndrome/Disease. The condition is inaccurately named a "syndrome"—implying that it is a "group of symptoms that collectively indicate or characterize a disease or disorder"; however, this condition—like fibromyalgia—has distinct clinical and histopathological findings and is therefore more accurately described and legitimized as a "disease", which it properly is.

Description/pathophysiology:

- **Autoimmune condition affecting the exocrine glands; mucosal surfaces become dry, irritated and prone to microbial colonization.** Clinically manifested as "*sicca* syndrome" which implies a group of symptoms caused by *dryness* of mucosal surfaces.
- Like most conditions, it is generally described as "idiopathic" by medical textbooks and journal articles.[710] More common than SLE, less common than RA; Sjogren's syndrome is considered by some references to be as common as RA.
- Occurs in two general forms:
  - Primary—only Sjogren's/Sicca syndrome *without evidence of systemic autoimmunity*
  - Secondary—the occurrence of Sjogren's syndrome *along with another autoimmune disease*, especially rheumatoid arthritis, but also SLE, systemic sclerosis, primary biliary cirrhosis, polymyositis, Hashimoto's thyroiditis, polyarteritis, interstitial pulmonary fibrosis

Clinical presentations:

- Much more common in women—90% of patients with Sjogren's disease are female[711]
- Average age of onset is 50 years (typical range 40-60 years)
- **"Sicca syndrome"** denotes dryness of mucus membranes:
  - Dry eyes, keratoconjunctivitis sicca: Lymphocyte and plasma cells cause destruction of lacrimal glands; subjective complaints are more prominent than objective evidence: dry eyes, burning, itching, inability to wear contact lenses, thick mucus, photophobia, corneal ulceration—the latter can lead to infection, vision loss.
  - Dry mouth, xerostomia: this is generally more problematic than keratoconjunctivitis sicca; dental carries ("cavities") are greatly increased; 33% of patients will have parotid gland tenderness (can be treated with analgesics) and fluctuations in gland size.
  - Nose, throat, bronchi, and vagina may also be affected.
- Joint pain: Similar distribution to RA but less severe and nondestructive; minimal swelling: PIP and knees most common
- Classic presentation: Woman (90%) aged 40-60 years with dry mouth, dry eyes, and arthritis that mimics RA; other common presentations include:
  - Photosensitivity, skin rash, hair loss
  - Mouth lesions, carries
  - Chest pain (caused by pleurisy) or breathlessness
  - Raynaud's phenomenon

---

[710] "In spite of [the fact that we have no evidence-based solutions to the etiology and pathogenesis of autoimmune diseases], consensus is often taken as a truth, which may hamper the production, funding and/or publication of new and original ideas and views." Konttinen YT, Kasna-Ronkainen L. Sjogren's syndrome: viewpoint on pathogenesis. One of the reasons I was never asked to write a textbook chapter on it. *Scand J Rheumatol Suppl* 2002;(116):15-22
[711] Tierney ML. McPhee SJ, Papadakis MA. *Current Medical Diagnosis and Treatment 2006. 45th edition*. New York; Lange Medical Books: 2006, pages 842-843

Major differential diagnoses:

- Dehydration, exposure to excessively dry air (furnaces, dehumidifiers, etc.)
- Another autoimmune disease may mimic or occur concomitantly: RA, SLE, scleroderma, polymyositis, autoimmune thyroid disease, arteritis—none of these conditions by itself will cause sicca/dryness.
- Medication side effects (dry eyes and dry mouth are common side effects of many drugs)
- Systemic illness: HIV, lymphoma, sarcoidosis
- Hepatitis C—may possibly induce Sjogren's syndrome[712]
- Mumps (swollen parotid glands)
- Menopause
- Normal aging
- Salivary gland atrophy/fibrosis due to previous radiation to head and neck

Clinical assessments:

- **History/subjective**:
  - See clinical presentations
- **Physical examination/objective**:
  - Schirmer test: Use filter paper to assess adequacy of lacrimation for 5 minutes; less than 5 mm of wetness is abnormal
  - Rose Bengal staining: Used to assess the health of the cornea and to thus search for objective evidence of keratoconjunctivitis sicca
- **Laboratory assessments**:
  - ANA: positive in >95%
    - If ANA is negative, consider HIV, lymphoma, sarcoidosis, hepatitis C.
    - Supportive evidence with **anti-SS-A (anti-Ro)** and **anti-SS-B (anti-La),** neither of which are specific
    - Autoimmunity directed toward glands/tissues such as stomach, adrenal, and neurons may also be noted[713]
  - RF: Positive in 70%
  - ESR: Elevated in 70%
  - CBC: Shows anemia (33%), leukopenia and eosinophilia (25%)
  - Thyroid disorders: Thyroid autoimmunity is common in patients with Sjogren's syndrome; test anti-thyroid peroxidase antibodies and anti-thyroglobulin antibodies along with TSH, T4, and perhaps T3—see Chapter 1 for discussions on thyroid assessments and interventions.
  - HLA markers: DR2 and DR3 are more common in patients who have Sjogren's syndrome *without rheumatoid arthritis.*
  - Schirmer test: Measures quantity of tears and thus objectively quantifies keratoconjunctivitis sicca.
  - Salivary gland biopsy: Not commonly performed except for atypical presentations such as unilateral involvement and to exclude malignancy.
  - Anti-parietal cell antibodies: Noted in various autoimmune conditions (e.g., approximately 33% of patients with Hashimoto thyroiditis); leads to gastric atrophy and associated hypochlorhydria, cobalamin malabsorption, and microbial overgrowth.
  - Assess patient as indicated for other conditions and complications.
- **Imaging**: Used as indicated per patient; generally not part of assessment
- **Establishing the diagnosis**: Both of the following must be present:
  1. Autoantibodies—ANA or variant: Preferably in combination with the gold standard in allopathic medicine: salivary gland biopsy—this is necessary for "definite diagnosis" but is not necessary for clinical purposes based on "probable diagnosis."
  2. Evidence of exocrine damage: keratoconjunctivitis sicca and/or xerostomia.

---

[712] Siegel LB, Gall EP. Viral infection as a cause of arthritis. *Am Fam Physician* 1996 Nov 1;54(6):2009-15
[713] Rehman HU. Sjogren's syndrome. *Yonsei Med J.* 2003 Dec 30;44(6):947-54 eymj.org/2003/pdf/12947.pdf

Complications:
- Vision impairment, vision loss due to corneal lesion, ulceration and secondary infection
- Dental carries
- Malnutrition, especially vitamin B-12 deficiency
- Inflammatory polyarthropathy
- Salivary stones
- Pneumonia: can be fatal
- Pancreatitis
- Raynaud's phenomenon is seen in ~20%
- Sensory neuropathy, peripheral neuropathy: immune complex neuropathy, nutrient/B12 deficiencies
- Renal tubular acidosis
- Renal insufficiency and failure: can be fatal
- Nephritis (immune complex disorder)
- Vasculitis (immune complex disorder)
- Cryoglobulinemia (immune complex disorder)
- **Lymphoma: Up to 3-10% of patients with Sjogren's syndrome develop lymphoma**; risk is increased in patients with severe dryness and systemic complications such as vasculitis, splenomegaly, and cryoglobulinemia.
- Waldenstrom's macroglobulinemia

Clinical management:
- <u>Medical treatment</u>: "Treatment is symptomatic and supportive."[714] "There is no specific [allopathic] treatment for the basic process. Local manifestations can be treated symptomatically."[715]
- Referral if clinical outcome is unsatisfactory or if serious complications are possible.

Treatments:
- Drug treatments include pilocarpine (5 mg 4 times daily) and/or cevimeline (30 mg three times daily) to promote salivation. Associated rheumatic diseases are treated as indicated; prednisone is commonly used.
- <u>Eye drops</u>: Consider vitamin-A-containing eye drops, available OTC or by a compounding pharmacist
- <u>For dry mouth</u>:
  - Sip fluids throughout the day.
  - Chew sugarless gum to promote saliva flow; xylitol chewing gum can stimulate saliva flow and inhibit the growth of cariogenic bacteria.
  - Saliva substitute with carboxymethylcellulose.
  - Fastidious oral hygiene (brushing, flossing, oral antiseptics) and regular dental care are important.
  - Liquid folic acid supplementation swished in the mouth may help alleviate mouth sores; likewise, topical vitamin E and glutamine may help (as they do with chemotherapy-induced mucositis); chewable deglycyrrhizinated licorice benefits some patients.
  - Acupuncture improves salivary flow rates in patients with Sjogren's syndrome.[716,717]

- **FOOD & NUTRITION: 5-part "supplemented Paleo-Mediterranean diet" (SPMD)** The 5-part "supplemented Paleo-Mediterranean diet" (SPMD—reviewed in Chapter 4) consists of ❶ foundational plant-based low-carbohydrate diet of fruits, vegetables, nuts, seeds, berries and lean sources of protein, ❷ multivitamin and multimineral supplementation, ❸ physiologic doses of vitamin D3 (range 2,000-10,000 IU/d), ❹ combination

---

[714] Tierney ML. McPhee SJ, Papadakis MA. *Current Medical Diagnosis and Treatment. 35ᵗʰ edition*. Stamford: Appleton and Lange, 1996 page 749 and Tierney ML. McPhee SJ, Papadakis MA. *Current Medical Diagnosis and Treatment 2006. 45ᵗʰ edition*. New York; Lange Medical Books: 2006, pages 842-843

[715] Beers MH, Berkow R (eds). *The Merck Manual. Seventeenth Edition*. Whitehouse Station; Merck Research Laboratories 1999 Page 424

[716] "CONCLUSIONS: This study shows that acupuncture treatment results in statistically significant improvements in SFR in patients with xerostomia up to 6 months. It suggests that additional acupuncture therapy can maintain this improvement in SFR for up to 3 years." Blom M, Lundeberg T. Long-term follow-up of patients treated with acupuncture for xerostomia and the influence of additional treatment. *Oral Dis* 2000 Jan;6(1):15-24

[717] "A majority of the patients subjectively reported some improvement after treatment, and a significant increase in paraffin-stimulated saliva secretion was found after treatment." List et al. The effect of acupuncture in the treatment of patients with primary Sjogren's syndrome. A controlled study. *Acta Odontol Scand* 1998 Apr;56(2):95-9

fatty acid therapy (CFAT) with n3-ALA, n6-GLA, n3-EPA, n3-DHA, and phytochemical-rich olive oil which contains n9-oleate, and ❺ probiotics.

- o Avoidance of allergenic foods: Any patient may be allergic to any food, even if the food is generally considered a health-promoting food. Generally speaking, the most notorious allergens are wheat, citrus (especially juice due to the industrial use of fungal hemicellulases), cow's milk, eggs, peanuts, chocolate, and yeast-containing foods. **Patients with celiac disease have an increased prevalence of Sjogren's syndrome[718], and patients with Sjogren's syndrome have an increased prevalence of celiac disease.[719] In one study, the estimated prevalence of celiac disease in Sjogren's patients was nearly 1 in 20.[720]** Celiac disease can present with inflammatory oligoarthritis that resembles rheumatoid arthritis and which remits with avoidance of wheat/gluten; the inflammatory arthropathy of celiac disease has preceded bowel symptoms and/or an accurate diagnosis by as many as 3-15 years.[721,722] Clinicians must explain to their patients that celiac disease and wheat allergy are two different clinical entities and that exclusion of one does not exclude the other, and in neither case does mutual exclusion obviate the promotion of intestinal bacterial overgrowth (i.e., proinflammatory dysbiosis) by indigestible wheat oligosaccharides.

- o Broad-spectrum fatty acid therapy with ALA, EPA, DHA, GLA and oleic acid: Fatty acid supplementation should be delivered in the form of combination therapy with ALA, GLA, DHA, and EPA. Given at doses of 3,000 – 9,000 mg per day, ALA from flax oil has impressive anti-inflammatory benefits demonstrated by its ability to halve prostaglandin production in humans.[723] Patients with Sjogren's syndrome have lower levels of GLA/DGLA[724] and fatty acid supplementation—particularly with GLA (along with vitamin C)—is safe and may be beneficial (positive reports[725,726], neutral report[727], negative report[728]).

- o Vitamin D3 supplementation with physiologic doses and/or tailored to serum 25(OH)D levels: Vitamin D insufficiency has been reported in patients with Sjogren's syndrome, presumably due to reduced intake and/or malabsorption. Vitamin D deficiency is common in the general population and is even more common in patients with chronic illness and chronic musculoskeletal pain.[729] Correction of vitamin D deficiency supports normal immune function against infection and provides a clinically significant anti-inflammatory[730] and analgesic benefit in patients with back pain[731] and limb pain.[732] Vitamin D status is inversely associated with inflammation in patients with Sjogren's syndrome.[733,734] Reasonable daily doses for children and adults are 2,000 and 4,000 IU, respectively, as defined by Vasquez, et al.[735] Deficiency

---

[718] "Sjogren's syndrome occurred in 3.3% of coeliac patients and in 0.3% of controls." Collin et al. Coeliac disease—associated disorders and survival. *Gut.* 1994 Sep;35:1215-8.

[719] "Further, our study shows that anti-tTG is more prevalent in SS than in other systemic rheumatic diseases." Luft et al. Autoantibodies to tissue transglutaminase in Sjogren's syndrome and related rheumatic diseases. *J Rheumatol.* 2003 Dec;30(12):2613-9

[720] "The frequency of CD in the SS population was significantly higher than in the non-SS European population (4.5:100 vs 4.5-5.5:1,000)." Szodoray et al. Coeliac disease in Sjogren's syndrome--a study of 111 Hungarian patients. *Rheumatol Int.* 2004 Sep;24(5):278-82

[721] "We report six patients with coeliac disease in whom arthritis was prominent at diagnosis and who improved with dietary therapy. Joint pain preceded diagnosis by up to three years in five patients and 15 years in one patient." Bourne et al. Arthritis and coeliac disease. *Ann Rheum Dis.* 1985 Sep;44(9):592-8

[722] "A 15-year-old girl, with synovitis of the knees and ankles for 3 years before a diagnosis of gluten-sensitive enteropathy, is described." Pinals RS. Arthritis associated with gluten-sensitive enteropathy. *J Rheumatol.* 1986 Feb;13(1):201-4

[723] Adam et al. Effect of alpha-linolenic acid in the human diet on linoleic acid metabolism and prostaglandin biosynthesis. *J Lipid Res.* 1986 Apr;27(4):421-6

[724] "We found MD levels of 20:3n6 (dihommo-gamma-linolenic acid), and basal and indomethacin-enhanced NK cell activity significantly reduced, in 10 primary Sjogren's syndrome patients as compared with 10 healthy controls." Oxholm P, Pedersen BK, Horrobin DF. Natural killer cell functions are related to the cell membrane composition of essential fatty acids: differences in healthy persons and patients with primary Sjogren's syndrome. *Clin Exp Rheumatol.* 1992 May-Jun;10(3):229-34

[725] "An attempt to treat humans with Sjogren's syndrome by raising endogenous PGE1 production by administration of essential fatty acid PGE1 precursors, of pyridoxine and of vitamin C was successful in raising the rates of tear and saliva production." Horrobin DF, Campbell A. Sjogren's syndrome and the sicca syndrome: the role of prostaglandin E1 deficiency. Treatment with essential fatty acids and vitamin C. *Med Hypotheses.* 1980 Mar;6(3):225-32

[726] "Efamol treatment improved the Schirmer-I-test..." Manthorpe R, Hagen Petersen S, Prause JU. Primary Sjogren's syndrome treated with Efamol/Efavit. A double-blind cross-over investigation. *Rheumatol Int.* 1984;4(4):165-7. The duration of this study was ridiculously short—only 3 weeks.

[727] "The objective ocular status, evaluated by a combined ocular score, including the results from Schirmer-I test, break-up time and van Bijsterveld score, improved significantly during Efamol treatment when compared with Efamol start-values (p less than 0.05), but not when compared with placebo values (p less than 0.2)." Oxholm P, Manthorpe R, Prause JU, Horrobin D. Patients with primary Sjogren's syndrome treated for two months with evening primrose oil. *Scand J Rheumatol.* 1986;15:103-8

[728] "There was no significant improvement in any of the patients during the treatment period compared to assessments done pre and post treatment." McKendry RJ. Treatment of Sjogren's syndrome with essential fatty acids, pyridoxine and vitamin C. *Prostaglandins Leukot Med.* 1982 Apr;8(4):403-8

[729] Plotnikoff GA, Quigley JM. Prevalence of severe hypovitaminosis D in patients with persistent, nonspecific musculoskeletal pain. *Mayo Clin Proc.* 2003 Dec;78(12):1463-70

[730] Timms PM, et al. Circulating MMP9, vitamin D and variation in the TIMP-1 response with VDR genotype. *QJM.* 2002 Dec;95(12):787-96

[731] Al Faraj S, Al Mutairi K. Vitamin D deficiency and chronic low back pain in Saudi Arabia. *Spine.* 2003 Jan 15;28(2):177-9

[732] Masood H, Narang AP, Bhat IA, Shah GN. Persistent limb pain and raised serum alkaline phosphatase the earliest markers of subclinical hypovitaminosis D in Kashmir. *Indian J Physiol Pharmacol.* 1989 Oct-Dec;33(4):259-61

[733] "In conclusion the inverse correlations found between levels of 25 OH D and measures of clinical and immunoinflammatory status support the notion that vitamin D metabolism may be involved in the pathogenesis of primary SS." Bang B, Asmussen K, Sorensen OH, Oxholm P. Reduced 25-hydroxyvitamin D levels in primary Sjogren's syndrome. Correlations to disease manifestations. *Scand J Rheumatol.* 1999;28(3):180-3

[734] "Among patients with increased concentrations of IgM rheumatoid factor there was a significant negative correlation between the serum titres of IgM rheumatoid factor and 25-OHD3 concentrations." Muller K, et al. Abnormal vitamin D3 metabolism in patients with primary Sjogren's syndrome. *Ann Rheum Dis.* 1990 Sep;49(9):682-4

[735] Vasquez et al. The clinical importance of vitamin D: a paradigm shift with implications for all healthcare providers. *Altern Ther Health Med.* 2004 Sep-Oct;10(5):28-36

and response to treatment are monitored with serum 25(OH)vitamin D while safety is monitored with serum calcium; inflammatory granulomatous diseases and certain drugs such as hydrochlorothiazide greatly increase the propensity for hypercalcemia and warrant increment dosing and frequent monitoring of serum calcium.

- o <u>Green tea, green tea extract (EGCG), and other phytonutritional antioxidants and anti-inflammatories</u>: Very interestingly, an *in vitro* study[736] showed that epigallocatechin gallate inhibited the expression of major autoantigens, including those which are characteristic of Sjogren's syndrome: SS-B/La, SS-A/Ro. Given its antioxidant properties and anti-inflammatory actions (specifically via inhibition of NFkB[737]), green tea and related supplements may prove beneficial for patients with Sjogren's syndrome.

- o <u>High-dose short-term oral vitamin A</u>: Szocsik et al[738] administered vitamin A 100,000 IU per day for two weeks and obtained improved immune function, such as improved natural killer cell function, in patients with Sjogren's syndrome. Vitamin A is necessary for induction of T-regulatory cells; see Chapter 4.3.

- **INFECTIONS & DYSBIOSIS:** ❶ **antimicrobial treatments,** ❷ **immunorestoration,** ❸ **immunotolerance via Treg induction** Essentially all autoimmune/rheumatic disorders are associated with microbial colonization and intolerance to same; the presence of persistent microbial colonization is *prima facie* evidence of immunosuppression. The eight areas of dysbiosis (multifocal) are: ❶ sinorespiratory, ❷ orodental, ❸ gastrointestinal, ❹ urogenital/genitourinary, ❺ parenchymal/tissue, ❻ microbial, ❼ dermal/cutaneous, and ❽ environmental.

  - o <u>T-cell epitope mimicry between Sjögren's syndrome Antigen A (SSA)/Ro60 and oral, gut, skin and vaginal bacteria (*Clin Immunol.* 2014 May[739])</u>: "Amongst these, a peptide from the von Willebrand factor type A domain protein (vWFA) from the oral microbe *Capnocytophaga ochracea* was the most potent activator. Further, Ro60-reactive T cells were activated by recombinant vWFA protein and whole *Escherichia coli* expressing this protein. These results demonstrate that peptides derived from normal human microbiota can activate Ro60-reactive T cells."

  - o <u>Epstein-Barr virus in Sjögren's syndrome salivary glands drives local autoimmunity (*Nat Rev Rheumatol.* 2014 Jul[740])</u>: Paraphrasing from the original article: "Ectopic lymphoid structures (ELS) within the salivary glands of patients with Sjögren's syndrome serve as niches for latency and reactivation of EBV and contribute to the activation and differentiation of plasma cells. ... EBV is aberrantly expressed in the salivary glands of patients with Sjögren's syndrome, specifically in those glands that displayed ELS, as revealed by the presence of EBV-encoded small RNA (EBER) transcripts and EBER+ cells within infiltrating cells. ... EBV reactivation occurs in a substantial proportion of perifollicular plasma cells that produce anti-Ro52 antibodies."

  - o <u>Epstein-Barr Virus Infection in Disease-Specific Autoreactive B Cell Activation in Ectopic Lymphoid Structures of Sjögren's Syndrome (*Arthritis Rheumatol.* 2014 Sep[741])</u>: "Active EBV infection is selectively associated with ELS in the salivary glands of patients with SS and appears to contribute to local growth and differentiation of disease-specific autoreactive B cells."

  - o <u>Epstein-Barr Virus Infection, Vitamin D Deficiency, and Steps to Autoimmunity: A Unifying Hypothesis (*Autoimmune Dis.* 2012[742])</u>: Per this model, "Autoimmunity is postulated to evolve in the following steps: (1) CD8+ T-cell deficiency, (2) primary EBV infection, (3) decreased CD8+ T-cell control of EBV, (4) increased EBV load and increased anti-EBV antibodies, (5) EBV infection in the target organ, (6) clonal

---

[736] "EGCG inhibited the transcription and translation of major autoantigens, including SS-B/La, SS-A/Ro, coilin, DNA topoisomerase I, and alpha-fodrin. These findings, taken together with green tea's anti-inflammatory and antiapoptotic effects, suggest that green tea polyphenols could serve as an important component in novel approaches to combat autoimmune disorders in humans." Hsu et al. Inhibition of autoantigen expression by (-)-epigallocatechin-3-gallate (the major constituent of green tea) in normal human cells. *J Pharmacol Exp Ther*. 2005 Nov;315(2):805-11

[737] "In conclusion, EGCG is an effective inhibitor of IKK activity. This may explain, at least in part, some of the reported anti-inflammatory and anti-cancer effects of green tea." Yang et al. The green tea polyphenol (-)-epigallocatechin-3-gallate blocks nuclear factor-kappa B activation by inhibiting I kappa B kinase activity in the intestinal epithelial cell line IEC-6. *Mol Pharmacol*. 2001 Sep;60(3):528-33

[738] "Patients with Sjogren's syndrome were treated with vitamin A (100,000 U) daily during a two-week period. The vitamin treatment significantly elevated their ADCC and NK activity." Szocsik et al. Effect of vitamin A treatment on immune reactivity and lipid peroxidation in patients with Sjogren's syndrome. *Clin Rheumatol*. 1988 Dec;7(4):514-9

[739] Szymula et al. T cell epitope mimicry between Sjögren's syndrome Antigen A (SSA)/Ro60 and oral, gut, skin and vaginal bacteria. *Clin Immunol*. 2014 May-Jun;152(1-2):1-9

[740] Onuora S. Connective tissue diseases: Epstein-Barr virus in Sjögren's syndrome salivary glands drives local autoimmunity. *Nat Rev Rheumatol*. 2014 Jul;10(7):384

[741] Croia et al. Implication of Epstein-Barr Virus Infection in Disease-Specific Autoreactive B Cell Activation in Ectopic Lymphoid Structures of Sjögren's Syndrome. *Arthritis Rheumatol*. 2014 Sep;66(9):2545-57

[742] Pender MP. CD8+ T-Cell Deficiency, Epstein-Barr Virus Infection, Vitamin D Deficiency, and Steps to Autoimmunity. *Autoimmune Dis*. 2012;2012:189096

expansion of EBV-infected autoreactive B cells in the target organ, (7) infiltration of autoreactive T cells into the target organ, and (8) development of ectopic lymphoid follicles in the target organ [which drive the tissue damage and autoantibody production as recently demonstrated per *Nat Rev Rheumatol* 2014 Jul[743] and *Arthritis Rheumatol* 2014 Sep[744]]. It is also proposed that deprivation of sunlight and vitamin D at higher latitudes facilitates the development of autoimmune diseases by aggravating the CD8+ T-cell deficiency and thereby further impairing control of EBV." Congratulations to this author—Pender—for predicting two years in advance the research that would later support this model.

o <u>Aryl hydrocarbon receptor-mediated induction of EBV reactivation as a risk factor for Sjögren's syndrome</u> (*J Immunol* 2012 May[745]): This is very impressive research, connecting xenobiotic exposure with viral reactivation. "The aryl hydrocarbon receptor (AhR) is a ligand-activated transcription factor that mediates a variety of biological effects by binding to environmental pollutants, including 2,3,7,8-tetrachlorodibenzo-p-dioxin (TCDD or dioxin). ... This study evaluated the possibility that ligand-activated AhR reactivates EBV. ... TCDD enhanced BZLF1 transcription, which mediates the switch from the latent to the lytic form of EBV infection in EBV-positive B cell lines and in a salivary gland epithelial cell line. Moreover, TCDD-induced increases in BZLF1 mRNA and EBV genomic DNA levels were confirmed in the B cell lines. Saliva from SS patients activated the transcription of both CYP1A1 and BZLF1. Additionally, there was a positive correlation between CYP1A1 and BZLF1 promoter activities. AhR ligands elicited the reactivation of EBV in activated B cells and salivary epithelial cells, and these ligands are involved in SS." This is stunning research: it provides direct links between infections, xenobiotic exposure, and autoimmunity; further, by extension, this research also suggests that xenobiotic exposure could also enhance transcription of HERVs (directly, or indirectly via viral transactivation) which also contributes to autoimmunity.

o <u>Assess for and treat dysbiosis</u>: Insufficient flow of saliva and other fluids promotes microbial colonization of mucosal surfaces, particularly the digestive and respiratory tracts. Gastrointestinal infection/dysbiosis can cause nutrient malabsorption, and the resultant nutritional insufficiencies can exacerbate the sicca symptoms.[746] Patients with Sjogren's syndrome may have an increased prevalence of infection/colonization with *H. pylori*[747], an organism known to incite systemic inflammation and to produce pro-inflammatory endotoxin and antigens; eradication of this microbe—or others per patient—may alleviate clinical manifestations by addressing one of the inciting causes. Of particular note is that *H. pylori* promotes gastric autoimmunity, sicca syndrome, as well as intestinal lymphoma—all of which are noted in Sjogren's syndrome.

▪ <u>*H pylori* and gastrointestinal cancer</u>: "*H. pylori* infection is a major cause of gastric (stomach) cancer, specifically non-cardia gastric cancer (cancer in all areas of the stomach, except for the top portion near where it joins the esophagus). *H. pylori* infection also causes gastric mucosa-associated lymphoid tissue (MALT) lymphoma. *H. pylori* infection is associated with a decreased risk of some other cancers, including gastric cardia cancer (cancer in the top portion of the stomach) and esophageal adenocarcinoma."[748]

- | **NUTRITIONAL IMMUNOMODULATION: Treg induction for modulation of Th-1/2/17 inflammation** |
Nutrients and therapeutic approaches that promote Treg or IL-10 induction and/or Th-17, IL-17 suppression include 1) mitochondrial optimization and mTOR suppression, 2) biotin, 3) vitamin E, 4) sodium avoidance, 5) transgenic/GMO food avoidance, 6) probiotics, 7) lipoic acid, 8) vitamin A, 9) inflammation reduction, 10) vitamin D, 11) fatty acid supplementation with GLA and n3, 12) infection and dysbiosis remediation, 13) green tea EGCG. Acronym: MiBESTPLAIDFIG (2014) and MiBESTPLAIDFIGNaC (2016)—as reviewed in Chaper 4.3.

[743] Onuora S. Connective tissue diseases: Epstein-Barr virus in Sjögren's syndrome salivary glands drives local autoimmunity. *Nat Rev Rheumatol*. 2014 Jul;10(7):384
[744] Croia et al. Implication of Epstein-Barr Virus Infection in Disease-Specific Autoreactive B Cell Activation in Ectopic Lymphoid Structures of Sjögren's Syndrome. *Arthritis Rheumatol*. 2014 Sep;66(9):2545-57
[745] Inoue et al. Aryl hydrocarbon receptor-mediated induction of EBV reactivation as a risk factor for Sjögren's syndrome. *J Immunol*. 2012 May 1;188(9):4654-62
[746] Bosman et al. Sicca syndrome associated with Tropheryma whipplei intestinal infection. *J Clin Microbiol*. 2002 Aug;40(8):3104-6
[747] "Patients with SS are more prone to have H. pylori infection in comparison to other connective tissue diseases. Serum antibody titer to H. pylori correlated with index for clinical disease manifestations, age, disease duration and CRP." El Miedany et al. Sjogren's syndrome: concomitant H. pylori infection and possible correlation with clinical parameters. *Joint Bone Spine*. 2005 Mar;72(2):135-41
[748] cancer.gov/cancertopics/factsheet/Risk/h-pylori-cancer

- o <u>IL-17-producing T cells are expanded in the peripheral blood, infiltrate salivary glands and are resistant to corticosteroids in patients with primary Sjogren's syndrome</u> (*Ann Rheum Dis*. 2013 Feb[749]): "It has been recently observed that a T-cell subset, lacking of both CD4 and CD8 molecules and defined as double negative (DN), is expanded in the blood of patients with systemic lupus erythematosus, produces IL-17 and accumulates in the kidney during nephritis. Since IL-17 production is enhanced in salivary gland infiltrates of primary Sjögren's syndrome (SS) patients, we investigated whether DN T cells may be involved in the pathogenesis of salivary gland damage. ... CD3(+)CD4(-)CD8(-) DN T cells were major producers of IL-17 in SS and expressed ROR-γt. They were expanded in the peripheral blood, spontaneously produced IL-17 and infiltrated salivary glands. In addition, the expansion of $\alpha\beta$-TCR(+) DN T cells was associated with disease activity. Notably, IL-17-producing DN T cells from SS patients, but not from healthy controls, were strongly resistant to the in vitro effect of dexamethasone." Readers should by now (following discussion in Chapter 4) appreciate that IL-17 production and tissue infiltration are synonymous with autoimmune-type tissue damage and inflammation.

- • **DYSMETABOLISM: MitoDys, ERS-UPR, mTOR inhibition** The major clinical considerations in this section are mitochondrial dysfunction, endoplasmic reticulum stress, unfolded protein response, TLR activation, and the dysmetabolic effects of sustained hyperglycemia and hyperinsulinemia and resultant oxidative stress, inflammation, RAGE activation, and accumulation of AGE, palmitate and ceramide. The review of this information in Chapter 4 covered approximately 30 interventions relevant to dysmetabolism, mitochondrial dysfunction, ERS-UPR, etc; these will not be reviewed here except to mention those most commonly, easily, empirically, synergistically, and effectively used: 1) low-carbohydrate diet with 2) moderate exercise, 3) CoQ-10, 4) acetyl-carnitine with 5) lipoic acid, 6) NAC, 7) resveratrol, and 8) melatonin.

- • **STYLE OF LIVING (LIFESTYLE) & SPECIAL CONSIDERATIONS** This is a buffet of mostly lifestyle-based interventions yet also including considerations such as additional supplementation and surgery.
  - o <u>Individualized homeopathy</u>: A small randomized placebo-controlled trial found homeopathy beneficial for xerostomia.[750]
  - o <u>Replacement of gastric HCL</u>: Tablets/capsules of betaine HCL may improve digestion, nutrient assimilation, and also alleviate intestinal microbial overgrowth; antiparietal cell antibodies may be noted.

- • **ENDOCRINE IMBALANCE & OPTIMIZATION: Prolactin, Insulin, Estrogen, DHEA, Cortisol, Testosterone, Thyroid** Common hormonal imbalances seen among autoimmune/inflammatory patients are: ❶ *elevated* prolactin, ❷ *elevated* estrogen, ❸ *elevated* insulin, and ❹ *reduced* DHEA, ❺ *reduced* cortisol, and ❻ *reduced* testosterone; see Chapter 4 for discussion of these hormones and respective interventions. Thyroid evaluation should be comprehensive, as discussed in Chapter 1, with a low threshold for empiric treatment.
  - o <u>Endocrine alterations in primary Sjogren's syndrome</u> (*J Autoimmun*. 2012 Dec[751]): "Heightened serum and salivary gland tissue prolactin levels in primary SS patients have been also suggested as contributors in disease pathogenesis. Finally, autoimmune thyroid disease (ATD) occurs quiet commonly in the setting of primary SS and subclinical hypothyroidism is the main functional abnormality observed in these patients."
  - o <u>DHEA in Sjogren's syndrome—a hormonal deficiency and potential treatment in search of clinical significance</u>: Generally, the finding of low DHEA and the correction/normalization of low DHEA in patients with autoimmunity/inflammation/autoinflammation correlates with clinical improvement; such has not been the situation with Sjogren's syndrome, which has been consistently resistant to improvement following DHEA administration, a fact which I have noted since the first publication of *Integrative Rheumatology* in 2006. I think what is likely here is that the DHEA deficiency is important, but that isolated DHEA supplementation is insufficient to elicit a significant clinical improvement as monotherapy.

---

[749] Alunno et al. IL-17-producing CD4-CD8- T cells are expanded in the peripheral blood, infiltrate salivary glands and are resistant to corticosteroids in patients with primary Sjogren's syndrome. *Ann Rheum Dis*. 2013 Feb;72(2):286-92
[750] "Our results suggest that individually prescribed homeopathic medicine could be a valuable adjunct to the treatment of oral discomfort and xerostomic symptoms." Haila et al. Effects of homeopathic treatment on salivary flow rate and subjective symptoms in patients with oral dryness: a randomized trial. *Homeopathy*. 2005 Jul;94(3):175-81
[751] Mavragani et al. Endocrine alterations in primary Sjogren's syndrome: an overview. *J Autoimmun*. 2012 Dec;39(4):354-8

- Low serum dehydroepiandrosterone sulfate in women with primary Sjögren's syndrome as an isolated sign of impaired HPA axis function (*J Rheumatol*. 2001 Jun[752]): "The results show that women with pSS have intact cortisol synthesis but decreased serum concentrations of DHEA-S and increased cortisol/DHEA-S ratio compared with healthy controls. The findings may reflect a constitutional or disease mediated influence on adrenal steroid synthesis. The thyroid axis and gonadotropin secretion were similar in patients and controls."
- DHEA versus placebo for Sjögren's syndrome (*Arthritis Rheum*. 2004 Aug[753]): "A 24-week randomized, double-blinded, pilot trial of oral DHEA (200 mg/day) versus placebo was conducted. ... Apart from changes over the trial in dry mouth symptoms, no significant differences were noted between the DHEA and placebo groups for dry eye symptoms, objective measures of ocular dryness, stimulated salivary flow; IgG, or ESR. ... DHEA showed no evidence of efficacy in SS. Without evidence for efficacy, patients with SS should avoid using unregulated DHEA supplements, since long-term adverse consequences of exposure to this hormone are unknown."
- Dehydroepiandrosterone (DHEA) treatment for severe fatigue in DHEA-deficient patients with primary Sjögren's syndrome (*Arthritis Care Res* 2010 Jan[754]): "A multicenter, investigator-based, powered, randomized controlled clinical trial (crossover, washout design) using fatigue as the primary outcome measure was performed on patients with primary SS (n = 107) who had a general fatigue score > or =14 on the 20-item Multiple Fatigue Inventory (MFI-20), combined with age- and sex-adjusted serum DHEAS values below the mean. .. Similar to earlier results using pharmacologic doses, substitution treatment with 50 mg of DHEA in DHEA-deficient and severely tired primary SS patients does not help against fatigue better than placebo."

- **XENOBIOTIC ACCUMULATION & DETOXIFICATION: Chemical avoidance, nutritional support for detoxification pathways, urine alkalinization** | The clinical relevance and pathogenic mechanisms of xenobiotic accumulation are irrefutably well documented and described. Clinical assessments include history, physical examination, and laboratory assessment (using serum, whole blood, urine or—rarely yet accurately— fat biopsy), and response to treatment. Treatments include nutritional support for Phases 1 and 2 of detoxification (e.g., oxidation and conjugation) and excretion via bile and urine; for the latter, urinary alkalinization is generally recommended. Chemical toxins can be bound in the gut using activated charcoal, cholestyramine, or *Chlorella*—all of these three treatments have documented safety and effectiveness; clinically and empirically, phytochelatin (plant-derived peptides that bind toxic metals) concentrates appear safe and effective despite lack of conclusive published data supporting clinical use.
  - Aryl hydrocarbon receptor-mediated induction of EBV reactivation as a risk factor for Sjögren's syndrome (*J Immunol* 2012 May[755]): This is very impressive research, connecting xenobiotic exposure with viral reactivation. "The aryl hydrocarbon receptor (AhR) is a ligand-activated transcription factor that mediates a variety of biological effects by binding to environmental pollutants, including 2,3,7,8-tetrachlorodibenzo-p-dioxin (TCDD or dioxin). ... This study evaluated the possibility that ligand-activated AhR reactivates EBV. ... TCDD enhanced BZLF1 transcription, which mediates the switch from the latent to the lytic form of EBV infection in EBV-positive B cell lines and in a salivary gland epithelial cell line. Moreover, TCDD-induced increases in BZLF1 mRNA and EBV genomic DNA levels were confirmed in the B cell lines. Saliva from SS patients activated the transcription of both CYP1A1 and BZLF1. Additionally, there was a positive correlation between CYP1A1 and BZLF1 promoter activities. AhR ligands elicited the reactivation of EBV in activated B cells and salivary epithelial cells, and these ligands are involved in SS." This is stunning research: it provides direct links between infections, xenobiotic exposure, and autoimmunity; further, by extension, this research also suggests that xenobiotic exposure could also enhance transcription of HERVs (directly, or indirectly via viral transactivation) and thereby contribute to autoimmunity.

[752] Valtysdóttir et al. Low serum dehydroepiandrosterone sulfate in women with primary Sjögren's syndrome as an isolated sign of impaired HPA axis function. *J Rheumatol*. 2001 Jun;28(6):1259-65
[753] Pillemer et al. Pilot clinical trial of dehydroepiandrosterone (DHEA) versus placebo for Sjögren's syndrome. *Arthritis Rheum*. 2004 Aug 15;51(4):601-4
[754] Virkki et al. Dehydroepiandrosterone (DHEA) substitution treatment for severe fatigue in DHEA-deficient patients with primary Sjögren's syndrome. *Arthritis Care Res* (Hoboken). 2010 Jan 15;62(1):118-24
[755] Inoue et al. Aryl hydrocarbon receptor-mediated induction of EBV reactivation as a risk factor for Sjögren's syndrome. *J Immunol*. 2012 May 1;188(9):4654-62

Raynaud's Phenomenon

Introduction:
Raynaud's Phenomenon is a disorder of periodic vasoconstriction mainly affecting the hands/fingers; it is a manifestation of autonomic dysfunction associated with and often preceding autoimmune diseases, especially scleroderma. Per the 2010 criteria for fibromyalgia (FM), Raynaud's is now associated with that condition as well; this may be absurd except that both Raynaud's and FM are causatively associated with microbial dysbiosis, especially in the intestines, i.e., *Helicobacter pylori* with Raynaud's and SIBO with FM. The condition responds poorly to medical/pharmacologic treatment that focuses on vasodilation; the condition responds very well to integrative treatment, especially that which focuses on dysbiosis eradication, antioxidant supplementation, hormonal correction/supplementation, and other components of the Functional Inflammology protocol. I am increasingly interested in approaching Raynaud phenomenon from the perspective of alleviating neurogenic inflammation.

Introduction and Diagnosis

- Introduction and terminology: Raynaud's phenomenon is periodic recurrent severe vasoconstriction-induced hypoperfusion accompanied by discomfort most commonly affecting the fingers.
  - Primary Raynaud's phenomenon—formerly "Raynaud's disease": Not associated with a concomitant disease; therefore, in this case the vasospasm is considered its own problem, hence the previously used term "disease" when describing primary Raynaud's phenomenon.
  - Secondary Raynaud's phenomenon—formerly "Raynaud's syndrome": Associated with a concomitant disease, especially autoimmunity, especially scleroderma.
- Diagnosis and Evaluation: Assessment for the presence/absence of systemic disease is important; Raynaud's can precede systemic autoimmunity by several years, for example in scleroderma.
  - Digital artery blood pressure: A decrease of > 15 mmHg is consistent with vasoconstriction.
  - Doppler ultrasound: Can be used to measure blood flow.
  - Routine labs: CBC, chemistry/metabolic panel, ANA, CRP, and the full thyroid evaluation in Chapter 1..
  - Nailfold capillaroscopy: Reveals microvascular changes consistent with autoimmunity and autoimmune-expedited cardiovascular disease. Per Cutolo et al[756], "Raynaud's phenomenon (RP) represents the most frequent clinical aspect of cardio/microvascular involvement and is a key feature of several autoimmune rheumatic diseases. Moreover, RP is associated in a statistically significant manner with many coronary diseases. In normal conditions or in primary RP (excluding during the cold-exposure test), the normal nailfold capillaroscopic pattern shows a regular disposition of the capillary loops along with the nailbed. On the contrary, in subjects suffering from secondary RP, one or more alterations of the capillaroscopic findings should alert the physician of the possibility of a connective tissue disease not yet detected. Nailfold capillaroscopy (NV) represents the best method to analyze microvascular abnormalities in autoimmune rheumatic diseases. Architectural disorganization, giant capillaries, hemorrhages, loss of capillaries, angiogenesis and avascular areas characterize >95% of patients with overt scleroderma (SSc)."
- Complications: Long-term recurrent vasoconstriction can result in atrophy of the skin and subcutaneous tissues including muscle; digital ulceration and ischemic gangrene can result. Recurrent vasospasm-induced tissue hypoxia appears to increase inflammation via oxidative stress and possibly via elaboration of damage-associated molecular patterns.

Clinical Applications and Interventions

- Raynaud's phenomenon—specific treatments: Treatment of Raynaud's phenomenon should not be trivialized as merely symptomatic; the pain experienced by some patients with Raynaud's phenomenon is truly excruciating. Additionally, a wonderfully insightful comment by Simonini et al[757] in 2000 stated that the tissue

---

[756] Cutolo et al. Nailfold capillaroscopy is useful for the diagnosis and follow-up of autoimmune rheumatic diseases. A future tool for the analysis of microvascular heart involvement? *Rheumatology* (Oxford). 2006 Oct;45 Suppl 4:iv43-6 rheumatology.oxfordjournals.org/content/45/suppl_4/iv43.full.pdf

[757] "…daily episodes of hypoxia-reperfusion injury, produces several episodes of free radicals-mediated endothelial derangement. These events results in a positive feedback effect of luminal narrowing and ischemia and therefore to the birth of a vicious cycle of oxygen free radicals (OFR) generation, leading to endothelial damage, intimal thickening and fibrosis." Simonini et al. Emerging potentials for an antioxidant therapy as a new approach to the treatment of systemic sclerosis. *Toxicology*. 2000 Nov 30;155(1-3):1-15

ischemia induced by Raynaud's phenomenon is *pathogenic* because it promotes oxidative stress and the vicious cycle of inflammation; the recurrent ischemia and reperfusion of hypoxic Raynaud's phenomenon could be thought of somewhat as a "recurrent, mild heart attack [or stroke] of the hands" causing tissue damage and cell apoptosis/necrosis leading to release of damage-associated molecular patterns (DAMP) and the resultant immune activation, systemic inflammation, mitochondrial dysfunction, proinflammatory immunophenotype switch toward Th1/Th2/Th17 and resultant fibrosis and autoimmunity. Remarkably, Mahoney et al[758] proposed a similar model in 2011 when they wrote, "We propose that a recent change in the conception of the role of type 1 interferon and the identification of adventitial stem cells suggests a unifying hypothesis for scleroderma. This hypothesis begins with vasospasm. Vasospasm is fully reversible unless, as proposed here, the resulting ischemia leads to apoptosis and activation of type 1 interferon. The interferon, we propose, initiates immune amplification, including characteristic scleroderma-specific antibodies." Thus, treatments to maintain vasodilation and quench the free radicals resultant from recurrent hypoxic events are necessary. Antioxidants have been discussed previously and should be common knowledge to readers of this text. Vasodilation in Raynaud's phenomenon can be supported with any/all of the following:

- o Eradication of *Helicobacter pylori*: Eradication of *Helicobacter pylori* is one of the most effective treatments of Raynaud's disease/syndrome/phenomenon and should therefore be pursued in all affected patients.

  - Helicobacter pylori eradication ameliorates primary Raynaud's phenomenon (*Dig Dis Sci* 1998 Aug[759]): "Forty-six patients affected by primary Raynaud's phenomenon were evaluated. *H. pylori* infection was assessed by [13C]urea breath test. Eradication therapy was given to infected patients for seven days. … **Attacks of Raynaud's phenomenon completely disappeared in 17% of the patients with *H. pylori* eradication. Discomfort and the duration and frequency of attacks of Raynaud's phenomenon were significantly reduced in 72% of the remaining patients.** … The study shows that *H. pylori* eradication causes a significant decrease in clinical attacks of Raynaud's disease. The reduction of vasoactive substances determined by the eradication of the bacterium may be the pathogenetic mechanism underlying the phenomenon."

- o Inositol hexaniacinate: 3,000-4,000 mg/d *po* in divided doses[760,761,762]

- o *Ginkgo biloba*: Ginkgo reduces the number of daily Raynaud's attacks in patients with primary Raynaud's disease[763], and it is also an excellent antioxidant with potent anti-inflammatory benefits.

- o Magnesium: 300-500 mg/d or bowel tolerance; systemic alkalinization to achieve urine alkalinity of 7.5 promotes renal retention of magnesium and systemic cellular uptake.

- o Combination fatty acid therapy: must include GLA (minimum 500 mg) and EPA (minimum 2,000 mg)

- o L-arginine: L-arginine is the biochemical precursor to nitric oxide, which has vasodilating actions. L-arginine supplementation in patients with Raynaud's phenomenon showed benefit in one study[764] and no benefit in another.[765] However, arginine supplementation was tremendously beneficial in 4 case reports of scleroderma patients with Raynaud's-induced digital necrosis.[766] Excess arginine supplementation may lead to an overproduction of nitric oxide, which can be harmful in excess due to its free radical behavior and its contribution to peroxynitrite. Additionally, metabolism of arginine requires methyl groups, and therefore supplementation with methyl donors such as methylfolate/folinate, cobalamin, betaine, et al should be used anytime supplemental arginine is used for long periods of time; homocysteine levels should occasionally be measured.

---

[758] Mahoney et al. A unifying hypothesis for scleroderma: identifying a target cell for scleroderma. *Curr Rheumatol Rep*. 2011 Feb;13:28-36

[759] Gasbarrini A et al. Helicobacter pylori eradication ameliorates primary Raynaud's phenomenon. *Dig Dis Sci*. 1998 Aug;43(8):1641-5

[760] "It appears to be a safe and well tolerated drug, which, together with other symptomatic measures, merits to be used in the management of vasospastic disease of the extremities even in the presence of partial obliteration of the microcirculation." Holti G. An experimentally controlled evaluation of the effect of inositol nicotinate upon the digital blood flow in patients with Raynaud's phenomenon. *J Int Med Res*. 1979;7(6):473-83

[761] "Although the mechanism of action remains unclear Hexopal is safe and is effective in reducing the vasospasm of primary Raynaud's disease during the winter months." Sunderland et al. A double blind randomised placebo controlled trial of hexopal in primary Raynaud's disease. *Clin Rheumatol*. 1988 Mar;7(1):46-9

[762] "It is suggested that long-term treatment with nicotinate acid derivatives may produce improvement in the peripheral circulation by a different mechanism than the transient effect detected by short-term studies." Ring et al. Quantitative thermographic assessment of inositol nicotinate therapy in Raynaud's phenomena. J Int Med Res. 1977;5(4):217-22

[763] "Ginkgo biloba phytosome may be effective in reducing the number of Raynaud's attacks per week in patients suffering from Raynaud's disease." Muir et al. The use of Ginkgo biloba in Raynaud's disease: a double-blind placebo-controlled trial. *Vasc Med*. 2002;7(4):265-7

[764] "After therapy, patients with Raynaud's phenomenon secondary to systemic sclerosis showed: (1) higher digital vasodilation after local warming, (2) cold-induced digital vasodilation, and (3) increase of plasma levels of tissue-type plasminogen activator." Agostoni et al. L-arginine therapy in Raynaud's phenomenon? *Int J Clin Lab Res*. 1991;21(2):202-3

[765] "L-arginine supplementation, however, had no significant effect on vascular responses to acetylcholine and sodium nitroprusside." Khan F, Belch JJ. Skin blood flow in patients with systemic sclerosis and Raynaud's phenomenon: effects of oral L-arginine supplementation. *J Rheumatol*. 1999 Nov;26(11):2389-94

[766] "We report two cases in which oral L-arginine reversed digital necrosis in Raynaud's phenomenon and two additional cases in which the symptoms of severe Raynaud's phenomenon were improved with oral L-arginine." Rembold et al. Oral L-arginine can reverse digital necrosis in Raynaud's phenomenon. *Mol Cell Biochem*. 2003 Feb;244:139-41

- o <u>NAC 500-1,500mg *po tid ic*</u>: NAC is pleiotropically beneficial, via antiviral, antioxidant, GSH-supporting, and mTOR inhibiting actions.
  - <u>Intravenous N-acetylcysteine for treatment of Raynaud's phenomenon secondary to systemic sclerosis</u> (*J Rheumatol* 2001 Oct[767])—paraphrased/quoted as follows: "Twenty-two patients with RP secondary to SSc were enrolled in a multicenter, open clinical trial lasting 11 weeks and conducted in winter. Primary outcome measures were frequency and severity of RP attacks, and number of digital ulcers. Secondary outcome measure was improvement in digital cold challenge test assessed by photoelectric plethysmography. Patients received a continuous 5 day intravenous infusion of NAC starting with a 2 h loading dose of 150 mg/kg subsequently adjusted to 15 mg/kg/h. RESULTS: ... Both frequency and severity of RP attacks decreased significantly compared to pretreatment values. Active ulcers were significantly less numerous at all follow-up visits (25% of baseline count on Day 33 from the beginning of infusion). In the cold challenge test, mean recovery time fell by 69%, 67%, 71%, and 71% on Days 12, 19, 33, and 61 from the beginning of treatment. Side effects were minor, easily controlled, and reversible. CONCLUSION: N-acetylcysteine appears to be safe for the treatment of RP secondary to SSc. These preliminary data warrant further controlled studies."
- o <u>Acupuncture, biofeedback, counseling, stress reduction, cold avoidance, smoking cessation</u>: Since stressful events, cold exposure, and cigarette smoking are all vasoconstrictive, these should be avoided/modified to the highest extent possible. Stress reduction and modification of inter- and intra-personal socioemotional exchange would be beneficial for anyone.
  - <u>Biofeedback treatment of Raynaud's disease and phenomenon</u> (*Biofeedback Self Regul.* 1981 Sep[768]): "Six Raynaud's disease [primary] and four Raynaud's phenomenon [secondary] patients were treated with 12 sessions of finger temperature biofeedback. The mean frequency of vasospastic attacks was reduced to 7.5% of that reported during the pretreatment baseline and was maintained for a 1 year follow-up period. ... Raynaud's phenomenon [secondary] patients showed significantly greater temperature increases during feedback periods than Raynaud's disease [primary] patients."
- o <u>Hormonal interventions</u>: Annotated below:
  - <u>Treatment of Raynaud's phenomenon with large doses of triiodothyronine [T3]</u> (*Ann Rheum Dis.* 1987 Dec[769]): Triiodothyronine was prescribed at a dosage of 80 mcg/d to 9 female patients with autoimmunity (SLE, SSc, RA, overlap syndrome [OS]); they all experienced safe and significant remission of their Raynaud's symptoms. Patients who could not tolerate 80 mcg/d due to anticipated heat intolerance and palpitations were treated with lower doses of 40-60 mcg/d. "In all patients, blood pressure, pulse pressure, and pulse rate remained essentially unchanged and thyroid function tests were confirmatory of drug compliance. ... In the first place, every one of them described a substantial, if not dramatic, improvement in their condition. ... Large dosages of T3 were found in this study to be a highly effective treatment for Raynaud's phenomenon and one principally free from side effects."
  - <u>Treatment of Raynaud's phenomenon with triiodothyronine [T3] corrects co-existent autonomic dysfunction</u> (*Postgrad Med J* 1992 Apr[770]): Nine female patients with autoimmunity and Raynaud's phenomenon showed a high prevalence of cardiovascular autonomic dysfunction as assessed by five standard non-invasive tests (3 of heart rate and 2 of blood pressure). "The subjects were given triiodothyronine, 60 to 80 micrograms per day, for vasospastic attacks. ... Test results [of autonomic function] showed a considerable improvement. ... Adverse side effects to triiodothyronine occurred in a single subject and were readily controlled. ... Triiodothyronine may have corrected autonomic dysfunction by increasing blood flow to ischemic peripheral nerves or by acting on the autonomic system more directly."

---

[767] Sambo et al. Intravenous N-acetylcysteine for treatment of Raynaud's phenomenon secondary to systemic sclerosis: a pilot study. *J Rheumatol.* 2001 Oct;28(10):2257-62
[768] Freedman et al. Biofeedback treatment of Raynaud's disease and phenomenon. *Biofeedback Self Regul.* 1981 Sep;6(3):355-65
[769] Dessein PH, Gledhill RF. Treatment of Raynaud's phenomenon with large doses of triiodothyronine: a pilot study. *Ann Rheum Dis.* 1987 Dec;46(12):944-5
[770] Gledhill et al. Treatment of Raynaud's phenomenon with triiodothyronine corrects co-existent autonomic dysfunction. *Postgrad Med J.* 1992 Apr;68(798):263-7

- Successful treatment of Raynaud's phenomenon with L-thyroxine [T4] (*Med Hypotheses* 2003 Mar[771]):"A 50-year old patient a 15-year history of Raynaud's phenomenon developed thyroid deficiency with exacerbation of the symptoms of Raynaud's. After substitution therapy with L-thyroxine, the patient became euthyroid and the symptoms of Raynaud's phenomenon disappeared. Similarly, several patients with Raynaud's phenomenon were found to be hypothyroid and replacement therapy again eliminated the symptoms."
- 7-oxo-DHEA contra Raynaud's phenomenon (*Med Hypotheses* 2003 Mar[772]): The authors of this report basically provide a review of the literature on Raynaud's phenomenon—its assessments and treatments—and then provide a single case report of improvement; the dose and duration of treatment are not provided. "An initial result is encouraging. A 46-year old patient had increasingly frequent vasospastic attacks accompanied by pain and pallor in her left fingers except the thumb. Precipitating factors included being in an excessively air-conditioned environment, touching cold objects, and digging in cold, wet earth. The episodes were less than 10 min duration. The patient had no other complaints, denied other illnesses, and does not take any prescription medications. The patient does not smoke, and consumes minimal amounts of alcohol occasionally. On examination, her hands were without any abnormalities with normal skin and color appearance. These vasospastic attacks did not occur after taking 7-oxo-DHEA but returned within one week of discontinuing the medication, and disappeared again on resuming the medication." Obviously that is a pretty weak case report, but nonetheless, clinicians might consider using this generally considered as safe nonprescription agent in conjunction with the treatments aforementioned.

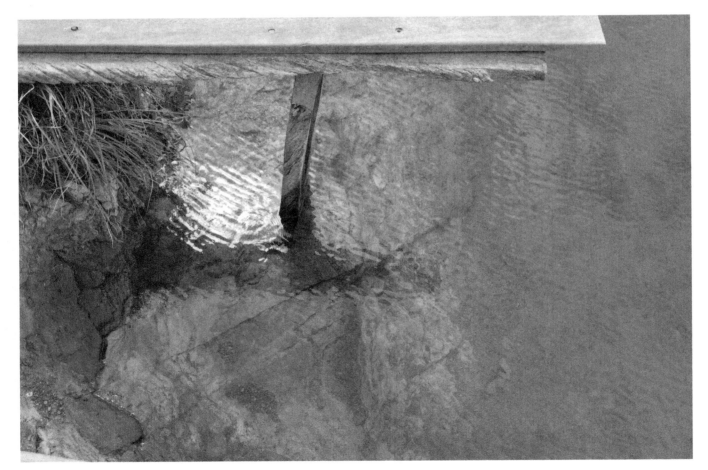

Lago Azul (Blue Lake) near Villa de Leyva, Colombia: 2014 photo by DrV

---

[771] Ihler et al. 7-oxo-DHEA and Raynaud's phenomenon. *Med Hypotheses*. 2003 Mar;60(3):391-7
[772] Ihler et al. 7-oxo-DHEA and Raynaud's phenomenon. *Med Hypotheses*. 2003 Mar;60(3):391-7

Clinical Notes on Additional Conditions:
Behçet's Disease, Sarcoidosis, Dermatomyositis and Polymyositis

Introduction:

The sections that follow are original to *Integrative Rheumatology* 2006/2007; later versions of my books were too large to allow inclusion of these sections per limitations of the publisher's printing capacity, and thus the sections were not updated. Here, they are presented with few modifications, mostly the removal of redundant material presented in the previous sections. The overall clinical approach is generally as outlined previously since all autoimmune/autoinflammatory diseases have the same basic components as recalled per the F.I.N.D.S.E.X.® acronym. I strongly agree with Threoau's statement that "What is once done well is done forever" (*Civil Disobedience*, page 13), and I consider the previous reviews to be at least reasonable and the research from which it was derived no less valuable simply because it has acquired a few years without updated reinforcement; the updates made to the overall protocol should generally suffice, along with the following details and nuances.

Behçet's Disease/Syndrome

Description/pathophysiology:
- **A relapsing systemic/multiorgan autoimmune disease associated with vasculopathy and ulcerations of the oral and genital mucosa**
- "Idiopathic"[773]; etiopathogenic associations include:
  - Occult **bacterial**/viral/fungal/parasitic infections with resultant molecular mimicry and stimulation of autoreactive T-cells[774]: as summarized by Verity et al[775], "…the evidence indicates that **the underlying immune events in BD are triggered by a microbial antigen** and subsequently driven by genetic influences which control leukocyte behavior and the coagulation pathways."
  - Associated with HLA-B51 in Japan and Mediterranean areas
- Considered **uncommon in the US**

Clinical presentations:
- Two-fold more common in men than in women
- Age of onset is generally in 20's and 30's; may occur in children
- Painful oral and genital ulcers: resembles recurrent aphthous stomatitis, most commonly the first manifestation of the disease
- Ocular complaints: pain, photophobia, blurred vision, iridocyclitis
- Skin lesions in 80% of patients: papules, pustules, vesicles, folliculitis, erythema nodosum-like lesions, "exaggerated" inflammatory reactions to minor skin trauma
- Joint pain: nondestructive arthritis in 50% of patients
- Vasculitis and thrombophlebitis: can affect any organ
- Neurocognitive disturbances and central nervous system involvement
- Abdominal pain and intestinal involvement: some patients have evidence of enteropathy

Major differential diagnoses:
- Aphthous stomatitis (DDX: oral herpes)
- Autoimmunity in general, vasculitis in particular
- Infection: conceivably possible to confuse oral ulcers with Koplic's spots
- Crohn's disease—multisystemic disease, oral ulcerations

[773] Beers MH, Berkow R (eds). *Merck Manual. 17th Edition*. Whitehouse Station; Merck Research Laboratories 1999 Page 424
[774] Sakane et al. Etiopathology of Behcet's disease: immunological aspects. *Yonsei Med J*. 1997 Dec;38(6):350-8 eymj.org/1997/pdf/12350.pdf
[775] Verity et al. Behcet's disease: from Hippocrates to the third millennium. *Br J Ophthalmol*. 2003 Sep;87(9):1175-83 bjo.bmjjournals.com/cgi/reprint/87/9/1175

Clinical assessments:
- **History/subjective**:
  - See clinical presentations
- **Physical examination/objective**:
  - Oral, ocular, and genital examinations
  - Other examinations as indicated
- **Laboratory assessments**:
  - ESR: elevated
  - CBC: mild leukocytosis
  - HLA-B51: may or may not be positive, but is associated with increased likelihood of the disease
  - Homocysteine: Patients with Behcet's syndrome have elevated homocysteine which exacerbates arterial and venous occlusion which underlies many of the clinical complications of the disease.[776,777]
  - Lactulose/mannitol assay: Patients with Behcet's disease have increased intestinal permeability.[778] Whether this is due in an individual patient to gastrointestinal dysbiosis or is simply a gastrointestinal reflection of systemic inflammation should be determined on a per-patient basis. Dysbiosis is so common in patients with the combination of 1) autoimmunity and 2) "leaky gut" that such patients should be presumed to have dysbiosis until proven otherwise by comprehensive parasitology assessment by a specialty laboratory.
  - Oxidant/antioxidant assessment: Numerous studies have documented increased oxidative stress and decrease antioxidant defenses in patients with Behcet's disease.[779] Vitamin C deficiency has been documented.[780] Broad-spectrum antioxidant therapy with diet and supplements is indicated.
  - Assessment for occult infections and dysbiosis: Research suggests the probability that Behcet's disease is stimulated by occult bacterial/viral/fungal/parasitic infections with resultant molecular mimicry and stimulation of autoreactive T-cells.[781] **Bacteria that have been most consistently associated with this disease are *Streptococcus sanguis*, *Escherichia coli*, *Staphylococcus aureus*[782], and *Chlamydia pneumoniae*,** as discussed in the Treatment section that follows. **The fact that antimicrobial/penicillin administration reduces the severity and frequency of the disease clearly indicates that the disease is perpetuated at least in part by an occult infection.**[783] Additional support for a microbial contribution to the pathogenesis of this disease comes from studies showing **exacerbations of the disease following exposure to streptococcal antigens.**[784] There is no consistent evidence of *B. burgdorferi*[785] (Lyme disease), varicella zoster[786], or viral hepatitis[787] in most patients with Behcet's.
  - Xenobiotic depurition: Impairment in acetylation has been demonstrated[788] and may contribute to the pathogenesis of Behcet's disease by leading to the accumulation of xenobiotics or the haptenization of

---

[776] "CONCLUSION: Homocysteine may play a role in ocular involvement of BD. Chronic inflammation can induce hyperhomocysteinemia, thereby leading to thrombosis in the retinal vascular bed in a way similar to that recently proposed for the pathogenesis of coronary artery disease." Okka et al. Plasma homocysteine level and uveitis in Behcet's disease. *Isr Med Assoc J.* 2002 Nov;4(11 Suppl):931-4

[777] "CONCLUSION: Hyperhomocysteinaemia may be assumed to be an independent risk factor for venous thrombosis in BD. Unlike the factor V Leiden mutation, hyperhomocysteinaemia is a correctable risk factor. This finding might lead to new avenues in the prophylaxis of thrombosis in BD." Aksu et al. Hyperhomocysteinaemia in Behcet's disease. *Rheumatology* (Oxford). 2001 Jun;40(6):687-90 rheumatology.oxfordjournals.org/cgi/reprint/40/6/687

[778] "The intestinal permeability in BS was significantly more than that seen among the healthy controls." Fresko et al. Intestinal permeability in Behcet's syndrome. *Ann Rheum Dis.* 2001 Jan;60(1):65-6 ard.bmjjournals.com/cgi/reprint/60/1/65

[779] Kose et al. Lipid peroxidation and erythrocyte antioxidant enzymes in patients with Behcet's disease. *Tohoku J Exp Med.* 2002 May;197(1):9-16 jstage.jst.go.jp/article/tjem/197/1/9/_pdf

[780] Noyan et al. The serum vitamin C levels in Behcet's disease. *Yonsei Med J.* 2003 Oct 30;44(5):771-8 eymj.org/2003/pdf/10771.pdf

[781] Sakane et al. Etiopathology of Behcet's disease: immunological aspects. *Yonsei Med J.* 1997 Dec;38(6):350-8 eymj.org/1997/pdf/12350.pdf

[782] Direskeneli H. Behcet's disease: infectious aetiology, new autoantigens, and HLA-B51. *Ann Rheum Dis.* 2001 Nov;60(11):996-1002 ard.bmjjournals.com/cgi/reprint/60/11/996

[783] "CONCLUSION: Penicillin treatment was demonstrated to offer adjunctive benefits in the prevention of arthritis episodes which are not obtainable with colchicine monotherapy. This finding could provide additional evidence for antigen triggering in the pathogenesis of Behcet's disease." Calguneri et al. The effect of prophylactic penicillin treatment on the course of arthritis episodes in patients with Behcet's disease. A randomized clinical trial. *Arthritis Rheum.* 1996 Dec;39(12):2062-5

[784] "Interestingly, the induction of systemic Behcet's disease symptoms was observed after the streptococcus skin test in 15 of 85 cases tested, but no case of induction by the other bacteria was observed. Our study supports the possible pathogenetic role of certain streptococcal antigens in Behcet's disease." Behcet's Disease Research Committee of Japan. Skin hypersensitivity to streptococcal antigens and the induction of systemic symptoms by the antigens in Behcet's disease. *J Rheumatol.* 1989 Apr;16(4):506-11

[785] "CONCLUSION: These results suggest no association between Behcet's disease and B. burgdorferi infection." Onen et al. Seroprevalence of Borrelia burgdorferi in patients with Behcet's disease. *Rheumatol Int.* 2003 Nov;23(6):289-9

[786] "The serological positivity for VZV IgG and IgM antibodies in BD was not statistically different from other skin diseases." Akdeniz et al. The seroprevalence of varicella zoster antibodies in Behcet's and other skin diseases. Eur J Epidemiol. 2003;18(1):91-3

[787] "HGV-RNA was detected in two patients with BD and in none of the healthy controls. In conclusion, BD does not seem to be associated with hepatitis viral infections including hepatitis B, C, or G." Ozkan et al. Is there any association between hepatitis G virus (HGV), other hepatitis viruses (HBV, HCV) and Behcet's disease? *J Dermatol.* 2005 May;32(5):361-4

[788] "As a result of this study we conclude the NAT2 slow acetylator status may be a determinant in susceptibility to Behcet's disease. This finding may have implications for the theories of the pathogenesis of the disease as well as for therapeutic aspects." Tamer et al. N-acetyltransferase 2 polymorphisms in patients with Behcet's disease. *Clin Exp Dermatol.* 2005 Jan;30(1):56-60

endogenous antigens by reactive intermediates. Assessment of detoxification with caffeine-benzoate-aspirin-acetaminophen challenge may provide therapeutic insight when working with individual patients, particularly those with a history of xenobiotic exposure and/or multiple chemical sensitivity.

- **Imaging**:
  - Only for monitoring complications and excluding other diseases
- **Establishing the diagnosis**: Clinical assessment based on published criteria[789]
  - Recurrent oral/genital mucosal lesions: at least 3 times in one 12-month period, *plus two of the following*:
    - Eye lesions: Anterior uveitis, posterior uveitis, or retinal vasculitis
    - Skin lesions: Erythema nodosum, pseudofolliculitis, papulopustular lesions, or acneiform nodules
    - Positive pathergy test: Exaggerated inflammatory skin response 24–48 hours following otherwise benign injury/trauma to the skin
  - Diagnosis is additionally supported by:
    - Elevated ESR
    - Systemic/multiorgan relapsing disease, and associated clinical presentations and findings
    - Exclusion of other diseases: this is "relative" rather than "absolute" due to the nonspecific nature of Behcet's disease

Complications:

- **Blindness**: Patients with ocular involvement are at risk for blindness—urgent/emergency referral/immunosuppression may be necessary
- Paralysis
- Vena cava obstruction

Clinical management:

- Referral if clinical outcome is unsatisfactory or if serious complications are evident.
- Medical approach per *Merck Manual* up to 1999: "The syndrome is generally chronic and manageable... Symptomatic treatment is relatively successful." [790]

Treatments:

- Medical/pharmaceutical treatments:
  - Colchicine: 0.5 mg BID or TID for the treatment of oral/genital ulcers[791]
  - Topical corticosteroids: For oral and ocular involvement; oral corticosteroid therapy does not alter the course of the disease[792]
  - High-dose oral prednisone: 60-80 mg/d is indicated for severe uveitis, CNS involvement, or other urgent complications; cyclosporine immunosuppression is indicated for patients who do not respond to prednisone[793]
- Antioxidant therapy: Such as with mixed tocopherols[794] or Chinese herbal formula called "BG-104"[795] and any combination of antioxidants such as lipoic acid and phytonutrients. Recall that the Paleo-Mediterranean diet is inherently antioxidative due to the low glycemic indexes and loads and the additive and synergistic effects of phytonutrients from fruits, vegetables, nuts, seeds, and berries.[796]
- Orthoendocrinology: On an individual basis, clinicians and patients may find it valuable to assess prolactin, cortisol, DHEA, free and total testosterone, serum estradiol, and thyroid status (e.g., TSH, T4, *and* anti-thyroid peroxidase antibodies). Some studies have shown that patients with Behcet's disease have higher levels of

---

[789] Verity et al. Behcet's disease: from Hippocrates to the third millennium. *Br J Ophthalmol.* 2003 Sep;87(9):1175-83 bjo.bmjjournals.com/cgi/reprint/87/9/1175
[790] Beers MH, Berkow R (eds). *Merck Manual. 17th Edition.* Whitehouse Station; Merck Research Laboratories 1999 page 425
[791] Beers MH, Berkow R (eds). *Merck Manual. 17th Edition.* Whitehouse Station; Merck Research Laboratories 1999 page 425
[792] Beers MH, Berkow R (eds). *Merck Manual. 17th Edition.* Whitehouse Station; Merck Research Laboratories 1999 page 425
[793] Beers MH, Berkow R (eds). *Merck Manual. 17th Edition.* Whitehouse Station; Merck Research Laboratories 1999 page 425
[794] Kokcam I, Naziroglu M. Effects of vitamin E supplementation on blood antioxidants levels in patients with Behcet's disease. *Clin Biochem.* 2002 Nov;35(8):633-9
[795] "The treatment with BG-104 and/or vitamin E significantly enhanced the plasma SSA in all disorders studied. Both the erythrocyte sedimentation rates, the absolute number of neutrophils, as well as C-reactive protein levels were significantly lower in patients treated with BG-104 and/or vitamin E than those without these drugs." Pronai et al. BG-104 enhances the decreased plasma superoxide scavenging activity in patients with Behcet's disease, Sjogren's syndrome or hematological malignancy. *Biotherapy.* 1991;3(4):365-71
[796] Liu RH. Health benefits of fruit and vegetables are from additive and synergistic combinations of phytochemicals. *Am J Clin Nutr.* 2003 Sep;78(3 Suppl):517S-520S

proinflammatory prolactin than do normal controls[797], while other groups have contradicted these findings.[798,799]

- Antimicrobial treatments and assessment for dysbiosis: **Assess for occult infections; treat as indicated.** In patients for whom no specific microbes are detected with specialty testing such as stool testing or mucosal culture, clinicians should treat for presumptive bacterial overgrowth of the small bowel.

  o Orodental dysbiosis: Since **oral infection with variant strains of** *Streptococcus sanguis* **are the most likely and most consistently identified single source of antigenic stimulation in patients with Behcet's disease**[800], all patients should use potent antimicrobial mouthwashes daily. Obviously, extracts from berberine-containing botanicals such as *Hydrastis canadensis* are first-line therapy due to their potency against oral *Streptococcus* species.[801] Since non-berberine constituents—flavonoids—from *Hydrastis* are synergistically antimicrobial and increase the effectiveness of berberine against oral pathogens[802], the ideal antimicrobial in this regard would be a broad-spectrum extract standardized for its content of berberine. Berberine/Hydrastis powder can be used in a "swish, hold, and swallow" mouth rinse—the initial taste is quite bitter but it becomes tolerable; patients may prefer a comparatively better-tasting antimicrobial mouthwash such as Listerine or its generic equivalent. Warm water nasal lavage with Berberine/Hydrastis powder, salt and baking soda (sodium chloride and sodium bicarbonate) can be used twice daily and is well-tolerated. **Patients with orodental/sinus dysbiosis should get into the habit of ❶ cleaning their sinuses (ie, nasal lavage) when ❷ brushing their teeth and ❸ using antimicrobial mouthwash, a tripartite event that should occur at least twice daily.**

  o Gastrointestinal dysbiosis: Although patients with Behcet's disease appear to have a similar prevalence of *Helicobacter pylori* as the rest of the population, **eradication of gastrointestinal** *H. pylori* **infection leads to clinical improvement and resolution of genital and oral ulcers in these patients, thus showing that gastrointestinal dysbiosis is an underlying pathoetiologic factor in this condition.**[803]

  o Sinorespiratory dysbiosis: **Recent research has clearly demonstrated evidence of chronic** *Chlamydia pneumoniae* **infections in Behcets patients.**[804] Per Ben-Yaakov et al[805], "Because there is as yet no standardization of serological criteria for persistent infection, we considered antibody titers of > 1/20 in the IgA fraction, together with **IgG titers of 1/64 to 1/256, to be indicative of persistent infection."**

| Chlamydia pneumoniae IgG | >1:256 | High | Neg:<1:16 |
| Chlamydia pneumoniae IgM | <1:10 | | Neg:<1:10 |

Elevated titers to *Chlamydia/Chlamydophila pneumoniae* **suggesting chronic persistent infection— improvement with azithromycin and NAC**: Following detection of the elevated antibody titer, the patient started on azithromycin and NAC, which resulted in a short-term (12-hour) exacerbation of symptoms followed by complete and sustained resolution of sinus congestion and improved energy levels and exercise endurance.

  o Cutaneous dysbiosis: Recent research implicates the skin as a loci of dysbiosis: **pustules of patients with Behcet's disease are not sterile**[806] and are contaminated with bacteria that are distinct from those seen in regular acne and which are productive of antigens and superantigens that are capable of perpetuating

---

[797] "The mean prolactin levels in all subgroups of patients with BD were higher than normal, but no statistically significant difference was shown between these subgroups. CONCLUSION: Hyperprolactinemia occurred in a small number of patients with BD and its significance remained unclear. Serum PRL level did not correlate with disease manifestations and activity." Houman et al. Prolactin levels in Behcet's disease: no correlation with disease manifestations and activity. *Ann Med Interne* (Paris). 2001 Apr;152(3):209-11

[798] "However, we found no such correlation in Behcet's disease. On the contrary, prolactin levels were lower in attacks than in remissions." Apaydin et al. Serum prolactin levels in Behcet's disease. *Jpn J Ophthalmol*. 2000 Jul-Aug;44(4):442-5

[799] "We found that mean PRL levels in patients with clinically active BS, were not significantly higher than patients with clinically inactive BS and healthy controls." Keser et al. Serum prolactin levels in Behcet's Syndrome. *Clin Rheumatol*. 1999;18(4):351-2

[800] Direskeneli H. Behcet's disease: infectious aetiology, new autoantigens, and HLA-B51. *Ann Rheum Dis*. 2001:996-1002 ard.bmjjournals.com/cgi/content/full/60/11/996#B26

[801] "Thus, berberine sulfate interferes with the adherence of group A streptococci by two distinct mechanisms: one by releasing the adhesin lipoteichoic acid from the streptococcal cell surface and another by directly preventing or dissolving lipoteichoic acid-fibronectin complexes." Sun et al. Berberine sulfate blocks adherence of Streptococcus pyogenes to epithelial cells, fibronectin, and hexadecane. *Antimicrob Agents Chemother*. 1988 Sep;32(9):1370-4

[802] "Berberine (3) exhibited an additive antimicrobial effect when tested against S. mutans in combination with 1." Hwang et al. Antimicrobial constituents from goldenseal (the Rhizomes of Hydrastis canadensis) against selected oral pathogens. *Planta Med*. 2003 Jul;69(7):623-7

[803] "In 13 patients with BD, the number and size of oral and genital ulcers diminished significantly and various clinical manifestations regressed after the eradication of HP. CONCLUSION: HP may be involved in the pathogenesis of BD." Avci et al. Helicobacter pylori and Behcet's disease. *Dermatology*. 1999;199(2):140-3

[804] "These finding provide serological evidence of chronic C. pneumoniae infection in association with Behcet's disease." Ayaslioglu et al. Evidence of chronic Chlamydia pneumoniae infection in patients with Behcet's disease. *Scand J Infect Dis*. 2004;36(6-7):428-30

[805] Ben-Yaakov et al. Prevalence of antibodies to Chlamydia pneumoniae in an Israeli population without clinical evidence of respiratory infection. *J Clin Pathol*. 2002 May:355-8

[806] "At least one type of microorganism was grown from each pustule. Staphylococcus aureus (41/70, 58.6%, p = 0.008) and Prevotella spp (17/70, 24.3%, p = 0.002) were significantly more common in pustules from BS patients, and coagulase negative staphylococci (17/37, 45.9%, p = 0.007) in pustules from acne patients. CONCLUSIONS: The pustular lesions of BS are not usually sterile." Hatemi et al. The pustular skin lesions in Behcet's syndrome are not sterile. *Ann Rheum Dis*. 2004 Nov;63(11):1450-2

the disease via proinflammatory immunodysregulation. Furthermore, there is **a direct relationship between number of pustules and the severity of arthritis**[807] which suggests that proinflammatory immunodysregulation may result from microbial antigens and superantigens from cutaneous dysbiosis.

o <u>Clinical implementation</u>: In patients with established Behcet's disease, clinicians may be faced with the task of simultaneously treating numerous dysbiotic loci—mouth and gastrointestinal tract, sinus and lungs, and skin. Indeed, treatment should be orchestrated to address different loci with as few treatments as possible and as broadly as possible—**all loci should be treated simultaneously**. This may require co-administration of botanical and pharmaceutical antimicrobials, with the latter chosen for their systemic bioavailability. Patients should generally implement the alkalinizing supplemented Paleo-Mediterranean diet (with broad-spectrum fatty acid supplementation, probiotics, vitamin D, etc.) to effect a down-regulation of inflammation for the purpose of gaining some stability before facing aggressive antimicrobial treatment, which can trigger a "die off" Herxheimer-type reaction due to increased microbial (endo)toxin production.[808] Since the treatment of large/systemic bacterial infections can lead to a dramatic increase in endotoxin release[809], prophylactic treatment with NFkB inhibitors, or other potent anti-inflammatory treatments (such as single-dose prednisone) might be considered.

- <u>Treatments to lower homocysteine</u>: Patients with Behcet's syndrome have elevated homocysteine which exacerbates arterial and venous occlusion which underlies many of the clinical complications of the disease.[810,811] See previously detailed section—most recently updated in sections on migraine and fibromyalgia.

- *Ginkgo biloba*: Ginkgo may be of therapeutic value due to its anticoagulant, vasodilating, antioxidant, and anti-inflammatory actions. *In vitro* studies demonstrate an antioxidant benefit of ginkgo in erythrocytes of Behcets patients.[812]

---

[807] Diri et al. Papulopustular skin lesions are seen more frequently in patients with Behcet's syndrome who have arthritis: a controlled and masked study. *Ann Rheum Dis.* 2001 Nov;60(11):1074-6 ard.bmjjournals.com/cgi/reprint/60/11/1074

[808] "There is clear experimental evidence that antibiotics increase the bioavailability of endotoxin from Gram-negative bacteria." Hurley JC. Antibiotic-induced release of endotoxin. A therapeutic paradox. *Drug Saf.* 1995 Mar;12(3):183-95

[809] "A three- to 20-fold increase in the total concentration of endotoxin occurs as a consequence of antibiotic action on gram-negative bacteria both in vitro and in vivo." Hurley JC. Antibiotic-induced release of endotoxin: a reappraisal. *Clin Infect Dis.* 1992 Nov;15(5):840-54

[810] "CONCLUSION: Homocysteine may play a role in ocular involvement of BD. Chronic inflammation can induce hyperhomocysteinemia, thereby leading to thrombosis in the retinal vascular bed in a way similar to that recently proposed for the pathogenesis of coronary artery disease." Okka et al. Plasma homocysteine level and uveitis in Behcet's disease. *Isr Med Assoc J.* 2002 Nov;4(11 Suppl):931-4

[811] "CONCLUSION: Hyperhomocysteinaemia may be assumed to be an independent risk factor for venous thrombosis in BD. Unlike the factor V Leiden mutation, hyperhomocysteinaemia is a correctable risk factor. This finding might lead to new avenues in the prophylaxis of thrombosis in BD." Aksu et al. Hyperhomocysteinaemia in Behcet's disease. *Rheumatology* (Oxford). 2001 Jun;40(6):687-90 rheumatology.oxfordjournals.org/cgi/reprint/40/6/687

[812] "These data indicate that an oxidative damage is present in erythrocytes obtained from Behcet's patients, and EGb 761 [Ginkgo biloba extract], which may strengthen the antioxidant defense system, may contribute to the treatment of BD." Kose et al. In vitro antioxidant effect of Ginkgo biloba extract (EGb 761) on lipoperoxidation induced by hydrogen peroxide in erythrocytes of Behcet's patients. *Jpn J Pharmacol.* 1997 Nov;75(3):253-8

Sarcoidosis

Description/pathophysiology:

- A multisystem granulomatous disease; symptoms are dependent upon the site of involvement, most common of which is the mediastinum as well as central and peripheral lymph nodes.
- Sarcoidosis is not a *classic* autoimmune disease except that 1) endogenous immune mechanisms contribute to tissue destruction and clinical manifestations, and 2) approximately 20% of patients have endocrine autoimmunity.[813]
- Spontaneous improvement and resolution may occur in as many as 50-80% of patients.
- Like many inflammatory conditions, sarcoidosis was considered "idiopathic"[814]; new research is suggesting that—as with other disorders of sustained inflammation—occult infections (i.e., dysbiosis) are the underlying trigger.[815] The proposal that the condition has an infectious etiology is somewhat supported by cure of the disease in two case reports following administration of melatonin[816], which has potent immunostimulatory and anti-infective actions.[817]

Clinical presentations:

- Typical age of onset is between 20-40 years
- More common in Northern Europeans and African Americans (two groups with pandemic vitamin D deficiency)
- Typical autoimmune systemic manifestations: fatigue, malaise, low-grade fever, anorexia, and weight loss
- Hypercalcemia—due to a combination of hyperparathyroidism and granulomatous conversion of 25-hydroxycholecalciferol (the less active form of vitamin D) to 1,25-dihydroxycholecalciferol (the much more active form of vitamin D)
- Hyperparathyroidism
- Lymphadenopathy
- Dermal plaques and nodules in chronic disease
- Erythema nodosum—a nonspecific dermatologic manifestation characterized by erythema and subcutaneous nodules—this is considered a positive/beneficial finding in sarcoidosis because it is the best predictor of benign course of disease
- Hepatic granulomas are found in 70% of patients and may be present despite normal levels of serum liver enzymes
- **Granulomatous uveitis occurs in 15% of patients and can result in bilateral blindness—this must be treated as a medically urgent condition.**
- Cardiac involvement—seen in 5-10% of patients—can result in heart failure
- Peripheral polyarthropathy or oligoarthropathy
- CNS involvement and cranial nerve palsies: **neurosarcoidosis has been associated with a 10% mortality[818] and must therefore be treated as a medically urgent condition.**

Major differential diagnoses:

- Lymphoma
- Tuberculosis

---

[813] "In conclusion, a high frequency of endocrine autoimmunity in patients with sarcoidosis, occurring in about 20% of the cases, was demonstrated. Thyroid autoimmunity and polyglandular autoimmune syndromes occurred most frequently." Papadopoulos et al. High frequency of endocrine autoimmunity in patients with sarcoidosis. *Eur J Endocrinol* 1996 Mar;134(3):331-336

[814] Beers MH, Berkow R (eds). *Merck Manual. 17th Edition*. Whitehouse Station; Merck Research Laboratories: 1999, pages 2482-85

[815] "But now the inflammation of sarcoidosis has succumbed to antibiotics in two independent studies. This review examines the cell wall deficient (antibiotic resistant) bacteria which have been found in tissue from patients with sarcoidosis." Marshall TG, Marshall FE. Sarcoidosis succumbs to antibiotics--implications for autoimmune disease. *Autoimmun Rev*. 2004 Jun;3(4):295-300

[816] Cagnoni et al. Melatonin for treatment of chronic refractory sarcoidosis. *Lancet*. 1995 Nov 4;346(8984):1229-30

[817] Gitto et al. Effects of melatonin treatment in septic newborns. *Pediatr Res*. 2001 Dec;50(6):756-60 pedresearch.org/cgi/content/full/50/6/756

[818] "Neurosarcoidosis carries a mortality of 10 per cent, over twice that of sarcoidosis overall." James DG. Life-threatening situations in sarcoidosis. *Sarcoidosis Vasc Diffuse Lung Dis* 1998 Sep;15(2):134-9

- **Fungal infection of the lungs: histoplasmosis, coccidioidomycosis, aspergillosis, cryptococcosis**—appropriate management of sarcoidosis requires exclusion of these conditions before the administration of prednisone or other immunosuppressants.
- **Rheumatoid arthritis with pulmonary involvement**
- **Idiopathic pulmonary fibrosis**

<u>Clinical assessments</u>:
- **<u>History/subjective</u>**: See clinical presentations.
- **<u>Physical examination/objective</u>**:
  - As indicated—see clinical presentations
  - Skin examination
  - Cardiopulmonary examination
- **<u>Laboratory assessments</u>**:
  - <u>Leukopenia</u>: common
  - <u>Elevated serum uric acid</u>: without gout
  - <u>Alkaline phosphatase and GGT</u>: elevated with liver involvement
  - <u>Assessment for any and all types of dysbiosis</u> and/or the implementation of empiric clinical trials of systemic antimicrobial treatments appears warranted based on emerging evidence that occult infections are a primary perpetuating factor in this disease.[819]
  - <u>Creatine kinase</u>: may be elevated in patients with sarcoid myopathy
  - <u>Intestinal permeability (IP) assessment with lactulose and mannitol</u>: Increased intestinal permeability in patients with active sarcoidosis has been documented.[820] The clinical implications of this are not perfectly clear, since the increased mucosal permeability may simply reflect systemic inflammation and does not necessarily point to an enterogenic problem. However, as discussed previously in Chapter 4, increased intestinal permeability alone is sufficient to perpetuate systemic inflammation via increased antigen absorption and bacterial translocation. Some doctors use IP testing as a barometer of overall health and thus IP testing can be used to objectively quantify overall health.
  - <u>Endocrine autoimmunity</u> is very common (20%) in patients with sarcoidosis[821] and is detected by appropriate serologic tests and clinical assessments:
    - <u>Hashimoto's thyroiditis</u>: elevated anti-thyroid peroxidase enzymes, normal or elevated TSH
    - <u>Grave's disease</u>: elevated thyrotropin-receptor antibodies; suppressed TSH, elevated T4
    - <u>Addison's disease</u>: increased ACTH, low cortisol, failure to increase cortisol production following ACTH injection, anti-adrenal antibodies[822]
    - <u>Insulin-dependent diabetes mellitus</u>: hyperglycemia with hypoinsulinemia
    - <u>Premature ovarian failure</u>: anovulation, hypoestrogenemia, infertility, elevated FSH and LH
- **<u>Imaging and biopsy</u>**:
  - **Chest radiographs are abnormal in 90% of patients and are an excellent and commonly employed screening test**—characteristic findings include mediastinal lymphadenopathy and "ground glass" pulmonary infiltration
  - **Biopsy results** of pulmonary nodules, liver, or lymph nodes
  - **Whole-body gallium scanning shows pathognomonic signs**—false negative results due to prednisone/immunosuppression should be avoided

---

[819] "But now the inflammation of sarcoidosis has succumbed to antibiotics in two independent studies. This review examines the cell wall deficient (antibiotic resistant) bacteria which have been found in tissue from patients with sarcoidosis." Marshall TG, Marshall FE. Sarcoidosis succumbs to antibiotics—implications for autoimmune disease. *Autoimmun Rev*. 2004 Jun;3(4):295-300

[820] "Patients with active pulmonary sarcoidosis exhibited a marked increased IP to 51Cr-EDTA (4 +/- 0.54%), which was not found in patients with inactive sarcoidosis." Wallaert et al. Increased intestinal permeability in active pulmonary sarcoidosis. *Am Rev Respir Dis*. 1992 Jun;145(6):1440-5

[821] "In conclusion, a high frequency of endocrine autoimmunity in patients with sarcoidosis, occurring in about 20% of the cases, was demonstrated. Thyroid autoimmunity and polyglandular autoimmune syndromes occurred most frequently." Papadopoulos et al. High frequency of endocrine autoimmunity in patients with sarcoidosis. *Eur J Endocrinol* 1996 Mar;134(3):331-336

[822] "Autoantibodies in patients with isolated Addison's disease are directed against the enzymes involved in steroid synthesis, P45oc21, P45oscc and P45oc17." Martin Martorell et al. Autoimmunity in Addison's disease. *Neth J Med*. 2002 Aug;60(7):269-75. Review. Erratum in: *Neth J Med*. 2002 Oct;60(9):378 zuidencomm.nl/njm/getpdf.php?id=159

- **Establishing the diagnosis**: any one of the following:
  - Characteristic radiographic findings and clinical presentation
  - Biopsy results of pulmonary nodules (50-80% positive), liver (70% positive), or palpable lymph nodes (> 85% positive)
  - Pathognomonic signs with whole-body gallium scanning
- **Complications**: 10% of patients develop serious disability, including or due to pulmonary insufficiency, cardiac insufficiency, blindness, fatigue and debility. Granulomatous uveitis occurs in 15% of patients with sarcoidosis and can result in bilateral blindness—this must be managed as a medically urgent condition.

Clinical management:

- Serial pulmonary function tests are recommended—consider referral to pulmonologist or other specialist.
- **Pulmonary fungal infections should be conclusively excluded—referral to pulmonologist or other specialist is advised.**
- **Granulomatous uveitis occurs in 15% of patients with sarcoidosis and can result in bilateral blindness**—this must be managed as a medically urgent condition.
- Referral if clinical outcome is unsatisfactory or if serious complications are evident.

Therapeutic considerations:

- Drug treatments[823]:
  - Prednisone may be initiated at 20-60 mg/d po and tapered to 5 mg/d po for relief of symptoms; this treatment does not alter long-term outcome. **Prednisone and any immunosuppressant medication must only be employed following exclusion of an infectious differential diagnosis—administration of corticosteroids to a patient with occult pulmonary infections could result in a fatal outcome.**
  - Methotrexate at 2.5 mg per week can be initiated in patients unresponsive to prednisone; CBC and liver enzymes are measured every six weeks.
- Vitamin D3 supplementation tailored to serum 25(OH)D levels and serum calcium levels: **Sarcoidosis is the classic exemplification of a granulomatous disease that can cause hypercalcemia due to "vitamin D hypersensitivity."** [824,825] **Vitamin D supplementation—if used at all in these patients—must be supervised with care to avoid hypercalcemia.** Deficiency and response to treatment are monitored with serum 25(OH)vitamin D while **safety is monitored with serum calcium; inflammatory granulomatous diseases—** *sarcoidosis being the classic example—* **and certain drugs such as hydrochlorothiazide greatly increase the propensity for hypercalcemia and warrant incremental dosing and frequent monitoring of serum calcium.**
- Orthoendocrinology: No characteristic patterns of hormonal abnormalities have been described nor researched in patients with sarcoidosis. However, on an individual basis, clinicians and patients may find it valuable to assess prolactin, cortisol, DHEA, free and total testosterone, serum estradiol, and thyroid status (e.g., TSH, T4, *and* anti-thyroid peroxidase antibodies). **Melatonin (20 mg hs) appears to have cured two patients with drug-resistant sarcoidosis.** [826] Immunostimulatory anti-infective action of melatonin was demonstrated in a clinical trial wherein septic newborns administered 20 mg melatonin showed significantly increased survival over nontreated controls[827]; given that sarcoidosis is associated with many subclinical infections, melatonin may provide therapeutic benefit by virtue of its anti-infective properties.
  - Melatonin is a safe and effective treatment for chronic pulmonary and extrapulmonary sarcoidosis. (*J Pineal Res.* 2006 Sep[828]): "Melatonin was given for 2 yr (20 mg/day in the first year, 10 mg/day in the second year) to 18 CS patients. Pulmonary function tests, chest X rays, pulmonary computed tomography, Ga(67) scintigraphy and angiotensin-converting enzyme (ACE) were assayed at baseline and in the follow-up. Normalization of ACE, improvement of pulmonary parameters and resolution of skin involvement were found in the patients given melatonin. After 24 months of melatonin therapy, hylar adenopathy completely resolved in eight patients and parenchymal lesions were markedly improved in all patients;

[823] Beers MH, Berkow R (eds). *Merck Manual. 17th Edition*. Whitehouse Station; Merck Research Laboratories: 1999, pages 2482-85
[824] Vasquez et al. The clinical importance of vitamin D: a paradigm shift with implications for all healthcare providers. *Altern Ther Health Med*. 2004 Sep-Oct;10(5):28-36
[825] Sharma OP. Vitamin D, calcium, and sarcoidosis. *Chest*. 1996 Feb;109(2):535-9 http://www.chestjournal.org/cgi/reprint/109/2/535
[826] Cagnoni et al. Melatonin for treatment of chronic refractory sarcoidosis. *Lancet*. 1995 Nov 4;346(8984):1229-30
[827] Gitto et al. Effects of melatonin treatment in septic newborns. *Pediatr Res*. 2001 Dec;50(6):756-60 http://www.pedresearch.org/cgi/content/full/50/6/756
[828] Pignone et al. Melatonin is a safe and effective treatment for chronic pulmonary and extrapulmonary sarcoidosis. *J Pineal Res*. 2006 Sep;41(2):95-100

in the five patients with reduced diffusion capacity of the lung for carbon monoxide, the values normalized after 6 months of therapy and remained stable until month 24. After 24 months, Ga(67) pulmonary and extra-pulmonary uptake was totally normalized in seven patients and, at month 12 months, ACE was normalized in six patients in which the values were high at the baseline. Skin lesions, present in three patients, completely disappeared at month 24 months. No side effects were experienced and no disease relapse was observed during melatonin treatment. Melatonin may be an effective and safe therapy for CS when other treatments fail or cause side effects."

- Antibacterial therapies with systemic bioavailability: The 2004 monograph by Marshall and Marshall[829] reviewed research implicating cell wall deficient (antibiotic resistant) bacteria as the major causative factor in sarcoidosis, evidenced by remission of the disease following antimicrobial treatment and the incitement of a rather **severe Jarisch-Herxheimer reaction** as the bacteria increase their production of endotoxin in response to exposure to antimicrobial agents. Also in 2004, Bachelez et al[830] published results of a small clinical trail using minocycline and/or doxycycline in 12 patients with sarcoidosis—ten of twelve patients showed a positive response.

  - **Minocycline: The study by Bachelez et al used 200 mg/d minocycline for 12 months for the treatment of sarcoidosis.**

  - **Doxycycline: Alternate treatment by Bachelez et al was 200 mg/d doxycycline for the treatment of sarcoidosis.**

  - *Artemisia annua*: Artemisinin has been safely used for centuries in Asia for the treatment of malaria, and it also has effectiveness against anaerobic bacteria due to the pro-oxidative sesquiterpene endoperoxide.[831,832] I commonly use artemisinin at 200 mg per day in divided doses for adults with dysbiosis. Whether from dried herb, teas, or standardized extracts, **artemisinin is systemically bioavailable** and has an excellent record of safety. However, its usefulness in sarcoidosis based on the treatment of occult infections has not been documented.

  - St. John's Wort (*Hypericum perforatum*): Hyperforin from *Hypericum perforatum* shows *in vitro* antibacterial action, particularly against gram-positive bacteria such as *Staphylococcus aureus*, *Streptococcus pyogenes*, *Streptococcus agalactiae*[833] and perhaps *Helicobacter pylori*.[834] Up to 600 mg three times per day of a 3% hyperforin standardized extract is customary in the treatment of depression, and such **high doses may result in serum hyperforin levels that are systemically antimicrobial.** The safety and antidepressant effectiveness of Hypericum extracts are exceedingly well documented. The usefulness of hyperforin in sarcoidosis based on the treatment of occult infections has not been documented.

- Fumaric acid esters: **Three patients with drug-resistant cutaneous sarcoidosis were successfully treated with fumaric acid esters** (Fumaderm®).[835] Adverse effects of oral fumarate have been reported, namely renal failure.[836]

- Oral enzyme therapy with proteolytic/pancreatic enzymes: Polyenzyme supplementation is used to ameliorate the pathophysiology induced by immune complexes.[837] Approximately 60% of sarcoid patients have CIC (circulating immune complexes)[838] and these are particularly relevant in patients with concomitant vasculitis.[839]

---

[829] "But now the inflammation of sarcoidosis has succumbed to antibiotics in two independent studies. This review examines the cell wall deficient (antibiotic resistant) bacteria which have been found in tissue from patients with sarcoidosis." Marshall TG, Marshall FE. Sarcoidosis succumbs to antibiotics--implications for autoimmune disease. *Autoimmun Rev*. 2004 Jun;3(4):295-300

[830] Bachelez et al. The use of tetracyclines for the treatment of sarcoidosis. *Arch Dermatol*. 2001 Jan;137(1):69-73

[831] Dien et al. Effect of food intake on pharmacokinetics of oral artemisinin in healthy Vietnamese subjects. *Antimicrob Agents Chemother*. 1997 May;41(5):1069-72

[832] Giao et al. Artemisinin for treatment of uncomplicated falciparum malaria: is there a place for monotherapy? *Am J Trop Med Hyg*. 2001 Dec;65(6):690-5

[833] Schempp et al. Antibacterial activity of hyperforin from St John's wort, against multiresistant Staphylococcus aureus and gram-positive bacteria. *Lancet*. 1999 Jun 19;353(9170):2129

[834] "A butanol fraction of St. John's Wort revealed anti-Helicobacter pylori activity with MIC values ranging between 15.6 and 31.2 microg/ml." Reichling et al. A current review of the antimicrobial activity of Hypericum perforatum L. *Pharmacopsychiatry*. 2001 Jul;34 Suppl 1:S116-8

[835] "CONCLUSIONS: On the basis of our findings FAE therapy seems to be a safe and effective regimen for patients with recalcitrant cutaneous sarcoidosis." Nowack et al. Successful treatment of recalcitrant cutaneous sarcoidosis with fumaric acid esters. *BMC Dermatol* 2002 Dec 24;2(1):15 http://www.biomedcentral.com/1471-5945/2/15

[836] "The case of a 38 year old woman who was treated with fumaric acid (420 mg bid) for 5 years before she complained of fatigue and weakness. According to clinical laboratory she had developed severe proximal tubular damage." Raschka C, Koch HJ. Longterm treatment of psoriasis using fumaric acid preparations can be associated with severe proximal tubular damage. *Hum Exp Toxicol* 1999 Dec;18(12):738-9

[837] Galebskaya et al. Human complement system state after wobenzyme intake. *Vestnik Moskovskogo Universiteta (Seriya 2: Khimiya)*. 2000:41(6 Suppl): 148-149 chem.msu.ru/eng/journals/vmgu/00add/148.pdf

[838] "Complexes were detected in 29 (58%) patients." Johnson et al. Circulating immune complexes in sarcoidosis. *Thorax*. 1980 Apr;35(4):286-9

[839] "Circulating immune complexes were demonstrated and may have been important in the pathogenesis of both types of skin lesion." Johnston C, Kennedy C. Cutaneous leucocytoclastic vasculitis associated with acute sarcoidosis. *Postgrad Med J*. 1984 Aug;60(706):549-50

Polymyositis, Dermatomyositis, Dermatopolymyositis, Dermatomyositis sine myositis

Description/pathophysiology:

- **Autoimmune disease associated with immune complexes, autoantibodies, and cell-mediated muscle destruction.** Although both conditions are characterized by polymyopathy, skin involvement is a characteristic of **dermatomyositis (DM)** and not **polymyositis (PM)**. Unless articles/textbooks specifically refer to either PM or DM, the hyphenation PM-DM will be used to acknowledge that data probably applies to both conditions. The term **dermatopolymyositis** is somewhat outdated and not commonly used in contemporary literature. **Dermatomyositis sine myositis** is a rare variant of dermatomyositis characterized by inflammation of the skin *without overt myopathy.* Endogenous antigens targeted for autoimmune attack include human **Glycyl-tRNA synthetase**[840] and—not surprisingly—**myosin** from skeletal muscle.[841]

- Tissue damage is caused in large part by muscle infiltration by lymphocytes and macrophages. Lymphocytes from patients with PM-DM produce a "lymphotoxin" that causes muscle necrosis.[842]

- Despite the *idiopathic* label which is inappropriately applied to these disorders, several medical textbooks and numerous journal articles readily acknowledge that underlying viral infections[843,844], bacterial infections[845], parasitic infections[846], and malignancy[847] can contribute to the development of PM-DM. Interestingly and specifically supportive of the hypothesis that dysbiosis plays an etiologic role in the development of PM-DM, two of the endogenous autoantigens in PM share amino acid homology (molecular mimicry) with **histidyl-tRNA synthetase** and **alanyl-RNA synthetase** from *E. coli.*[848] Furthermore, myosin in human skeletal muscle shares amino acid homology with M5 protein from *Streptococcus pyogenes.*[849] Limited evidence suggests that DM may be triggered or exacerbated by bacterial infections/dysbiosis—particularly with *Staphylococcus aureus*[850,851] and *Streptococcus pyogenes.*[852,853] Patients with DM have an exaggerated response to streptococcal M5 protein[854] as well as streptococcal M12 protein.[855] Streptococcal infections may precipitate or exacerbate DM via mechanisms including molecular mimicry[856,857]; furthermore, streptococcal M protein acts as a superantigen and

Microorganisms causatively or molecularly associated with induction of polymyositis and dermatomyositis
• *Streptococcus pyogenes*
• *Staphylococcus aureus*
• *Toxoplasma gondii*
• *Mycoplasma pneumoniae*
• *Borrelia burgdorferi*
• *Coxsackie B virus*
• *Mycoplasma hominis*
• *Haemophilus influenzae*
• *Helicobacter pylori*
• *Escherichia coli*
• *Bacillus subtilis*

[840] Ge et al. Primary structure and functional expression of human Glycyl-tRNA synthetase, an autoantigen in myositis. *J Biol Chem.* 1994 Nov 18;269(46):28790-7 jbc.org/cgi/reprint/269/46/28790

[841] Massa et al. Self epitopes shared between human skeletal myosin and Streptococcus pyogenes M5 protein are targets of immune responses in active juvenile dermatomyositis. *Arthritis Rheum.* 2002 Nov;46(11):3015-25

[842] Ichimiya et al. Association between elevated serum antibody levels to streptococcal M12 protein and susceptibility to dermatomyositis. *Arch Dermatol Res.* 1998 Apr;290(4):229-30

[843] Beers MH, Berkow R (eds). *Merck Manual. 17th Edition.* Whitehouse Station; Merck Research Laboratories 1999 Page 434

[844] Siegel LB, Gall EP. Viral infection as a cause of arthritis. *Am Fam Physician* 1996 Nov 1;54(6):2009-15

[845] Massa et al. Self epitopes shared between human skeletal myosin and Streptococcus pyogenes M5 protein are targets of immune responses in active juvenile dermatomyositis. *Arthritis Rheum.* 2002 Nov;46(11):3015-

[846] "We report a case of polymyositis and myocarditis in a 13-year old immunocompetent girl with toxoplasmosis. The patient presented with proximal muscle weakness, dysphagia, palms and soles rash and elevated serum levels of muscle enzymes, with liver and myocardial involvement." Paspalaki et al. Polyomyositis and myocarditis associated with acquired toxoplasmosis in an immunocompetent girl. *BMC Musculoskelet Disord.* 2001;2:8. Epub 2001 Nov 20 biomedcentral.com/1471-2474/2/8

[847] Tierney ML. McPhee SJ, Papadakis MA (eds). *Current Medical Diagnosis and Treatment 2006. 45th edition.* New York; Lange Medical Books: 2006, pages 840-842

[848] "The amino acid sequences of Escherichia coli histidyl-tRNA synthetase and alanyl-tRNA synthetase, two proteins recently identified as autoantigens in polymyositis, were compared by a computer alignment procedure with those of the 3600 proteins tabulated in the National Biomedical Research Foundation protein sequence database. Both proteins contain sequences long enough to function as epitopes that match sequences on viral and muscle proteins." Walker EJ, Jeffrey PD. Polymyositis and molecular mimicry, a mechanism of autoimmunity. *Lancet.* 1986 Sep 13;2(8507):605-7

[849] Massa et al. Self epitopes shared between human skeletal myosin and Streptococcus pyogenes M5 protein are targets of immune responses in active juvenile dermatomyositis. *Arthritis Rheum.* 2002 Nov;46(11):3015-25

[850] Lane et al. Dermatomyositis following chronic staphylococcal joint sepsis. *Ann Rheum Dis.* 1990 Jun;49(6):405-6

[851] Moore et al. Staphylococcal infections in childhood dermatomyositis--association with the development of calcinosis, raised IgE concentrations and granulocyte chemotactic defect. *Ann Rheum Dis.* 1992 Mar;51(3):378-83

[852] Massa et al. Self epitopes shared between human skeletal myosin and Streptococcus pyogenes M5 protein are targets of immune responses in active juvenile dermatomyositis. *Arthritis Rheum.* 2002 Nov;46(11):3015-25

[853] Ichimiya et al. Association between elevated serum antibody levels to streptococcal M12 protein and susceptibility to dermatomyositis. *Arch Dermatol Res.* 1998 Apr;290(4):229-30

[854] Massa et al. Self epitopes shared between human skeletal myosin and Streptococcus pyogenes M5 protein are targets of immune responses in active juvenile dermatomyositis. *Arthritis Rheum.* 2002 Nov;46(11):3015-25

[855] Ichimiya et al. Association between elevated serum antibody levels to streptococcal M12 protein and dermatomyositis. *Arch Dermatol Res.* 1998 Apr;290(4):229-30

[856] Ichimiya et al. Association between elevated serum antibody levels to streptococcal M12 protein and dermatomyositis. *Arch Dermatol Res.* 1998 Apr;290(4):229-30

[857] Ichimiya et al. Association between elevated serum antibody levels to streptococcal M12 protein and dermatomyositis. *Arch Dermatol Res.* 1998 Apr;290(4):229-30

may enhance expression of endogenous autoantigens.[858] Young patients with calcific dermatomyositis have at least one immune defect (impaired granulocyte chemotaxis) that impairs their ability to fight *Staphylococcus aureus* infections/colonization/dysbiosis; this defect in chemotaxis is associated with and may be caused by elevations in serum IgE, some of which is specific for *Staphylococcus aureus*.[859] A relatively complete list of microorganisms associated with induction of PM-DM in humans includes *Staphylococcus aureus*[860,861], *Streptococcus pyogenes*[862,863], *Toxoplasma gondii*[864,865,866,867], *Mycoplasma pneumoniae*[868,869], *Borrelia burgdorferi*[870,871], and Coxsackie B virus.[872] Microorganisms that share amino acid homology with human skeletal muscle myosin include *Streptococcus pyogenes, Borrelia burgdorferi, Mycoplasma hominis, Haemophilus influenzae, Helicobacter pylori, Escherichia coli,* and *Bacillus subtilis.*[873]

- Like other disorders, PM-DM may occur with other autoimmune diseases, in which case it is described as an **overlap syndrome.** This is not surprising since the underlying characteristic of all autoimmune disorders is *immune dysfunction*; the protean consequences of immune dysfunction can morph without regard for the anthropocentric labels that we affix to different patterns of disordered expression. As with all autoimmune disorders, the course is variable and marked by exacerbations and remissions; yet the general trend is one of progressive decline. Spontaneous remission may occur.

- These conditions are commonly described as "idiopathic." The 2006 edition of *Current Medical Diagnosis and Treatment* refers to these two disorders as "idiopathic inflammatory myopathies"—a title no longer worthy of codification since 1) we have clear evidence of microbial induction/exacerbation of these disorders, 2) the hormonal aspects of these disorders (like most other autoimmune disorders) is increasingly recognized (for the most recent example, see Sereda and Werth[874]), and 3) the intentional overuse of the term *idiopathic* is leveraged by drug companies and other pharmaceutical/medical interests to justify endless medicalization in lieu of more profound assessments and effective treatments. One of the consequences of the pharmaceutically-influenced *idiopathicization* of otherwise understandable and treatable diseases is that doctors are no longer trained to *cure* disease by addressing the underlying problems; rather, they are trained to *medicate* disease indefinitely by *additive and infinite pharmacotherapy* and **symptom exchange**—trading symptoms of the disease for the side

[858] Ichimiya et al. Association between elevated serum antibody levels to streptococcal M12 protein and dermatomyositis. *Arch Dermatol Res.* 1998 Apr;290(4):229-30
[859] Moore et al. Staphylococcal infections in childhood dermatomyositis--association with the development of calcinosis, raised IgE concentrations and granulocyte chemotactic defect. *Ann Rheum Dis.* 1992 Mar;51(3):378-83
[860] Lane et al. Dermatomyositis following chronic staphylococcal joint sepsis. *Ann Rheum Dis.* 1990 Jun;49(6):405-6
[861] Moore et al. Staphylococcal infections in childhood dermatomyositis--association with the development of calcinosis, raised IgE concentrations and granulocyte chemotactic defect. *Ann Rheum Dis.* 1992 Mar;51(3):378-83
[862] Massa et al. Self epitopes shared between human skeletal myosin and Streptococcus pyogenes M5 protein are targets of immune responses in active juvenile dermatomyositis. *Arthritis Rheum.* 2002 Nov;46(11):3015-25
[863] Ichimiya et al. Association between elevated serum antibody levels to streptococcal M12 protein and susceptibility to dermatomyositis. *Arch Dermatol Res.* 1998 Apr;290(4):229-30
[864] "The case of a patient who developed an acute dermatomyositis-like syndrome upon infection by Toxoplasma gondii is reported." Saberin et al. Dermatomyositis-like syndrome following acute toxoplasmosis. *Bull Soc Sci Med Grand Duche Luxemb.* 2004;(2):109-19
[865] "We report a case of polymyositis and myocarditis in a 13-year old immunocompetent girl with toxoplasmosis. The patient presented with proximal muscle weakness, dysphagia, palms and soles rash and elevated serum levels of muscle enzymes, with liver and myocardial involvement." Paspalaki et al. Polyomyositis and myocarditis associated with acquired toxoplasmosis in an immunocompetent girl. *BMC Musculoskelet Disord.* 2001;2:8. Epub 2001 Nov 20 biomedcentral.com/1471-2474/2/8
[866] "The patient improved over the next six months and has been followed for approximately a five year period. During this time, antibody levels to the toxoplasma antigen have significantly decreased but the patient has developed a chronic myositis indistinguishable from polymyositis." Adams EM, Hafez GR, Carnes M, Wiesner JK, Graziano FM. The development of polymyositis in a patient with toxoplasmosis: clinical and pathologic findings and review of literature. *Clin Exp Rheumatol.* 1984 Jul-Sep;2(3):205-8
[867] "The serologic data suggested that inflammatory muscle disease was associated with recent active toxoplasma infection in certain patients." Phillips PE, Kassan SS, Kagen LJ. Increased toxoplasma antibodies in idiopathic inflammatory muscle disease. A case-controlled study. *Arthritis Rheum.* 1979 Mar;22(3):209-14
[868] "We describe the case of a 10-year-old girl who developed polymyositis associated with a Mycoplasma pneumoniae infection." Aihara Y, Mori M, Kobayashi T, Yokota S. A pediatric case of polymyositis associated with Mycoplasma pneumoniae infection. *Scand J Rheumatol.* 1997;26(6):480-1
[869] "Polymyositis, transverse myelitis, ascending polyneuritis, bilateral optic neuritis, and hearing loss developed in a patient with high complement-fixing antibody titers to Mycoplasma pneumoniae." Rothstein TL, Kenny GE. Cranial neuropathy, myeloradiculopathy, and myositis: complications of Mycoplasma pneumoniae infection. *Arch Neurol.* 1979 Aug;36(8):476-7
[870] "Lyme disease with muscle involvement can mimic or trigger dermatomyositis and should be considered in the differential diagnosis of dermatomyositis." Hoffmann et al. Lyme disease in a 74-year-old forest owner with symptoms of dermatomyositis. *Arthritis Rheum.* 1995 Aug;38(8):1157-60
[871] "We report the first case of dermatomyositis that appears to have been triggered by B. burgdorferi. This case involved an individual from Westchester County, NY, who presented with skin lesions suggestive of erythema migrans and who was seropositive for Lyme disease. He soon developed a clinical syndrome suggestive of dermatomyositis: periorbital edema, dysphagia, proximal muscle weakness, and a markedly elevated level of creatine phosphokinase." Horowitz et al. Dermatomyositis associated with Lyme disease: case report and review of Lyme myositis. *Clin Infect Dis.* 1994 Feb;18(2):166-71
[872] "These data suggest that the host response to coxsackie B virus might be related to the pathophysiology of JDM." Christensen et al. Prevalence of Coxsackie B virus antibodies in patients with juvenile dermatomyositis. *Arthritis Rheum.* 1986 Nov;29(11):1365-70
[873] Massa et al. Self epitopes shared between human skeletal myosin and Streptococcus pyogenes M5 protein are targets of immune responses in active juvenile dermatomyositis. *Arthritis Rheum.* 2002 Nov;46(11):3015-25
[874] "Using antiestrogen medication in women with DM may result in a significant improvement in their rash, possibly via the inhibition of TNF-alpha production by immune or other cells." Sereda D, Werth VP. Improvement in dermatomyositis rash associated with the use of antiestrogen medication. *Arch Dermatol.* 2006 Jan;142(1):70-2

effects of the drugs used to treat the disease.[875] Consequently, the top questions that doctors ask themselves during clinical encounters are 1) "What is the cause of symptom X?", 2) "What is the dose of the 'appropriate' drug?", and 3) "How should I manage disease or finding X?"[876] Notice that the internal dialogue of the allopathically trained physicians centers on symptoms, drugs, and management rather than any attempt to discover and address the underlying cause(s) of the symptoms or any attempt at authentic cure. Convincing doctors that *endless additive medicalization* is synonymous with *effective patient care* has been the major goal of the pharmaceutical companies[877] and is one that they accomplish by influencing medical school curricula[878,] sources of biomedical information[879], and by 'educating' doctors and patients with an incessant barrage of infomercials.[880]

<u>Clinical presentations</u>:
- **Bilateral symmetrical proximal muscle weakness most commonly affecting the shoulders, neck, and hips:** This weakness is reflective of the underlying autoimmune myopathy and may not be markedly present at the beginning of the disease process although it is eventually noted in all PM-DM patients. Characteristic difficulties include rising from a chair or squatting position (indicating weakness of glutei, quadriceps, and other intrinsic hip muscles), and upholding the arms (such as to comb hair) or lifting objects overhead (deltoids and rotator cuff muscles).
- **Skin/dermatologic abnormalities:**
  - <u>**Heliotrope/purple facial/cheek rash:**</u> "Periorbital edema with a heliotrope hue (purplish appearance) is pathognomonic."[881]
  - <u>**Gottron's sign:**</u> **scaly patches over the metacarpophalangeal (MCP) and PIP joints of the hands**— considered highly suggestive (not quite pathognomonic) of the disease.
  - Generalized skin rash and erythema, particularly over the shoulders ("shawl sign") and eyelids
  - Cuticular telangiectasias
  - Photosensitivity
- Polyarthralgia: pain and swelling, generally mild
- Muscle tenderness
- Raynaud's phenomenon: most commonly in patients with other autoimmune disease
- Fatigue
- Weight loss
- Soft tissue calcification: seen in PM-DM and scleroderma
- Cardiac involvement
- 2:1 more common in women than in men
- More common in persons of African descent, which is probably due at least in part to the higher incidence of vitamin D deficiency in this population. Vitamin D insufficiency predisposes toward inflammation, immune dysfunction, autoimmunity, and increased susceptibility to infections.
- Seen in children (5-15 years: "juvenile dermatomyositis/polymyositis") and adults (40-60 years)
- Rapid or slow onset; often preceded by infection

---

[875] "It begins on the first day of medical school… It starts slowly and insidiously, like an addiction, and can end up influencing the very nature of medical decision-making and practice… Attempts to influence the judgment of doctors by commercial interests serving the medical industrial complex are nothing if not thorough." Editorial. Drug-company influence on medical education in USA. *Lancet.* 2000 Sep 2;356(9232):781

[876] ""What is the cause of symptom X?" "What is the dose of drug X?" and "How should I manage disease or finding X?"" Ely et al. Analysis of questions asked by family doctors regarding patient care. *BMJ.* 1999 Aug 7;319(7206):358-61 http://bmj.bmjjournals.com/cgi/content/full/319/7206/358

[877] Angell M. *The Truth About the Drug Companies: How They Deceive Us and What to Do About it.* Random House; August 2004

[878] "It begins on the first day of medical school… It starts slowly and insidiously, like an addiction, and can end up influencing the very nature of medical decision-making and practice… Attempts to influence the judgment of doctors by commercial interests serving the medical industrial complex are nothing if not thorough." Editorial. Drug-company influence on medical education in USA. *Lancet.* 2000 Sep 2;356(9232):781

[879] "…despite lush advertisements from companies with obvious vested interests, and authoritative testimonials from biased investigators who presumably believe in their own work to the point of straining credulity and denying common sense… (translate: economic improvement, not biological superiority)." Stevens CW, Glatstein E. Beware the Medical-Industrial Complex. *Oncologist* 1996;1(4):IV-V theoncologist.alphamedpress.org/cgi/reprint/1/4/190-iv.pdf

[880] "…many ads may be targeted specifically at women and older viewers. Our findings suggest that Americans who watch average amounts of television may be exposed to more than 30 hours of direct-to-consumer drug advertisements each year, far surpassing their exposure to other forms of health communication." Brownfield et al. Direct-to-consumer drug advertisements on network television: an exploration of quantity, frequency, and placement. *J Health Commun.* 2004 Nov-Dec;9(6):491-7

[881] Beers MH, Berkow R (eds). *Merck Manual. 17th Edition.* Whitehouse Station; Merck Research Laboratories 1999 Page 435

<u>Major differential diagnoses</u>:
- <u>Cancer</u>: All patients with PM-DM must be screened (in a patient-specific manner) for cancer.
- <u>Celiac disease, gluten sensitivity</u>
- <u>Corticosteroid myopathy</u>
- <u>Drug toxicity</u>: Numerous drugs can cause muscle weakness and elevated serum levels of muscle enzymes. All of the following drugs can cause proximal muscle weakness, and the drugs that are underlined can also cause elevated muscle enzymes: corticosteroids, alcohol, clofibrate, penicillamine (very commonly reported cause of polymyositis), hydroxychloroquine, <u>colchicine</u> (especially in older patients with renal failure), <u>HMG-CoA reductase inhibitors—"statins"</u>, especially when combined with gemfibrozil, cyclosporine, niacin, erythromycin, azole antifungals, and protease inhibitors, <u>Zidovudine</u>, and <u>AZT</u>.
- <u>Hepatitis and viral hepatitis</u>: Elevated AST and ALT may be seen in PM-DM and hepatitis.
- <u>Hypothyroidism</u>: Hypothyroidism can almost perfectly mimic PM-DM with periorbital edema, dermatitis, and "hypothyroid myopathy" with proximal muscle weakness, and elevated CK.[882]
- <u>Inclusion body myositis (IBM)</u>: Earlier editions of some medical books discussed inclusion body myositis as a subset of polymyositis; more recent editions clearly distinguish inclusion body myositis as a distinct entity, hence its inclusion here under the category of differential diagnoses. Clinically, **IBM tends to present with *distal* muscle involvement rather than the *proximal* localization of early PM-DM**. Furthermore, muscle involvement is likely to be *asymmetrical* with IBM, differentiating IBM from PM-DM in which muscle involvement is typically symmetric.
- <u>Infection</u>: viral infection, bacterial infection, toxoplasmosis, HIV polymyositis, postviral rhabdomyolysis.
- <u>Lambert-Eaton myasthenic syndrome</u>: A disorder with pathophysiology similar to myasthenia gravis—autoantibodies directed to neuromuscular junction (voltage-gated calcium channels at terminal of alpha motor neuron); clinical presentation similar to PM-DM with proximal limb weakness. May also present with dry mouth and dry eyes (DDX: **Sjogren's syndrome**), eye ptosis and diplopia (DDX: **myasthenia gravis**), and exacerbations caused by heat (DDX: **multiple sclerosis**). Lambert-Eaton myasthenia is like PM-DM commonly associated with occult malignancy (especially small cell lung cancer) and therefore all patients with Lambert-Eaton myasthenia must be comprehensively screened for cancer. Diagnosis of Lambert-Eaton myasthenia is performed with serum tests for antibodies, supported by EMG, and followed with comprehensive cancer screening, which should include CT of lungs and biopsy of suspicious lung lesions.
- <u>Multiple sclerosis</u>: Diagnosis based on clinical presentation, findings such as internuclear ophthalmoplegia and optic neuritis, and characteristic MRI brain lesions. DDX: celiac encephalopathy.
- <u>Myasthenia gravis (MG)</u>: Presents with muscle weakness; however MG presents with facial and ocular weakness which are not characteristic of PM-DM; caused by autoantibodies directed to neuromuscular junction (acetylcholine receptor of the motor end plate).
- <u>Myocardial infarction</u>: Both MI and PM-DM have elevated CK-MB.
- <u>Neuropathy and radiculopathy</u>: Both can cause muscle weakness that can mimic PM-DM.
- <u>Polymyalgia rheumatica</u>: In these patients, muscle pain predominates over muscle weakness.
- <u>SLE</u>: Both SLE and DM can present with systemic inflammation, fatigue, butterfly heliotrope facial rash, and positive ANA. Elevated CK and aldolase are characteristic of DM but are uncommon in SLE.

<u>Clinical assessments</u>:
- **<u>History/subjective</u>**: See clinical presentations
- **<u>Physical examination/objective</u>**:
  - Assess muscle strength
    - Shoulders: flexion and abduction.
    - Neck: flexion, extension, and lateral bending.
    - Hips: use a combination of direct muscle testing as well as functional assessments such as "squat and rise" and rising from a chair.

---

[882] Bowman et al. Bilateral adhesive capsulitis, oligoarthritis and proximal myopathy as presentation of hypothyroidism. *Br J Rheumatol* 1988;27(1):62-4

- **Laboratory assessments**:
  - ○ ESR/CRP: Normal in 50% of patients.
  - ○ CBC: Assess for anemia (uncommon), infection, and possible nutritional deficiencies
  - ○ Metabolic/chemistry panel: Elevated AST and ALT may be seen and can be confused with hepatitis.
  - ○ Muscle enzymes: These are useful for establishing the diagnosis and monitoring the course of disease and response to treatment. Both tests should be performed together, especially at the initial evaluation.
    - ▪ Creatine kinase (CK) (previously called creatine phosphokinase (CPK): CK is generally elevated but may normalize in patients with active disease and widespread muscle atrophy[883] in a manner similar to the reduction of liver enzymes with the progression of hepatic cirrhosis.
    - ▪ Aldolase
  - ○ ANA: Positive in many patients[884] especially those with another autoimmune disorder—overlap syndrome.[885]
  - ○ Anti-Jo-1: Seen mostly with lung disease.
  - ○ Serum IgE: Young DM patients affected by calcinosis have elevated serum IgE.[886]
  - ○ Serologic testing for *Toxoplasma gondii*: Serologic testing for *Toxoplasma gondii* has been recommended because of the association between this infection and the development of PM-DM.[887]
  - ○ Testing for celiac disease: This is especially important in PM-DM patients who have malabsorption.[888]
  - ○ Dysbiosis testing: Assess for multifocal dysbiosis.
- **Imaging and biopsy**:
  - ○ **Skin/muscle biopsy is necessary for definitive diagnosis**.
  - ○ Imaging is not generally indicated except when looking for complications or concomitant disease, such as chest radiographs for associated interstitial lung disease.
  - ○ Electromyographic assessment may be used to support the diagnosis and to exclude/evaluate concomitant disorders; this is generally unnecessary.
- **Establishing the diagnosis**:
  - ○ The following should be present:
    - ▪ Proximal muscle weakness
    - ▪ Skin rash
    - ▪ Increased levels of muscle enzymes in serum
    - ▪ Muscle biopsy findings—specific, mandatory for definite diagnosis
    - ▪ EMG abnormalities are supportive

Complications:

- Occult malignancy—up to 25% of patients with dermatomyositis have an occult malignancy. Evaluation for underlying/occult malignancy is mandatory in all adult patients with dermatomyositis.[889] Assessment for malignancy should include complete physical examination and routine blood tests (CBC, chemistry/metabolic panel, serum protein electrophoresis, serum ferritin); additional assessments are chosen per the patient's individual profile based on age, gender, family history, and other risk factors. Measuring PSA in middle aged and older men and CA-125 in adult women would be very reasonable, as would a colonoscopy in any PM-DM patient over age 40 years. Radiographs and CT imaging are warranted for any PM-DM patient with pulmonary symptoms or history of exposure to inhaled carcinogens, including asbestos and tobacco smoke.
  - ○ **Up to 20% of women with dermatomyositis develop ovarian cancer**
  - ○ **Breast cancer** and **lung cancer** are also more common

[883] Klippel JH (ed). *Primer on the Rheumatic Diseases. 11th Edition*. Atlanta: Arthritis Foundation. 1997, page 277
[884] Tierney ML. McPhee SJ, Papadakis MA (eds). *Current Medical Diagnosis and Treatment 2006. 45th edition*. New York; Lange Medical Books: 2006, pages 840-842
[885] Tierney LM. Saint S, Whooley MA (Eds). *Current Essentials of Medicine. 3rd Edition*. New York; Lange Medical Books: 2005, page 165
[886] Moore et al. Staphylococcal infections in childhood dermatomyositis--association with the development of calcinosis, raised IgE concentrations and granulocyte chemotactic defect. *Ann Rheum Dis*. 1992 Mar;51(3):378-83
[887] "We report a case of polymyositis and myocarditis in a 13-year old immunocompetent girl with toxoplasmosis. The patient presented with proximal muscle weakness, dysphagia, palms and soles rash and elevated serum levels of muscle enzymes, with liver and myocardial involvement." Paspalaki et al. Polyomyositis and myocarditis associated with acquired toxoplasmosis in an immunocompetent girl. *BMC Musculoskelet Disord*. 2001;2:8. Epub 2001 Nov 20 .biomedcentral.com/1471-2474/2/8
[888] "Based on our findings, we further emphasize that an evaluation for celiac disease, including anti-gliadin antibodies, anti-endomysium antibody and tissue trans-glutaminase antibodies should be considered in PM/DM patients presenting with unusual and unexplained gastrointestinal features." Marie I, Lecomte F, Hachulla E, Antonietti M, Francois A, Levesque H, Courtois H. An uncommon association: celiac disease and dermatomyositis in adults. *Clin Exp Rheumatol*. 2001 Mar-Apr;19(2):201-3
[889] Tierney ML. McPhee SJ, Papadakis MA. *Current Medical Diagnosis and Treatment 2006. 45th edition*. New York; Lange Medical Books: 2006, pages 840-842

- o Associated cancers have **poor prognosis**
- o **Appropriate screening includes the following**[890]:
  - History
  - **Physical examination**
  - **CBC**
  - **Chemistry/metabolic panel**
  - **Serum protein electrophoresis**
  - **Urinalysis**
  - **Age-, gender-, and risk-appropriate screening tests**
  - **Follow-up for cancers that become evident within the next few months**
- Vasculitis with necrosis of internal organs, especially intestines
- Dyspnea due to weakness of respiratory muscles may progress to respiratory failure
- Dysphagia due to weakness of muscles of upper pharynx
- Cardiac involvement
- Renal failure secondary to rhabdomyolysis
- Intestinal ulcerations with bleeding
- Corticosteroid myopathy
- Muscle inflammation begins with weakness and progresses to fibrosis and contractures

Clinical management:
- Referral if clinical outcome is unsatisfactory or if serious complications are possible or evident.

Treatments:
- *Medical/drug treatments*[891,892]
  - o <u>Prednisone</u>: Generally started at 40-60 mg/g, then tapered.
  - o <u>Methotrexate</u>, <u>azathioprine</u>, or <u>intravenous immune globulin</u>: Used for patients who do not respond to corticosteroids.
- <u>Vitamin E</u>: Several articles have shown benefit of vitamin E supplementation in different autoimmune conditions. Conditions that may respond to vitamin E supplementation include scleroderma, discoid lupus erythematosus[893], porphyria cutanea tarda, **polymyositis**, and vasculitis.[894,895,896] Given that vitamin E is not a single compound but rather a family of closely related tocopherols, most clinicians prefer to use a source of "mixed tocopherols" inclusive of alpha, beta, delta, and—perhaps most importantly—gamma tocopherol.[897] Vitamin E has a wide margin of safety and although daily doses are kept in the range of 400-1200 IU, doses up to 3,200 IU are generally considered non-toxic.
- <u>Avoidance of allergenic foods</u>: **Celiac disease can present with a clinical picture that closely mimics polymyositis; the '"disease" remits with gluten avoidance.**[898] Any patient may be allergic to any food, even if the food is generally considered a health-promoting food. Generally speaking, the most notorious allergens are wheat, citrus (especially juice due to the industrial use of fungal hemicellulases), cow's milk, eggs, peanuts, chocolate, and yeast-containing foods. According to a study in patients with migraine, some patients will have

[890] Tierney ML. McPhee SJ, Papadakis MA. *Current Medical Diagnosis and Treatment 2006. 45ᵗʰ edition*. New York; Lange Medical Books: 2006, pages 840-842
[891] Tierney ML. McPhee SJ, Papadakis MA. *Current Medical Diagnosis and Treatment 2006. 45ᵗʰ edition*. New York; Lange Medical Books: 2006, pages 840-842
[892] Tierney LM. Saint S, Whooley MA (Eds). *Current Essentials of Medicine. 3ʳᵈ Edition*. New York; Lange Medical Books: 2005, page 165
[893] "Despite conflicting opinions, our personal experience and a number of reviewed clinical reports indicate that vitamin E, properly administered in adequate doses, is a safe and effective treatment for chronic discoid lupus erythematosus, and may be of value in treating other types of the disease." Ayres S Jr, Mihan R. Lupus erythematosus and vitamin E: an effective and nontoxic therapy. *Cutis*. 1979 Jan;23(1):49-52, 54
[894] "She then made a dramatic improvement when large doses of vitamin E (d, alpha-tocopheryl acetate) were administered." Killeen RN, Ayres S Jr, Mihan R. Polymyositis: response to vitamin E. *South Med J*. 1976 Oct;69(10):1372-4
[895] "Casually, vitamin E (600 mg daily) was added. After 6 months, clinical manifestations of heart failure were disappeared and the echocardiogram showed a normally-sized left ventricle with normal wall motion." Morelli et al. Systemic sclerosis (scleroderma). A case of recovery of cardiomyopathy after vitamin E treatment. *Minerva Cardioangiol*. 2001 Apr;49(2):127-30
[896] "Among the diseases that were successfully controlled were a number in the autoimmune category, including scleroderma, discoid lupus erythematosus, porphyria cutanea tarda, several types of vasculitis, and polymyositis." Ayres S Jr, Mihan R. Is vitamin E involved in the autoimmune mechanism? *Cutis*. 1978 Mar;21(3):321-5
[897] Jiang Q, Christen S, Shigenaga MK, Ames BN. gamma-tocopherol, the major form of vitamin E in the US diet, deserves more attention. *Am J Clin Nutr*. 2001 Dec;74:714-22
[898] "Treatment with gluten-free diet resolved all clinical and laboratory abnormalities." Evron et al. Polymyositis, arthritis, and proteinuria in a patient with adult celiac disease. J Rheumatol. 1996 Apr;23(4):782-3

to avoid as many as 10 specific foods in order to become symptom-free.[899] **Several cases of co-existent celiac disease with PM-DM have been reported.**[900] Regardless of the absence of allergy in a particular patient, clinicians must explain to their patients that celiac disease and wheat allergy are two different clinical entities and that exclusion of one does not exclude the other, and in neither case does mutual exclusion obviate the promotion of intestinal bacterial overgrowth (i.e., pro-inflammatory dysbiosis) by indigestible wheat oligosaccharides.

- o <u>Dermatomyositis associated with celiac disease responsive to a gluten-free diet. (*Can J Gastroenterol.* 2006 Jun[901])</u>: "A … case of concomitant dermatomyositis and celiac disease in a 40-year-old woman is presented. After having been diagnosed with dermatomyositis and iron deficiency anemia, this patient was referred to the gastroenterology clinic to exclude a gastrointestinal malignancy. Blood tests revealed various vitamin deficiencies consistent with malabsorption. The results of gastroscopy with duodenal biopsy were consistent with celiac disease. After she was put on a strict gluten-free diet, both nutritional deficiencies and the dermatomyositis resolved. The patient's human leukocyte antigen haplotype study was positive for DR3 and DQ2, which have been shown to be associated with both juvenile dermatomyositis and celiac disease. It is suggested that patients with newly diagnosed dermatomyositis be investigated for concomitant celiac disease even in the absence of gastrointestinal symptoms."

- <u>Vitamin D3 supplementation with physiologic doses and/or tailored to serum 25(OH)D levels</u>: Vitamin D deficiency is common in the general population and is even more common in patients with chronic illness and chronic musculoskeletal pain.[902] Correction of vitamin D deficiency supports normal immune function against infection and provides a clinically significant anti-inflammatory[903] and analgesic benefit in patients with back pain[904] and limb pain.[905] Reasonable daily doses for children and adults are 1,000-2,000 and 4,000 IU, respectively.[906] Deficiency and response to treatment are monitored with serum 25(OH)vitamin D while safety is monitored with serum calcium; inflammatory granulomatous diseases and certain drugs such as hydrochlorothiazide greatly increase the propensity for hypercalcemia and warrant increment dosing and frequent monitoring of serum calcium. Vitamin D2 (ergocalciferol) is not a human nutrient and should not be used in clinical practice.

- **<u>Assessment for dysbiosis</u>: Given the numerous links between PM-DM and various microorganisms, testing for and treating multifocal dysbiosis (as outlined in Chapter 4) is strongly encouraged.** Yeast, bacteria, and parasites are treated as indicated based on identification and sensitivity results from comprehensive parasitology assessments. Patients taking immunosuppressant drugs such as corticosteroids/prednisone have increased risk of intestinal bacterial overgrowth and translocation.[907,908] Other dysbiotic loci should be investigated as discussed in Chapter 4 in the section on multifocal dysbiosis.

Microorganisms causatively or molecularly associated with induction of polymyositis/dermatomyositis
• *Streptococcus pyogenes*
• *Staphylococcus aureus*
• *Toxoplasma gondii*
• *Mycoplasma pneumoniae*
• *Borrelia burgdorferi*
• Coxsackie B virus
• *Mycoplasma hominis*
• *Haemophilus influenzae*
• *Helicobacter pylori*
• *Escherichia coli*
• *Bacillus subtilis*

- <u>Orthoendocrinology</u>: Assess prolactin, cortisol, DHEA, free and total testosterone, serum estradiol, and thyroid status (e.g., TSH, T4, *and* anti-thyroid peroxidase antibodies).

- o <u>Prolactin (excess)</u>: The role of prolactin in PM-DM has not been studied. However, prolactin is increasingly well-known as a proinflammatory and

---

[899] Grant EC. Food allergies and migraine. *Lancet*. 1979 May 5;1(8123):966-9

[900] "Based on our findings, we further emphasize that an evaluation for celiac disease, including anti-gliadin antibodies, anti-endomysium antibody and tissue trans-glutaminase antibodies should be considered in PM/DM patients presenting with unusual and unexplained gastrointestinal features." Marie et al. An uncommon association: celiac disease and dermatomyositis in adults. *Clin Exp Rheumatol*. 2001 Mar-Apr;19(2):201-3

[901] Song et al. Dermatomyositis associated with celiac disease: response to a gluten-free diet. *Can J Gastroenterol*. 2006 Jun;20(6):433-5

[902] Plotnikoff GA, Quigley JM. Prevalence of severe hypovitaminosis D in patients with persistent, nonspecific musculoskeletal pain. *Mayo Clin Proc*. 2003 Dec;78(12):1463-70

[903] Timms et al. Circulating MMP9, vitamin D and variation in the TIMP-1 response with VDR genotype: mechanisms for inflammatory damage in chronic disorders? *QJM*. 2002 Dec;95(12):787-96 qjmed.oxfordjournals.org/cgi/content/full/95/12/787

[904] Al Faraj S, Al Mutairi K. Vitamin D deficiency and chronic low back pain in Saudi Arabia. *Spine*. 2003 Jan 15;28(2):177-9

[905] Masood et al. Persistent limb pain and raised serum alkaline phosphatase the earliest markers of subclinical hypovitaminosis D in Kashmir. *Indian J Physiol Pharmacol*. 1989 Oct-Dec;33(4):259-61

[906] Vasquez et al. The clinical importance of vitamin D: a paradigm shift with implications for all healthcare providers. *Altern Ther Health Med*. 2004 Sep-Oct;10(5):28-36

[907] "A 63-year-old man with systemic lupus erythematosus and selective IgA deficiency developed intractable diarrhoea the day after treatment with prednisone, 50 mg daily, was started. The diarrhoea was considered to be caused by bacterial overgrowth and was later successfully treated with doxycycline." Denison H, Wallerstedt S. Bacterial overgrowth after high-dose corticosteroid treatment. *Scand J Gastroenterol*. 1989 Jun;24(5):561-4

[908] "These bacteria also translocated to the mesenteric lymph nodes in mice injected with cyclophosphamide or prednisone." Berg et al. Immunosuppression and intestinal bacterial overgrowth synergistically promote bacterial translocation. *Arch Surg*. 1988 Nov;123(11):1359-64

immunodysregulatory hormone. Serum levels of prolactin tend to be higher in patients with autoimmunity, and therapeutic lowering of prolactin levels results in clinically significant anti-inflammatory benefits. Among women with hyperprolactinemia, 75% of them show serologic evidence of asymptomatic autoimmunity.[909] As discussed elsewhere, patients with RA and SLE have higher basal and stress-induced levels of prolactin compared with normal controls[910,911], and men with RA have higher serum levels of prolactin that correlate with the severity and duration of the disorder.[912,913] Serum prolactin is the standard assessment of prolactin status. Since elevated prolactin may be a sign of pituitary tumor, assessment for headaches, visual deficits, and other abnormalities of pituitary hormones (e.g., GH and TSH) should be performed; CT or MRI must be considered. Patients with prolactin levels less than 100 ng/mL and normal CT/MRI findings can be managed conservatively with effective prolactin-lowering treatment and annual radiologic assessment (less necessary with favorable serum response).[914, see review 915]

> **Antiestrogen treatments are generally antiinflammatory**
>
> "Using **antiestrogen medication** in women with **dermatomyositis** may result in a significant improvement in their rash, possibly via the inhibition of TNF-alpha production by immune or other cells."
>
> Sereda D, Werth VP. *Arch Dermatol*. 2006 Jan

o Estrogen (excess): Men with rheumatoid arthritis show an excess of estradiol and a decrease in DHEA, and the excess estrogen is proportional to the degree of inflammation.[916] Estrogen status can be assessed using serum estradiol or a 24-hour urine sample. Interventions to combat high estrogen levels may include any effective combination of the following:

- Anastrozole/Arimidex: In a 2006 case report, administration of anastrozole lead to clinical improvement in a woman with dermatomyositis; per the (lack of) details in the case report, the dose was not provided but was likely 1 mg/d since this is the standard dose for the treatment of breast cancer, with which the patient was diagnosed in 2003 after developing dermatomyositis in 1998.[917] In our office, we commonly measure serum estradiol in men and administer the aromatase inhibitor anastrozole/arimidex 1 mg (2-3 doses per week) to men whose estradiol level is greater than 32 picogram/mL. The Life Extension Foundation[918] advocates that the optimal serum estradiol level for a man is 10-30 picogram/mL. Clinical studies using anastrozole/arimidex in men have shown that aromatase blockade lowers estradiol and raises testosterone[919]; generally speaking, this is exactly the result that we want in patients with severe systemic autoimmunity. Our practice has been to use the 1 (one) mg dose, with the frequency of dosing based on serum and clinical response.

o Thyroid (insufficiency or autoimmunity): Because PM-DM can be convincingly mimicked by asymptomatic hyperthyroidism, hypothyroidism, and thyroid autoimmunity (including Grave's disease and Hashimoto's thyroiditis), all patients with PM-DM should receive a comprehensive thyroid evaluation including thyroid gland palpation and serum measurements of TSH, T4, anti-thyroid peroxidase antibodies, and possibly free T3. Overt or imminent hypothyroidism is suggested by TSH

---

[909] "Twenty-five of 33 (75.7%) HPRL women were found to have at least one autoantibody, while none of the 19 women with normal PRL had any. Yet none of the HPRL women whose serum was found to contain high titers of autoantibodies presented with symptoms related to the respective autoimmune disorders." Buskila et al. Autoantibody profile in the sera of women with hyperprolactinemia. *J Autoimmun*. 1995 Jun;8(3):415-24

[910] Dostal et al. Serum prolactin stress values in patients with systemic lupus erythematosus. *Ann Rheum Dis*. 2003 May;62(5):487-8 ard.bmjjournals.com/cgi/content/full/62/5/487

[911] "RESULTS: A significantly higher rate of elevated PRL levels was found in SLE patients (40.0%) compared with the healthy controls (14.8%). No proof was found of association with the presence of anti-ds-DNA or with specific organ involvement. Similarly, elevated PRL levels were found in RA patients (39.3%)." Moszkorzova et al. Hyperprolactinaemia in patients with systemic lupus erythematosus. *Clin Exp Rheumatol*. 2002 Nov-Dec;20(6):807-12

[912] "CONCLUSION: Men with RA have high serum PRL levels and concentrations increase with longer disease evolution and worse functional stage." Mateo et al. High serum prolactin levels in men with rheumatoid arthritis. *J Rheumatol*. 1998 Nov;25(11):2077-82

[913] "Male patients affected by RA showed high serum PRL levels. The serum PRL concentration was found to be increased in relation to the duration and the activity of the disease. Serum PRL levels do not seem to have any relationship with the BMD, at least in RA." Seriolo et al. Serum prolactin concentrations in male patients with rheumatoid arthritis. *Ann N Y Acad Sci*. 2002 Jun;966:258-62

[914] Beers MH, Berkow R (eds). *Merck Manual. 17ᵗʰ Edition*. Whitehouse Station; Merck Research Laboratories 1999 Page 77-78

[915] Serri et al. Diagnosis and management of hyperprolactinemia. *CMAJ*. 2003 Sep 16;169(6):575-81 cmaj.ca/cgi/content/full/169/6/575

[916] "RESULTS: DHEAS and estrone concentrations were lower and estradiol was higher in patients compared with healthy controls. DHEAS differed between RF positive and RF negative patients. Estrone did not correlate with any disease variable, whereas estradiol correlated strongly and positively with all measured indices of inflammation." Tengstrand et al. Abnormal levels of serum dehydroepiandrosterone, estrone, and estradiol in men with rheumatoid arthritis: high correlation between serum estradiol and current degree of inflammation. *J Rheumatol*. 2003 Nov;30(11):2338-43

[917] "Using antiestrogen medication in women with DM may result in a significant improvement in their rash, possibly via the inhibition of TNF-alpha production by immune or other cells." Sereda D, Werth VP. Improvement in dermatomyositis rash associated with the use of antiestrogen medication. *Arch Dermatol*. 2006 Jan;142(1):70-2

[918] Male Hormone Modulation Therapy, Page 4 Of 7: lef.org/protocols/prtcl-130c.shtml Accessed October 30, 2005

[919] "These data demonstrate that aromatase inhibition increases serum bioavailable and total testosterone levels to the youthful normal range in older men with mild hypogonadism." Leder et al. Effects of aromatase inhibition in elderly men with low or borderline-low serum testosterone levels. *J Clin Endocrinol Metab*. 2004 Mar;89(3):1174-80 jcem.endojournals.org/cgi/reprint/89/3/1174

greater than 2 mU/L[920] or 3 mU/L[921], low T4 or T3, and/or the presence of anti-thyroid peroxidase antibodies.[922] Hypothyroidism can cause an inflammatory myopathy that can resemble polymyositis, and hypothyroidism is a frequent complication of any and all autoimmune diseases. Specific treatment considerations are detailed in Chapter 1:

- Comprehensive antioxidation: Patients with PM-DM may have reduced antioxidant defenses amenable to antioxidant supplementation.[923] Oxidative stress results from and contributes to systemic inflammation because 1) increased immune activity results in elaboration of oxidants, and 2) oxidative stress upregulates NFkB (and other pathways) for additive immune activation. *Antioxidant supplementation* alone is clinically and biochemically inferior to a *comprehensive program* that includes both antioxidant supplementation and dietary modification (i.e., the supplemented Paleo-Mediterranean diet, as described previously) that includes heavy reliance upon fruits, vegetables, low-glycemic juices, nuts, seeds, and berries for their additive and synergistic antioxidant benefits.[924]
- Sunscreen: To protect against photosensitivity.

[920] Weetman AP. Hypothyroidism: screening and subclinical disease. *BMJ*. 1997 Apr 19;314(7088):1175-8 bmj.bmjjournals.com/cgi/content/full/314/7088/1175
[921] "Now AACE encourages doctors to consider treatment for patients who test outside the boundaries of a narrower margin based on a target TSH level of 0.3 to 3.0. AACE believes the new range will result in proper diagnosis for millions of Americans who suffer from a mild thyroid disorder, but have gone untreated until now." American Association of Clinical Endocrinologists (AACE). 2003 Campaign Encourages Awareness of Mild Thyroid Failure, Importance of Routine Testing aace.com/pub/tam2003/press.php November 26, 2005
[922] Beers MH, Berkow R (eds). *Merck Manual. 17th Edition*. Whitehouse Station; Merck Research Laboratories 1999 Page 96
[923] "Fifty patients with low GSH-Px levels were treated with tablets containing 0.2 mg selenium as Na2SeO3 and 10 mg tocopheryl succinate. The GSH-Px levels increased slowly within 6-8 weeks of treatment." Juhlin et al. Blood glutathione-peroxidase levels in skin diseases: selenium and vitamin E treatment. *Acta Derm Venereol*. 1982;62(3):211-4
[924] Liu RH. Health benefits of fruit and vegetables are from additive and synergistic combinations of phytochemicals. *Am J Clin Nutr*. 2003 Sep;78(3 Suppl):517S-520S

Do the Benefits of Botanical and Physiotherapeutic Hepatobiliary Stimulation Result From Enhanced Excretion of IgA Immune Complexes?

This article was originally published in *Naturopathy Digest* 2006
InflammationMastery.com/reprints/2006IgAhepatobiliary.html

Antigen-IgA complexes are phagocytized by hepatocytes and delivered largely intact directly into the bile. This is the most efficient means of disposing of antigens resistant to hydrolytic degradation due either to their size or physiochemical configuration. IgA immune complexes are taken up by hepatocytes and then secreted into the bile for elimination. The fact that bile duct obstruction retards systemic clearance of IgA immune complexes and that restoration of bile flow reduces serum IgA levels by enhancing biliary IgA excretion in animals and humans proves the importance of ensuring optimal hepatobiliary function and supports the use of botanical and physiological therapeutics that facilitate bile flow. Evidence from journals such as the *Archives of Internal Medicine* suggests the primary physiotherapeutic intervention for the stimulation of bile flow is the enema. Enemas are differentiated from colonics in that enemas generally are delivered as a single insertion of water with a modest volume (generally 1-2 quarts [1-2 liters]), whereas colonics generally employ numerous insertions and removals of water, the total volume of which might exceed several gallons (>4-8 liters). Relatedly, the purpose of an enema is to stimulate normal function, while colonics are used to mechanically cleanse the bowel of debris in a manner analogous to the removal of dirt by hand-washing under running water. Colon irrigations were endorsed by the American Medical Association for the adjunctive treatment of numerous health problems as late as 1932, when Bastedo published a review in *Journal of the American Medical Association* endorsing and encouraging their use. In that same year, the *New England Journal of Medicine* documented the value of colon irrigation in the treatment of mental disease. In 1939, Snyder wrote a review article published in the prestigious *Medical Clinics of North America* in which he extolled the clinical benefits of colonics and enemas and lamented the decline in their use, which he attributed to doctors and nurses not having the time or inclination to administer the procedure.

Treatments to reduce the adverse effects of autoantibodies and immune complexes: a conceptual overview with interventional considerations

Goal	Strategic means	Technical means
Reduce *de novo* formation of autoantibodies	→ Biological immunomodulation	→ Orthoendocrinology, particularly supraphysiologic DHEA supplementation → Anti-inflammatory hypoallergenic diet → Anti-inflammatory nutrition: ALA, GLA, EPA, DHA, cholecalciferol, antioxidants, NFkB inhibitors, and anti-inflammatory botanicals → Xenobiotic detoxification
	→ Pharmacologic immunosuppression	→ Prednisone and other corticosteroids → Antibiologics such as hydroxychloroquine which exert their clinical benefits via interfering with normal immunologic function, not by improving overall health or addressing underlying etiologic factors
	→ Removal/correction of primary stimuli for antibody formation *per patient*	→ Orthoendocrinology → Xenobiotic detoxification → Mitochondrial resuscitation → Antidysbiotic interventions: assessment and correction of multifocal dysbiosis
Reduce effects of autoantibodies	→ Anti-inflammatory treatments	→ Anti-inflammatory nutrition: ALA, GLA, EPA, DHA, cholecalciferol, antioxidants, NFkB inhibitors, and anti-inflammatory botanicals

Goal	Strategic means	Technical means
Reduce effects of autoantibodies —*continued*	→ Proteolytic enzymes	→ Proteolytic/pancreatic enzymes appear to reduce *de novo* formation of immune complexes
Enhance clearance of autoantibodies	→ Allopathic interventions	→ Immunoadsorption[925] → Plasmapheresis[926,927]
	→ Naturopathic interventions (theoretical[928])	→ Choleretic and cholagogic botanicals: beets, ginger[929], curcumin[930], *Picrorhiza*[931], milk thistle[932], *Andrographis paniculata*[933] and *Boerhaavia diffusa*.[934] → Low-volume enemas to stimulate bile flow and liver clearance[935]

Multifocal Dysbiosis: Pathophysiology, Relevance for Inflammatory and Autoimmune Diseases, and Treatment With Nutritional and Botanical Interventions

This article was originally published in *Naturopathy Digest* 2006
The complete text is available at InflammationMastery.com/reprints/2006dysbiosis.html

At least 70 percent of patients with chronic arthritis are carriers of "silent infections," according to a 1992 article published in the peer-reviewed medical journal *Annals of the Rheumatic Diseases*. A 2001 article in that same journal which focused exclusively on five bacteria showed that 56 percent of patients with idiopathic inflammatory arthritis had gastrointestinal or genitourinary dysbiosis. Indeed, published research strongly and consistently indicates that bacteria, yeast/fungi, amoebas, protozoa, and other "parasites" (rarely including helminths/worms) are underappreciated causes of neuromusculoskeletal inflammation. In my own clinical practice, gastrointestinal dysbiosis is so common in patients with autoimmune/inflammatory disorders that I consider all of these patients to have dysbiosis until proven otherwise. We perform stool testing with a specialty laboratory, and I am rarely "disappointed" with the finding of normal stool analysis and parasitology. Overall, including patients without autoimmune/inflammatory disorders, I estimate that in my practice, approximately 80 percent of stool and parasitology examinations return with at least one clinically relevant abnormality that, when corrected, provides either subjective or objective improvement in the patient's primary complaint. My experience is consistent with that of other authors and researchers, who note a prevalence of dysbiosis in the range of 70 percent to 100 percent in patients with inflammatory disorders. Recognizing the need to appreciate and transcend the contributions by Koch and Pasture, I've defined dysbiosis as "a relationship of non-acute non-infectious host-microorganism interaction that adversely affects the human host." When used without additional specification, the term "dysbiosis" generally is meant to imply "gastrointestinal dysbiosis." However, as research has continued to progress in this arena, clinicians are now obligated to appreciate the concept of "multifocal dysbiosis" because patients might have dysbiosis in extra-intestinal sites, namely their skin, mouth, sinuses, respiratory tract, genitourinary tract, surrounding environment, and parenchymal tissues. We might reasonably describe multifocal dysbiosis as "a

[925] Braun et al. Immunoadsorption onto protein A induces remission in severe systemic lupus erythematosus. *Nephrol Dial Transplant*. 2000 Sep;15(9):1367-72

[926] Santos-Ocampo AS, Mandell BF, Fessler BJ. Alveolar hemorrhage in systemic lupus erythematosus: presentation and management. *Chest*. 2000 Oct;118(4):1083-90

[927] Choi BG, Yoo WH. Successful treatment of pure red cell aplasia with plasmapheresis in a patient with systemic lupus erythematosus. *Yonsei Med J*. 2002 Apr;4):274-8

[928] Vasquez A. Do Benefits of Botanical and Physiotherapeutic Hepatobiliary Stimulation Result From Enhanced Excretion of IgA Immune Complexes? *Naturo Digest* 2006 Jan

[929] "Further analyses for the active constituents of the acetone extracts through column chromatography indicated that [6]-gingerol and [10]-gingerol, which are the pungent principles, are mainly responsible for the cholagogic effect of ginger." Yamahara et al. Cholagogic effect of ginger and its active constituents. *J Ethnopharmacol*. 1985;13:217-25

[930] "On the basis of the present findings, it appears that curcumin induces contraction of the human gall-bladder." Rasyid A, Lelo A. The effect of curcumin and placebo on human gall-bladder function: an ultrasound study. *Aliment Pharmacol Ther*. 1999 Feb;13(2):245-9

[931] "Significant anticholestatic activity was also observed against carbon tetrachloride induced cholestasis in conscious rat, anaesthetized guinea pig and cat. Picroliv was more active than the known hepatoprotective drug silymarin." Saraswat B, Visen PK, Patnaik GK, Dhawan BN. Anticholestatic effect of picroliv, active hepatoprotective principle of Picrorhiza kurrooa, against carbon tetrachloride induced cholestasis. *Indian J Exp Biol*. 1993 Apr;31(4):316-8

[932] Crocenzi et al. Preventive effect of silymarin against taurolithocholate-induced cholestasis in the rat. *Biochem Pharmacol*. 2003 Jul 15;66(2):355-64

[933] Shukla B, Visen PK, Patnaik GK, Dhawan BN. Choleretic effect of andrographolide in rats and guinea pigs. *Planta Med*. 1992 Apr;58(2):146-9

[934] Chandan BK, Sharma AK, Anand KK. Boerhaavia diffusa: a study of its hepatoprotective activity. *J Ethnopharmacol*. 1991 Mar;31(3):299-307

[935] Garbat AL, Jacobi HG. Secretion of Bile in Response to Rectal Installations. *Arch Intern Med* 1929; 44: 455-462

clinical condition characterized by a patient's simultaneously having more than one foci/location of dysbiosis; generally the adverse physiologic and clinical consequences are additive and synergistic." Although different foci of dysbiosis generally require different types of treatment (e.g., oral versus topical versus environmental), the pathophysiologic mechanisms and clinical consequences are largely identical. Thus, sinorespiratory dysbiosis or genitourinary dysbiosis can be just as devastating as gastrointestinal dysbiosis, and therefore requires appropriate clinical consideration, particularly in patients with autoimmune/inflammatory disorders such as lupus, rheumatoid arthritis, psoriasis, polymyositis, ankylosing spondylitis, and various types of vasculitis.

Dysbiotic Emphases and Therapeutic Prioritization and Contextualization

With the concepts and data that I have presented in Chapters 1, 4, and here in 5, readers are hopefully gaining an appreciation of 1) the great importance of dysbiosis in inflammatory and autoimmune disorders, and 2) the relative importance of the various types and combinations of dysbiosis that are more compellingly implicated in various conditions. Hopefully, clinicians will also not lose sight of the fact that patient-specific variations on these themes clearly exist; yet despite the importance of patient specificity and biochemical individuality, clear patterns do exist, and I have roughly represented these emphases and relationships in the image that follows. Again, clear delineations are impossible in complex living systems affected simultaneously by all of these (and other) variables.

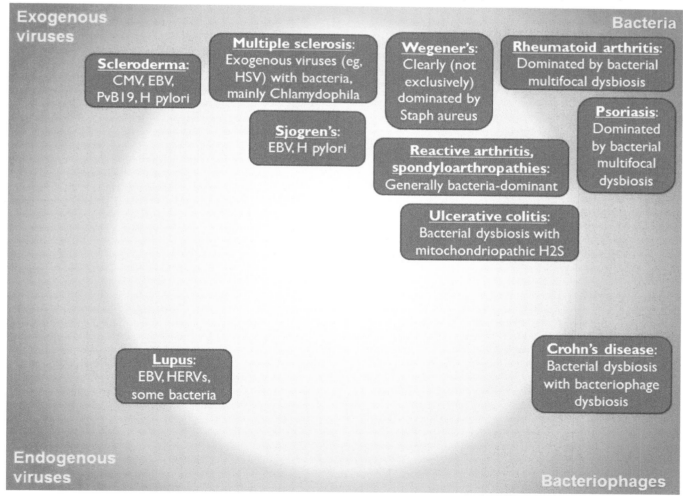

Dysbiotic emphases in various disease states: A rough estimates based on overview of research literature and clinical experience; my hope is that readers will appreciate the disease-specific information presented in this book within its disease-specific context and then break free from that context to see how the information applies to other diseases generally and individual patients specifically.

The End
<ul><li>"It was during the years of my lowest vitality that I ceased to be a pessimist. The instinct of self restoration forbade me a philosophy of poverty and discouragement. As it were, that is how those years appear to me now. I soon discovered life anew...including myself. I turned my will to health, to life, into a philosophy....into the will to power."</li><li>"The time is now past when accidents could befall me; and what **could** now fall to my lot which has not already be my own!? It returns only, it comes home to me at last—mine own Self. And such of it as has been long abroad, and scattered among things and accidents. And one thing more do I know: I stand now before my last summit, and before that which has been longest reserved for me."</li><li>"You have within you the power to merge everything you have lived through – attempts, false starts, errors, delusions, passions, your loves and your hopes – into your highest goal, with nothing left over."</li><li>"At every step one has to wrestle for truth; one has to surrender for it almost everything to which the heart, to which our love, our trust in life, cling otherwise. That requires greatness of soul: the service of truth is the hardest service..."</li><li>"With your love go into your isolation and with your creativity, my brother; and only later will justice limp after you.</li><li>"What makes a person heroic?" Answer: "To simultaneously face one's greatest fear and one's highest hope."</li><li>"My principle article of faith is that one can only flourish among people who share the identical ideas and the identical will."</li><li>"Not around the inventors of new noise but around the inventors of new values does the world revolve."</li></ul>Friedrich Nietzsche (German classical Scholar, Philosopher and Critic of culture, 1844-1900)

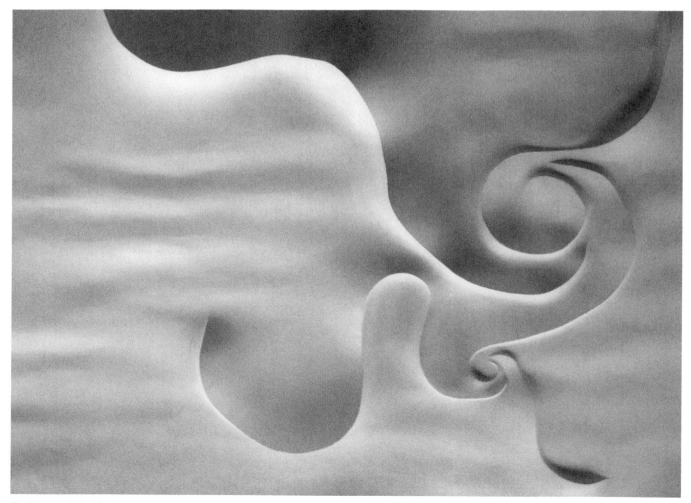

Ceiling of Café de La Pedrera in Barcelona: 2014 photo by DrV

How did Colombians overturn laws mandating the destruction of their grains, their mining, (ie, their food and ways of living)?

- Organization, protests and strikes in many cities
- 648 arrests of protesters, 262 detentions (overturned)
- 660 human rights violations
- 485 wounded
- 12 people killed during protests

That is the cost of freedom from GMO monopolization, more accurately described as GMO neocolonization. See reporting at youtube.com/watch?v=9Vz0tiRKvD0

ICHNFM.org • Colombia • Spain • United States

"Early in September, 2013, the Colombian government was forced to partially concede to the demands of a nationwide general strike instigated by farmers of the largely agrarian nation. The three week long protests and blockades that shut down much of the nation were supported by thousands of miners, truckers, students, bus drivers, and Colombian citizens, blocking roads and clashing with police. Close to 650 arrests were made, 485 injuries were reported, 12 people killed, and over 600 cases of human rights violations reported. Coverage of the nationwide protests feature rural peoples and urban demonstrators in the typical contest against body-armor clad, state riot police armed with gas, rubber bullets, flash-bang grenades and batons, beating people and dispersing women and children in clouds of smoke. ... Implementation of seed control was described by Colombian president Juan Manuel Santos as 'having Colombia tuned up to international reality.' This statement is, of course, completely true. The trending international reality is exactly this, trojan horse conquest of national food sovereignty by means of international corporate/government treaties and agreements sponsored by international governing bodies and the bottomless coiffeurs of the companies that benefit directly from such trade agreements. The shift to this international model of farming simply does not make economic or common sense for the people of most nations. Author and self-proclaimed 'economic hitman' John Perkins wrote about this type of imperial foreign occupation by corporate influence in his critical book, '*Confessions of an Economic Hitman*.' It is the newest means of international conquest. The international drive toward the monopolization of seed, the global reduction of seed diversity, and the abolishment of small scale farming is being seen all over the world."

globalresearch.ca/colombians-successfully-revolt-against-seed-control-and-agricultural-tyranny/5352534

"Tensions have been rising between the Colombian government and the agricultural sector since the regulations imposed by the **U.S.-Colombia Free Trade Agreement**, which went into effect in May 2012. ... But farmers have bristled at the **requirement that they use genetically modified seeds, engineered by international conglomerates like Monsanto and Du Pont, and pay an annual fee to do so.**"

rollingstone.com/politics/news/will-colombias-farmers-get-what-they-want-20131118

The question that needs to be asked is: "Why is the US government enforcing the international adoption of genetically modified/manipulated foods, when this is clearly in the interest of private industry (unless corporate interests now rule international politics) and at the risk of destabilizing other countries (unless the goal is to destabilize those countries)?"

Index:

11-beta hydroxysteroid dehydrogenase, 737

12-hydroperoxyeicosatetraenoic acid, 370

12-R-HETE, 370

12-R-lipoxygenase, 375

12-S-HETE, 370

12-S-lipoxygenase, 375

13-S-HODE, 369

15-hydroperoxyeicosatetraenoic acid, 370

15-hydroxy-eicosatrienoic acid, 368

15-lipoxygenase-1, 375

15-lipoxygenase-2, 375

15-S-HETE, 370

2,4-dichlorophenol, 237

2,5-dichlorophenol, 236

2010 ACR guidelines for the diagnosis and assessment of FM, 910

25(OH) vitamin D, 59, 745

2-hydroxyestrone, 693

3-3-hydroxyphenyl-3-hydroxypropionic acid, 442, 935

5-HETE, 370

5-hydroperoxyeicosatetraenoic acid, 369

5-hydroxytryptophan, 960

5-lipoxygenase, 374

5pSPMD, 717

8-lipoxygenase, 375

8-S-HETE, 370

Abducens, 23

Acacia catechu, 535

ACEi, 807

Acetaminophen, 913

Acetyl-L-carnitine, 789

Acetyl-L-carnitine, 970

Acinetobacter spp, 94

Acupuncture, 791, 973

Acute nontraumatic monoarthritis, 122

Acute red eye, 119

Acute-onset HTN, 752

Adenosine monophosphate (AMP), 571

Adipokines, 205, 822

Adipose, 205, 822

ADP, dosing and clinical use, 493, 720

Adrenic acid, 367

Adverse food reactions, 379, 984

African American, 807

ALA, 359

Alcohol, 413, 460, 929

Aldolase, 1146

Aldosterone:renin ratio, 748

Aldosterone-to-renin ratio, 748

Algal chlorovirus ATCV-1, 441, 935

Alginate, 1093

Alkalinization, 267, 770

Allergy diagnosis, 391

Allium sativum, 779

Alpha-2 agonists, 813

Alpha-adrenergic receptor class-2 agonist, 813

Alpha-adrenergic receptor type-1 antagonist, 812

Alpha-linolenic acid, 359

Alveolar hemorrhage, 1062

Alzheimer's disease, 92

Amitriptyline, 912

Amlodipine, 810

Amoxicillin, 496

ANA - interpretation, 78

ANA - overview, 26

Analgesia (natural), 266, 267

ANCA, 1103

ANCA-associated vasculitis (also called "granulomatosis with polyangiitis", formerly Wegener's granulomatosis, 428

Andrographis paniculata, 537

Anesthetics, 298

Anethum graveolens, 535

Aneurysm (intracranial), 875

Angiotensin-2 converting enzyme inhibitors, 807

Anise, 534

Ankylosing spondylitis, 1110

Anti-autoantibody interventions, 1071

Antibiotic/antifungal drugs, 495

Anticardiolipin antibodies, 1064

Anti-CCP antibodies, 81, 1024

Anticitrullinated protein antibodies, 81

Anticyclic citrullinated peptide, 1024

Anti-double stranded (DS, native) DNA antibodies, 1064

Antidysbiotic lifestyle, 489

Antifibrillarin antibodies, 1092

Anti-histone antibodies, 1064

Antihistorical, 196

Anti-inflammatory & analgesic treatments, 255

Anti-Jo-1, 1146

Antimetabolites, 413, 415, 928

Antimicrobial treatment of SIBO, 963

Antimutagenesis as a direct antiviral strategy, 573, 582

Anti-nuclear antibodies, 1064

Antinuclear antibody - interpretation, 78, 79

Antioxidant capacity of fruits and vegetables, 209

Antiphospholipid and Anticardiolipin antibodies, 1064

Antiphospholipid syndrome, 427

Antiphospholipid/ anticardiolipin/ Hughes syndrome, 85

Anti-Ro antibodies, 1064

Anti-Sm (anti-Smith) antibodies, 1064

Antiviral (phyto)nutrition, 723

Aortic coarctation, 735

Arachidonate avoidance, 769

Arachidonic acid metabolites formed by cyclooxygenase, 368

Arachidonic acid, 366

Arginine, 775, 776

Arginine, omega-3 fatty acids and nucleotide-supplemented enteral support, 585

Armour thyroid, 697

Aromatase, 693

Aromatase, 828

Artemisia annua, 494, 533, 722

Artificial sweeteners, colors and other additives, 212

Ascorbic acid, 587, 770

Aspartame, 212

Asthma & Reactive Airway Disease, 1001

Atlantoaxial instability in AS and RA, 1111

Atlantoaxial instability, 120, 121

Atlas vertebra realignment, 795

Augmentin, 496, 964

Authentic living, 221

Autism, 414, 415, 483, 484, 485, 530

Auto-brewery syndrome, 459

Autoimmune hepatitis, 85

Autoimmune thyroid disease, 85

Autointoxication, 459

Autonomization, 224

Avascular necrosis of the femoral head, osteonecrosis, 123

Azithromycin for psoriasis, 1048

Azithromycin, 496

Babesia, 93

Bacterial allergy, 434

Bacterial DNA, 409

Bacterial overgrowth, 473

Bacteriophage therapy, 497

Bacteriophages, 556, 1059

Balance shoes, 294

Barrett's esophagus, 1078

Bed rest, 254

Beets, 537

Behcet's Disease, 1133

Behcet's Syndrome, 1133

Berberine, 533, 781

Berberine: dosing and clinical use, 720

Beta-adrenergic receptor blockers, "beta blockers", 809

Beta-glucuronidase, 104, 488

Betaine, 576

Betulina, 534

Bile flow, 706

Biochemical Individuality - overview, 216

Biochemical individuality, 195

Biofilms, 439

Bioflavonoids in the treatment of allergy, 388, 994

Biotin, 611

Bismuth, 494, 534, 722

Blastocystis hominis, 493, 525, 720

Bleach bath, 515

Blood Dysbiosis, 511

Blood pressure measurement, 743

Body mass index (BMI) for predicting amount and duration of weight loss, 744

Body Mass Index, 204, 822

Boerhaavia diffusa, 537

Bone necrosis caused by NSAIDs, 250

Borrelia burgdorferi, 93

Boswellia serrata, 259
Bowel-associated dermatitis-arthritis syndrome (BADAS), 434
Bradycardia, 807
Breath testing, 487
Bromocriptine, 691, 692
Brucea javanica, 535
Buchu/betulina, 534
Butyrate, 415
BVG-LOC profile, 753
Bystander activation, 428
Cabergoline, 691
Caffeine, 212
Calcium channel blockers (dihydropyridine class), 810
Calcium pyrophosphate dihydrate deposition disease, 124, 125
Campylobacter, 93
Canadian Hypertension Education Program recommendations, 761
C-ANCA, 1103
Candida albicans, 526
Candida hypersensitivity, 434
Cannabis sativa and related variants, 261
Caprylic acid, 535
Capsicum annuum, Capsicum frutescens, 260, 1049
Carbohydrate loading for supercompensation, 211
Carboxy-methyl-lysine, 904
Cardiopulmonary examination, 743
Carica papaya ("papaya"), 567
Carnitine Insufficiency Caused by Aging and Overnutrition, 789
Carnitine, antiinflammatory effects, 1049
Carpal bones myofascial release, 290
Carpal tunnel syndrome - clinical management, 286
Carpal tunnel syndrome - manipulative treatment, 292
Carrageenan, 212
Cartilage destruction caused by NSAIDs, 250
Casokinins, 773
Catecholamine-O-methyltransferase, 737
Cat's claw, 259
Cauda equina syndrome, 2, 120
Cayenne pepper - monograph, 1049
Cayenne pepper, 260
CBC – overview, 25
CCB, 810
CCP, 81, 1024
Celiac disease and autoimmunity, 492
Celiac disease and autoimmunity, 719
Celiac disease, 85, 429
Cell wall-deficient bacteria, 408
Centella asiatica, 1088
Central neurogenic hypertension, 738
Cephalexin, 497, 516
Cervical spine dysfunction, 742
Cervical Spine: Rotation Emphasis, 280

CH50, 1064
Chemistry panel – overview, 25
Chemistry/metabolic panel, 745
Chiropractic model of illness and healing, 152
Chiropractic spinal manipulative therapy, 792, 794
Chiropractic, 973
Chiropractic-supervised water-only fasting in the treatment of borderline hypertension, 668, 669, 763
Chlamydia trachomatis, 93
Chlamydia/Chlamydophila pneumoniae, 93, 517, 918
Chlorella pyrenoidosa, 673, 725
Chlorella, 673, 725, 979
Chlorovirus ATCV-1, 441, 935
Chlorpyrifos, 236
Chocolate, 771
Chondroitin, 270
Chronic fatigue syndrome, 94
Chronic inflammatory disease, sustained inflammatory response, 398
Churg-Strauss syndrome, 1099
CIC (circulating immune complexes), 1141
Ciprofloxacin, 497
Citrate synthase, 890
Citrobacter freundii, 526
Citrobacter rodentium, 526
Clinical Assessments for HTN, 742
Clinical Case: 45yo HLA-B27+ woman with recurrent UTIs and a 7-year history of ankylosing spondylitis, 501
Clinical Case: Abnormal lactulose-mannitol ratio in a patient with idiopathic peripheral neuropathy, 499
Clinical Case: Elevated hsCRP (high-sensitivity C-reactive protein) in a male patient with metabolic syndrome and rheumatoid arthritis, 500
Clinical Case: Elevated plasma ammonia in the absence of liver disease, 461
Clinical Case: Exemplary case of clinical and laboratory evidence of reversal of "severe, aggressive, drug-resistant" rheumatoid arthritis, 402
Clinical Management, 752
Clinical practice involves much more than "diagnosis and treatment", 114
Clonidine, 813
Clostridium, especially in autism, 485
Clove, 534
Cluster headache - differential diagnosis of head pain, 875
Cluster headache, 874

Cluster headaches, treatment with melatonin, 899
Cocaine, 735
Cockcroft-Gault formula, 740
Cocoa, 771
Cod liver oil, 588
Coenzyme Q10 (CoQ10) in cardiac disease, 788
Coenzyme Q-10, 787, 966
Coffee as a gastrointestinal stimulant, 495
Cold and stretch treatment for MFTP, 277
Colonization, 399
Combination of streptococcal antigen with bacterial DNA, 410
Combinatorial inflammology, 478
Combinatorial multifocal polydysbiosis, 398
Commiphora molmol, 533
Complement, 84
Complements C3 and C4, 54
Composite seropositivity, 1024
Composite seropositivity, 81
Comprehensive parasitology, 102
Comprehensive parasitology, 102, 501, 529
Compression - use in injury management, 255
Conn's syndrome, 739
Conscious living, 196
Consciousness-raising, 224
Consent to treatment, 110
Contemplation, 194
Contraceptives, 735
Controlled breathing, 791
CoQ-10 in the treatment of allergy, 388, 994
CoQ-10 treatment for migraine, 890
CoQ10, 420, 787, 969
Corrective experience, 224
Cortef, 695
Cortical spreading depression, 866
Cortisol, 694
Cosmetics, 979
Cough headache - differential diagnosis of head pain, 875
Counterthrust, 279
CPDD, 125
CPPD, 124, 125
Cranberry, 534
Cranial nerve V, pain sensation in migraine, 863
Cranial nerves, 22, 23
C-reactive protein - interpretation, 27
Creatine kinase, 1146
Creatine monohydrate, 970
CREST syndrome, 1074
Cross-reactivity, 423
CRP - interpretation, 52
Cryoglobulinemia, 1098
Curcumin requires piperine for absorption, 308, 377, 389, 996
Curcumin, 537
Cushing's disease/syndrome, 735

Cutaneous dysbiosis/colonization—introduction to assessment, 90
Cyclic citrullinated protein antibodies, 81, 1024
Cyclobenzaprine, 913
Cyclooxygenase (COX), 373
Cymbalta, 912
Cytochrome-c-oxidase, 890
Cytomegalovirus (CMV), 1054
Cytomegalovirus (CMV), 548
Cytomegalovirus (CMV), 92
Cytomegalovirus—Induction of vasculopathy, 1084
Cytomegalovirus—Induction of vasculopathy, 549
Cytomel, 697
Daily living, 190
DAMP, 417
Danazol, 1066
Danger/damage-associated molecular patterns—DAMP—receptors, 417
Dark Chocolate, 771
DASH: Dietary Approaches to Stop Hypertension, 758
DDE, 235
DDT, 235
Deep tendon reflexes, 24
Definition of dysbiosis, 396
Deglycyrrhizinated licorice, 1122
Delta-4-desaturase, 373
Delta-5-desaturase, 373
Delta-6-desaturase, 372
Dengue virus, 567
Dental care, 505
Depuration, 238, 239
Dermatomyositis sine myositis, 1142
Dermatomyositis, 1142
Dermatopolymyositis, 1142
Detoxification defects caused by leaky gut, 486
Detoxification programs are a necessity, 235
Detoxification, 239, 921
Detoxification, problems and solutions, 704
Detoxification: An Ultracondensed Clinical Review, 699
Devil's claw, 259
DGLA metabolites formed by 15-lipoxygenase, 368
DGLA metabolites formed by cyclooxygenase, 367
DGLA, 365
DHA, 257
DHA, 361
DHEA, 1108
DHEA, 695
Diabetes mellitus type 1.5, 85
Diabetes, 512
Dientamoeba fragilis, 526
Diet optimization, 957
Dietary haptenization, 382, 988
Dietary molecular mimicry, 383
Dietary molecular mimicry, 988
Differential Diagnoses of HTN, 734
Diffuse idiopathic skeletal hyperostosis, 1114

Diffuse systemic sclerosis, 1074
Diflucan, 965
Dihomo-gamma-linolenic acid, 365
Diindolylmethane, 693
Dill (antimicrobial actions), 535
DIM, 693
Dimercaptosuccinic acid, 709, 920
DISH, 1114
D-lactic acid intestinal bacteria in chronic fatigue syndrome, 413, 929
D-lactic acid, 924
D-lactic acidosis, 414
D-lactic acidosis, 929
DMSA, 709
DMSA, 920
DNA methylation and "folic acid"*, 577
DNA methylation and histone acetylation, 449
DNA methylation as an antiviral antireplication strategy, 576
DNA methylation, 1058, 582
Docere, 131
Docosahexaenoic acid, 361
Docosapentaenoic acid, 361, 367
Docosatrienes, 308, 362
Dostinex, 691
Double hit model of microbe synergism for autoimmunity induction, 427
DPA, 361
D-ribose, 970
Drop thrust, 283, 607
Drug treatments for chronic HTN, 805
Drug-induced lupus, 428
Drugs for intestinal bacterial overgrowth, 495
Dry needling or injection of local anesthetic or saline
Duloxetine, 912
Dysbiosis can be distinguished based on the location(s) of the dysbiotic foci/focus, 396
Dysbiosis in scleroderma, 553
Dysbiosis treatments, 532
Dysbiosis—introduction to concepts and testing, 86
Ear lobe crease, 743
Ebola virus infection, 544, 572
ECG, 749
Eicosanoid modulation, 267
Eicosapentaenoic acid, 360
Eicosatetraenoic acid, 360, 366
Eicosatrienoic acid, 365
EKG, 749, 750
Electrocardiography, 749
Elimination and challenge technique, 391, 999
Elongase, 373
Emergencies, 119
Emotional literacy, 224
Emotional, mental, and social health, 221
Endocrinologic activity of adipose tissue, 205
Endolimax nana, 493, 527, 720

Endoplasmic reticulum (ER) and ER stress (ERS), 651
Endotoxins (lipopolysaccharide) from gram-negative bacteria, 404
Enemas, 537
Enhanced processing of autoantigens, 425, 441, 934
Entamoeba hartmanni, 493, 720
Entamoeba histolytica, 471, 479, 527
Enterococcus, 527
Enteropathic spondylo-arthropathy, enteropathic arthritis, 1110
Enterovirus D68, 544
Enthesopathies, 1111
Environmental dysbiosis, 517
Environmental dysbiosis/colonization—introduction to assessment, 90
Enzyme therapy, 594
Enzymes in fatty acid metabolism, 372
EPA - review, 360
EPA, 257
Epicatechin, 772
Epigenetic dysbiosis/eubiosis, 448
Epigenetic dysfunction, 448
Epigenetic silencing of viral sequences, 543
Epinephrine and norepinephrine, 749
Epstein-Bar virus (EBV), 92, 548, 1054, 1085
Erythromycin, 496, 722
Esophageal dysfunction and GERD in scleroderma, 1092
ESR - interpretation, 54
Essay: Common Oversights and Shortcomings in the Study and Implementation of Nutritional Supplementation, 315
Essay: Five-Part Nutritional Wellness Protocol That Produces Consistently Positive Results, 310
Essay: Implementing the Five-Part Nutritional Wellness Protocol for the Treatment of Various Health Problems, 312
Essay: Twilight of the Idiopathic Era and The Dawn of New Possibilities in Health and Healthcare, 814, 858
Essential fatty acid, 358, 365
Estrogen, 692, 735
Ethanol, 460, 736
Eucalyptus oil, 521
Exceptional living, 195
Exercise, 201, 791
Eye and fundoscopic examination, 743
Facial nerve, 23
Faecalibacterium, 472
Family health history, 13
Fasting (short-term water-only), 762
Fatty Acid Modulation of Eicosanoid Production and Genetic Expression, 309
Fatty acid supplementation, 769
Fatty acids, 588
Fecal transplant, 497

Ferritin - interpretation, 54
Ferritin - overview, 26
Feverfew, 897
Fibromyalgia clinical criteria: description and contrast of the 1990 criteria and the 2010 criteria, 909
Fibromyalgia disease, 902
Fibromyalgia initiated by dysbiosis, 463
Fibromyalgia, 901
Fibrosis of the skin and internal organs, 1074
Fish oil, 769
Fish oil, EPA with DHA - rationale for use in basic conservative care, 257
Flax seed oil, 359
Flossing, including use of "floss picks", 505
Fluconazole, 965
Folate deficiency and cervical dysplasia, 576
Food allergen avoidance, 763
Food allergens, 213
Food allergy diagnosis, 391, 999
Food allergy in the induction and perpetuation of autoimmunity, 986
Food allergy, 379, 985
Food challenges, 391, 999
Formula SF722, 493, 720
Fructose avoidance, 767
Fumaderm, 1141
Fumaric acid esters, 1141
Functional assessment, 19
Functional Medicine (FxMed) perspectives, 916
Fundoscopic examination, 743
Furosemide, 811
Gamma delta T cells, 610
Gamma strep, 527
Gamma-linolenic acid, 257, 365
Garlic, 534, 779
Gastric ulceration and gastrointestinal bleeding caused by NSAIDs, 250
Gastrointestinal dysbiosis, 471
Gastrointestinal dysbiosis/colonization—introduction to assessment, 88
Gene products - amplification by NF-kappaB, 376
Genital mucosal lesions, 1135
Genitourinary dysbiosis/colonization—introduction to assessment, 89
GERD in scleroderma, 1092
Gestational hypertension, 736
Giant Cell (Temporal) Arteritis, 1097
Giant Cell Arteritis (previously Temporal Arteritis), 1100
Giant cell arteritis, 119
Giardia lamblia, 527, 528
Ginger, 258, 537
GLA - review, 365
Glial activation, 441, 935
Gliotoxin, 438

Glossopharyngeal, 23
Glucosamine, 270
Glutamate and the NMDA receptor in headache, 870, 872
Glutamate/NMDA receptor, 442, 935
Glutamine, 589
Gluten avoidance, SLE treatment, 1066
Glycolytic pathways, 894
Glycyrrhiza glabra, 565, 737
Goldhamer, 762
Gottron's sign, 1144
Gotu cola, 1088
Gout, 124
Granulomatosis with polyangiitis, formerly Wegener's granulomatosis, 429
Granulomatous disease (sarcoidosis), 1138
Granulomatous uveitis, 1138
Grape seed extract (GSE), 308, 377, 389, 571, 996
Green tea, 308, 377, 389, 618, 996
Group A streptococci, 531
Gulf War Illness, 94
H2S—hydrogen sulfide, 924, 929
Haemophilus influenzae, 427
Haptenization, 428
Harpagophytum procumbens, 259
HCTZ, 811
Helicobacter pylori, 94, 528, 1085
Heliotrope/purple facial/cheek rash, 1144
Hematocolpos, 1113
Hemochromatosis, 160
Hemochromatosis, 919
Hemoglobin A1c, 747
Henoch-Schonlein purpura, 1099
Hepatic and renal injury and failure caused by NSAIDs, 250
Hepatic encephalopathy in the absence of liver disease, 459
Hepatitis B virus (HepB, HBV), 92
Hepatitis C virus (HepC, HCV), 92
Hepatobiliary stimulation for IgA-complex removal, 536
Herpes simplex virus type-2 (HSV-2), 560
Herpes simplex virus types 1 and 2 (HSV1, HSV2), 92
Herpes zoster. The treatment and prevention of neuralgia with adenosine monophosphate, 571
HERV, 554, 1055
HFE mutation, 167
Hgb-A1c, 747
Hierarchy of Therapeutics, 131
High glycemic foods, 255
High-dose mannose-binding lectin therapy for Ebola virus infection, 572
High-fructose corn syrup, 737
High-risk pain patients, 109
History taking, 8
HLA-B27, 425

Homologs, 423, 427
Hormones in the treatment of allergy, 390, 998
Hospital/physician errors, 253
HPHPA, 442, 935
HPV, 1054
HPV, 548, 561, 1054
HTLV (human T-lymphotropic virus) in SLE, 549, 1055
HTN prevalence, 732
HTN, CVD, 730
Hughes syndrome, 85
Human endogenous retroviruses (HERVs) play a role in autoimmune diseases, 554
Human herpes virus type-6 (HHV-6), 92, 560
Human immunodeficiency virus (HIV), 92, 558
Human papilloma virus (HPV), 548, 561, 1054
HVLA, 279
Hydralazine, 813
Hydrochlorothiazide (HCTZ), 811
Hydrogen sulfide, 413, 474, 924, 929
Hydrosoluble coenzyme Q10, 789
Hydroxocobalamin, 883
Hyperaldosteronism, 739
Hypercalcemia, 736
Hyperglycemia adversely impacts the innate immune system, 599
Hypericum perforatum shows impressive antibacterial action, 494, 533, 722
Hyperinsulinemia, 211, 736
Hyperprolactinemia, 689
Hypersensitivity/allergic dysbiosis, 474
Hypertension, see also HTN, 728
Hypertensive emergency, 752, 752
Hyperthyroidism, 742
Hypochlorite, 516
Hypoglossal nerve, 23
Hypomethylation, 577
Hypothyroidism, 742, 801, 917
I3C, 693
Iatrogenic neurosis, 265
Ice/heat, 254
Idiopathicization, 1143
IgE and IgG assays, 999
Immune complex formation and deposition, 430, 1053
Immune complexes, 1141
Immunodysregulatory dysbiosis, 479
Immunonutrition (against dysbiosis), 536
Immunonutrition, 585
Immunophenotype determination, 610
Immunostimulation by bacterial DNA, 409
Immunosuppression via gliotoxins, 438
Immunosuppressive dysbiosis, 474
Immunotoxicity, 699

Inadequacies in musculoskeletal education and training among physicians, 247
Inclusion body myositis, 1145
Increased intestinal permeability caused by NSAIDs, 250
Individualize treatment - importance, 255
Individuation, 196
Indole, 413, 929
Indole-3-carbinol, 693
Inflammation promotes more inflammation, 376
Inflammatory bowel disease-- laboratory testing, 85
Inflammatory dysbiosis, 475
Informed consent, 110
Inhibition of detoxification by dysbiosis, 434
Insufficiency dysbiosis, 432
Insulin resistance and gut dysbiosis, 481
Insulin resistance, 211, 512, 736
Insulin, 747
Internal locus of control, 226
Intestinal/mesenteric vasculitis, 1062
Intracranial aneurysm, 875
Intracranial mass lesion, 876
Intradependence, 224
Introduction to Injection Therapies, 298
Iodine, 697
Iodine/iodide—oral administration of pharmacologic doses, 569
Iron overload as a cause of headaches, 877
Iron Overload, 160, 876, 919
Juvenile spondylo-arthropathy, 1111
Kawasaki disease, 552, 1099
Keflex, 497
Keratoconjunctivitis sicca, 1120
Klebsiella pneumoniae, 471, 528
Koch's Postulates, 399
LA, 365
Labile support surface, 294
Laboratory assessments: general considerations, 25
Lactoferrin, 104, 488
Lactokinins, 773
Lactulose-mannitol assay evaluates paracellular/pathologic and transcellular/physiologic absorption, 487
Lactulose-mannitol assay, 26, 487
LADA, 85
Lambert-Eaton myasthenic syndrome, 1145
L-Arginine, 775
Lasix, 811
Latent autoimmune diabetes in adults, 85
Laxatives promote eradication of intestinal microbes, 495
L-carnitine, 789
Lead accumulation, 748
Lead and HTN, 77, 748
Lead, 920

Leaky gut diagram, 486
Leaky gut, 101, 416
Lemon balm (Melissa officinalis), 568
Leukotriene B4, 370
Leukotriene B-5, 362
Levothyroxine, 696
L-form, 408
Licorice, 565, 737
Lifestyle habits, 191
Limited cutaneous scleroderma, 1074
Linoleic acid metabolites formed by lipoxygenases, 369
Linoleic acid, 365
Linolenic acid, 359
Liothyronine, 697
Liotrix, 697
Lipoic acid, 308, 377, 389, 578, 996
Lipoxygenases (LOX), 374
Lisinopril, 808
Liver biopsy in iron overload, 167
Low starch diet, 492, 719
Low-back pain: differential diagnostic considerations, 1113
Low-carbohydrate (low fermentation) supplemented Paleo-Mediterranean diet, 491
Low-carbohydrate (low fermentation) supplemented Paleo-Mediterranean diet, 718
LOX, 374
LPS triggers TRL4 to activate mitochondrial hyperpolarization, 421
LT-C4, 370
LT-D4, 370
LT-E4, 370
L-tryptophan, 949
L-tyrosine and iodine, 697
Lugol's solution against influenza, 569
Lumbar Roll, 284
Lupus and Epstein-Barr, 549
Lupus, 1053
Lyme disease, 93
Lyrica, 912
Lysine, 570
Madecassol, 1088
Magnesium, 767, 961
Malignant HTN, 752
Manipulation of the Costovertebral Junction, 282
Manipulation, mobilization, and massage, 266
ManKind Project, 224
Manual Medicine, 278
Marshall protocol, 452
Mask-like face, 1075
Massage, 263
Mechanisms of autoimmune disease induction by microorganisms, 403
Mechanistic dysbiosis, 479
Mechanistic Target of Rapamycin, 656
Medical history, 13
Meditation, 791
Melatonin, 200, 592, 802, 969
Melissa officinalis, 568
Melzack and Wall, 908

Meningitis, 876
Mentha piperita, 494, 534, 722
Mercurial myopathy, 920
Mercury impairs catecholamine degradation, 737
Mercury toxicity, 237, 702, 737, 920
Metabolic dysbiosis, 479
Metabolism of omega-3 fatty acids and related eicosanoids - illustration, 364
Metabolism of omega-6 fatty acids and related eicosanoids - illustration, 371
Methylation of DNA, 582, 1058
Metoprolol, 810
Metronidazole, 495
Metronidazole, 722
MFTP - clinical management, 274
Microbial colonization, 86
Microbial dysepigenetics, 448
Microbial hypersensitivity, bacterial allergy, 434
Microbial Induction of Noninfectious Systemic Disease, 403
Microglial activation, 441, 935
Migraine - differential diagnosis of head pain, 876
Migraine with aura, 874
Milk protein-derived peptide inhibitors of angiotensin-I-converting enzyme, 775
Milk thistle, 537
Milnacipran, 913
Mimotopes, 423, 427
Mind-Body Approaches, 791
Minimize factors that promote disease, 241
Minocycline, 496
Mitochondrial DAMPs, 417
Mitochondrial dysfunction and mTOR activation, 420
Mitochondrial dysfunction promotes central sensitization, 928
Mitochondrial dysfunction, 904, 905
Mitochondrial impairment is the origin of migraine and cluster headache, 864
Mitochondrial myopathy, 905
Mitophagy, 906, 925, 949, 951, 965, 966
Mixed connective tissue disease, 1074
Mobilization, 266
Molecular mimicry, 423
Monoarthritis, 122
Mononeuritis multiplex, 1101
Mononucleosis, 92
Motivation, 193
Motivation: moving from theory to practice, 194
mTOR, 420, 656
Mucuna pruriens, 690
Multifocal Dysbiosis, 396, 1152
Multifocal polydysbiosis, 86
Multiple chemical sensitivity, 436
Multiple sclerosis (MS), 93, 94, 514

Multivitamin/multimineral
supplementation, 600
Muscle strength – grading scale, 24
Musculoskeletal emergencies, 119
Musculoskeletal Manipulation, 278
Mycoplasma species including
pneumoniae, fermentans, hominis,
penetrans, genitalium, 94
Mycoplasma species, 918
Myelopathy, 2, 120
Myofascial trigger points - clinical
management, 274
Myrrh, 533
NAC, 580
N-acetyl-cysteine (NAC), 580
NADH-cytochrome-c-reductase, 890
NADH-dehydrogenase, 890
Nail pitting, 1039
National Heart, Lung, and Blood
Institute (NHLBI), 818
Nattokinase, 781
Naturopathic model of illness and
healing, 129, 130
Neisseria gonorrhoeae, 427
Neoantigens/neoautoantigens, 428
Neomycin, 964
Neurogenic hypertension, 738
Neurologic deficit in the evaluation of
head pain - clinical management,
877
Neurologic examination, 19, 744
Neuronal autoimmunity, 94
Neuropsychiatric lupus is a medical
emergency, 1061
Neuropsychiatric lupus, 119
Neurotoxic dysbiosis, 483
NF-kappaB, 417, 418, 419
NFkB and its phytonutritional
modulation, 376
NFkB inhibition as an antiviral
antireplication strategy, 578
Niacinamide, 270
NLRP3 inflammasome is activated in
fibromyalgia, 419
NLRP3 inflammasome is activated in
fibromyalgia, 969
NMDA receptor, 442, 935
NMDA-type glutamate receptor
(NMDAr), 871
NOD-like receptors (NLR), 419
Nonsteroidal anti-inflammatory drugs,
739
Nuclear transcription factor kappa
beta, 376, 419
Nucleotide-binding oligomerization
domain, 419
Nucleotides, 590
Nutrigenomics, 217
Nutrition and Physical Degeneration,
textbook by Weston Price,, 206
Nutritional Genomics, 217
Nutritional immunomodulation, 307,
609
Nystatin, 496, 723

O'Keefe and Cordain in Mayo Clinic
Proceedings, 206
Obesity, 204, 822
Objective means for the identification
of allergens, 999
Occult infections, 918
Octreotide, 1083
Oculomotor, 23
Oil pulling/swishing, 505
Olfactory, 23
Omega-3 fatty acids - review, 359
Ophthalmic, 23
Opioid epidemic, 245
Oral contraceptives, 735
Oregano oil, 533, 720
Organic foods rather than industrially-
produced foods, 212
Orodental dysbiosis, 88, 503
Orthoendocrinology, 688
Orthomolecular Immunomodulation,
386, 993
Orthomolecular Medicine - overview,
216
Orthopedic/musculoskeletal
examination: concepts and goals,
20
Orwellian newspeak, 249
Osteochondritis dissecans, 123
Osteomyelitis, 2, 121
Osteopathic manipulation, 798, 973
Osteopathic manipulative treatment
for adult pneumonia, 606
Osteopathic Medicine, 149
Overlap syndromes, 1074
Oxygen, for cluster headaches, 892,
970, 973
PABA, 1088
Pain/fatigue syndromes and SIBO,
480
Paleo-, 758
Paleo-Mediterranean Diet, 219, 492,
597, 756
Pancreatic and proteolytic enzymes,
273, 594
Papaya, 567
PAR, 110
Paradigms, and their reasonable
alternatives, 197
Parasitelogy, 102
Parasiteology, 501, 529
Parasites, 525
Parenchymal dysbiosis/colonization—
introduction to assessment, 91
Parenchymal/Blood Dysbiosis, 511
Parvovirus B-19 (PvB19), 548, 561,
1054, 1085
Pasteurian paradigm, 399
Pathophysiologic responses, 416
Patient (mis)education in standard
medicine, 914
Pattern recognition receptors—PRRs,
417
P-cresol, 415
Penicillin treatment of psoriasis, 1048
Pentosedine, 904

Peppermint, 494, 534
Peppermint, 722
Peptidoglycans and exotoxins from
gram-positive bacteria, 406
Peripheral neurogenic hypertension,
738
Pesticide exposure, 237
Phenolic content, 209
Pheochromocytoma, 739
Phlogenzym, 595
Phospholipase-A2, 373
Physical examination, 19, 743
Physical exertion, 201
Physical medicine: spinal
manipulation, mobilization, 605
Physician errors, 253
Phytochelatins, 711
Phytochemicals, 208
PI3K/Akt/mTOR pathway, 422
Picrorhiza, 537
Plasminogen activator inhibitor, 362
Pleomorphic, "cell wall-deficient"
bacteria, 408
Political and social action, 238
Polyarteritis nodosa, 1098
Polymicrobial dysbiosis in
scleroderma, 553
Polymyalgia Rheumatica, 1100
Polymyositis, 1142
Polyphenolics and phytonutrients, 581
Porphyria cutanea tarda, 162
Post-isometric stretching treatment for
MFTP, 276
Potaba, 1088
Potassium supplementation, 764
Potassium-sparing diuretic:
spironolatone, 812
Povidone iodine, 515
Prazosin, 813
Pre-contemplation, 194
Preeclampsia, 736
Pregabalin, 912
Preparation, 194
Primary biliary cirrhosis, 85
Primary sclerosing cholangitis, 85
Primary/Genetic Hemochromatosis,
160
Primum Non Nocere, 130
Probiotic supplementation, 535
Probiotics, 490, 603, 782, 962
Progressive Systemic Sclerosis, 1074
Proinflammatory and endocrinologic
activity of adipose tissue, 205
Pro-inflammatory foods, 255
Prolactin, 689
Prolotherapy, 298
Propionic acid, 414
Propolis, 308, 377, 389, 996
Proprioceptive rehabilitation and
retraining, 293, 300
Proprioceptive retraining, 266
Prostacyclin, 368
Prostaglandin D2, 368
Prostaglandin E-1, 367
Prostaglandin E2, 308, 368

Prostaglandin E-3, 362
Prostaglandin F2-alpha, 369
Prostaglandin G2, 369
Prostaglandin G-3, 362
Prostaglandin H2, 369
Prostaglandin H-3, 362
Prostaglandin I2, 368
Prostaglandin I-3, 362
Prostaglandin synthase complex, 373
Protect & prevent re-injury, 254
Protein - calculation of daily intake, 206, 268, 328
Proteolytic enzymes (used in the treatment of dysbiosis), 535
Proteolytic enzymes, 273, 594
Proteus mirabilis, 471
PRRs, 417
Pseudomonas aeruginosa, 94, 471
Psoriasis, main chapter, 1038
Psoriatic rheumatism, 1038
Putrescine, 413, 929
Pyridoxine lowers serum/blood glutamate levels, 886
Pyridoxine, 288, 689, 885
Pyruvate dehydrogenase complex, 894
Qigong, 791, 973
Quorum sensing, 439
Raynaud's phenomenon in scleroderma, 1094, 1129
Raynaud's phenomenon, 94, 1129, 1133
Reactive arthritis, 93, 466, 1110
Reasons to avoid the use of nonsteroidal anti-inflammatory drugs (NSAIDs), 247, 249
Referred pain with compression, 274
REFLEXES – grading scale, 24
Relative rest - definition and application in basic holistic care, 254
Renal artery (renovascular) stenosis, 740
Renal disease survey, 743
Renal failure, cause of death in patients with SLE, 1061
Renal injury and failure caused by NSAIDs, 250
Resolvins, 363
Restless leg syndrome, 949
Retinal vasculitis, 1062
Review of systems, 12
Rheumatic psoriasis, 1038
Rheumatoid Factor - interpretation, 80
Rib manipulation, 282
Riboflavin, 290
Rifaxamin, 496
Rifaximin as treatment for SIBO and IBS, 954
Rifaximin, 954, 964
ROS: review of systems, 12
Rosacea, 482
Rose Bengal staining, 1121
Roseburia intestinalis, 427
Rosemary, 308, 377, 389, 996
Saccharomyces boulardii, 492, 719
SAD: Standard American Diet, 757

S-adenosyl-methionine, 576, 962
Safe patient + safe treatment = safe outcome, 110
Salivary gland biopsy, 1121
Salmonella, 93
SAMe, 576
Sarcoidosis, 1138
Savella, 913
Schirmer test, 1121
Schober test, 1114
Scleraderma, 741
Scleroderma secondary to xenobiotic immunotoxicity, 1074
Scleroderma, 1074
Screening laboratory tests in the evaluation of patients with musculoskeletal complaints, 25
Secondary Hemochromatosis, 160
Secretory IgA, 103, 488
SEID, 479
Selective estrogen receptor modulators inhibit Ebola virus infection, 572
Selenium, 573
Septic arthritis, 121, 125, 126
Septic arthritis, in rheumatoid arthritis, 1023
Seropositivity, 81, 1024
Serotonin synthesis, 211
Serum IgE and IgG assays, 391
Shigella, 93
Short-chain fatty acids, 104, 488
SIBO, 922
Sicca syndrome, 1120
Sick role, 265
Silibinin/silybin from Silymarin marianum, 593
Silymarin, 168
Sinorespiratory dysbiosis, 508
Sjögren Syndrome/Disease, 550, 1120
Skatole, 413, 929
Skin taping to increase afferent stimuli, 296
Skin-prick testing, 391, 999
SLE, 1053
Sleep apnea, 741
Sleep, 199
Slipped capital femoral epiphysis, 124
Small intestinal bacterial/microbial overgrowth, 473
Small intestine bacterial overgrowth in fibromyalgia, 923
Social history, 13
Sodium avoidance, 613
Sodium benzoate, 212
Sodium chloride, 763
Sodium hypochlorite, 516
Somatic dysfunction, 149
Somatostatin analog, 1083
Special considerations in the evaluation of children, 112
Spinal accessory nerve, 23
Spinal cord compression, 2, 120
Spinal manipulation, 605
Spironolatone, 812
SPMD, 717

Sporothrix schenckii, 570
St. John's Wort, 533
Standard Medical Treatment for Fibromyalgia, 912
Staphylococcus aureus, 531
Stearidonic acid, 360
Stool analysis and comprehensive parasitology, 487
Stool analysis, 103
Streptococcal infections, 94
Streptococcus pyogenes, 531
Stress is a "whole body" phenomenon, 222
Stress management and authentic living, 221
Subluxation, 742
Superantigens, 411
Supercompensation (carbohydrates), 211
Supplemented Paleo-Mediterranean Diet, 219, 256
Syndemic obesity, inflammation, cardiometabolic syndrome, and brain dysfunction, 652
Synthroid, 696
Systemic exertion intolerance disease, 479
Systemic Lupus Erythematosus, main chapter, 1053
Systemic Sclerosis, 741, 1074
Systolic hypertension, 788
Syzygium species, 534
Takayasu arteritis, 1098
Tanacetum parthenium, 897
Tartaric acid, 413, 929
Tartrazine, 212
Television, 191
Temporal arteritis, 119, 1100
Testing for Occult Infections and Dysbiosis, 86
Testosterone, 694
Tetanus toxoid, 427
Tetracycline, 497
Th17 cells, 609
Therapeutic dependency - defined, 265
Therapeutic exercise, 266
Therapeutic Interventions, 956
Therapeutic passivity - defined, 265
Thrombocytopenia, 719
Thromboxane A-2, 368
Thromboxane A-3, 362
Thromboxane B2, 368
Thrust vectors, 279
Thyme, 534
Thymus vulgaris, 534
Thyroid (insufficiency or autoimmunity), 696, 697
Thyroid disease, 742
Thyroid glandular—nonprescription T3, 697
Thyroid hormone, 689
Thyroid stimulating hormone - interpretation, 64
Thyroid testing, 745
Thyrolar, 697
Tinidazole, 495

Tissue/Parenchymal/Blood Dysbiosis, 511
Tolle Causam, 130
Toll-like receptors (TLR), 417
Toll-like receptors (TLR, e.g., TLR2 and TLR4), 651
Toll-like receptors, 418
Total inflammatory load (TIL), 479
Total microbial load (TML), 479, 1054
Toxic oil syndrome, 1076
Toxicant Exposure and Detoxification/Depuration, 705
Toxoplasma gondii, 1086
Tramadol, 913
Transcendental meditation, 791
Transgenic food avoidance, 613
Transient synovitis, irritable hip, 123
Treatment for MFTP, 277
Treatment-resistant hypertension, 731
T-regulatory cells, 609
Tricycline, dosing and clinical use, 494, 720
Trigeminal nerve, pain sensation in migraine, 863
Trigeminal, 23
Tripterygium wilfordii Hook F, 690
Triptolide, 690
Trochlear, 23
Truncated self, 226
Tryptamine, 413, 929
Tryptophan, 960
TSH: thyroid stimulating hormone - interpretation, 64
Turmeric, 537
Twitch response, 274
Tyramine, 413, 483, 929
Una de gato, 259
Uncaria guianensis and Uncaria tomentosa, 259
Undecenoic acid, 493, 720
Undecylenic acid, 535
Undecylenic acid, dosing and clinical use, 493, 720
Unfolded protein response (UPR), 650
Unhistorical, 196

Uric acid reduction, 767
Uric acid, 746
Urinalysis (UA), 745
Urinary alkalinization, 770
Urine pH, 746
Urine sodium and potassium, 746
Uva Ursi, 534
Vagal stimulation, 443, 923
Vancomycin, 964, 496
Varicella zoster virus (VZV), 561
Varicella zoster virus in giant cell arteritis, 552
Varicocele, 693
Vasculitic Diseases, 1095
Vasculitis, 464, 508
Vasodilators, 813
Vegetarian diet for fibromyalgia, 958
Vegetarian diet, 758
Vestibulocochlear, 23
Vinyl chloride disease, 1076
Viruses, part 1—Known/popular "epigenomic" viruses, 1054
Viruses, part 2—Human endogenous retroviruses (endoretroviruses, HERVs or ERVs), 1055
Viruses, part 3—Bacteriophages of the gastrointestinal bacteria, 1059
Viruses, part 4—Bacterial synergism via NFkB activation and immunosuppression, 1060
Vis Medicatrix Naturae, 130
Viscous Agents, 298
Visual analog scale, 23
Vitamin A for all patients with measles, 587
Vitamin A, 587
Vitamin A, retinoic acid, RA, 615
Vitamin B-12 in the treatment of allergy, 388
Vitamin B-12 in the treatment of allergy, 995
Vitamin B-6, 288
Vitamin C (ascorbic acid), 587
Vitamin C in the treatment of allergy, 388, 994
Vitamin C purge, 494, 720

Vitamin C, 273, 770
Vitamin D - antiinflammatory benefits, 378, 450
Vitamin D deficiency - assessment in patients with musculoskeletal pain, 26, 916
Vitamin D status testing, 59
Vitamin D, 728, 742, 746, 769, 770, 801, 815, 816
Vitamin D, 982, 983
Vitamin D3 (cholecalciferol, not ergocalciferol), 586
Vitamin E in the treatment of allergy, 388, 994
Vitamin E, 612
Vitex astus-cagnus, 690
Wall, neurophysiology researcher, 908
Wall-less bacteria, 408
Waterhouse, 456
Wegener's granulomatosis, 428, 1097, 1102
Weight optimization, 265, 791
Wellness, 4
Whey peptides, 773
Whey protein isolate, 591
Williams, Roger J, 195
Willow bark, 258
Wobble board, 294
Wobenzym, 595
WomanWithin, 224
Work ethic, 198
Xenobiotic Immunotoxicity, 699
Xenobioticcs, 920
Xerostomia, 1120
Xifaxan, 496, 964
Yellow dye #5, 212
Yersinia, 93
Yoga, 290
Zeff, Jared N.D., 189
Zingiber officinale, 258
Zonulin, 404
Zygomycosis, 570

Appendix—2015 media and excipients for common vaccines from the US Centers for Disease Control (CDC): Observance is made here—with selected highlights of common allergens and immunogens—of potential allergens to which patients may respond; by use of this information, clinicians can make better choices regarding the selection or avoidance of particular vaccines in patients with known allergies or possible hypersensitivity reactions. For example, according to the recent study by Zug et al[1], among 883 North American children approximately 60% have positive (ie, allergic) responses to substances via patch testing, and neomycin sulfate (a component of come vaccines) sensitivity is one of the more common allergies/hypersensitivities. Thus this list helps clinicians identify potential hypersensitivity reactions that might be triggered by vaccine ingredients. This document is available as of early 2016 via the CDC website at this location: http://www.cdc.gov/vaccines/pubs/pinkbook/downloads/appendices/B/excipient-table-2.pdf

Vaccine Excipient & Media Summary
Excipients Included in U.S. Vaccines, by Vaccine

This table includes not only vaccine ingredients (e.g., adjuvants and preservatives), but also substances used during the manufacturing process, including vaccine-production media, that are removed from the final product and present only in trace quantities. In addition to the substances listed, most vaccines contain Sodium Chloride (table salt).

Last Updated February 2015

All reasonable efforts have been made to ensure the accuracy of this information, but manufacturers may change product contents before that information is reflected here. If in doubt, check the manufacturer's package insert.

Vaccine	Contains	Source: Manufacturer's P.I. Dated
Adenovirus	sucrose, D-mannose, D-fructose, dextrose, potassium phosphate, plasdone C, anhydrous lactose, micro crystalline cellulose, polacrilin potassium, magnesium stearate, cellulose acetate phthalate, alcohol, acetone, castor oil, FD&C Yellow #6 aluminum lake dye, human serum albumin, fetal bovine serum, sodium bicarbonate, human-diploid fibroblast cell cultures (WI-38), Dulbecco's Modified Eagle's Medium, monosodium glutamate	March 2011
Anthrax (Biothrax)	aluminum hydroxide, benzethonium chloride, formaldehyde, amino acids, vitamins, inorganic salts and sugars	May 2012
BCG (Tice)	glycerin, asparagine, citric acid, potassium phosphate, magnesium sulfate, Iron ammonium citrate, lactose	February 2009
DT (Sanofi)	aluminum potassium sulfate, peptone, bovine extract, formaldehyde, thimerosal (trace), modified Mueller and Miller medium, ammonium sulfate	December 2005
DTaP (Daptacel)	aluminum phosphate, formaldehyde, glutaraldehyde, 2-Phenoxyethanol, Stainer-Scholte medium, modified Mueller's growth medium, modified Mueller-Miller casamino acid medium (without beef heart infusion), dimethyl 1-beta-cyclodextrin, ammonium sulfate	October 2013
DTaP (Infanrix)	formaldehyde, glutaraldehyde, aluminum hydroxide, polysorbate 80, Fenton medium (containing bovine extract), modified Latham medium (derived from bovine casein), modified Stainer-Scholte liquid medium	November 2013
DTaP-IPV (Kinrix)	formaldehyde, glutaraldehyde, aluminum hydroxide, Vero (monkey kidney) cells, calf serum, lactalbumin hydrolysate, polysorbate 80, neomycin sulfate, polymyxin B, Fenton medium (containing bovine extract), modified Latham medium (derived from bovine casein), modified Stainer-Scholte liquid medium	November 2013
DTaP-HepB-IPV (Pediarix)	formaldehyde, gluteraldehyde, aluminum hydroxide, aluminum phosphate, lactalbumin hydrolysate, polysorbate 80, neomycin sulfate, polymyxin B, yeast protein, calf serum, Fenton medium (containing bovine extract), modified Latham medium (derived from bovine casein), modified Stainer-Scholte liquid medium, Vero (monkey kidney) cells	November 2013
DTaP-IPV/Hib (Pentacel)	aluminum phosphate, polysorbate 80, formaldehyde, sucrose, gutaraldehyde, bovine serum albumin, 2-phenoxethanol, neomycin, polymyxin B sulfate, Mueller's Growth Medium, Mueller-Miller casamino acid medium (without beef heart infusion), Stainer-Scholte medium (modified by the addition of casamino acids and dimethyl-beta-cyclodextrin), MRC-5 (human diploid) cells, CMRL 1969 medium (supplemented with calf serum), ammonium sulfate, and medium 199	October 2013
Hib (ActHIB)	ammonium sulfate, formalin, sucrose, Modified Mueller and Miller medium	January 2014
Hib (Hiberix)	formaldehyde, lactose, semi-synthetic medium	March 2012
Hib (PedvaxHIB)	aluminum hydroxphosphate sulfate, ethanol, enzymes, phenol, detergent, complex fermentation medium	December 2010

---

[1] Zug et al. Patch testing in children from 2005 to 2012: results from the North American contact dermatitis group. *Dermatitis.* 2014 Nov-Dec;25(6):345-55

Vaccine	Contains	Source: Manufacturer's P.I. Dated
Hib/Hep B (Comvax)	yeast (vaccine contains no detectable yeast DNA), nicotinamide adenine dinucleotide, hemin chloride, soy peptone, dextrose, mineral salts, amino acids, formaldehyde, potassium aluminum sulfate, amorphous aluminum hydroxyphosphate sulfate, sodium borate, phenol, ethanol, enzymes, detergent	December 2010
Hib/Mening. CY (MenHibrix)	tris (trometamol)-HCl, sucrose, formaldehyde, synthetic medium, semi-synthetic medium	2012
Hep A (Havrix)	aluminum hydroxide, amino acid supplement, polysorbate 20, formalin, neomycin sulfate, MRC-5 cellular proteins	December 2013
Hep A (Vaqta)	amorphous aluminum hydroxyphosphate sulfate, bovine albumin, formaldehyde, neomycin, sodium borate, MRC-5 (human diploid) cells	February 2014
Hep B (Engerix-B)	aluminum hydroxide, yeast protein, phosphate buffers, sodium dihydrogen phosphate dihydrate	December 2013
Hep B (Recombivax)	yeast protein, soy peptone, dextrose, amino acids, mineral salts, potassium aluminum sulfate, amorphous aluminum hydroxyphosphate sulfate, formaldehyde, phosphate buffer	May 2014
Hep A/Hep B (Twinrix)	formalin, yeast protein, aluminum phosphate, aluminum hydroxide, amino acids, phosphate buffer, polysorbate 20, neomycin sulfate, MRC-5 human diploid cells	August 2012
Human Papillomavirus (HPV) (Cerverix)	vitamins, amino acids, lipids, mineral salts, aluminum hydroxide, sodium dihydrogen phosphate dehydrate, 3-O-desacyl-4' Monophosphoryl lipid A, insect cell, bacterial, and viral protein	November 2013
Human Papillomavirus (HPV) (Gardasil)	yeast protein, vitamins, amino acids, mineral salts, carbohydrates, amorphous aluminum hydroxyphosphate sulfate, L-histidine, polysorbate 80, sodium borate	June 2014
Human Papillomavirus (HPV) (Gardasil 9)	yeast protein, vitamins, amino acids, mineral salts, carbohydrates, amorphous aluminum hydroxyphosphate sulfate, L-histidine, polysorbate 80, sodium borate	December 2014
Influenza (Afluria)	beta-propiolactone, thimerosol (multi-dose vials only), monobasic sodium phosphate, dibasic sodium phosphate, monobasic potassium phosphate, potassium chloride, calcium chloride, sodium taurodeoxycholate, neomycin sulfate, polymyxin B, egg protein, sucrose	December 2013
Influenza (Agriflu)	egg proteins, formaldehyde, polysorbate 80, cetyltrimethylammonium bromide, neomycin sulfate, kanamycin, barium	2013
Influenza (Fluarix) Trivalent and Quadrivalent	octoxynol-10 (Triton X-100), α-tocopheryl hydrogen succinate, polysorbate 80 (Tween 80), hydrocortisone, gentamicin sulfate, ovalbumin, formaldehyde, sodium deoxycholate, sucrose, phosphate buffer	June 2014
Influenza (Flublok)	monobasic sodium phosphate, dibasic sodium phosphate, polysorbate 20, baculovirus and host cell proteins, baculovirus and cellular DNA, Triton X-100, lipids, vitamins, amino acids, mineral salts	March 2014
Influenza (Flucelvax)	Madin Darby Canine Kidney (MDCK) cell protein, MDCK cell DNA, polysorbate 80, cetyltrimethlyammonium bromide, β-propiolactone, phosphate buffer	March 2014
Influenza (Fluvirin)	nonylphenol ethoxylate, thimerosal (multidose vial–trace only in prefilled syringe), polymyxin, neomycin, beta-propiolactone, egg proteins, phosphate buffer	February 2014
Influenza (Flulaval) Trivalent and Quadrivalent	thimerosal, formaldehyde, sodium deoxycholate, egg proteins, phosphate buffer	February 2013
Influenza (Fluzone: Standard (Trivalent and Quadrivalent), High-Dose, & Intradermal)	formaldehyde, octylphenol ethoxylate (Triton X-100), gelatin (standard trivalent formulation only), thimerosal (multi-dose vial only), egg protein, phosphate buffers, sucrose	2014

Centers for Disease Control and Prevention
Epidemiology and Prevention of Vaccine-Preventable Diseases, 13th Edition

April, 2015

From: http://www.cdc.gov/vaccines/pubs/pinkbook/downloads/appendices/B/excipient-table-2.pdf on 2016 January

Vaccine	Contains	Source: Manufacturer's P.I. Dated
Influenza (FluMist) Quadrivalent	ethylene diamine tetraacetic acid (EDTA), monosodium glutamate, hydrolyzed porcine gelatin, arginine, sucrose, dibasic potassium phosphate, monobasic potassium phosphate, gentamicin sulfate, egg protein	July 2013
Japanese Encephalitis (Ixiaro)	aluminum hydroxide, Vero cells, protamine sulfate, formaldehyde, bovine serum albumin, sodium metabisulphite, sucrose	May 2013
Meningococcal (MCV4-Menactra)	formaldehyde, phosphate buffers, Mueller Hinton agar, Watson Scherp media, Modified Mueller and Miller medium, detergent, alcohol, ammonium sulfate	April 2013
Meningococcal (MCV4-Menveo)	formaldehyde, amino acids, yeast extract, Franz complete medium, CY medium	August 2013
Meningococcal (MPSV4-Menomune)	thimerosal (multi-dose vial only), lactose, Mueller Hinton casein agar, Watson Scherp media, detergent, alcohol	April 2013
Meningococcal (MenB – Bexsero)	aluminum hydroxide, E. coli, histidine, sucrose, deoxycholate, kanomycin	2015
Meningococcal (MenB – Trumenba)	polysorbate 80, histodine, E. coli, fermentation growth media	October 2015
MMR (MMR-II)	Medium 199 (vitamins, amino acids, fetal bovine serum, sucrose, glutamate) , Minimum Essential Medium, phosphate, recombinant human albumin, neomycin, sorbitol, hydrolyzed gelatin, chick embryo cell culture, WI-38 human diploid lung fibroblasts	June 2014
MMRV (ProQuad)	sucrose, hydrolyzed gelatin, sorbitol, monosodium L-glutamate, sodium phosphate dibasic, human albumin, sodium bicarbonate, potassium phosphate monobasic, potassium chloride, potassium phosphate dibasic, neomycin, bovine calf serum, chick embryo cell culture, WI-38 human diploid lung fibroblasts, MRC-5 cells	March 2014
Pneumococcal (PCV13 – Prevnar 13)	casamino acids, yeast, ammonium sulfate, Polysorbate 80, succinate buffer, aluminum phosphate, soy peptone broth	January 2014
Pneumococcal (PPSV-23 – Pneumovax)	phenol	May 2014
Polio (IPV – Ipol)	2-phenoxyethanol, formaldehyde, neomycin, streptomycin, polymyxin B, monkey kidney cells, Eagle MEM modified medium, calf serum protein, Medium 199	May 2013
Rabies (Imovax)	Human albumin, neomycin sulfate, phenol red indicator, MRC-5 human diploid cells, beta-propriolactone	April 2013
Rabies (RabAvert)	β-propiolactone, potassium glutamate, chicken protein, egg protein, neomycin, chlortetracycline, amphotericin B, human serum albumin, polygeline (processed bovine gelatin), sodium EDTA, bovine serum	March 2012
Rotavirus (RotaTeq)	sucrose, sodium citrate, sodium phosphate monobasic monohydrate, sodium hydroxide, polysorbate 80, cell culture media, fetal bovine serum, vero cells *[DNA from porcine circoviruses (PCV) 1 and 2 has been detected in RotaTeq. PCV-1 and PCV-2 are not known to cause disease in humans.]*	June 2013
Rotavirus (Rotarix)	amino acids, dextran, sorbitol, sucrose, calcium carbonate, xanthan, Dulbecco's Modified Eagle Medium (potassium chloride, magnesium sulfate, ferric (III) nitrate, sodium phosphate, sodium pyruvate, D-glucose, concentrated vitamin solution, L-cystine, L-tyrosine, amino acids solution, L-glutamine, calcium chloride, sodium hydrogenocarbonate, and phenol red) *[Porcine circovirus type 1 (PCV-1) is present in Rotarix. PCV-1 is not known to cause disease in humans.]*	May 2014
Smallpox (Vaccinia – ACAM2000)	human serum albumin, mannitol, neomycin, glycerin, polymyxin B, phenol, Vero cells, HEPES	September 2009

Centers for Disease Control and Prevention
Epidemiology and Prevention of Vaccine-Preventable Diseases, 13th Edition

April, 2015

Vaccine	Contains	Source: Manufacturer's P.I. Dated
Td (Decavac)	aluminum potassium sulfate, peptone, formaldehyde, thimerosal, bovine muscle tissue (US sourced), Mueller and Miller medium, ammonium sulfate	March 2011
Td (Tenivac)	aluminum phosphate, formaldehyde, modified Mueller-Miller casamino acid medium without beef heart infusion, ammonium sulfate	April 2013
Td (Mass Biologics)	aluminum phosphate, formaldehyde, thimerosal (trace), ammonium phosphate, modified Mueller's media (containing bovine extracts)	February 2011
Tdap (Adacel)	aluminum phosphate, formaldehyde, glutaraldehyde, 2-phenoxyethanol, ammonium sulfate, Stainer-Scholte medium, dimethyl-beta-cyclodextrin, modified Mueller's growth medium, Mueller-Miller casamino acid medium (without beef heart infusion)	March 2014
Tdap (Boostrix)	formaldehyde, glutaraldehyde, aluminum hydroxide, polysorbate 80 (Tween 80), Latham medium derived from bovine casein, Fenton medium containing a bovine extract, Stainer-Scholte liquid medium	February 2013
Typhoid (inactivated – Typhim Vi)	hexadecyltrimethylammonium bromide, formaldehyde, phenol, polydimethylsiloxane, disodium phosphate, monosodium phosphate, semi-synthetic medium	March 2014
Typhoid (oral – Ty21a)	yeast extract, casein, dextrose, galactose, sucrose, ascorbic acid, amino acids, lactose, magnesium stearate, gelatin	September 2013
Varicella (Varivax)	sucrose, phosphate, glutamate, gelatin, monosodium L-glutamate, sodium phosphate dibasic, potassium phosphate monobasic, potassium chloride, sodium phosphate monobasic, potassium chloride, EDTA, residual components of MRC-5 cells including DNA and protein, neomycin, fetal bovine serum, human diploid cell cultures (WI-38), embryonic guinea pig cell cultures, human embryonic lung cultures	March 2014
Yellow Fever (YF-Vax)	sorbitol, gelatin, egg protein	May 2013
Zoster (Shingles – Zostavax)	sucrose, hydrolyzed porcine gelatin, monosodium L-glutamate, sodium phosphate dibasic, potassium phosphate monobasic, neomycin, potassium chloride, residual components of MRC-5 cells including DNA and protein, bovine calf serum	February 2014

A table listing vaccine excipients and media *by excipient* can be found in:

Grabenstein JD. *ImmunoFacts: Vaccines and Immunologic Drugs* – 2013 (38th revision). St Louis, MO: Wolters Kluwer Health, 2012.

From: http://www.cdc.gov/vaccines/pubs/pinkbook/downloads/appendices/B/excipient-table-2.pdf on 2016 January

Lightning Source UK Ltd.
Milton Keynes UK
UKOW07f0258050117
291383UK00008B/32/P